Nursing Older People

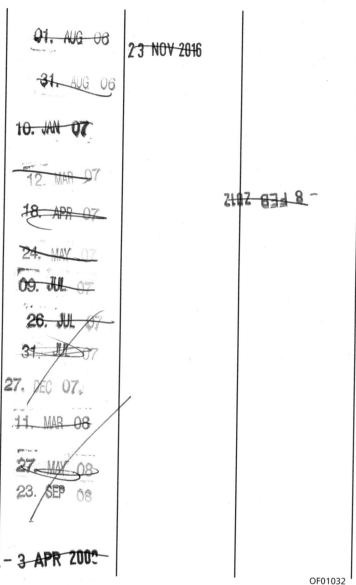

For Elsevier:

Senior Commissioning Editor: Ninette Premdas
Project Development Manager: Mairi McCubbin
Project Manager: Emma Riley
Designer: Erik Bigland
Illustrator: David Graham

Nursing Older People

Fourth edition

Edited by

Sally J. Redfern BSc PhD RGN

Emeritus Professor of Nursing, Nursing Research Unit, King's College London, London, UK

Fiona M. Ross BSc PhD RGN DN

Professor of Gerontological Nursing in Primary Care and Director, Nursing Research Unit, King's College London, London, UK

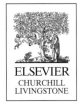

ELSEVIER
CHURCHILL
LIVINGSTONE

EDINBURGH LONDON NEW YORK OXFORD PHILADELPHIA ST LOUIS SYDNEY TORONTO 2006

ELSEVIER
CHURCHILL
LIVINGSTONE

First edition 1986
Second edition 1991
Third edition 1999
Fourth edition 2006

ISBN 0 443 07459 3

British Library Cataloguing in Publication Data
A catalogue record for this book is available from the British Library

Library of Congress Cataloging in Publication Data
A catalog record for this book is available from the Library of Congress

Notice
Knowledge and best practice in this field are constantly changing. As new research and
experience broaden our knowledge, changes in practice, treatment and drug therapy
may become necessary or appropriate. Readers are advised to check the most current
information provided (i) on procedures featured or (ii) by the manufacturer of each
product to be administered, to verify the recommended dose or formula, the method
and duration of administration, and contraindications. It is the responsibility of the
practitioner, relying on their own experience and knowledge of the patient, to make
diagnoses, to determine dosages and the best treatment for each individual patient,
and to take all appropriate safety precautions. To the fullest extent of the law, neither
the publisher nor the editors assumes any liability for any injury and/or damage.

The Publisher

ELSEVIER your source for books,
journals and multimedia
in the health sciences
www.elsevierhealth.com

Working together to grow
libraries in developing countries
www.elsevier.com | www.bookaid.org | www.sabre.org
ELSEVIER | BOOK AID International | Sabre Foundation

The
Publisher's
policy is to use
**paper manufactured
from sustainable forests**

Printed in China

Contents

Contributors

Joan Adams BSc MSc RCNT RGN
Lecturer, Florence Nightingale School of Nursing and Midwifery, King's College London, London, UK
18 Maintaining body temperature

Barry Aveyard BA MA CertEd RNT RMN RGN
Lecturer in Nursing, University of Sheffield, Sheffield, UK
24 Person-centred dementia care

Suzanne Bench BSc MSc PGDipHE ENB100, 998
Lecturer, Critical Nursing Care, Florence Nightingale School of Nursing and Midwifery, King's College London, London, UK
15 Breathing

Helen Brett MSc DipN(Lond) CertEd RGN IFPA AMBAcR
Senior Lecturer, Faculty of Health, Canterbury Christ Church University College, Canterbury, UK
31 Complementary therapies

Margaret Bruce BA MPhil CertEd DPodM
Senior Lecturer, School of Health Professions, Faculty of Health and Social Work, University of Plymouth, Plymouth, UK
14 Care of the foot

Avril Charnock DBO(D) Dip
Head Orthoptist, Orthoptic Department, The Western Eye Hospital, London, UK
12 Eyesight and older people

S. José Closs BSc MPhil PhD RGN
Professor of Nursing Research, School of Healthcare, University of Leeds, Leeds, UK
20 Sleep and rest

Angela Cotter BSc PhD Dip Health Ed RN
Ferguson Fellow, Woodbrooke Quaker Study Centre, Birmingham and Jungian analytic psychotherapist in private practice, London
21 Sexuality and relationships in later life

Sarah Cowley BA PhD PGDE RGN RHV HVT
Head of Public Health and Health Services Research Section, Florence Nightingale School of Nursing and Midwifery, King's College London, London, UK
30 Health promotion for older people

Maureen Crane MSc PhD RGN RMN
Research Fellow, Sheffield Institute for Studies on Ageing, University of Sheffield, Community Sciences Centre, Northern General Hospital, Sheffield, UK
29 Health care for older homeless people

Sue Davies BSc MSc PhD RGN RHV
Senior Lecturer in Gerontological Nursing, University of Sheffield, Sheffield, UK
24 Person-centred dementia care

Tina Day BSc MSc CertEd RNT ENB100
Lecturer, Critical Care, Florence Nightingale School of Nursing and Midwifery, King's College London, London, UK
15 Breathing

Andrei Dunn BSc Adult Nurs, MSc DipHE Nurs Studies
Specialist Nurse for Older People, Elderly Care Day Hospital, Guy's Hospital, London, UK
8 Nursing older people in hospital

Denise Forte MSc DipAppSci PGCEA RGN RSCN
Principal Lecturer, Gerontology, Faculty of Health
and Social Care Sciences, Kingston University
and St George's, University of London, UK
21 Sexuality and relationships in later life

Claire Goodman BSc MSc PhD RN DN
Professor of Health Care Research, University of
Hertfordshire, Hatfield, UK
*9 Intermediate and long-term care provision for
older people*

Dinah Gould BSc MPhil PhD CertEd RGN RNT
Professor of Applied Health, School of Nursing,
City University, London, UK
27 Drugs and older people

Christine Hanks
Principal Lecturer, School of Nursing
and Acute Care, University of Plymouth,
Plymouth, UK
14 Care of the foot

Rosamund A. Herbert BSc MSc CertEd RGN
Healthcare Education Consultant, London, UK
5 The biology of human ageing
18 Maintaining body temperature

Colin Hughes MA(Cantab) PGCE CPNCert RMN
Consultant Nurse – Older People (Mental
Health), Chesterfield Primary Care Trust,
Walton Hospital, Chesterfield, Derbyshire, UK
25 Depression in older people

Margaret Johnson BA MEd
Formerly Lecturer in Nursing, Florence
Nightingale School of Nursing and Midwifery,
King's College London, London, UK
26 Dying, bereavement and loss

Diana T. F. Lee MSc PhD PRD(HCE) RM RN RTN
Professor, Nethersole School of Nursing and
Assistant Dean, Faculty of Medicine, The Chinese
University of Hong Kong, Shatin, New
Territories, Hong Kong
33 Carers and lay caring

Andrée C. le May BSc PhD RGN PGCE(A)
Professor, School of Nursing and
Midwifery, University of Southampton,
Southampton, UK
10 Communication challenges and skills

Ann Mackenzie MA PhD DN RGN
Professor of Gerontological Nursing, Faculty of
Health and Social Care Sciences, St. George's,
University of London, UK
33 Carers and lay caring

Jill Manthorpe MA
Professor of Social Work, Social Care Workforce
Research Unit, King's College London,
London, UK
*6 Policy developments in the organization of
support for older people*

Claudine McCreadie MA DipSocAdmin (LSE)
Research Fellow, Institute of Gerontology,
King's College London, London, UK
32 Abuse of older people

Susan M. McLaren BSc PhD RGN
Professor of Nursing and Director of the Centre
for Leadership and Practice Innovation, Faculty
of Health and Social Care, London South Bank
University, London, UK
16 Eating and drinking

Elaine New MSc GradDipPhys MCSP SRP
Healthcare Ergonomist, Occupational
Health Department, St George's Healthcare
NHS Trust, London, UK
13 Promoting safe mobility

Ian J. Norman BA MSc PhD RN DipASS CQSW RNT RMN
RNMH RGN
Professor of Interdisciplinary Care,
Florence Nightingale School of Nursing
and Midwifery, King's College London,
London, UK
23 Delirium (acute confusional states) in later life
24 Person-centred dementia care

Christine Norton MA(Cantab) PhD RN
Burdett Professor of Gastrointestinal Nursing,
Florence Nightingale School of Nursing and
Midwifery, King's College London and Nurse
Consultant, St Mark's Hospital, Middlesex, UK
17 Eliminating

Claire O'Tuathail DipGerontology, MSc PGCE(HE) REN
Lecturer, Centre for Nursing Studies,
National University of Ireland, Galway, Ireland
28 Assessment of older people

Gillian E. Pedley BSc MSc PGCEA ILTM RN ENB148
Principal Lecturer, School of Nursing, Faculty of
Health and Social Care Sciences, Kingston
University and St George's University of
London, UK
19 Maintaining healthy skin

Bridget Penhale
Senior Lecturer in Gerontology, School of
Nursing and Midwifery, University of Sheffield,
UK
32 Abuse of older people

Maria T. Ponto BA MSc PhD CertCouns CertEd RGN RM
Senior Lecturer, Faculty of Health and Social
Care Sciences, Kingston University and
St George's University of London, UK
4 The psychology of human ageing

Sally J. Redfern BSc PhD RGN
Emeritus Professor of Nursing, Nursing Research
Unit, King's College London, London, UK
1 Introduction
*9 Intermediate and long-term care provision for
  older people*
34 Reflections

Fiona M. Ross BSc PhD RGN DN
Professor of Gerontological Nursing in Primary
Care and Director, Nursing Research Unit, King's
College London, London, UK
1 Introduction
*7 Health and social care for older people in the
  community*
28 Assessment of older people
34 Reflections

Kate Seers BSc PhD RGN
Head of Research, RCN Institute, Radcliffe
Infirmary, Oxford, UK
22 Pain and older people

Janet M. Simpson BSc MSc PhD FCSP AFBPsS
Honorary Senior Lecturer, Centre for
Research and Rehabilitation, St George's
University of London, UK
13 Promoting safe mobility

Iain R. C. Swan MD ChB FRCS
Senior Lecturer in Otolaryngology, University
of Glasgow, Glasgow, UK
11 Hearing

Hamish Thomson BSc MSc RGN DipNEd RNT
Lecturer, Florence Nightingale School of Nursing
and Midwifery, King's College London, London,
UK
23 Delirium (acute confusional states) in later life

Debbie Tolson BSc MSc PhD RGN
Professor of Gerontological Nursing, Director of
the Calidonian Nursing & Midwifery Research
Centre, School of Nursing, Midwifery and
Community Health, Glasgow Caledonian
University, Glasgow, UK
11 Hearing

Christina R. Victor BA MPhil PhD HonMFPH AcSS
Professor of Gerontology and Health Services
Research, Head of School of Health and Social
Care, University of Reading, UK
2 What is old age?
3 Demographic and epidemiological trends in ageing
*7 Health and social care for older people in the
  community*

Anthony M. Warnes BSc PhD AcSS
Professor of Social Gerontology, Sheffield
Institute for Studies on Ageing, University of
Sheffield, Sheffield, UK
29 Health care for older homeless people

Diane Wells BA MPhil RGN RNT DipSocStud DipN DSR
CertPsychosocial Nursing
Senior Lecturer, Faculty of Health and
Social Care Sciences, Kingston University and
St George's, University of
London, UK
21 Sexuality and relationships in later life

Preface

This fourth edition has been reorganized, expanded and largely rewritten because major policy initiatives and organizational change in health and social care since publication of the third edition in 1999 have influenced nursing care of older people. Important policy initiatives that have shaped our approach to this fourth edition include the Royal Commission on the Funding of Long-Term Care; care standards arising from the *National Service Framework for Older People*; and the patient and public involvement agenda.

We hope this book will continue to be a key text for students on diploma and degree courses in nursing and health care, and at a post-registration level for nurses and other practitioners working in the community, care home and independent sectors specializing in the care of older people. That the book is now in its fourth edition is testimony to its success over the years, since the first edition was published in 1986. Reviewers have identified it as the textbook of choice in many nursing curricula in universities across the UK. It has stood the test of time and each new edition has enlisted the expertise of contributors from many different disciplines to ensure the content has kept up to date with developments in health policy, practice and research.

In this edition, many of our contributors have changed. They continue to come from different disciplines concerned with the care of older people – nurses, therapists, social workers, social scientists and gerontologists – and we are pleased to include new contributors who are expert practitioners and consultant nurses. Others we have retained because of their acknowledged expertise in their respective fields, and all have strong connections with practice.

Each chapter ends with a list of recommended reading to guide readers to other sources if they wish to explore a topic further. More photographs and case studies have been included in this edition to enliven the text with illustrative vignettes and examples of good and, sometimes, not-so-good practice.

For this fourth edition our specific thanks go to our patient contributors who have given this book its reputation. Once again, they have done a great job in adapting their ideas to our specification. We are indebted, too, to Gian Brown for her meticulous attention to detail and her mastery of the production process.

London, 2005

Sally J. Redfern
Fiona M. Ross

ACKNOWLEDGEMENTS

We are grateful to all those who have contributed unattributed photos: Barbara Kuyper, Denise Forte, Louise Hirschhauser, Aasta Vasstrand, Maria Ponto and Eleanor Hall. We thank our families and friends for inspiration and support, particularly Margaret Ross, John Tatam, Hugo and Jonny Ross-Tatam and Pat Shipley.

Chapter 1

Introduction

Sally J. Redfern and Fiona M. Ross

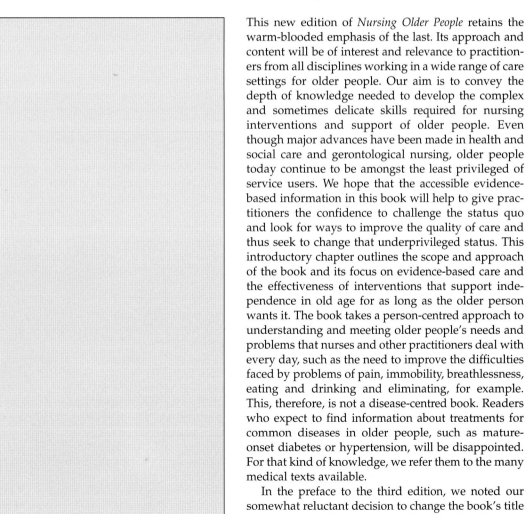

This new edition of *Nursing Older People* retains the warm-blooded emphasis of the last. Its approach and content will be of interest and relevance to practitioners from all disciplines working in a wide range of care settings for older people. Our aim is to convey the depth of knowledge needed to develop the complex and sometimes delicate skills required for nursing interventions and support of older people. Even though major advances have been made in health and social care and gerontological nursing, older people today continue to be amongst the least privileged of service users. We hope that the accessible evidence-based information in this book will help to give practitioners the confidence to challenge the status quo and look for ways to improve the quality of care and thus seek to change that underprivileged status. This introductory chapter outlines the scope and approach of the book and its focus on evidence-based care and the effectiveness of interventions that support independence in old age for as long as the older person wants it. The book takes a person-centred approach to understanding and meeting older people's needs and problems that nurses and other practitioners deal with every day, such as the need to improve the difficulties faced by problems of pain, immobility, breathlessness, eating and drinking and eliminating, for example. This, therefore, is not a disease-centred book. Readers who expect to find information about treatments for common diseases in older people, such as mature-onset diabetes or hypertension, will be disappointed. For that kind of knowledge, we refer them to the many medical texts available.

In the preface to the third edition, we noted our somewhat reluctant decision to change the book's title from *Nursing Elderly People* to *Nursing Older People* to pre-empt criticism from readers who regard 'elderly' as a pejorative word. That it has become so continues, in our view, to be cause for regret because of its pedigree and origins in the Anglo-Saxon word 'eld' which forms the root of words that convey wisdom on account of age and experience. An example is the old term 'alderman', meaning an elected councillor in local government. We do not condone use of 'the elderly' as a collective noun because of its erroneous and ageist assumption of homogeneity and denial of individual differences. It seems, though, that 'elderly' has gone the way of 'geriatrics' – another misused and banished word. Although we would prefer to use words in their original meaning we continue in this fourth edition to go with the tide of opinion by referring to senior citizens as older people. Older is not as specific as elderly because it is a relative term that applies to any age; a 5-year-old child is older than a 4-year-old. As underlined in the earlier editions, misuse of language is a serious issue because it creates stereotypes of identity and behaviour which have a powerful and often damaging effect on those so labelled. We are not suggesting that words should never change; language naturally evolves over time. But when a collective term is needed – and some question whether one is ever needed – a return to the magnificent word 'elders' would be welcome and would help those of us who have not yet got there and may never do so to recognize the wisdom of those who have, and to learn from them.

There are four sections in this edition which are arranged differently and, we think more appropriately, than in the last edition. Section 1, on ageing and old age, contains four updated and rewritten chapters on what it means to be old, demographic and epidemiological trends in ageing, and the psychology and biology of human ageing. Chapter 2 explores the meaning of old age from biological, psychological, social and political perspectives. It draws on the sociological and gerontological literature to discuss influences of the life course on roles of older people in the family and society, integration and isolation, and intergenerational challenges. Chapter 3 updates information on demographic and epidemiological trends in ageing with particular emphasis on the four countries of the UK. Chapter 4 reviews psychological theories of ageing and discusses factors that influence successful ageing, adaptation and satisfaction in later life. It contains an additional section on the role of emotions in later life. Biological theories of ageing, highlighting the incidence and prevalence of some common diseases, are covered in Chapter 5. This chapter also includes discussion on the biological components of frailty.

Section 2, on policy changes and contexts of care for older people, contains four chapters. Chapter 6 is new. It reviews the major policy changes that have influenced health and social care service development and delivery for older people, including community care policies and the *National Service Framework for Older People*. The chapter also discusses the modernization agenda, citizenship and the role of older people in the policy-making process and the policy response to meeting the needs of difference and diversity with the attendant challenge for practitioners to develop cultural competence. Chapter 7, on health and social care, is a new chapter that combines Chapters 5 and 6 from the third edition. It reviews components of service provision for older people in primary health care and social care, outlines roles of practitioners in the field and describes some key principles for care-giving practice in primary care nursing. Some examples are given of partnership-working between health and social care that have developed innovative models of service delivery. Chapter 8, on nursing older people in hospital, has been rewritten to provide an overview of key quality issues arising from the organization of hospital services and nursing care, new nursing roles in hospital nursing, including the consultant nurse and modern matron, benchmarking and standards of care, patient assessment, patient care pathways, rehabilitation, team-working and discharge from hospital arrangements. Chapter 9 has been rewritten to include intermediate and long-term care for older people in care homes. The chapter describes the kinds of long-term provision available to older people, changes in funding arrangements for nursing care and legislative changes in the regulation of care homes. It discusses why institutional care is viewed with such suspicion, and the transition from home to care home, which can be so traumatic if handled inappropriately. Also discussed are health needs of older residents and access to health and palliative care, a brief look at assessment in long-term care and a discussion of changes in nursing, particularly with respect to nurse-led units and new roles in nursing, so expanding on the overview in Chapter 8.

Section 3, on nursing care of older people, emphasizes independence, autonomy and self-fulfilment. It contains 18 chapters, all updated from those of the third edition or rewritten. Chapter 10 is a new chapter that combines Chapters 10 and 17 of the previous edition. It includes the factors that shape and influence communication between older people and nurses, and focuses on communication challenges that older people face and strategies caregivers can use to improve their communication skills. Chapter 11 continues the discussion of communication but with particular focus on the experiences of people with hearing impairment and disability. The chapter highlights the stigma of deafness, describes assessment of hearing loss in some detail and shows what can be done to help people manage their hearing loss by using personal and environmental aids. Chapter 12 covers the prevalence, causes and treatment of common sight problems among older people and how the nurse can help. Promoting safe mobility is discussed in Chapter 13, which considers factors affecting mobility, assessment and management with a focus on preventing falls, Parkinson's disease and stroke. The importance of a physiotherapist working with the nurse in achieving shared rehabilitative goals is emphasized. Chapter 14 continues the theme of mobility by addressing care of the foot. Nurses can do a lot to help older people remain mobile before referral to the chiropody/podiatry services becomes necessary. People with breathing problems have mobility difficulties, too, and Chapter 15 shows what can be done to assess and improve the quality of life for those with breathing difficulties and chronic airways disease in particular.

Chapter 16, on eating and drinking, contains comprehensive information on nutritional assessment, common nutritional problems for older people and techniques for helping them. As we see from Chapter 17, many older people have less than perfect control over their elimination processes and nurses, working in collaboration with other members of the multiprofessional team, whether in a patient's own home, in a care home or in hospital, can do much to alleviate suffering and restore people's dignity. Deaths of old people from hypothermia hit the headlines and Chapter 18 covers early detection and management of hypothermia. Given the very hot spells of summer weather in recent years, the chapter also discusses heat and its effects. With increasing numbers of people surviving into very old age, many people are at risk from pressure sores. The assessment and management of prevention of pressure sores are major components of Chapter 19, on maintaining healthy skin, and the chapter contains an additional section on wound care. Sleep and rest are of paramount importance to the restoration of health and maintenance of well-being. This is often overlooked by nurses and other practitioners. Chapter 20 discusses the physiological, psychological and social components of sleep, evidence-based interventions for nursing and practical strategies that may make a difference to the comfort and rest of older people who are receiving care in institutional settings.

Expressing sexuality for older people, the subject of Chapter 21, continues to be plagued by myths, stereotypes and discrimination. As we learn from this chapter, older service users of the future are likely to be more assertive about their needs and rights and it is our responsibility to ensure we are educated and equipped to fulfil our obligations to them, wherever they are living. Pain, the subject of Chapter 22, is often assumed to be an inevitable consequence of old age because of the prevalence of chronic disease and multiple pathology, but this need not be so. Thorough assessment and treatment can lead to a painfree life.

Acute confusional states (delirium) and dementia occupy two chapters, Chapters 23 and 24 respectively. Delirium is a common symptom of disease in older people and is reversible if treated early. Dementia is more complex. It is seen in Chapter 24 as arising from medical pathology but also as an illness socially constructed by professional carers and by society. Nurses can do much to improve the quality of life of people with dementia and their carers, as well as for people with depression, the subject of Chapter 25. Though very common in older people, depression often goes undetected. If left untreated the prognosis is poor. Nurses have a major role in its assessment, management and prevention. Grief, loss and bereavement may underlie depression and are the subject of Chapter 26. This chapter shows how nurses can support dying people and their families, making this final phase of living a positive experience. The final chapter in this section, Chapter 27, on drugs and older people, has been updated. It includes the development in current thinking towards the use of 'adherence' or 'concordance' to drug treatments that promote the idea of partnership between the provider of medication and the recipient, rather than the coercive notion of 'compliance', with its emphasis on power lying in the hands of the professional.

Section 4 focuses on current issues and reflections on caring for older people. It contains seven updated or rewritten chapters, including one new chapter (Chapter 29). Chapter 28 covers assessment and care planning and has been updated to include the single multiprofessional assessment process recommended by the *National Service Framework for Older People*. Chapter 29, on working with marginalized groups, considers the care needs of homeless people in particular. Health promotion for older people, Chapter 30, reviews different ways of looking at the concept of health and different approaches to promoting health. It places autonomy and choice centre-stage, so enabling people to create health on their own terms – particularly important if health education and health promotion are to be successful. Choice is fundamental to the use of complementary therapies, the subject of Chapter 31, which looks at the range and use of complementary therapies with older people. There is a review of the use of massage, including discussion of the evidence for its effectiveness. Chapter 32 provides an important review of the literature on the characteristics of abusing situations involving older people. Risk assessment and methods of early identification and prevention are discussed.

Lay caring and carers have occupied an increasingly high profile in the UK and, as discussed in Chapter 33, particularly nurses who work in the community have privileged access to people's homes and can see at first hand the difficulties that some family carers face. This chapter emphasizes the importance of culturally appropriate strategies to support family carers by drawing from research with Chinese communities.

Readers may be surprised to find no chapter in this book entitled 'rehabilitation'. Our view is that rehabilitation is too huge a subject for any single chapter to do it justice. Instead, we see rehabilitation as a continuous thread that is more explicit in some chapters – on mobility, care of the foot, hearing, sight, nutrition, elimination, for example – than others,

The final chapter, Chapter 34, has given us an opportunity to draw together and reflect on themes that run throughout the book and that provide pointers to future action. Throughout the narrative we intersperse photographs, extracts from literature and poetry as well as stories that highlight our themes. We set out to draw attention to important issues for older people: images of ageing, the importance of valuing personal relationships, balancing rights and risk-taking, rehabilitation, empowerment and involvement of older people. We discuss key issues for workers, including interprofessional working, emerging roles for nurses working with older people, education and the importance of ensuring service user perspectives in evaluating high-quality care. We hope that this book will be useful, stimulating and make a contribution to the development of services for older people and their families that improve both their experience and clinical outcomes of care.

SECTION 1

Ageing and old age

SECTION CONTENTS

Chapter 2

What is old age?

Christina R. Victor

This chapter considers some of the background issues relevant to nursing older people. First, definitions of old age are discussed, followed by consideration of the stereotypes and attitudes that are commonly held about both old age and the ageing process. Finally, we consider some of the methodological problems that confront the student of ageing.

WHAT IS OLD AGE?

What is old age? When does it start? These apparently simple questions are, in reality, rather complex and the answers are not as straightforward as might be expected. In this section we look at the main approaches to the definition of old age.

The *Shorter Oxford Dictionary* defines age as 'a naturally distinct period or stage of life; especially old age'. A further definition is 'to grow or make old'; however, this dictionary definition is of only limited value as it neither defines the attributes that define old age nor describes the criteria that make it distinct from other phases of life. This provides the first hint that defining the criteria that may identify and delineate old age is rather more problematic than we might first expect. There are four main approaches to the identification and definition of old age and each of these is discussed briefly. This short review illustrates the very arbitrary way in which old age is defined and counsels us to be cautious about how such terms are used within the health care context.

Biological definitions of old age

The study of the biological aspects of ageing is discussed in detail in Chapter 5. This section highlights some of the main issues that have influenced work in the general area of biological definitions of old age. Clearly this is a very challenging area of research for there is no agreement as to the definition of human ageing nor are there any precise measures of ageing. The main point to note here is that there is no readily available, easy-to-operationalize and measure 'biological' definition of old age. Hence all the definitions that we tend to use, in research, policy development and the provision of services, are essentially indirect and largely socially constructed. As such they have only a very tenuous relationship to the biological 'ageing' of both individuals and populations. It is therefore important that all those working with older people (or working with specialist services for older people) recognize the fundamentally arbitrary nature of the definitions used to identify and define their client group and the fluidity of such definitions both culturally and historically.

Normal ageing is characterized by progressive and irreversible changes in both structure and function with time (Kirkwood 1999). Age-related changes (termed senescence) are not observed in all biological populations because of the influence of disease or predatory action. Some populations do not live long enough to grow old. Within a population the chance (or probability) of death increases with age. Put another way, the percentage of survivors (hence this form of analysis is known as survivorship analysis) from a given population decreases with time (i.e. there is an increasing chance or probability of death with age). This type of analysis illustrates two important concepts in ageing research: life expectancy and maximum lifespan. Life expectancy is the number of years an individual can expect to live from a given point. Expectation of life is often calculated from birth but can be calculated from any age (e.g. expectation of life from, for example, age 60). Life expectancy varies between populations, within populations and over time. In the UK expectation of life at birth has increased by approximately 22 years for men and 25 years for women, to 71 and 77 years respectively, since 1900. This increase is largely due to improvements in infant survival resulting from improvements in public health such as the control of common infectious diseases.

Life expectancy at birth has increased consistently over the course of the twentieth century in most western societies. However, we should note that increases in life expectancy resulting from improved public health are fragile and not inevitable. In eastern Europe, most notably, but not exclusively, in Russia, the collapse of the public health system has resulted in the increase in prevalence of common infectious diseases and other harmful health behaviours. This has resulted in a decrease in the expectation of life at birth. Survivorship curves allow for the theoretical possibility of maximum lifespan. This is best defined as the greatest age that a member of a population can attain under optimal conditions. It remains a matter of contention as to whether there is a maximum lifespan for humans and what this 'theoretical maximum' could be (Kirkwood 1999).

Chronological age

In modern society we use chronological age, i.e. the length of time (usually counted in years) that a person has lived, as a key social indicator. Age is extensively used as a social gatekeeper and social regulator across the life course. For example, in the UK children have to go to school from the age of 5 and should remain there until they are 16 years old. At 17 people may obtain a driving licence; the age of 10 is used to determine criminal responsibility for rape and at 18 people may vote, marry or purchase alcohol. However, there is considerable variation between countries in the age, for example, at which children have to go to school, when they are considered capable of consenting to sexual intercourse or when they can purchase and consume alcohol. Hence there is no unanimity across countries (and we may infer over time) in the chronological ages used to define when (and when not) people can (or must) undertake particular activities. Furthermore we can only use chronological age as a social differentiator when there is a reliable system for recording and authenticating age, usually via universal birth certification. It is worth noting that it is only for the last 150 years that the UK has had a systematic, comprehensive and reliable system for the registration of births and deaths.

The chronological age used to define 'old age' is largely arbitrary and varies both culturally and historically. Most biological and physiological parameters show a gradual decline with age, rather than a clear break point at which we could identify old age. Hence the ages used to define old age are rarely biologically or physiologically based. Rather they are rooted in the cultural values and norms of each society. In the UK we often use the age of 65 years and over to signal the start of old age. However, there is immense variation in the age used, both within the UK and across the globe (Bytheway 1994).

It is not the age itself that is important, but the ageing process that it represents that is the issue of interest to the gerontologist and health care practitioners. Given the diversity of the population in terms of race, class and gender we must be aware that biological ageing will vary between groups and thus the identical age may not have the same link with biological processes for different types of people. For example, the health status of males aged 65–69 from unskilled occupations is similar to that of men aged 80+ from professional and managerial occupations (Victor 1991). We must be aware of the diversity within specific age groups. Therefore, rather than concentrating on examining in detail the various ages in order to define old age, it is important simply to note the variation and the arbitrary way such ages are arrived at. The issue of the diversity of the ageing experience and the heterogeneous nature of the older population is examined further in Chapter 3.

The highly arbitrary relationship between chronological age and biological ageing has implications for the development and provision of health services for older people (Chapters 6 and 7). However, it is important to note that services for older people that use chronological age as an entry criterion are using only a very crude proxy measure for biological ageing. For example, the selection of the age of 75 years for routine screening of older people in primary care introduced in the 1990s was essentially a pragmatic one. Similarly, there is little uniformity across the country in the age at which specialists in the medicine of old age treat patients. This diversity within the fabric of service provision highlights the difficulties involved in using age as a criterion for the provision (or withdrawal) of services and is now linked to the *National Service Framework for Older People* and policies for antidiscriminatory practice.

One interesting area of research is the relationship (or lack of it) between chronological age and how old people perceive themselves to be (known as subjective age identity). Individuals may not perceive themselves as being 'old' despite having achieved a specified number of calendar years. For example, a woman in her mid-40s may be defined by others as 'middle-aged' (or by the medical profession as premenopausal), yet she may still consider herself 'young' and entirely reject this view of herself. At earlier points in our history, and in other societies, a woman of this age may well have been considered 'old'. Similarly, many older people will feel themselves still to be young. Evidence for this is provided by Ward (1984). A survey of 1134 Americans reported that 20% of those aged 60–69 defined themselves as old, while a third of those aged 80 and over described themselves as middle-aged or young. This disjunction between chronological and felt age may well have its roots in our negative views of ageing and a reluctance of older people to accept a stigmatized and damaged identity. However, it does have implications for nurses as it means 'the old lady' for whom they are caring may well not accept this label and not respond positively to being addressed as such. We return to this area in the section on attitudes and stereotypes of ageing.

Old age as a stage in the life cycle

The idea that life is divided up into a series of distinct stages or phases is not new. Bytheway (1995) observes that it was common in the Middle Ages to divide the lifespan into a series of phases and to allocate individuals to a phase according to the age reached. Shakespeare in *As You Like It* describes the classic 'seven ages' of men, with old age a distinct phase. With this life-cycle approach, chronological age is loosely related to each of the phases; hence we can both classify the life course and divide the population into very approximate age groups. This approach is very pervasive and forms part of popular discourse in how individuals make sense of the pattern of their lives. Research has shown that people have clear ideas as to how major role transitions, such as marriage, parenthood or retirement, relate to some 'ideal' chronological age and how their own life has followed (or deviated from) this ideal pattern, as evidenced by such common statements as 'I married early (or late)' and 'I had my children (child) late (or early)' (Victor 2005).

However, there are, again, problems with this type of approach, which are not just theoretical or conceptual. For example, it is difficult to operationalize this type of definition of old age. Developing and implementing specialist nursing and health services would be problematic, as it would be difficult to identify potential patients easily. Furthermore there are difficulties in deciding how many phases the life cycle is divided into. Shakespeare offered us a seven-stage model of the ideal life course of an upper-class male, while Erikson proposed eight phases (Erikson 1980). This model is well established within the psychology of ageing and is considered in detail in Chapter 3. Thomas (1977) proposed, on the other hand, a more modest four-phase model (infancy, youth, maturity and decline). While we may have some confidence in distinguishing childhood from adulthood it is more difficult to determine further subdivisions. For example, when does mid-life change into old age? When does childhood move to adolescence? It is not always clear that the phases are sequential and that an individual should progress in linear fashion through each segment, neither can we presume a homogeneous pattern across the different subgroups within the population.

A development of this life-course approach to the study and definition of ageing has been the identification of the 'third and fourth ages'. Neugarten (1974) was the first to draw the distinction between the 'young old' (those aged up to about 75 years) and the 'old old' (those aged over 75 years). This segmentation of later life (or old age) has reappeared as the third and fourth ages proposed by Laslett (1996). The third age is seen as a time of opportunity and activity. People are typified as mature adults freed from child care and labour market responsibilities and who have sufficient resources to take advantage of this 'free time'. In contrast, the fourth age is seen as 'final dependence, decrepitude and death'. Empirically it is clear that the experience of old age is much more complex than the simple divisions into third and fourth age. Indeed, the *Carnegie Inquiry into the Third Age* (Banks 1992) described the complexity encapsulated within what at first sight is an apparently homogeneous group. Such global categories are an oversimplification of the complex experience that is later life (see Chapter 3 for further discussion of this issue).

Political economy approach

This perspective on construction of old age relates it to participation in the labour market (Phillipson 1986). The definition of old age is linked to formal (and often legally sanctioned) withdrawal from the formal labour market via the universalization of the concept of retirement. Under this approach old age is defined neither by chronological age nor life-cycle stage. Rather it is defined by people's relationship to (or withdrawal from) the means of production. Thus it is clearly linked to both the concept of retirement and the availability of pensions to support those who are no longer gainfully employed. Here the concept of retirement is linked to the needs of the economy for labour: in times of labour shortage retirement is discouraged, while in times of depression older workers are encouraged to make way for younger ones (Laczko & Phillipson 1991). Entry into retirement is linked to the availability of pensions. As these are usually less than wages or salaries, older people, once they have left the labour market, experience financial dependence upon the state and other pension providers. Retirement policies mark the boundary and, as such, age of eligibility for pensions has become used as a prevalent proxy, albeit a rather arbitrary one, for the onset of old age. Such theories have been revised in the light of criticism that they are both too mechanistic and do not reflect the heterogeneous nature of the population (Phillipson 1998).

THEORETICAL PERSPECTIVES ON OLD AGE

The theoretical basis for the social study of ageing is limited. Much of the focus of gerontological research has been upon the documentation of 'the facts' about ageing. The majority of work in this field has been ori-

ented towards empirical study rather than theoretical development. While this area of research is not rich in theoretical perspectives, there are a number of theoretical concepts and developments that have influenced the nature and content of the study of ageing and these have implications for the provision of nursing (and indeed other) services for older people. These major theoretical perspectives are briefly outlined (see Victor 1994 for a more detailed discussion and analysis of the role of theory in gerontological research) and the key assumptions underlying them are exposed. Identification of the values and assumptions underpinning research concerned with ageing (and indeed other areas) is important because it highlights the limitations of the way that the questions were posed and answered (or indeed why they were asked in the first place).

Structural–functionalist theories

This perspective is concerned with developing theory at the macro (or societal) level. Hence the basic unit of analysis is society. Society is conceived as a set of interrelated parts (or social institutions or structures) that are integrated into a (relatively) stable structure. These parts are studied both as individual units and as elements for the maintenance of society. It is assumed that each element of the system has functional consequences for society overall. It is the task of the researchers to analyse the individual social elements, their relationship to other parts and the role they play in preserving society.

This perspective has been very influential in the area of ageing research. Two important theories (activity theory and disengagement theory) are essentially functionalist in nature. Other theories from this tradition (but not considered for reasons of space) include modernization theory, role transition theory, continuity theory and social integration theory. A key element of the functionalist perspective is the emphasis upon maintaining equilibrium, which neglects the important areas of social change and social conflict. Furthermore it is a research perspective that accords little power to individuals; rather they are theorized as passive social actors. Much of the research in social gerontology is concerned with how people respond to ageing (the search for successful ageing) and how they adapt and integrate into society. This is exemplified by the plethora of work concerned with personal and social adjustment, quality of life and role transitions. An example of this approach is much (but not all) of the literature concerned with informal care, which has focused on documenting the prevalence and nature of such care (Chapter 33). Extensive research therefore now exists to provide empirical answers to such questions as 'Who provides informal care? What (tasks) do they do? What are the costs to families and the individual of providing care? What are the implications of demographic change?' Such research has not, however, challenged (or examined) why families continue to be the main providers of help to those with long-term care needs, often in circumstances that are very challenging. This illustrates how the theoretical perspective influences the nature of the questions posed and the way that such questions are answered.

Activity theory

Havinghurst (1963) developed the activity theory of ageing, which, put at its most reductionist, states that adjustment (or adaptation) is the key concern of individuals. This is best achieved by those who adapt to ageing by remaining as active as they had been in mid-life. Hence this theory represents a mirror image of the disengagement view of ageing, which is described later. This activity could be achieved either via the maintenance of pre-existing roles/activities or by the adoption of new ones. In order to militate against the overwhelmingly negative societal view of age, the individual must deny the existence of old age by remaining 'middle-aged' for as long as possible. Following this theory, old age is seen as a time in which people maintain activity and successful ageing is achieved when roles are maintained (or new ones added). The underlying premise of this perspective is that there is a positive relationship between activity and life satisfaction. Social and health policies derived from this theoretical view on ageing would stress activity and interaction as the vehicles for 'successful ageing' (Rowe & Kahn 1997).

There are several theoretical problems with this approach to the study of ageing. It makes the easy, but not empirically verified, assumption that old age is a time of psychological and social adjustment. It is assumed that people have the resources to reconstruct (or maintain) middle-aged lifestyles (or to substitute new roles for older, lost roles) in later life. This does not allow for those who cannot replace roles, either because of financial limitations or because they are not easily replaced (e.g. widowhood). Nor is there any relationship between the lost and substituted roles. Can one easily replace the lost roles of parent or marriage? Furthermore the empirical data do not conform to the theoretical postulates. It has been demonstrated that older people can demonstrate high satisfaction without maintaining high levels of activity (or in the face of declining levels of activity). Like other theories on ageing, this one is highly prescriptive and value-laden: the 'use it or lose it' view of ageing.

Disengagement theory

Cumming & Henry (1961) developed this theory, which is diametrically opposed to the implicit assumptions of the activity theorists, who strongly proposed the idea that activity, engagement and involvement were the keys to successful ageing. Disengagement theory proposes that successful ageing (for both the society and the individual) is best achieved by the progressive loss of social roles and relationships with age and the withdrawal of older individuals. This facilitates the smooth transfer of power to the young with the minimum of disruption to society as a whole. From this perspective disengagement is seen as necessary because of the inevitability of death, the presumed decline in abilities with age, the value placed upon youth and the need for society to continue to function efficiently. To age successfully the individual is required to reduce activity and involvement and hand over responsibility to the next generation. At the same time that the individual withdraws from society, society also withdraws from the individual. This theory derives (as indeed does activity theory) from the structural–functionalist approach and is based on the assumption that society is a system that is in equilibrium and that disengagement is one mechanism by which this stability is achieved (or via activity for the protagonists of activity theory).

Again there are obvious limitations to this theory. Disengagement (as indicated by variables such as widowhood or retirement) is not often voluntary, inevitable or universal. The term 'disengagement' is not defined and can be subject to variability of interpretation; one person's disengagement may well be another's engagement and activity – what is the reference point against which disengagement is measured? Both activity and disengagement theory assume that the solution to the (social) problem of ageing will be via 'successful' ageing. These two approaches assume a consensus as to what constitutes successful ageing that in reality does not exist. Ageing is a diverse experience that these types of theories do not readily take into account. Furthermore, such approaches to ageing, and indeed the whole orientation of research aimed at identification and definition of successful ageing, can be used to blame older people for the often marginal condition they find themselves in. The logic of these approaches is that older people are in poor circumstances because they have not been successful in adapting to the challenge of ageing (and is conveniently nothing to do with the provision of support and benefits for older people).

Age stratification theory

The activity and disengagement approaches to theorizing about old age are concerned with adaptation at the individual level. Age stratification theory, while it is still an essentially functionalist approach which is concerned with social integration, operates at the collective level. This perspective views age as a universal criterion for the allocation of social roles (Riley et al 1972). At its most simplistic this is a theory concerned with social age grading. Age is conceptualized as the crucial factor in the allocation of social roles and the accompanying rights and privileges. The focus of attention is on relationships between and within different age strata. People are divided according to chronological age (or life stage) such as 'middle-aged' or 'young' or in terms of cohort experiences, e.g. 'baby boomers'. Each stratum can then be analysed in terms of the roles played and the value ascribed to such roles by society. Again this is an approach which is limited. The key assumptions inherent in this approach are that: (1) vertical stratification is inherent in all social systems; and (2) the inequalities created as a result of this stratification are both inevitable and politically acceptable. Again the heterogeneous nature of this approach does not encapsulate the diversity of older people nor recognize the importance of class, gender and ethnicity.

Conflict theory

Conflict theory is concerned with the ways that social structures and social change affect ageing at both individual and collective levels. Researchers from this theoretical perspective are of the view that conflict and instability are central to social life and are the prime factors in the organization of people into groups. Hence this approach places emphasis on what divides groups rather than the values that they share.

These types of approach to the study of ageing remain fairly rare and novel. 'Inequality' theory has developed out of the conflict theory approach. This theory argues that the inequalities characteristic of other stages of life are maintained into later life. Hence those who were poor in mid-life remain so in old age, while the wealthy maintain their privileged lifestyle. One manifestation of this approach in the field of gerontology is the notion of 'structured dependency' (Townsend 1981). Townsend argues that the dependency of older people so frequently documented is 'socially constructed'. He is concerned with how and why society restricts the life chances of older people and argues that institutions such as retirement and pensions are tools for the management of the economy but ones that result in the marginalization and dependence of older people. He also argues that we must recognize that there are (potential) conflicts of interest between older people and the not so old, especially over the allocation of 'scarce' health and social welfare resources; for example, the so-called 'intergenerational conflict' (Johnson et al 1989).

The analysis and explanation that this approach produces are at a macro, rather than an individual, level. Criticisms of this approach have largely focused on its Marxist manifestations. It is dominated by economic factors, gives little credit to other influences, is highly deterministic, and suggests that older people are compelled (or coerced) into particular positions, which gives the impression of a 'conspiracy' theory applied to social policy. Phillipson (1998) has refined the theory to take account of these criticisms and it still retains an appeal for the school of critical gerontologists.

Interpretative theories

These theories operate at the microsociological level and assume that choice (or free will) is the most basic aspect of human behaviour. These types of approach are usually concerned with social interaction within specific settings, and with communication (usually language) as the key to the understanding and analysis of society. The focus is on understanding the way that individuals perceive their world and others in it, and the meaning that they attribute to these experiences. Therefore explanations for the issue of informal care for older people would be different, using this theoretical framework, from the functionalist perspective noted earlier. The functionalist, for example, would examine the role of the carer of parent or spouse as a behaviour 'imposed' on the individual by external social norms. The interpretative perspective, on the other hand, would investigate the meaning of such terms as 'obligation', 'duty' and 'responsibility' and look at how caregiving is negotiated between the parties involved.

Labelling theory is an illustration of this theoretical approach. Labels (such as 'mad' or 'old') are linguistic descriptions that are a shorthand for the characteristics illustrated by a group and others apply such labels to groups or individuals. This approach draws heavily from deviance theory, in which labels are used negatively to confer stigma or deviant status and to marginalize individuals. The most well-known proponent of this view was Goffman (1961), who showed how the behaviour of former mental patients was always under scrutiny once they had been given the label of 'mental patient'. In the case of older individuals, their behaviour is always being watched for signs of physical and/or mental decline and the challenge for the older person is to maintain independence and social competence.

Another approach in the interpretative tradition is social exchange theory. The assumption here is that human beings seek to influence each other via social interaction. This is achieved by the exchange of rewards. Social exchange theory has several underpinning assumptions. First, individuals opt for interactions from which they will benefit. Second, interactions will be sustained if the benefits outweigh the costs. Finally, it is assumed that power is derived from imbalances in the social exchange. If one individual is dependent on another the one gains power while the other loses it. Several authors and researchers have used social exchange theory to understand the process of ageing (De Beauvoir 1972, Dowd 1975, 1980). Martin (1971) used this approach to family visiting patterns of older people and concluded that most older people had little 'power' in this situation and were largely in a dependent or deferent position to their family (unless they had a large inheritance, which greatly enhanced their power). Similarly, Dowd (1975) argues that reciprocity is the key to understanding human relationships. With age the potential for reciprocity decreases, as older people have few resources (other than experience) and hence they lose autonomy and control over their environment. However, Finch (1989) indicates how this is a very limited approach as she argues that reciprocity needs to be understood within a lifecourse perspective.

The main criticism of these approaches is the level of analysis. These types of theory are often concerned with the minute details of daily life rather than dealing with the large-scale structures and processes of society. Therefore, although interesting insights may be identified, the structural or institutional dimensions of the process of ageing are not addressed. However microlevel approaches can be very illuminating tools when studying the process of care and care giving.

Old age as social problem

This is not a theory of ageing but it is an approach that has been very influential in the development of British gerontological research work (Victor 2005). At its most simplistic it has concentrated on identifying and enumerating the problems experienced in old age (a humanitarian approach) and on 'the burden' that this poses for society (an institutional perspective). Work in these areas has concentrated on looking at health and service issues (especially quality of life, health status and use of services) as well as looking at retirement and employment. This typically views older people as 'a problem' and is concerned with determining the burden this poses for society as well as the individual. Hence there are numerous studies of who provides care and help to older people but comparatively few about how much help older people provide, either to other older people or to younger family members (e.g. collecting children from school so that their mother can work). Hence, while this is not a particular theory of ageing, it is an approach that has influenced the types of question posed and hence the knowledge base of British gerontology. For example, work on loneliness and old age has presumed that this is a problem unique to older people and has sought to establish the prevalence and risk factors for loneliness (Townsend 1957, Tunstall 1966). It is only recently that researchers have sought to include the views of older people and to investigate the factors that 'protect' against loneliness (Victor et al. 2005).

It is evident from the comments so far that there is no single theoretical approach that may be universally applied to the study of ageing. For all its limitations, biological work in ageing has been very influential in the development of ageing research. Within the fields of medicine and nursing, in particular, the biomedical approach has been enormously influential. This approach to the study of ageing has concentrated on determining physiological and biological explanations of ageing (and the health of older people). However, such a model denies the importance of psychological or social factors in determining people's health experience (or indeed other aspects of ageing). Hence no account is taken of factors such as class, gender and ethnicity in explaining the existence of disease and illness and in the utilization of health services. The preeminence of the biomedical approach has resulted in the relative neglect of issues such as health promotion and prevention in favour of an emphasis on illness, treatment and management. Furthermore, by denying the importance of social and psychological factors in understanding ageing, we portray the individual as a passive entity who has little influence on the events which happen to him/her. However, it is evident that the experience of ageing is not a fixed and inevitable consequence of chronological age. Rather it is a multifaceted experience that results from the complex interrelationship between psychological, social and biological variables. Indeed Rowe & Kahn (1997) argue that social factors may be more important than biological or genetic factors in influencing the quality of later life. This complexity needs to be recognized in the enterprise of ageing research, which is almost always multidisciplinary in nature.

OLD AGE: ATTITUDES, MYTHS AND STEREOTYPES

Old age, however we define it, is a part of the life-course about which myths and stereotypes abound. Nurses, like other segments of the population, illustrate many of the commonly held, highly negative views about old age. Old age and ageing are, in a modern western society that is highly youth-dominated, associated with highly undesirable negative traits such as poor health, mental frailty and social isolation. These negative or undesirable traits result in the stigmatization and marginalization of old people. This rather negative image of the old and ageing is often contrasted with some previous 'golden age' in which reverence for older people was the norm. To draw such an extreme comparison is to overstate the case. There is no doubt that some societies at some times venerated older people. However, this is not necessarily the norm and we should be wary of wearing rose-coloured spectacles when examining other cultures or times from our own past.

Surveys of both adults and children have consistently reported 'old age' as the least desirable phase of the life cycle, characterized by financial, health, social and other problems (Aiken 1995). These types of study consistently reinforce the negative images and stereotypes of old age. A stereotype is a caricature-type summary of the attributes (either positive or negative) of specific social groups, such as older people, adolescents or asylum-seekers. Old age is presented as a time of physical, mental and social decline. Older people are perceived as in poor health, with impaired sight/hearing, mentally frail and socially isolated and neglected by their family. Implicit within this set of images is the notion that older people are passive and unable to exert any control or autonomy over their lives or to maintain their independence, regardless of their social competence before 'old age'. Such negative views of older people are identifiable in health care professionals working with older people in the UK, Australia (Morris & Minicheillo 1992) and the USA (Aiken 1995). There is the view that nurses (and doctors, and probably related professionals such as physiotherapists and occupational therapists) hold negative views of older people and that these influence their career decisions. Negative images of older people discourage nurses from entering gerontological nursing. Too often working with older people is seen as unchallenging: older people are slow to respond to treatment and 'there is no cure' for ageing. Furthermore this area of work is seen as blocking career development and enhancement. Negative images of older people held by health staff may also result in less than optimal care being received by patients. The ten-dency to infantalize older people and treat them as if in a 'second childhood' is documented (Hockey & James 1993). This approach can also promote poor-quality care by encouraging patients to become dependent rather than independent.

The UK in the 1990s saw the development of a new, positive stereotype of ageing. The new image of old age is of a population of carefree, financially secure people, free from the demands of participation in the labour market. This is just as much a distorted representation of many of the realities of ageing and later life as the more traditional negative stereotypes. This view of older people spawned a variety of descriptive acronyms including GLAMs (grey, leisured, affluent, middle-class), OPALs (older people with affluent lifestyles) and JOLLIEs (jet-setting oldies with loads of loot). Such a view can be easily used as an argument to withdraw public services from older people on the grounds that they are not needed because: (1) older people are 'really in good health'; or (2) those who require services can afford to pay for them. It is not clear that the development of these more positive images of older people has improved their image with health professionals or proved effective in attracting high-calibre staff to work with older people.

Ageism

One important manifestation of this negative stereotyping of older people has been the development of the notion of ageism. Like racism and sexism, this implies wholesale stereotyping and discrimination against a specific subgroup in society. Ageism describes the discrimination against people simply on the basis of their chronological age and as such it may be implicit or explicit. The term was first coined by Butler in the late 1960s (Butler 1975), although others had argued along similar lines (e.g. Rosenfelt 1965, De Beauvoir 1972, Comfort 1977). Bytheway (1995) deconstructs the various issues involved within the broad term of 'ageism'. He identifies, in particular, the way that age is used as a barrier (or entry criterion) for access to services. Age discrimination in access to health care services has been the subject of recent debate in both the UK (Williams & Evans 1997) and North America (Callahan 1987). In the absence of research demonstrating the outcome of providing specific health care services to older people (or indeed other segments of the population), age-based barriers to services (e.g. not providing dialysis to people aged over 65) appear to be rooted in a negative ideology concerning the worth of an older person's life (in comparison to a younger person). As such, the arbitrariness of such decisions should be exposed and debated. Indeed the recent *National Service Framework for Older People* (Department of Health 2001) includes the statement that age should not be a barrier to the receipt of services.

Older women

Old age and later life is predominantly a female experience. As the demographic data described in Chapter 3 illustrate, there is a marked imbalance in the number of old men and old women, although this is decreasing as male mortality rates improve. Men are much less likely to reach old age because of their elevated mortality rates. Hence the majority of older people are women. It is only recently that the predominantly female nature of the ageing experience has been noted and enumerated (Arber & Ginn 1991, 1995). The importance of gender in shaping the experience of old age is now recognized. Compared with men, older women are more likely to experience poor health, social isolation, widowhood and poverty (Arber & Ginn 1991, 1995). However, the importance of studying the experience of older men within a predominantly female experience is also important.

For women the experience of ageism is often linked with sexism and sexist attitudes. Older women may be discriminated against because they are both old and female. This double disadvantage was termed 'the double standard of ageing' by Sontag (1978). However its pedigree significantly predates the development of the term. Both Plato and Hippocrates agreed that 'old age' started earlier for women than men. More recent social research confirms this idea – that women become 'old' 5–10 years earlier than men (Victor 2005). The roots of this concept appear to lie in the differential social value ascribed to men and women. Men are valued for their competence, power and authority, while women are valued for their child-rearing and reproductive functions. Nowhere is the double standard of ageing so clearly visible than in the area of reproduction and sexuality. Older men are seen as desirable, whereas older women are not. Older men may marry (or associate with) much younger women, while for older women this is frowned upon. Women taking advantage of fertility treatments to have children after the onset of the menopause are 'irresponsible', while older fathers are not the recipients of such negative social sanctions and, indeed, are admired for their continued virility.

It is undoubtedly true that gender is an important determinant of the experience of old age. It is a variable that has, until recently, been rather neglected in the analysis of later life. However this reflects a wider problem of the failure, until recently, of gerontological work to acknowledge the importance of social factors such as gender, class and race in the experience of old age. Nurses need to acknowledge the diversity presented by the older population and respond and devise appropriate services and interventions. Hence we need to look not only at gender but also at class and, increasingly, the ethnic profile of older people and consider how these dimensions of social differentiation intersect and interact to influence the experience of old age and ageing.

METHODOLOGICAL ISSUES IN THE STUDY OF AGEING

As has already been observed, the study of later life and ageing is theoretically, conceptually and methodologically challenging. In this section we examine some of the key methodological issues that should be addressed by the student of ageing (see Jamieson & Victor 2002 for a detailed analysis of this field). The aim here is not to produce fully-fledged researchers but rather to equip nurses and other health professionals working with older people to be able to evaluate critically the research evidence concerning the care of older people. This is a skill that all health practitioners will need to develop as we move towards the provision of evidence-based health care (Muir-Gray 1996).

Identifying age differences

Gerontology is concerned with the study of ageing and with the identification of age-related changes (senescence) and age differences. For example, the gerontologist may be interested in studying physiological functions such as changes in respiratory function or muscle strength. Nurses may be interested in changes in wound-healing rates with age or in investigating susceptibility (or risk factors) for infection rates with age. This task is not quite as straightforward as it sounds. Observed differences between people of different age groups (age differences) in, for example, physical health status, dementia, sexual or smoking behaviour may arise either because of ageing (i.e. they are age effects) or because of other reasons such as cohort or period effects (or, even more confusing, some combination of these). We consider these different constructs in more detail to illustrate the complexity of this area of research. Further, this serves to emphasize that practitioners need to be very cautious in inferring that patients' problems are due to their age or because of ageing. The research approaches described here are largely concerned with quantitative types of study. Later in this chapter we consider the role of qualitative and biographical research traditions within 'ageing' research.

Age effects

These may be either intrinsic (i.e. changes produced as a true result of the ageing process) or reactive (i.e. changes produced as a result of the socioenvironmental context). However, in reality it is difficult to distinguish between these. Indeed, it is extremely difficult to identify 'true' age effects. Strehler (1982) proposed four criteria that could be used to determine if observed biological changes are displayed in order to be classed as part of normal ageing (as opposed to a pathological or disease process). These were: (1) universality (it must happen to everyone regardless of their social and physical environment); (2) progressiveness (it should happen gradually and not as a result of a catastrophic event); (3) intrinsicness (it should be the result of 'natural' processes rather than the result of harmful environmental exposures of agents); and (4) that the process was deleterious (it reduced the ability of the person to cope). Hence for dementia (or grey hair or wrinkles) to be a 'true' age effect it should happen to everyone regardless of their social and cultural context. This test for universality in particular is an important way of distinguishing pathology from ageing. Most of the health problems and disease which older people may experience are often tritely attributed by health professionals and older people themselves as being 'due to ageing'. The requirement for universality illustrates how superficial such analyses of the health problems of older people are. In the field of social gerontology universality, progressiveness and deleteriousness would be important tests for the veracity of an observed age difference (in, for example, quality of life) to be accepted as a true age effect.

Cohort effects

These reflect the influence of historical time and are attributes specific to a particular generation (or cohort). As well as being defined by age, cohorts may be defined on the basis of social class, ethnicity or other variables. For example, we might study a group (or cohort) of students applying to medical school or a group of débutantes who had been presented at court. Good examples of cohort rather than age effects are the very high number of spinster (never married) older women resulting from the high male death rates during the First World War, and the large-scale adoption of smoking (during the First World War for men and the Second World War for women). However we need to note that a particular historical event (such as the First World War or the postwar period) is not experienced uniformly by everyone of the same age (because of the effect of class or gender),

and that the same event will be experienced by people of different ages. Hence the experience of a particular event/period will differ between and within different cohorts.

Looking at the current generation of older people, it must be acknowledged that cohort effects may be important in shaping their experience of ageing and in the types of health care problems presented. People aged 80 or more will have experienced the First World War as infants/young children, the Great Depression as young adults and another world war and then the implementation of the welfare state as middle-aged adults. How many of the attributes currently ascribed to the effects of ageing are, in fact, reflections of the experiences of these varying historical events and their ramifications such as poverty, poor nutrition and lack of access to health and welfare services? Will the so-called 'baby boomer' generation, who are the children of the postwar welfare state, present a similar (or radically different) profile when they reach old age? We cannot answer these questions with any degree of certainty. Hence we must always be aware that the patterns and problems seen among older people today may reflect cohort rather than age effects and, as such, may not be repeated by subsequent generations.

Period (or time) effects

These are changes resulting from wholesale societal changes in attitude towards, for example, the role of women, marriage, sexual behaviour, homosexuals or the role of religion in society. These can be difficult to differentiate from cohort effects. In reality it is often difficult to establish if age, period or cohort differences (or indeed some combination of these) are responsible for any observed age differences.

However, it is important to be aware that the simple observation of age differences, such as the reluctance of older people to learn to use computers, may reflect a real decrease in the ability of older people to learn new skills because of reductions in blood supply to the brain (an age effect), the limited education received by older people (a cohort effect) or the widespread availability and familiarity of computers within modern society from which older people have been excluded (a period effect).

APPROACHES TO THE STUDY OF AGEING

What types of research design are used in order to determine and describe age differences? Irrespective of the research question (e.g. evaluating diet and health status or describing attitudes towards retirement or grandparenting), there are three main types of study design that are used in the study of ageing and the identification of age-based differences (Table 2.1). These are considered in turn.

Cross-sectional studies

These involve comparing people of different ages at the same point in time on the variable of interest. For example, we might investigate the prevalence of chronic illness and disability among different age groups by comparing prevalence rates between people of different ages. In this type of approach we would survey people aged 45–54, 55–64, 65–74 and 75 years and over at a single point in time. The rationale for this approach is that any differences we observe would represent the result of ageing. While this can demonstrate differences between age groups it cannot unambiguously determine whether any observed differences represent the result of ageing. It is virtually impossible to determine from this type of study

Table 2.1 Schema of major research designs used in the study of ageing

Year of birth	Dates of data collection		
	1970	1980	1990
1910	A	B	C
1920	D	E	
1930	F		G

Cross-sectional study (study of people of different ages at single point in time) = comparison of cells A, D, F (ages 60, 50, 40).
Longitudinal study (study of cohort over several time points) = comparison of cells A, B, C (ages 60, 70 and 80).
Time-lag study (comparison of people of same age but measured at different time points) = comparison of cells A, E, G (ages 60). These effects are confounded or impossible to distinguish from cohort effects. For example, if a cross-sectional study demonstrated that older people performed less well on standard psychological memory-type tests, what inferences could we draw from this result? Such a result may indicate that memory deteriorates with age. Alternative but equally plausible explanations include the possibility that this group of older people had bad memories, even when they were young, or that they were so intimidated by the test situation that they underperformed. The main advantage of this type of research method is that these studies are relatively cheap and straightforward to administer and provide fairly rapid results. Also, if all we are interested in is establishing the existence or otherwise of age differences (rather than age effects) then this approach is perfectly valid.

whether observed differences reflect age, cohort or period differences.

Longitudinal studies

These involve individuals who, after initial identification, are followed over time and repeated measurements are made for the variable(s) of interest. In the hypothetical example in Table 2.1 we would first identify a group of 60-year-olds and then follow them up every 10 years for further data to be collected. This method could be used to look at changes in mental health with ageing, quality of life or attitudes towards work and retirement. This is a very powerful research tool that has been used to look at development (especially child development) over time. It is the most scientifically rigorous way of studying ageing but it is expensive and difficult to administer. Loss to follow-up because of death, refusal or inability to trace subjects is a major methodological problem, as the sample may become less representative (or biased because of the systematic exclusion of particular groups such as the very frail or very fit) of the population and that will limit the inferences that can be drawn from the study. Also there are more technical limitations to this approach, as study participants may become familiar with the testing regimen because of repeated exposure to the measurement techniques. Consequently longitudinal studies can be compromised because of selection effects (i.e. loss of sample members), history effects (the events which individuals experience between testing periods) and testing effects (the result of repeated exposure to the testing regimen). Furthermore it is not clear if longitudinal studies, which are usually based on a single cohort, are generalizable. If each cohort may present a different profile of ageing, can we generalize from studies based on a single group?

Time-lag design

This involves collecting data from several cohorts of people but at different points in time, although the individuals are of the same age. Hence the subjects studied are of the same age when the research is undertaken but they were born at different times (i.e. they belong to different cohorts) and are measured at different time points.

Examples of cross-sectional and longitudinal research

There are numerous examples of cross-sectional studies that have documented age differences within the population. In the UK some of the best-known and most widely used surveys are conducted by the Office of National Statistics (ONS) and include the General Household Survey (GHS) and the Health Survey for England. These two surveys contain a wealth of health-related data about all age groups within the population; they are described further in Chapter 3. There are several well-known longitudinal studies of ageing. Among the better known are the Duke University and Berlin ageing studies. In the UK we have, as yet, no nationally based longitudinal study of ageing, although we have a series of National Child Development Studies and the English Longitudinal Study of Ageing is now underway.

While it is not the role of this chapter to dwell in detail on the more practical issues of research, it is important to identify some of the key issues that readers should consider when examining data from any type of research design. These issues all relate to the confidence with which we can make generalizable inferences from the research population studied to the wider population. Hence nurses may wish to determine how much confidence they can place in evaluating the effectiveness of, for example, a programme to manage arthritis in primary care or a programme that supports older people at home and prevents admission to residential or nursing homes. The identification of the sources upon which these studies are based can place important limitations on the utility of the findings. For example, routine surveys often classify all people aged 65 years and over as a single group. This makes identification of the subgroups within these broad age bands problematic. Researchers should carefully define the subjects of study. It is easy to assume that a Longitudinal Study of Ageing is concerned with older people when, in fact, it has a much broader remit and included people aged from 20 to 80 years.

The sources of the sample and method of recruitment are also important. The GHS is based on those living in the community. This therefore excludes all those resident in institutions. As this is about 20% of those aged 85 years and over, this is an important omission and may well influence estimates concerning the health of this age group. More difficult is the source used to generate our sample. This applies especially to situations in which we study a sample of the population of interest rather than the whole group. Regardless of the objectives of the study, the population researched should be representative of the population under consideration. This enables us to make inferences from the sample studied to the wider population. For example, we may wish to study older car drivers or people married to a much younger spouse. If our sample is not representative then our results will be subject to bias because some groups may be systematically excluded. Hence the source from which the sample was generated is of considerable importance. As yet there is no national population register with data about age from which we can select samples. A variety of sources are used to generate general samples of the population, including general practitioners' lists, electoral rolls and postcode address files. It is usually slightly easier to study populations of service users (e.g. older people treated as day patients) as there are usually case records/administrative lists that can be used. However, we should not make inferences about the general population from samples of service users/group members. For example, carers who belong to a carers' group may well be quite different from the general population of informal carers of older people. Hence inferences made about carers based upon samples derived from group membership are not necessarily applicable to all carers. Similarly, we should be wary of studies based on volunteer samples and those that rely on non-random methods of recruitment.

Data on participation in the Baltimore Longitudinal Study of Aging (Sharma et al 1989) illustrate some of the loss to follow-up issues mentioned earlier and raise the issues of non-response and non-participation rates. Of the 1088 subjects initially recruited for the study in 1958, 658 (60%) were still actively participating in June 1977. Of those lost to study, 177 had died and 253 were alive but had dropped out of the study. These attrition rates are not exceptional but serve to illustrate how what may once have been a representative sample can quickly become unrepresentative (or biased, which means that some elements of the sample such as the very healthy or the very frail are systematically excluded from the study).

Much research in social gerontology, especially in the health-related field, includes a survey element. The issue of minimizing bias is one of the central concerns of survey research. Bias can be introduced into a study both by the systematic failure to include certain groups (e.g. minority elders) in the sample or by the systematic failure of certain groups to participate; for example, the frail or the visually/hearing impaired may be less likely to participate in studies. Therefore it is important that response rates are maximized in order to minimize bias and increase the confidence we can have in the results. A target of 90% is desirable. Non-response bias is less problematic if we have some basic information (e.g. age, sex) about the characteristics of the sample. We can then compare responders and non-responders and determine the extent and nature of non-response bias and statistically adjust the results. However such information is rarely available.

In both cross-sectional and longitudinal studies a variety of measures may be used to collect the data we are interested in. These can be questions included in a survey, or physiological measures such as blood samples. In survey research it is important to adopt 'best practice' in question design, such as not asking leading questions or asking double-negative questions (see De Vraus (1993) for a good review of the survey method).

Whatever the measures used, we need to consider two factors: reliability and validity. Reliability relates to the stability of a measure. For example, does a blood pressure machine give stable readings or do answers to questions about health service use or quality of life remain constant (assuming of course that the individual's circumstances have not changed)? Validity is concerned with whether the measure actually records the factor we are interested in or not. For example, do questions on smoking really measure the true prevalence of smoking? Normally we determine the validity of a measure by comparison with an established gold standard; however, in many areas, especially those concerned with attitudes or quality of life, this is not possible.

In research with older people there are problems because many of the measures used, especially in psychological/health outcome research, have not been validated or tested for reliability with older people. This naturally reduces the scientific rigour of the instruments. For example, many of the widely used measures of social support were measured and tested on American college students. By using such samples to develop these measures we may not capture the issues that are pertinent to older people. For example the SF36, a widely used quality-of-life measure, is very concerned with work (as defined by paid employment). This makes it difficult to use with older people. Even when a measure is developed with older people we still need to be wary. The Barthel index, which is a widely used 'disability' measure, was actually developed to determine nursing care needs for older people in rehabilitation wards following a stroke, therefore its usefulness as a general-population measure may be limited. Hence we need to look at the measures and how they were developed before using them with older people.

The most efficient research design for the study of ageing

None of the most commonly used designs (cross-sectional or longitudinal studies) by themselves enables researchers confidently to identify age effects free from the confounding effects of cohort and time of measurement. Cross-sectional studies confound age with cohort differences, longitudinal studies confound

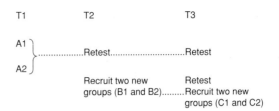

Fig. 2.1   Most 'efficient' research design for studying ageing. T, time.

ageing effects with differences due to time of measurement, and time lag designs confound time of measurement with cohort differences. In response to this research conundrum Schaie (1977) has proposed a sequential research design that includes aspects of both longitudinal and cross-sectional studies within a single study (Fig. 2.1). The study starts with a standard cross-sectional design. A group of two (or more) age groups is identified and data are collected. These subjects are then followed up and resurveyed 5 years later, for example. This provides data about longitudinal change in a specific cohort. At the second testing point another two age groups are added and the process can be repeated. Such a design provides data on cross-sectional differences (by comparing people of different ages at specific time points), longitudinal differences (by following people over time) and cohort changes (by comparing people of the same age but from different cohorts). This method of study is complex both analytically and in design but it has been used in the Seattle Longitudinal Study (Schaie 1983) and the Australian Longitudinal Study of Ageing (Andrews et al 1989).

QUALITATIVE RESEARCH AND THE STUDY OF AGEING AND LATER LIFE

In the UK the majority of the work undertaken into the experience of ageing and later life has been empirical and quantitative in nature. This largely reflects the applied nature of much research in this area. Much gerontological research in the UK has largely been concerned with counting and classifying older people. However this research tradition does not have a monopoly on the study of old age and ageing. Qualitative research has the potential to make a significant contribution to our understanding of later life (Gubrium & Santiar 1994), especially in examining the experience of 'old age'. It is easy to dichotomize the quantitative/qualitative research debate. Clearly the two traditions differ in their approach, the types of question posed and the type of material that researchers would classify as data. However it is simplistic to see these two approaches as being in conflict; rather they should be considered as complementary. Qualitative research is concerned with understanding meanings and values and experiences of older people. As such, questions which could be approached from a qualitative perspective would include: What is the meaning of marriage? What is the meaning and experience of widowhood? How do older people understand and define loneliness? What do older people think about their own and others' health? There are now good examples of qualitative health-related research with older people (Sydell 1995). Such research can often have major policy significance. The qualitative approach blends in with the development of life history and biographical approaches to the study of ageing and later life. This approach proposes that to understand old age we need to review the biographies of individuals. For example, we cannot hope to understand the meaning of marriage to an older couple without first locating it within the biography (or life history) of the parties concerned. This is an approach which is still developing but which locates ageing within a dynamic of biography. As such it clearly offers a very fruitful and stimulating perspective on the study of ageing and the experience of old age.

CONCLUSION

The terms 'old people', 'older' and 'geriatrics' are widely used in popular and professional discourse. In this chapter we have demonstrated the conceptual and methodological complexity that underpins these apparently simple, and highly pejorative, terms. There is no good, easily available definition of old age. Nurses and other health professionals need to recognize the highly arbitrary and socially constructed way that such groups are defined and labelled. Health care workers, like other segments of society, often hold highly negative, unjust (and often patronizing) views of older people. Such stereotypes do not recognize the complexity that is the modern experience of ageing. Older people are as diverse a social group as any other segment of society. They are not 'all alike' and health care workers need to recognize the highly limited and distorted views of older people that are prevalent in society and start to recognize the individuals they are caring for.

Recommended reading

Bytheway W 1994 Ageism. Open University Press, Buckingham.
This is a good résumé of the issues surrounding the use of chronological age.

De Vraus DA 1993 Surveys in social research practice. Heinemann, London.
A comprehensive and accessible book covering all aspects of survey research.
Jamieson A, Victor CR (eds) 2002 Researching ageing in later life. Open University Press, Buckingham
This book focuses on the theory and practice of doing research, drawing from a range of methodologies and illustrated by case studies.
Kitwood T (1999) The time of our lives. Weidenfeld and Nicholson, London
A stimulating book examining biological and social perspectives on ageing.
Peace SM (ed) 1990 Researching social gerontology. Sage, London.
An examination of theories, concepts and methods that aim to understand, explain and study old age.
Victor CR 1994 Old age in modern society, 2nd edn. Chapman & Hall, London.
This overview of social aspects of ageing with a particular focus on the UK is widely used by students, professionals and researchers in gerontology.
Wallace RB, Woolson RF 1992 The epidemiologic study of the older. Oxford University Press, Oxford.
This book covers epidemiological methods for the study of ageing, e.g. case-control studies and cross-sectional studies.

Useful websites

www.ace.org.uk
Age Concern UK and links to a wide range of resources about ageing.
www.agenet.ac.uk
Summary of major UK longitudinal studies concerned with older people and ageing.
www.bbc.co.uk/radio4/reith2001/
The transcript of the 2001 Reith lectures by Tom Kirkwood, examining attitudes and perspectives on ageing.
www.bgs.org.uk/
British Geriatrics Society.
www.bsra.org.uk/
British Society for Research into Ageing – the biology of ageing.
www.doh.gov.uk/publich/health/healtholderpeople2000.htm
Reports and data from the 2000 health survey for England, providing a wealth of data concerning the mental and physical health of older people in community and residential/nursing homes.
www.gad.gov.uk
For actuarial data about life expectancy and population projections.
www.geron.org
Gerontological Society of America.
www.soc.surrey.ac.uk/
British Society for Gerontology.
www.statistics.gov.uk/
Gateway to a wealth of vital statistics data and ad-hoc surveys for the UK.
www.who.int
For mortality, life expectancy and other comparative health data.

References

Aiken LR 1995 Aging: an introduction to gerontology. Sage, London

Andrews G, Choek F, Carrs S 1989 The South Australian longitudinal study of ageing. Australian Journal of Ageing 8: 31–35

Arber S, Ginn J 1991 Gender and later life. Sage, London

Arber S, Ginn J (eds) 1995 Connecting gender and ageing. Open University Press, Buckingham

Banks T 1992 Foreword. Carnegie inquiry into the third age. Centre for Policy on Ageing, London

Butler RN 1975 Why survive: being old in America. Harper & Row, New York

Bytheway B 1994 Ageism. Open University Press, Buckingham

Bytheway B 1995 Ageism, 2nd edn. Open University Press, Buckingham

Callahan D 1987 Setting limits: medical goals in an ageing society. Simon & Schuster, New York

Comfort A 1977 A good age. Mitchell Beazley, London

Cumming E, Henry W 1961 Growing old: the process of disengagement. Basic Books, New York

De Beauvoir S 1972 Old age. Penguin, Harmondsworth

Department of Health 2001 National service framework for older people. Department of Health, London

De Vraus DA 1993 Surveys in social research practice. Heinemann, London

Dowd J 1975 Aging as exchange: a preface to theory. Journal of Gerontology 30: 584–594

Dowd J 1980 Stratification among the aged. Brooks Cole, Monterey

Erikson EH 1980 Identity and the life cycle. Norton, New York

Finch J 1989 Family obligations: a social change. Polity, London

Goffman E 1961 Asylums. Penguin, Harmondsworth

Gubrium J, Santiar A 1994 Qualitative methods in aging research. Sage, London

Havinghurst R 1963 Successful ageing. In: Williams RH, Tibbitts C, Donahoe W (eds) Process of aging. University of Chicago Press, Chicago, pp 311–315

Hockey J, James A 1993 Growing up and growing old. Sage, London

Jamieson A, Victor C 2002 Researching ageing and later life. Open University Press, Buckingham

Johnson P, Conrad C, Thomson D 1989 Workers versus pensioners. Manchester University Press, Manchester

Kirkwood T 1999 The time of our lives. Weidenfeld and Nicholson, London

Laczko F, Phillipson C 1991 Changing work and retirement. Open University Press, Buckingham

Laslett P 1996 A fresh map of life, 2nd edn. Weidenfeld & Nicholson, London

Martin JD 1971 Power, dependence and the complaints of the older: a social exchange perspective. Ageing and Human Development 2: 108–112

Morris M, Minicheillo V 1992 Why choose to work in geriatrics? Australian Journal of Physiotherapy 38: 21–28

Muir-Gray JA 1996 Evidence based health care. Macmillan, Basingstoke

Neugarten B 1974 Age groups in American society. Annals of the American Academy of Political and Social Science 415: 187–198

Phillipson C 1986 Capitalism and the construction of old age. Macmillan, Basingstoke

Phillipson C 1998 Reconstructing old age. Sage, London

Riley MW, Johnson M, Fones A 1972 A sociology of age stratification. Russell Sage, New York

Rosenfelt RH 1965 The older mystique. Journal of Social Issues 2: 37–43

Rowe JW, Kahn RL 1997 Successful ageing. Gerontologist 33: 433–440

Schaic KW 1977 Research designs in the psychology of ageing. In: Birren JE, Schaie KW (eds) Handbook of the psychology of ageing. Van Nostrand Reinhold, New York, pp 129–141

Schaie KW (ed) 1983 Longitudinal studies of adult psychological development. Guilford Press, New York

Sharma SK, Tobin JD, Brant LJ 1989 Attrition in the Baltimore longitudinal study of aging. In: Lawton MP, Herzog AR (eds) Special research methods for gerontology. Baywood, Amityville, NY, pp 233–248

Sontag S 1978 The double standard of ageing. In: Carver V, Liddiard P (eds) An ageing population. Open University Press, Milton Keynes, pp 72–80

Strehler BL 1982 Ageing: concepts and theories. In: Viiditc A (ed) Lectures on gerontology. Academic Press, London

Sydell M 1995 Health in old age. Open University Press, Buckingham

Thomas K 1977 Age and authority in early modern England. Oxford University Press, Oxford

Townsend P 1979 Poverty in the United Kingdom. Penguin, Harmondsworth

Townsend P 1981 The structured dependency of the older creation of social policy in the twentieth century. Ageing and Society 1: 5–28

Tunstall S 1966 Old and alone. Routledge & Kegan Paul, London

Victor CR 1991 Health and health care in later life. Open University Press, Buckingham

Victor CR 2005 The social context of ageing. Routledge, London

Victor CR, Scambler S, Bowling A, Bond J 2005 The prevalence of and risk factors for loneliness in later life. Ageing and Society 25 (in press)

Ward R 1984 The ageing experience. Harper & Row, New York

Williams A, Evans J 1997 The rationing debate: rationing health care by age. British Medical Journal 314: 20–25

Chapter 3

Demographic and epidemiological trends in ageing

Christina R. Victor

It was noted in Chapter 2 that the use of chronological age to determine the onset and definition of old age is highly arbitrary. In this chapter we take those aged 65+ years as being the older population. However, the limitations of this definition are fully acknowledged. This chapter examines the size and composition of the older population, reviews the epidemiological data for this age group and provides a public health perspective on the health care needs of this segment of the population.

POPULATION AGEING IN THE UK

Size of the older population

In examining demographic trends and population ageing we need to consider two separate dimensions: the absolute number of older people and the relative proportion of the total population represented by this group. The absolute number of older people in the current population reflects the interrelationship between births in 1938 (or earlier) and subsequent rates of mortality (plus a small effect of inward and outward migration). Fluctuations in the absolute number of older people in the population largely reflect variations in the original size of the birth cohort. For example, in the period 1900–1910 there were 900 000 births a year, compared with 600 000 in the 1930s (Grundy 1995). The percentage of the population this (or indeed any other age group) represents depends upon both the absolute numbers of older people and the size of the other age groups.

In 2001 the enumerated population of the UK was 58 789 194, of whom 9 340 999 (15.8%) were aged 65+ years (Table 3.1). When we define the population aged 65+ as 'older people' we are identifying a very large subgroup of the population as this can encompass a 40-year age span. Gerontologists are concerned with not treating this part of the population as a single homogeneous group (with an implied universal set of needs) but with disaggregating this population into its relevant constituent parts. One important distinction which is made is between the 'young old' (sometimes referred to as the third age: Laslett 1996) and the 'old old'. Very simply, the 'young old' are those aged under 75 years, while the 'old old' are usually defined as those aged 85+ years. Variations in the percentage of very old people within a population can have an important influence on the demand for care, as this is the group that presents the highest prevalence of disability. Nationally 1.9% of the population (or approximately 1 124 061 people) are aged 85+ years. When we identify the percentage of older people aged 85+ as a factor likely to influence the demand for nursing care we are using age as a proxy measure for need. However, as we shall see in the sections on health, not all very old people are frail or without resources. Therefore we must be careful not to treat all older people (or all those aged 85+) as a homogeneous group who will present a common set of health problems to which we can respond in an identical fashion.

A key feature of later life is that it is predominantly a female experience (Table 3.1). The predominance of women amongst the older age groups increases with age so that by the age of 85+ there are 260 women for every 100 men. Grundy (1996) observes that the predominance of women has decreased slightly in the last 20 years. However, although this trend is continuing, it is likely that women will continue to dominate within the older age groups well into the foreseeable future.

Changes in the size of the older population

The demographic structure of populations (be they countries or localities) is not static but rather subject to constant change. Populations may grow or decline and their internal age and sex composition changes. Overall the national population is growing at a fairly slow rate. By the year 2040 it is estimated that the population of the UK will peak at 64 million and decline slowly thereafter (assuming current trends in mortality and fertility continue, which is, of course, a fairly significant assumption). The most significant feature of the population in the next decades (as over the last 50 years) is the ageing of the population (Victor 1994). For example, for England and Wales in 1901, 4.7% of the population were aged 65+ and 0.2% were aged 85+ (the absolute numbers in these age groups being 1 376 000 and 44 000 respectively). This compares with 2001 when 15.8% of the population were aged 65+ and 1.9% were aged 85+. Over the 20 years 2001–2021 it is estimated that the population aged 60+ will increase by 32.9% (Table 3.2). This increase is not equally distributed across the age groups and is most pronounced amongst those 85 years and over (by 79%). However the actual increases in the numbers in these age groups is rather less spectacular. This 'ageing' of the older population reflects both variations in the size of the initial birth cohort – in absolute terms, the larger the initial birth cohort, then the larger will be the number entering old age – and significant reductions in late-life mortality.

This large percentage increase in the numbers of older people is often referred to as 'the demographic time bomb' as it is thought to be accompanied by a decrease in the number of young people (though we should be cautious about this, as it is notoriously difficult to predict when and how many children each generation will produce). While the increase in the numbers of older people is almost inevitable (as we are already born), barring any major changes in mortality patterns, we cannot predict with any certainty what sorts of demands such groups may make upon the caring services. It is this large percentage increase in the numbers of the very old that provokes alarm because of: (1) the greater prevalence of solo living amongst this group; and (2) the high levels of morbid-

Table 3.1   UK population by age and sex (000s)

Age (years)	M	F	Total	%	M:F
0–14	5688	5417	11 105	18.9	105
15–24	3636	3574	7210	12.2	101
25–34	4095	4265	8360	13.2	96
35–44	4334	4443	8771	14.9	98
45–59	5506	5610	11 116	18.9	98
60–64	1410	1470	2880	4.9	96
65–74	2301	2636	4937	8.4	87
75–84	1300	1980	3280	5.5	66
85+	310	814	1124	1.9	38
Total	28 580	30 209	58 789		

Source: 2001 Census website (www.statistics.gov.uk/Census 2001). Male: female ratio summarizes the sex balance of the population and is calculated thus: number of males/number of females × 100.

Table 3.2   England and Wales: population (thousands) aged 65+ 1901–2041

Year	Numbers aged			% of total population aged 65+
	65–74 years	75–84 years	85+ years	
1901	992	340	44	4.7
1921	1645	753	76	6.1
1941	2751	981	131	10.0
1961	3526	1678	309	11.9
1981	4619	2389	541	15.2
1991	4515	2787	812	15.9
2001	4367	2933	1012	15.9
2011	4814	2935	1304	
2021	5822	3607	1425	
2041	6339	5040	2274	

Source: Grundy (1996) and Government Actuary's Department 2001-based projects available online at www.gad.gov.uk/population/index.asp.

ity and disability amongst this population (discussed later in this chapter). However, it is a matter of speculation as to whether future generations of older people will illustrate the same patterns of morbidity as today's cohorts of elders who have experienced considerable privation over their life course. Future generations of elders may present a whole different set of needs because of the difference in experiences they will have had compared with older people we see today.

Family circumstances

Arber & Ginn (1991) have indicated that access to caring resources is an important factor in maintaining older people independently in the community. In considering access to caring resources we need to distinguish between caring resources provided by the formal service sector (e.g. health services, private services) and those provided by the informal sector (family, friends and neighbours). These issues are explored in detail in later chapters in this book. Wenger (1984, 1994) has clearly demonstrated that the social network available to older people is linked to their need for support from state services; those with wide social support networks are less likely to have to use state services than those with a very restricted network. Access to 'informal caring resources' is rather difficult to measure empirically. However, routinely available demographic data do provide information about two

variables which may be taken as 'indirect' proxy measures of the availability of informal carers. These are marital status and household composition. To some extent these two variables are clearly interrelated as the household circumstances of older people obviously reflect the interrelationship between age and civil status (see Chapter 33 for further discussion on carers and lay caring).

Civil status

The civil status of people aged 65+ in 2001 shows the oft-reported difference between older men and older women, resulting from sex differentials in mortality (higher for men than women) and the age difference between spouses (men usually older than women) (Table 3.3). For men aged 65+, three-quarters are married compared with one-third of women. Almost half of women are widowed. For women, the majority are widowed by the time they are aged 75, while for men the majority are not widowed until they are aged 85. Even in the very oldest age groups men are much more likely to be still married than women. This indicates that old men are likely to have a spouse to provide care, while for women this is not the case.

However, we cannot take distributions such as these as fixed and constant. The marital status of the older age groups (and indeed, other components of the population) is subject to change as social norms about marriage and divorce change within society. Over the 30 years 1971–2001 the civil status of people aged 65+ shows several major changes. First there is the demise of the spinster. In 1971 14% of women aged 65+ were classified as single (i.e. never married); this had almost halved by 2001 (7.1%). This decrease reflects an interesting cohort effect: the dying-out of the group (or cohort) of now older women who had never married because of the lack of available males in

Table 3.3   Marital status: % of those aged 65+ by age and sex: England and Wales 2001

Status	65–74 years		75–84 years		85+ years	
	M	F	M	F	M	F
Single	3.5	5.6	6.8	6.8	6.2	9.2
Married	75.1	55.6	65.5	31.2	44.9	9.8
Widowed	13.4	30.3	23.6	57.8	46.6	78.9
Divorced/ separated	8.0	8.5	4.1	4.2	2.3	2.1

Source: 2001 Census website (www.statistics.gov.uk/Census 2001).

the wake of the devastation brought about by the 1914–1918 war. This serves to remind us that we cannot take for granted that the current civil status patterns will be shown by future generations of elders. Second, it seems almost inevitable that there will be an increase in the percentage of older people who are divorced and in those in second and third marriages. Indeed, the table does hint at the increased prevalence of divorce amongst older people. It seems highly likely that future generations of older people will display more complicated household and family formation patterns as a result of these changes in society. However, as we know so little of what marriage means to older people it is difficult to predict what the effects of divorce and remarriage might be (Askham 1995).

Following on from the civil status of older people, Table 3.4 describes household composition. This indicates that the majority live either alone or with their spouse. Only a minority of older people live in 'other' types of complex household, such as with siblings or children. Again there is a very clear gender difference, with older women much more likely to be living alone than their male contemporaries. Additionally, older women appear more likely than men to live with children.

We also need to recognize that there are variations between areas in the household circumstances of older people and that this will influence their needs for state care. In particular the prevalence of older people living alone is markedly higher in urban areas compared with other parts of the country; it is especially high in inner London, where 42% of those aged 65+ live alone (see Victor 1996a for a more detailed description of the circumstances of older people in inner London).

Again the household circumstances of older people (and indeed other age groups) are not constant over time. The household situation of older people has changed markedly since 1945, when only 12% lived

alone (only a marginal increase on the 7% reported for 1851; Grundy 1995), compared with 30% in 1994–1995 (Central Statistical Office 1996). The increased prevalence of solo living is not confined to the older age groups but is a more general social trend. In 1961 14% of all households consisted of one person, compared with 30% in 2001, and the number of households increased by 43% over this period (16.2 million to 23.1 million). Similarly, in 1961 3% of all households consisted of a single person under pensionable age and 7% of single people of pensionable age; by 1994/1995 these percentages had increased to 16% and 14% respectively. Again it seems reasonable to expect that the percentage of older people living alone will increase in future decades and that this may result in further demands for social care, especially if family structures have been complicated and fragmented by the increased prevalence of divorce and remarriage.

Family circumstances of older people

What are the wider family circumstances of older people and how much contact do they have with friends, relatives and neighbours? Data from the 2001 General Household Survey (GHS) indicate that three-quarters of those aged 65+ saw their relatives or friends weekly and the majority saw their neighbours to chat to. However, levels of social contact are much lower amongst those in the oldest age groups. Of course we cannot infer from this that the friends, neighbours or relatives would be willing to contribute to the care of the older person simply because they are in contact with him or her. All these data do is indicate the social integration of older people and the potential support network available to them (Phillipson et al. 2001).

As we shall see in Chapter 33, the family is a major source of care for older people. Apart from the spouse, the next most important members of the caring

---

Table 3.4 Household composition (%) by age and sex: UK 2001

Lives	65–69 years		70–74 years		75–79 years		80–84 years		85+ years	
	M	F	M	F	M	F	M	F	M	F
Alone	15	30	24	39	27	51	27	63	54	69
Lives with spouse	66	52	59	42	61	37	63	21	37	10
Lives with spouse + others	14	8	11	6	7	3	4	3	3	2
Lives with siblings	1	1	1	2	2	1	1	2	0	2
Lives with children	1	4	1	5	1	2	0	5	1	8
Other	4	4	3	5	2	5	5	7	3	9

Source: General Household Survey 2001 available from: www.statistics.gov.uk/lib2001/section3730.html.

network are sons and daughters (including in-laws). However, it is not known how many older people have surviving children. Grundy (1995) estimates that in 1962 23% of those aged 65 had no surviving children, 51% had one or two children and the rest three or more children. She suggests that in 1986 slightly fewer older people had no surviving children (17%); 62% had one or two children and a much lower percentage had three or more children. This suggests that more older people had surviving, but fewer children. This reflects the decrease in average family size that has taken place over the last 40 years.

Ethnicity

The British population aged 65+ is predominantly white, with 3.5% of this age group identifying themselves as belonging to minority communities. In 2001 it was estimated that 17% of those who described themselves as white were aged 65, compared with 6% black/black British and 2.5% Asian/Asian British, and 3.9% other. However, in the coming decades we will see the ageing of the minority communities as the cohorts of those who came to this country for employment move into old age. This may result in the presentation of different types of health problem and will require services to adapt to the cultural variety presented by the ageing ethnic-minority population (see Chapter 6).

Geographical distribution

Nationally the percentage of the population aged 65+ is not equally distributed throughout the country. The urban areas generally have a lower percentage of older people than the shire counties. In outer London 14.7% of the population are aged 65+, compared with 16.8% of the population of the shire counties and 15.8% nationally. Furthermore there are clusters of areas in which the percentage of older people considerably exceeds the general norm. The south-west and East Anglia have the highest percentage of those aged over 60 and over 80. Such areas include the traditional 'retirement towns' of the south coast. This means that within each of the authorities responsible for providing health and social care there may be different levels of demand, which need to be acknowledged in both the planning and funding of nursing care services.

MATERIAL RESOURCES IN LATER LIFE

Only a small percentage (13%) of those aged 60–65+ are still in paid employment. Consequently job-related earnings are a comparatively unimportant element of pensioners' incomes. Older people are dependent on three main sources for their income: (1) state benefits/pensions (received by about 98% of older people, as benefits within this category are both universal and means-tested); (2) private (occupational/employment) pensions (received by 53% of older people); and (3) income from savings and investments (received by 65% of older people) (Victor 1996b).

There has been much discussion about the financial circumstances of older people (Johnson & Falkingham 1992). In particular it was suggested that older people were improving their financial circumstances relative to other segments of the population. This is true only in so far as older people were improving their position relative to other groups dependent on benefit, such as the long-term unemployed (Falkingham & Victor 1991). The gulf between older people and the rest of the employed population remains large, with only a very few very-well-off older people (Falkingham & Victor 1991). Overall it is estimated that 60% of pensioners' income is derived from the state, 20% from occupational pensions, 14% from savings and investments and 6% from earnings (Victor 1996b).

The relative importance of state and non-state sources of income varies within the older population. It is only amongst the younger components of the population at the top of the income distribution that non-state sources of income are of major significance (Hancock & Weir 1994, Victor 1996b). Women, those living alone, those over 80 and those from a background of unskilled manual jobs are most at risk of experiencing poverty and low income in later life (Townsend 1979, Arber & Ginn 1991, Johnson & Falkingham 1992, Victor 1996b, Ginn et al. 2001). It is precisely those elements of the older population experiencing the greatest health needs who have the least access to household caring resources and the least ability to pay for the care they need. Groves (1995) concludes that, on the basis of current research evidence, only a small minority of older people can realistically make a significant contribution towards the cost of their care.

Housing is another factor that is important for the material resources available to older people for two main reasons. First, the home provides the location within which older people live, and home has a very important meaning for older people (and indeed other age groups). Second, the quality, design and state of repair of the dwelling can obviously hinder (or promote) the ability of older people to live independently within the community. Additionally, for those who are home owners, this represents a significant financial asset which could, in theory at least, be released to provide resources to contribute to their care. In 1994

55% of those aged 65+ owned their home outright, while another 9% had an outstanding mortgage, compared with 42% and 5% respectively in 1980 (Jarvis et al. 1996). Over the same period, renting from the council decreased from 41% to 30% and private renting from 12% to 6% (Jarvis et al. 1996). The prevalence of home ownership is highest amongst the 'young old', with 72% of those aged 60–64 classed as home owners, compared with 57% of those aged 80+.

Most older people remain in their own homes during their later life. However 10% of those aged 65+ live in sheltered accommodation (Bennett et al. 1996). This ranges from 7% of those aged 65–69 to 18% of those aged 85+ (Office of Population Censuses and Surveys 1996).

EPIDEMIOLOGICAL ASPECTS OF AGEING

In this section we look at the major aspects of the epidemiology of health in later life. Before examining the empirical data concerning the health of older people it is first necessary to describe the key concepts underpinning epidemiological analysis.

Incidence and prevalence

In population-based (or epidemiological) research there are two key concepts: incidence and prevalence. The method of calculation of these two measures is shown in Box 3.1. Incidence describes the number of new cases of a specific disease (or disability) occurring within a defined population (e.g. a health authority area) during a given time period (e.g. a year). The incidence rate describes the number of new cases

which a health care agency, such as a district nursing service, might expect over a given period. Thus incidence can be used to estimate the 'expected' workload of a department and the potential requirement for resources.

Prevalence records the number of cases of a specific disease (e.g. stroke or coronary heart disease) in a defined population at a specific time point. Prevalence rates describe, for example, the total workload with which a community nursing service may be dealing at any one time.

Although incidence and prevalence rates are usually used to measure disease, we may calculate the number of new disabled older people (incidence rate) as well as the prevalence of disability in particular areas or populations. This would indicate both the number of new cases we might have to deal with each year, as well as enumerating the total workload for this client group.

Incidence rates are extremely useful measures for those concerned with needs assessment, as they indicate how many new cases of a disability, or particular form of behaviour (such as hospital admission), might be expected over a specified time period, e.g. a year. Changes in incidence rates indicate whether a certain problem is increasing (or decreasing) and also reflect the changing size of the 'population at risk' of particular social care problems. Incidence rates could form a useful measure for the evaluation of the effectiveness of health care and nursing activities. It may be inferred that decreasing incidence rates indicate the success of particular interventions. For example, a reduced incidence of admissions to nursing home care may be ascribed to the development of intensive home care services.

However, it is worth noting that the notions of both incidence and prevalence are questionable, because they assume that we may unambiguously categorize populations (or individuals) into two distinct and discrete groups: those with the disability and those without. For many conditions, especially those related to the health of older people, this is problematic because there are rarely situations in which individuals may be unequivocally described as presenting (or lacking) the condition under review. This is particularly so for chronic conditions such as dementia or disability where there is a continuum ranging from no impairment to total impairment.

Sources of information about health and disability

Information about the health status of older people may be derived from two main sources: (1) national data sets; and (2) locally based information such as health or disability surveys. Most of the examples described in this

---

Box 3.1   Method of calculation of incidence and prevalence rates

Incidence = the number of new cases in a given reference period/population at risk
e.g. calculation of incidence rate for stroke in those aged 65+
= number of new cases in 1 year/population aged 65+
= 20/2000
= 1% (or 10 per 1000)
Prevalence = total number of people aged 65+ with stroke/population at risk
e.g. calculation of stroke prevalence rate
= total numbers with stroke/population aged 65+
= 500/20 000
= 2.5% (or 25 per 1000)

section relate to national data but this does not mean that local data sets are unimportant, although their availability and quality do vary considerably. When using local surveys as a way of estimating the prevalence of specific conditions, such as disability, users need to evaluate critically the quality of data by examining sampling (i.e. were responders drawn from the general population or was the survey based on samples of service users?), response rate (are the data limited by non-response bias – the systematic underrepresentation of specific groups?) and the types of questions used (were leading questions used or were standardized assessment schedules modified, thereby undermining their scientific properties?).

Information about disability and disabling conditions

When attempting to assess the need of older people for community care we are interested in data that relate to the difficulties experienced by people in maintaining their independence. Hence we are predominantly interested in establishing the prevalence (and incidence) of disability, and disabling conditions (both mental and physical), in the population rather than in describing health status per se. The following describes sources of data available for use in needs assessment.

Mortality

It remains a paradox of epidemiological research that our most reliable source of information about the health of the older population relates to mortality data. Information about the numbers and causes of death is available for the UK and its constituent areas (see Victor 1995 for a review of sources of health data). Registration of death is compulsory and a doctor is required to certify the cause of death. The precision

with which cause of death is identified varies considerably and is generally much less accurate for older people than those in younger age groups. It is almost inevitable that some causes of death that carry a considerable social stigma, such as acquired immune deficiency syndrome (AIDS), are underreported.

Patterns of mortality in later life

In 2001 there were approximately 556 000 deaths in England and Wales, of which 80% were accounted for by people aged 65+. Mortality rates are high (about 6 per 1000) in the first year of life and then decrease to a very low level in childhood and early adulthood, rising inexorably from the mid-30s onwards into middle and old age (this is the J-shaped distribution of mortality).

The pattern of mortality in later life shows distinct variations between groups. Overall there is little difference between men and women but in later life there is a pronounced gender difference. At all ages over 65 years men illustrate mortality rates approximately 50% higher than their female contemporaries. This ranges from 70% for those aged 65–74 to 30% for those aged 85+ (Table 3.5). Social class variation in mortality in the UK population is well documented (Townsend 1979). Such analyses have traditionally excluded those aged 65+ but it is now clear that such class-based variations in mortality extend well into old age (Victor 1991b). It remains unclear whether ethnic-minority elders experience worse (or better) health than the host population (Blakemore & Boneham 1994).

One feature of the postwar period has been the decrease in late-age mortality rates. Over the period 1971–1995 there was only a modest change in overall male mortality, while rates for women increased very slightly (Table 3.6). However, there have been substantial reductions in mortality in later life – of

Table 3.5   Mortality rates: England and Wales 1971–2001 (rate per 1000 population)

Year	65–74 years		75–84 years		85+ years		All ages	
	M	F	M	F	M	F	M	F
1971	50.5	26.1	113.0	73.6	231.8	185.7	12.1	11.0
1981	45.6	24.1	105.2	66.2	226.5	178.2	12.0	11.3
1991	38.5	22.0	93.6	58.6	197.1	163.8	11.2	11.3
2001	30.4	18.35	78.4	52.2	190.0	158.8	10.0	10.4
% change 1971–2001	−40	−30	−31	−29	−18	−14	−17	−5

Source: Office of National Statistics 2003 – Health statistics quarterly 18, Table 6.1, available at www.statistics.gov.uk/downloads/theme-health/HSQ18.pdf.

Table 3.6 Expectation of life: England and Wales 1976–1991

Year	Birth		60 years		70 years		80 years	
	M	F	M	F	M	F	M	F
1961	68.1	74.0	15.11	19.1	9.3	11.8	5.2	6.4
1971	69.0	75.2	15.4	20.0	9.5	12.6	5.5	7.0
1981	71.0	77.0	16.4	20.9	10.1	13.4	5.8	7.5
1991	73.4	79.0		22.1		14.5		8.4
2000	75.6	80.3	19.6	23.1	12.3	15.1	7.0	8.6
Change in years	7.5	6.3	4.5	4.0	3.0	3.3	2.2	2.2

Source: Office of National Statistics (1996/2003 – Health statistics quarterly 18, Table 6.1, available at: www.statistics.gov.uk/downloads/theme-health/HSQ18.pdf.

30% for males aged 65–74 and 16% for women aged 85+ (Table 3.5).

Expectation of life

Another indicator of decreasing general and late-age mortality rates is change in life expectancy (Table 3.6). Between 1961 and 2000 there was an increase of 7 years in expectation of life at birth. The increases in the number of years older people may expect to live having reached aged 60 (or 70 or 80) are significant. For example, there has been an increase of approximately 4 years in expectation of life at age 60 and of 2 years at age 80. These data therefore suggest a real improvement in the health of older people.

What are the major health problems of old age?

The paucity of morbidity measures leads us to use mortality statistics because of their ready availability. This is justified by the view that, on the whole, when mortality is high then so is morbidity, a view broadly confirmed by research studies. While current patterns of mortality may identify the areas or groups (such as older people) with poor health, such data may give a very poor picture of the types of health problem experienced by these groups.

As defined by mortality, the main health problems of later life are circulatory disease, cancer and respiratory disease. These account for over 90% of deaths of those aged 65–74 and 80% of deaths of those aged 85+. These data expose the limitations of mortality data in shedding light on the main health problems of different groups, as many major causes of non-fatal ill health account for relatively few deaths. For example, data about the extent of mental health problems in the community are not well covered by mortality data. Mental illness is numerically a comparatively unim-

portant cause of death, accounting for about 2% of deaths amongst those aged 65+, but is the cause of considerable morbidity and disability within the population. Similarly, musculoskeletal diseases are a low-mortality but high-morbidity condition.

Sources of morbidity data

Morbidity statistics are concerned with the amount and types of disability and illness that occur within the population. As such, these would appear to be more appropriate measures to use when examining the health of older people. However, most routinely collected morbidity data suffer from serious shortcomings, partly because of the variable nature and imprecise diagnosis of many illnesses and partly because of inadequacies in the information system (Victor 1995).

Data about the national population are available from several sources. First, the 1991 censuses included a question about the number of individuals within households with 'long-term limiting illness'. This is a very broad indicator of the prevalence of chronic health problems within the population. At both local and national level it correlates very well with data about mortality.

The GHS, an annual social survey undertaken by the Office of National Statistics (ONS; previously the Office of Population Censuses and Surveys, OPCS), collects data about the prevalence of both acute and chronic health problems (using a question similar to that used in the 2001 census). However, the GHS only includes within its study population those adults resident in the community. Excluded from the study are those resident in institutions (e.g. nursing and residential homes and prisons). This may limit the usefulness of the data when we are trying to determine the 'true' health status of the total population. ONS also sponsors a variety of ad hoc surveys looking at health issues. For example, they undertook a survey of the prevalence of disability within the population (Martin et al. 1988). They are often a useful source of broad prevalence rates which can then be applied to a particular context and can provide an indication of the scale of different problems within the communities served. Similarly, the English Health Survey can provide information about the health status of the population; however, it has only a limited amount of information about disability issues as it has concentrated on enumerating risk factors for cardiovascular disease. Furthermore, almost all the data sources that are readily available relate to prevalence; comparatively little information is available about incidence and they usually relate to the population resident in the community.

Prevalence of chronic illness and disability

Mortality data show two distinct trends: (1) death rates increase with age; and (2) men illustrate higher mortality rates than women. Such an analysis would identify older men as therefore having the poorest health in later life. Is this pattern replicated when we examine the distribution of chronic health problems in later life? The age-related increase noted above is maintained from 20% at age 35–44 to 57% for those aged 75+ (Victor 1991a). However, the gender difference observed for mortality is reversed. Thus men are less likely than women to survive into old age. Those who do are generally in better health than their female contemporaries: females illustrate rates of chronic health problems approximately 20% higher than their male contemporaries. Those older people from professional occupation groups illustrate better health than their contemporaries from manual occupations (Victor 1991b).

Causes of disability

Martin et al. (1988) reported that, for adults, the major causes of disability were musculoskeletal disorders (46% in community and 37% in institutions), mental disorders (13% in community and 56% in institutions), nervous disorders (13% and 30%), circulatory (20% and 16%) and respiratory disease (13% and 16%). Neoplasms were the cause of disability for 2% of adults in the community and 4% in institutions (Martin et al. 1988). Hence a morbidity-based analysis reveals a different constellation of health problems from a mortality-based perspective. Such a different pattern of health problems may require different styles

and types of service from that based on a mortality-type analysis.

Functional ability: activities of daily living

Another way of looking at the health of older people is to look at their ability to perform various activities of daily living that relate directly to their ability to live independently in the community. Such activities broadly cover three aspects of daily life: (1) mobility; (2) self-care (such as dressing and feeding); and (3) domestic care tasks (such as shopping, cooking and cleaning). Within each category the percentage unable to manage these tasks increases with age. Highlighting those aged 85+, at least 20% are unable to manage one of the self-care tasks (compared with 4% of those aged 65–69), 60% cannot manage household shopping (8% of those aged 65–69) and 44% have at least one mobility problem (5% of those aged 65–69) (Table 3.7). Although there are gender differences in the reported prevalence of difficulties with activities of daily living, it is unclear whether this is a 'true' reflection of differences in chronic illness between men and women or the strong gender demarcation of household responsibilities and tasks in this age group (Arber & Ginn 1991, Wilson 1995).

One issue of considerable policy relevance is the degree to which observed age-related variations in health status reflect the influence of ageing or are a reflection of cohort effects. Given the biography of the current generation of elders (the experience of two wars and the privation of the interwar depression), we might speculate that much of the pattern of ill health seen in later life reflects these generational experiences. Future generations of elders, because of their experiences – especially in early childhood – may show a pattern of better health in later life. There are insufficient available data with which to examine this hypothesis. However, there were no significant changes in percentages able to undertake activities of daily living over the 1980–2001 period (Table 3.8). We may, therefore, assume, for the present, that we are unlikely to see significant changes in the immediate future in the percentages of older people unable to manage these types of activities. Bone (1996), in her analysis of patterns of dependency in the 1980s, arrived at a similar conclusion.

MENTAL HEALTH

A morbidity-based analysis indicates that dementia is a major health problem of later life; however, it is a relatively unimportant source of mortality, accounting for 1.8% of deaths. Dementia is an important

Table 3.7 UK population (%) unable to undertake activities of daily living: 2001

Activity	%					
	65–69	70–74	75–79	80–84	85+	All 65 +
Going out or walking down road	6	10	14	20	41	14
Getting up/down steps	5	7	10	16	24	10
Getting around house	1	0	2	2	2	1
Getting to the toilet	1	1	1	1	3	1
Getting in/out of bed	2	1	2	3	5	2
Wash all over	3	5	6	11	21	7
Dress/undress	2	2	2	4	8	3
Wash face/hands	0	0	0	1	2	0
Feeding	0	0	0	0	3	0
Cut toenails	18	29	34	43	64	31
Household shopping	5	9	14	21	41	13
Wash/dry dishes	1	2	3	3	9	3
Clean inside windows	9	13	20	29	48	19
Use vacuum	5	8	10	17	34	11
Wash clothes by hand	6	6	9	12	24	9
Cook main meal	3	4	5	9	15	5
Prepare snack	1	1	2	3	7	2
Make a cup of tea	0	1	1	2	5	1

Source: General Household Survey 2001 – available at www.statistics.gov.uk.

Table 3.8 Percentage of those aged 65+ unable to manage selected activities of daily living: UK 2001

Activity	1980	1985	1991	1994	2001
Going outdoors and walking down road	12	13	11	13	14
Getting up/down steps and stairs	8	9	9	9	10
Getting around house on level	2	2	2	1	1
Getting to the toilet	2	2	1	1	1
Getting in/out of bed	2	2	2	2	2
Wash face and hands	1	1	0	1	1
Feed self	0	1	1	0	0
Household shopping	14	16	19	16	13
Clean windows inside	17	19	16	20	19
Wash clothes by hand	7	8	8	7	9

Source: Goddard & Savage (1994); Bennett et al. (1996), General Household Survey 2001 – available online at www.statistics.gov.uk.

health problem that can result in a significant need for community care services (as well as health care services). Enumerating the number of older people suffering from dementia is problematic as it is particularly difficult to establish where along the continuum of behaviour dementia starts. Jorm et al. (1987) have undertaken a meta-analysis of the various studies that have attempted to determine the prevalence (and incidence) of dementia in the community. The prevalence of clinically significant dementia (i.e. a degree of impairment of intellectual function which would merit service interventions by health and social service agencies) approximately doubles every 5 years, from 0.5% of those aged 60–64 to 34% of those aged 90 and over (Table 3.9). There is no consensus as to whether dementia is more common in men than women, and the pattern amongst minority communities remains to be established. Nursing care of older people with dementia is discussed in detail in Chapter 24.

The above data relate to the prevalence of the condition; however, it is also useful to know its incidence. How many new cases are diagnosed each year? Brayne & Ames (1988) suggest we should use the 'guesstimate' of 1% per annum for the population aged 65+. This suggests that in the UK there are 90 650 clinically significant new cases of dementia annually.

HEALTH CARE NEEDS OF OLDER PEOPLE

It is now part of national policy that health service provision should be informed by the assessment of health needs (Pickin & St Leger 1993). In this context a population may range from a primary care trust locality or family doctor practice to the whole country. The development of health needs assessment was given its strongest impetus by the 1991 changes to the National Health Service, and the introduction of the purchaser/provider split. In order to purchase appropriate health care for its resident population, health commissioning agencies need to profile, or describe, the characteristics of their population and assess its need for health care, and then purchase appropriate health care (Victor 1995). Policies on assessment are now established through the recommendations of the *National Service Framework for Older People* (Department of Health 2001) for the single assessment process (discussed further in Chapter 28).

Table 3.9 Estimated number of people aged 60+ with dementia: UK 1996–2021

Age (years)	% with dementia	Total population	Total with dementia
60–64	0.5	2 544 754	12 723
65–69	1.1	2 292 482	25 217
70–74	3.9	2 074 550	80 907
75–79	6.7	1 755 023	17 586
80–84	13.5	1 178 314	159 072
85–89	22.8	676 678	154 282
90 +	34.1	535 727	182 682
All 60+			682 469

Source: Derived from Jorm et al. (1987).

Needs assessment: defining the terms

Prior to a substantive examination of needs assessment we must first clarify the terms that are being used in the discussion. McWalter et al. (1994) note that clear definitions of the terms used are required so that suitable tools may be developed to collect the relevant information.

We must first distinguish between three very important concepts: need, demand and supply. These terms are often used interchangeably in popular discourse but they have a very specific meaning when discussing population-level assessments of needs. Within this context the terms may be defined as follows:

- *Need* defines interventions/treatments or services from which people (either individuals or populations) would benefit
- *Demand* relates to what people would use in a free social care system (or pay for in a market-based system)
- *Supply* describes what is actually provided.

Each of these three terms is now considered in more detail.

Need

The *Shorter Oxford Dictionary* defines need as 'to be in want of'. Within a population health context, need has a more specific and technical meaning: the ability of an individual (or population) to benefit from a specific health care intervention (Stevens & Raferty 1994). Within the health care context such benefits are termed 'outcomes'. These are used to measure the success (or otherwise) of an intervention in achieving its stated goals. For example: How well does an early discharge scheme meet its desired objective of reducing length of stay? This, of course, requires that services have very clearly stated goals which they wish to achieve (we will return to this issue in the very brief consideration of evaluation later in this chapter).

If need is defined in terms of what people would benefit from, this raises the question of how we define benefit (or outcome). There is no consensus as to how benefit should be measured, although its multi-faceted nature is widely accepted in both the health and social care fields. In the health field it is usual to measure benefit (or outcome) in a variety of domains, including mortality (i.e. survival), morbidity (i.e. symptoms) and quality of life. In the fields of both morbidity measurement and quality-of-life measurement there has been considerable interest in the development of standardized outcome measures that can be used in a variety of different settings and with different population groups (e.g. older people) (Jinkinson 1994). It is worth noting here that many of the standardized outcome and assessment tools used in the evaluation of health services were not designed with older people in mind (Victor 1999).

It is also important to remember that need is a dynamic concept. Services that were 'needed' in the past, such as mass chest X-ray screening or the provision of mobile meals services to people whose houses had been bombed during the war, may outlive their usefulness. The development of new and worthwhile services and interventions will create new health care needs.

In the health field this very broad concept of need is usually further subdivided into four categories, depending on the mechanism by which needs are identified (Bradshaw 1972):

1. *Normative* needs are those defined or identified by an expert or professional. This involves the definition of a 'standard' below which people are described as being 'in need'. For example, a district nurse who considers that an older person needs help with bathing is making a normative-based needs assessment
2. *Felt* needs are those needs that are identified by users or carers, such as the need for help with bathing
3. *Expressed* needs are felt needs translated into action; for example, the demand from older people for a 'drop-in' centre or from minority elders for special dietary provisions from the home meals service
4. *Comparative* needs are defined by the comparison of health care provision received by the population (or subsection of the population) in one area with those elsewhere. If we do not know what the optimal pattern of service provision is then simple comparisons between groups and areas may highlight areas of unmet (or overmet) need.

Demand

Demand for social health care relates to needs translated into action. It is what is asked for. Demand may originate from users, carers, voluntary workers or professionals (or some combination of these). Demand for health (or indeed social care) services is not necessarily an accurate reflection of the need for services because demand for services is affected by:

- Knowledge of the existence of services. This very simply reflects the fact that an individual cannot use or demand a service if unaware of its existence. For example, older people cannot attend a 'drop-in' lunch club or for breast screening if they don't know the service exists or that they are eligible to use it. Inevitably publicity, whether at local or national level, about the existence of a service will increase demand for that service.
- The local availability of services. This means that if a service does not exist locally or is limited in its availability then demand is affected. For example, a respite care service that only operates in a very restricted manner is not likely to attract great use.

Supply

Supply relates to the availability of particular services, but again is not necessarily a surrogate for need. The level of supply of a particular service reflects numerous pressures and constraints, including historical patterns of supply as well as political, professional and public pressure.

The fact that some services are available may well stimulate use even though they may not be appropriate for meeting people's needs. The importance of supply factors in generating utilization of some services should not be underestimated, although its exact impact remains difficult to quantify, and probably varies between different services. However, one of the main features of the health care changes is to get away from a 'supply-based' identification and meeting of populations' identified needs.

Relationship between need, demand and supply

What is the relationship between need, demand and supply? As already hinted at, the relationship is far from perfect. The eight main combinations of the concepts of need, demand and supply are outlined below:

1. intervention or services needed, wanted and supplied
2. some services will be demanded and supplied but are not needed
3. some services may be provided but are not needed or demanded
4. some services will be needed and demanded but not supplied
5. services needed and supplied but not demanded
6. services which are needed but not demanded or supplied (known as unmet need; see below)
7. services may be demanded but are neither needed nor supplied.

These may be broadly divided into three main groups:

1. Unmet need: those where there is a need but no demand or supply. There may be extensive needs existing within the community which are neither identified by health care workers nor have services provided for them. This is well illustrated by surveys of older people living in the community which inevitably and universally identify extensive amounts of previously unrecorded illness, morbidity or need for services (Williamson et al. 1964, Victor 1996a)

2. Overmet need: this is where there is supply but either no demand or need. However, identifying such services can be problematic as there is often considerable professional investment in them and to reduce them is often very contentious, involving as it does a cut in provision

3. Those services where there is demand but no need or supply: this again highlights the contentious nature of needs assessment work because, as well as identifying areas where there is unmet need for services, unnecessary/inappropriate forms of provision may be identified, and challenging the status quo of service provision can be a difficult and uncomfortable experience.

EVALUATION OF HEALTH CARE

The whole underpinning of needs assessment is the provision to the users/clients/patients of services/therapies/interventions that are of proven benefit. This then raises the problem of what interventions are beneficial and how this is determined. Although much more interest is now being expressed in the importance of evaluation in health care (St Leger et al. 1992), it remains unfortunate that remarkably few health services have been evaluated. It has been estimated that only 20% of health service interventions have been evaluated and found to be of proven benefit (St Leger et al. 1992). This section raises some issues and questions about evaluation that are pertinent to a review of the provision of health care for older people but is obviously only the most sketchy introduction to this vast and complex area of research.

The first thing we need to determine is, what is evaluation? In this context evaluation relates to the 'scientific' assessment, in as rigorous a way as possible, of the extent to which health care services (or their constituent parts) achieve their stated goals. Thus a prerequisite of any evaluation is that the service/intervention under review should have clearly stated and measurable goals. For example, do domiciliary services prevent admission to long-stay care

or do respite care schemes reduce the burden felt by carers?

In attempting to evaluate any health care intervention Maxwell (1984) suggested that the following six issues need to be addressed:

1. *Effectiveness*: this is the key aspect of any evaluation, in that it describes the achievement in terms of specified outcomes resulting from the intervention. This measure tells us how successful (or otherwise) an intervention was in achieving its stated goals; for example, the number of older people 'prevented' from being admitted to long-stay care by the development of an intensive home care service. This, of course, requires that all services/interventions have clearly articulated and measurable goals. This is not always the case

2. *Efficiency*: this is an economically based measure and describes the relationship between the resources put into, and the outputs from, a service. This is a very difficult concept to measure. However, it is worth noting that services can be both efficient and also ineffective. For example, automated pathology testing may be very efficient (i.e. can do many tests per unit cost) but will be ineffective if the test being performed is not of proven benefit

3. *Equity*: this examines the degree to which the service/intervention is offered equally to all those who need it. For example, a home meals service, by only providing a limited range of foods, may exclude users from various cultural backgrounds

4. *Acceptability*: this is a neglected but important concept in both needs assessment work and evaluation studies, but is one which should be at the forefront. If the health care system is unacceptable to potential users, then regardless of its effectiveness or level of efficiency it will not be used. This dimension of evaluation deals with the way a treatment or service is delivered and is largely concerned with issues of quality. Is it delivered humanely? What do users think of the service? Would you be happy for one of your family to be cared for in this way? Issues such as providing culturally appropriate care fall within the broad concept of acceptability. This is a difficult but vital aspect of evaluation to measure

5. *Appropriateness*: this relates to the selection of the 'most appropriate' method of treatment or service delivery for a particular health care problem or client group. An intervention can

only be appropriate when certain criteria are met. The intervention should only be performed if appropriate and adequate resources are available and if it is undertaken in a way that is acceptable to the patient. For example, getting young offenders to undertake house maintenance for older people could be an inappropriate way of delivering a 'care and repair' service if the older people were not happy with the system or the service providers lacked the necessary skills

6. *Accessibility*: this relates to the access to services and considers whether individuals get the treatment that they need. Again this is a multi-faceted concept as it relates to the barriers which may (or may not) exist to people using services, such as distance to services, transport, access for disabled people and the operation and opening hours of offices. Other aspects of the concept of accessibility include access to the decision-making process and access to information about health care matters in general and the services offered. For the various aspects of access there are issues regarding the right of access, the ease of access and the cost of access that require consideration.

When looking at health services for older people we need to consider how far each of these issues is addressed. It is clearly difficult to define indicators to measure all of these aspects but a comprehensive evaluation study should try to assess these dimensions. When critically reviewing evaluative studies we also need to look at how these different areas have been assessed. It remains the case that comparatively few of the services used by older people (described in Chapter 7) have ever been rigorously evaluated. There is a major research agenda to be addressed.

CONCLUSION

The UK population includes a substantial percentage of older people. Future decades will see a continuation of the trend for the numbers of older people to increase. This trend is not unique to the UK but is a feature of most European countries. The nature of the older population is dynamic and reflects wider social trends. Old age is predominantly a female experience and this seems unlikely to change in the near future. However, we shall see an increase in the numbers of older people living alone and in the number of divorced/separated older people. It remains the subject of speculation as to how the changing pattern of family structure and rela-

tionships will influence the demands for care from older people and the role of the family in providing informal care. The ageing of the minority communities remains another issue about which we can only speculate and draw attention to the need for further research.

Older people are the main users of most of the elements of the health care system; however, there are as yet few evaluative data about the most effective ways of providing for their care. It is vital that such issues are addressed.

We have seen that, as measured by mortality and morbidity, health declines in later life. Men are less likely than women to achieve old age but those who do are less likely to experience chronic illness and disability than their female contemporaries. It is unclear what the future patterns of health in old age will look like. Fries (1980) offers an optimistic view of the future health of older people. He argues, from the premise of a fixed biological limit to the human lifespan, that the onset of morbidity will be delayed, while age of death will remain fixed. People would die after a short period of ill health; morbidity and disability would be compressed into a short period at the end of life. While this view has been strongly challenged, it has served to draw attention to two important features of health in later life: (1) the length of time for which people experience disability before death; and (2) the relationship between 'healthy' and 'unhealthy' life expectancy. The alternative view of the relationship between mortality and disability is more pessimistic. Greunberg (1977) has argued that reductions in late-age mortality have been achieved by medical interventions that result in the postponement of disability and disease and not their reduction. Following this line of argument would suggest that those surviving into old age are becoming frailer (Riley 1990). A third, intermediate, view is that older people are experiencing longer periods of disability than in the past but that the consequences of disability are less severe. We cannot determine which of these suggestions about future patterns of late age health status is correct. There is clearly a need for further research into the health status of older people and trends over time.

Recommended reading

Arber S, Ginn J 1991 Gender and later life. Sage, London.
An examination of age and the older woman from a sociological perspective. It is an informative text in an area that has previously had little literature.
Evandrou M 1997 Baby boomers: ageing in the 21st century. Age Concern, London.

This book has a good section on demography and an analysis of the social and economic circumstances of the ageing baby-boomer generation and its impact on society.

Jameson A, Victor C R (eds) 2002 Researching ageing and later life. Open University Press, London.

With contributions from leaders in the field of gerontology, this book has sections on using existing data sources to provide demographic social and epidemiological information for researchers and practitioners, as well as a discussion of research methods.

Jarvis C, Hancock R, Askham J, Tinker A 1996 Getting around after 60: a profile of Britain's older population. Age Concern Institute of Gerontology, London.

This book is a mine of helpful information and detail about the daily lives and experiences of older people.

Victor C 1991 Health and health care in later life. Open University Press, Milton Keynes.

This book provides a population overview. Although it is slightly dated, the principles are still relevant and useful.

References

Arber S, Ginn J 1991 Gender and later life. Sage, London

Askham J 1995 The married lives of older people. In: Arber S, Ginn J (eds) Connecting gender and ageing. Open University Press, Milton Keynes, pp 69–86

Bennett M, Haruis L, Rolands D 1996 Living in Britain: results from the 1994 General Household Survey. HMSO, London

Blakemore K, Boneham M 1994 Age, race and ethnicity. Open University Press, Milton Keynes

Bone M 1996 Trends in dependency in old people resident in England. OPCS, London

Bradshaw J 1972 The concept of social need. New Society 30: 640–643

Brayne C, Ames J 1988 The epidemiology of mental disorders in old age. In: Gearing B, Johnson M, Heller T (eds) Mental health in old age. Open University Press, Milton Keynes

Central Statistical Office 1996 Social trends 1996. HMSO, London

Department of Health 2001 National Service Framework for Older People. HMSO, London

Falkingham J, Victor CR 1991 The myth of the woopie. Ageing and Society 11: 471–493

Fries J 1980 Ageing, natural death and the compression of morbidity. New England Journal of Medicine 303: 130–135

Ginn J, Street D, Arber S (eds) 2001 Women, work and pensions, Open University Press, Buckingham

Goddard E, Savage D 1994 People aged 65 and over, Series EHS no. 22, supplement A. HMSO, London

Greunberg E 1977 The failures of success. Millbank Memorial Quarterly 55: 3–24

Groves D 1995 Costing a fortune: pensioners' financial resources in the context of community care. In: Allen I, Perkins E (eds) The future of family care for older people. HMSO, London, pp 141–162

Grundy E 1995 Demographic influences on the future of family care. In: Allen I, Perkins E (eds) The future of family care for older people. HMSO, London, pp 1–17

Grundy E 1996 Population review (5): population aged 60 and over. Population Trends 84: 14–20

Hancock R, Weir P 1994 More ways than means: a guide to pensioners' incomes. Age Concern Institute of Gerontology, London

Jarvis C, Hancock R, Askham J, Tinker A 1996 Getting around after 60: a profile of Britain's older population. Age Concern Institute of Gerontology, London

Jinkinson C (ed) 1994 Measuring health and medical outcomes. UCL Press, London

Johnson P, Falkingham J 1992 Ageing and economic welfare. Sage, London

Jorm AF, Korten A, Hendeson AS 1987 The prevalence of dementia: a quantitative integration of the literature. Acta Psychiatrica Scandinavica 76: 465–479

Laslett P 1996 A fresh map of life, 2nd edn. Macmillan, Basingstoke

Martin J, Meltzer H, Elliot D 1988 The prevalence of disability amongst adults. HMSO, London

Maxwell RJ 1984 Quality assessment in health. British Medical Journal 288: 1470–1473

McWalter G, Toner H, Croser A et al. 1994 Needs and needs assessment: their components and definitions with reference to dementia. Health and Social Care 2: 213–219

Office of Population Censuses and Surveys 1996 1992-based national population projections. HMSO, London

Phillipson C, Bernard M, Phillips J, Ogg J 2001 The family and community life of old people. Routledge, London

Pickin C, St Leger S 1993 Assessing health needs across the life cycle. Open University Press, Milton Keynes

Riley J 1990 The risk of being sick: morbidity trends in four countries. Population and Demographic Review 3: 403–432

St Leger S, Shneiden H, Walsworth Bell JP 1992 Evaluating health services' efficiency. Open University Press, Milton Keynes

Stevens A, Raferty J (eds) 1994 Introduction. In: Health care needs assessment. Radcliffe, Oxford

Townsend P 1979 Poverty in the United Kingdom. Penguin, Harmondsworth

Victor CR 1991a Health and health care in later life. Open University Press, Milton Keynes

Victor CR 1991b Continuity or change: inequalities in health in later life. Ageing and Society 11: 23–39

Victor CR 1994 Old age in modern society, 2nd edn. Chapman & Hall, London

Victor CR 1995 Information and health promotion. In: Pike S, Foster D (eds) Health promotion for all. Churchill Livingstone, Edinburgh, pp 69–80

Victor CR 1996a Old age in the inner city. Health and Place 2: 221–227

Victor CR 1996b The financial circumstances of older people. In: Bland R (ed) Developing services for older people and their families. Kingsley, London, pp 43–57

Victor CR 1996c How useful are health outcome measures with older people? Paper presented at joint BGS/BSRA/BSG conference, Manchester

Victor CR 1997 Older people and community care. Chapman & Hall, London

Victor CR, Henderson L, Lamping D 1999 Evaluating the use of standardised health measures with older people: the example of social support. Reviews in Clinical Gerontology 9: 371–382

Wenger GC 1984 The supportive network. Allen & Unwin, London

Wenger GC 1994 Understanding support networks and community care. Avebury, Aldershot

Williamson J, Stokoe IH, Gray S, Fisher M 1964 Old people at home: their unreported needs. Lancet i: 1117–1120

Wilson G 1995 I'm the eyes and she's the arms: changes in gender roles in advanced old age. In: Arber S, Ginn J (eds) 1995 Connecting gender and ageing. Open University Press, Milton Keynes, pp 98–113

Chapter **4**

The psychology of human ageing

Maria T. Ponto

INTRODUCTION

In order to understand the psychology of human ageing it is necessary to consider the consequences of ageing on individuals. These are likely to be different for various people and will depend on their state of health, both physical and mental, as well as on their individual, social, family and cultural circumstances. Psychological ageing is also likely to be influenced by individual life experiences and by societal expectations of age-graded behaviour. Because ageing is both an individual and a normative age-graded experience, it is a complex psychological phenomenon. Many developmental theories are concerned with the concept of 'age', but according to Kimmel (1980: 30), 'age is merely a measure of a number of revolutions that the earth has made around the sun since a person's birth. Thus, chronological age by itself may not be a very meaningful indicator of development. At best, age provides a convenient index of the passage of *time*.'

This chapter examines psychological explanations of human ageing from many perspectives. Initially sociopsychological theories of ageing are explored and thereafter ageing is considered from psychodynamic, humanistic, cognitive and behavioural perspectives. There is also a section that evaluates the explanations and contributions made by these four psychological perspectives on the changes in mental health occurring in old age. The transitions and tasks of old age, life review and reminiscence among older people as well as successful adaptation and adjustment to ageing are also debated. Finally, developmental approaches to ageing as well as satisfaction in later life are considered by examining the work of several developmental theorists.

The complexity of ageing has been recognized by developmental theorists (Gould 1978, Levinson et al. 1978, Erikson 1980; Erikson & Erikson 1997) who consider getting old as part of human development. The notion of development implies growth, movement, progression and maturity, and indeed human ageing can be considered from these perspectives. However, for the purpose of this chapter, ageing is considered in terms of social psychological theories and other major psychological perspectives.

SOCIAL PSYCHOLOGICAL THEORIES OF AGEING

There are two distinct and contrasting explanations of processes involved in ageing: social disengagement theory (Cumming & Henry 1961) and activity theory (Havighurst 1963).

Social disengagement theory

This theory proposes that, as individuals grow older, they gradually withdraw or disengage from society. At the same time there is a withdrawal of society from the individual. Social disengagement is mainly influenced by children leaving home, partners or friends dying and social circles decreasing. The theory is based on a 5-year study of 279 individuals aged 50–90 from Kansas City. The study involved interviewing participants on issues related to health, general activities and interactions with others. On the basis of what emerged from these interviews, Cumming & Henry came up with arguments for disengagement in old age. Whether these findings were representative of the rest of the population in the 1960s is unclear. It is also difficult to speculate on whether the 50-year-old participants interviewed in 1961 continued to disengage 10 years later.

The theory of social disengagement has been severely criticized almost from the moment it was introduced. Although it is true that, for most individuals, life revolves around work and, once retired, it becomes difficult to maintain work relationships, it is not necessarily true that all individuals disengage from society once retired. Some continue to be active and remain involved with society. The theory tends to imply that disengagement is desirable, thus almost condoning the separation of older people from mainstream society. Of course some people may choose to disengage in order to pursue a lifestyle which was not possible to adopt earlier because of family commitments. There is also a cultural dimension on disengagement, as in western society, retirement may impose disengagement for some people. That is not the case in China where government ministers are often in their 80s. Also, in some African tribes the elders become important members of the community who are valued for their life experience and wisdom.

A different explanation of disengagement is offered by Bromley (1990), who suggests that a tendency to disengage could be related to the personality type as well as being a characteristic of ageing. Current views acknowledge that lifespan development has an influence on how people adjust to old age (Baltes 1987) and that some older people may be more content with solitude after retirement than in earlier adulthood (Bee 1998).

Activity theory

Activity theory, proposed by Havighurst (1963), was introduced almost as an alternative to disengagement theory. Activity theory suggests that for individuals to age successfully they need on retirement to find substitutes for the activities and work of middle-age. However this theory is idealistic in nature as the maintenance of activity is not possible for all older people and will be influenced by personal, social, biological and economic circumstances. Furthermore, this theory is unidirectional as it implies that people who are active are more likely to be happy, but there is evidence that the opposite is true and that people who are happy are more likely to be active (Baltes & Baltes 1990). A more modern approach to ageing considers developmental changes during the lifespan and also focuses on changes in social relationships and how people adjust to these changes as they age (Lang & Carstensen 1994). Turner & Helms (1995) suggest that the best way of looking at human ageing is from the perspective of personality which influences styles of ageing. Since personality is considered to be an important variable in human ageing, it will be examined in some detail under each psychological perspective below.

PSYCHODYNAMIC AND HUMANISTIC PERSPECTIVES

Psychodynamic perspective

The psychodynamic perspective has its origins in the work of Sigmund Freud (1856–1939) and continues to be influential in psychology. It incorporates those psychological systems and theories that emphasize the processes of change and development and considers motivation and drive theories as central to human development. The influence of unconscious forces on most aspects of human behaviour is also highlighted. The psychodynamic perspective offers a holistic model of a person with behaviour and emotions resulting from the conflict of dynamic, unconscious forces (Kline 1993). The main concepts involve the development of personality and subsequent development of self. Freud considered development in late life to be similar to that of childhood. He believed that the narcissistic tendencies of early childhood return to people in old age. Most of Freud's work was concerned with early-childhood development and, according to him, one's personality develops during the first 5 years of life. Therefore, using a Freudian explanation, adult personality is influenced by the experiences of early childhood, in particular during the first three stages of psychosexual development. According to Freud, children pass through five stages of psychosexual development: (1) the oral stage; (2) the anal stage; (3) the phallic stage; (4) the latency stage; and (5) the genital stage. Difficulties experienced during any of these stages (fixation at any stage) will be reflected in the adult personality. Problems experienced by adults in later life may result in regression to the behaviour consistent with a stage of fixated childhood psychosexual development. Furthermore, adult neuroses could be the result of inadequate solutions to problems experienced during a particular stage of psychosexual development in childhood.

Although Freud's theory is difficult to confirm or refute, there has been some evidence to support it, in that the types of personality described by Freud do appear to exist (Hampson 1995). There is evidence for the existence of oral personality and Kline (1984) has found that characteristics associated with the oral personality tend to cluster in some individuals. Freud offered interesting explanations for the structure of personality, in that it consists of three components: (1) id (unconscious); (2) ego (preconscious and conscious); and (3) superego (conscious). The id is the most inaccessible part of our personality; it is governed by the pleasure principle and is driven by basic instincts that desire immediate gratification. The ego is governed by the reality principle and common sense, in contrast to the id, as id is influenced by emotions. Freud explains that the ego constantly influences the id and its instinctual tendencies by bringing it back to reality (Freud 1923).

The third component of personality is the superego, which is influenced by parental moral values. The superego is subdivided into conscience and ego-ideal. The development of the superego is shaped by the injunctions of significant others, parents, teachers and people in authority (Freud 1923). If we behave badly our conscience makes us feel guilty, but if we behave well our ego-ideal makes us feel good (Eysenck 1996).

There is a continuous struggle to maintain a dynamic equilibrium between the id, the ego and the superego and a degree of conflict is inevitable. For instance, it is normal for the id to demand instant gratification, while the ego fears the consequences of the id succeeding and this results in neurotic conflict. When the ego fears punishment from the conscience of the superego, the result is a moral conflict. Because it seems that the id and the superego constantly compete for dominance, the ego may use defence mechanisms for protection. According to Freud, the outcome of conflict can demonstrate itself in three ways: (1) in dreams; (2) in neurotic symptoms; or (3) in defence mechanisms.

There are a number of ego defence mechanisms and knowing about defence mechanisms may give us an insight into the behaviour of older people.

Denial occurs when the conscious mind refuses to accept the reality of a potential threat. For instance, a client may be diagnosed with cancer but refuse to accept it. *Repression* happens when a traumatic event is forced out of consciousness into the unconscious. *Regression* occurs when the individual is unable to deal with the current situation and reverts to an earlier stage of development, eating sweets when upset for example, particularly if sweets were used to make things better in childhood. *Rationalization* occurs when an individual finds an acceptable excuse for an unacceptable outcome in order to protect the self-image. For example, I failed the exam because I had a migraine and could not concentrate. *Projection* is evident when people attribute their faults to others. *Displacement* occurs when an individual is unable to demonstrate real (often angry) feelings towards someone and uses another person, animal or object as a substitute. *Reaction-formation* happens when the repressed impulse is held in check by exaggerating the opposite tendency, and individuals display behaviour which contrasts with what they feel unconsciously, for example, being extra nice to someone they dislike. *Isolation* is evident when an individual dissociates thinking from emotion, for example talking about an unpleasant personal experience without any evident emotion (Gross 2001).

There are widely recognized methodological flaws in Freud's work. His sample (middle-class, middle-aged women in Vienna) probably did not represent the rest of the population and his methods of collecting data may be considered unsound by today's standards. However, his ideas were original and have influenced not only developmental psychology but also western culture as a whole (Thomas 1990). Replicating Freud's original work is difficult as defence mechanisms, according to Freud, are unconscious. However, Fonagy (1995) argues that, while it is impossible to validate psychoanalytic ideas experimentally, the processes involved in psychoanalysis can be observed.

To summarize, Freud's ideas continue to be recognized as a major contribution to our understanding of ourselves and of others (Stevens 1995, Kline 1998). Furthermore, his work has influenced other psychologists and particularly those working in the psychodynamic tradition, for example, Erikson, whose work is discussed later.

Humanistic perspective

The humanistic perspective incorporates psychological theories that are concerned with higher human motives – self-development, self-awareness and understanding – with an emphasis on conscious experience. Humanistic theories utilize phenomenological and existentialist ideas, and are concerned with human experience, human needs, meaning and issues related to self-concept. Humanistic psychologists recognize that all individuals have a potential for personal growth which can culminate in self-actualization.

In order to evaluate the humanistic perspective this section examines contributions made by Maslow and Rogers. Abraham Maslow (1908–1970) is generally considered to be the creator of humanistic psychology and is best remembered for his 'hierarchy of needs', introduced in 1954 (Box 4.1). According to Maslow (1954), all human beings are motivated by two forces, the survival force and the self-actualization force, and have needs that reflect these forces. The survival force has priority and to fulfil it the needs on the lower levels of the hierarchy must be met. They include physiological needs, safety needs, love and belongingness and esteem needs. Once the lower needs are satisfied, attention can be given to the self-actualization force by striving for cognitive and aesthetic needs. These needs are much more difficult to achieve and are closely related to life experience. Maslow (1987) acknowledges that self-actualization means different things for different people and that we all have needs that are individual and person-specific. He also accepts that not everyone will self-actualize. Maslow's hierarchy of needs is a model that is very suitable for nursing and can be successfully applied when nursing older people.

Carl Rogers (1902–1987) also recognized the individuality of people and, like Maslow, considered self-actualization to be an innate predisposition. According to Rogers, people are predominantly good and have the potential to develop in every way. Rogers' main contribution to psychology is his theory on client-centred therapy and the concept of self. The concept of self can be explained in terms of self-image or how we perceive ourselves. When our self-image matches our ideal self we have the potential to self-actualize. If, however, there is a mismatch between our self-image and the ideal self, the chances for anxiety and emotional dissatisfaction increase (Atkinson et al. 2000). Rogers' client-centred therapy has contributed considerably to counselling theory. For counselling to be successful, Rogers (2002) recommends that the therapist offers unconditional positive regard to the client by being supportive, accepting and non-judgemental. Rogerian ideas have been accepted not only in counselling circles but have also inspired groups arising from the 'personal growth' movement. Opportunities for personal growth within such groups can be achieved if participants interact freely and openly with each other (Gross 2001).

COGNITIVE AND BEHAVIOURAL PERSPECTIVES

Cognitive perspective

The cognitive perspective in psychology incorporates those psychological theories that emphasize internal and mental processes. Mental processes or behaviours are often abstract in nature and may involve representation, belief, intention, expectancy, imagery and symbolizing. The cognitive perspective in psychology is also concerned with cognitive abilities, which involve thinking, reasoning and problem-solving, amongst others. In essence, cognitive functioning depends on the ability to process information. The information-processing model involves several operational mental stages: input, coding, storing, retrieval, decoding and output of the information. To put it simply, informa-

---

Box 4.1   Maslow's hierarchy of needs
• Self-actualization
Realizing one's potential, to find self-fulfilment
• Aesthetic needs
Beauty, order and symmetry
• Cognitive needs
To know, to explore, to search for meaning
• Esteem needs
To achieve respect from others, self-esteem, self-respect
• Love and belongingness needs
To be accepted, to be loved and to love
• Safety needs
To feel secure, safe and out of danger, physically and psychologically
• Physiological needs
Food, drink, rest, activity, survival needs

Based on Maslow (1954)

tion-processing is about organizing, interpreting and responding to incoming stimuli or information (Reber & Reber 2001). To be able to manipulate information successfully we need to use language, memory, attention, perception and intelligence. The research into cognitive changes associated with ageing has found that the speed with which older people process information declines with age, thus leading to higher reaction times (Salthouse 1996).

Although an increase in reaction time in older people has been well documented, there are a number of explanations that need considering. Often older people have difficulty in maintaining readiness prior to reaction-testing tasks, particularly when distracting stimuli are present. However if the participants are told where to focus their attention, differences are minimal (Madden & Gottlob 1997). Stuart-Hamilton (2000) proposes that being exposed to competing information also interferes with reaction time, which suggests that older people may find it difficult to divide their attention. Salthouse et al. (1995), on the other hand, report that, providing the tasks are not complicated, older and younger people have a similar range of ability when attending to simultaneous activities, for example having a conversation, watching TV and knitting. Cerella (1990) is critical of the focused testing used in studies that assess one aspect of information-processing. He proposes that deficits in information-processing result from defects distributed throughout the neural network and are determined biologically. This view is similar to that of Berk (1998), who believes that slowing in information processing could be due to degeneration of neural networks as the neurons in the brain die.

Irrespective of the explanations offered on cognitive decline, it has to be remembered that inevitably there will be individual variations, resulting from differences in ability and motivation. These differences may also be influenced by biological and physiological changes, for example high blood pressure, cardiac or cerebrovascular disorders and reduced activity in general (Schaie 1996). Apart from information-processing, problem-solving ability is another cognitive skill that has been reported to be affected by ageing, even with tasks adjusted to focus on practical cognition and practical problem-solving (Denney 1989). However, Santrock (2002) makes a relevant point regarding testing of problem-solving ability in the laboratory experiment, which may fail to demonstrate how individuals use a problem-solving approach in their everyday lives. Most tests into problem-solving rely on hypothetical, abstract thinking activities, which may not be relevant to practical problem-solving, but are frequently assessed by intelligence tests.

The concept of intelligence has been debated by psychologists since intelligence testing began. The main arguments concern definitions of intelligence and the nature/nurture debate. The question is whether intelligence is innate (that is, genetically acquired) or dependent on environmental factors, such as upbringing and education. In the early 1900s when the first tests were being developed, research was concerned with improving and validating the tests. Since then, intelligence testing has been used to predict educational performance as well as to explain many different aspects of intelligence. The popularity of intelligence testing has not declined even though the predictive value of the intelligence quotient (IQ) score is highly debatable. In relation to older people, we have to consider whether ageing affects intelligence. This is a controversial issue that has attracted a considerable amount of research. Most intelligence tests rely on testing general knowledge, comprehension, arithmetic and vocabulary within a specific time. Therefore the speed of information-processing is important for people to do well in such tests but, as previously stated, the research evidence points to a slowing in the speed of information-processing with age. This means that older people are likely to be disadvantaged in standard intelligence testing, unless the tests are standardized for older age groups.

To explore this point further, the methods used for intelligence testing also need to be considered. A number of studies use cross-sectional rather than longitudinal approaches to compare older and younger age-group participants. The problem with the cross-sectional approach is that it tests participants from different age groups on the same tests. Results from these groups are then compared, and generally the scores from older people will compare unfavourably. To explain this we need to consider differences in the educational opportunities that were available to a group of 30-year-olds as opposed to the educational opportunities that were available to the 70-year-old group. Without a doubt the research that uses longitudinal studies where the same individuals are tested over a long period of time is likely to offer more reliable information on changes in intelligence that occur with ageing. Schaie (1996) reports on the Seattle Longitudinal Study, which tested the primary mental abilities of over 500 adults aged 20–70 between 1956 and 1977. Schaie states that there were clear decreases in most primary abilities after the age of 60, although in relation to verbal intelligence they found that intellectual decline did not start until about 74 years of age. Schaie (1996) concludes that the results were cohort-specific, which could be explained in terms of differences in educational opportunities.

The appropriateness of the test is also very important. The most commonly used scale for testing adult intelligence is the Wechsler Adult Intelligence Scale (WAIS). This scale was originally developed in 1944 but has been revised twice since, most recently in 1981, and is now known as WAIS-R. The Wechsler adult scale (Wechsler 1981) has verbal and performance scales. The verbal scale tests people on the following: general knowledge, comprehension, arithmetic, similarities, vocabulary and digit span. The performance scale tests people on picture completion, picture arrangements, block design, object assembly and digit symbol (Gross 2001). Although the subtexts of the verbal scale are not timed, the performance scale is timed, so it could be argued that the speed of information-processing and problem-solving abilities are being tested and consequently that older people will score less favourably.

Another way of looking at the concept of intelligence is to consider fluid and crystallized intelligence. Fluid intelligence is similar to abstract intelligence and is characterized by the ability to solve unusual problems in a creative way. The speed of information-processing as well as problem-solving abilities and mental agility all contribute to fluid intelligence. Crystallized intelligence is characterized by the ability to manipulate factual information, which is acquired through education and life experience. There is evidence that fluid intelligence declines with age, whereas crystallized intelligence remains more static and might even improve with maturity (Baltes & Baltes 1990).

One of the factors that influence performance on intelligence tests is memory. There has been considerable research on the ageing memory. Many older people notice some memory deterioration, and complain about being forgetful. The majority of the research tends to make a distinction between short-term memory (primary memory), which involves holding information in consciousness, and working memory, which involves information-processing while dealing with other information or cognitive tasks at a conscious level (Backman et al. 2001). Most tests on short-term memory require participants to hold information passively and to recall it immediately, for example the recall of a name or a number of digits. Tests on working memory may involve tasks that require participants to process, transform, manipulate, reorganize and retain the information.

Since the majority of short-term memory testing relies on laboratory experiments, this makes it difficult to apply findings to everyday life. However, if aspects of long-term memory are examined separately, more realistic findings will result. A recent large longitudinal study of 711 people born in 1922, 1932, 1942 and 1952 by Laursen (1997) followed participants for 11 years between 1982–1983 and 1993–1994. Laursen tested many cognitive functions and reported a decline in non-verbal learning and memory, retention of verbal memory and concentration and reaction times. Laursen concludes that there is a greater variability in the older generation and that these abilities become more disseminated with age.

Tulving (1985) suggested that long-term memory could be divided into three systems: episodic, semantic and procedural. Episodic memory involves memory for personal experiences; semantic memory concerns general knowledge; and procedural memory involves memory for motor and cognitive skills such as playing the piano, driving or cycling (Fig. 4.1). The research into memory ageing has shown that there is virtually no decline in semantic memory, although retrieval from semantic memory is slower according to Light (1991). Well-learned motor skills such as typing (procedural memory) remain unaffected by ageing, although learning a new skill will take longer. Of the three components of long-term memory, episodic memory tends to be most vulnerable to impairment (Backman et al. 2001).

Findings from research into memory further elucidate cognitive functioning in late adulthood and enable us to understand the difficulties that can be experienced by older learners. Nowadays, access to education is possible for everyone and some older people may seek further education. Some people may want to learn about new technology, whereas others may wish to continue education as a means of self-actualization. The evidence that older people can maintain their cognitive abilities into old age is demonstrated by the activities of members of the House of Lords, clergy and the judicial system. Cohen et al. (1992) have examined the performance of the older students at the Open University and found that older students did well in the course work, gaining better grades than younger students. However, when they were under pressure of time in examinations, older students did less well than younger students. Maylor (1994) studied participants in the television programme *Mastermind*. He found that in the 'specialized subject' round there was no age effect, while in general knowledge, older participants did better than younger ones. The results from both studies demonstrate that the ability to learn and remember does not necessarily decline with age. Of course, it has to be recognized that both studies examined highly motivated older adults, who were probably also very intelligent. Schaie & Willis (1986) studied 4000 older adults and used individualized training to improve the partici-

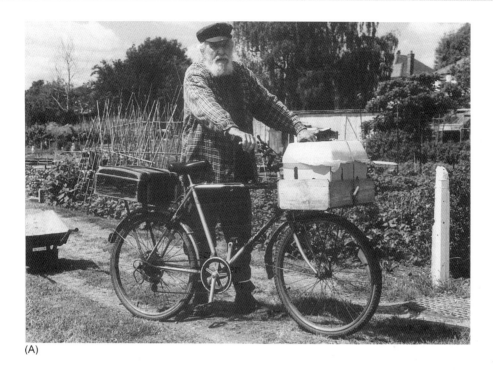

(A)

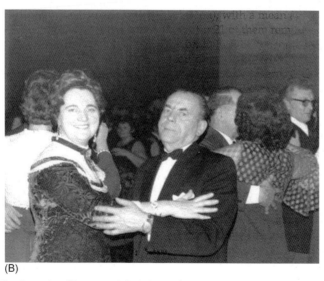

(B)

Fig. 4.1 (a, b) Keeping going. (Courtesy of Chris Rogers.)

pants' cognitive abilities. They found that, with training, declining cognitive abilities had returned to the levels found 14 years earlier. These findings demonstrate that cognitive decline not only can be arrested but also can be improved with training.

As we have seen, decline in cognitive competence affects older people, but the decline does not afflict everyone, may not be apparent until the mid-70s or 80s and may be reversible with training. When looking at the empirical evidence, it is important to remember individual differences in terms of education, occupation, lifestyle and nutrition as well as childhood influences on the individuals tested. Questions also need to be raised regarding the research tools used for testing cognitive abilities and, in particular, the suitability of general intelligence scales for older people. One has to agree with Sternberg & Lubart (2001), who believe that the research should focus on dimensions of practical intelligence, wisdom and creativity and on how age and experience interact to influence cognitive functioning.

Behavioural perspective

The behavioural perspective in psychology incorporates those psychological theories which are concerned with measurable and observable behaviour. The behavioural approach was first introduced to psychology by Watson in the 1920s (Gross 2001), but has been considerably influenced by Skinner (1974), amongst others. The emphasis of the behavioural perspective is on explanations of learning and in particular on the conditions that are necessary for learning to take place. The main empirical concepts within the behavioural perspective centre on conditioning, which can be either classical or operant. Classical conditioning is considered to be a most basic form of learning which involves actions and reactions without conscious control. An example of this would be when we salivate while going past a bakery or a fish-and-chip shop. In relation to older people we will consider another example. Mr Brown, who has meals on wheels, becomes very ill soon after eating his fish dinner. He may end up associating the meal with the illness (even if the meal was not the reason for his illness) and will consequently avoid such meals in the future; he has generalized the response from that particular situation to similar future situations. A slightly different example, but still demonstrating conditioning, is that of Mrs Smith, who is anxious about going upstairs at night and sleeps in the armchair downstairs. By sleeping downstairs, her fear is relieved and that relief acts as a reinforcer, maintaining her response (sleeping downstairs). Another reinforcer using the same example could be illustrated differently. For instance, Mrs Smith may be anxious about going upstairs because her neighbour, who is the same age, fell down the stairs and broke her leg, ending up in hospital. These explanations demonstrate the concept of generalization, which refers to the fact that once a response is learned, it may be applied to similar situations.

Operant conditioning explains the second type of learning, in which the actions are voluntary and conscious. Here, the individual operates on the environment to cause an effect. For instance, Mrs Rogers, who has no relatives or friends living nearby, feels lonely and isolated as nobody visits her. One day she accidentally leaves her milk on the doorstep and her neighbour calls to check on her that evening. She enjoys the chat as they have a cup of tea. In the weeks that follow, the neighbour notices that the milk is not collected two or three times a week. Mrs Rogers, who saw the first visit as a reinforcer, is reinforcing the visits from her neighbour by not collecting her milk. These examples illustrate the main claim made by behaviourist psychologists, that any behaviour can be shaped by its consequences or that any behaviour which is rewarded is likely to be repeated.

This discussion highlights the point that our behaviour is very much influenced by other people, by their rewards or punishments. We learn if our behaviour is acceptable by observing how other people react to it, whether they approve or disapprove. The learning which takes place in this way is best explained by a theory which derives from the behavioural perspective, known as social learning theory (Bandura 1977). According to this theory all behaviour is learned during interactions with others. While the behaviourist psychologists consider both classical and operant conditioning as important to learning, social-learning psychologists accept the importance of conditioning but do not believe that conditioning can explain all aspects of learning. They stress the importance of observational learning, which occurs without any reinforcement.

Observational learning (or modelling) occurs spontaneously – the observer does not make any obvious effort to learn but is usually able to reproduce or imitate the behaviour observed in others (Gross 2001). Apart from explaining modelling behaviours in children, social learning theory can be used to explain the differences between generations of people. The influence of parents, schools, peers and the media is powerful and has an impact on the behaviour of each generation. This also has an impact on the way the various groups are seen by others in society. The image of old people presented on television may influence the way in which some viewers perceive them (Slater 1995). This can be positive if older people are portrayed as active and helpful, but can be negative if they are portrayed as difficult and rude. In terms of nursing, the modelling or observational aspect of social learning theory can be used to teach older clients particular aspects of care – for example, giving insulin injections.

MENTAL HEALTH AND AGEING

We now consider the contributions made by the main psychological perspectives towards our understanding of lifelong human development, and the changes in mental health that can result from ageing. The term 'mental health' not only implies an absence of mental disorder but also refers to behavioural and emotional adjustment and adaptability in dealing with everyday life (Reber & Reber 2001). Vaillant (1990) offers a similar definition and states that mental health indicates the ability to deal with stress, grief, conflict and past failure as well as having good self-care and self-esteem. His definition is based on a review of a 45-year study, which followed 204 Harvard students since 1940. The study examined many aspects of psychosocial life adjustments and also considered mental health changes, which in this sample were minimal. This is an interesting study; however, its sample was biased towards successful ageing as all the participants were white, male, in good physical health and with high achievement records.

A comprehensive way of viewing mental health is provided by Jahoda (1958), who proposes a number of characteristics which are important for mental well-being. Jahoda considers the ability to cope with stress, the ability to introspect, being realistic about the world, and the ability to grow, to develop and to self-actualize as being as fundamental to mental health as the absence of mental illness. Whether we can meet all these criteria all of the time is highly debatable; for instance, it is widely accepted that not everyone will self-actualize (Eysenck 1996, Bee 1998).

Prevalent mental health changes in older people are depression, anxiety, acute confusional state and dementia, but they are not universal and therefore are not an inevitable consequence of ageing. All these changes can be detrimental to individual well-being and they are addressed in greater detail in Chapters 23–25. This chapter, however, considers anxiety from the psychological perspectives discussed earlier. Anxiety is a psychological disorder which produces an unpleasant emotional state, characterized by motor tension, which is displayed in the inability to relax and trembling (Reber & Reber 2001). Anxiety may also be characterized by hyperactivity with symptoms of dizziness, a racing heart and perspiration, as well as unreasonable apprehension, unexplained dread, distress and uneasiness (Santrock 2002). Anxiety is often seen as a symptom of depression and consequently less attention is paid to it. However, Lindesay et al. (1989) report that, out of 890 older people over 65, surveyed in inner London, 3.7% suffered from generalized anxiety disorder (10% with phobic anxiety and 13% with depression). According to Woods (1999), the incidence of anxiety in old age may be greater than previously thought and may involve as much as 10% of the older population. Anxiety as a disorder may be underreported, as older people may misconstrue the symptoms they are experiencing by confusing them with physical ill health. Older people may be anxious for a number of reasons. They may have a number of fears, such as a fear of falling in the house or in the street, fear of crime or fear of dying. The fear of falling is worrying to older people because of the consequences of a fall which could result in an individual being hospitalized and/or being dependent on others. Howland et al. (1993) found fear of falling to be the most common fear in the people they studied (Chapter 13). The fear of crime is real for most people nowadays, with so much crime being reported on a daily basis. Older people see themselves as vulnerable because they perceive themselves as less fit physically than they used to be. Fear of dying is another source of anxiety for some older people. Fry (1990) has shown that older people may fear the pain and suffering related to dying. Older people are likely to have suffered bereavement and loss as a result of spouses', friends' or neighbours' deaths, which could cause them anxiety. Anticipatory bereavement, when someone close is likely to die, can also contribute to generalized anxiety and grief. Loss, bereavement and grief can affect the mental health of older people, leading to distress and depression. The ability to deal with loss and grief is individual and Thompson et al. (1991) found that, although some bereaved people recovered 12 months after a loss, a significant number were still showing mental health distress 30 months later (see Chapter 26 for more on bereavement and loss).

To appreciate the psychodynamic and humanistic explanations, the contributions from both perspectives will be used to explain anxiety. In terms of Freudian theory, anxiety in later life originates from earlier experiences, possibly from childhood. Anxiety arises from the conflict between demands made on the ego, which has to balance the instinctual needs of the id with the constraints of the superego (Stevens 1995). Humanistic theories, using existentialist ideas, see anxiety as characterized by notions of the meaninglessness and incompleteness of the world. Both psychodynamic and humanistic approaches suggest that we should deal with anxiety by means of psychotherapy – psychoanalytic or client-centred.

In terms of mental health changes, both cognitive and behavioural perspectives can lead to successful psychotherapy. Behaviour therapy is generally sought when there is a need to change a maladaptive behaviour. Classical or operant conditioning can be utilized well in behaviour therapy, which focuses on treating the behaviour rather than the causes of that behaviour. Behaviour therapy has been favourably used, particularly with phobic anxiety (Woods 1999) and generalized anxiety (King & Barrowclough 1991).

DEVELOPMENTAL APPROACHES TO AGEING

While early developmental research in psychology centred mainly on childhood, more recently the transitions and tasks of adulthood and old age have been addressed. Although there are no distinct psychological theories that concentrate solely on ageing, a number of human development theories consider the psychological changes during early and late adulthood which are relevant to old age (Erikson 1973, Gould 1978, Levinson et al. 1978).

Erikson's theory of development

Erik Erikson's work follows the psychoanalytic tradition but places greater emphasis on psychosocial development. Erikson proposed that the human life follows a cycle of eight ages, from infancy to old age, as illustrated in Table 4.1. For each cycle there is an emphasis on ego development, which is underpinned by physical development and biological maturation. The stages are sequential, but no chronological age indicators are given for those in adulthood. Each cycle or stage is embedded in a social context and the outcome for each stage results in personal growth. According to Erikson, ego development during each stage centres on a crisis which involves the struggle between two opposing polarities, culminating in a

dynamic balance which is desirable for personal growth. Development during each stage also follows an 'epigenetic' process, meaning that the growth of the ego is gradual and progressive as well as unfolding.

To each stage, Erikson adds the lasting outcome, highlighting the basic advantages achieved – hope, willpower, purpose, competence, fidelity, love, care, wisdom. Erikson views these advantages (which he terms virtues) as necessary and re-emerging from generation to generation. His last two stages extend over a long time and Vaillant (1977) recommends that Erikson's theory should be expanded. An attempt to do that has been made by his widow (Erikson & Erikson 1997), who added the ninth stage – although not in the format of the eight stages. In essence Joan Erikson proposes that in the ninth stage individuals revisit all other stages and are challenged by the negative outcomes such as mistrust and shame as well as doubt and guilt, mainly due to not being sure of their own capabilities. For further discussion of the ninth stage see Erikson & Erikson (1997). Although sensitively written, the chapter on the ninth stage lacks clarity when compared with the work on the eight human stages.

Levinson's transitions in adult life

Levinson et al. (1978), in the book *The Seasons of a Man's Life,* offer an explanation of transitions in adulthood. The stages offered by Levinson et al. are not separated by chronological age but are concerned with transitions that occur as we move through the life cycle. In pursuing their research Levinson and his colleagues aimed to address the following questions: 'What does it mean to be an adult? What are the root issues of adult life – the essential problems and satisfactions, the sources of disappointment, grief and fulfilment?' (Levinson et al. 1978: ix). Levinson et al. interviewed 40 men aged 35–45 over a 2–3-month period and saw each subject for 10–20 h. Wives were also interviewed and, where appropriate, places of work were visited. On the basis of the data collected they proposed nine stages of adult development (Table 4.2).

The main interest for Levinson's team was a focus on the changes in mid-life, but they also describe transitions in old age. Each period of adult development has developmental tasks which must be mastered during that stage.

Gould's theory of the evolution of adult consciousness

Gould (1978) takes a different approach to adult development in his theory of the evolution of adult consciousness. Gould developed his theory whilst

Table 4.1 A cycle of eight ages		
Stages of development and their outcomes	**Virtue**	**Age**
8 Integrity versus despair, disgust	Wisdom	Old age
7 Generativity versus stagnation	Care	Maturity
6 Intimacy versus isolation	Love	Young adulthood
5 Identity versus role confusion	Fidelity	Adolescence
4 Industry versus inferiority	Competence	School age
3 Initiative versus guilt	Purpose	Play age
2 Autonomy versus shame, doubt	Willpower	Early childhood
1 Trust versus mistrust	Hope	Infancy

Based on Erikson (1973).

Table 4.2   Levinson's stages of development

Age (years)	Stage
17	Childhood and adolescence
22	Early-adult transition
28	Entering the adult world
33	Age-30 transition
40	Settling down
45	Mid-life transition
50	Entering middle adulthood
55	Age-50 transition
60	Culmination of middle adulthood

Based on Levinson et al. (1978).

working as a psychiatrist and he subsequently tested the theory on 524 people, aged 16–50 (not his patients). He proposed that growth and maturity involve a resolution of the separation anxiety which remains with us from childhood. This theory extends Freudian psychoanalytic theory, as it looks at adulthood but in terms of childhood influences. Gould's stages show approximate ages for each developmental stage, as is illustrated in Table 4.3.

Developmental theories in perspective

The last two stages of Erikson's theory and the corresponding stages of Levinson's and Gould's theories will now be discussed as they loosely reflect the mature time of life. Erikson did not use chronological age indicators against the eight stages but many psy-

Table 4.3   Gould's stages of adult development

Age (years)	Stage
16–18	Desire to escape parental control
18–22	Leaving the family; peer-group orientation
22–28	Developing independence; commitment to a career and children
29–34	Questioning self; role confusion; marriage and career vulnerable to dissatisfaction
35–43	Period of urgency to attain life's goals; awareness of time limitation; realignment of life's goals
43–53	Settling down; acceptance of one's life
53–60	More tolerance; acceptance of past; less negativism; general mellowing

Based on Gould (1978).

chologists interpret stage 7 as corresponding with middle adulthood and stage 8 as late adulthood. The age span for stage 7 is interpreted as 40–65 years and, for many people, these are their most productive years (Atkinson et al. 2000). During this stage, which Erikson calls maturity, people guide the next generation, either through their own children or through the young people at work. By helping young people become responsible and knowledgeable adults, 'generativity' – a valuable contribution to society – can be achieved. Some people who feel that they are stagnating in life may change the course of their life at this point.

Erikson's stage of 'generativity versus stagnation' is reflected in Levinson's 'middle adulthood' and Gould's stage of 'mid-life decade'. Levinson's 'middle adulthood' is a period of transition, when an individual is likely to review life so far. This involves some disillusionment, which may provide an opportunity to modify life and its structure. Gould's stage of 'mid-life decade' also suggests the end of illusion, as well as an awareness of one's mortality and a sense of urgency in realigning life's goals.

Erikson refers to the eighth stage as old age and this stage spans late adulthood, from 65 onwards to old age. The polarities for ego development at this stage are 'integrity versus despair'. During this stage people can look back and reflect on what they have achieved during their lives. To experience egointegrity, individuals must feel that they have achieved their major life goals and have no regrets about the past – the resulting virtue is then wisdom. However, if on reaching this last stage of development they find they are lacking a sense of fulfilment and that they regret many decisions which they have made in life, the outcome can be despair. Erikson's last two stages are reflected in Levinson's 'late adulthood transition' and 'late adulthood' stages. They concern transition to retirement and beyond. Levinson recognizes that this is a time for 'integrity versus despair', but also asserts that this could be a time for creative development.

In evaluating Erikson's, Levinson's and Gould's adult developmental theories one is aware of the similarities between them and the ways in which they complement each other. Research evidence to support human development theories is limited because of methodological difficulties and the unreliable nature of subjective reports (Bee 1998). Some psychologists also believe that the concepts proposed by Erikson are difficult to operationalize. However, Kogan (1990) and Keyes & Ryff (1998) argue that there is enough evidence that generativity is a concern for many middleaged and older people.

Before concluding this section it would be useful to consider a more recent approach to explaining development as proposed by Baltes (1987). According to Baltes, human development should be considered from the lifespan perspective and he suggests that development is lifelong, multidimensional, multidirectional, plastic, embedded in history, multidisciplinary and contextual. Most of us will agree that development follows a lifelong process and that we can develop in many dimensions and directions. By asserting that development is plastic, Baltes (1987) implies flexibility and adaptation to different life conditions. We will probably readily agree that development is embedded in history as many world and societal events will affect us all at some point. Human development during the lifespan is studied by many disciplines and thus it is multidisciplinary. The final contention made by Baltes is that development is contextual, meaning that it is influenced by the contexts in which we grow and develop. These contexts are biological, psychosocial, environmental and cultural and are individually experienced as well as influenced by normative age-graded, history-graded and non-normative life events. Normative age-graded experiences are common to all, for example starting school, puberty, menopause, retirement. Normative history-graded experiences are associated with history, for instance World War II, whereas non-normative life events provide individual experiences that influence development, for example, the death of a parent, diagnosis of a terminal illness or moving to live in another country.

The concept of wisdom

Wisdom is an outcome and a virtue of Erikson's last developmental stage. Wisdom is generally considered to be an attribute of old age and Erikson et al. (1986) suggest that it is a desirable outcome of the tension between integrity and despair. The sense of integrity must prevail for wisdom to emerge. Erikson et al. define wisdom as a point in life when a person realizes that, in spite of life experience and the ability to resolve many life-related tasks, one is aware of how very little one knows. A similar explanation of wisdom is proposed by Birren & Fisher (1990: 325), who assert that 'wisdom is an intellectual ability to be aware of the limitations of knowledge'. They also consider wisdom to be a balance between knowledge and doubt, action and inaction, and emotion and detachment. A different definition is proposed by Baltes & Kunzmann (2003: 131), who define wisdom as 'expert knowledge and judgement about important, difficult and uncertain questions associated with meaning and conduct of life. Wisdom-related knowledge deals with matters

of utmost personal and social significance.' Baltes & Kunzmann have designed a test for wisdom in which they present people with difficult hypothetical situations. Interestingly, they found that the wisdom-related knowledge emerges in late adolescence and early adulthood and that there is no further change in the level of wisdom during later adulthood beyond that level. Furthermore they found that high levels of wisdom-related knowledge are rare. They also assert that cognitive factors such as intelligence are not the most powerful predictors of knowledge-related wisdom, whereas personality factors are. These include having a sense of generativity, being creative and being open to new experience. Baltes & Kunzmann (2003) also state that there is a link between wisdom-related knowledge and the emotional style of individuals. This work is very interesting indeed, although some of the characteristics associated with wisdom which have been identified are not that different from those proposed earlier by Erikson et al. (1986), who believed that the possession of wisdom includes good judgement and the ability to deal with difficult life problems.

Developmental stages and the adult personality

Developmental stages, discussed earlier, provide a good framework for understanding the development of the adult personality. However, before they can be applied, we need to remember that individual differences influence the meaning and timing of each developmental stage. In examining the concept of personality in relation to ageing, the main issue concerns the nature of stability and change in personality. Approaches to the study of personality in ageing can be broadly divided into 'trait models', 'single construct models' and 'developmental models'. Developmental models, as discussed earlier, suggest that development continues throughout adulthood and that the changes that occur are reflected in the personality. On the other hand, single and multitrait approaches show statistically significant support for interindividual stability (Kogan 1990), meaning that personality traits acquired early in life remain stable until old age. Single construct models, instead of looking at traits, involve examining one construct of personality. An example of such a construct is 'locus of control' (Rotter 1966), discussed in the next section, which has been used successfully to assess possible changes in the perception of control that may occur with ageing.

In the past, most researchers have been mainly concerned with testing stability of the personality, using personality scales. More recent approaches focus on the individual variations that contribute to successful ageing and later life resilience. Ryff & Singer (2001) suggest that a better approach would be to explore how coping, goal orientations and self-evaluative processes of personality affect well-being, life satisfaction and adaptation in later life.

Locus of control

The term 'locus of control' is used to explain the perceived source of control over our behaviour. An internal locus of control attributes outcomes in life to internal factors which are under a person's control. Conversely, if outcomes in life are attributed to external factors outside one's control, the locus of control is external. Research shows stability in the locus of control construct, except for domain-specific scales of health and intelligence, where findings show a tendency to an increased external locus of control in older people (Kogan 1990).

The external orientation in locus of control may affect coping processes in older people. A sense of control over our destiny is important and, if not perceived, may result in a passive rather than active way of coping with everyday problems. Acceptance of help from community services or admission to a nursing home may be perceived as admitting to incompetence, which can lead to loss of control. Passive acceptance of the situation can result in a state of 'learned helplessness' (Seligman 1975) and can lead to depression. Seligman argues that depression can arise when individuals believe that life events are beyond their control. By late adulthood many people will have experienced some role transitions, losses and changes; they may feel that they are unable to influence events and will therefore feel helpless. For example, people who move to a nursing home may judge their situation as unsatisfactory but as unavoidable and inescapable and may, therefore, act in a passive and helpless way. However, if they reappraise the situation, they may discover that options do exist relating to how they cope. Depending on the option chosen, outcomes may be negative or positive. A positive outcome can be explained in terms of the concept of 'self-efficacy' (Bandura 1977). Self-efficacy requires a cognitive change towards positive beliefs regarding the outcomes of our behaviour and involves efficacy expectations and outcome expectations. An example of this for the newly institutionalized person could be in contemplating the question: What are the chances that I will be happy here? Believing that social support resulting from participation in the activities provided will lead to satisfaction and happiness can influence a reappraisal of the situation which is then perceived as satisfying. Interestingly, more recent research has shown that social support can influence self-efficacy and can stimulate feelings of control (Bandura 1997, Bisconti & Bergeman 1999).

REVIEW AND REMINISCENCE AMONG OLDER PEOPLE

Recalling the past and reminiscing are popular mental activities amongst most groups of people, especially during family gatherings. We all have stories to tell about past experiences and reactions to various events. To engage in a life review is a normal activity and a psychological pursuit not exclusive to older people but open to all. Recalling stories can be a pleasurable experience for the person telling the story as well as for the listener. Interestingly, according to Rubin et al. (1998), most autobiographical memories come from a period between 10 and 30 years old. Some recollections can be cathartic or therapeutic and structured reminiscence has been reported to increase self-esteem and life satisfaction (Haight 1992). Haight (1991) reviewed 97 papers and found that only seven reported negative outcomes from reminiscence. Coleman (1989) acknowledges the value of reminiscence, but disagrees that everyone benefits from it. Coleman (1986) studied 50 people (27 men and 23 women), with a mean age of 80, for 2 years. He found that for 21 of them reminiscence was a positive experience. However, 8 people found no satisfaction and 15 could not see the point.

Generally, the terms 'life review' and 'reminiscence' are used interchangeably, but Haight & Burnside (1993) distinguish between them. According to them, the term 'life review' is used when the client is being offered assistance by the therapist to achieve a sense of integrity. This may involve recalling events and experiences in a one-to-one session, resembling counselling, with the therapist acting as a therapeutic listener. A similar description of life-review therapy is offered by Garland (1994). This form of therapy involves working through painful memories and contains elements and principles of psychodynamic therapy.

The term 'reminiscence', on the other hand, is generally applied to a group activity which has a number of goals, including socialization, communicating and entertainment. If sad memories emerge, the leader and the group will act as a support. Reminiscence may be a starting point for contact and interest with older people in day centres or in long-stay institutions and may contribute to life satisfaction. Cook (1998) found that older women in a residential home reported increased levels of life satisfaction after participating in organized group reminiscence. Reminiscence is often used in reality-orientation sessions and with depressed patients, as well as with those who suffer from dementia.

SUCCESSFUL ADAPTATION, ADJUSTMENT AND SATISFACTION IN LATER LIFE

It has been suggested earlier that individuals' personality is influential in determining adaptation and adjustment to ageing. There is also evidence that some personality types may be better adapted to early adulthood than later adulthood and vice versa. For instance, individuals with type A personalities who are very competitive, impatient and hard-driving may find it difficult to adjust to a slower, more sedentary lifestyle with fewer responsibilities. Conversely, individuals with type B personalities who are easy-going and care-free may find later adulthood much easier to adjust to than earlier adulthood (Stuart-Hamilton 2000).

There has been some research evidence on the possible link between cognitive and personality factors in later life (Woods 1999). It seems that older people who have intact cognitive abilities will preserve their personality and will consequently be more satisfied and will adjust better to old age. However, there are some older people who have not adjusted well to old age and may therefore be cantankerous, withdrawn or hostile and shunned by their neighbours and families. Hostility is a personality trait which is characterized by having a negative orientation towards others. This attitude may be less problematic in earlier adulthood, even though it has been linked to increased coronary heart disease and other illnesses (Meesters et al. 1996, Ranchor et al. 1997); however in late adulthood it has been associated with being mistreated (Comijs et al. 1999).

Apart from personality factors discussed above, the experience of negative life events and stresses also affects adjustment to ageing. The experience of life events and the ability to cope with stress may provide some answers as to why some people cope better than others. The first point to make is that not all life events affect well-being in the same way. Normative life events, which affect most people during adult life, are often perceived as less stressful, whereas non-normative events tend to cause more stress. When life events defy the natural order of development, they may be perceived as more stressful. For instance, the death of a child may cause more psychological stress than the death of a spouse in old age (Davies 1996). There is evidence that older adults rate the death of a spouse as less stressful than do younger adults, particularly if the deceased has suffered from a long-term illness (Wells & Kendig 1997). The explanation for this may be linked to the social expectations for adult behaviour during each developmental stage in life, many of which involve some gains and some losses. The concept of loss is very often used to describe the experience of ageing. Indeed, older people experience many losses, involving loss of friends, neighbours, relationships, family, places, work as well as aspects of functioning which may result in a loss of independence. Apart from the experience of loss and life events there are other causes of stress. According to Holahan et al. (1984), daily hassles may cause more psychological stress for older people than major life events. Retirement may be stressful for some older people, especially through loss of income and of meaningful activities. Of course, it could be argued that being involved in meaningful activities is desirable and satisfying at any time in life. However, this becomes more important in later life when work and family responsibilities no longer take up most of the time and meaningful activities might help to structure time as well as maintain particular identities and roles in life. Interestingly, recent research shows that workers in more physically demanding jobs retire earlier than those in less physically demanding jobs (Ucello 1998). Conversely workers who are employed in less physically demanding jobs and more cognitively demanding jobs are less likely to retire early (Czaja 2001).

From this brief examination of literature it becomes evident that good adaptation and adjustment in late life may depend on a person's personality and ability to maintain a high level of self-esteem and self-acceptance, which can be achieved by gradually adjusting expectations (Dittmann-Kohli 1990). Self-esteem can be nurtured to become more resilient by maintaining interest not only in family members but also in other people (Coleman et al. 1993). Having a perception of control over events boosts self-esteem and promotes better adjustment. Conversely, loss of a perceived control can lead to low self-esteem, poor morale and even ill health (Schulz & Heckhausen 1998).

Satisfaction in late life also seems to be correlated with personality. People who have a relaxed, emotionally stable personality have been found to be more satisfied in late life. Marital adjustment, involvement with social organizations and positive health are also good predictors of later life satisfaction. However, adjustment to ageing is a very individual experience and therefore generalizations are inappropriate.

In drawing this section to a conclusion, it is evident that people do not age in the same way, nor do they necessarily have similar experiences of ageing. Some people enjoy the freedom of their later years, as they have fewer responsibilities and more leisure time. Most advice for successful ageing suggests keeping active in body and mind (Figs 4.2 and 4.3).

CONCLUSION

This chapter has examined human ageing from a number of psychological perspectives. The evidence presented suggests that a developmental approach offers the best explanation for transitions which occur throughout the lifespan. This approach helps us to understand adaptation and adjustment, which are part of normal and healthy ageing. The process of ageing should not be seen as a negative experience but as a time to enjoy the freedom from constraints of work

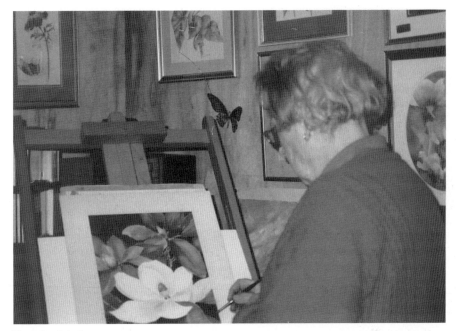

Fig. 4.2   Painting.

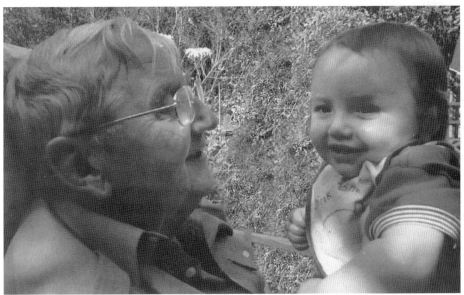

(A)

Fig. 4.3   (a–c) Bridging the generations.

Continued

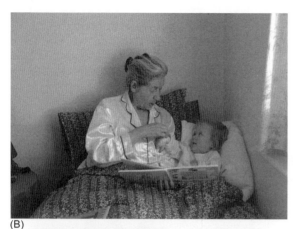

(B)

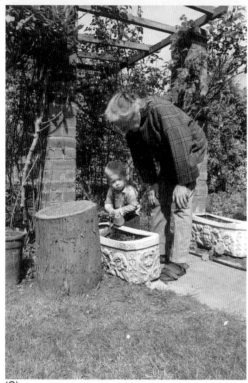

(C)

Fig. 4.3   *Continued*

and family responsibilities. The psychological changes in ageing should not be considered in isolation but must be viewed from biological, social, environmental and historical contexts.

Recommended reading

Baltes PB, Baltes MM 1990 (eds) Successful aging. Perspectives from behavioural sciences. Cambridge University Press, Cambridge

This book considers many longitudinal data in order to identify indicators for successful ageing. Questions on strategies of coping as well as on the characteristics of individuals who age most successfully are also addressed.

Bee H 1998 Lifespan development, 2nd edn. Longman, New York

This text presents a review of developmental theories throughout the lifespan. It is very easy to read and offers summaries and critical reviews of the chapters, some of which are very colourful and cheerful.

Birren JE, Schaie KW (eds) 2001 Handbook of the psychology of ageing, 5th edn. Academic Press, London

This book offers a comprehensive review of theory, research and interventions which help to explain the psychology of ageing. The book addresses the environmental influences on ageing and also examines gender differences in ageing. A chapter on wisdom and creativity is particularly useful.

Santrock JW 2002 Life-span development, 8th edn. McGraw-Hill, New York

This text is well laid out and presented and logically follows development during the life cycle. The book examines a number of theories of adult development and supplements these with relevant and up-to-date research.

Stuart-Hamilton I 2000 The psychology of ageing: an introduction, 3rd edn. Jessica Kingsley, London

A comprehensive approach to psychology of ageing is evident in this book. The review of cognitive psychology of ageing is particularly good. The text considers psychosocial and biological theories relevant to ageing and changes that occur in old age as well as examining the future of ageing.

Useful websites

There are a number of useful websites which offer explanations of psychological concepts and findings from past and current research. Some of these websites are listed below:

www.mentalhealth.com/main.htlm
www.mentalhelp.net/psyhelp/
www.ncbi.nlm.nih.gov/entrez/query.fcgi
www.psych.ucsb.edu/research/cep/new.htlm
www.socialpsychology.org

References

Atkinson RL, Atkinson RC, Smith EE, Bem DJ, Nolen-Hoeskema S 2000 Hilgard's introduction to psychology, 13th edn. Harcourt Brace Jovanovich, London

Backman L, Small BJ, Wahlin A 2001 Aging and memory: cognitive and biological perspectives. In: Birren JE, Schaie KW (eds) Handbook of the psychology of ageing, 5th edn. Academic Press, London, pp 349–377

Baltes PB 1987 Theoretical propositions of life-span developmental psychology: on dynamics of growth and decline. Developmental Psychology 23: 611–626

Baltes PB, Baltes MM 1990 (eds) Successful aging. Perspectives from behavioural sciences. Cambridge University Press, Cambridge

Baltes PB, Kunzmann U 2003 Wisdom. Psychologist 16: 131–133

Bandura A 1977 Social learning theory. Prentice-Hall, Englewood Cliffs, NJ

Bandura A (ed) 1997 Self-efficacy: the exercise of control. WH Freeman, New York

Bee H 1998 Lifespan development, 2nd edn. Longman, New York

Berk LE 1998 Development through the lifespan, Allyn & Bacon, London

Birren JE, Fisher LM 1990 The elements of wisdom: overview and integration. In: Sternberg RJ (ed) Wisdom: its nature, origin and development. Cambridge University Press, Cambridge, pp 317–332

Bisconti TL, Bergeman CS 1999 Perceived social control as a mediator of the relationships among social support, psychological well-being and perceived health. Gerontologist 39: 94–101

Bromley DB 1990 Behavioural gerontology. John Wiley, Chichester

Cerella J 1990 Ageing and information-processing rate. In: Birren JE, Schaie KW (eds) Handbook of the psychology of ageing, 3rd edn. Academic Press, London, pp 201–221

Cohen G, Conway MA, Stanhope N 1992 Age differences in the retention of knowledge by young and older students. British Journal of Developmental Psychology 10: 153–164

Coleman PG 1986 The past in the present: a study of older people's attitudes to reminiscence. Oral History Journal 14: 50–59

Coleman PG 1989 Ageing and reminiscence processes: social and clinical implications. Wiley, Chichester

Coleman PG, Ivani-Chalian C, Robinson M 1993 Self-esteem and its sources: stability and change in later life. Ageing and Society 13: 171–192

Comijs HC, Jonker C, van Tilburg W, Smit JH 1999 Hostility and coping capacity as risk of elder mistreatment. Social Psychiatry and Psychiatric Epidemiology 34: 48–52

Cook EA 1998 Effects of reminiscence on life satisfaction of older female nursing home residence. Health Care for Women International 19: 109–118

Cumming E, Henry WE 1961 Growing old: the process of disengagement. Basic Books, New York

Czaja SJ 2001 Technological change and the older worker. In: Birren JE, Schaie KW (eds) Handbook of the psychology of ageing, 5th edn. Academic Press, London, pp 547–568

Davies ADM 1996 Life events, health adaptation and social support in the clinical psychology of late life. In: Woods RT (ed) Handbook of clinical psychology of ageing. Wiley, Chichester, pp 115–140

Denney NW 1989 Everyday problem-solving: methodological issues, research findings, and a model. In: Poon LW, Rubin DC, Wilson BA (eds) Everyday cognition in adulthood and later life. Cambridge University Press, New York, pp 330–351

Dittmann-Kohli F 1990 The construction of meaning in old age: possibilities and constraints. Ageing and Society 10: 279–294

Erikson EH 1973 Childhood and society. Penguin, Harmondsworth

Erikson EH 1980 Identity and the life cycle. Norton, New York

Erikson EH, Erikson JM 1997 The life cycle completed. Norton, New York

Erikson EH, Erikson JM, Kivnick HQ 1986 Vital involvement in old age. Norton, London

Eysenck M 1996 Simply psychology. Psychology Press, Hove

Fonagy P 1995 Psychoanalysis. In: Coleman AM (ed) Applications of psychology. Longman, London, pp 76–96

Freud S 1923 On metapsychology: the theory of psychoanalysis. In: Richards A (ed) 1984 The Pelican Freud library, vol. 11. Penguin, Harmondsworth

Fry PS 1990 A factor analytic investigation of home-bound older individuals' concerns about death and dying, and their coping responses. Journal of Clinical Psychology 46: 737–748

Garland J 1994 What splendour, it all coheres: life-review therapy with older people. In: Bornat J (ed) Reminiscence reviewed; evaluations, achievements, perspectives. Open University Press, Buckingham, pp 21–31

Gould RL 1978 Transformations: growth and change in adult life. Simon & Schuster, New York

Gross RD 2001 Psychology: the science of mind and behaviour, 4th edn. Hodder & Stoughton, London

Haight BK 1991 Reminiscing: the state of the art as basis for practice. International Journal of Aging and Human Development 33: 1–32

Haight BK 1992 Long-term effects of a structured life review process. Journals of Gerentology: Psychological Sciences 47: 312–315

Haight BK, Burnside I 1993 Reminiscence and life review: explaining the differences. Archives of Psychiatric Nursing 7: 91–98

Hampson SE 1995 The construction of personality: an introduction, 2nd edn. Routledge, London

Havighurst RJ 1963 Successful ageing. In: Williams RH, Tibbitts C, Donahue W (eds) Process of ageing, vol 1. Atherton, New York, 299–320

Holahan CK, Holahan CJ, Belk S 1984 Adjustment in aging: the roles of life stress, hassles and self-efficacy. Health Psychology 3: 315–328

Howland J, Peterson EW, Levin WC, Fried L 1993 Fear of falling among the community dwelling older. Journal of Aging and Health 5: 229–243

Jahoda M 1958 Current concepts of positive mental health. Basic Books, New York

Keyes CLM, Ryff CD 1998 Generativity in adult lives. Social structural contours and quality of life consequences. In: McAdams DP, de St. Aubin E (eds) Generativity and adult development: psychosocial perspectives on caring for and contributing to the next generation. American Psychological Association, Washington, DC

Kimmel DC 1980 Adulthood and ageing: an interdisciplinary, developmental view. Wiley, New York

King P, Barrowclough C 1991 Clinical pilot study of cognitive-behavioural therapy for anxiety disorders in the older. Behavioural Psychotherapy 19: 337–345

Kline 1984 Psychology and Freudian theory: an introduction. Methuen, London

Kline P 1993 Personality: the psychometric view. Routledge, London

Kline P 1998 The new psychometrics. Routledge, London

Kogan N 1990 Personality and aging. In: Birren JE, Schaie KW (eds) Handbook of the psychology of aging, 3rd edn. Academic Press, New York, pp 330–346

Lang FR, Carstensen LL 1994 Close emotional relationships in later life: further support for proactive aging in social domain. Psychology and Aging 9: 315–324

Laursen P 1997 The impact of aging on cognitive functioning: an 11 year follow-up study of four age cohorts. Acta Neurologica Scandinavica Supplementum 172: 7–86

Levinson DJ, Darrow DN, Klein EB, Levinson MH, McKee B 1978 The seasons of a man's life. Knopf, New York

Light LL 1991 Memory and aging: four hypotheses in search of data. Annual Review of Psychology 42: 333–376

Lindesay J, Briggs K, Murphy E 1989 The Guys/Age Concern survey: prevalence rates of cognitive impairment, depression and anxiety in an urban older community. British Journal of Psychiatry 155: 317–329

Madden DJ, Gottlob LR 1997 Adult age differences in strategic and dynamic components of focused visual attention. Aging, Neuropsychology and Cognition 4:185–210

Maslow A 1954 Motivation and personality. Harper & Row, New York

Maslow A 1987 Motivation and personality, 3rd edn. Harper Collins, New York

Maylor EA 1994 Ageing and the retrieval of specialized and general knowledge: performance of 'masterminds'. British Journal of Psychology 85: 105–114

Meesters CMG, Muris P, Backus IPG 1996 Dimensions of hostility and myocardial infarction in adult males. Journal of Psychosomatic Research 40: 21–28

Ranchor AV, Sanderman R, Bouma J et al. 1997 An exploration of the relation between hostility and disease. Journal of Behavioural Medicine 20: 223–240

Reber AS, Reber ES 2001 The Penguin dictionary of psychology, 3rd edn. Penguin, London

Rogers CR 2002 Client centred therapy. Constable, London

Rotter JB 1966 Generalized expectancies for internal versus external control of reinforcement. Psychological Monographs 30: 1–26

Rubin DC, Rahhal TA, Poon LW 1998 Things learned in early adulthood are remembered best. Memory and Cognition 26: 3–19

Ryff CD, Singer BM 2001 Emotion, social relationships and health. Oxford University Press, Oxford

Salthouse TA 1996 The processing-speed theory of adult age differences in cognition. Psychological Review 103: 403–428

Salthouse TA, Fristoe NM, Lineweaver TT, Coon VE 1995 Aging and attention. Does the ability to divide decline? Memory and Cognition 23:59–71

Santrock JW 2002 Life-span development, 8th edn. McGraw-Hill, New York

Schaie KW 1996 Intellectual development in adulthood: the Seattle longitudinal study. Cambridge University Press, New York

Schaie KW, Willis SL 1986 Can decline in adult intellectual functioning be reversed? Developmental Psychology 22: 223–232

Schulz R, Heckhausen J 1998 Emotion and control: a life-span perspective. Annual Review of Gerontology and Geriatrics 17: 185–205

Seligman MEP 1975 Helplessness: on depression, development and death. WH Freeman, San Francisco

Skinner BF 1974 About behaviourism. Knopf, New York

Slater R 1995 The psychology of growing old: looking forward. Open University Press, Buckingham

Sternberg RJ, Lubart TI 2001 Wisdom and creativity. In: Birren JE, Schaie KW (eds) Handbook of the psychology of ageing, 5th edn. Academic Press, London, pp 500–522

Stevens R 1995 Freudian theories of personality. In: Hampson SE, Coleman AM (eds) Individual differences and personality. Longman, London, pp 59–76

Stuart-Hamilton I 2000 The psychology of ageing: an introduction, 3rd edn. Jessica Kingsley, London

Thomas K 1990 Psychodynamics: the Freudian approach. In: Roth I (ed) Introduction to psychology, vol 1. Lawrence Erlbaum/Open University, Hove/Milton Keynes, pp 131–184

Thompson LW, Gallagher-Thompson D, Futterman A, Gilewski MJ, Peterson J 1991 The effects of late-life spousal bereavement over a 30 month interval. Psychology and Aging 6: 434–441

Tulving E 1985 How many memory systems are there? American Psychologist 40: 385–398

Turner JS, Helms DB 1995 Lifespan development, 5th edn. Harcourt Brace College Publishers. Fort Worth, FL

Ucello CE 1998 Factors influencing retirement: their implications for raising retirement age. American Association of Retired Persons. Washington Public Policy Institute, Washington

Vaillant GE 1977 Adaptation to life. Little Brown, Boston

Vaillant GE 1990 Avoiding negative life outcomes: evidence from a 45 year study. In: Baltes PB, Baltes MM (eds) Successful aging. Perspectives from behavioural sciences. Cambridge University Press, Cambridge

Wechsler D 1981 Wechsler adult intelligence scale (revised). Harcourt Brace Jovanovich, New York

Wells YD, Kendig HL 1997 Health and well-being of spouse caregivers and the widowed. Gerontologist 37: 666–674

Woods RT 1999 Mental health problems in late life. In: Woods RT (ed) Handbook of the clinical psychology of ageing. Wiley, Chichester, pp 73–110

Chapter 5

The biology of human ageing

Rosamund A. Herbert

INTRODUCTION

In the past research into the biology of human ageing has always seemed to emphasize the loss or deterioration of function as a person gets older, and so most of us tend to have a pessimistic view of ageing. Ageing is often seen as synonymous with reduced biological efficiency. However, we can adopt a more positive approach, since evidently the majority of older people function very adequately in a biological sense and so this negative view of biological ageing is unwarranted.

Undoubtedly, with the passage of time over the adult period, profound changes in appearance and function do occur in all organisms, including humans. However, what tends to be forgotten is that these changes result from a combination of possible influences, including genetics, early life factors and environmental risks and lifestyle in mid and late life (Huppert et al. 2000). Nutrition and state of physical fitness and presence of disease will also play a part. The health of an individual from a physiological viewpoint, of any age, ultimately depends on the efficient functioning of the individual cells and tissues in all systems of the body. Many factors are known to influence health: diet, exercise, personal habits (e.g. smoking) and psychosocial factors all play an important role in determining one's state of health at any age – whether 8, 18 or 80! The ageing process is a continual process during life (not just in the latter stages of life) and is a reflection of numerous exogenous and endogenous factors and related medical, social and inherent characteristics.

Another issue that is widely debated is what is meant by 'normal ageing'. One of the most obvious findings in gerontology is the enormous variability between individuals, even if they are of a similar chronological age. For instance, some 70-year-olds may be able to run a marathon or to windsurf, whilst others are hardly able to perform the daily activities of living. Acknowledging this variability is important, as it makes generalizations about an older person's capabilities virtually impossible. The explanation for this variability relates to the many factors influencing the ageing process.

There is a strong association between the length of life of parents and that of their offspring and this again reflects the combination of genetic, lifestyle and environmental factors. There is definitely a genetic component to ageing: recent research has identified genes involved in ageing processes (see later). Studies comparing identical and non-identical twins show that age of death is closer in identical twins. The consistent sex difference in longevity, with females living longer than males, is yet further indication of genetic influences. Similarly evidence from centenarians (people living to 100) is supporting a strong genetic influence upon longevity (Perls et al. 2002). Gerontologists now also recognize the importance that variations in lifestyle, such as diet, patterns of activity and smoking, have on health status and lifespan. Socioeconomic factors are also relevant, as are disease-related factors such as exposure to infectious diseases.

For all these reasons chronological age is a relatively weak indicator of physiological age. The enormous variability, or heterogeneity as it is often known, is one issue that complicates discussion of normal ageing and also makes research into the study of human ageing more problematic. In order to be able to make any meaningful comments about the biological ageing process, researchers need to study large numbers of people. The realization of the extent of variability within human ageing has also led to further clarification of what is meant by 'old'; for instance, 65–75 might be referred to as young old age/old; 75–85 as middle old age/old; and 85+ as old old age/very old. Another term used increasingly is 'frail' older people. The term is self-explanatory, and refers to people who are vulnerable as a result of health problems (such as stroke or dementia) often combined with social care needs (Department of Health 2001). Frailty is often experienced in late old age.

Another problem in discussing normal ageing is the difficulty in determining whether any changes observed in people are in fact due to ageing itself or due to a disease process superimposed upon ageing. In an attempt to overcome this, Strehler (1962), an American gerontologist, proposed that any physiological phenomenon must meet four criteria before it can be unequivocally stated to be a component of the overall ageing process: the change must be shown to be *universal* (identifiable in all members of a species), *intrinsic* (occurring from within the organism), *progressive* and *deleterious*. This last factor is controversial, but these are useful criteria to consider when thinking about changes observed in older people; for example, loss of hearing caused by shingles or an ototoxic drug is not an age-related change, whereas loss of hearing due to age-related decline in sensory nerve cells in the auditory pathway is. Ageing itself is not a disease: it is a normal part of the life cycle (Kirkwood 2003).

Some physiological changes that are observed in older people are simply due to the fact that they have become less fit. We are aware that if we reduce our habitual activity levels for some reason – maybe illness, bedrest, temporary injury or apathy – then our physical capabilities are reduced. However, we can build up our fitness again and this cycle applies to older people too. Thus Strehler's criteria, that change must be progressive and universal before it can be classified as an age change, can be helpful in distinguishing the cause of change – in this example, change is due to the individual's deconditioning or just becoming less fit, rather than to an intrinsic change.

Thus, in many ways the term 'normal ageing' has limitations. Rowe & Kahn (1987) suggested an alternative: namely, 'usual and successful' rather than 'normal' ageing. As Rowe & Kahn point out, the use of the term 'normal' in this context neglects the heterogeneity of older people in the non-diseased group and also implies that the changes are harmless or without risk; we tend to think of 'normal' as somehow natural and therefore beyond purposeful modification. Accordingly, Rowe & Kahn describe people who age successfully as those having minimal physiological loss when compared with the average of their younger counterparts, i.e. those broadly successful in physiological terms (the marathon runners would certainly be in this category). People who show typical non-pathological age-linked losses demonstrate usual ageing. Together, 'successful' and 'usual' define the heterogeneous category of 'normal' (i.e. non-diseased) in any age group. This approach is most constructive, particularly with regard to health promotion for older people: the aim would be to move people from the usual age category 'up' into the successful ageing group.

THE STUDY OF HUMAN AGEING

Knowledge and understanding about the biology of ageing (biological gerontology) have been gained from many different areas of research. Much work is done studying the changes of ageing cells in cultures – isolated groups of cells, e.g. fibroblasts, artificially grown in vitro (literally, in glass). Research on ageing animals, from rats to primates, attempts to gain knowledge from suitable animal models; often this information is extrapolated into an analogy with humans. There are obvious inadequacies with cell cultures and animal studies in telling us about human ageing, but they are still invaluable in increasing general understanding of the ageing process.

In addition to animal studies, many studies are performed on people across a wide age range and the findings for different age groups are then compared. Two main approaches have been used to study human ageing, namely cross-sectional and longitudinal studies. Both approaches have their own particular strengths and limitations but information gained from these two methods together has given us considerable knowledge about human ageing.

Cross-sectional studies involve taking a sample of people in any one population at one time from a wide age range (e.g. 20-, 40-, 60-, 80-year-olds) and assessing their physiological function to look for changes that seem to occur with increasing age. Much of the early work on ageing in the 1950s and 1960s was done using this approach and produced findings that indicated a deterioration in function. Using this approach it is impossible to control for variables like nutrition and lifestyle that are known to influence the ageing process. The problem of looking at different age groups and directly comparing their responses is that people from different age decades have lived through very different circumstances, e.g. wars, economic depression, food shortages and changes in diets, access to health and medical care. If these factors affect the variable under consideration (this is called the 'cohort effect'), differences in average values may wrongly be attributed to ageing.

To avoid some of the pitfalls and limitations of cross-sectional studies, many longitudinal studies have been set up: the advantage that longitudinal studies have is that they follow the same individuals over a long time span. These are obviously very costly studies to run and so there are fewer undertaken; often, financial constraints can lead to their discontinuation. Several large-scale longitudinal studies have been underway for some years in the USA (for instance, the Baltimore Longitudinal Study of Aging or BLSA) and in the UK and other parts of Europe. Some studies have been running for a long time while others have been set up relatively recently: a multidisciplinary investigation of old people aged 70 plus who live in former Berlin was started in 1990 (Berlin Ageing Study (BASE): Steinhagen-Thiessen & Borchelt 1999). There are also many mini-longitudinal studies that follow a group of people for, say, 5–10 years over key periods. This approach also requires researchers

with altruistic tendencies: unlike studies on rats, where ageing changes occur in a period of 2–3 years, longitudinal studies on human ageing may not yield results within the working life of the researchers.

Longitudinal studies are not without their problems, which must be considered when assessing the significance of the results. For example, until 1978 the sample for the early BLSA was only made up of male subjects (which, given the fact that females live longer than males, may be somewhat inappropriate). Also, the fact that the participating subjects must be interested and motivated enough to take part in a longitudinal programme involving considerable commitment on their part often leads to a sample biased towards higher social classes and those with a particular sympathy for research. The BLSA does have an excess of subjects with better-than-average educational backgrounds and socioeconomic status.

The inference drawn from averages based on the early cross-sectional studies that physiological functions generally decline over the entire adult lifespan has been contradicted by longitudinal studies; for example, a substantial number of subjects aged 65 and over showed no decline in health status or intellectual function and some actually showed improvement in health over a number of years (Maddox & Douglass 1974). Even subjects who had substantial impairment of physical functioning, electroencephalogram abnormalities, cardiovascular disease or impairment in vision and hearing often remained active in the community, living fairly mobile and independent lives.

Longitudinal observations have shown that the rate of change with age for some variables observed in individual subjects did not differ significantly from the mean rates derived from analysis of cross-sectional observations. On the other hand, many individuals followed patterns of ageing that could never have been identified from cross-sectional data alone. For example, many subjects experienced periods of 5–10 years during which their kidney function showed no sign of change, while the average curve (from cross-sectional data) was declining. In a few individuals, kidney function actually improved over a 10-year interval when average values were falling. Conversely, there were some people whose decrement was greater than that predicted from cross-sectional studies (Shock 1985).

It is often difficult to find human subjects for research and some of the early studies on human ageing used a population that was easy to access, namely institutionalized older people. These people were obviously not representative of the 'normal' older population. Using samples like this may have been one reason for the skewing of research findings towards decrements in function. Again, because of very real practical constraints, studies were often carried out on small samples of older people and the variability of individuals often makes meaningful interpretation very difficult. Perhaps it is easy to see why the results of ageing research sometimes seem contradictory. Rigorous attention to methodology is essential. It is much easier to study ageing in rats than in humans! (Greig et al. (1994) clearly demonstrate the problems of recruiting 'fit' older people to study the effects of exercise and ageing.)

The general conclusion from longitudinal studies is that relatively few individuals follow the pattern of age changes predicted from averages based on measurements made on different subjects. Chronological age is a poor predictor of performance, and ageing is so highly individualized that average curves give only a rough approximation of patterns of ageing followed by individuals. Gerontologists now appreciate the importance of lifestyle in the ageing process, but very little is understood about how critical events such as retirement, onset of pathology, loss of mobility and death of a spouse affect performance. The links between different psychological states and their effects on physiology (the so-called mind–body links) are being increasingly recognized and acknowledged – especially the effects on the immune system – and may be very pertinent to studies on older people.

So different methods for studying ageing all contribute to our understanding, but they have their own advantages and disadvantages; by critically combining data from a variety of sources, a fuller picture of the biology of ageing can be gained. Research approaches to ageing are also discussed in Chapter 2.

MAINTENANCE OF HOMEOSTASIS IN OLDER PEOPLE

In the study of human ageing there is a tendency to compartmentalize, considering changes in single systems within the body (e.g. blood glucose control or kidney function) without thinking of the function of the individual as a whole. However, it is whole-body function that matters ultimately, i.e. can the individual manage an independent life? From a physiological viewpoint, the health of a person depends on the efficient functioning of the individual cells and tissues in all systems of the body, i.e. on maintaining the stability of the internal environment. The maintenance of this steady state (despite variations in both internal and external environments), or homeostasis, involves a complex series of physiological and biochemical changes and responses and almost all organs and systems in the body participate in this process, albeit to different degrees.

Is homeostasis maintained in older people? The simple answer is yes, as most older people are able to live a normal independent life, and most processes in the body appear to function adequately under basal or resting conditions. However, it is true to say that most physiological processes in the body become less effective under certain circumstances with increasing age and it is generally accepted that with ageing there is a decline in the functional competence of the individual. This decline in function may be due in part to the progressive loss of functioning body cells – i.e. there is a gradual loss of body tissue in many systems with age. The age-related deficits that exist are only apparent when the body or system is physiologically stressed, e.g. by illness, strenuous exercise or exposure to extreme environmental temperatures. So, values for body temperature, blood glucose, and so on do not change significantly under resting conditions but, if these values are increased for some reason, changes are often greater in older people than younger ones and more time is required to return the parameter back to its original value.

Older people do become more susceptible to disturbances of fluid and electrolyte balance. Reflexes that maintain blood pressure when going from lying to standing positions become less efficient and some older people are prone to develop postural hypotension (this is probably one of the factors associated with an increase in the incidence of falls in older people). Liver and renal function are less efficient and so metabolism and drug excretion are altered, and drugs can accumulate in the body more easily and reach toxic levels.

Therefore, disorders of homeostasis with age can be considered to arise not by virtue of changes in equilibrium levels, but in the efficiency with which these steady states can be re-established once displacement has occurred. This is sometimes described as a decline in the adaptive ability of the body to cope with changes or stress imposed. Frail older people who are compromised in several ways may be at greater risk of problems. Thus, homeostasis is still maintained, but with increasing difficulty as the years pass.

FUNCTIONAL RESERVE WITHIN SYSTEMS

It is characteristic of many biological systems that each has a certain amount of 'spare capacity' or functional reserve. An obvious example is that we can manage perfectly well with one kidney although we are born with two. This is an important concept because it relates to the decline in function shown by researchers to occur with ageing; because of this reserve a decline in function may proceed for many years without lowering the functional capacity below that required for homeostasis (Fig. 5.1). It is only when the functional capacity can no longer meet homeostatic needs that failure becomes evident (Johnson 1985). So system failure only occurs when the spare capacity or functional reserves are depleted below the levels required for homeostasis – and this may only happen after years of continual loss of function.

An example of reduction in functional capacity is coronary arteriosclerosis (the thickening and loss of elasticity of the arterial walls) which begins in childhood and in many individuals is well advanced by the age of 30. This steady loss of coronary vessel function usually goes unnoticed because there is still an adequate perfusion of the myocardium – in other words, because there is no effect on homeostatic function.

Flexibility and adaptability

Another complicating factor in studying homeostasis is that the decline in function of the various systems of the body is not uniform, and some aspects do not appear to deteriorate to any great extent. For instance, velocity of nerve conduction does not decline greatly, whereas muscle strength does show a measurable decline in function.

The complexities of looking at homeostasis are illustrated by a study by Rodeheffer et al. (1984), who examined cardiac function under resting and exercise conditions in fit subjects ranging in age from 26 to 79. It had been widely stated in the literature that cardiac output (the output of the heart per minute) decreased with increasing age. However, Rodeheffer et al. found that resting cardiac output in these fit subjects was not age-related and that with exercise there was no age-related decline in cardiac output, even at high levels of exercise. There were, however, differences in the way the younger and older subjects achieved the increased cardiac output under exercise stress. Cardiac output can be increased by increasing either the heart rate or stroke volume (the amount of blood ejected per beat by the ventricle) or both. The young subjects achieved the improved cardiac output primarily by increasing the heart rate, whereas the older people, whose maximum achievable heart rate had decreased with age, achieved the increase primarily by increasing the stroke volume.

This study demonstrates a key feature of the body's response to ageing: there is considerable inherent flexibility and adaptability of the physiological processes in the body, so that if one organ or system is compromised (or perhaps has 'aged' more), then other systems and mechanisms can take over to compensate. This adaptability is seen in many circumstances.

Physical capacity

One aspect of ageing that is often very obvious is a decline in the physical capacities affecting exercise, agility and mobility. These depend on coordination between many systems in the body; for example, muscles, joints, the cardiovascular and respiratory

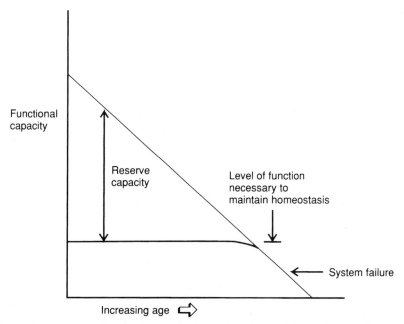

Fig. 5.1 System failure only occurs when functional reserve is depleted and homeostatic needs can no longer be met.

systems, balance, neural factors and skill all affect the ability to perform physical activity. Often in older people (this is again a generalization) you can see a decline in fitness, stamina and muscle strength. Some of these changes are due to the ageing process itself and some are due to the harmful or negative effects of inactivity. Ageing changes in joints, cartilage and collagen, and an increase in osteoporosis and a decline in the number of muscle cells could account for some of the observed changes. The cardiovascular system is not thought to be the limiting factor normally, and certainly skill factors are retained and can often compensate for the decline in strength. Structural and functional changes in the respiratory system seem to be important in restricting severe exercise and the psychological factors of decreased confidence, self-esteem and motivation probably account for some of the decline (Young 1986).

Jarvis et al. (1996), in their profile of an older population in the UK, reviewed the activities and abilities of a British 60+ population based on the 1991 General Household Survey. Although most older people managed adequately, this survey illustrates the types of problem that develop with increasing age. For instance, close to 95% of men and women aged 65–69 years found no difficulty with tasks such as washing themselves all over and preparing a hot meal. However, within the age group 85–87 years, only 69% of women and 54% of men experienced no difficulties in washing themselves all over and only 63% of women (57% of men) could prepare a hot meal without some difficulty.

Aniansson et al. (1980) looked at simpler movements, including activities of living, rather than at exercise capacity per se. They investigated, for instance, manual dexterity (e.g. putting a plug in a socket or a key in a lock), aspects of hygiene and dressing activities, ability to get up from a stool, function in the kitchen (e.g. lifting objects on to shelves, pouring water from a jug), stepping on to a platform on a bus and the most comfortable walking speed across pedestrian crossings. Studies like these, evaluating activities of living, can form the basis for recommendations to create an environment that is adapted to the needs of older people – an environment that would provide, among other things, strategically placed handrails, well-designed furniture and pedestrian 'walk' signals that would give older people enough time to cross the road.

By the time they are in their 80s, the maximum contraction that many older people can generate in their quadriceps (thigh muscles) is just enough to get up from a chair without using their arms; if they use their arms to help push up, then they need less strength in their quadriceps. The classic 'armless chair' is the toi-

let – this is why handrails are so useful for some older people.

Once at this stage the ageing changes then greatly interfere with the ability to lead a normal independent life. This brings us back to the point discussed earlier about maintaining activity levels in older people. So often with the change in lifestyle that accompanies advancing age, physical activity in general declines and cardiorespiratory and muscular systems in particular become deconditioned. Physical deconditioning will accentuate age-related declines in performance, particularly in response to physiological stress. So appropriate activity and exercise (be it simply standing to do the washing up, walking upstairs to the toilet, attending appropriate keep-fit classes or hill-walking in the Lake District) should be encouraged for all older people; there is still likely to be an overall decline in capacity but it will be less if the individual is fitter. (This is a message to all of us who have a tendency to 'do things' for older people, thinking we are helping them; we may not be helping at all.) See the section on health and disease later in this chapter for a further discussion of these issues.

FUNCTIONAL CHANGES WITH AGEING

The previous section emphasized the importance of considering the interrelationships between ageing in the various systems of the body as a whole. It is still valuable to consider more discrete individual systems too, provided the reader remembers that a decline in function may not mean impaired homeostasis (see Functional reserve within systems, above). A detailed and comprehensive review of ageing changes is beyond the scope of this chapter. However, the discussion below selects some important aspects for further consideration.

Nutrition and gastrointestinal tract

The relationship of nutrition to the ageing process in humans is complex but nutritional factors almost certainly have an influence; the role of nutrition in maintaining normal body function and also in prevention of negative changes is now well accepted for all ages. Malnutrition is common in older people and may broadly be divided into protein-energy malnutrition and vitamin deficiency (Olde Rikkert & Rigaud 2003).

One of the earliest findings in experimental gerontology was that food restriction significantly increased the length of life of rats; this was work done by Clive McCay and colleagues in the 1930s (McCay et al. 1935), and these findings have been repeatedly confirmed. In McCay's early work, dietary restriction prolonged the life of rats – in many instances, because of the delayed onset of chronic diseases – and was accompanied by better retention of many physiological functions. With any experiments on laboratory-kept animals one must keep in mind the fact that controlled laboratory conditions bear little relation to normal situations in the wild, where the animals would hunt for food and get exercise. More work looking at the effects of calorie restriction is being done (see section on Theories and mechanisms of ageing, below).

As already seen, there is a progressive decline throughout adult life in many physiological functions, which are accompanied by changes in body composition (Fig. 5.2) and in metabolism of nutrients. There is little evidence, in many instances, relating human nutrition directly to fundamental ageing changes; one exception is the role of diet in the development of osteoporosis. Many dietary factors (calcium, phosphorus, vitamin D both from the diet and skin, protein, fluoride and fibre) are implicated in determining the extent of osteoporotic bone loss, as is the extent of weight-bearing use. Taking vitamin D supplements has been shown to reduce the incidence of fractures in people aged over 65. Participants who received one capsule containing 100 000 international units of vitamin D_3 every 4 months had a 22% lower risk of a fracture at any site, and had 33% fewer fractures at osteoporotic sites (Trivedi et al. 2003). An increase in antioxidant consumption would help mop up free radicals (see section on Theories and mechanisms of ageing, below) and might have an impact on the ageing processes; this is

another example of a direct link between diet and ageing. The interrelationships between nutrition, diet and ageing are complex and often link with the development of health problems/diseases such as atherosclerosis or diabetes, rather than to 'normal ageing' processes. Being either overweight or underweight can have a detrimental effect on an older person's health and well-being (Department of Health 2001). Being underweight can predispose to developing pressure sores and these will take longer to heal. Most frail older people tend to be undernourished and need foods with a high calorie content to maintain or gain weight and provide energy (Tolson et al. 2002). Certainly the increase in obesity in the population as a whole will have adverse health effects on older people and lead to a significant increase in morbidity.

It is well established that food intake in many older people diminishes with age, but little is directly known about the nutrient requirements of older people and whether their reduced intakes fall below desirable levels. The study by McGandy et al. (1966), which looked at the reduction in energy intake with age, showed that there was a reduction in basal metabolic rate (approximately 200 kcal) which parallels the decline in lean body mass resulting mainly from a reduced muscle mass. The reduction in energy intake is also due to a much larger decline in physical activity undertaken by older people (400 kcal reduction in energy expenditure). Exton-Smith (1980), in a study of 70–80 year-olds, showed a more rapid reduction in energy intake in later years due to disabilities limiting the physical activity of the ageing person. Studies of energy intakes of nursing-home patients, whose immobility is often considerable, confirm this.

As a consequence of this decreased energy requirement, energy intake (i.e. the amount of food eaten) throughout adult life declines, and so the essential nutrients present in the energy source (food) are liable to be eaten in smaller amounts by the ageing individual. Studies have shown varying results; for example, McGandy et al. (1966) only found a slight reduction in intake of iron, thiamine, riboflavin and niacin, and no reduction in intake of calcium, vitamin A and ascorbic acid as age increased. However, other studies looking at older people from less privileged groups (Exton-Smith & Stanton 1965) have shown that intakes of all nutrients underwent extensive reductions during the period of 70–80 years of age.

However, it is not known whether this reduced intake brings the older person to levels below the levels of adequacy. The specific recommended dietary allowances (RDAs) are just not known for older people. Does the need of older people for individual nutrients become less, remain the same, or possibly even

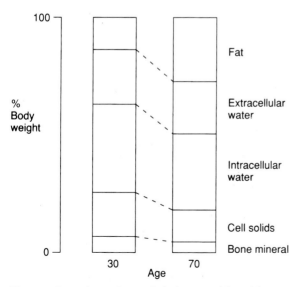

Fig. 5.2 Approximate changes in body composition with ageing. (Individual variations are large.)

increase, from factors such as malabsorption? This again underlies the desirability of remaining physically active into old age, with the double advantage of maintaining energy expenditure and physical fitness.

There are many changes in the gastrointestinal tract, some of which are briefly described below. However, despite all these changes, the function of the gut is usually adequate. This is another illustration of there being reserve capacity within biological systems, so that loss of function does not necessarily impair function.

In the oral cavity, dental decay and gum recession can lead to inadequate dentition; this in itself may have a negative impact on food intake. Salivary flow, too, is reduced in individuals after the age of 50. Atrophic gastritis, reducing gastric secretion, is common in older people but there is debate as to whether this is a pathological process. In the small intestine the villi shorten and become broader which significantly reduces the surface area for absorption, but there is no evidence that absorption of major nutrients is impaired in a healthy older person. Amino acid absorption does not appear to be impaired, although lipid absorption is reduced. The liver is reduced in size and weight and in the number of hepatocytes, which leads to some reduced storage capacity and function. The digestive functions of the pancreas are well conserved. In the colon there is atrophy of mucosa and muscle layers leading to reduced and weaker peristaltic action. There is an increased incidence of diverticula and reduced elasticity of the rectal wall, which gives a reduced maximal tolerance to faeces.

Throughout the gut and associated organs (liver, pancreas, etc.) there is a reduction in perfusion and in the coordination of the enteric nerve reflexes which synchronize events in the gut. Despite all these changes, function in 'healthy' older people remains adequate. Constipation is a frequent occurrence in old age and has a multifactorial aetiology: loss of muscle tone and motor activity in the colon, a low-fibre diet, reduced mobility, a rise in the threshold of stimulation for initiation of defecation reflexes and damage by laxative abuse all contribute. A diet containing wholegrain cereals and more fruit and vegetables has the potential to reduce constipation (Department of Health 2001).

Malnutrition does occur in older people and its causes are wide-ranging – from ignorance regarding the need for a balanced diet, to social isolation, poverty (which restricts the range of food available to some old people), mental disorders such as depression and confusion, excessive intake of alcohol and use of therapeutic drugs which can interfere with nutrient utilization, as well as changes in the gastrointestinal tract itself. For a fuller discussion of the nutritional requirements of older people, see Chapter 16, the Department of Health report (1992) and Tolson et al. (2002).

Immune system

It is well established that there is a general decline in immunocompetence with ageing, which could be an important contributor to senescence and to the development of chronic diseases and disorders. Certainly, due to the age-related changes in the immune system, older people are more susceptible to microbial infections than the young (Schroder & Rink 2003) and both latent and acute viral infections lead to increased morbidity and mortality in older people (Effros 2003). The decline in immunity in older people has largely been attributed to the impairment of T-cell mechanisms (see below). The evidence of a role for the immune system in ageing is more convincing for the diseases of old age than it is for the normal processes of ageing. As immunological efficiency decreases, there is an increased incidence of infections, autoimmune diseases and cancer. However, some theories suggest that normal ageing is the consequence of a developing immunodeficiency; these are attractive theories, as they imply that the process might then be potentially accessible to manipulation!

The immune system, which is distributed throughout the body and interacts with all other systems, provides a vital aspect of defence of the internal environment. The immune system recognizes foreign molecules (antigens) and acts to immobilize, neutralize or destroy them. When it operates effectively, this system protects the body from a wide variety of infectious agents as well as from abnormal body cells. When it fails, malfunctions or is disabled, some of the most serious diseases, such as cancer, rheumatoid arthritis and acquired immune deficiency syndrome (AIDS) may result.

Humoral and cell-mediated immunity are the two main components of a functioning immune system and the responsiveness of both declines with increasing age. With ageing, lymphoid tissue is lost from the thymus, spleen, lymph nodes and bone marrow. One major change in the system is in the T cells or T lymphocytes that mature in the thymus gland. T cells are the non-antibody-producing lymphocytes that constitute the cell-mediated arm of immunity. These T cells directly attack and lyse body cells infected by viruses or other intracellular parasites, cancer cells and foreign grafts, and release chemical mediators that enhance the inflammatory response or help to activate lymphocytes or macrophages. There is a blunted T-cell response with ageing and increased production of proinflammatory cytokines (Luz et al. 2003). Changes in the B cells which are responsible for the humoral response (i.e. by circulating antibodies) are smaller and often secondary to changes in T-cell population.

The involution of the thymus gland during the first half of life may explain the altered formation and function of the immune system observed during the second half of life. The thymus gland is at its maximum size at sexual maturity, and after puberty its size decreases; by the age of 45–50 only 5–10% of the cellular mass of the thymus remains. The concentration of thymic hormones in the serum begins to decline between the ages of 20 and 30 years and thymic hormones can no longer be detected after 60 years of age (Lewis et al. 1978). The thymus is the site of differentiation of immature lymphocytes from the bone marrow; the lymphocytes then enter the cortex of the thymus gland and eventually become T lymphocytes.

The level of natural antibodies also decreases with age and there is an increase in autoantibodies (i.e. antibodies which react against an antigenic component of the individual's own tissues). Autoantibodies to nucleic acids (e.g. DNA, RNA), smooth muscle, mitochondria, lymphocytes, gastric parietal cells, immunoglobulins and thyroglobulin have all been found with increased frequency in old people.

Almost all studies show a decline in the antibody response with age. Abundant evidence exists to show how the immune system changes with age. To summarize, cell-mediated and humoral immune response to foreign antigens decreases, while response to autologous (belonging to the same organism) antigens increases. The changes are undoubtedly complex, and one problem is that age-associated changes in the immune system do not always distinguish between an immune system impaired by age (i.e. an ageing change itself) and an immune system compromised by the environment within an older host (i.e. a consequence of other ageing changes within the individual). Environmental factors known to influence immune competence include disease, nutrition and exposure to ionizing radiation.

The possible relationship between nutrition and immunity in older people is interesting. It is known that both undernutrition and overnutrition suppress immune responses in the body. Chandra & Puri (1985) have studied the effects of dietary intake, nutritional status and risk of infection in old age; they argue that impairment of the immune response is not an inevitable part of ageing, as some older people are as immunocompetent as young people. Chandra & Puri have demonstrated that both nutritional supplementation and regular moderate exercise can positively influence immune competence. Also, the duration of illness in those older people taking nutritional supplementation was found to be reduced – people taking supplements were ill for a shorter time.

Respiratory and cardiovascular systems

The respiratory and cardiovascular systems work together to ensure that an adequate supply of oxygen is delivered to the tissues and that carbon dioxide is removed from the body. The cardiovascular system also has a more general role in transporting heat and substances such as nutrients, hormones and waste products around the body.

A variety of structural changes occur in the thorax and lung with ageing and have an adverse effect on function (see also Chapter 15). For example, there are changes in lung volume and capacity that result in a reduced surface area being available for gas exchange, e.g. the fraction of lung volume occupied by the airways increases at the expense of alveolar space and the alveoli become smaller. The lung tissue seems to lose its elasticity, primarily as a result of stiffening changes in the collagen. More muscular work is required to move air in and out of the lungs, because of the stiffening of ribs and other joints in the thorax and the structural changes in the lung tissue.

One of the main defence mechanisms in the lungs that protects against inhaled particulate matter is sometimes described as the 'mucociliary escalator'. This depends on particles being trapped in the layer of mucus lining the larger airways, after which the mucus is 'wafted' up to the larynx by beating movements of the cilia (hair-like projections) situated on the bronchial epithelium. With ageing, cilia are lost from the airways and the vigour of the remaining cilia is reduced. Thus the mucociliary escalator is less effective in removing debris. Macrophages that form the last line of defence further down the airways, at the alveolar levels, also become less efficient. These changes partly account for the increased incidence of respiratory infections in older people.

Thus there is an age-related loss of respiratory function. In a range of studies, between 30% and 60% of older adults report having symptoms such as cough, wheeze and breathlessness, much of which was probably related to smoking in earlier life (Connolly 1996). The loss of function is substantially greater in smokers than in non-smokers and some return in function does occur if smokers give up; this is a strong reason for advising cessation of smoking at any age, but particularly for older people, when a decline in respiratory function can already be compromising.

The study of ageing changes in the cardiovascular system has been dogged by methodological problems. It is difficult to get a 'coronary artery disease-free' population for study so that ageing changes rather than disease-induced changes can be investigated. It is also particularly important when comparing the cardiovascular function of young and older subjects to ensure that the level of physical conditioning or fitness is similar in subjects of all ages; heart rate, blood pressure and other cardiorespiratory parameters vary substantially according to the amount of physical activity normally undertaken.

The notion that there is a substantial obligatory decline in cardiovascular function at rest is not supported by the research. It has been shown that in subjects living independent (i.e. non-institutional) lives, cardiac output (i.e. heart rate by stroke volume) is not markedly affected by age (see Rodeheffer et al.'s (1984) work, discussed earlier). However, there are changes in the various components of the cardiovascular system. The heart and blood vessels are highly dependent for their normal function on the physical properties of connective tissue and muscle, namely distensibility, contractility and elasticity, and these alter with ageing, leading to increased stiffness generally. Heart weight, as a fraction of body weight, tends to increase slightly. Sometimes a moderate left ventricular hypertrophy develops as an adaptive response to the changes in aortic compliance that occur (due to changes in collagen in blood vessel walls; Cheitlin 2003). There is a change in the character of the connective tissue matrix which leads to some stiffness of the myocardium. There is also a dropout of atrial pacemaker cells, resulting in a decrease in intrinsic heart rate (Cheitlin 2003). The blood vessels undergo changes with ageing, too. There are major structural alterations in the arteries, due to an increase in collagen and smooth muscle, which lead to increased arterial stiffness and reduced compliance with increasing age. As elsewhere in the body, collagen tends to become cross-linked and calcium is deposited in the framework. Veins become increasingly tortuous, the walls become weaker due to loss of elastic tissue and varicosities occur in veins subjected to high pressure. The basement membrane of the capillary endothelium becomes thicker and the fenestrations (windows) of the endothelium become fewer. These changes in the capillary structure, in association with the increased density of ground substance of connective tissues, impair the diffusion of gases and nutrients to and from the cells. Bruising is more common due to the fragility and altered structure of the vessels and supporting tissues.

The work done by the heart tends to reduce slightly with age, while the total peripheral resistance increases at a rate of approximately 1% per year from the age of 40 onwards (Kenney 1989). Thus, there is a tendency for perfusion of the organs in the body to be reduced, although the extent of this reduction varies considerably. Blood flow to the kidneys is reduced by up to 50% and there are also large decreases in the splanchnic and cutaneous circulations. Cerebral blood flow is thought to reduce by 20%. Changes in resting blood flow to the myocardium and skeletal muscle are less marked; however, the ability to increase blood flow to these tissues when required, e.g. following tissue hypoxia, is reduced in older people.

Many of the factors mentioned above would be expected to increase arterial pressure. Both longitudinal and cross-sectional studies have shown an increase in systolic pressure with age with a smaller rate of increase in the diastolic pressure. In the very old, diastolic pressure may fall. The elevation in systolic pressure increases left ventricular work and the risk of left ventricular hypertrophy, whereas the decrease in diastolic blood pressure may compromise coronary blood flow (Basile 2002). There is debate, however, as to whether this increase in blood pressure is an inevitable consequence of normal healthy ageing. Individuals who live in isolated, primitive societies do not show an increase in blood pressure as they age, nor do chronic psychiatric patients who grow old in a protected institutional environment (Kenney 1989). It may well be that the age-related rise in pressure is a consequence of other factors such as diet and social stresses. Whatever the reasons behind its development, systolic hypertension is a known risk factor for developing coronary heart disease and heart failure and strokes, and so treatment now tries to ensure that systolic pressures in middle-aged and older people are kept down to 140 mmHg (Basile 2002).

As discussed above, some early research showed a reduced ability of the cardiovascular system to adapt to stress or exercise with increasing age, but the extent of the changes have been exaggerated due to effects of deconditioning and undiagnosed coronary artery disease; physical endurance of many older people is much greater than some earlier studies indicated. There is a true age-related decline in the maximum heart rate that can be achieved with age mainly due to loss of pacemaker cells and the decline seems to be approximately linear. Several equations are used to predict this decline; one proposed by Astrand & Rodahl (1977) is:

$$\text{Maximum heart rate} = 210 - (0.65 \times \text{age}).$$

So, for a person aged 75, it would be approximately 162.

The decline in achievable maximum heart rate has been suggested to be due to a change in the number of beta-adrenergic receptors, a reduced release of neurotransmitters or changes in the sinoatrial node. There is decreased responsiveness to beta-adrenergic receptor stimuli, which is in part compensated for by an increase in circulating catecholamines adrenaline (epinephrine) and noradrenaline (norepinephrine) (Cheitlin 2003). There is also decreased reactivity to baroreceptors and chemoreceptors. The diminished target-organ responsiveness to beta-adrenergic stimulation could be a key mechanism for the age-related differences in many facets of the stress response (Lakatta 1983). For a fuller discussion of the cardiovascular changes with ageing, see Cheitlin (2003).

Endocrine and nervous systems

Many common problems encountered in an ageing individual can be related to neuroendocrine phenomena (Rehman & Masson 2001), and so changes in these systems are implicated in both 'normal' ageing changes and common health problems. The endocrine system plays a central role in many of the body's regulatory and adaptive responses. Some of the studies in this area give conflicting information on age-related changes in endocrine function; as with other systems in the body, there are many complicating factors or influences that need to be taken into consideration. For instance, disease, medication, smoking, alcohol, diet, exercise, percentage body fat, social factors and methodological factors which may bias findings in research studies can all influence hormone levels and so make it difficult to say whether any changes observed are due to ageing or reflect alterations in some other parameter. At one time the thyroid gland was thought to be implicated in ageing, as some of the features of hypothyroidism are similar to observations in ageing (e.g. drying of skin, loss of hair); however, the capacity to maintain a euthyroid ('normal') state continues during ageing in many older people despite some changes in overall secretion and metabolism, and there is no significant change in plasma thyroid hormone levels.

Ageing affects the endocrine system by altering endocrine cells, the hormones produced by these cells and hormone receptors or postreceptor processes in the target cells; Rehman and Masson (2001) review many of the changes with ageing, especially the hypothalamic neuroendocrine system. Studies on the endocrine system extend beyond the simple measurement of blood hormone levels under different physiological stresses, as it is appreciated that the plasma levels of a particular hormone depend upon many factors, for instance secretion of regulatory hormones, transport around the body, binding with receptors on target cells and the clearance of the hormones from the blood. Figure 5.3 shows some of these stages.

Many of the endocrine glands do seem to decrease in weight and to develop a patchy atrophic appearance accompanied by vascular changes and fibrosis. Basal (resting) hormonal levels are generally not influenced by age, but some older people have reduced serum levels of the most active forms, e.g. renin, aldosterone, triiodothyronine (T_3) and, in men, an androgen known as dihydroepiandrosterone. There does seem to be a decline in the secretion rate of many hormones with advancing age, but at the same time there is a reduced clearance rate from the circulation, with the net result being 'normal' hormone levels. Thus the body seems to retain the capacity to adjust hormone secretion in order to maintain stable plasma levels of hormones.

A range of effects are apparent in the endocrine system with ageing. For instance, there is no major impact of ageing on some important endocrine functions, e.g. the reserve capacity to secrete cortisol appears unchanged with advancing age. However, growth hormone secretion is reduced in certain situations; in particular, there is a decline in its normal secretion during sleep. Changes in neuroendocrine controls of salt and water homeostasis with age may make some older people more susceptible to fluid and electrolyte disturbances such as dehydration and overhydration (Phillips et al. 1993). The thirst mechanism may become less sensitive in older people and problems of hydration can be an issue for people in hospital. However the majority of healthy older people maintain an adequate hydration status most of the time (Kenney and Chiu 2001).

On the other hand, ageing may mimic a disorder with a major morbidity. For instance, carbohydrate intolerance leads to a progressive increase in blood glucose levels with ageing; although this may share

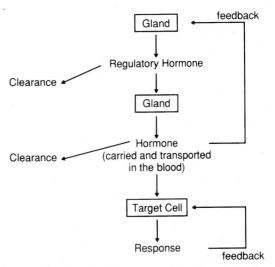

Fig. 5.3 The sequence of hormone action and regulation. Clearance refers to removal from the blood, and feedback is usually negative.

certain common mechanisms or clinical complications, it can be distinguished from clinical diabetes. What may be happening is that ageing is eroding the physiological reserve of the endocrine systems; this may in turn be related to the expression of disease or the increased mortality known to be associated with certain other stresses, such as from burns and surgery, in advancing age. The sympathoadrenal system is a modifier of much of the endocrine system and ageing appears to be associated with an enhanced sympathetic response (see later). This may in turn influence other endocrine functions such as carbohydrate tolerance. Healthy ageing is associated with significant distress and activation of the hypothalamic–pituitary–adrenal axis, and complex psychoneuroendocrine relationships involved with cytokine production during ageing (Luz et al. 2003).

The age-related impairment in the capacity to maintain carbohydrate homeostasis after a glucose challenge, e.g. in a glucose tolerance test, has been known for years. Some clinical studies indicate a progressive increase in plasma glucose levels with increasing age (Holmes 1994) but the most striking change is the elevation in blood glucose levels after oral or intravenous glucose loads (Fig. 5.4). This age-related impairment in glucose metabolism is less marked but still present after careful screening for fac-

tors, such as diet, lack of exercise and increased adiposity, that influence blood glucose metabolism. Ageing does seem to be associated with marked insulin resistance, possibly due to loss of insulin receptors, but the precise mechanisms for insulin insensitivity with ageing are still unknown. There also seems to be a marked impairment in the ability to dispose of glucose with increasing age. So there is some genuine impairment of glucose utilization with age, partly due to explainable changes but possibly also from ageing changes. There is also evidence that some of the well-known ageing changes are linked with high levels of glucose in the body; there is a similarity between tissue changes in diabetes and in ageing, e.g. senile cataracts, joint stiffness and atherosclerosis (Furth & Harding 1989). This is discussed further under Theories and mechanisms of ageing, below.

The general picture of the ageing nervous system is of declining efficiency, although, as with other systems, function is maintained. There are enormous inconsistencies in research findings on the ageing brain, often due to methodological problems. Some of the losses or decrements observed in the central nervous system may in fact reflect an age-dependent decline in the need for or use of certain circuits. Brain weight and volume have been shown to decline with age (this seems to occur more rapidly after the age of 60), but in care-

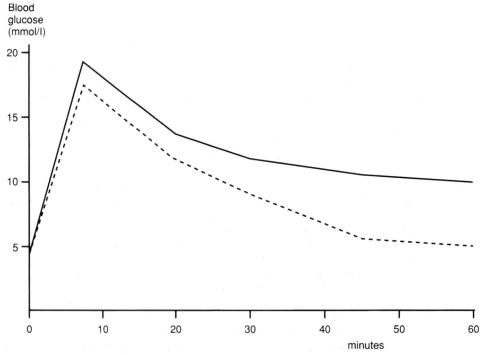

Fig. 5.4 Effect of glucose administration on young (------ age 20–30 years) and older (——— age 60–70 years) subjects.

fully screened, mentally normal older individuals these declines are probably not significant. Some investigators have reported neuronal loss in selected layers and regions of the ageing human cortex, but not in most brainstem structures (where the vital centres that control functions such as heart rate, blood pressure and respiration are located). Neurofibrillary tangles and senile plaques are seen in the brains of aged normal people and patients with neuropathology (Chapter 24). Results are available that support almost any type of age-dependent change in central nervous system circuitry – loss of synapses, increases or no change at all! Synaptic growth and remodelling probably occur well into old age and can repair small injuries or 'nicks' in brain circuitry. Anderton (2002) discusses further some of the changes in the brain with ageing.

As mentioned previously, cerebral blood flow does decrease with age, but adequate oxygen delivery is maintained as oxygen extraction from the blood is increased (more oxygen is released from the haemoglobin). The vertebral arteries that deliver blood to the brain tend to become tortuous with ageing due to changes in the vertebrae and intervertebral discs and may become kinked with movements of the neck. This can lead to transient ischaemic attacks, to which many old people are prone.

There are changes in patterns of neurotransmission with changes in synthesis, storage and release of neurotransmitters. Changes in the metabolism of neurotransmitters can have profound effects on both behavioural and regulatory systems. The cholinergic system has been studied because of its involvement in memory and disorders such as parkinsonism and Alzheimer's disease. Alzheimer's-type dementia is discussed in detail in Chapter 24. There is also reduced velocity of conduction of nerve impulses with age. Some of the reflexes, e.g. Achilles tendon reflex, are depressed and reaction time is longer by about 30% (i.e. slower reactions) in old subjects; some of this deterioration is due to nerve changes, but some to a reduction in muscle power and stiffer joints.

The autonomic nervous system is clearly affected by age in humans (Collins et al. 1980). Autonomic dysfunctions are implicated in many pathophysiological changes of age, including postural hypotension, impaired thermoregulation and gastrointestinal function, urinary incontinence and impaired penile erection in men. It is not known whether these changes stem from central control (i.e. within the brain) or from a lower level.

A relatively consistent picture of sympathetic activity has begun to emerge, showing that plasma noradrenaline levels increase in ageing humans. It has not yet been resolved whether this is due to release of more noradrenaline or whether clearance (removal from the blood) of noradrenaline is reduced (this type of shift in metabolism was also discussed under Endocrine and nervous systems, above). Thus plasma noradrenaline appears to rise more readily in response to most stimuli, seems to require longer periods to return to its baseline and may well exhibit higher baseline levels.

In contrast to this trend toward increased activity of the sympathetic nervous system, many tissues and organs seem to become less responsive to sympathetic stimulation with ageing. For instance, blood pressure and cardiovascular responses to stimuli such as tilting, standing or exercise, which test the function of sympathetic reflexes, are often significantly reduced with ageing. The whole area is complex, as not all tissues become less responsive with age, and the extent of decline varies among individuals. The decrease in cardiac responsiveness with age is also probably due to a decrease in sensitivity to adrenergic stimulation.

Although less is known about the parasympathetic nervous system, age-correlated impairments are also reported in this system. Thus, substantial alterations in autonomic function occur during ageing; these changes are likely to play an important role in the decline of normal physiological homeostasis.

Special senses

Hearing is at its most efficient in both acuity (clearness) and range of perceived frequencies at age 10 and it becomes gradually impaired with advancing age. There is a particular decline in sensitivity for higher frequencies and this loss contributes significantly to difficulty in understanding speech. There are changes in all parts of the ear. The tympanic membrane becomes more rigid and there is an increased rigidity of the bones in the middle ear, along with some loss of muscle fibres. In the inner ear there are changes in the Reissner's and basilar membranes and a significant loss of hair cells in the organ of Corti. It has also been shown that there is a gradual loss of ganglion cells and fibres of the auditory nerve and that neurons are lost throughout the auditory pathway in the brain. The auditory orienting reflex, i.e. the location of sounds, becomes slower and less accurate with age, perhaps contributing to the confusion that some older people show when in a three- or four-way conversation. It is no wonder, with all these changes, that there is a marked hearing loss with age: presbycusis is the term used for these changes (see Chapter 11 for more information on hearing in older people).

Vision is affected by age, too. There is a loss of retro-orbital fat around the eye, which leads to recession of the eye; loss of elastic tissue of the eyebrow and upper lid can lead to ptosis and occlusion of the upper visual field, while loss of elastic tissue in the lower lid may allow the lid to fall forwards, separating the lid from the eye and interfering with the normal drainage of tears. Tear production also diminishes, which can lead to dry eyes. The cornea and conjunctiva become thinner. The diameter of the pupil is at a maximum in the early teens and gets smaller, to a minimum around the age of 60. Changes in the fibrous network of the iris fixes the pupil at this small size and substantially impairs the amount of light admitted. This leads to a rise in the threshold for light perception and an increase in the level of illumination necessary for reading. An arcus senilis (a white ring encircling about 1 mm within the corneal margin) is a corneal degeneration that is often apparent, but does not itself damage sight.

Presbyopia, the loss of ability to accommodate for near vision, is well known, and is essentially due to loss of flexibility of the lens, making it unable to adapt its shape appropriately and so focus the image on the retina properly. The lens continues to grow throughout life by laying down new cells on its surface; consequently the lens becomes thicker with increasing age. The near point (the distance from the eye at which print can be read) begins to recede; at the age of 20 it is about 10 cm from the eye, but by the age of 70 is about 100 cm. This explains the common experience of having to hold books further and further away in order to be able to read them. Cataracts (due to clouding of the lens) are very common in older people, giving blurred vision.

Receptors are lost from the retina, mainly the rods of the peripheral retina, and this reduces the size of the visual field. There are minor losses of receptors at the fovea or macula (the area of clearest vision), which lead to loss of visual acuity. Macular degeneration is not uncommon in older people. The chemical processes of vision involving photochemical pigments become impaired, so that adaptation to dark/light conditions occurs more slowly and to a lesser extent (see Chapter 12 for more information in older people).

The senses of taste and smell undergo deteriorative changes, too. The taste papillae on the tongue degenerate and the number of taste buds is reduced. Some reports have shown a reduction by two-thirds in the number of taste buds between childhood and age 80. Loss of taste sensation is also exacerbated by a reduced saliva flow and reduced content of amylase, which starts the digestive process. This can lead to the pleasure of eating being diminished, with possible nutritional consequences. A decrease in taste sensation may also result in excessive sugar and salt being used,

which is undesirable. Also, the sense of taste acts as a protective mechanism and this too is diminished.

Maintenance of balance relies on an integration of responses from the visual system, the vestibular system in the inner ear and from proprioceptors in muscles and joints. Older people require greater angular movements in the joints for proprioceptor perception to be achieved. The increased sway seen when older people stand still with their eyes closed demonstrates the reduced efficiency of vestibular and proprioceptor systems.

Skin

All tissues in the skin, including the hair, undergo regressive changes and, although there is no 'skin failure' as such with ageing, old skin can and does impair the quality of life.

Very little is known about the changes that occur in the hair, despite grey hair being one of the most obvious signs of ageing. Paradoxically, the hair on the head thins but there is an increase in hairs in the nose, ears and eyebrows. Scalp hair growth rate decreases, with noticeable thinning past the age of 65; most people over 40 have some greying of the hair. The tendency to go grey is inherited, as is baldness.

The structure of the skin is altered with ageing. There are two components to ageing in the skin; intrinsic ageing, which is largely genetically determined, and extrinsic ageing, caused by environment exposure, primarily ultraviolet light (Jenkins 2002). The process of intrinsic skin ageing resembles that seen in most internal organs and is thought to involve decreased proliferative capacity leading to cellular senescence. The net result is that the skin becomes thinner, more translucent and often becomes dry and scaly; it is more easily damaged, slower to heal and older people have an altered early inflammatory response (Benbow 2002). Older people have reduced sebum production and perspiration which leads to this drier, coarse and itchy skin. Sweat glands become less effective and blood flow through the skin diminishes, which reduces the individual's ability to lose heat. Sensitivity to the effects of the sun increases in older people; less melanin is produced and the skin becomes paler. Some melanocytes produce extra melanin, resulting in age spots in areas exposed to the sun (Benbow 2002).

The epidermis flattens because of the loss of papillae; the papillae are responsible for the undulating contour (rather like egg boxes) which ensures good adhesion between the layers of the skin. This loss of papillae reduces the strength of attachment between the dermis and epidermis. Consequently, a shearing force produced, say during poor lifting techniques, will more readily peel off the epidermis in ageing skin; this is one of the contributing factors to the predisposition of older individuals to develop pressure sores (Chapter 19). The precise cause of the 'wrinkle', one of the most tell-tale signs of ageing, is probably due to some changes in the collagen and elastin components of the dermis. Figure 5.5 shows the difference between young and old skin.

Throughout the skin are a large number of nerve endings that are sensitive to temperature, pain, touch and pressure, and some of these nerve endings are affected by age. Observations suggest that pain and thermal sensation are diminished and this increased threshold of pain sensation means that some older people are less capable of sensing danger, for instance hot surfaces, and may not act appropriately. Tactile sensitivity diminishes with age as well. In the very old, sensitivity to pain seems to increase again and it has been suggested that this is due to the excessive thinning of the skin which allows a greater number of nerve endings to be stimulated.

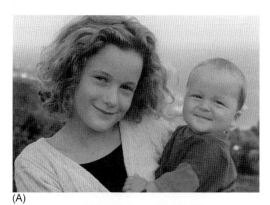

(A)

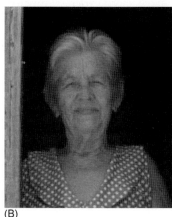

(B)

Fig. 5.5 (a) Young and (b) old skin.

There is regression and disorganization of small blood vessels and capillaries in the skin and, as this will reduce the supply of fluid and nutrients to the skin, it may account for thinning hair and reduced sweating. This degeneration of the small vessels is almost certainly an intrinsic age change and progresses relentlessly even in protected skin. Topical therapy, where drugs are absorbed into the body via the skin, may not be as effective in older people as it is in younger people due to these changes in the microcirculation. The changes in the connective tissue in the dermis result in a loss of support for the cutaneous vessels, leading to increased fragility and the easy or spontaneous bruising often seen in older people. This will be compounded if the person is also taking aspirin or other anticoagulant therapy.

The acute inflammatory reactions in the skin are reduced in older people and this again leads to a decrease in obvious danger signals. Surgical experience clearly shows that even the very old (beyond 85) can effectively repair extensive wounds, but on the whole, the wounds do take longer to heal. The tensile strength of 5-day wounds is considerably reduced in older people and collagen deposition is slower (Sandblum et al. 1953). This is important to remember when caring for old people after surgery. Wound dehiscence is more common in older people. With regard to more superficial wounds, re-epithelialization takes twice as long for 75-year-olds as it does for 25-year-olds (Orentreich & Selmanowitz 1969). As usual, there is considerable variation amongst older people with respect to ageing and changes in the skin.

Supporting tissues

Connective tissue, cartilage and bone are the three major supporting tissues of the body, and changes in these tissues are widespread with ageing. Connective tissue has two major components: the ground substance, which consists of mucopolysaccharides in the form of a hydrated gel, and fibrous proteins (collagen, elastin and reticular fibres). With age there is an increased density of fibres, meaning that the volume occupied by the ground substance is reduced. The gel also becomes less hydrated. Consequently, the diffusion of material through the connective tissue is impaired and mobility of cells (e.g. macrophages) is reduced. These changes threaten both the nutrition of cells and the repair processes. The collagen fibres increase in size and number and cross-linkage occurs between fibres, and so the collagen becomes more stable. The elastic fibres also undergo cross-linkage and become more rigid.

The normal elastic properties of cartilage are lost, too, as it loses water and fibres are deposited. The increased fibre density in connective tissue and cartilage provides a 'mesh' for the deposition of calcium and this accounts for the increased calcification seen with ageing.

Connective tissue is widespread – it is found just about everywhere in the body and so the changes in connective tissue affect every part of the body. As we have already seen, skin loses its elasticity and becomes wrinkled, the lungs lose their elastic recoil and the costal cartilages become increasingly rigid, making breathing harder, and joints in the body become stiffened by the increase in fibrous tissue. The loss of hydration in the cartilage in the intervertebral discs leads to compaction of the vertebrae and shrinkage in stature. The cardiovascular system, which depends to a great extent on the properties of distensibility and elasticity, is adversely affected: the chambers of the heart become less distensible; there is reduced contractility; the valves of the heart become stiffer; and the elastic arteries become more rigid.

Bone tends to lose mineral as it ages – this process is known as osteoporosis. The bone tends to erode from within, while deposition occurs at a slower rate on the outer surface. Thus, the external diameter of the bone increases, but the walls become thinner. This thinning of the cortex of the long bones weakens them and fractures can occur even under slight loads. Bone mass steadily declines at a rate of almost 1% per year from around the mid-30s.

The loss of bone mass is greater in women than in men. Longitudinal studies, starting just before the subjects reached menopause, found that the rate of loss of bone is most rapid within 5–10 years after the menopause and after that there is a fall in the rate of loss (Johnston et al. 1979). There are many factors involved in this bone loss, including the size of the initial bone mass, which depends on genetic factors, the individual's sex, the amount of physical activity undertaken and nutritional factors in early life. Girls at the age of 18 have a 20% lower bone mass in relation to body weight than males. Thus females start off with less bone; together with the rapid loss after the age of 50, this means that there is likely to be a higher prevalence of osteoporosis in older women. Known risk factors for osteoporosis include menopause (especially early menopause), family history of osteoporosis, inactivity, toxins (e.g. lead), certain drugs, smoking and excessive alcohol intake, and poor nutrition with a lack of vitamins C, D and K (Kirkwood & Wolff 1995).

It is not oestrogen deficiency alone that determines postmenopausal osteoporosis. Several other hormones are believed to be involved, namely parathyroid hormone, vitamin D, calcium and possibly also progesterone and corticosteroids. Oestrogen deficiency may accelerate bone loss by increasing the sensitivity of bone to the resorbing (breakdown) action of parathyroid hormone, which leads to an increase in calcium released from the bone and increased renal excretion of calcium. Hormone replacement therapy (HRT) measurably decreases bone loss by suppressing bone turnover.

Calcium and vitamin D play a role in determining age-related bone loss. Calcium absorption from the gut may fall with age and vitamin D levels are sometimes low. Low vitamin-D levels are believed to be due primarily to a lack of exposure to sunlight, limiting vitamin D synthesis in the skin and leading to a further decrement in calcium absorption. Whether calcium intake is inadequate in older women is debatable but inadequate intake could at least be part of the cause of postmenopausal bone loss.

The more sedentary lifestyle (or periods of immobility) common among older people certainly does contribute to bone loss, i.e. disuse leads to atrophy of the bone. There is significant bone loss from the vertebrae in both sexes, but this is more marked in females and leads to increased spinal curvatures. Shortening of the cervical vertebrae can also lead to kinking of the vertebral arteries – a contributing factor in transient ischaemic attacks experienced by some old people.

Reproductive system

The reproductive organs in both sexes undergo many age-related changes which are similar to those occurring in other organs and tissues. The function of the reproductive organs is greatly influenced by a hierarchy of hormones from the hypothalamus, anterior pituitary and the gonads (ovaries and testes) and many changes are influenced by these hormones.

Females have a more or less abrupt end to their reproductive lifespan, with the menopause occurring at an average age of 50–51 years. It is often difficult to study the decline in reproductive capacity in women due to the widespread use of contraceptive devices and decreased frequency of intercourse. From the age of 30 onwards, ovarian weight decreases, the amount of connective tissue increases and perfusion diminishes. There is a reduction in the number of follicles that undergo normal growth and development. Women have lower fertility and a higher rate of miscarriage in the years before onset of the menopause.

The other reproductive organs undergo changes mainly as a result of a decrease in the quantity of female hormones. The uterus atrophies and shrinks to a small proportion of its premenopausal size. The vagina becomes smaller in length and diameter; the protective cornified layer of epithelium can be lost and the glandular secretions that are under the influence of the ovarian hormones are often inadequate. This can lead to reduced lubrication during intercourse and cause dyspareunia. The alterations in vaginal secretions produce changes in the vaginal flora, leading to symptoms of vaginitis which can progress to ulceration and bleeding. Weakness in the pelvic floor muscles is common and is one of the contributory factors in urinary incontinence. Breast tissue atrophies and relaxation of ligaments and loss of muscle tone occur.

Some of the impact of a reduced level of ovarian hormones after the menopause can be reversed if the woman takes HRT, but HRT is not suitable for all women and many questions still remain to be answered about the longer-term effects of HRT. Oestrogens have also been shown to relieve some of the symptoms of Alzheimer's disease in older women.

Men do not show the same sharp cut-off in reproductive function: reduction in reproductive capacity seems to be a more gradual process, and some men retain full reproductive capacity into extreme old age. Helgason et al. (1996) studied the sexual function of men in Sweden and found that in their oldest subject group (70–80 year-olds) 46% reported orgasm at least once a month. Sperm production continues into old age, but the rate of spermatogenesis slows down and there is an increase in the number of abnormal sperm. Testosterone and androgen secretions from the Leydig cells in the testes diminish, although the extent of decline varies.

The prostate gland shows many different histological, biochemical and functional changes with ageing, resulting in an enlargement of the gland. This is known as benign prostatic hypertrophy and is present to some extent in all men. Connective tissue accumulates and this leads to the familiar problems with micturition so common among older men – namely frequency, urgency and a poor stream of urine. The changes in the prostate gland are related to alterations in the sex hormone levels of ageing men. Enlargement of the prostate gland and reduced testosterone levels are considered to be factors in the increase of urinary tract infections in older men (Bissett 2004). Changes also occur in other male reproductive organs: the capacity of seminal vesicles decreases and sclerotic changes occur in the erectile tissue in the penis.

THEORIES AND MECHANISMS OF AGEING

Why ageing occurs and what causes ageing are questions that have fascinated people for years. Much of the early interest in the ageing process was directed at finding the 'elixir' of life and ways of increasing longevity. Much progress has been made over the last 50 years in understanding the processes underpinning ageing, but fundamental questions still remain.

Many different theories have been proposed in an attempt to explain ageing; some of these theories can be grouped together, as they incorporate similar approaches. For example, some theories have looked at the genetics of ageing and these can be linked in with evolutionary aspects. Some researchers have investigated changes in whole-body function or in one particular system, while others have concentrated on changes in cell structure and function. More recently, research has been directed at the molecular basis of ageing and changes in DNA and these again may link up with the genetics of ageing. Fortunately, many of the theories about ageing are not mutually exclusive – they just seek to explain ageing in a different way. As discussed earlier, knowledge about the biology of ageing has come from many different sources – from cell culture work, from studies using animals as models for human ageing, or from investigations of conditions with some features similar to those of ageing, for example Werner's syndrome (see below). Mathematical models and predictions based on accepted biological principles have also been proposed. It is not possible in a chapter of this nature to consider or do justice to all the theories of ageing; however, a few interesting issues will be considered briefly. Kirkwood (2001, 2002) and Martin (2001) give useful reviews of the theories of ageing.

It is an attractive proposition to look for one single explanation for all features of ageing; however, research to date has not suggested that there is a unitary cause of ageing, or indeed that all cells and tissues age in the same way. It is likely that different tissues in an animal not only age at different rates but possibly also age for different reasons. Each ageing individual may have a mix of changes and/or impairments at the cellular or tissue level and these together contribute to the common manifestations of ageing. Often it can be hard to work out whether particular events are a cause of ageing or simply a correlate of ageing (Martin & Loeb 2004).

Some classic early work with human fibroblasts (immature connective tissue cells) was done by Hayflick and colleagues. Hayflick (1985) showed that normal animal cells have a fixity of lifespan that indicates a kind of genetic programme of ageing in the cell – a programme that could underlie ageing of the whole body. Healthy cells taken from a human fetus divide normally enough in culture if supplied with food and a place to grow, but they divide only 50 times or thereabouts. Cells from a short-lived species were shown to double less often than cells from longer-lived species. Hayflick originally proposed that there was a finite predetermined number of times that a cell could replicate even under the most favourable conditions. (This is not the case for cancer cells – these abnormal cells seem to become immortal and have an infinite lifespan.) However, in the light of more recent work it now seems likely that, although normal cells do have a finite capacity for replication, this limit is very rarely reached in vivo (i.e. in the body). Other functional problems occur prior to the cessation of capacity to divide, i.e. before the normal cells have reached their maximum proliferative capacity (Hayflick 1985). Apoptosis (or programmed cell death) is one area of investigation to help understand the ageing process.

As discussed at the beginning of the chapter, it has been known for a long time that the lifespans of animals (most of the work has been done on rodents but it has been shown to apply to many other species too) can be consistently increased (by up to 40%) by restricting calorie intake (Martin 2001). The effect is most marked when the calorie restriction is started from weaning, but significant extensions of lifespan are also produced when adult animals are subjected to calorie restriction. Many of the changes that are characteristic of ageing also seem to be influenced and there is also a striking reduction in certain diseases commonly seen in ageing rodents. Certainly work has identified several genes involved in the control of energy metabolism (especially via the insulin signalling pathway) that seem to be centrally involved in ageing (Kirkwood 2002). Differences in energy metabolism may be associated with changes in longevity (Speakman et al. 2004). There is increasing interest in this area as it relates to humans and is obviously linked with the current concerns about increasing obesity levels in many countries.

It has been suggested that evolutionary pressures would lead to a programmed ageing of species and that there are genes that determine ageing, i.e. genes that in one way or another programme for ageing. Certainly heredity plays a part, as we know from familial data, and ageing and longevity are indeed governed by genetic factors. Twin studies have been very helpful; the lifespan of monozygotic (identical) twins (who have exactly the same genetic make-up) are statistically more similar than lifespans of dizygotic twins, the magnitude of the difference indicating that approximately one-quarter to one-third of what determines lifespan is genetic (Kirkwood 2002). Some human genetic disorders display features of accelerated ageing, for example Werner's syndrome. Werner's syndrome (or progeria of the adult) is a rare disease where people age very prematurely and can be 'old' by the time they reach their late 20s. People with Werner's condition may have premature cataracts, skin changes, greying and loss of hair, osteoporosis, diabetes, hypogonadism and neoplasia. They often die from atherosclerosis and heart disease in their late 40s and 50s. Research into Werner's syndrome has shown that it is due to a single gene defect, an autosomal recessive condition, where people carry two copies of the defective gene WRN. The gene concerned codes for a helicase enzyme which is involved in DNA replication; helicase enables repair enzymes to weed out random mutations that threaten the integrity of genes and chromosomes (Concar 1996). So although it is acknowledged that genetic factors play a part, evolutionary theory now argues strongly against programmed ageing, suggesting that organisms (and that includes humans) are programmed for survival, not death (Kirkwood 2002). There are unlikely to be specific genes that program for ageing, but it is likely that (because genes ultimately control all body processes anyway) genes are of particular importance in influencing ageing and longevity by their ability to determine normal maintenance and repair processes in the cells. Chance or random events also seem to play a part in the ageing process and would help to explain the unpredictable nature of ageing at the level of the individual.

In contrast to the idea that ageing is predetermined or preprogrammed, there are error theories which suggest that function carries on until some catastrophe occurs and only then is normal function lost. This might occur suddenly or as a result of wear and tear, or of, simply, an accumulation of different minor deteriorations. For instance, one small error in the long chain of reactions during protein synthesis would produce an imperfect structural protein or enzyme which in turn might interfere with cell function. There is evidence that DNA, proteins and lipids do all accumulate damage during ageing. Some enzymes do show signs of ageing and protein synthesis does slow down, but it is by no means universal and there are many instances of normal biochemical processes in the body at all ages. There is currently a great deal of research on DNA damage and mutation in mitochondrial DNA with implications for the oxidative damage theory of ageing (see below) (Martin 2001). In fact, dozens of functional changes are seen in ageing cells and some of these may lead to a loss of 'normal' cell function and play a role in the expression of ageing – but are they a cause or a result of ageing? Failure in part of the immune system and increasing levels of autoantibodies have also been implicated in the aetiology of ageing.

Various theories have been concerned with changes in DNA. Some work suggests that with ageing there is a failure of the cell's ability to repair damaged DNA or that random genetic damage accumulates despite the existence of repair processes (which are themselves imperfect) in the cell. Any accumulation of errors in protein synthesis would result in abnormal proteins and these are found in ageing cells. There may also be a failure to remove abnormal proteins. One theory along these lines links the changes seen in proteins in diabetic people with those seen in ageing individuals, as in both instances there is an accumulation of glycosylated proteins (proteins that have become associated with glucose). For example, glycosylated proteins are thought to be implicated in the development of cataracts and atherosclerosis. Thus some changes seen in diabetic people are rather like premature ageing effects (Furth & Harding 1989, Concar 1996).

There is increasing support for the view that ageing results from the accumulation during life of damage in cells and tissues. The body is not able to maintain normal cell function and to repair damage and these are possibly the main factors resulting in the manifestations of ageing. Kirkwood (2002) proposes that the principal genes determining longevity and rate of senescence are genes that specify the levels of maintenance functions (for example, DNA repair genes, antioxidant enzymes, stress proteins) and not specific genes that 'program' for ageing. These ideas are considered further in the section on the disposable soma theory of ageing, below.

Another cluster of ageing theories relates to the accumulation of cross-linkages in macromolecules. As we have already seen, collagen changes with age; it becomes much stiffer and loses its usual properties due to an increase in cross-linkages. Cross-linking of some cellular macromolecules, e.g. proteins and lipids, produces fluorescent chemical compounds, collectively called age pigments or lipofuscin. (These age pigments are not the same as the common changes in skin pigmentation seen with advancing age.) Age pigments seem to accumulate, particularly in cardiac muscle and the nervous system. The role of these pigments is disputed, although it is accepted that they are a good indicator of the degree of ageing; regardless of its function, lipofuscin accumulation is used as an index of physiological ageing. It has been suggested that age pigment accumulation may impair cell function, although there is no direct evidence for this. These substances may result from the correction of free radical damage (see below).

Oxidative damage theory of ageing

All the theories mentioned above beg the question of what actually causes the changes in ageing. The oxidative damage theory, also known as the free radical theory of ageing, first discussed by Harman (1956) and developed considerably since then (for example, Harman 1988, 1992, Martin 2001), attempts to overcome this issue; it proposes that free radicals are central agents in producing changes at tissue, cellular and subcellular levels. Free radicals are normally produced during some metabolic processes in the body. Free radicals are highly reactive unstable molecules owing to the presence of an unpaired electron; this results in a large increase in free energy which allows them to attack adjacent molecules. According to the theory, free radicals damage important biological molecules and accumulation of this damage leads to the decline in function seen with ageing. The superoxide molecule, an excited form of oxygen, is one such free radical. (Some reactive oxygen forms, e.g. single oxygen atoms, are not free radicals but are capable of causing oxidative damage, hence the currently preferred terminology of oxidative damage theory of ageing: Martin 2001.)

Organisms have evolved enzymes (e.g. superoxide dismutase and catalase) and non-enzymatic systems (e.g. vitamins C and E) for scavenging free radicals and destroying potentially harmful products before further damage can occur. Normally, any superoxide radicals that form during metabolism are inactivated by superoxide dismutase found naturally in the cells. Enzymes like these seem to have evolved specifically to help to protect important substances in the cells; thus if there is a defect in these protective mechanisms, oxidative damage could result. According to the theory, accumulated damage due to free radicals leads to an age-related decrease in function.

Membrane lipids, both on the cell surface and within the cells in organelle membranes, seem to be particularly vulnerable to free radical attack. The damage caused can take many forms, e.g. it can cause cross-linkage in collagen, nucleic acids, proteins and membrane phospholipids. If this occurs, the normal function of the molecule is impaired. It is known that when these molecules are attacked in this way fluorescent pigments are produced; hence the link with the so-called age pigments.

It has been known for some time that irradiation also causes life-shortening and seems to lead to an increased incidence of age changes. Whether changes due to radiation are the same as 'normal' ageing changes is a matter of some debate; life-shortening induced by ionizing radiation or mutagenic compounds appears to differ both quantitatively and qualitatively from the normal process of ageing. However, it does seem that the harmful effects of radiation are also due to the formation of free radicals. Thus free radical reactions are suggested to be the cause of many degenerative changes in ageing cells.

A major attraction of the oxidative damage theory is that it makes ageing potentially treatable: chemical antioxidants should be able to prevent this oxidative damage to important molecules. Vitamins C and E are examples of chemical antioxidants that are capable of interrupting free radical reactions. When this theory was first proposed, it did in fact lead to substantial sales of vitamins C and E; this may be the reason why the theory has become so popular! Some animal experiments have suggested that antioxidants do extend the lifespan, but others have shown no effect on the rate of ageing or on lifespan. There is currently little evidence in humans for these vitamins having any direct benefit. However, it has been suggested that average life expectancy at birth can be increased by 5 years or more by nutritious low-calorie diets and antioxidant supplements (Harman 1992).

Disposable soma theory of ageing

Kirkwood & Holliday (1986) suggest that two theoretical approaches may be taken in explaining the evolution of ageing: namely, that ageing can be said to be either adaptive or non-adaptive. The former approach implies that ageing is a beneficial trait in its own right and 'good' for the species. For example, ageing prevents overcrowding and promotes evolutionary change through the generations with turnover of genetic material. But if ageing is adaptive, i.e. is such a good thing, it is strange that it is rarely seen in wild populations. Another difficulty with the idea is that ageing is clearly disadvantageous to the individual, although possibly beneficial to the species.

The non-adaptive theories are currently favoured (remember, theories do go in and out of vogue). In these theories ageing is said to occur because natural selection is either unable to prevent the deterioration of old organisms or it is a byproduct of selection for other adaptive qualities. Ageing is thus detrimental or at best neutral, and so its evolution must be explained indirectly.

One non-adaptive theory considers the alleged exhaustion of physiological energy reserves; this looks at the association between the rate of living and longevity – those with a high rate have a shorter lifespan. There are known to be specific instances where sexual activity hastens senescence: in the *Drosophila* fruit fly, for example, copulation and egg-laying shorten life. It is obviously not easy to assess this in humans but Kirkwood & Austad (2000) give some possible evidence for this in human populations.

Kirkwood & Holliday (1986) proposed a non-adaptive theory along these lines, which they have called the 'disposable soma theory' (Fig. 5.6). In this theory an organism is considered rather like a 'black box' which takes up energy from the environment in the form of nutrients and then transforms this energy into progeny (offspring). However, in order to maintain life, part of the energy input must be allocated to and used for normal maintenance and repair of the non-reproductive bodily tissue (i.e. the soma). Maintenance and repair include prevention and removal of DNA damage, protein synthesis, breakdown of defective or unwanted molecules, wound healing, immune responses, and so on. In this theory the more energy the organism allocates to somatic maintenance, the less is available for reproduction, and vice versa; hence the name, disposable soma theory. In other words, there is a trade-off between normal maintenance and repair, and reproduction. So a balance must be struck between the com-

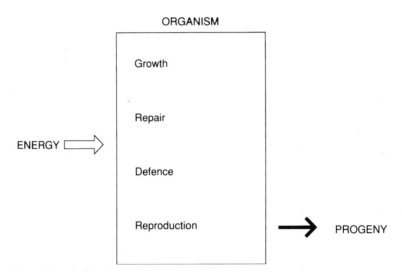

Fig. 5.6   The disposable soma theory of ageing.

peting benefits of living longer (by allocating resources to cope with random damage) or reproducing at a greater rate. Grimley Evans (1993) uses the analogy of 'metabolic switches' where, in simple terms, energy is switched from one area of metabolic activity to another.

Kirkwood & Holliday (1986) have demonstrated mathematical support for this theory; they also suggest that it explains some of the special features of human ageing that are not generally seen in other animals; survival well into the post reproductive period, the menopause and the slow development of children are predominantly human phenomena. Something similar to the menopause may be seen in some primates but it does not exist in lower animals.

Humans certainly do have a significant expectation of survival into the senescent phase or post reproductive phase of their lifespan. The complex social behaviour seen in human society affords significant protection against environmental hazards, but at the cost of greatly delaying maturation and prolonging the dependence of children on parents. As a female grows older, the hazards of further pregnancies increase and beyond the age of 40–50 years it may be more advantageous for a woman to cease to reproduce while she is bringing up her children (i.e. to direct energy towards maintenance and repair). Thus the advent of the menopause is 'good' since it stops fertility and allows energy to be directed towards maintenance and repair and so extends the lifespan (Kirkwood 2002).

Part of the attractiveness of this theory is that it allows other theories to be incorporated; for instance, ideas that postulate particular kinds of somatic damage as the cause of ageing. Thus, damage by free radicals, somatic mutation, errors in protein synthesis, macromolecular cross-linkage and so on could all be included. It could also encompass the idea that senescence is due to wear and tear – not because wear and tear is inevitable, but because it arises as the indirect result of optimizing the balance between somatic maintenance and repair with reproduction.

As the above discussion shows, many of the theories of ageing are not mutually exclusive: some can indeed be integrated and the findings can and do complement each other. In the final analysis, whatever the mechanisms or causes prove to be, ageing is likely to result from a combination of genetic and random processes.

HEALTH AND DISEASE IN OLDER PEOPLE

It should be apparent from the previous discussions that human ageing is malleable (Kirkwood 2003): if approximately 25% of ageing is genetically determined, 75% is not! And thus promoting health, preventing or delaying the onset of ageing changes, is possible to some extent. Promotion of physical health in later life requires attention to the same factors as at any age; for instance, regular exercise, a balanced diet and a healthy lifestyle (e.g. avoiding smoking and so on). The situation with older people may be more complex as often manifestations of ageing intermingle with symptoms of disease. A growing body of evidence suggests that diseases and conditions that are the primary cause of loss of function and independence in later life are preventable and certainly physical activity can play an important part (Department of Health 2004).

The importance of maintaining regular activity is frequently acknowledged, but not acted upon. As discussed earlier in the section on physical capacity, it is sometimes difficult to differentiate the effects of disuse, i.e. physical deconditioning, from those of ageing; as a consequence, old age is often considered to be synonymous with disability, but there is much evidence to dispute this: a decline in levels of physical fitness is not inevitable. The amount of physical activity undertaken can be low for many reasons: genuine disability, disease, a desire to 'take it easy' or a lack of energy, fear of falls, lack of appropriate facilities and lack of companionship for exercise are some possibilities. Crombie et al. (2004) found that even though levels of knowledge about the specific benefits of physical exercise in their sample of older people was good, many still did not participate in leisure-time activity. A study by Jarvis et al. (1996) gives a detailed and fascinating profile of the activities and functional abilities of the older population in the UK, both in terms of leisure activities and activities such as getting around the home.

However, the evidence of research studies is very convincing (and has been for some time) – even a minimal amount of regular physical activity has a significant effect on aspects of health. For instance, undertaking the 'right' exercise can have a positive effect on bone mass, help to maintain joint flexibility, reduce joint stiffness, improve balance, and increase muscle tone and strength. It can also help with bowel movements and incontinence. Exercise can sharpen alertness, help insomnia, increase self-confidence, alleviate depression and enhance mood, and may improve some aspects of cognitive function (Department of Health 2004). Many, many studies have been done showing the health benefits of exercise for older people. Participation in regular exercise has a beneficial effect on cardiovascular disease, type 2 diabetes and obesity as well. Dionne et al. (2003) review the impact of cardiovascular fitness and physical activity level on health outcomes in older people.

Of course, some older people would not be able to undertake strenuous activity; however, even regular seated exercise (i.e. performing exercises while sitting down) has been shown to benefit even very old residents of old people's homes and to improve their functional capacity (McMurdo & Rennie 1993). Some of the studies looking at exercise and the elderly have used expensive specialized training equipment but, while this is valuable in research terms, if exercise is to be widely adopted by older people it should ideally be enjoyable, inexpensive and achievable by most old people (McMurdo & Johnstone 1995). There are many sources now of recommended exercise regimes for older people suitable for all levels of fitness and ability (see Useful sources and websites section, below).

It has been suggested that older people who are active may also adopt a lifestyle that promotes overall health through proper sleeping habits, regular meals, moderate alcohol consumption, maintenance of normal weight and abstinence from smoking. Such a lifestyle has also been associated with increased longevity.

The results of participation in a physical conditioning regimen are measurable in people at any age, at least up to the time that senescence makes exercise most difficult. Obviously not every older person is in a position to be active in the sense of going for a walk or going swimming, but knitting, sitting in a chair and doing ankle exercises, walking to the toilet or the telephone may be appropriate exercise to encourage in other instances. The type of exercise that is encouraged will obviously depend on the individual's capabilities, but generally, rhythmic exercise involving the use of a large muscle mass is recommended: walking is one of the ideal activities.

Certainly, the functional alterations brought about by regular exercise blunt the downward trends commonly associated with ageing. Creative approaches are required to counter the rather negative perceptions among many older people of the desirability of physical activity. One great disservice we can do to an older person, even if for the best of intentions, is to reduce the amount of physical activity undertaken; it may be as little as stopping her standing up at the sink to wash up, or going to fetch something for her to save her the effort. What regimens of inactivity we inflict on old people in many care settings does not bear thinking about. No wonder that older people when discharged after a stay in hospital have difficulty in coping because of a loss of fitness during the hospital stay. It may be simplistic, but if you don't use it, you lose it! Approximately two-thirds of older patients have been shown to lose mobility during an acute illness, and two-thirds of these individuals will not have fully regained their abilities by the time of discharge (MacKnight & Rockwood 1995). One study in the USA looked at changes in activities of daily living in people aged 70 and above before and after hospitalization and found that 35% of patients had a decline in overall activities of daily living between admission and discharge, caused by excessive bedrest, inadequate nutrition, multidrug regimes and sleep deprivation (Covinski et al. 2003).

While aiming to optimize an individual's physical health, it is perhaps unrealistic to refer only to 'healthy' older people; the interaction between ageing and disease is complex, with a continuum between 'normal' ageing changes and pathology or disease. At one end of the spectrum there are instances where there is little or no interaction between ageing and disease (as in skin cancer, for example), while at the other extreme the changes that occur with age actually represent or mimic disease, e.g. an altered glucose tolerance, or the development of cataracts. Many of the important diseases of old age, including Alzheimer's disease and osteoporosis, show interaction and overlap with normal ageing; for example the bone loss that causes osteoporosis in susceptible individuals is seen to some degree in all older people (Kirkwood 2003). Similarly the characteristic changes seen in Alzheimer's disease (amyloid plaques and neurofibrillary tangles) are sometimes found in older people even if there was no clinical evidence of dementia. Some physiological changes that occur with ageing can increase the likelihood or severity of disease; normal ageing is associated with a decline in pulmonary function, for instance, and this together with reduced efficiency of the immune system may mean that a respiratory tract infection could lead to a marked loss of lung function. The same infection in a younger person may not have such a debilitating effect.

Multiple pathology is also common in older people. Here the decline in function within several systems might interact to increase the likelihood of a problem. The classic example of this is falling in older people. Falls are a major cause of disability and the leading cause of mortality due to injury in older people over 75 in the UK (Department of Health 2001). The higher incidence of falls in older people is due to a combination of factors: increased postural sway and poor balance, postural hypotension, poor eyesight and reduced muscle strength might all make a contribution. The prescription of tranquillizers, certain cardiovascular medications and anti-inflammatory drugs has also been shown to increase the risk of falls (Koski et al. 1996). In addition to these intrinsic risk factors associated with ageing, environmental factors such as poor lighting, loose carpets, badly fitting shoes or lack of handrails also increase the likelihood of falls. Attention to these factors will minimize falls, but also exercising has been shown to be effective in falls prevention (Hainsworth 2004), by improving balance and muscle strength. A more novel approach is now recommended too: t'ai chi taught in 15-week courses has been shown to improve muscle strength and balance and reduce the risk of falls (NICE 2004). So, reducing the incidence of falls requires attention to both physiological aspects and to environmental considerations (Legge 2003, Perdue 2003).

Some physiological changes that are aspects of normal ageing clearly have adverse clinical consequences. For instance, the menopause is 'normal' but increases the risk of osteoporosis; similarly, the endocrine changes in men that result in benign prostatic hypertrophy frequently lead to urinary tract problems. Thus, some normal age-related changes certainly increase the risk or likelihood of health problems. To add further to the complexities, the presentation of the disease or problem may also be altered in older people; consider, for example, the classic painless myocardial infarction, or the reduction in elevation of temperature with infections in older people.

So it seems that individuals born with a particular genetic complement of strengths and weaknesses in maintenance and repair systems are exposed to a range of environmental challenges and eventually develop, on one hand, somatic alterations which we recognize as old age, and on the other hand, structural and functional changes which we recognize as disease processes (Ruse & Parker 2001).

This chapter has considered some of the important aspects of the biology of human ageing and the implications of these physiological changes. Clearly, the changes observed in ageing are not all as bad as they are often portrayed; quite the opposite – most older people, in a biological sense, cope very adequately. What must be remembered is the enormous variability amongst older people; what is normal for one 80-year-old might be quite inappropriate for another. Similarly, there are ways of promoting or optimizing the health and physical capacities of an older person, just as there are for a younger individual.

Recommended reading

Department of Health 2004 At least five a week: evidence on the impact of physical activity and its relationship to health. London: Department of Health.
Discussion on the importance of physical activity in maintaining health and preventing disease, including a specific chapter (Chapter 6) on the benefits for older adults.

Kirkwood TBL 1999 Time of our lives: the science of human ageing. Weidenfeld and Nicholson, London.
Easily readable and informative look at ageing.
Kirkwood TBL 2002 Evolution of ageing. Mechanisms of Ageing and Development 123 : 737–745.
A fascinating discussion on the theories surrounding the evolution of human ageing. It considers the genetic aspects, looks at the evidence for problems in cellular maintenance and repair and studies specialist aspects such as menopause and longevity in humans.
Kirkwood TBL 2003 The most pressing problem of our age. British Medical Journal 326:1297–1299.
A discussion of what we know about ageing and the reasons for infirmity in old age.

Useful journals:

- Mechanisms of Ageing and Development: a multidisciplinary journal aimed at revealing the mechanisms that underlie the processes of ageing.
- Age and Ageing: the journal of the British Geriatrics Society that includes much research on normal ageing changes and those associated with age-related diseases.

Useful sources and websites

Age Concern 2004 Staying healthy in later life. Fact sheet 45. Age Concern, London. Also available from www.ageconcern.org.uk/AgeConcern/media/FS45SEPT04.
British Heart Foundation Active for Later Life. British Heart Foundation, London (available in book form or via) www.bhfactive.org.uk-Active for Later Life.
Resource produced to help professionals involved in physical activity programmes for older people of all ages and abilities.
www.extend.org.uk
Extend: a network of teachers providing movement to music for over 60s and people with disabilities. Classes can be held in nursing homes, sheltered housing developments and hospitals.
www.napa-web.co.uk
National Association for Providers of Activities for Older People (NAPA) provides information for organizers of activities in care homes and day-care settings.

References

Age Concern 2004 Staying healthy in later life. Fact sheet 45. Age Concern, London. Also available from www.ageconcern.org.uk/AgeConcern/media/FS45SEPT04
Anderton BH 2002 Ageing of the brain. Mechanisms of Ageing and Development 123: 811–817
Aniansson A, Rundgren A, Sperling L 1980 Evaluation of functional capacity in activities of daily living in 70 year old men and women. Scandinavian Journal of Rehabilitation Medicine 12: 145–154

Astrand P, Rodahl K 1977 Textbook of work physiology. McGraw-Hill, New York

Basile JN 2002 Systolic blood pressure: it is time to focus on systolic hypertension – especially in older people. British Medical Journal 325: 917–918

Benbow M 2002 The skin: its structure and function. Nursing Times 98:43–46

Bissett L 2004 The control of urinary tract infection in hospitalised older people. Nursing Times 100:54–56

Chandra RK, Puri S 1985 Nutritional support improves antibody response to influenza virus vaccine in the older. British Medical Journal 291: 705–706

Cheitlin MD 2003 Cardiovascular physiology – changes with aging. American Journal of Geriatric Cardiology 12: 9–13

Collins KJ, Exton-Smith AN, James MH, Oliver DJ 1980 Functional changes in autonomic nervous responses with ageing. Age and Ageing 9: 17–24

Concar D 1996 Death of old age. New Scientist 2013: 24–29

Connolly MJ 1996 Obstructive airway disease: a hidden disability in the aged. Age and Ageing 25: 265–267

Covinski KE, Palmer RM, Fortinsky RH et al. 2003 Loss of independence in activities of daily living in older adults hospitalised with medical illnesses: increased vulnerability with age. Journal of the American Geriatrics Society 51: 451–458

Department of Health 1992 The nutrition of older people. HMSO, London

Department of Health 2001 National service framework for older people. London, Department of Health

Department of Health 2004 At least five a week: evidence on the impact of physical activity and its relationship to health. London, Department of Health

Dionne IJ, Ades PA, Poehlman ET 2003 Impact of cardiovascular fitness and physical activity level on health outcomes in older persons. Mechanisms of Ageing and Development 124: 259–267

Effros RB 2003 Genetic alterations in the ageing immune system: impact on infection and cancer. Mechanisms of Ageing and Development 124: 71–77

Exton-Smith AN 1980 Nutritional status: diagnosis and prevention of malnutrition. In: Exton-Smith AN, Caird FI (eds) Metabolic and nutritional disorders in the older. Wright, Bristol

Exton-Smith AN, Stanton BR 1965 Report of an investigation into the diets of older women living alone. King Edward's Hospital Fund, London

Furth A, Harding J 1989 Why sugar is bad for you. New Scientist 1683: 44–47

Greig CA, Young A, Skelton DA et al. 1994 Exercise studies with older volunteers. Age and Ageing 23: 185–189

Grimley Evans J 1993 Metabolic switches in ageing. Age and Ageing 22: 79–81

Hainsworth T 2004 The role of exercise in falls prevention for older people. Nursing Times 100: 28–29

Harman D 1956 Ageing: a theory based on the free radical and radiation chemistry. Journal of Gerontology II: 298–300

Harman D 1988 Free radicals in ageing. Molecular and Cellular Biochemistry 84: 155–161

Harman D 1992 Free radical theory of ageing. Mutation Research 275: 275–266

Hayflick L 1985 The cell biology of ageing. Clinical Geriatric Medicine 1: 15–27

Helgason AR, Adolfsson J, Dickman P et al. 1996 Sexual desire, erection, orgasm and ejaculatory functions and their importance to older Swedish men: a population-based study. Age and Ageing 25: 285–291

Holmes S 1994 Nutrition and older people. Nursing Times 90: 31–33

Huppert FA, Brayne C, Jagger C, Metz D 2000 Longitudinal studies of ageing: a key role in the evidence base for improving health and quality of life in older adults. Age and Ageing 29: 485–486

Jarvis C, Hancock R, Askham J, Tinker A 1996 Getting around after 60: a profile of Britain's older population. HMSO, London

Jenkins G 2002 Molecular mechanisms of skin ageing. Mechanisms of Ageing and Development 123: 801–810

Johnson HA 1985 Relations between normal ageing and disease. Raven Press, New York

Johnston CC, Norton JA, Khairi RA, Longscope C 1979 Age-related bone loss. In: Barzel US (ed) Osteoporosis II. Grune & Stratton, New York

Kenney HA 1989 Physiology of ageing: a synopsis, 2nd edn. Year Book, Chicago

Kenney WL, Chiu P 2001 Influence of age on thirst and fluid intake. Medicine and Science in Sports and Exercise 33: 1524–1532

Kirkwood TBL 2001 Biological origins of ageing. In: Grimley Evans J, Williams TF, Beattie BL, Michel JP, Wilcock GK (eds) Oxford textbook of geriatric medicine, 2nd edn. Oxford University Press, Oxford

Kirkwood TBL 2002 Evolution of ageing. Mechanisms of Ageing and Development 123: 737–745

Kirkwood TBL 2003 The most pressing problem of our age. British Medical Journal 326: 1297–1299

Kirkwood TBL, Austad SN 2000 Why do we age? Nature 408: 233–238

Kirkwood TBL, Holliday R 1986 Ageing as a consequence of natural selection. In: Bittles AH, Collins KJ (eds) The biology of human ageing. Cambridge University Press, Cambridge

Kirkwood TBL, Wolff SP 1995 The biological basis of ageing. Age and Ageing 24: 167–171

Koski K, Luukinen H, Laippala P, Kivelä S-L 1996 Physiological factors and medications as predictors of injurious falls by older people: a prospective population-based study. Age and Ageing 25: 29–38

Lakatta EG 1983 Determinants of cardiovascular performance: modification due to ageing. Journal of Chronic Disease 36: 15–30

Legge A 2003 Breaking the fall. Nursing Times 99: 22–25

Lewis VM, Twomey JJ, Bealmear P, Goldstein G, Good RA 1978 Age, thymic involution and circulating thymic hormone activity. Journal of Clinical Endocrinology and Metabolism 47: 145–150

Luz C, Dornelles F, Preissler T et al. 2003 Impact of psychological and endocrine factors on cytokine production of healthy older people. Mechanisms of Ageing and Development 124: 887–895

MacKnight C, Rockwood K 1995 A hierarchical assessment of balance and mobility. Age and Ageing 24: 126–130

McCay CM, Crowell MF, Maynard LA 1935 The effect of retarded growth upon the length of life span and upon the ultimate body size. Journal of Nutrition 10: 63–79

Maddox GL, Douglass GB 1974 Ageing and individual differences: a longitudinal analysis of social, psychological and physiological indicators. Journal of Gerontology 29: 555–563

Martin GM 2001 Biological mechanisms of ageing. In: Grimley Evans J, Williams TF, Beattie BL, Michel JP, Wilcock GK (eds) Oxford textbook of geriatric medicine, 2nd edn. Oxford University Press, Oxford

Martin GM, Loeb LA 2004 Ageing: mice and mitochondria. Nature 429: 357–359

McGandy RB, Barrows CM, Spanias A et al. 1966 Nutrient intakes and energy expenditure in men of different ages. Journal of Gerontology 21: 551–558

McMurdo MET, Johnstone R 1995 A randomized controlled trial of a home exercise programme for older people with poor mobility. Age and Ageing 24: 425–428

McMurdo MET, Rennie L 1993 A controlled trial of exercise by residents of old people's homes. Age and Ageing 22: 11–15

NICE 2004 Falls: the assessment and prevention of falls in older people. www.nice.org.uk/pdf/Falls_FULLguideline_2ndconsultation.pdf

Olde Rikkert MGM, Rigaud A 2003 Malnutrition research: high time to change the menu. Age and Ageing 32:241–243

Orentreich N, Selmanowitz VJ 1969 Levels of biological functions with ageing. Transactions of the Academic Science Series B 31: 992–1012

Perdue C 2003 Falls in older people: taking a multidisciplinary approach. Nursing Times 99: 28–30

Perls T, Levenson R, Regan M, Puca A 2002 What does it take to live to 100? Mechanisms of Ageing and Development 123: 231–242

Phillips PA, Johnson CI, Gray L 1993 Disturbed fluid and electrolyte homeostasis following dehydration in older people. Age and Ageing 22: 26–33

Rehman HU, Masson EA 2001 Neuroendocrinology of ageing. Age and Ageing 30:279–287

Rodeheffer RJ, Gerstenblich G, Becker LC et al. 1984 Exercise cardiac output is maintained with advancing age in healthy human subjects: cardiac dilatation and increased stroke volume compensate for a diminished heart rate. Circulation 69: 203–213

Rowe J, Kahn R 1987 Human ageing – usual and successful. Science 237: 143–149

Ruse CE, Parker SG 2001 Molecular genetics and age-related disease. Age and Ageing 30: 449–454

Sandblum PH, Peterson P, Muren A 1953 Determination of the tensile strength of healing wounds as a clinical test. Acta Chirurgica Scandinavica 105: 252–257

Schroder AK, Rink L 2003 Neutrophil immunity of the older. Mechanisms of Ageing and Development 124: 419–425

Shock N 1985 Longitudinal studies of ageing in humans. In: Finch CE, Schneider EL (eds) Handbook of the biology of ageing, 2nd edn. Van Nostrand Reinhold, New York

Speakman JR, Talbot DA, Selman C et al. 2004 Uncoupled and surviving: individual mice with high metabolism have greater mitochondrial uncoupling and live longer. Aging Cell 3: 87–95

Steinhagen-Thiessen E, Borchelt M 1999 Morbidity, medication and functional limitations in very old age. In: Baltes PB, Mayer KU (eds) The Berlin ageing study: ageing from 70–100. Cambridge University Press, New York

Strehler BL 1962 Time, cells and ageing. Academic Press, New York

Tolson D, Schofield I, Booth J, Ramsay R 2002 Nutrition for physically frail older people. Nursing Times 98: 38–40

Trivedi DP, Doll R, Khaw KT 2003 Effect of 4 monthly oral vitamin D_3 (cholecalciferol) supplementation on fractures and mortality in men and women living in the community: randomised double blind controlled trial. British Medical Journal 326: 469–472

Young A 1986 Exercise physiology in geriatric practice. Acta Medica Scandinavica Supplement 711: 227–232

SECTION 2

Policy change and contexts of care

Chapter 6

Policy developments in the organization of support for older people

Jill Manthorpe

INTRODUCTION

This chapter centres on policy for older people, focusing on the organization of support for older people in health and social care (Fig. 6.1). This is not to say that other policy areas are unimportant, but they will be covered more briefly. This chapter also considers some key themes evident in government responses to an ageing population, in relation to specific groups of older people and policy developments or 'hot spots', notably around difference and diversity. The chapter ends with an analysis of the power and influence of older people in the policy-making process, since it is often forgotten that many older people are highly active in social and political debates and have much to say about what they think is wrong and what should be done. New policy debates will have to acknowledge older people's human rights and their expression of these.

CARE IN THE COMMUNITY AND BEYOND

The building blocks of today's systems of health and social care in the UK, and indeed some parts of pension provision and housing, owe much to the legislation laid down in the 1940s and the compromises made to implement the welfare state. Older people's needs and circumstances were evident to the founding fathers of the welfare state. They had become starkly visible in planning for the Second World War and in designing the welfare state, particularly the needs of older people living in hospital and the reliance of older people on their families, especially their daughters. Many current services have their origins in the thinking of that time and in ideas developed as wartime stopgaps. These include the development of meals services, home helps and the setting-up of local

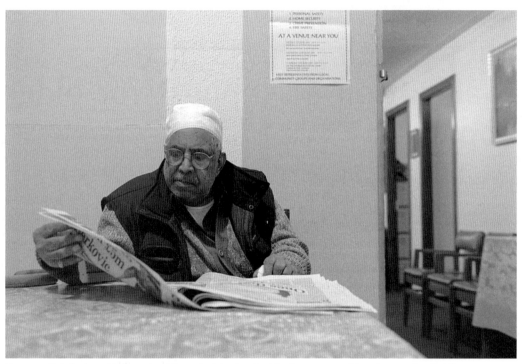

Fig. 6.1 Keeping up with the news. (Photograph by Jon-Paul Davis, courtesy of Age Concern Scotland.)

organizations and initiatives to meet needs (Local Old People's Welfare Committees, now called Age Concern groups). A familiar issue of pre-war policy is the pressure to remove older people from occupying hospital beds, now discussed in terms of 'bed blocking'. The community elements of the National Health Service (NHS) and Community Care Act (1990) have similar roots in government concern that older people were posing a social problem in their excessive consumption of the welfare budget, particularly residential care. The charging (or fining) of local authorities for failing to arrange hospital discharge for patients reflects similar concerns.

The NHS and Community Care Act 1990 provides a useful starting point to set the context for recent health and social care policies. This Act combined two sets of thinking: one in the White Paper *Working for Patients* (Department of Health 1989a), the other in the White Paper *Caring for People*, with its often forgotten subheading: *Community care in the next decade and beyond* (Department of Health 1989b).

Working for Patients

This White Paper had three key aims: (1) to extend patient choice; (2) to provide value for money; and (3)

to alter responsibilities in the NHS. Bearing in mind the public's great attachment to the principles of the NHS, the White Paper confirmed that the NHS would continue to be open to everyone, no matter what their income, and would still be funded mainly out of general taxation. The Conservative government was troubled however by the rising costs of the NHS, mindful of the growing numbers of older people with higher expectations for health care, and attracted to other ways in which health care could be provided, especially by ideas that gave greater power at local level and introduced market ideas to the organization of health care, including notions that more people might be willing to take out private health insurance. Moving the centre of gravity from a system whereby central government provided money to a centralized NHS into a new organizational structure proved difficult. Allowing self-governing hospitals (trusts) and permitting general practitioners (GPs) to have more control over the budgets of their practice were seen as ways by which greater efficiency could enter the NHS. Many GPs took advantage of these new systems and became fund-holding practices, with contracts being set up with local hospitals in respect of patient care. The description of a quasi or 'almost' market was used to describe the idea that a purchaser/provider relationship could be applied to health care, with GPs purchasing on behalf of patients from a range of potential providers, such as hospitals. Fund-holding GPs were also able to run more services in their own practices, such as counselling.

What was less obvious at the start was the consequences for increases in inequality, rising costs in terms of setting up contracts, difficulties in monitoring payment and delivery systems and a suspicion that these reforms were undermining the NHS. The position of patients as consumers was not as simple as it sounded: older people in particular had needs that were not easily solved by shopping around for the cheapest or quickest operation or treatment. In the event, the concept of consumerism at that stage had to be considerably watered down because of professional and public resistance (Glennerster 2000). Nonetheless, many of the changes of *Working for Patients* (Department of Health 1989a) have remained, although in an altered form. These include trusts and the central role of primary care trusts (broader than GP fund-holding bodies) in commissioning health services from a range of possible providers.

Caring for People

Caring for People (Department of Health 1989b) was an associated White Paper that set out the basis for community care of adults. It was one of the first documents to use community care as a term to cover support for disabled people outside hospitals, acknowledging that many long-stay hospitals had closed or were winding down. Geriatric hospitals and psychogeriatric hospitals had been places where older people with long-term or chronic health care problems received care if they could no longer live in their own homes, or if they were considered too disabled for local-authority old people's homes. The hospital closure programmes were themselves a response to dismay about the poor quality of care in such settings (often revealed in scandals: see Stanley et al. 1999), anxieties about their rising costs and need for repair, and general scepticism that patients were in fact receiving decent health care. Classic reports, such as *Sans Everything* (Robb 1967), fuelled public and political concern by pointing to the deprivations of such long-stay wards.

Caring for People also confirmed new policy trends, in particular that of targeting, or awarding priority to those in greatest need. Its first policy objective stated: 'In future the Government will encourage the targeting of home-based services on those people whose need for them is greatest' (Department of Health 1989b: para 1.11). How this would be done was later explained:

- need would be assessed
- people with 'slight' needs would receive advice and information
- priority would be given to those whose needs were greatest.

The advantages of this were judged to make financial and political sense. The system of social care would be fairer as it would be clear why people were to receive help or not. The system would be affordable, in that care managers (typically social workers, but sometimes nurses employed by social services) would target resources and coordinate care, making the most of other helping networks (such as families), and the new system would be efficient in that instead of local authorities providing services, such as home helps, old people's homes and day care, this type of activity could be provided by commercial or voluntary organizations if they were cheaper and more flexible, in other words if they provided best value. The new system would not be led by services, but needs-led, and individual and flexible support would be available. Box 6.1 sets out six key aims for community care set out in *Caring for People*.

The Royal Commission on the Funding of Long-Term Care (1999) provides evidence of some of the consequences of this approach. Social care has been targeted, in that more very disabled people are receiving greater support at home. On the other hand, fewer people are receiving low-level support to help them with practical matters or social contact. Since the Act was implemented, there has been an overturn in the type of provider of social care and cuts in wages and other staff costs have produced some of the desired efficiencies. Most residential and home care is now provided by private or commercial organizations,

---

Box 6.1   Six policy aims of *Caring for People* (Department of Health 1989b, paras 1.11 and 1.12)

1. To promote the development of home care, day care and respite services to help people live at home as long as is possible and sensible
2. To give practical support for carers high priority
3. To provide a proper assessment of need and care management
4. To make maximum use of the independent sector of care
5. To clarify who is responsible for what and how they will be accountable
6. To set up different funding arrangements for public funding of social care

with a small amount provided by local authorities and some by voluntary or not-for-profit organizations. Many staff receive the minimum wage, care homes have borrowed money to expand and to improve facilities, and some chains of homes are taking over when smaller homes close or their owners retire. Examples of different scenarios are given in Case studies 6.1–6.3.

Case study 6.1

Mrs Dunne lives in a care home that was previously owned and run by a local authority in England. It is now under the ownership and management of an independent not-for-profit trust. The local authority has a contract with this trust for 25 places and pays a set fee for each place. Mrs Dunne pays part of the cost, her Attendance Allowance pays for some and the local authority makes up the remainder. If she were in Scotland, she would receive further financial assistance to pay for the personal care provided by the home but would still have to contribute towards her food and living costs. The home is part of a group of homes, and considerable sums have been borrowed to modernize the building. Now most residents do not have to share a bedroom. Staff receive training and over half have a basic qualification. Over the past few years the home has moved from having no inspections (when it was under the local authority), to inspection by the local authority's inspection unit, then by the National Care Standards Commission, and more recently (in 2004) by the Commission for Social Care Inspection.

Case study 6.2

Mrs Eden lives in a nearby care home that is owned and run by a former nurse. It is a small home with only seven residents, and the owner is wondering how long she will keep the business. She has had to make extensive changes to comply with new standards and very few of her staff are interested in training. All the residents have their fees paid by the local authority, which has assessed everyone financially and calculated the amounts they must pay, but there is little contact between their care managers and the home-owner. The local community nurses are regular visitors to the home to help with the treatment of leg ulcers and other conditions.

Case study 6.3

Mrs Fox goes to a care home every weekday while her daughter is at work; this home is run by a large commercial company and the arrangement is that Mrs Fox will receive a bath every week, and stay until after supper time when her daughter can collect her. The home provides respite care so Mrs Fox's daughter gets a break. Staff are offered training but their turnover is high as the area has little unemployment and there are many jobs available in the local supermarkets and health services. Mrs Fox has considerable savings and pays for her own care.

In England, the Commission for Social Care Inspection (in Scotland, the Scottish Commission for the Regulation of Care) registers and inspects care homes. Under the Care Standards Act 2000 in England, national minimum standards apply to care homes for older people (section 23(1)) and these standards insist that homes must focus on users (residents), must be fit for purpose, must meet assessed needs, must provide quality standards and employ a quality workforce (for Scotland, see the Regulation of Care (Scotland) Act 2001). As will be evident from Chapter 32 on elder abuse, this is not always easy to do.

These examples indicate the variety of care homes and the potential for high turnover of owners, staff and residents. Ninety per cent of all care homes are in the independent sector (private or voluntary organizations), providing care for 85% of people in care homes. Levels of disability in most care homes are high, with many residents having mental health problems such as dementia and depression. More discussion of nursing care in care homes can be found in Chapter 8.

Despite this diverse picture of care homes, they still accommodate a minority of older people, about 20% of those over 80 years old. Most older people live in their own homes and support for them continues to be provided by family, support that they arrange and pay for themselves, with some (15%) receiving help from social care services, arranged for and charged for by local authorities (on a means-tested basis). For local authorities, the White Paper *Modernising Social Services* (Department of Health 1998: p. 111) repeated the government's objectives:

- to promote independence, in people's own home wherever possible
- to enable people to live as healthy, safe, full and normal a life as possible

- to work with the NHS, other agencies and carers to avoid unnecessary hospital and inappropriate care home admission
- to enable carers to continue to care for as long as they and the disabled person wish
- to identify and assess needs, plan care, purchase care, review and monitor it for those who are eligible for local-authority support.

It will be evident that many of these aims fit neatly with the *National Service Framework for Older People* (NSFOP) (Department of Health 2001a), itself a policy document setting out a plan for 10 years of activity and a firm list of standards and priorities. Fitting services to needs is but a repetition of the aims of *Caring for People* and person-centred care has much in common with needs-led care, not least a certain vagueness and distance from the language of lay people. Rooting out age discrimination, standard 1 of the NSFOP, is new, however, and represents growing understanding across the 1990s that older people remained disadvantaged in the new systems of community care by limits on the resources available to their support and a lack of systems to respond in a timely and appropriate way to individual needs, as well as concerns that their care in the NHS was awarded lower priority than other patients'.

At the level of individuals and their families, evidence about the issues that remain can be illustrated by a report by the Audit Commission (2000) on the difficulties experienced by older people with mental health problems when using home care services to continue to live at home and to enable families to continue to care. These issues include:

- a complicated mixture of agencies (commercial, some voluntary-sector and some social services provision)
- a lack of continuity of home care workers (high turnover and problems with quality)
- continued restrictions of availability over the time of day and the days of the week
- a lack of experienced or specialist workers
- continued problems with coordination
- limited short-break care services at home (e.g. sitting services)
- a lack of useful information about service users to inform care staff.

This report concluded that residential care still dominates service provision and professional options. It has proved more difficult to switch funding from this sector to other more individually designed support that could 'wrap around' people, despite rising expectations and the known problems and inconsistencies

with existing services. This raises the issue about the difficulty of translating the policy aims of government for the NHS and health care into plans for practical implementation.

National Service Framework for Older People

This central government policy initiative aimed to improve service quality and service design. The NSFOP (Department of Health 2001a), like other national service frameworks developed by the Labour government since 1997, sets out key standards (Box 6.2) and targets, with details of how these are to be implemented in local contexts. The NSFOP centres on England, though a similar framework is likely to emerge in Wales. Philp et al. (2000: 99) have described the NSF as 'an innovative mechanism which is intended to produce a nationally uniform standard of care, to eliminate unacceptable practice, to reduce local variations and to drive up the quality of care'. At local level, local implementation teams, assisted by champions from the professions, but also from councils, trust non-executive boards and patients' fora, have been established to keep up momentum and to report back to central government whether milestones are being achieved. A 'tsar' (National Director for Services for Older People) continually encourages local improvement, the spreading of good practice and the building-up of evidence but also monitors localities. This role also argues the case for resources within central government, particularly around further investment from the Treasury.

All the NSF standards expose the interdependency between health and social care services, as well as the importance of other public services, and community networks. Intermediate care (standard 3), for example,

---

Box 6.2   The eight standards of the *National Service Framework for Older People*

1. To root out age discrimination
2. To develop person-centred care
3. To develop intermediate care services
4. To provide specialist hospital care
5. To improve stroke services
6. To develop falls services
7. To improve mental health services
8. To promote health and active life in old age

A further standard sets out targets for improving the management of medicines, such as reviews of medication at regular intervals.

can be misunderstood as a medical or nursing intervention but rehabilitation may involve a host of practitioners, family members and older people themselves. The new focus on early identification of dementia, set out as a policy goal under standard 7, will impact upon individuals and their families who may have to live with this diagnosis but find that services are underdeveloped for people who do not respond to medication or whose symptoms are not presenting major problems. As this chapter explores, the emphasis on challenging age discrimination (standard 1) is a continuing thread in current policy for an ageing society (Box 6.3).

Fair access to care

The changes in health and social care set in place by the NHS and Community Care Act 1990 had immediate but also long-term effects. Adjustments have been made to resolve particular difficulties and to respond to the pressures for structural change across organizations. For example, the pendulum has swung:

- From local authority to independent (private sector) provider residential care and home care
- From low-level support for large numbers of older people to more support for fewer older people (only 15% of older people receive support from social services: Association of Directors of Social Services/Local Government Association 2003)
- A variety of local thresholds for services and charging systems has emerged, resulting in differences between places.

The latter problem has been addressed by a new set of eligibility criteria for social care services. These were set up under the Fair Access to Care initiative established by the White Paper *Modernising Social Services* (Department of Health 1998). This new system is meant to be 'fair' in respect of removing local variations (the postcode lottery) and it is also designed to explain to the public the basis for social services' deci-

sions. In some respects these classifications of need sit comfortably with criteria used in mental health services for adults of working age under the Care Programme Approach. Both systems are designed to target resources on those in more need or with highest levels of risk. There are many convincing arguments for such a focus:

- Help goes to those in most need
- Evidence is that this enables people to stay at home
- Carers appear to find this approach helpful
- It acknowledges that resources are limited and hard decisions have to be made
- Most people manage well without high levels of services.

However, other views suggest that targeting leads to the following:

- a focus on crisis help
- limited ability to prevent problems getting worse
- pressure on families
- too great an emphasis on assessment and the threshold for services
- the removal of professional discretion
- a focus on risk that is negative and controlling.

Below are summaries of the four bands for service eligibility that determine service use at the time of writing. When reading this section we suggest that you may find it helpful to obtain a copy of the public information leaflet from your area giving greater details and the current position.

Priority: critical
Individuals who have a serious disability, impairment or condition that can result in a serious risk to safety or self or others and/or is preventing them from looking after themselves might count as being in critical need. Indicators might include:

- life is/will be threatened
- significant health problem(s)
- little/no choice or control
- serious abuse/neglect
- unable to carry out personal care/domestic routines
- no social support.

In this category, the phrase 'immediate risk' of harm or of danger is commonly quoted in the guidance.

Priority: substantial
Individuals who have a serious disability, impairment or condition that affects their ability to look after

---

Box 6.3 Some older people's feelings of age discrimination in health care

- Finding it difficult to obtain medical care
- Being denied medical treatment
- Receiving inferior care
- Being disbelieved when describing problems or being misdiagnosed (Harding 2004)

themselves and/or results in risk that can usually be predicted and managed might be assessed as having substantial need. Indicators include:

- being unable to carry out many daily routines or personal care without assistance
- being unable to make/act on many decisions without help
- having limited control over environment
- having some difficulties in mobility and restricted movements around home.

The difference between critical and substantial priority is therefore a matter of degree and urgency, and several practitioners may be asked to provide their professional opinion.

Priority: moderate

Indicators for moderate needs include:

- inability to carry out several personal care/domestic tasks
- several social support systems and relationships cannot be sustained.

Examples might include some memory problems, intermittent ill health, communication problems with limited risk to independence, potential need for equipment, some assistance needed with personal care and domestic routines.

This banding suggests the importance of assessment in negotiating the thorny areas of 'inability' and 'can do with assistance'. The single assessment process discussed in Chapter 28 will be a key document in providing evidence of these 'grey' areas as well as confirming elements that are more clear-cut.

Priority: low

Individuals with low levels of need may be referred to other organizations or to other parts of the local authority or health services. It is unlikely that they will receive a detailed assessment. For those who feel they are unfairly placed in this category, the existence of advocacy services may be helpful. However, for older people, advocacy services are variable geographically and in respect of their priorities (Dunning 1998). Individuals in this category may of course benefit from low-level services and prevention of ill health, disability or social stresses. Although of course the concept of prevention has proved attractive to policy-makers and professionals, it has been criticized for taking a narrow focus on avoiding expense and demand for services. Wistow et al. (2003) have argued that it needs to take on some of the root causes of inequalities and can play a major role in improving quality of life for older people. As the Audit Commission (2004) pointed out, inde-

pendence for older people has to be fostered by wider supports than simply those provided by health and social care services (Box 6.4).

Admission and discharge from hospital

For decades, problems have been identified in the hospital care of older people, many of them leading to policy rather than clinical reforms. Particular problems may arise when older people are discharged from hospital at night or over the weekend and have no one to support them, and delays in leaving hospital have resulted in the development of services such as intermediate care (see Chapter 8). Leaving hospital without sufficient or appropriate support may simply result in a person's rapid return to hospital, with needless distress or disability, or precipitate a move to a care home as a community care 'failure'. Naturally not all hospital discharges result in problems; over two-thirds of hospital beds are occupied by older people according to the *National Beds Inquiry* (Department of Health 2000a) and for many, their treatment and care are highly satisfactory. However, both admissions and discharges have been put under the spotlight in attempts to respond to the problems that may arise if they are inappropriate and of course the suffering that might be felt by other older people who need treatment in hospital and whose health is deteriorating while they wait. Chapters 6–8 discuss initiatives such as intermediate care that attempt both to reduce the need for hospital admission and to rehabilitate older people on their return home, hospital-at-home schemes where care, treatment or observation can be provided at home, and continuing care funding that enables people to receive free nursing care outside hospital settings.

In England, the Community Care (Delayed Discharges etc.) Act (2003) has taken a different emphasis by setting up a system of cross-charging or reimbursement for cases where a local authority is judged to have delayed a person's discharge by not setting up social care to enable a safe discharge home or to

---

Box 6.4   What helps older people remain independent (Audit Commission 2004)?

- Suitable housing in good repair
- Safe and friendly neighbourhoods
- Being able to get out and about
- Adequate money
- Timely and relevant information
- Health and healthy living

another setting. The effects of this system have yet to emerge but there are fears of its potential to antagonize relationships and to undermine joint working. The government has been influenced by a system in Sweden where older people now spend 30% less time in hospital since a similar system was introduced in 1992. From 2004, local authorities have been charged £100 per day (£120 in London and south-east England) if they fail to set up a care package for a person in hospital 3 days after the hospital has declared that the person is ready to be discharged (excluding people under the care of a consultant psychiatrist). Other money has been provided to encourage local authorities and the NHS to work together to explore why delays are happening and to invest in services that can reduce delayed discharges. Delayed discharge has been on the decline in any event and so it may be that the new system of reimbursement only continues this downward trend; for example, the number of delayed discharges fell from 5700 in July 2002 to 3220 in December 2003. Research on the effect of this policy on community services, on older people and carers, and on other parts of the care system is eagerly awaited.

Direct payments

Originally, older people were excluded from a system of support that had at its heart the empowerment of disabled people using services to support them at home. The Community Care (Direct Payments etc.) Act (1996) enabled those eligible to receive money from the local authority to live independently and to spend this money in ways that would promote this. Most commonly, disabled people employed people to act as their personal assistants, providing help with activities of daily living, but also with a range of other activities that disabled individuals saw as important, such as accompanying them on visits or to leisure activities. In 1999 direct payments were extended to older people (in response to pressure that their exclusion was flagrantly ageist) and from 2002 local authorities have had a duty to offer direct payments to eligible service users.

The potential of such a system was set out by Ann Macfarlane, an older service user, who argued that direct payments may result in an improved self-image and a more individualized and thus effective and acceptable system of support (Help the Aged 2002a). Other advantages are that service users have greater control and can employ whom they like, and get things done the way they like and when. Some people have found that a support service can be useful with the paperwork and it can be helpful to hear from a person who has already used such a scheme. Despite the challenges of such a system, and apparent lack of

enthusiasm for it among some professionals, such schemes may be a way of giving greater choice to older people and those who are experienced in their use often report on them extremely positively. Under the Family and Disabled Children Act (2000), carers are eligible for direct payments but there is little evidence as yet of how this is working.

FROM CARE TO CASE MANAGEMENT?

Some have argued that case management is the way forward to make sure that older people with high health needs receive a proactive service which can prevent continual readmission to hospitals, crises in care and support, and optimize rehabilitation and quality of life. The Wanless report (2002), for example, considered that 'properly targeted assessment and active care management' would promote independence, prevent deterioration and manage risk, and even potentially reduce service demand. The government's interest in US systems of enhanced case management, such as Evercare (promoted by the company United Healthcare), where nurses play a key role in home support for a small minority of older people with high levels of need, sometimes termed 'at risk', has been enhanced by positive early evaluations, such as that by the National Primary and Care Trust Development Programme (2004). Such a move would perhaps counter some nurses' feelings that they have lost control over their own activities and practice (Kesby 2002). This leads to the vexed question of terminology, such as the difference between case management and care management (for an overview of definitions, see Lee et al. 1998). It also brings in other concepts and definitions that can reveal barriers to understanding and good practice. A helpful framework that clarifies a raft of common terms and ideas arising from policy developments in the care of older people is provided by the Personal Social Services Research Unit (Kesby 2002: p. 360):

- 'Continuity is the ideal that all patients/users will need to some degree
- Integrated care occurs where health and social care inputs are organized and delivered in the same care package, consistently over time and working towards jointly agreed objectives and outcomes
- Coordinated care occurs where services are linked together to ensure continuity within a pathway of care with jointly agreed objectives and outcomes
- Parallel care occurs where two or more services are providing care to the same users or client

groups, but pursuing their own objectives and outcomes. It can be assumed here that the user does not require either integrated or coordinated care and not that there has been a failure to set up integrated or coordinated care so that parallel care is the accidental and inappropriate result.'

MODERNIZING CARE

Many of the changes in health and social care services for older people brought about by the Labour government can be seen as part of its promised modernizing agenda. Put simply, this is an approach to joining up services, or even integrating them, to resolve problems caused by service or professional boundaries and disputes, and to create services that can give choice and flexibility, by using markets, regulating competition and spreading the cost. *The NHS Plan* (Department of Health 2000b), *Modernising Social Services* (Department of Health 1998) and the *NSFOP* (Department of Health 2001a) are good examples of such renegotiations around boundaries and illustrate how systems such as intermediate care bridge (temporarily) traditional health and social care divides, often making use of the private sector to assist with problems in the NHS. In other parts of the NHS, the private finance initiative and the Local Improvement Finance Trust (LIFT) initiatives are ways in which capital for buildings in the main is being funnelled into the NHS, with the consequences of this being passed to future generations. The concordat with the private sector and the compact with the voluntary sector are agreements at a national level that will have an impact on traditional public services as much as widening the ability of people to make choices about provision of care and its location. So, will more voluntary groups employ nurses to provide nursing care? Will private companies offer screening and treatment, moving into more areas of the health service?

National perspectives

While this chapter has concentrated on England, it is important to note that older people's experiences are being affected by political devolution. Private or commercial care, for example, is far more common in England than in Scotland and Wales. Community Care Works (www.gla.ac.uk/Nuffield), with its database of good practice in community care, is exposing different priorities in Scotland, a country with less developed community care than other parts of the UK, but one which has chosen to provide 'free' personal care, at considerable government cost, following the recommendations of the Royal Commission on the Funding

of Long-Term Care (1999) (see Scottish Executive 2002). Scotland has also reformed its law in respect of mental capacity – Adults with Incapacity Act in Scotland (2000), which has particular importance for people with dementia, well in advance of England, where the Mental Capacity Bill was published in 2004. In Scotland the Adults with Incapacity in Scotland Act (2000) requires that anything done on behalf of adults with incapacity must benefit them (such as spending their money), must take account of the person's wishes (current or past) and those of family or appointed guardian, and must be as minimally restrictive as possible (for full details, see the legal statute and regulations).

In Wales, smaller and closer working relationships between health and social services, aided perhaps by coterminous boundaries, suggest that it will be able to focus on its predicted growth in older people (currently 17% of the population) and decline in numbers of younger people (Welsh Assembly Government 2003). Free bus passes for older people in Wales may reflect its Assembly's interest and commitment to rural communities' needs and the generally lower levels of income among older people in Wales. The Strategy for Older People in Wales (Box 6.5) is an early example of efforts to 'join up' policies for older people.

Partnerships

An emphasis on partnership was clearly set out in the modernization agenda of the White Paper *The New NHS: Modern and Dependable* (Department of Health 1997). New duties for the NHS in this respect replaced its focus on the internal market developed out of *Working for Patients*, although separation of planning

---

Box 6.5   The Strategy for Older People in Wales (Welsh Assembly Government 2003)

- Aims to tackle age discrimination, promote positive images of ageing and give older people a stronger voice
- Will develop older people's capacity to continue to work and make an active contribution to society
- Will plan integrated services to promote health and well-being
- Will promote independence through a safe, supportive and responsive service
- Will fund changes and improvements and planning across sectors

and provision and the continued priority of developing primary care remained. Partnership in the new NHS was to be a way of reducing bureaucracy, getting rid of secrecy and inefficiencies and replacing them by cooperation, unified budgets, long-term agreements and openness. In place of GP fund-holders and health authorities primary care groups (primary care trusts or PCTs) were set up, representative of all GP practices, with powers to commission secondary (hospital) care and strategic health authorities, to which PCTs would be accountable. For all NHS trusts, partnership was to become a duty, most notably with local-authority partners. A small number of areas have taken advantage of this encouragement of closer working to bring together NHS trusts with local authorities into care trusts under the Health and Social Care Act (2001). The ways in which they will be truly integrated and what will be the advantages and disadvantages for patients/service users are yet to be fully evaluated. In the meantime, partnership boards are bringing together work in some areas between PCTs and local authorities, starting in the main with learning disability and mental health services. This relationship has the advantages of pooling budgets and avoiding some duplication of services, but it has the drawback of requiring change and reorganization. The implications for nursing older people in primary care settings are further discussed in Chapter 7.

Partnerships may have equal relevance *inside* health services, and the White Paper *Primary Care: Delivering the Future* (Department of Health 1996) outlined the potential for practitioners within primary care to develop new roles and to promote team-working or closer working between professionals, for example collaboration between primary care services and optometrists and ophthalmologists to monitor the eye health of people with diabetes. The development of shared-care protocols around supporting people with dementia, for example, has similar potential to help reduce waiting times and multiple sources of advice.

Partnership can be seen as an important strand in the relationship between older people and nurses. The principle of nurses working in partnership with older people has been taken up by the Royal College of Nursing (2004) and it plans to form alliances with older people to be 'true partners' in care planning and delivery (p. 8) and to work with older people in developing professional training, in eliminating negative stereotypes and in developing positive images.

THE IMPORTANCE OF HOME

The National Health Service and Community Care Act (1990) led to a close examination of the borders between services, professionals and structures. Many of these had their origins in the welfare state established piecemeal after the Second World War. But older people have other needs and resources, and housing is a policy area where sporadic interest from health and social care means that the area is sometimes forgotten. Place however matters to older people, as do their neighbourhoods and communities, and above all, the home is important as a place where individuality, choice and relationships can be exercised. Since the Second World War major changes in housing have occurred. Older people have witnessed immense growth and then decline in local-authority (council) housing; they have been amongst the leaders in changing the majority of housing type in the UK to owner occupation. They have seen attention oscillate from residential care, to sheltered housing, to very sheltered housing or housing with care. Some have been excluded from housing improvements, remaining in poor facilities in the private rented sector or facing homelessness. As nurses will recognize, the home of an older person matters in any assessment and in the delivery of treatment, care and support.

Many older people live in housing that is unsuitable for a variety of reasons and this has an impact on their quality of life and their ability to cope with disability. The law acknowledges the vulnerability of older people and local authorities are obliged to accommodate older homeless people (over 55 years) in ways in which they do not have to for other adults (except those with young families, pregnant women or disabled individuals). Generally, at local level links with housing advice agencies in the voluntary sector are useful for nurses with concerns over the housing of an older person or groups of older people to consult. Studies of projects that work with older homeless people indicate that long-standing psychological and social problems often lie behind homelessness and that responses need to be intensive, personalized and sustained (Pannell et al. 2002). Older homeless people may experience general facilities for homeless people as violent or dangerous and as unable to respond to their needs. Residential care moreover is unlikely to be considered appropriate. Developing links between nurses and housing support staff may be a way of promoting support for this highly vulnerable group of older people. Homelessness and older people are discussed in terms of the policy and evidence base in Chapter 29.

Below, three new developments that illustrate the importance of linking housing and health care are briefly described to indicate the potential for thinking about accommodation and its links to health.

The smart home

Such names may be given to demonstration sites that provide individuals, carers and professionals with an idea of the ways in which technology can assist people with disabilities. In the situation of a person with dementia, for example, technology can switch off gas cookers, can monitor the level of bath water (to avoid flooding) and can provide prompts to check that door chains are on or medication is due. Even more simply, large-scale clocks and calendars are popular and reportedly effective (Chapman 2001). Such adaptations may be expensive but local systems may be able to meet such needs through the use of direct payments, carers' support monies or sums for aids to independent living that are joint-funded between health and social services partnerships.

The safe home

Many older people report feeling that crime and disorder in their communities make their lives difficult and sometimes miserable. Community safety initiatives, often linked to regeneration programmes, are locally led partnerships that aim to provide visible demonstrations that it is safe to go outside the house, and that harassment of older people, or anyone else, will not be tolerated. Research has found that particularly in inner-city areas, many older people do not feel safe and think that the community is dangerous and out of control. Evidence of neglect, such as rubbish and graffiti, is being targeted by joint initiatives, sometimes including older people and seeking their views, but sometimes not. Scharf et al.'s (2002) study of the impact of social exclusion on older people living in highly deprived urban areas (in parts of London, Liverpool and Manchester) found high levels of poverty, fear and experience of crime, concerns about the decline of areas to which they are often greatly attached, and risks of loneliness and isolation. Those working in such areas will no doubt recognize the multiple risks to health and well-being that such areas pose, as well as the resilience of many social networks.

The home with care

The view that there is nothing between living independently and life in residential care has been challenged by the development of 'extra care' or 'very sheltered housing'. Although this has been promulgated for some time, new developments have only recently occurred, making use of complex funding systems involving grant aid to housing associations in the voluntary sector, funds from individuals' benefits and rents, and assistance from local authorities. In such accommodation, tenants may have the ability to draw on support as their needs change, for example, receiving extra hours of home care on returning from hospital, or taking their meals in a restaurant if they are no longer able to cook or eat without support. Other possible changes may emerge with greater development of different types of housing with care, such as very sheltered housing, as alternatives to care homes. Here, older people have the status of tenants, not residents, and although many are likely to be very disabled, tenants may have symbolic as well as real power over important aspects of daily life, such as the key to their door. In addition they potentially have greater involvement in determining who will work in their homes, rather than whether they will be considered suitable for entry into a care home. For more information about sheltered housing, see Chapter 9.

'Staying put' at home

Nonetheless, older people mostly live in their own homes and in many areas of the UK owner occupation is the majority form of housing tenure. This has advantages, and older people often wish to grow older at home, in familiar neighbourhoods, in familiar surroundings. For many the advantage of owner occupation provides capital that can be passed to younger generations. The disadvantages are also evident, especially if disability occurs. Homes may be difficult or expensive to adapt, and maintenance and repairs may be hard to afford when income is low and capital diminishes. In response, private-sector schemes offer people the ability to raise money on the basis of the capital of their home, while other agencies at local level can assist older people to take advantage of loans and grants to repair their homes or to make adaptations (for example, housing improvement agencies or staying-put schemes). While in the past such schemes have concentrated on alterations and facilities to help people with physical disabilities, some schemes are now considering ways in which they can provide support to people with long-term conditions such as dementia. As with most voluntary-sector activity, there is much local variation and nurses may find that information on specific local resources is best obtained from groups such as the local Age Concern. This variation illustrates one of the dilemmas of local initiatives: they may be able to respond to local needs but great variations between areas may be confusing and inequalities will occur. A centrally controlled organization like the NHS, if it becomes fragmented with greater local decision-making powers, will exchange some inflexibility for greater diversity, but not necessarily equality.

SUPPORTING THE SUPPORTERS

Caring for People (Department of Health 1989b) outlined the central role of carers in providing support to older people. The full title of the *National Service Framework for Older People and their Carers* confirmed their importance. A separate policy document, the *National Carers Strategy* (Department of Health 1999), summed up government views that carers should be free to take up caring or not, that they themselves may require help and support at various stages, and that care is often provided at high cost to carers' own health and social and economic well-being (Box 6.6).

Older people (aged over 70) caring for their adult children with learning disabilities have also been identified as having particular needs and yet they may be invisible to services. The White Paper *Valuing People* (Department of Heath 2001b) noted their need for support and charged local partnership boards with finding these older carers, through surveys for example, offering them assistance with current and future needs, involving them in planning services and supporting others, assessing their needs and developing good practice. The little available knowledge about carers tends to be scattered across different agencies. While the emphasis of such work is on making plans for people with learning disabilities living with their parents, the needs of such parents may be for reassurance and support, such as short-break care. Equally, policy is clear that people with learning disabilities are often providing care to their ageing parents and they too may need assistance in this role.

Older carers are now more visible overall in policy terms. It is evident that spouses provide more hours of care than other carers, not surprisingly, since they are most likely to live with the disabled older person, and that between a third to a half of all unpaid care provided to older people is from other older people, in the main, partners or spouses (Milne et al. 2001). Support to older carers needs to be tailored to their circumstances, so, for example, respite care when a couple is separated, or home care that provides domestic assistance to the disabled person living alone.

Valuing People then has some overlap with the *NSFOP*, which was critical of the inappropriate placement of people with learning disabilities in care homes for older people, who are often many years their senior and with very different support needs. As is evident, both documents relate to the *National Carers Strategy*. This means that practitioners have to join up to several policy threads and communicate with other agencies and services working with other adult groups. The implications of an ageing population mean that knowledge, skills and resources will have to be shared with colleagues who have previously seen themselves as not working with older people. There is further discussion of carers in Chapter 33.

DIFFERENCE AND DIVERSITY

Policies for an ageing population need to reflect the growing diversity of older people; they are a group that is increasingly hard to 'lump together' as homogeneous. This section briefly outlines some of the strategies that are emerging to respond to this increasing divergence of identity, experiences, preferences, values and beliefs and ethnicity. Huge differences exist, moreover, between older people of different sexes, age cohorts and income brackets, as well as sexual identity, location and health status. For policymakers this diversity makes it increasingly difficult to establish comprehensive policies for older people or an ageing society.

Any discussion of race, ethnicity and culture encounters terminology that is subjective and evolving as well as confused, ambivalent, emotive and contested (Aspinall 2002). Aspinall's catalogue of collective terminology used in the UK reflects the variety of terms used within popular discussion, policy documents and surveys, and political arguments. Briefly summarized, the author suggests that certain descriptors are so imprecise as to lose meaning or utility, such as pan-ethnic terms like 'Asian', or 'mixed-race' and that binary terms such as black or white make white minorities invisible, such as older people from Irish or Polish backgrounds.

Much debate within health and social care services continues to refer to the difficulty of responding to small numbers of older people from minority ethnic groups (Daker-White et al 2002). Some parts of the UK are said to have particularly low levels of minority communities (Daker-White et al. 2002), prompting con-

---

Box 6.6   The four main themes of the Carers Strategy
1. Carers need better information
2. Carers need support from a number of sources
3. Carers need care themselves: in looking after their own health, and in making choices
4. Carers need to be able to continue in employment and to get back to work if they want

cern that practitioners in such areas lack the confidence and experience to be responsive. The assumption that minority groups 'look after their own' is now widely questioned. A larger policy question remains, however, about the advisability of developing separate services for ethnic-minority older people and whether these would inevitably be beneficial, responsive or practical. While we do not know the extent of such services in the UK, some directories give an idea of their scope (Help the Aged 2002b) and, while numbers are still small, in some areas proportions of older people from minority ethnic groups are now similar to white groups.

The 2001 census (White 2002) observed that there are now twice as many older people aged 65 years and over from black and minority ethnic communities (350 000) than there were in 1991 in the UK. Over half live in London (for details of the variety of voluntary-sector projects in London, see Help the Aged 2002b), and the rise mainly reflects the move into retirement age of migrants from Caribbean and South Asian communities. Like many other people from black and minority ethnic communities, they continue to experience multiple inequalities and discrimination. Strategic or policy responses need to respond to older people's experiences of racism, reported in the Growing Older study undertaken by Butt et al (2003), but progress seems limited since older people still form a minority among most black and minority ethnic communities, resources are scarce and targets are unclear. While some local authorities have begun to work in partnerships with local agencies such as PCTs to consider local services and planning (Manthorpe 2004a), much of such developments focuses on a narrow range of activities. Translation and interpreting services, for example, may be in short supply in many areas but many older people from black or minority groups do not need these, and not everyone may view specialist services positively. The Race Relations (Amendment) Act (2000) not only reminds public bodies of their duties to eliminate racial discrimination, but sets out a duty to promote equality of opportunity in service provision. Strategies for older people need to reflect this legal imperative but also need to be aware of local contexts, and overall global influences. In the UK this can extend to the support given to relatives abroad, the wishes of many older people to spend time overseas as well as in the UK, and the increases in mobility among young people who may find it convenient to seek short-term work in health and social care sectors, as well as informally to provide support for older people.

Cultural competence may be a way for nurses to acquire skills and confidence in working with older people but this runs the risk of seeing culture as something that makes groups different and glosses over individuals' relationship with their own culture (for example, people may be strong adherents to a religion or they may not). For older people, other characteristics such as socioeconomic position and the accumulations of age and experience are very important. The policy response to older people from black and minority ethnic groups is therefore increasingly likely to have to tackle disadvantage and to recognize that there are more differences between ethnic groups (intra) than between them (inter). The poverty of older people from Bangladeshi backgrounds, for example, may be far greater that that of other migrant groups even in similar areas and specific public health measures may be needed to assist this group as well as greater attention by nurses to ensuring that welfare benefits are maximized in such communities.

WORK IN LATER LIFE

Much emphasis in health and social care is on the minority of older people who are major users of services. It is easy to forget that many older people make significant contributions to society and the economy. A report from Age Concern (2004) outlined that:

- Older workers (over 50) contribute about a quarter of the total economic output
- Older workers are just as productive as anyone else, with only a few exceptions
- Three million people aged over 50 are carers
- A quarter of families rely on grandparents for child care.

From 2006, age discrimination in employment will be illegal in the UK. For the first time age discrimination in work and in training may be challenged with some 'teeth'. Barriers do not just exist in getting work but are experienced by older people in access to training and in being considered 'past it' when other opportunities arise. Research into the experiences of nurses over 50 (Watson et al. 2003) found that, even in a profession where it is widely acknowledged that there are significant shortages of staff, ageist attitudes exist and more attention is given to recruiting younger people than to retaining older nurses or providing ways for older nurses to return to their profession. The European Union Council Directive on Equal Treatment in Employment and Occupation of 2000 (Official Journal of the European Communities 2000) means that the UK will have to make a law prohibiting age discrimination in employment. A single equalities body, the proposed Commission for Equality and Human Rights, will be established to monitor equal opportunities across a range of areas such as sex, disability, sexual orientation and age (Office for the Deputy Prime Minister 2002).

One key issue raised by many older people and those coming up to retirement age is the mandatory retirement age, which means people can be forced to retire at a certain age. A variety of views are evident. On the one hand, organizations such as Age Concern (Lishman 2004) argue that mandatory retirement ages should be illegal and that people should not be made to retire on the grounds of age. Instead they should be judged on their ability to do the job. Others argue that the mandatory retirement age could perhaps be raised, say to 70. Or is it best to leave the system as it is, in recognition of the fact that many older people on low incomes and already in poor health will not benefit from delayed retirement and that the type of work they will have to undertake in later life will perhaps be menial and low-paid? Such an argument is cynical about the new-found interest in older workers, seeing this discovery as simply a way of making up for labour shortages and not really increasing older people's quality of life. One compromise that may emerge is the idea of phased or flexible retirement, though any such moves would require major changes in tax, pension and disability benefits. However, the nature of employment itself will also have to change so that older people with health or disability-related needs can stay in work, or retrain, and work contracts may have to be more flexible to allow for greater part-time working, for example. Nurses working in health promotion and those working with people with long-term conditions may play greater parts in the support of older people maintaining their roles in employment: such roles may require close collaboration with professionals allied to medicine who have experience in occupational settings.

This debate over age discrimination at work and the advantages and disadvantages of a fixed retirement age relate to ageism more generally (Box 6.7). A series of choices are available to policy-makers and older people will be able to influence what is chosen to a degree, as well as those 'baby boomers' (born in the 1950s and 1960s) who may be more articulate and who may have particular interests. Hornstein et al. (2001) have outlined the need for hard choices between legislation that is clear and prescriptive and that which is

flexible. The balance between individuals' rights will also have to be weighed against those of other age groups. There will need to be some agreement over the ways in which such equal-opportunities legislation is enforced, together with an emphasis on promoting good practice, monitoring or scrutinizing activities.

Work in later life is also unlikely to resolve the growing divides between older people who have adequate or substantial resources in later life and those who are poor. Those who have worked in low-paid jobs, and/or have been unemployed or made redundant, those who have had long-term health problems or who have provided care for family members are those who enter retirement on low incomes and often experience old age as a time of poverty, disadvantage and exclusion from social activities and community life. These 'harsh times' (Cook et al. 2004) mean that older people in poverty are at risk of unhealthy diets, isolation and anxiety. Low take-up of means-tested benefits may be one issue that nurses are able to address, by focusing on the personal factors that mean people fear charity and its stigma, or lack information or confidence, as well as process issues, such as difficulty in understanding technological systems or information (Cook et al. 2004). Numerous initiatives from the Pension Service, and proposals to set up a third-age service to help address such problems, abound. Locating advice and support in primary health settings is one established way of promoting benefit take-up, particularly if professionals such as nurses encourage referrals. Among disabled older people, Attendance Allowance (non-means-tested) is underclaimed, and among carers of working age, Carers Allowance is underclaimed, although this is restricted to certain carers and means-tested.

OLDER PEOPLE IN THE POLICY–MAKING PROCESS

One-third of the votes cast in the 2001 UK general election were by people aged over 50, making the 'grey vote' significant. In the UK there has not been much sign of a retired person's political party but in the European context there are 'grey' parties and 'grey/green' representatives. As Ginn (1993) noted, in the UK, most organizations of older people have had few numbers and have been middle-class in membership and their interests. The National Pensioners Convention, with its links to the trades union movement, has had a chequered influence on political decisions, but the future may see more coming together of groups representing interests of common concern to many older people. As older people are so different in their current and past circumstances, it might be

---

Box 6.7   What is age discrimination?

Age discrimination is the [potential] manifestation of ageism, which is a form of prejudice like racism or sexism. Age discrimination can be a barrier to older people seeking access to employment, goods and services, and an equal part of society (Help the Aged 2002c)

impossible for any one organization to represent them all. Nonetheless, political images of older people are changing. Previous stereotypes of them as the deserving poor (grateful for Christmas bonuses or concessions), largely homogeneous and thus easy to sway with simple measures or promises; as lacking influence because they cannot withdraw their labour; as always voting as they have done; as not seeing themselves as having age-related interests (such as the protection of pension funds and entitlements) are being undermined. Vincent (1999) has argued that these images are set to change and that politicians ignore older voters at their peril.

The notion of increasing citizen participation challenges health and social care services to find out the views of and consult older people. Several models are evident, such as working with local senior citizens' or older people's fora (Help the Aged 2002d), drawing on the experiences of patients and former patients (through the annual national surveys of patient experiences), examining concerns raised with the Patient Advice and Liaison Services and the independent complaints advocacy services, and using emerging local patients fora. Some older people themselves have taken on roles in research and development to bring their perspectives and ideas to the area of health care (Warren et al. 2003, Bright & Green 2004). While the Expert Patient Programme has been constructed to encourage people to help themselves (Audit Commission 2004) by breaking the cycle of symptoms, trying pain management techniques and improving their health generally, this too may have potential for people to tell service commissioners and providers how they can provide better support.

Choice is one key concept that is being applied in many ways. As an ideal, it is seen as integral to citizens' ambitions for themselves and their own care. In health policy the concept is being translated into choice over provider of health care and in respect of choice about care homes. The latter has been available for some time, in that people entering care homes are theoretically offered a range of care homes from which they can choose. In reality, such choice is often not available, care home vacancies are in short supply in many places and many care homes can be selective in the residents they accept (Rowland & Pollock 2004). The Choice initiative in the NHS is being rolled out into choice of hospital for treatment if a local service cannot meet a target date for the procedure (such as an operation). This initiative may be particularly relevant to older people on waiting lists for procedures, such as cataracts and hip or knee replacements, and the commitment in the 5-year plan for the NHS (Department of Health 2004) to a further reduction of waiting lists is

designed to provide accessible and responsive care to groups who have been highly critical of harmful delays. For some people the proximity of a local hospital may be worth the wait, while for others having the surgery as soon as possible may be more important. The NHS will no doubt be challenged by problems in organizing the movement of patient notes, the smooth transfer of aftercare details, and so on. Evidence about the preferences and desires for this type of choice among older people is not yet conclusive and is likely to reflect their diversity, and of course many report great difficulty with current achievement of continuity of care in the health service. While choice may be extended in this way, it is also being restricted, as older people will be expected to accept interim care home placements, even if they would prefer another solution (Rowland & Pollock 2004). It seems that choice is not as important as other policy goals. Further discussion of choice in relation to primary and social care can be found in Chapter 7.

Older people are not only involved as voters but also often play an important part in local democracy (Fig. 6.2). In the health service, where democratic structures are not developed, older people may be appointed to membership of trust boards and some have used their own and their family's experiences as ways of thinking about and influencing older people's provision. This example from a non-executive director of a PCT who was a champion for older people illustrates this potential:

> I am now over 60 and so have a vested interest. Older people can get a rough deal, particularly in hospital/homes. I would like to be able to assist in securing better things for older people. Modern society does not seem to value the knowledge, experience and skills of older folk (cited in Manthorpe 2004b: p. 11).

The inspection process of health and social care services has made some moves to include older people as

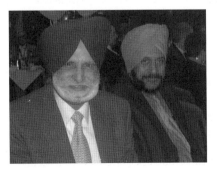

Fig. 6.2 Community participation: local councillors.

lay observers. Other means of having some influence and control include innovative ways of seeking the views of individual older people; for example, Allen (2001) has described how staff working in service development can involve people with dementia through communication and consultation. Given the right kind of support, Allen found that individual staff could find out more about residents' feelings, for example, than by asking some people what they felt about living in the home; some residents might respond better or be more expansive if asked what they thought someone else might feel on moving into the care home. Individual relationships were reported to be important, time and trust were necessary and items such as photos could be useful prompts. Such work suggests that there is more room for older people, even if very disabled, to set out their feelings and for these to be considered and reflected on.

Outside party politics, older people are involved in a variety of local community activities. These include sports, arts, environmental, and other civic or community groups. They are active in faith groups. They are involved in volunteering. New debates over social capital have provided a way of looking at such contributions to society. Riseborough & Jenkins (2004: p. 22), for example, declared that 'older people represent a large part of the productive capacity within communities' within both urban and rural communities but they found that this was not consistently acknowledged in regeneration strategies.

It is unusual to end a chapter on older people and policy with observations that older people are contributors to society rather than problems and that their citizenship may be a key theme in policy debates, rather than their status as patients or service users. In exercising more control over their own health and social care, quality of life and participation, older people will challenge practitioners and managers, as well as politicians, by their differences and demands (Fig. 6.3). Understanding the development of policy can be helpful in appreciating that policy is as much a matter of implementation as it is the declaration of new systems and structures.

Recommended reading

Adams T, Manthorpe J (eds) 2003 Dementia care. London, Arnold.
This edited book considers services in health and social care for people with dementia and their families in a policy and practice context. Questions are asked about why some areas have been comparatively neglected, such as care of people who are dying and the bodily care of people with dementia. Other areas provide examples of innovative services and new ideas in practice and how these link to the context of service systems.

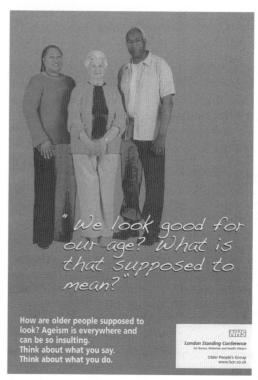

Fig. 6.3 "We look good for our age? What is that supposed to mean?" (Reproduced with permission from a series of images produced by the London Standing Conference for Nursing, Health Visiting and Midwifery to counter ageism in nursing).

Glasby J, Littlechild R 2004 The health and social care divide: the experiences of older people. Bristol, Policy Press.
This book is a clear overview of services at the frontline and their moves to become more integrated. The historical perspective sets out the pressures and multiple demands on social care and the authors are dubious about the way in which some initiatives will actually improve relationships between health and social care.

Royal Commission on the funding of long-term care 1999 With respect to old age: long-term care rights and responsibilities. London, Stationery Office.
This report and the accompanying two volumes of research provide a state-of-the-art overview of policy and the evidence considered by the Royal Commission. The differences between the majority and minority reports encapsulate debates about means-testing and the most effective way of distributing resources.

References

Adults with Incapacity (Scotland) Act 2000 Edinburgh, HMSO
Age Concern Greater London 2004 The economy and older people. Age Concern, London

Allen K 2001 Communication and consultation. Policy Press, Bristol

Aspinall PJ 2002 Collective terminology to describe the minority ethnic population. Sociology 36: 803–816

Association of Directors of Social Services/Local Government Association 2003 Inverting the triangle of care. Local Government Association, London

Audit Commission 2000 Forget me not. Audit Commission, London

Audit Commission 2004 Supporting frail older people: independence and well being 3. Audit Commission, London

Bright L, Green B 2004 Older people as research colleagues. Quality in Ageing 7: 14–16

Butt J, Moriarty J, Brockmann M, Hoong Sin C, Fisher M 2003 Quality of life and social support among older people from different ethnic groups. ESRC Growing Older Programme, University of Sheffield, Sheffield

Care Standards Act 2000 HMSO, London

Chapman A 2001 There's no place like a smart home. Journal of Dementia Care 9: 28–31

Community Care (Direct Payments) Act 1996 HMSO, London

Community Care (Delayed Discharges etc.) Act 2003 HMSO, London

Cook G, Reed J, Childs S, Hall A 2004 Does money matter? Older people's views of their monetary resources. York Publishing Services, York

Daker-White G, Beattie A, Means R, Gilliard J 2002 Serving the needs of marginalised groups in dementia care: younger people and minority ethnic groups. University of the West of England, Bristol

Department of Health 1989a Working for patients. HMSO, London

Department of Health 1989b Caring for people: community care in the next decade and beyond. Cmnd 849. HMSO, London

Department of Health 1996 Primary care: developing the future, Cm 3512. Stationery Office, London

Department of Health 1997 The new NHS: modern and dependable. Department of Health, London

Department of Health 1998 Modernising social services. Department of Health, London

Department of Health 1999 National carers strategy. Department of Health, London

Department of Health 2000a Shaping the future NHS long term planning for hospitals and related services (national beds inquiry). Department of Health, London

Department of Health 2000b The NHS plan: a plan for investment, a plan for reform. CM4818–1. Department of Health, London

Department of Health 2001a National service framework for older people. Department of Health, London

Department of Health 2001b Valuing people. Department of Health, London

Department of Health 2004 The NHS improvement plan. HMSO, London

Dunning A 1998 Advocacy, empowerment and older people. In: Phillips J, Bernard M (eds) The social policy of old age. Centre for Policy on Ageing, London, pp 200–222

Ginn J 1993 Grey power: age-based organizations' responses to structured inequalities. Critical Social Policy 38: 23–47

Glennerster H 2000 British social policy since 1945, 2nd edn. Blackwell, Oxford

Harding T 2004 Everyday age discrimination: what older people say. Help the Aged, London

Health and Social Care Act 2001 HMSO, London

Help the Aged 2002a Direct payments, direct control: enabling older people to manage their own care. Help the Aged, London

Help the Aged 2002b Working with minority ethnic older people in London. Help the Aged, London

Help the Aged 2002c Age discrimination in public policy. Help the Aged, London

Help the Aged 2002d Senior citizens' forums: a voice for older people. Help the Aged, London

Hornstein Z, Encel S, Gunderson M, Neumark D 2001 Outlawing age discrimination. Policy Press, Bristol

Kesby S 2002 Nursing care and collaborative practice. Journal of Clinical Nursing 11: 357–366

Lee D, Mackenzie A, Dudley-Brown S, Chin T 1998 Case management: a review of definitions and practices. Journal of Advanced Nursing 27: 933–939

Lishman G 2004 Letter. Financial Times 25 June

Manthorpe J 2004a Strategies for black and minority older people. Better Government for Older People, London

Manthorpe J 2004b Older people's champions: a survey of 208 champions. Better Government for Older People, London

Mental Capacity Bill 2004 HMSO, London

Milne A, Hatzidimitriadou E, Chryssanthopoulou C, Owen T 2001 Caring in later life: reviewing the role of older carers. Help the Aged, London

National Health Service and Community Care Act 1990 HMSO, London

National Primary and Care Trust Development Programme 2004 Implementing the evercare programme: interim report. www.natpact.nhs.uk (accessed 20 August 2004)

Office for the Deputy Prime Minister 2002 Equality and diversity: making it happen. Office for the Deputy Prime Minister, London

Official Journal of the European Communities 2000 Council directive 2000 78/EC 27 November L.303/16-L.303/22. European Union, Brussels

Pannell J, Means R, Morbey H 2002 Surviving at the margins: older homeless people and the organizations that support them. Help the Aged, London

Philp I, Ashe A, Lothian K 2000 Designing and implementing a national service framework. In: Warnes A, Warren L, Nolan M (eds) Care services for later life. Jessica Kingsley, London, pp 89–102

Race Relations (Amendment) Act 2000 HMSO, London

Regulation of Care (Scotland) Act 2001 HMSO, Edinburgh

Riseborough M, Jenkins C 2004 Now you see me ... now you don't: how are older citizens being included in regeneration? Age Concern England, London

Robb B 1967 Sans everything. Nelson, Edinburgh

Rowland D, Pollock A 2004 Choice and representativeness for older people in the 'patient centred' NHS. British Medical Journal 328: 4–5

Royal College of Nursing 2004 Caring in partnership: older people and nursing staff working towards the future. Royal College of Nursing, London

Royal Commission on the funding of long-term care 1999 with respect to old age (chair Stewart Sutherland). HMSO, London

Scharf T, Phillipson C, Smith A, Kingston P 2002 Growing older in socially deprived areas: social exclusion in later life. Help the Aged, London

Scottish Executive 2002 Adding life to years: report of the expert group on healthcare of older people. Scottish Executive, Edinburgh

Stanley N, Manthorpe J, Penhale B (eds) 1999 Institutional abuse: perspectives across the life course. Routledge, London

Vincent J 1999 Politics, power and old age. Open University Press, Buckingham

Wanless D 2002 Securing our future health: taking a long-term view. HM Treasury, London

Warren L, Cook J, Clarke N et al. 2003 Working with older women in research: some methods-based issues. Quality in Ageing 4: 24–31

Watson R, Manthorpe J, Andrews J 2003 Nurses over 50: options, decisions and outcomes. Policy Press, Bristol

Welsh Assembly Government 2003 The strategy for older people in Wales. Welsh Assembly Government, Cardiff

White A 2002 Social focus on ethnic minorities. Office for National Statistics, London

Wistow G, Waddington E, Godfrey M 2003 Living well in later life: from prevention to promotion. Nuffield Institute for Health, Leeds

Chapter 7

Health and social care for older people in the community

Fiona M. Ross and Christina R. Victor

INTRODUCTION

Staying at home, being with family and friends in the familiar and the known is important for most of us, because home represents something of ourselves and as people grow older preserving independence becomes more important. Older people mostly live at home supported by family, friends and local community networks. Primary health and community care services are available to provide support for older people to manage recovery from acute illness, promote rehabilitation and function in chronic disease and enhance independence. Policies promoting primary health and community care are not new: they have been around for nearly four decades, expounding the need to take into account the preferences and choices of older people themselves, although the extent to which this has been realized is questionable.

Radical policy and organizational changes in primary health and community care (since the late 1980s) are reflected in the shifting balance of care from hospital to community, the decentralization of services, the patient and public involvement agenda and partnership working between health and social care. This chapter discusses the implications of these changes for nursing care of older people, with a particular emphasis on primary health care and the interface with secondary and social care. Current issues for nursing care of older people in the community will be discussed and the consequences of policy implementation will be examined, such as use of services, length of hospital stay, readmission, the emergence of new services and innovation in the development and delivery of care. In addressing these issues we pose some questions: how far are real choices available for older people? In what ways do agencies and professionals work together?

DEFINITIONS

Primary care is the term used to describe, variously and somewhat confusingly, first contact services, processes, levels of care and even strategies for organizing the health system (Peckham & Exworthy 2003). The World Health Organization (1978) defines primary health care somewhat idealistically as essential care based on practical, scientifically sound and acceptable methods and technology, made universally available to individuals and families in the community through full participation and at affordable cost. These objectives, although laudable, perhaps lose some of their significance because of the attempt to be universal and thus relevant across all health systems. In contrast to this there are some who define primary care more narrowly in terms of general *medical* care, albeit based in a wider population health context (Starfield 1998).

A more inclusive and broad-ranging definition of primary health care describes it as the first point of contact for people seeking advice, support and treatment for health problems. This definition encapsulates the responsibilities of primary health care to encourage people to participate in the planning and organization and management of their own health care at home, school, work and in the general practice surgery. It includes surveillance, health promotion, acute and continuing care and covers a wide range of specialist and generalist services with the nature of care ranging from the episodic to the long-term, incorporating social as well as family support. This broad view of primary care has been described by Gordon & Plampling (1996) as a community-based health service linked to a wide social network, embracing user-led initiatives and a range of services, and going beyond the confines of the general practitioner (GP) service. In this chapter we adopt this approach to primary health and community care as it seeks to be comprehensive, multidisciplinary and inclusive of older people and their carers.

THE ORGANIZATION AND UTILIZATION OF PRIMARY CARE SERVICES BY OLDER PEOPLE

The development of health and social care policy has to be seen within the wider context of demographic changes, new patterns of disease, inequalities in health, rising public expectations and technological innovation, discussed further in Chapter 6. In recent years there have been a plethora of policy documents and initiatives to develop primary care. This chapter refers to some of the recent policy documents (Department of Health 1996a, 1996b, 2000, Audit Commission 2004) and discusses the changes in general practice that have consequences for the organization of services for older people. The year 1996 was important because for the first time policy documents reflected the view that primary care was not synonymous with general practice. The 1996 White Papers on primary care emphasized the need to develop appropriate and sensitive services to meet needs, as well as promoting teamwork, partnerships in care, professional knowledge and organizational flexibility.

Organizational reforms in primary care in the UK since 1997 reflect political devolution, geographical variation and the respective health policies of England, Scotland, Wales and Northern Ireland. While the four countries in the UK are developing primary care policies with common themes, in England general primary care organizations or primary care trusts (PCTs) were set up in 2002 to commission services to address population needs in partnership arrangements with social care. The specific goals of PCTs are to:

- improve the health of the local population
- develop primary care
- secure health services for their population.

A major recent change has been the introduction of a new General Medical Services (GMS) contract for general practice (Department of Health 2003). For the first time it has changed the basis of funding from per-capita and fee-for-service payments to a system based on needs and quality outcomes. The GMS contract recognizes the importance of:

- changing to needs-based funding of general practice
- allowing practices to manage their own workload and enabling primary care professionals to exercise more flexibility and choice
- including a quality framework, which is evidence-based and widely supported by doctors and others
- retaining the strength of organizing services for registered patients, enabling coordination and continuity of care
- enabling expansion of primary medical services capacity
- guaranteed increased investment (Audit Commission 2004).

Although GPs retain their independent contractor status (a cherished feature of the 1948 National Health Service Act), which sets them apart from their hospital colleagues and fellow members of the primary care team, this contract does provide some levers for change in the quality of care. Encapsulated within *The NHS Plan* (Department of Health 2000), *The National*

Service Framework (NSF) for Older People (Department of Health 2001a) and the agenda of National Health Service (NHS) improvement (Department of Health 2004a), there are key areas of policy that focus on service improvement, which will have an impact on services for older people:

- improving the patient experience (person-centred services)
- management of long-term conditions
- public health and reducing inequalities
- access to treatment and support
- investment in service development and workforce capacity.

Primary health care is perhaps one of the key services for achieving the objective of government policy for the care of older people: the maintenance of older people in their own homes for as long as possible. Several of the standards defined in the NSF for older people, such as the development of services to prevent falls and falls-related injuries, are beginning to challenge the traditional organization of the workforce in primary care (the NSF standards are outlined in Chapter 6). District nurses, health visitors and practice nurses often work together in an integrated nursing team providing specialist skills and supporting the wider primary care team (Ross et al. 2000, Furne et al. 2001). The primary care team has a key role in the surveillance and monitoring of older people and in determining unmet needs for care. GPs are important because of their 'gatekeeper' function, whereby they can control the entry of older people into the care system by referrals to appropriate agencies. They are also important in making referrals to hospital- and community-based services. The attitudes of the primary care team, to how they evaluate and prioritize the health needs of older people, are, therefore, an important aspect of the access older people have to services.

What use do older people make of the primary care team? This is slightly difficult to answer as data are not routinely collected about consultations between older people and all members of the constantly evolving primary care team. However, national data are available for three principal members of the team: the GP, the practice nurse and the community nurse.

Consultations with general practitioners

It is estimated that approximately 75% of those aged 65+ will visit their family doctor each year (Victor 2004). Data from the 2002–2003 General Household Survey (GHS) (Rickards et al. 2004) report that 21% of males aged 75+ and 27% of females in this age group consulted their GP in the 14 days before interview.

Annually people in this age group consult their GP on average eight times per year. Taking a slightly shorter time frame, 53% of those aged 65+ consulted their GP at the surgery and 6% had a home visit in the 3 months before interview (Table 7.1). One important dimension of the utilization of the family doctor's service by older people is the location of the consultation. For those aged 65–69, 3% had a home visit, as did 25% of those aged 85+ years (Table 7.1). At all ages, except those aged between 70 and 74 years, women are more likely to have a home consultation than their male contemporaries. Older people are much more likely than any other group within the population to see their GP at home. Forward projection of current trends implies a potential increase in demand for home consultations.

How have consultation rates with GPs changed over time? The most complete data about time trends in GP consultations are available from the GHS. This provides data on the percentage of people consulting a GP in the previous 14 days for the period 1972 to 2002–2003 and shows little evidence of increase for males aged 75+ (increasing from 19% to 21%) but a slight increase for women of the same age (from 20% to 27%; Victor 2005). These data show only limited evidence of increased demand for GP services from older people over the past three decades. However, if future generations of elders show the same patterns of service use then GP services will experience increased demands for their services simply because of the demographic changes noted in Chapter 3.

Community nursing services

The primary care nursing workforce represents 17% of the nurses, midwives and health visitors employed in the NHS in England. In 2002 there were 49 651 whole-time-equivalent nurses and health visitors working in primary care (Department of Health 2002, Drennan et al. 2004). Although the practice nurse and registered nurse workforce has grown throughout the 1990s (Atkin et al. 1994), the focus of the practice nurse's work lies with treatments and health promotion work in general practice, comprising clinics for immunizations, well woman, diabetes, respiratory disease, coronary heart disease, smoking cessation and wound care (Audit Commission 2004). In contrast, there has been little change overall in the numbers of district nurses and health visitors and it is from these groups, which have a significantly higher age profile, that approximately half the current staff will retire within the next 10 years (Drennan et al. 2004). This has implications for the future service development for older people, because with the exception of some extended practice nurse roles in the management of chronic disease such as diabetes and chronic obstructive airways disease, the majority of care interventions and supportive rehabilitation for older people in the home is carried out by district nursing and intermediate care teams (Goodman et al. 2003). The nature and type of nursing care for older people in primary care is outlined in Box 7.1.

Box 7.1   The nature and type of nursing care for older people in primary care

- Available 24 h/day 365 days a year
- Works in partnership and supportive of individuals through major life events
- Establishes close relationships with clients and carers
- Has a knowledge of the local environment and social context
- Provides care for sick people in their own homes
- Ambulatory and domiciliary health promotion and the management of chronic disease
- Provides a link between agencies and professionals
- Identifies and manages risk of vulnerable clients

District nursing and, to a lesser degree, health-visiting services are important for older people as part of the framework of primary health care services. Overall about half (47%) of visits undertaken by district nurses are to those aged 65+, compared with 10% of health visitor contacts (Victor 1991). Over 80% of the district nursing budget is accounted for by work with those aged 65+.

Data provided by the 1994 GHS do not distinguish between district nurses and health visitors. In 2001 6% of those aged 65+ were in receipt of district nursing/health-visiting services (Table 7.1). So, although older people form the main client group for the community nursing service and account for the majority of the budget, the service actually only covers a small minority of the older population. This remains true even though utilization rates increase significantly with age. For example, 2% of those aged 65–69 are in receipt of district nursing/health visitor care, compared with about 19% of those aged 85+.

Services are provided to only a minority, even when considering those in greatest need. Of those who need help with walking outdoors, 23% receive district nursing visits (Fig. 7.1), as do 16% of those who need help getting out of bed, 17% of those who need help showering and 15% of those who need help dressing (Bennett et al. 1996). Of those who live alone and need help getting outdoors, getting up steps or with bathing, less than one-fifth receive visits from the district nurse (11%, 15% and 12% respectively; Victor 1997).

Table 7.1   Consultation with primary care team: UK 2001

	Age (years)											
	65–69		70–74		75–79		80–84		85+		65+	
	M	F	M	F	M	F	M	F	M	F	M	F
Last 3 months												
General practitioner at surgery	49	48	52	55	57	55	60	56	56	42	53	52
General practitioner at home	2	4	4	6	9	9	11	14	18	28	6	10
Nurse at surgery	25	28	27	30	31	33	34	28	31	19	29	29
Last month												
District nurse/ health visitor	1	2	4	3	4	6	7	11	17	21	4	7
Local authority home help	1	1	2	2	2	3	5	8	6	23	3	5
Private home help	5	6	7	6	9	11	17	18	19	32	9	12
Meals on wheels	1	0	0	0	0	2	5	3	5	8	1	2

Values are percentages.
Source: Walker et al. (2002).

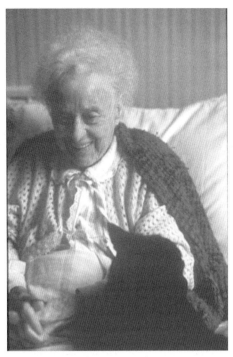

Fig. 7.1 A centenarian (with her cats), who is cared for by district nurses.

Older people are also extensive users of the practice nursing service (Table 7.1). In a 3-month reference period, 29% of those aged 65+ have seen a practice nurse: this is a substantial increase on the 17% reported a decade earlier. Indeed, the importance of practice nurses is illustrated by the fact that consultations with practice nurses are routinely included within the main section of the GHS. In the 14 days before interview, 11% of men aged 75+ and 12% of women had seen a practice nurse: respectively these groups have three and four consultations per year with the practice nurse. Practice nurses appear to be especially heavily involved with those in the 75–79-year age range. Not surprisingly, the demands for more health promotion in the GP contract have resulted in a rapid increase of practice nurses employed in general practice. This has aroused interest in the role and characteristics of practice nurses and their training needs in relation to health promotion, home visiting and counselling (Atkin et al. 1994, Ross et al. 1994) and their role in relation to the assessment of older people (Victor 1991). NHS Direct, the national nurse-led telephone helpline established in the late 1990s, was intended to widen access to confidential professional health care advice, 24 h a day, to support self management at home. However, early evaluation has found that it is popular with young families, but uptake by older people is low (Munro et al. 2000).

INVOLVEMENT OF OLDER PEOPLE

One of the many challenges facing primary care organizations is how to offer more choice for older people and to address and realize the opportunities for patients, carers and communities to shape local health care services (Alborz et al. 2002). Since the 1990s rapid policy development has steered the NHS towards recognizing and responding to the needs of its 'customers' (Department of Health 2001b, 2004b, Crawford et al. 2002). This is a complex area with a rapidly growing literature (Cooper et al. 2002). Selected examples of policy implementation are outlined here to illustrate the different levels at which service user and carer involvement may be achieved in health and social care.

Patient and public involvement framework

In England a new system of patient and public involvement has recently been established. The Community Health Councils were abolished in 2003 and in their place patient and public fora and patient advice and liaison services (PALS) were set up in every NHS trust. The work of these new bodies is in their infancy and we are yet to see how PALS and patient fora as well as the independent complaints and advocacy services (ICAS) and local-authority overview and scrutiny of health decision-making make a difference to the way in which the consultation process operates and the extent to which there are genuine opportunities for older people to contribute and provide feedback to their local NHS in order to improve services overall. The policy developments outlined above are currently supported by a new Commission for Patient and Public Involvement in Health (Fig. 7.2).

Achieving choice through care pathways

Care pathways describe the journey, across acute and community services, that most patients can expect to follow whilst receiving treatment for a particular illness or health need. Although many older people experience disjointed care planning between services and poor communication between sectors, the aim of care pathways is that they will provide a framework for involving patients, their carers and the public in decisions about the care they receive. Independent-sector treatment centres are being established in England to provide selected services, for example hip replacement and cataract surgery. The assumption is

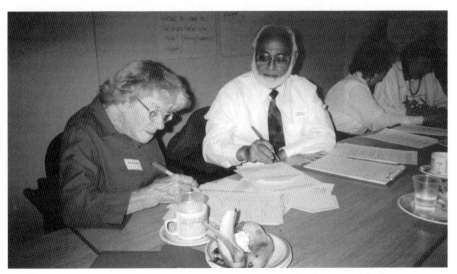

Fig. 7.2 Participation in falls prevention research: meeting of a consumer panel. (Reproduced with permission of Muriel Wood and Saleem Ullah Sheikh MBE.)

that users will be empowered by providing alternative treatment options and the choice between waiting to go to a local hospital or go to an independent provider (possibly outside the local area). This raises several questions about how to take account of individual need, diversity of expectation and appropriate methods of eliciting views and experiences of older people about what having choices means for them.

Current issues in patient and public involvement in primary care

Biggs (1993) points out the inherent inequalities that exist between users and professionals which limit the possibilities of true choice and participation. He identifies these as different interests, priorities and cultural concerns, as well as effective exclusion from the negotiating arena of commissioning. This then raises the question of the extent to which current policy is internally consistent, particularly in the discussion of choice and health care. In primary and social care the issue of involvement is complex, because of the diversity of generalist and specialist services, the uncertainty and long-term nature of many care pathways and the inconsistent use of terms for 'service user', 'patient', 'public', 'consumer' and 'lay person' (Warren 1999). A recent study of six primary care organizations in London showed that effective strategies to involve patients and local communities rarely follow any single model (Gillam et al. 2002). This perhaps reflects the importance of taking into account variation in context and priorities of different groups of older people, par-

ticularly minority ethnic groups. For nurses, as for other professionals, there are practical issues such as money, time and training for professionals to be able to support service user involvement (Smith et al. 2005) to develop meaningful partnerships rather than just expounding it as an 'article of faith' (Pattison 2001).

NURSING OLDER PEOPLE IN THE COMMUNITY

The role and allocation of tasks between community nurses are changing rapidly as new teams and working practices are designed to meet the targets of the new GP contract and the modernization agenda. Although historically the district nurse has had a key role in providing nursing care and support of older people in their own homes, and will continue to provide specialist expertise (Goodman et al. 2003), over the next few years in PCTs there will also be opportunities for newly qualified nurses, experienced registered nurses, specialist nurses and community matrons to contribute to an expanding mix of skills within the nursing team. It is likely that there will be a mixed economy of employers and the independent sector will provide care services in tandem with primary care services. Thus the focus of the next section is to draw attention to some of the current issues and challenges for the provision of good-quality care for older people in the community.

The expectations that patients have for appropriate and timely interventions, friendly services that involve people in decision-making, clear information that communicates with other parts of the system

(Ross et al. 2004) provide a framework for research priorities that can be translated into priorities for the delivery and organization of nursing care. Dieppe et al. (2002) discuss the importance of improving the patient's experience of the clinical encounter, which includes the following four elements:

1. values and attitudes of both professionals and patients (including expectations)
2. time spent in the encounter, balancing listening and talking
3. trust between professionals and patients
4. context in which the clinical encounter takes place, that may influence its nature (Dieppe et al. 2002: p. 280).

Case study 7.1 illustrates the importance of respect, thinking about the needs of the whole person and the nursing role operating within a wider community network.

Nurses working in the community need to be able to adapt to meet the needs of a wide spectrum of individuals, ethnic groups and social contexts. The home circumstances may pose constraints and limitations on the implementation of nursing care. Adaptation and improvisation in the home depend on the patient's condition, the environment and the available equipment (Fig. 7.3). Circumstances may be such that, for example, in the final stage of a terminal disease a decision not to carry out an insensitive and probably unnecessary dressing using a meticulous antiseptic technique would be wise because it would cause anxiety to the patient and additional stress for the family. Improvisation and the imaginative use of available equipment and resources are important – for example,

---

Case study 7.1

Freda is looking forward to her 90th birthday. She lives in a peaceful and comfortable corner terraced house with a garden full of carefully tended flowers. She is surrounded by books, photos and the treasures of a lifetime. She is physically frail, there is not an ounce of fat on her and she is unsteady on her feet. She is seriously deaf and her eyesight is poor. She potters about the house with a walking frame. Getting out of a chair is an effort, but Freda cooks and manages her personal business affairs with determination. She has no living relatives, but a close friend who lives 200 miles away. The friend cares and worries, but is not easily available. The community around her visit, bring shopping and organize the washing. Freda has worked out a careful paced daily routine to minimize exertion, practical difficulties and accidents, accepting uncomplainingly that many tasks are painful to do and very slow.

Freda is exceptionally determined to maintain her independence and avoid going into any sort of retirement or nursing home at almost all costs. Apart from the district nurse, who comes to dress a slow-healing leg wound over several months and has become quite a friend, she rigorously fends off community services and medical people. Although local friends and the community services are of help, Freda is an exceptionally private person and it is important for her sense of independence and dignity to be in control.

Freda had looked after a mentally frail neighbour and dear friend, who had become increasingly dependent on her and drifted into her house to be looked after on a near-permanent basis. This came to an abrupt end when Freda collapsed one day and was admitted to hospital as an emergency. The friend was taken into care, which was a loss to Freda and a source of guilt. She had tried to protect her neighbour from too much outside 'interference' and was horrified to think that she might have let her down in this respect. She felt that her hospitalization was the cause of her friend's going into care. Feelings of guilt and blame got in the way of the friendship, which was never the same again.

Freda carried on, a fragile leaf that could be knocked down easily. The district nurse visited regularly to 'keep an eye' on her and together with a supportive GP helped Freda.

This story is about the struggle for independence, friendship, a strong community and mutual caring that continues until let down by physical breakdown. It is about the community services supporting, unobtrusively perhaps, with visits that aim to spot the early signs of failing to cope and to anticipate the need to put in extra help at the right time – neither too early, which may be rejected as 'fussing', nor too late, when a crisis is full-blown. Above all, it is about the reality of community care; friendship and reciprocity that must be recognized and integrated into the services that form only a part of the jigsaw.

Freda hoped to die in her own home but had a fall in her sitting room and lay there for 9 h before being taken off by ambulance for her last week in hospital, where she felt bewildered, uncomfortable and defeated. There was little sense of helping her to die with peace and dignity, but a constant invasion of medical attention, gadgetry, drugs and noise. The manner of speech used to her, although meant kindly, was more appropriate for a backward child. It was all that she had dreaded!

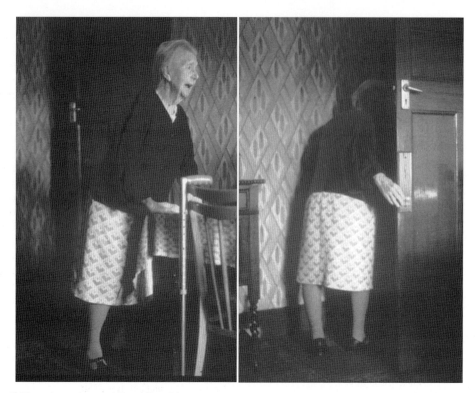

Fig. 7.3 (a, b) Managing at home with mobility aids.

using a wire coat hanger to make a catheter stand. Suggesting or making too many changes at once, particularly in a new, complex and personal situation, may be stressful for the patient. It may also be interpreted as interference or a painful reminder of the loss of independence and deterioration in health, or it may threaten the balance of a relationship where the carer's role is sustained by looking after a dependent member of the family. Case study 7.2 illustrates the difficulties faced by older people and their families in making decisions about appropriate placements for care, especially when under pressure from external constraints.

Chronic disease management

There are 17.5 million adults living with chronic disease and most of these are people aged 75 years and over, who receive support and treatment from health and social care (Department of Health 2004c). Community nursing has a long-established, if low profile in chronic disease management; for example, district nurses teach patients and their carers to manage insulin administration and recommend aids and adaptations and coping strategies to patients with rheumatoid arthritis as well as the practice nurse's role in managing coronary heart disease risk, providing advice to patients about exercise, stress reduction and diet.

The NHS improvement agenda sets out policies for developing chronic disease management using nurse-led case management systems. This has been informed by the experience of health maintenance organizations in the USA, e.g. Kaiser Permanente (North California) and Group Health (Washington state), which have implemented successful models of nurse-led disease management. These have had an impact on reducing costs, admissions to hospital and long-term care. Evercare is an example of a US health care programme which is being piloted in the UK to improve care (assessment, management and home care treatment) for vulnerable older people with chronic disease. Although there are a number of models operating with different populations, the approach has been summarized by Dixon et al. (2004) as:

- mobilizing community resources to meet the needs of patients
- cultural change in health care organizations from reactive to proactive models of care

Case study 7.2

Mary had fallen in her garden and fractured her femur. In hospital it was found that she had advanced breast cancer with bony metastases. Her femur was pinned and plated and she returned to her flat with a package of care from both the district nursing service and home care. But things did not work out. Mary relied on home carers to get her up and put her to bed. She was put to bed at 6 p.m. most nights and got up at around 10 a.m. She could not manage the toilet at night and wet the bed. She was given incontinence pads and at night lay on a wet pad. She told her sister that she wished she were dead. Her only comfort was her cat.

Her sister Ethel, who was 87, decided to move in with her. She managed to get Mary on the commode at night, helped her during the day and did the shopping, but this quickly became too much for her and she developed angina.

Mary was admitted to hospital as an emergency, where she was told she had only a short time to live. She decided that she wanted to spend her last days at home. She was discharged home with the combined support of the MacMillan team, district nurses and her GP. Management of pain, personal care, hygiene, nutrition and hydration were provided at visits twice a day. Taking time for a cup of tea and listening on the door step to Ethel was a central part of the supportive role of all professional carers.

- promoting self-management and the expert patient model
- designing delivery systems that encompass assessment, case management, interprofessional and collaborative processes as well as review
- evidence-based clinical pathways
- clinical information systems.

Case management and its role in chronic disease management are complex and requires clear definition in terms of the organizational context in which it operates, relationships and working systems between professional groups and the role of the service user and carer in assessment and self-care. There is the potential for conceptual confusion with *care* management policies, which were embedded in the community care reforms of the early 1990s and located within local-authority social services, which we discuss later in this chapter.

There is some growing evidence to suggest that nurse-led chronic disease management is effective, although more work needs to be done; for example, a meta-analysis of trials of intensive nurse home visiting support programmes of a general population of older people demonstrates a relationship with reductions in admissions to long-term care, but no significant reduction in hospital admission or improvement in functional status (Elkan et al. 2001). Other approaches that could be facilitated by nurses is the expert patient model and the findings from Lorig et al. (1987, Lorig 2000) that lay leaders can positively develop patient self-management skills in arthritis, specifically in relation to coping, functional ability and the use of hospital services. Lorig's work has emerged from a programme of research with people with both rheumatoid and osteoarthritis. The self-care and development of coping mechanisms have been developed to address outcomes of these conditions (Lorig et al. 1993), which are not, however, necessarily transferable across a range of other complex conditions with different disease trajectories, treatment interventions and health and social outcomes. Further there is growing evidence from the USA that team-based interventions in chronic disease are associated with better patient outcomes – the involvement of nurses in assessment, treatment, self-management support and follow-up have been linked to improved professional adherence to guidelines, patient satisfaction, clinical and health status and use of health services (Wagner 2000).

Health promotion

The ideas of chronic disease management should be linked to Caplan's (1961) classic classification of health promotion and prevention as primary, secondary and tertiary. Community nurses are involved to a varying degree in all three. The following discussion will focus on the nurse's role in the prevention and management of ill health and chronic disease in older people.

Primary prevention entails intervention to prevent the incidence of disease, for example by immunization. An old person with an abrasion from a fall may alert the nurse, at an encounter either in the home or health centre, to organize tetanus toxoid administration through the GP and to initiate a falls risk assessment.

Secondary prevention involves the early detection of illness using tested screening techniques, for instance, measuring blood pressure or testing the urine for glucose. This may take place routinely at a first visit or if a clinical problem is suspected. Community nurses increasingly participate in multidisciplinary screening programmes. In addition to undertaking some technical procedures, such as venepuncture for haemoglobin levels, sight testing and electrocardiographs, they may be involved in promoting health advice on diet, exercise and leisure activities. The obligation on GPs to screen all people over 75 years, introduced in 1990, has now been quietly removed in the new contract and replaced with the targeted approach to chronic disease management discussed earlier.

Tertiary prevention is defined as the measures taken to alleviate an existing condition, prevent complications and modulate the effects of illness. The community nurse uses this preventive approach in many ways:

- implementing a rehabilitation programme for the aftercare of a stroke patient at home, helping with adjustment to disability and preventing complications
- identifying the risk of falls in partnership with the older person and teaching patient safety, such as measures to prevent accidents and falls caused by unsuitable footwear, torn floor coverings and unlit passages
- teaching older people about environmental problems that may cause ill health, such as the risks of hypothermia, the problems of muscle wastage caused by immobility and constipation owing to a low-roughage diet and insufficient exercise
- teaching carers how to prevent pressure sores, and demonstrating the principles of safe lifting to ensure comfort to the carer and prevent damage to the patient's delicate skin tissues.

Health promotion, such as a falls exercise class, may take place in the home at an individual level with the patient or carer, or in a group in a health centre, community centre, day centre or residential home. It may be provided by an occupational therapist, physiotherapist or lay leader. The community nurse is in a unique position to promote health as an accepted visitor in the home. She may become a well-known and trusted figure over time and therefore will be in a position to influence and change existing behaviour. However, for some black and ethnic-minority (BEM) groups there may be perceived barriers to the uptake of health promotion or exercise. For example, in the aftermath of terrorist attacks it may be that older people from BEM fear for their safety in open spaces, or it may be that some individuals lack knowledge about community facilities, feel uncomfortable if they are the only black person in a mixed-sex group or may be concerned about the lack of privacy in many changing areas.

Gould (1999) suggests some practical strategies to encourage participation of BEM in exercise and activity:

- Value their experiences and encourage them to help as well as participate
- Include physical activity in a wider health promotion package
- Acknowledge and build on existing attitudes and health beliefs such as (for Muslims) praying being a form of exercise and that sweating is regarded by many older Asians as beneficial to health
- Use existing community groups such as church lunch clubs and BEM community leaders
- Promote a range of activities which people will enjoy, including traditional dances, yoga and brisk walking
- Use BEM media and networks to advertise activities.

Further information on health promotion can be found in Chapter 30 (see Fig. 7.4).

SHIFTING THE BALANCE OF CARE

The resourcing and development of primary care cannot be discussed in isolation from acute hospital care. Shifting the balance of care between hospital and com-

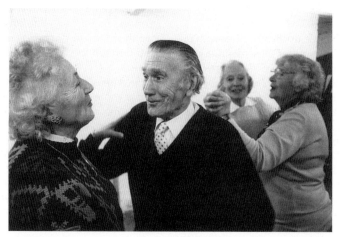

Fig. 7.4   Dancing. (Reproduced with permission of Age Concern England.)

munity has been a policy seesaw for 30 years. Harrison (1993) has identified a number of forces working to change the pattern of service provision in such a way as to reduce the role of the acute hospital:

- Users are seeking greater involvement in service provision, in some areas making their preferences known for patterns of care which reduce hospital use
- Chronic conditions are becoming more important in terms of caseload than acute illness, so that more care has to be provided on a continuing basis
- Technological change is making it possible to shift care from the hospital (which hitherto was the only provider) by, for example, making it possible for patients to monitor their own condition and for GPs to carry out tests in surgeries and health centres.

These pressures lead to questions about how primary and secondary care should relate to each other and what the division of functions should be as PCTs develop their commissioning role. This debate is being carried out at all levels, particularly in relation to commissioning, and has resulted in changing patterns of service delivery such as intermediate care, integrated care pathways and the development of specialist community nursing services. The increase in day care for surgical techniques such as hernia repair, but also for invasive investigations such as cardiac catheterization, inevitably has consequences for the nature of work being done in the community by the primary health care team.

Discharge from hospital back to the community

The increased utilization of health services by older people has been achieved by increased bed occupancy, significant reductions in the length of time people spend as inpatients and by the growth of day-case treatment (Harrison 1993). However, the average length of stay in hospital for older people is usually longer than that for a young person with a similar medical condition. This reflects the multiple pathology which is often a feature of older people presenting with specific medical conditions. Intensive inpatient treatment regimens may result in 'sicker' patients being discharged back to the community, with the resultant increased strain on community care services. For many patients, irrespective of age, admission to an acute hospital constitutes only one phase of their health career. Many patients need continuing care, follow-up or rehabilitation. A constant theme in research concerned with the hospital care of older people is the discharge from hospital back to the community. Discharge is, perhaps, the

wrong term to use. This implies a severing of relationships, when many will need continuing care; perhaps the term 'transfer' is a more accurate representation of the concept involved.

Research has consistently demonstrated that the transfer of older patients from hospital to the community can be problematic, with older people sent home without adequate arrangements having been made for their continuing medical and community care (see Marks 1994 for a comprehensive review). In spite of the policy focus on discharge arrangements, there are still problems in the information provided by hospitals to primary care staff on the discharge of older patients (Tierney et al. 1994, Closs 1997) and the referral to practitioners such as district nurses (Audit Commission 1999). However, there are few examples of interventions that have resulted in improved discharge outcomes (Parkes & Shepherd 2003). Discharge policies are discussed further in Chapter 8.

Delayed discharge and the 'inappropriate' use of acute beds

Alongside the debates about the most effective methods of discharge planning are concerns about the 'blocking' of acute beds by older people who no longer need the facilities provided by an acute setting but who, for other reasons, cannot be discharged. Such patients are sometimes given the pejorative label 'bed blockers', which implies that it is the older person's fault that he or she cannot be discharged. This is highly inaccurate as it is almost always the case that people cannot be discharged because they are waiting to be assessed or because the appropriate services are not supplied for them. This problem is not inconsiderable. The House of Commons Health Committee (2002) estimated that, in 2002–2003 in the second quarter there were 7000 people 'delayed' in hospital, accounting for 6% of all acute beds at an annual cost of £720m per annum. The majority of these delayed-transfer patients are older people, as this survey indicated that 12% of those aged 75+ in hospital were 'inappropriately' located. Preventing delayed discharge from hospital is now a key NHS priority, as indicated by the introduction of the Community Care (delayed discharges) Act (House of Commons 2002), which charges social services departments for hospital beds 'blocked' by those awaiting social care provision.

The issue of bed-blocking is not new. As early as 1948 the British Medical Association commented: 'unless sufficient residential homes are provided for old people ... hospital beds will inevitably become "blocked" and the whole service will break down' (Means & Smith 1985: p. 175). Hence, almost since the creation of the postwar welfare state, there has been a concern that the hospital–social care interface could, very easily for older people, become a bottleneck which would bring down the whole system if not managed effectively. Consequently a number of studies have sought to define methods of empirically identifying 'inappropriate' patients, describing their characteristics and the reasons why such patients could not be discharged, with the presumed aim of improving services so that such problems could be avoided. Such studies have varied in the methodologies employed to undertake this type of research and the populations studied. Consequently this makes comparison across studies problematic and makes it difficult to assess whether the introduction of community care has made things worse or better (Glasby 2003).

Those older patients identified as being inappropriately placed within an acute unit almost always have a very real need for care. Indeed, their health characteristics highlight the types of problems that often occupy the interface between acute and community care. Typically, patients identified as 'inappropriate' present problems such as incontinence, immobility, problems with self-care and dementia which are likely to present considerable nursing care demands but which do not necessarily require continued inpatient care of the type provided by an acute unit (Victor 1990).

This serves to highlight, yet again, one of the most persistent problems to have dogged the British welfare state since its creation: the boundary between health and social care. The architects of the original welfare state and the recent community and health service changes made an assumption that it is easy to distinguish between these two different types of need and therefore formulated services accordingly. For older people the distinction is not clear-cut and, as they represent the largest single group using these welfare services, problems of demarcation and definition abound (Means & Smith 1985). Means & Smith (1985: p. 183) quote Marjorie Warren, an eminent pioneer geriatrician, in 1951 as stating: 'the elderly frequently fall between the two bodies – the individual not being sick enough to justify admission to hospital and yet too disabled for a vacancy in a [residential] home'. In a similar vein they quote a member of parliament as identifying older people falling in the 'no man's land' between the NHS and local authority because 'they are not sick enough for hospital yet need more care and attention than can be given to them in their own homes' (Means & Smith 1985: p. 183). We discuss the interface between primary health and social care later in this chapter.

Services that support the transition between hospital and community care have been developed in many places. They provide important multidisciplinary care, medical and nursing interventions to prevent admission or to provide support over the recovery period following discharge.

The day hospital

Day hospitals provide a bridge between hospital and the community. They are often located within the geriatric department of a general hospital. The aim is to provide a therapeutic environment during office hours, supported by a multidisciplinary team, including occupational therapy, physiotherapy, speech therapy and chiropody. The aims of referral to a day hospital include continuity of care on discharge, rehabilitation, treatment to maintain the progress of an intensive hospital programme, the provision of medical and nursing procedures that cannot be carried out at home and social care. There are excellent models of day hospitals that provide a focus for hospital and community staff to implement local clinical plans flowing from the *NSF for Older People* (Department of Health 2001a). Arranging transport at convenient times for collection and return home is one of the challenges for day-hospital provision.

Intermediate care

Intermediate care is a broad term that includes nurse-led care, the community hospital model and hospital-at-home schemes. The concept of the community or general practice hospital is not new but is becoming fashionable again as a way of providing intermediate care between the 'high tech' hospital and the home. The aim of the community hospital is to provide a service for rehabilitation, respite care, terminal care and for patients with acute medical problems not requiring intensive treatment. It is estimated that in the UK there are approximately 10 000 beds in 30 hospitals accessed by roughly 15% of GPs (Steiner 1997). Usually community hospitals are nursing-led, with medical support provided primarily by GPs with access to specialist care. With earlier discharges of older people from acute hospitals, some community hospitals provide 'convalescence' and the careful planning necessary for a good discharge. These developments are discussed in Chapter 9.

It is nearly 30 years since the Peterborough hospital-at-home scheme was introduced in 1978. Despite the claims made for the importance of primary care, it is ironic that this type of programme has been so slow to develop, and there are even now remarkably few schemes established in mainstream care (Haggard & Bosma 1996). This is probably due to a number of factors: resistance to supporting the transfer of funds and power from the secondary to primary care sectors, and the lack of purchasing incentives to develop the service.

Broadly there are two organizational models for hospital-at-home. One is the creation of a specialized team, hospital-based, often linked to a surgical specialty; the other model is based in a primary care organization, staffed by community teams with specialist input. Most hospital-at-home schemes have been set up to deal with the needs of complex acute conditions, for example renal failure, acquired immune deficiency syndrome (AIDS) and paediatric cases, and for the acute crises predominantly affecting older people: cerebrovascular accidents, congestive cardiac failure, early discharge of hip replacement patients 3 days after operation, respite care and terminal care. The range of possibilities is expanding as outreach develops.

The benefits of a hospital-at-home service to patients and carers are, in theory at least, a choice of service specific to their own lifestyle, allowing more choices and autonomy in care and recovery. The underlying rationale is to reduce long periods spent in hospital and bed-blocking, to prevent admission and to improve cost-effectiveness. Some evaluation of individual schemes has been carried out (Gould & Iliffe 1995, Sims et al. 1997). Patients and carers report positive views of this type of care, but it is not clear if such schemes save money overall. Lack of standardized evaluation tools makes comparisons across schemes difficult. In the absence of more rigorous methods of investigation of cost–benefit it is not likely that there will be widespread service development.

CARE IN THE COMMUNITY: LOCAL-AUTHORITY SERVICES

Community care has existed as a broad political goal for 30 years; however, until the late 1980s there was no concerted political or professional will to implement the stated objectives. The change in direction was influenced by the pressure that came from the reports of the government's watchdog Audit Commission (1986) and political advisor on health (Griffiths 1988). In brief, these reports argued that community care lacked a coherent policy framework, and the delivery of services was fragmented, which endorsed a prevailing culture that 'community care is a poor relation; everybody's distant relative but nobody's baby' (Griffiths 1988: p. iv). Following this, local authorities changed their role to be enablers and organizers of care as well as providing direct services which include home care (home help) services, day care, social work,

meals services, occupational therapy and home aids/adaptations. In 2004 the government launched a review of adult services in social care, which may change the shape of local-authority social services again. A brief description of each service will be considered in turn.

Social work services

Social workers are employed by, and normally based in, the social services department of the local authority. Their role as care manager is as a broker or purchaser of services. In the past social workers have been criticized for not giving priority to work with older people (Stevenson 1996); however, Lewis & Glennerster (1996) argue that this is changing now as a result of the community care reforms. A number of different services may be offered through social services in packages of care: these include special advice for the blind, respite care, laundry for the incontinent and welfare benefit advice. Over the past 15 years there have been a number of organizational models for social workers in primary care, for example co-location or attachment to a GP or based in a health centre, which has been shown to facilitate communication and more appropriate referrals and a faster response rate (Cumella 1995, Ross & Tissier 1997). However, there is only limited evidence that formal arrangements for collaboration have improved outcomes for older people (Kharicha et al. 2004).

Domiciliary occupational therapists

Domiciliary occupational therapists are based in social work departments. They assess older people's potential for independence and needs for aids for daily living and may function as care managers as well. The Chronically Sick and Disabled Person's Act 1970 obliges local authorities to make necessary adaptations to the home, such as installing ramps, handrails, hoists and stair-lifts. Other services provided under this act include help in obtaining radios and televisions, the allocation of telephones and enabling older people to have holidays.

Home care services

Traditionally the home help service (now called home care) provided regular help with domestic and household tasks, including shopping, collecting prescriptions, cleaning and the preparation of meals. Increasingly the provision of domiciliary services is organized through the local authority contracting with the independent sector to provide a mixed economy of personal care and domestic services. In order to support dependent people at home and avoid admission to residential care, the intensity of home care provision has increased: average hours per household more than doubled since 1992, from 3.2 to 7.6 in 2001 (Knapp et al. 2001), although its coverage is reduced. Domiciliary services are now subject to regulation from the National Care Standards Commission. In an interesting study that looked at the motivations of domiciliary care providers in England, Kendall and colleagues (2003) highlighted the importance of the personal relationship and trust involved in establishing effective contracts between providers and local-authority purchasers.

Although local-authority provision is still the largest in this sector, there has been an increase from the private sector, which has been in line with government policy. However, there is some evidence that most users of the home care service appear to receive a minimal level of service (Victor 1997). Table 7.1 shows that local-authority services are only received by a minority of older people, and overall there is little gender difference in levels of receipt of these services. It is interesting to note the use of private home helps, which may reflect an unmet need for help with home care which is not being accepted by the local authority (perhaps because of their targeting and eligibility criteria; Victor 1997).

Provision of home meals

Home meal provision is, as it sounds, a way of providing a hot, two-course meal for people who are otherwise unable or unlikely to cook for themselves. Meals on wheels has been a feature of most local-authority provision, with a significant contribution from the voluntary sector; originally the provider was the Women's Royal Voluntary Service (WRVS). The voluntary sector remains a key provider, serving 31% of meals provided and 36% of recipients (Department of Health 1995). Like the home help service, there is variable provision of meals on wheels service across local authorities. In some areas older people are restricted to meals once a week, and in others clients may receive meals 7 days a week, according to need. Most receive three meals or fewer a week, although this may be an overestimate, given current cuts in spending. Special diabetic or low-roughage diets can be arranged on request. The meals service also often fulfils a surveillance function. If an old person fails to answer the door or

suddenly deteriorates, then the appropriate agency can be informed.

Social day care

Day care is provided by the local authority or a voluntary organization. Day centres offer a hot lunch, entertainment, diversionary activities, adult education, bathing, a chiropody service and facilities for self-help or health education groups. The majority of older people do not attend day centres and there has been much speculation as to why this is the case. It may be that low uptake may be related to the difficulties of arranging transport. It is for the house-bound, isolated older person that day-centre provision is important and it is for precisely this group that places are restricted, because of the shortage and unpredictability of transport. Many old people are frustrated by long circuitous journeys, the uncertainty of picking-up times and the uncomfortable seating. This illustrates the frequent absence of collaboration among services when planning new programmes. Although day care is often offered as a means of providing some respite for carers, it may be that the older person may become more confused by being taken to a day centre and therefore need more support from the carer on return (Fig. 7.5).

HEALTH AND SOCIAL CARE: BOUNDARIES AND PARTNERSHIP WORKING

Health and social care have historically operated side by side, separated by an arbitrary boundary. The health system is still mostly free at the point of use, whereas social care is subject to rationing and is means-tested. It is interesting that there are a number of services for older people that have shifted from the health to social services, for example aids and equipment and the 'social bath'. For some older people this may in practice mean that the service is no longer available, because of the need to meet eligibility criteria.

Care management

Assessment and care management in social care were introduced as the cornerstone of the community care reforms. It was driven by value for money considerations, the need to provide integrated and 'seamless' care, and the intent to reflect user and carer concerns in the assessment and delivery of care. Many conceptual and operational difficulties about care management in social care exist, not only for individual professional groups, but also between disciplines and participating agencies. Some of these difficulties

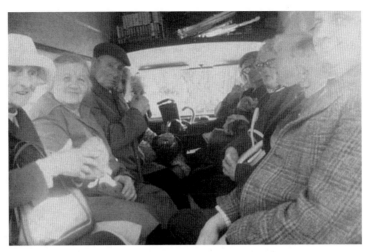

Fig. 7.5   Community transport to the day centre.

include confusion over the definition of case/care management, the role in relation to assessment, definitions of eligibility, referral, decision-making, resource allocation, interprofessional and interagency work, confidentiality and the interpretation of the role in relation to various client groups and settings in community and primary care.

The term 'care management' originated from case management. During consultation on the policy guidance for community care, 'case' was regarded as demeaning to the individual and misleading, in that it is the care and not the person that is being managed. Both terms are referred to in the literature on this subject, and, to make matters even more confusing, case management is the term currently used in the implementation of policy on chronic disease discussed earlier. The concept originated in the USA. The only extensively evaluated scheme in the UK at the time of the community care changes was the Kent community care scheme (Challis & Davies 1986), which had been replicated in Gateshead (Challis et al. 1990) and Darlington (Challis et al. 1989). Care management as a concept is subject to widely differing interpretations but these schemes were targeted at frail older people to reduce admission to institutional care. In Kent and Gateshead the case manager was a social worker performing the core tasks of care management: case-finding, screening, assessment, care-planning, monitoring, review and holding control of the resources. The findings indicated increased morale and quality of care. The Darlington project extended the concept, with the care manager being a member of a multidisciplinary team, the nursing input intrinsic to the process, and

using multipurpose health care assistants. The findings again showed an improvement in morale and a reduction in the incidence of depression in older people.

The *care manager* has been defined as any practitioner who undertakes all, or most of, the core tasks of care management, who may carry budgetary responsibility, but is not involved in any direct service provision. It is intended that the care manager should act as a broker for services across the statutory and independent sectors. It is not expected that the care manager should be involved in direct service delivery, or carry management responsibility. This therefore separates the process of procuring services from delivery, in order to remove any possibility of conflict of interest. At the present time there are many interpretations of the above, and it is not surprising if there is some confusion over the nature of the role, and how it relates to the notion of the assessor, key worker and coordinator and now the case management role developing for community matrons in the management of chronic disease.

Care management emphasizes routine approaches to assessment and agency-centred targeting of need (mainly for social care) based on eligibility criteria, which paradoxically may have increased the risk of resources being used inappropriately (Richards 2000, Parry-Jones & Soulsby 2001). It has been criticized for overlooking the central needs of users and carers (Hardy & Wistow 1999), and not contributing to the drive for 'seamless care' through improved interprofessional and interagency collaboration (Glendinning & Rummery 2003).

Partnership working

A key thrust of the public sector modernization agenda is the policy intention to work towards seamless and coordinated care. Clearly, in a system of care delivery with a diversity of providers, ranging from health and social care to the independent and voluntary sectors, it is vital to pay attention to mechanisms of partnerships and joint working. There has been much emphasis in the policy guidance about collaboration, and specifically between the local authority, PCTs and the independent sector. Since central government was careful not to be prescriptive about how policy should be implemented at local level, it is not surprising that there has been some activity in developing collaborative projects around care management and assessment, for example developing agreed criteria for the assessment of health and social need, core assessment tools and hospital discharge arrangements. Although there has been some progress in developing relationships between social service departments and PCTs, GPs have been slow to participate in community care planning (Leedham & Wistow 1992, Henwood 1995).

The government has put in place new powers to support partnership working between health and social care agencies (the Health Act Flexibilities 1999). This removed legal and financial constraints, and now enables the NHS and local authorities to provide and commission more integrated services. These include pooled budgets, lead roles for commissioning and integrated provision. Poxton's study (1996) for the King's Fund reports on some positive initiatives for older people in five sites and identifies some key features that need to be in place for effective joint commissioning (Box 7.2).

Some examples are given below of partnership in practice:

- Nurses working in a care manager and purchaser role with social services
- Joint development of single assessment process

Box 7.2   Key issues in joint commissioning (derived from Poxton 1996)

Achieving a better quality of life: sharing aims, objectives and underpinning values
- Being clear about what really makes a difference to older people's lives
- Involving older people in decisions
- Ensuring a better understanding by older people of the health and social care systems

Obtaining better services: developing an agreed programme of service change and development
- Effectiveness: meeting needs clearly identified through user involvement
- Efficiency: avoiding duplication of effort, reducing costs associated with 'non-client contact' (e.g. overheads, travelling time)
- Accessibility: simplifying the ways in which people make use of the health and social care systems
- Innovative ways of meeting needs: beyond the traditional public-sector way of thinking and responding
- Equity: adopting a system-wide approach to the allocation of resources

Jointness: being clear about the extent to which working together will influence decision-making
- 'Joint' or 'collaborative' commissioning: being clear about whether decisions are to be taken together
- Resource implications: being clear about the source and use of budgets
- Impacting upon services: coordination or integration – the importance of having a clear view of the aims

Commissioning: understanding what is involved and the extent of local application
- Involves decision-making ranging from needs assessment to determining appropriate responses, on an individual, locality or service basis (or some mix of all three)
- Including both strategic and operational elements
- On a rigorous and systematic basis with clear timescales and responsibilities
- Based on the statutory responsibilities of health and social care commissioners
- Also involving providers, users, carers, advocates and others who can bring an 'added value' to the process
- With users, carers and other members of local communities having an important role in decision-making
- Having inbuilt mechanisms for monitoring and review

- Respite services that provide personal and health support
- Advice and resource centre involving inputs from health, social services and the district council
- Improved information provision
- Provision of safety equipment in homes
- Development of a stroke rehabilitation programme
- Expansion of the warden alarms scheme
- Development of a joint bathing service
- Development of day care for older people with a mental frailty
- Transfer of health funds to the district council for targeted work on aids and adaptations for highly dependent older people.

An example of an innovation in community care involving partnership between professional groups and agencies is the Sheffield neighbourhood support unit (NSU) (Walker & Warren 1996). The aim of NSUs is to break down the traditional division between domiciliary, day and residential care and to make services more user-oriented with respect to older people and their carers. The units were locally situated and were the physical base for services that were delivered in older people's homes as well as being a day centre and a community resource. The services provided from the unit itself included a weekly lunch club, twice-weekly meals on wheels, twice-weekly day care, a club for older people with mental disabilities, a laundry service, bathing facilities and shopping trips. Teams of community support workers replaced the traditional warden and home-help role. They undertook caring duties based on a holistic assessment of needs and resources and demonstrated the shift from charring to caring. In one of the units there was also joint work with the primary health care team. The evaluation of this initiative suggests that, although the individuals were generally older, even severely disabled, they were supported in remaining in their own home – 'ageing in place' (Walker & Warren 1996: p. 152). Carers provided the bulk of care but they were no more involved in care-planning than in the usual form of care. Clearly there were political and resourcing issues that prevented the continued existence of this experiment beyond the initial funding, although the authors note that many of its characteristics are to be found in the Elderly People's Integrated Care System that has developed in several parts of the UK.

Another example of partnership innovation is the Bromley by Bow Centre (cited in Peckham & Exworthy 2003: p. 236). The Bromley by Bow Centre is a community organization which runs a variety of projects in an integrated way, linking health with education and enterprise in a way that will provide a focus for regeneration in the local area. It incorporates a health centre and is integrating the work of GPs and other health professionals with community projects. There is a café and nursery and the Centre runs a wide range of activities including art training, employment skills, community care services for older people and sports. The Centre is funded from regeneration monies and the new Opportunities Fund with some statutory agency revenue.

SUMMARY

Responding to the needs of older people remains one of the biggest challenges for primary health and community care and nursing has an important part to play in meeting these. It is perhaps easier to see where policy and service development has come from than what it will look like in the future. On the whole it seems that service provision is thinly spread and that in order to receive care it is necessary to be very old and dependent. The move towards targeting services for those at risk, motivated by cost containment, is likely to be an enduring feature of provision. However, the ping-pong ball between health and social care is bewildering to clients and time-wasting for professionals and it is encouraging to see signs of flexibility in the allocation of resources. Cultures of professional practice need to change to ensure that priority is given to individuals rather than systems and to provide care that is respectful as well as effective.

Recommended reading

Gordon P, Hadley J (eds) 1996 Extending primary care. Radcliffe, Oxford.

This book contains five short chapters with an introduction that redefines primary care as a network of community-based health services and challenges some of the common assumptions that primary care is synonymous with general practice. There are also chapters that describe innovative ways of extending primary care to hospital-at-home, polyclinics and resource centres.

Leathard A (ed) 2003 Interprofessional collaboration: from policy to practice in health and social care. Brunner-Routledge, Hove.

This new edition on interprofessional collaboration collects together key contributions from leading writers on teamwork. It takes a broad sweep and covers policy, professional and practice issues with chapters on user perspectives, and service development for older people.

Littlejohns P, Victor C (eds) 1996 Making sense of a primary care-led health service. Radcliffe, Oxford.

This short and accessible book raises for discussion the key policy and management issues that flow from the primary care-led NHS. There are contributions from a range of experts from management, general practice and health services research and evaluation. Although books on policy quickly become out of date, this will continue to be useful, because it puts the changes in context.

Peckham S, Exworthy M (2003) Primary care in the UK: policy, organization and management. Palgrave Macmillan, Basingstoke.

This is a clearly written and contemporary analysis of recent policy developments in primary care. There are useful chapters on commissioning, management and delivery of services. Although there is not a specific focus on older people, the book explores relevant issues such as partnership working, patient involvement and collaboration between professionals to provide effective care.

Rummery K, Glendinning C 2000 Primary care and social services: developing new partnerships for older people. Radcliffe Medical Press, Oxford.

This short concise book provides useful examples of partnership working in projects for older people and draws out the lessons for patients and professionals. There is a helpful final chapter on the evaluation of frontline collaboration projects that asks how to define and recognize success.

Victor C 2004 The social context of ageing. Routledge, London.

Christina Victor's book is an up-to-date text on ageing drawing from demographic, epidemiological and health and social care policy.

References

Alborz A, Wilkin D, Smith K 2002 Are primary care trusts consulting local communities? Health and Social Care in the Community 10: 20–27

Atkin K, Hirst M, Lunt N, Parker G 1994 The role and self perceived training needs of nurses employed in general practice: observations from a national census of practice nurses in England and Wales. Journal of Advanced Nursing 20: 46–52

Audit Commission 1986 Making a reality of community care. HMSO, London

Audit Commission 1999 First assessment: a review of district nursing work. Audit Commission, London

Audit Commission 2004 Transforming primary care. Audit Commission, London

Bennett M, Haruis L, Rolands D 1996 Living in Britain: results from the 1994 general household survey. HMSO, London

Biggs S 1993 User participation and interprofessional collaboration in community care. Journal of Interprofessional Care 7: 151–159

Caplan G 1961 An approach to community mental health. Tavistock, London

Challis D, Davies B 1986 Case management in community care: implications for the implementation of caring for people. King's Fund, London

Challis D, Darton R, Johnson L et al. 1989 Supporting frail elderly people at home: the Darlington community care project. Personal Social Services Research Unit, Kent University, Kent

Challis D, Chessum R, Chesterman J, Luckett R, Traske K 1990 Case management in social and health care: the Gateshead community care scheme. Personal Social Services Research Unit, Kent University, Kent

Closs SJ 1997 Discharge communications between hospital and community care. Health and Social Care in the Community 5: 181–197

Cooper M, Parahoo K, McKenna H, Thompson K 2002 User participation in primary care: a literature review. Royal College of General Practitioners, Northern Ireland. University of Ulster, Ulster

Crawford M, Rutter D, Manley C et al. 2002 systematic review of involving patients in the planning and development of health care. British Medical Journal 325

Cumella S 1995 Researching general practice-based social work. CAIPE Bulletin 10: 23–24

Department of Health 1995 Health and personal social service statistics for England. HMSO, London

Department of Health 1996a Primary care: the future choice and opportunity. HMSO, London

Department of Health 1996b Primary care: delivering the future. HMSO, London

Department of Health 2000 The NHS plan. HMSO, London

Department of Health 2001a The national service framework for older people. HMSO, London

Department of Health 2001b Involving patients and public in healthcare. A discussion document. Department of Health, London

Department of Health 2001c The expert patient: a new approach to chronic disease management for the 21st century. Department of Health, London

Department of Health 2002 NHS hospital and community health services non-medical workforce census England. www.doh.gov.uk/public/nhsworkforce.htm/nonmed

Department of Health 2003 Delivering investment in general practice: implementing the new GMS contract. Department of Health, London

Department of Health 2004a The NHS improvement plan: putting people at the heart of public services. Department of Health, London

Department of Health 2004b Patient and public involvement in health: the evidence for policy implementation. A summary of results of the health in partnership research programme. Department of Health, London

Department of Health 2004c Improving chronic disease management. Department of Health, London

Dieppe P, Rafferty AM, Kitson A 2002 The clinical encounter – the focal point of patient centred care. Health Expectations 5: 279–281

Dixon J, Lewis R, Rosen R, Finlayson B, Gray D 2004 Managing chronic disease: what can we learn from the US experience? King's Fund, London

Drennan V, Andrews S, Sidhu R 2004 Flexible entry to primary care nursing project: improving recruitment and retention in primary care. Primary Care Nursing Research Unit, University College London, London

Elkan R, Kendrick D, Dewey M et al. 2001 Effectiveness of home based support for older people: systematic review and meta-analysis. British Medical Journal 323: 1–9

Furne A, Rink E, Ross F 2001 The integrated nursing team in primary care: views and experience of participants exploring ownership, objectives and a team orientation. Primary Health Care Research and Development 2: 187–195

Gillam S, Anderson W, Florin D, Mountford L 2002 Every voice counts: primary care organizations and public involvement. King's Fund, London

Glasby J 2003 Hospital discharge – integrating health and social care. Radcliffe Medical Press, Abingdon

Glendinning C, Rummery K 2003 Collaboration between primary health and social care: from policy to practice in developing services for older people. In: Leathard Λ (ed) Interprofessional collaboration: from policy to practice in health and social care. Brunner-Routledge, Hove, pp 186–200

Goodman C, Ross F, Mackenzie A, Vernon S 2003 A portrait of district nursing: its contribution to primary health care. Journal of Interprofessional Care 17: 97–107

Gordon P, Plampling D 1996 Primary health care – its characteristics and potential. In: Gordon P, Hadley J (eds) Extending primary care. Radcliffe Medical Press, New York, pp 1–15

Gould M 1999 Care of black and ethnic minority elders. In: Redfern S, Ross F (eds) Nursing older people. Churchill Livingstone, Edinburgh

Gould M, Iliffe S 1995 Hospital at home: a case study in service development. British Journal of Health Care Management 1: 809–812

Griffiths R 1988 Community care: agenda for action. HMSO, London

Haggard L, Bosma E 1996 Hospital care at home. In: Gordon P, Hadley J (eds) Extending primary care. King's Fund, London

Hardy B, Young R, Wistow G 1999 Dimensions of choice in the assessment and care management process: the views of older people, carers and care managers. Health and Social Care in the Community 7(6): 483–491

Harrison A 1993 Health care UK 1992/93. King's Fund, London

Henwood M 1995. Making a difference? Implementation of the community care reforms ten years on. King's Fund, London

House of Commons Health Committee 2002 Delayed discharges: third report. Stationery Office, London

Kendall J, Matosevic T, Forder J et al. 2003 The motivations of domiciliary care providers in England: new concepts, new findings. Journal of Social Policy 32: 489–511

Kharicha K, Levin E, Iliffe S, Davey B 2004 Social work general practice and evidence-based policy in the collaborative care of older people – current problems and future possibilities. Health and Social Care in the Community 12: 134–141

Knapp MRJ, Hardy B, Forder J 2001 Commissioning for quality: ten years of social care markets in England. Journal of Social Policy 30: 283–306

Leedham I, Wistow G 1992 Community care and general practitioners. Paper no. 6. Nuffield Institute of Health Service Studies, University of Leeds, Leeds

Lewis J, Glennerster M 1996 Implementing the new community care. Open University Press, Milton Keynes

Lorig K (ed) 2000 Living a healthy life with a chronic condition, 2nd edn. Bull Publishing, Boulder

Lorig K, Kankol L, Gonzalez V 1987 Arthritis patient education: a review of the literature. Patient Education and Counselling 10: 207–252

Lorig KR, Mazonson PD, Holman HR 1993 Evidence suggesting that health education for self-management in patients with chronic arthritis has sustained health benefits while reducing health care costs. Arthritis and Rheumatism 36: 439–446

Marks L 1994 Seamless care or patchwork quilt: discharging patients from acute hospital care. Research report 17. King's Fund, London

Means R, Smith R 1985 The development of welfare services for elderly people. Croom Helm, Beckenham

Munro J, Nicholl J, O'Cathain A, Knowles E 2000 Evaluation of NHS Direct first wave sites. School of Health and Related Research, University of Sheffield, Sheffield

Parkes J, Shepherd S 2003 Discharge planning from hospital to home (Cochrane review). Cochrane Library issue 1. Update Software, Oxford

Parry-Jones B, Soulsby J 2001 Needs-led assessments: the challenges and the reality. Health and Social Care in the Community 9(6): 414–428

Pattison S 2001 User involvement and participation in the NHS: a personal perspective. In: Heller T, Murston R, Sidell M, Lloyd C (eds) Working for health. Open University Press, London

Peckham S, Exworthy M 2003 Primary care in the UK: policy organization and management. Palgrave, Macmillan, Basingstoke

Poxton R 1996 Joint approaches for a better old age. King's Fund, London

Richards S 2000 Bridging the divide: elders and the assessment process. British Journal of Social Work 30: 37–49

Rickards L, Fox K, Roberts C 2004 Living in Britain: number 31. Results from the 2002 General Household Survey. The Stationary Office, London

Ross F, Tissier J 1997 The care management interface with general practice: a case study. Health and Social Care in the Community 5: 153–161

Ross F, Bower P, Sibbald B 1994 Practice nurses: characteristics, workload and training needs. British Journal of General Practice 44: 15–18

Ross F, Rink E, Furne A 2000 Integration or pragmatic coalition: an evaluation of nursing teams in primary care. Journal of Interprofessional Care 11: 259–267

Ross F, Smith E, Mackenzie A, Masterson A 2004 Identifying research priorities in nursing and midwifery service delivery and organization: a scoping study. International Journal of Nursing Studies 41: 547–558

Sims J, Rink E, Walker R, Pickard L 1997 The introduction of a hospital at home service: a staff perspective. Journal of Interprofessional Care 11: 217–224

Smith E, Ross F, Donovan S 2005 Current issues for patient and public involvement in primary care. National Association of Primary Care Annual Review 2005, London

Starfield B 1998 Primary care: balancing health needs, services and technology. Oxford University Press, New York

Steiner A 1997 Intermediate care: a conceptual framework and review of the literature. King's Fund, London

Stevenson O 1996 Changing practice – professional attitudes, consumerism and empowerment. In: Bland R (ed) Developing services for older people and their families. London: Jessica Kingsley, pp 204–215

Tierney A, Worth A, Closs A, King C, Macmillan M 1994 Older patients' experiences of discharge from hospital. Nursing Times 90: 36–39

Victor CR 1990 A survey of the delayed discharge of elderly people from hospital in an inner city health district. Archives of Gerontology and Geriatrics 4: 117–124

Victor C 1991 Health and health care in later life. Open University Press, Milton Keynes

Victor C 1997 Community care and older people. Thorne, Cheltenham

Victor CR 2004 The social context of ageing. Routledge, London

Wagner E 2000 The role of patient care teams in chronic disease management. British Medical Journal 320: 569–572

Walker A, Warren L 1996 Changing services for older people. Open University Press, Milton Keynes

Walker A, O'Brian M, Traynor J et al. 2002 Living in Britain: results of 2001 GHS. The Stationery Office, London. Also available at www.statistics.gov.uk/lib2001/resources/file attachments/GHS2002.pdr

Warren L 1999 Conclusion: empowerment: the path to partnership? In: Barnes M, Warren L (eds) Paths to empowerment. The Policy Press, Bristol

World Health Organization 1978 Primary health care. WHO/UNICEF, Geneva

Chapter 8

Nursing older people in hospital

Andrei Dunn

INTRODUCTION

The UK *National Service Framework (NSF) for Older People* notes that, over the past 70 years, people over the age of 65 years have grown in numbers by more than 200% (Department of Health 2001a). The NSF estimates that between 1995 and 2025 the population of 90-year-olds and older will double. To address this increase in demand, *The NHS Plan* (Department of Health 2000) recommended that the National Health Service (NHS) should have an increase of 7800 more nursing staff to provide care and support for older people. This is supported by the Medical Research Council's Cognitive Function and Ageing Study and the Resources Implications Study (Melzer et al. 1999) from their interviews of people over the age of 65 from four areas in the UK between 1991 and 1992.

The *NSF for Older People* recognizes that the care needs for older people admitted to hospital are complex and require prompt access to specialist care. The management of the complex needs that older people have requires an early assessment to identify further treatment required. This assessment should be at a multidisciplinary level, so providing early access to the full range of specialist care. When in a surgical or a general medical ward in hospital, care for older individuals may involve controlling their fluid management and pain levels, preventing pressure sores, orienting them to their environment, preventing falls and improving their mobility. Older people are more likely to need a longer stay in hospital than younger people because of the impact the acute phase of illness has on them, requiring complex interventions to facilitate a safe discharge from the ward. Following discharge they may need personal care at home, equipment or adjustments to the home and extensive rehabilitation, and so will require intermediate care services or long-term care. Rehabilitation is often hindered by the patient's medical condition. Many are admitted to hospital in a physically weak and dependent state. This may present as a loss of mobility, loss of dexterity, delirium or a fall, risking fracture of the hip or wrist. These problems can be caused by a systemic infection worsening an underlying chronic condition and may affect the level of recovery made. In hospital the older patient's rehabilitation potential is evaluated together with the risks involved in returning home. Nursing older people in hospital has recently focused on rehabilitation involving the multidisciplinary team, promoting patient-centredness in the approach to care, and patients' participation in their own care.

In the UK, the Department of Health's (now the Department of Health and Social Care or DHSC) publications influence the way in which hospitals interpret best practice for the older patient. The underlying principles for best practice include:

- to provide an early assessment of the patient by the multidisciplinary team
- to involve patients in the planning and decision-making process by ensuring that they have sufficient information to make an informed decision at both a personal and strategic level
- to provide an efficient and equitable service for older people
- to remove ageism from the decision-making process at all levels.

The hospital service is identified in *The NHS Plan* (Department of Health 2000) as being service-led rather than patient-centred. Since the *NSF for Older People* (Department of Health 2001a) and *The Essence of Care* (Department of Health 2001b) targets were published, hospitals and primary care NHS trusts have been striving to become more patient-centred in their service delivery. This is resulting in greater access by patients to decision-making fora that address the operation of service provision for older people. This decision-making process is led by primary care trusts and acute hospital trusts in the NHS.

The Department of Health has identified eight key aspects of care that need addressing by hospitals: (1) personal and oral hygiene; (2) privacy and dignity; (3) pressures sores; (4) continence of bladder and bowel; (5) nutrition and food; (6) record-keeping; (7) safety of people with mental health illnesses; and (8) promoting self-care (Department of Health 2001a, 2001b).

This chapter provides an overview of care of older people in hospital. It focuses particularly on policies and guidelines that have emerged from the DHSC in recent years, including the organization of hospital services and nursing care, benchmarking and standards of care, patient assessment, rehabilitation, team-

working and discharge from hospital. Stroke illness and falls are selected as examples to illustrate the policy issues and cross-reference is made to other chapters which cover some of these in more detail.

ORGANIZATION OF HOSPITAL SERVICES

Hospital services in the UK vary in the extent to which they address the needs of older people. Some hospitals provide nurse-led units for the care of older people or an elderly care unit (ECU) that specializes in the treatment of older people (known as specialist services). In other hospitals care for older people is not designated as a specialist area of care and older people join younger patients in the general medical unit (known as integrated services). Each ward may have a specialty within the ECU, such as mental health or orthopaedic and rehabilitation care, with access to acute care when necessary. Some services may include a multidisciplinary assessment and rehabilitation service for people as outpatients. These outpatient facilities are often provided in a day-hospital setting, but may also be based in an intermediate care setting (Forster et al. 1999).

Specialist services

Specialist services for older people in hospital consist of wards that specialize in the management of older people, day hospital care and supported discharge services. Two major conditions that the *NSF for Older People* expects these units and services to address are those associated with stroke illness (cerebrovascular accident) or falls. The NSF includes targets for prevention of falls and managing stroke illness. Both conditions require early assessment and intervention from the multidisciplinary team. This process is coordinated with the accident and emergency service so that the patient receives prompt specialist treatment. Either a specialist is available in the accident and emergency department to assess the patient immediately, or a referral process to a specialist is made that is prompt and accessible. Detailed discussion of the single assessment process can be found in Chapter 28. Prevention and management of mobility deficits and falls are covered in Chapter 13 and stroke illness, with a particular emphasis on nutrition, in Chapter 16. Specialist units are seen as the centres for best practice because of their coordinated and comprehensive approach to the management of older people and stroke patients.

Integrated services

Integrated services provide care for patients regardless of their age, and so old and younger adults are nursed in the same ward. Equally, acutely ill patients may be cared for in the same ward as patients requiring rehabilitation or long-term care. *The NSF for Older People* (Department of Health 2001a) argues that, regardless of setting, care should be of the same standard as in a specialist area. Therefore, patients would have access to consultant geriatricians, therapists, consultant nurses and nurse specialists for older people. The process of access and care in an integrated service depends on the workload of individual professionals and on the efficiency of the communication process within the organization. If key professionals are diverted to younger patients with life-threatening conditions, the needs of the older patient may have to wait. The presence of designated specialist rehabilitation wards for the older patient to gain access from the acute care setting will ensure a high standard of service provision for older people.

ORGANIZATION OF NURSING CARE

Nursing care in specialist wards for older patients is usually organized as 'team nursing' or 'primary nursing' or a combination of both (Waters & Easton 1999). 'Task allocation' was once the dominant style of organizing nursing care whereby patient care was divided into a number of tasks, each carried out for all patients by a different member of the nursing staff. Over the past 50 years, nursing in the UK has moved away from task allocation to a more individualized approach to patient care. Individualized patient care within a team-nursing or primary-nursing approach is supported by a care plan for each patient based on assessment, goal-setting, implementation and evaluation of care (Waters & Easton 1999).

Team nursing

In team nursing the nurses in the ward are allocated to small groups and work together. Each team is responsible for planning and providing care for a group of patients. Each team includes nurses and care assistants with varying degrees of skill and knowledge led by the team leader (Waters 1985). The combined efforts of the team with good communication between each member ensure an effective process of patient care. Waters & Easton (1999) suggest that team nursing promotes good communication between nurses and creates continuity of care for the patient. However, they report that an inadequate skill-mix can impair the quality of the individualized care process.

Primary nursing

In primary nursing an experienced nurse has overall responsibility and accountability for the nursing care of the patient from the time of admission to the ward to discharge from it. The nurse's key role is to coordinate and deliver the patient's care supported by other nurses and care assistants (Wright 1990, Ersser & Tutton 1991). Difficulties can arise when the primary nurse is absent if the deputy nurse has not been properly briefed. When this happens, the patient's care may not be re-evaluated and necessary changes to care may not be made. The success of primary nursing depends on the level of communication between nurses in the ward. This process requires the primary nurse to have a manageable caseload and be the main point of contact for the patient's family and other professionals. Primary nursing requires an adequate number of nurses with good clinical and care management skills.

Person-centred care

Person-centred care involves removing the boundaries between professionals that can obstruct the provision of care so that appropriate intervention is provided as quickly as possible to support the older person. The emphasis is always to treat patients with respect and to involve them, if they wish, in the decision-making process concerning their care. The guidance from *The NSF for Older People* (Department of Health 2001a) recommends that health care workers and managers should: listen to older people; respect their dignity and privacy; recognize cultural and religious differences; encourage patients to make an informed decision about their care; and involve and support the carers when needed. Sometimes older patients prefer to be passive during the decision-making process regarding their own care (Biley 1992, Litva et al. 2002) but are willing to participate in discussions regarding the service at patient fora or citizens' panels (Walker & Dewar 2001). It is important that the nurse, the patient and the carer, if necessary, share information and that the carer and patient feel included in the decision-making process. In Walker & Dewar's (2001) study, carers were not satisfied that they had been adequately involved. The carers attributed their dissatisfaction to the hospital's systems and processes which, they said, hindered their involvement and their relationship with the nurses. The policy document, *Improvement Leaders' Guide to Involving Patients and Carers* (NHS Modernisation Agency 2002), argues that it is essential to involve patients in the decision-making process if health services and social services are to improve. Holmes-Rovner et al. (2001) regard the ideal situation as one in which patients are given research-based information and the opportunity to decide their own health interventions. However, patients may see this as having too much responsibility if the outcome is poor. The *Improvement Leaders' Guide to Involving Patients and Carers* suggests that patient involvement in care will improve the quality of the service, make policy and planning decisions more patient-focused, improve communications between organizations and communities and give patients control and greater understanding of the services they use.

New nursing roles

Nursing education in the UK is now based in universities. It focuses on the promotion of evidence-based practice and understanding of research within nursing's field of expertise. The *Agenda for Change* policy document (Department of Health 2003) plans to change the pay structure for nurses in the UK, based on performance measured against 16 competence criteria. The implication of this change is that nurses' roles will be more clearly defined with an extended clinical career structure. A nurse may, for example, aspire to the level of consultant nurse, a role that was introduced by the Department of Health in 2000. Consultant nurses for older people have expertise in nursing practice specific to care of this age group and have strategic leadership skills in introducing improvements to practice, in educating and supervising students and staff and in evaluating practice and keeping up-to-date with research in their field. They promote a culture for learning at an interdisciplinary level, they provide clinical consultancy for patients, families and the organization, and are champions for patient-centred care (Manley & Dewing 2002).

A national evaluation of the establishment of the role of consultant nurse, midwife and health visitor has been completed (Guest et al. 2001, 2003, Redfern et al. 2003) and a follow-up study by the same team is in progress, both funded by the DHSC. The findings from the preliminary study revealed typical teething problems that so often occur when establishing a new role. There was considerable uncertainty about who should provide resources and support and how the role should be structured. The national role specification is helpful but the consultants' perception that they should be deeply engaged in expert practice, leadership, education and research and development activities has led to strong evidence of work overload. There is a risk that the job is simply too big. The research group anticipated that, as the consultants became more experienced in their roles, they would prioritize the most important elements and work overload would ease. In practice, they found the opposite. It may be that an average job tenure of 6 months was too short to assess this issue, but there needs to be careful monitoring of workload over

time t̶ ̶ ̶ ̶ ̶k pressures fall or increas̶ ̶ ̶ ̶ ̶ ̶ ̶out and ill health in the con̶ ̶ ̶ ̶ ̶ ̶following the consultant̶ ̶ ̶ ̶ ̶ ̶many have been in the job for 2 years, ̶ ̶ ̶ ̶on the workload issue and its consequences for the ̶ ̶ell-being of consultants and their patients. The study is also investigating how consultants are 'crafting' their roles, why some posts are more successful than others, what leadership means in this context, and is exploring the impact of the role on patient care and outcomes.

The role of nurse specialist for older people emerged alongside the drive for greater integration of NHS acute hospital trusts with primary care trusts. This nurse is a specialist clinical resource and provides educational support to nurses working with older people. A major part of the role is to carry out comprehensive assessments of older people to ensure they receive the full range of services they require. Promotion and maintenance of access and equity in health and social care are important aspects of the role. The nurse specialist for older people promotes links between hospitals and primary care trusts and is a major player in the development of intermediate care services and continuing care (see Chapter 9 for more information on intermediate and continuing care, and on new roles in nursing). Active involvement in all decision-making stages of the service is, therefore, essential. Nurse specialists and the consultant nurse working together make a formidable team in developing and improving the quality of service provision for older people. Although there is some overlap in their roles, the specialist focuses more on direct care of patients/clients and their families, while the consultant's role is broader and more strategic.

The new role of 'modern matron' was proposed in *The NHS Plan* (Department of Health 2000) and elaborated further in a Health Service circular (Department of Health 2001c). The role was set up in response to apparent public demand to 'bring back matron' as a way of strengthening nursing leadership at ward level, improving fundamental aspects of care and ensuring a swift response to problems experienced by patients and their families. The Department of Health (2002) specified the following 10 components as crucial to the modern matron's role:

1. act as a role model by demonstrating the high standard of nursing care patients expect
2. ensure that patients receive a high standard of care
3. ensure their nutritional needs are met
4. prevent patients developing hospital-acquired infection

5. ensure environmental budgets are spent appropriately
6. empower nurses to improve patient care
7. ensure that dignity and privacy of patients are maintained at all times
8. resolve problems for patients and their relatives
9. ensure an appropriate number of staff in the clinical environment to meet patients' needs.

Readers may wonder why a new role of this kind is needed when these components surely fall within the responsibility of the current ward sister/charge nurse/clinical manager roles. High standards do not, it seems, always follow and central policy decision-makers have responded to falling standards (reported, for example, by *The NHS Plan*) by introducing this senior ward sister/charge nurse role. The new role was evaluated by an independent research group at Sheffield University and the Royal College of Nursing (Read et al. 2004). This study identified three working models for the role: (1) the clinical model; (2) the managerial model; and (3) the mixed model – partly clinical and partly managerial. The researchers recommended that the role needed to be clarified by each trust, including on its role in the management of complaints. The role also requires support managerially, professionally, with educational development and with supporting resources (Read et al. 2004).

As well as the role developments mentioned above, some NHS trusts have established nurse practitioner posts – the 'falls nurse practitioner' for example, recruited in response to the NSF. Responsibilities of this role include screening people entering the accident and emergency department and working closely with those who have fallen. Finding the cause of the fall is a priority for falls nurse practitioners before onward referral. If the cause is mechanical, referral is likely to be to the primary care therapy team or an outpatient service. If the cause is underlying medical pathology, the nurse will investigate further, request blood and other tests for pathological scrutiny and refer the patient to the appropriate hospital unit.

BENCHMARKING AND STANDARDS OF CARE

The NHS Plan (Department of Health 2000) identifies wide variations in the standards of care provided across the country. The plan proposes to identify examples of best practice and facilitate dissemination of these practices to other sites. Targets for achieving best practice are identified in the expectation that less successful services can raise the standard of care in their localities and improve service provision. For this process to occur, the DHSC has developed an administrative structure to monitor the changes within the service and to identify where best practice is being achieved and where the service is failing to reach its targets. For older people, the local delivery of services is to be measured against clearly defined standards of practice specified in *The NSF for Older People* (Department of Health 2001a) and *The Essence of Care* document (Department of Health 2001b). An important part of monitoring targets is to involve patients and the public in decision-making much more than has been the case in the past.

The following eight standards of care for older people are identified as priorities by the NSF: (1) identifying and removing age discrimination in organizations; (2) promoting person-centred care; (3) developing intermediate care; (4) improving general hospital care; (5) improving the service for patients with stroke illness; (6) those who have fallen; (7) improving mental health services for older people; and (8) promoting a healthy and active life. The reader is referred to Chapters 9, 13, 24, 30 and 32 which discuss these issues in more detail.

The Essence of Care (Department of Health 2001b) focuses on what has been identified from a number of large surveys as fundamental and essential aspects of care and identifies eight key issues: (1) personal and oral hygiene; (2) privacy and dignity for the patient; (3) prevention and reduction of pressure ulcers; (4) continence and bladder and bowel care; (5) food and nutrition; (6) safety of people with mental health illness; (7) principles of self-care and (8) record-keeping. *The Essence of Care* recommends the development of standards through the process of benchmarking. Benchmarking requires each clinical area to be audited and scored using the A–E (best to worst) grades specified in *The Essence of Care*. Comparisons are made between clinical units and those scoring less well are encouraged to learn from high-scoring units and introduce changes to improve their practice. The clinical auditing process is seen as a continuous cycle that is repeated over time in an attempt to monitor, improve and sustain good practice. Best practice needs strong support with policies, procedures, guidelines and efficient record-keeping. It follows that all staff, both clinical and non-clinical, need to be aware of the policies and procedures, and what is expected of them. They need supervision, training and support from management. Improving deficiencies in service provision may range from a need for efficient communication and information-giving procedures with patients, better record-keeping, enough equipment of the right sort, to better partnership-working with patients and their families.

The Essence of Care benchmark for record-keeping has complex requirements for achieving best practice. These include patients being involved in planning their care if they wish, having access to their notes and integrating the separate notes from each health care professional into one comprehensive document in order to improve communication (a practice that has been more common in maternity services than in acute hospital medicine). Time is needed to adjust to the changes.

Achieving the benchmark for continence and bladder and bowel care involves providing patients with information and direct access to professional advice, assessment, planning, implementation of treatment and evaluation of outcome. Nurses providing the service in acute NHS trusts need education and training so that they can advise primary care nurses about patients' needs for continuing care and supplies. Some acute trusts have the necessary services in place, whilst others have had to develop new services to ensure the benchmark is achieved (see Chapter 17 for information on incontinence and constipation).

The benchmark for personal and oral hygiene requires individual assessment and easy access to toilets and washing facilities, together with assistance and advice as required. Provision of accessible toilet facilities in older hospitals may be difficult unless the buildings are redesigned or modified.

The benchmark for hospital-based services to prevent and treat pressure ulcers focuses on early assessment, involving patients in planning and evaluating the care, providing them with information that will help and advising primary care services and aftercare agencies on continuing care needs. Further information on the prevention and care of pressure ulcers is given in Chapter 19.

The benchmark for food and nutrition includes similar attention to the assessment and patient care process and also the need to consider the presentation of food and its availability for patients outside normal hours. Patients who want to eat at night because they have missed the scheduled mealtime through late admission to the ward or absence for investigations, treatment or surgery should have access to food (see Chapter 16 for a detailed discussion of nutritional care).

The privacy and dignity benchmark emphasizes how important it is for patients to feel valued. They need personal time to themselves without feeling neglected, and respect for their modesty, dignity and privacy when receiving intimate care (see Chapter 21 for a discussion of intimacy and relationships).

The benchmark for achieving safety of a person with mental health needs requires health care workers to protect them from harming themselves without restricting their movements unreasonably.

Finally, the benchmark for achieving self-care has direct relevance to rehabilitation and care of older people in hospital. The benchmark promotes patient choice and emphasizes the importance of respecting their views. Assessing patients' abilities to be self-caring is fundamental and providing them with knowledge, skills and resources to be so is essential.

Early assessment and a patient-centred approach to care are common themes throughout all the benchmarks in *The Essence of Care* and the standards specified in the *NSF for Older People*. Regular audits in all clinical units monitor grades achieved over time so that progress is made transparent. The DHSC expected plans to be in place to meet any shortfall in achieving the benchmarks and standards by March 2004 (Department of Health 2001a).

Patient involvement

Patients' involvement in decision-making has become an important component of health care in the UK, continental Europe, Canada and the USA (Crawford et al. 2002). The aim is to improve treatment outcomes and the quality of care provided. Walker & Dewar (2001) identified four markers of satisfactory involvement: (1) sharing information between nurse and patient; (2) ensuring that the patient feels included in the decision-making process; (3) helping patient and carer to report whether the service has responded to their needs or not; and (4) acting as a satisfactory contact for the patient. Patient involvement is advocated by the NHS Modernisation Agency (2002) as a mechanism for improving health and social care services and increasing patient satisfaction.

Crawford et al.'s (2002) systematic review of the literature examines the involvement of patients in the planning and development of health care services. The researchers identified patient involvement as operating at two different levels, that is, in their own individual care and in service development decisions.

Walker & Dewar (2001) report that carers in their study felt dissatisfied with the level of involvement they were permitted to have. They identified two main causes for their dissatisfaction: inefficient organizational bureaucracy and lack of information necessary for knowing whom to contact and how to access services. Patients cannot make an informed decision regarding their treatment without the necessary knowledge. As Holmes-Rovner et al. (2001) suggest, if patients are given explicit information – preferably evidence-based – before they make a choice about their care, they will understand the benefits and risks they face and can contribute to decisions about choices on an equal footing with health care professionals. More information on involvement of the public in health service policy and provision can be found in Chapter 6.

ASSESSMENT

The single assessment process was mentioned earlier in relation to falls and stroke care, and the evidence-based rationale for streamlining and coordinating assessment is discussed in Chapter 28. This section introduces some general principles for the hospital nurse that provide the context for care planning. An early multidisciplinary assessment is essential, once the patient has been stabilized, to identify future care needs. Older people with complex illness typically require a comprehensive assessment so that they can benefit from the treatment and therapeutic care they need. Assessment of the hospital patient will vary depending on setting, i.e. inpatient or outpatient (Reuben et al. 1999).

The NHS Plan's (Department of Health 2000) recommendation for a single multidisciplinary assessment process for older people is intended to achieve transferability across health and social care. The aims of the single assessment process are to:

- raise the standard of the assessment
- standardize the process across all aspects of health and social care
- organize the time needed for assessment more effectively to meet the patient's needs
- improve the sharing of information between professionals
- encourage team-working to an agreed level of best practice for assessment and care.

The time it takes to complete the single assessment process is flexible. It may be a concentrated process completed over one session or require part-assessments over a number of occasions. An essential goal is to achieve a comprehensive, multidisciplinary assessment that avoids duplication and does not exhaust the patient (Department of Health 2001a).

Function versus pathology

During the past 25 years or so, there has been a shift of emphasis away from a 'pathology' view of the patient to a functional assessment of the patient's ability to carry out activities of daily living. Hall (1976) illustrated this well almost by pointing out that many disabilities commonly seen in a population, such as anaemia, cardiac failure, urinary symptoms, deafness and defective vision, could coexist in a single individ-

ual and yet that person may lead a satisfying life with no functional problems in terms of activities of daily living. It is important, therefore, that the assessment of the older patient in hospital should not simply focus on a medical diagnosis. For example, the patient's ability to perform the fine finger movements necessary for dressing is as important as the medical diagnosis of rheumatoid arthritis.

The assessment can start with a health history. This step normally includes gathering biographical information, reason for the hospital visit, current health status, medications taken, past history of health, allergies, previous hospital outpatient and inpatient episodes, family history of illnesses and how the patient functions at home on a day-to-day basis (Bowers & Thompson 1992). To avoid overwhelming patients, it is sometimes better to start by asking why they have come to the hospital and what has changed since becoming ill. This approach to the interview establishes rapport, aids communication, clarifies expectations of the hospital stay and the role that nursing can play and enables information to be gathered for formulating the care plan. There is no better source of information than the patients themselves but sometimes they may be too ill or too weak to respond to questions, or have profound communication problems such as dysphasia or deafness. Consequently, interviewing the spouse, children, friends, neighbours or any 'significant other' such as a home carer is invaluable. Applegate et al. (1990) warn, however, that older people tend to rate themselves as having more functional ability than do their carers. A person's health is primarily one's own concern and not everyone wants another person present during such a discussion.

Direct observation is an essential part of assessment and the patient's vital signs are recorded and explained to the patient to ensure understanding. The medical component of the assessment will ensure that each of the patient's physiological systems is examined to identify problems that require treatment (Bowers & Thompson 1992). Samples of body fluids (blood and urine) are taken if necessary for pathological testing and other investigations (X-ray and electrocardiogram) are ordered if required. After the initial assessment, reassessments continue throughout the patient's stay in hospital to monitor progress and evaluate the effectiveness of the interventions. Further information on the nurse's assessment of the patient, including assessment tools, is provided in Chapter 28.

Care plans

It has become common practice for care plans to be agreed with older patients or their carer to illustrate the importance of prescribed treatments and care in the recovery process (Cegala et al. 2000). Planning care together enables the nurse and patient to share information and identify the patient's problems together. The nurse will discuss treatment options with the patient and start the agreed programme of care. Not all older patients expect to be involved in making decisions about their care and they may need encouragement to express their views (Anell et al. 1997). Patients who truly understand that they have a choice are likely to take control and participate fully in decisions about their care. Patients who have a clear understanding of their own health are in a good position to manage their own recovery. As with patient assessment, *The Essence of Care* (Department of Health 2001b) recommends that patients' care plans and progress records should be integrated, multidisciplinary and accessible to the patient. The purpose is to improve the level of communication between health care professionals by ensuring that each person's notes about the patient are kept in the same place. The integrated, multidisciplinary care plan is a comprehensive source containing insights from all team members. Case study 8.1 describes the management of a patient that followed an effective multidisciplinary care plan.

Patient care pathways

Patient care pathways for older people have been developed for the management of stroke and falls patients, amongst others. Care pathways are designed to standardize practice and service provision. The guidelines from *The NSF for Older People* (Department of Health 2001a) for these two conditions are outlined below.

Stroke

The stroke care pathway examines three groups in the management of stroke (cerebrovascular accident): (1) people at risk of developing a stroke who have been identified by the primary care team; (2) people who are suspected of having had a transient ischaemic attack; and (3) those suspected of having had a stroke.

The pathway recommends immediate admission of the patient suspected of having had a stroke to a hospital-based stroke unit for assessment. After multidisciplinary assessment, it is recommended that they should immediately start the planned rehabilitation programme, which should be agreed with the patient. After recovery from the acute phase, the patient should be discharged with a secondary prevention programme so that rehabilitation continues in an

---

Case study 8.1

Mrs Brown, aged 83 years, was admitted to an elderly care ward with Parkinson's disease having been transferred from an orthopaedic ward after receiving a right total hip screw. She had fallen and fractured her right hip. After arriving in the ward, she was assessed by members of the multidisciplinary team who met and discussed their recommendations for treatment. The nurse in charge of Mrs Brown's care discussed the treatment options and decisions made were agreed with her and her daughter. Mrs Brown remained in the ward for 2 months receiving treatment and rehabilitation therapy from the team. The doctor changed the medication for her Parkinson's and prescribed a calcium supplement to promote healing of the fracture. The physiotherapist provided exercises to improve Mrs Brown's balance and strength. The ward nurses ensured that she continued the exercises every day and monitored her progress. They referred her to social services for a home help and meals on wheels to be provided when she was discharged home. Handrails were fitted to Mrs Brown's bed at home and a stool was provided by the occupational therapist for Mrs Brown to sit on while washing. As part of her discharge plan, she was booked for an appointment at the falls clinic and a tilt-table test 2 weeks after discharge from the ward in order to establish the cause of her fall and prevent further fractures. Arrangements were made to transport her from home to the clinic and back on the day of the appointment.

---

intermediate care setting or at home. The pathway recommends that the specialist stroke team follows up the patient together with the primary care team.

The patient suspected of having had a transient ischaemic attack should be referred to a neurovascular clinic or specialist stroke team for assessment before being referred to the general practitioner for preventive care and surveillance.

The patient identified as being at risk of a stroke, with high blood pressure or atrial fibrillation, for example, would be referred to the general practitioner who would plan a prevention programme with the patient and primary care team. Case study 8.2 illustrates the successful use of a patient care pathway.

Falls

The NSF's guidelines for the management of falls recommends a patient care pathway for patients who arrive at the accident and emergency department that starts with an immediate triage for risk of further falls.

Case study 8.2

Dorothy Moses, aged 76 years, was taken to an inner-city accident and emergency department with left-sided weakness and slurred speech. She was suspected of having had a stroke and a computed tomography brain scan taken shortly after she was seen in the accident and emergency department confirmed a small infarct in the right corona radiata. After she had become medically stable, she was transferred to a stroke ward and assessed by the specialist medical team consisting of nurse, physiotherapist and occupational therapist. The recommended plan of care was discussed and agreed with Mrs Moses and her husband. The medical team prescribed antiplatelet therapy and treatment for hypertension to reduce the risk of another stroke. Over the following 2 weeks in the ward, the nurses, the physiotherapist and occupational therapist provided intensive rehabilitation therapy to restore her ability to function independently (exercises, nutritional and hygiene care to restore independence in activities of everyday living and to build up her confidence). Home help and meals on wheels were arranged to be in place when she was discharged home. An appointment was made for her to attend the stroke clinic 4 weeks after the discharge date. Mrs Moses had her bed moved downstairs and a commode provided because she was no longer able to climb the stairs. The specialist stroke team worked closely with the general practitioner and district nurse in the primary care team to provide follow-up care and to reassess Mrs Moses' progress in regaining independence in activities of daily living.

After this, the assessment and investigative processes (X-rays and blood examination) can proceed.

The falls pathway recommends that people who have not fallen but are identified as at high risk of falling should be referred to the general practitioner, who would review them and provide immediate treatment as required and continuing care together with nurses and therapists in the primary care team. The patient would be encouraged to participate fully in the single assessment process. If still considered to be at high risk of falling, the therapist would plan care to improve the patient's motor skills and investigations would be made for the risk of osteoporosis, followed by preventive treatment if necessary. Referral to the hospital-based falls service would be made if a more detailed multidisciplinary assessment is needed. Admission to hospital may be indicated to give the patient access to all parts of the falls service and secondary prevention measures would be set up well before the patient is discharged home. Such measures may include provision of equipment in the home to promote independence and rearrangement of the home environment to improve safety. Continued rehabilitation would be available to patients at home or in other settings (such as intermediate care units and day hospitals).

The falls pathway recommends that patients entering the accident and emergency department with a history of falls who are then discharged home should be referred to an intermediate care centre or the general practitioner for a rapid assessment of their environment and available support. They would then be referred for a specialist assessment of their falls which would confirm their level of risk. At the same time, investigation for osteoporosis would be made, followed by treatment if necessary to reduce the risk of hip and wrist fractures and vertebral collapse. Once the patient's needs have been identified then referrals are made to specialist therapists and nurses who would coordinate the supply of equipment and services needed for the patient to be independent at home or at an intermediate care centre or day hospital. The primary care team would take responsibility for follow-up and continuing care with the option of referral to more specialist services if needed.

The patient attending the accident and emergency department, having fallen and fractured a limb, may be admitted to a hospital ward, perhaps a surgical ward at first, followed by transfer to a rehabilitation ward after recovery from the acute phase, as happened with Mrs Brown (Case study 8.1). The falls service would coordinate the discharge when the patient is ready to go home and so the ward would refer the patient to the falls service if the risk of falling again had not been addressed during the hospital stay (Brown 1999). During this time the patient should be screened for osteoporosis and given treatment if needed. The patient's home would be assessed and any adaptations or equipment needed would be put in place in the home, preferably before the date of discharge, but otherwise within 3 weeks of the discharge date. In some cases, a move to other accommodation, such as sheltered housing or a care home, may be recommended. The falls team will decide with the patient whether rehabilitation at home is indicated or whether benefit would be gained at an intermediate care centre or day hospital. Again, the primary care team would review progress with the older person and evaluate the services received.

Hu & Woollacott (1996) reviewed the literature on the rehabilitation of frail fallers and highlighted the importance of a comprehensive assessment of the patient's balance, including full history, a medical review, a neuromuscular examination, a mobility test and balance control. The reviewers recommend that patients should receive balance training, how to get up after falling, and should have their medication regularly reviewed for side-effects that affect balance. The review includes the need to attend to environmental saftety and preventive aids and adaptations, and also footwear worn by the patient.

Additional aids available to reduce the risk of injury from falling are hip and limb protectors. Hip protectors have been shown to reduce the risk of hip fracture when worn in institutional settings (Parkkari et al. 1998, Kannus et al. 2000). Persuading the patient to wear hip protectors when recommended can be difficult; for some they may be inappropriate and negotiating adherence can be difficult (Tracey et al. 1998). Those who do wear the hip protector have been reported as feeling more confident in completing their daily activities safely (Cameron et al. 2000).

Fear of falling is a complex concept linked to physical, social and psychological factors, and can be responsible for recurrent falls (Peterson et al. 1999, Velozo & Peterson 2001) together with loss of gait and confidence, resulting in decreased activity (Dyer et al. 1998). Risk factors have been identified as taking the wrong medication, inappropriate footwear and poor vision (Dyer et al. 1998). It should be noted, however, that multifactorial interventions with cognitively impaired individuals and people with dementia fail to reduce the risk of falling (Shaw et al. 2003). Identifying all the patient's needs can be complex and it has been suggested that assessment and care in the patient's home by a primary care professional – an occupational therapist for example – may help to reduce falls (Cumming et al. 1999). A coping strategy that can be used after a fall includes teaching the older person how to get up from the floor (Reece & Simpson 1996).

Preventing and treating falls in the older population are priorities in the political health agenda, as stated in the *NSF for Older People* (Department of Health 2001a). The literature confirms the need for a multidisciplinary approach to the assessment and planning of care over a lengthy period of time with intervention programmes, including exercise, tailored to the individual patient's needs. Care programmes of this kind have been shown to reduce the risk of falls (Province et al. 1995, Campbell et al. 1997, Gillies et al. 1999). The literature tends to focus on management of falls and reduction of risk to the patient but the patient's perspective is often missing. Information leaflets can help, such as the Department of Trade and Industry's (1999) *Avoiding Trips, Slips and Broken Hips* designed for patients, friends, neighbours, relatives and carers. The NSF urges greater involvement by patients and their families in care programmes and research evaluations. Case study 8.3 describes the management of a widower with a history of falling.

REHABILITATION

Young et al. (1999) identified a third of all people over the age of 85 years as having their lives affected by impaired mobility (more detail on mobility can be

---

Case study 8.3

Widower Albert Spencer, aged 93 years, was referred by his general practitioner to the local hospital-based falls clinic after having sustained three falls within the last 3 months. He was seen in the falls clinic within 4 weeks of the referral and assessed by the multidisciplinary team. He had been experiencing dizziness prior to falling. One fall had involved a trip on the pavement but with the other two he could not remember hitting the floor. Previously fiercely independent, refusing help from family and neighbours, he reported feeling increasingly anxious about going out and doing things for himself at home. He also suffered from diabetes and hypertension. The assessment and management strategy was devised in careful consultatation with Mr Spencer and included the following actions. The physiotherapist provided him with a walking stick, some exercises to do at home and arranged for him to visit the centre twice a week for group exercises to improve his strength and balance. The doctor reduced his medication for the management of hypertension and advised him to stop taking sedatives. He also prescribed vitamin B_{12} injections and vitamin D supplementation. The nurses monitored his blood pressure and diabetes and continued to help him with the exercises recommended by the physiotherapist. They also helped him to practise getting up from the floor without help. The occupational therapist conducted a home visit with Mr Spencer and his two sons, who both lived close by and were keen to support his wish to stay at home. Rails were installed in his hallway at home, as was a bath seat which the occupational therapist showed him how to use. A tilt-table test confirmed syncope. Therapy continued at the outpatient clinic for 8 weeks with all members of the team. Mr Spencer's general practitioner was informed of the treatment and discharge date from the outpatient clinic so that follow-up monitoring and review could continue by the primary care team.

found in Chapter 13). Rehabilitation is often classified into two types: active and maintenance rehabilitation. Active rehabilitation is advocated when the multidisciplinary team expects the patient to improve functionally, though it may not restore patients to their former level of function. Maintenance rehabilitation is provided to prevent deterioration in the patient who is unlikely to regain lost functioning. Patients with a variety of acute illnesses, such as congestive heart failure, stroke, falls or chest or urinary tract infections, can benefit from active rehabilitation. Rehabilitation may start within hours of the diagnosis or later on, depending on the stability of the patient's health in the acute phase (Oram 1997).

Bowman & Easton's (2000) review of the literature shows rehabilitation to be a complex process consisting of four types: (1) restorative rehabilitation; (2) maintenance rehabilitation; (3) adaptive and reconciliative rehabilitation; and (4) preventive rehabilitation. Restorative rehabilitation involves a comprehensive assessment of the older person and focuses on hospital and nursing home-based rehabilitative care. Maintenance rehabilitation includes exercise programmes to be used at home, reinforced with home visits. Adaptive and reconciliation rehabilitation includes provision of home adaptations and equipment and review and modification of the patient's medication.

Further discussion of rehabilitation relevant to specific conditions (problems of nutrition, elimination and mobility, for example) can be found in other chapters.

TEAMWORK

There is a plethora of terms used to describe teamwork in clinical care (multdisciplinary, multiprofessional, interdisciplinary and interprofessional teamwork). Barr (2002) points out the crucial distinction: that interprofessional learning relies on interaction, and therefore terms such as multidisciplinary and multiprofessional ('multi' meaning many) are not as positive about change as interdisciplinary and interprofessional ('inter' meaning between). This interactive, collaborative view is supported by Leathard (2003).

Within a multidisciplinary team there is often an overlap in role responsibility for clinical assessment and intervention with patients (Young et al. 1999). The nurse's role is a prime example. Physiotherapists promote mobility, for example, so that patients are able to perform tasks in everyday life. The occupational therapist encourages patients to carry out activities and, with them, works out how to cope in spite of their difficulties. The nurse's role overlaps with both. Nurses assess patients' mobility and ability to cope with daily activities, and they assess patients more broadly, including their psychological and social well-being. The overlaps between roles may duplicate the assessment and planning process unneccessarily and submit the patient to long and repetitive assessments before interventions can start.

In view of this role overlap, there has been growing interest in the development of the single assessment process and, in some cases, in introducing generic health care professionals to reduce duplication (Young et al. 1999). The idea is that the genericist will complete a broad overall assessment and the therapist will use the information collected as part of a more specialist assessment of a specific problem. It is proposed, but not yet supported by evidence, that assessments will be comprehensive and specialist but less repetitive and time-wasting for the patient. It is also proposed that generic health care workers can fulfil a range of skills that encompass nursing, physiotherapy and other therapy roles. The policy report by the NHS Modernisation Agency, *Pursuing Perfection: Raising the Bar in Healthcare* (2003), examines how teams work and whether they meet patients' needs. The examination process includes mapping the services provided and identifying service failures and underlying causes. The Modernisation Agency scrutinizes how the team works and then facilitates improvements in interdisciplinary working, so advocating a move away from multiprofessional working and changing the focus to patients and their needs. This process advocates integrated team-working, where skills are shared and coordinated by team members for the benefit of the patient. Sharing skills can be difficult for some health care professionals to accept; the blurring of boundaries between roles can cause interprofessional and intraprofessional tension (Strasser et al. 1994) through fear of loss of autonomy and status. It follows that, as highlighted by Young et al. (1999), success of this team-working initiative will depend on sensitive leadership and a process of open communication between all the members of the team so that they feel involved and part of the decision-making process.

Good teamwork goes further than just coordinating skills. It requires clear communication about goals of care and decision-making that is open and enables genuine participation by all team members who have a contribution to make, whatever their position in the hierarchy. Nurses play a key role in teamwork; they are central to the coordination of patient care. If their communication and negotiation skills are poor the patient's care and discharge plan can be hindered, especially for older people whose physical and, possibly, psychological dependence requires complex discharge plans and effective interagency working (Young et al. 1999).

DISCHARGE FROM HOSPITAL

Discharge from hospital can be preplanned and arranged with the nurse for standard procedures such as elective orthopaedic surgery and cardiac angioplasty. In these cases, patients know before admission when they will be discharged. A preadmission assessment is made in an outpatient clinic to identify potential risks and to tell the patient about the surgical procedure and subsequent care.

A recent systematic review of the literature on discharge arrangements for older people concluded that, although there is little evidence to suggest that improved arrangements have an effect on mortality or length of hospital stay, there are beneficial effects on subsequent readmission rates (Parker et al. 2002). Chapter 28 has a fuller discussion of the role of assessment and clinical teams in discharge planning.

Older people who are admitted to hospital for inpatient care are likely to be discharged to one of four destinations: their own home, an intermediate care unit, a residential care home or a nursing home (Department of Health 2001a). Some patients are discharged home with no need for aftercare from the health services or for equipment to be installed. If personal care and equipment are required, which may take time to install, these should be organized as soon as possible after admission to hospital to avoid delaying the discharge. *The NSF for Older People* (Department of Health 2001a) emphasizes the importance of completing an assessment of risk before discharge. Too often, discharge dates have to be postponed because planning and preparation and coordination with social services departments and other agencies have been inadequate.

In the event that the patient has had to wait a long time before being discharged, the hospital may offer transfer to a bed in a recovery unit in the primary care trust which will provide the care needed. These beds can be based in nursing homes or in an intermediate care centre. Some patients require longer-term care in a residential unit. This may be a residential care home, which may be indicated to maintain the safety of the older person, or an intermediate care bed may be more appropriate if restorative rehabilitation is the goal. It may be appropriate to provide extensive care at home with nurses visiting several times a day to attend to the patient's personal hygiene needs, pressure areas and medication. For patients who are very dependent and need 24-h care, discharge may be to a residential home, a nursing home or a home specializing in the care of older people with mental health needs. Further

information on intermediate and long-term institutional care is given in Chapter 9.

To monitor and support the patient through the discharge process, many hospitals have invested in discharge coordinators. Their role is to identify patients with complex discharge needs and to support staff in solving problems that may arise. Discharge coordinators will audit the discharge process, will reinforce best practice with the hospital staff and help to improve poor practice, particularly practice that delays patients' discharge from hospital.

Hospital-supported discharge

Another available service is the hospital-supported discharge team which supports the patient outside hospital even when intensive rehabilitation is required. This means that the patient can be discharged whilst also receiving skilled care, and the hospital can meet its discharge target. The team may operate from accident and emergency departments so that admission as an inpatient can be avoided and the accident and emergency departments meet their 4-h waiting-time target. If the patient is medically fit, reasonably mobile and partially independent in personal care activities, then the hospital-supported discharge team is an ideal solution for supporting the patient at home. The team consists of nurses and therapists and is available to support the patient for a short period of 4–6 weeks. If the patient cannot manage at home alone after this period, the team will arrange alternative care provision that avoids hospital admission if possible.

Rapid-response team

The rapid-response team is another service that is available for patients who need a short period of intensive care in order to avoid inpatient admission. The team is often based in the accident and emergency department and can effectively reduce the time patients are kept waiting there. The team attends to patients coming into the department who require physiotherapy or occupational therapy assessment and treatment before being deemed safe to go home. The team consists of physiotherapists, occupational therapists and sometimes a nurse. After assessment, they decide whether the patient requires specialist help in the primary care sector or basic support from the rapid-response team. Each patient would be mobile and able to carry out some self-care activities. Team members may visit the patient at home to assess the environment, complete a risk assessment and show the patient how to cope. Referral to the primary care team or social worker would follow if the patient is not coping or is deteriorating. Rapid-response teams for older people are relatively new services in the UK and have yet to be evaluated for their effectiveness.

Day hospital

Day hospitals are an important link between the acute hospital environment and the patient's own home. They provide active treatment and rehabilitation to maintain independence (Booth & Waters 1995) and they bridge the gap between the hospital and primary care services (Ames & Hastie 1995). Older people attending day hospitals are assessed by the multidisciplinary team as a day patient. Day hospital care can prevent acute hospital admission or support early discharge, though questions over their cost-effectiveness, given their small capacity, remain (National Audit Office 1994). They are staffed by nurses, physiotherapists, occupational therapists and care assistants who provide the range of treatment and care available to the acute hospital patient. Referral to the patient's general practitioner is made if medical attention is required.

CONCLUSION

With the new political agenda in the UK health service (following *The NHS Plan* and *The NSF for Older People*), implementing and managing change in services for older people is timely. Stringent guidelines and targets from the DHSC have to be met. The skills and competence of nurses are under increasing scrutiny which, together with greater participation of health service users in decision-making processes, should ensure a better quality of service. Patients are knowledgeable and demanding about the care and treatment they want and are prepared to take responsibility for their own health. Nursing in hospitals may look very different in the future given the development of shared education of health care students, the blurring of professional boundaries and continuing rapid developments in information technology. The hospital, too, may no longer exist in its current form.

Recommended reading

Creek J (ed) 1997 Occupational therapy and mental health. Churchill Livingstone, New York.
Although intended for use by occupational therapists, this book provides an insight into the assessment of older patients in the rehabilitation phase of care. The book describes various methods of assessment which can be of value to nursing.
Evans JG, Williams TF, Beattie BL, Michel J-P, Wilcock GK (eds) 2000 Geriatric medicine. Oxford University Press, Oxford.

This book provides useful information on illnesses within each physiological system and their medical management.
Fawcus R. (eds) 2000 Stroke rehabilitation: a collaborative approach. Blackwell Science, Oxford.
This book provides an overview of the management of stroke and the planning of care from a nursing perspective. The book addresses mobility and communication and how they can be managed in everyday living.
Gulanick M, Klopp A, Galanes S, Gradishar D, Puzas MK (eds) 1998 Nursing care plans: nursing diagnosis and intervention. Mosby, St Louis.
Provides information on how to individualize care plans and how to incorporate assessment findings into the plan. The care plans promote continuous assessment. The reader has access to over 50 care plans as useful illustrative examples.

References

Ames D, Hastie IR 1995 Geriatric day hospitals: the future? Postgraduate Medical Journal 71: 260–261

Anell A, Rosen P, Hjortsberg C 1997 Choice and participation in the health services: a survey of preferences among Swedish residents. Health Policy 40: 157–168

Applegate W, Blaas J, Wilhelms T 1990 Instruments for the functional assessment of older patients. New England Journal of Medicine 322: 1207–1214

Barr H 2002 Interprofessional education: today, yesterday and tomorrow. Learning and Teaching Support Network for Health Services and Practice, London

Biley FC 1992 Some determinants that affect patient participation in decision-making about nursing care. Journal of Advanced Nursing 17: 414–421

Booth J, Waters K 1995 The multi-faceted role of the nurse in the day hospital. Journal of Advanced Nursing 22: 700–706

Bowers AC, Thompson JM 1992 Clinical manual of health assessment, 4th edn. Mosby, St Louis

Bowman C, Easton P 2000 Rehabilitation in long-term care. Reviews in Clinical Gerontology 10: 75–79

Brown AP 1999 Reducing falls in elderly people: a review of exercise interventions. Physiotherapy Theory and Practice 15: 59–68

Cameron ID, Stafford B, Cumming RG et al. 2000 Hip protectors improve falls self-efficacy. Age and Ageing 29: 57–62

Campbell AJ, Robertson MC, Gardner MM et al. 1997 Randomised controlled trial of a general practice programme of home based exercise to prevent falls in elderly women. British Medical Journal 315: 1065–1069

Cegala DJ, McClure L, Marinelli TM, Post DM 2000 The effects of communication skills training on patients' participation during medical reviews. Patient Education and Counselling 41: 209–222

Crawford MJ, Rutter D, Manley C et al. 2002 Systematic review of involving patients in the planning and development of health care. British Medical Journal 325: 1263–1271

Cumming RG, Thomas M, Szonyi G et al. 1999 Home visits by an occupational therapist for assessment and modification of environmental hazards: a randomised trial of falls preventions. Journal of the American Geriatric Society 47: 1397–1402

Department of Health 2000 The NHS plan: a plan for investment, a plan for reform. Cmnd 4818-1. HMSO, London

Department of Health 2001a The national service framework for older people. HMSO, London

Department of Health 2001b The essence of care. HMSO, London

Department of Health 2001c Implementing the NHS plan – modern matrons: strengthening the role of ward sisters and introducing senior sisters. Health Service circular 2001/010. HMSO, London

Department of Health 2002 Modern matrons in the NHS: a progress report. HMSO, London

Department of Health 2003 Agenda for change. Department of Health, London

Department of Trade and Industry 1999 Avoiding slips, trips and broken hips. Department of Trade and Industry, London

Dyer CAE, Watkins CL, Gould C, Rowe J 1998 Risk-factor assessment for falls: from a written checklist to the penless clinic. Age and Ageing 27: 569–572

Ersser S, Tutton E 1991 Primary nursing in perspective. Scutari, London

Forster A, Young J, Langhome P 1999 Systematic review of day hospital care for elderly people. British Medical Journal 318: 837–841

Gillies E, Aitchison T, MacDonald J, Grant S 1999 Outcomes of a 12-week functional exercise programme for institutionalised elderly people. Physiotherapy 85: 349–356

Guest D, Redfern S, Wilson-Barnett J et al. 2001 A preliminary evaluation of the establishment of nurse, midwife and health visitor consultants. Report to the Department of Health by a team from King's College London and Birkbeck College. Management Centre, King's College, London (website: www.kcl.ac.uk/nursing/nru/nru.html)

Guest D, Redfern S, Wilson-Barnett J et al. 2003 An evaluation of a newly created job: an analysis of the introduction of nurse, midwife and health visitor consultants in the UK National Health Service. In: Hellgren J, Naswall K, Sverke M, Soderfeldt M (eds) New organizational challenges for human service work. Rainer Hampp Verlag, Munchen

Hall MRP 1976 The assessment of disability in the geriatric patient. Rheumatology and Rehabilitation 15: 279–291

Holmes-Rovner M, Llewellyn-Thomas H, Entwistle V et al. 2001 Patient choice modules for summaries of clinical effectiveness: a proposal. British Medical Journal 322: 664–667

Hu M-H, Woollacott MH 1996 Balance evaluation, training and rehabilitation of frail fallers. Reviews in Clinical Gerontology 6: 85–99

Kannus P, Parkkari J, Nieml S et al. 2000 Prevention of hip fracture in elderly people with use of a hip protector. New England Journal of Medicine 343: 1506–1513

Leathard A 2003 Interprofessional collaboration: from policy to practice in health and social care. Brunner-Routledge, Hove

Litva A, Coast J, Donovan J et al. 2002 The public is too subjective: public involvement at different levels of health-care decision making. Social Science and Medicine 54: 1825–1837

Manley K, Dewing J 2002 The consultant nurse role. NHS Journal of Healthcare Professionals May: 8–9 (available through http:www.nhsonline.net)

Melzer D, McWilliams B, Brayne C, Johnson T, Bond J 1999 Profile of disability in elderly people: estimates from a longitudinal population study. British Medical Journal 318: 1108–1111.

National Audit Office 1994 National Health Service day hospitals for elderly people in England. HMSO, London

NHS Modernisation Agency 2002 Improvement leaders' guide to involving patients and carers. Department of Health, London

NHS Modernisation Agency 2003 Pursuing perfection: raising the bar in healthcare. Department of Health, London

Oram JJ 1997 Caring for the fourth age. Armelle Press, Artegraf

Parker S, Peete S, McPherson A et al. 2002 A systematic review of discharge arrangements for older people. Health Technology Assessment 6: 1–195

Parkkari J, Heikkila J, Kannus P 1998 Acceptability and compliance with wearing energy-shunting hip protectors: a 6 month prospective followup in a Finnish nursing home. Age and Ageing 27: 225–229

Peterson E, Howland J, Kielhofner G et al. 1999 Falls self-efficacy and occupational adaptation among elders. Physical and Occupational Therapy in Geriatrics 16: 1–16

Province MS, Hadley EC, Hombrook MC et al. 1995 The effects of exercise on falls in elderly patients: a preplanned meta-analysis of the FIGSIT trials. Journal of the American Medical Association 273: 1341–1346

Read S, Ashman M, Scott M, Savage J 2004 The introduction of the modern matron role in the NHS. Available online at: http://www.shef.ac.uk/snm/research/modern_matron_evaluation.html

Redfern S, Guest D, Wilson-Barnett J et al. 2003 Role innovation in the NHS: a preliminary evaluation of the new role of nurse, midwife and health visitor consultant. In: Dopson S, Mark A (eds) Leading health care organizations. Palgrave Macmillan, Basingstoke, Hampshire, pp 153–172

Reece AC, Simpson JM 1996 Preparing older people to cope after a fall. Physiotherapy 82: 227–235

Reuben DB, Frank JC, Hirsch SH, McGuigan KA, Maly RC 1999 A randomized clinical trial of outpatient comprehensive geriatric assessment coupled with an intervention to increase adherence to recommendations. British Medical Journal 47: 269–276

Shaw FE, Bond J, Richardson DA et al. 2003 Multifactorial intervention after a fall in older people with cognitive impairment and dementia presenting to the accident and emergency department: randomised controlled trial. British Medical Journal 326: 73–75

Strasser DC, Falconer JA, Martino-Saltzmann D 1994 The rehabilitation team: staff perceptions of the hospital environment, the interdisciplinary team environment and the interprofessional relations. Archives of Physical Medicine and Rehabilitation 75: 177–181

Tracey M, Villar A, Hill P, Inskip H 1998 Will elderly rest home residents wear hip protectors? Age and Ageing 27: 195–198

Velozo CA, Peterson EW 2001 Developing meaningful fear of falling measures for community dwelling elderly.

American Journal of Physical Medicine and Rehabilitation 80: 662–673

Walker E, Dewar BJ 2001 How do we facilitate carers' involvement in decision making? Journal of Advanced Nursing 34: 329–337

Waters K 1985 Team nursing. Nursing Practice 1: 7–15

Waters KR, Easton N 1999 Individualised care: is it possible to plan and carry out? Journal of Advanced Nursing 29: 79–87

Wright SG 1990 My patient, my nurse: primary nursing in practice. Scutari, London

Young J, Brown A, Forster A, Clare J 1999 An overview of rehabilitation for older people. Reviews in Clinical Gerontology 9: 183–196

Chapter 9

Intermediate and long-term care provision for older people

Claire Goodman and Sally J. Redfern

INTRODUCTION

The move into a long-term care setting is often seen as a failure of care and a solution of last resort, the decision having been made because the older person is unable to continue living at home or the family caregiver cannot continue as before. Within our society there is a deeply rooted and widely held belief that living at home is always to be preferred to institutional care; a belief supported by a review of the literature on long-term care (Vetter 1999). Vetter reports the rates of usage of residential homes as being much lower in the UK compared with other European countries, particularly France and the Netherlands, so confirming the widespread belief of resistance to residential long-term care in this country. However, it is not always possible or appropriate to provide continuing individual support to older people in their own homes. Despite the growth in different types of provision of long-term care for older people that aim to cross the health and social care divide, many writers have observed that older people have low expectations of the health and social services that they should receive and that frequently their needs do not match what is offered (Twigg & Atkins 1994, Boaz et al. 1999). Also, their experience of care in the last years of life is often characterized by being passed between different services (Reed & Payton 1996).

Of the total population in England and Wales aged over 65, only 4% are resident in care homes, though the proportion rises progressively from age 75, with 30% of people aged over 90 resident in care settings (Wanless 2001). Changes in family circumstances that have made caring by the family more difficult, coupled with projections of the health status of the very old, a rise in dementias and neurodegenerative disorders, all contribute to recognition by policy-makers that it is essential to provide a range of care options to support people in old age. Furthermore, subsequent generations of older people are likely to have higher expectations than their predecessors of what services should be available for them and are less likely to put up with inadequate care (Wanless 2001).

This chapter considers the experience and needs of older people who are recipients of intermediate or long-term care within care homes that offer nursing care and/or residential care. The chapter includes a review of policy on intermediate and long-term care provision for older people in the UK, a discussion of why institutional care is viewed with such suspicion, what kinds of long-term provision are available to older people, their known health needs, a brief look at assessment in long-term care and a discussion of changes in nursing, particularly with respect to nurse-led units and new roles in nursing.

THE POLICY CONTEXT OF INTERMEDIATE AND LONG-TERM CARE

Two reviews of the history of long-term care in the UK argue powerfully that the economic imperative has been a significant factor in determining its provision (Stanley & Reed 1999, Vetter 1999). Stanley & Reed highlight how labour-intensive and expensive residential care is and that, despite a lack of evidence, the policy argument has consistently been that non-institutional alternatives are cheaper and better.

Care provision in institutional settings for older people in the UK has been actively discouraged by policy initiatives from the late 1980s. Increasing the availability of alternative forms of care outside the nursing home has become common in other European countries too, such as Belgium, Denmark, Germany and the Netherlands (Meijer et al. 2000). In the UK, the Care in the Community reforms emphasized that older people should be supported in their own homes whenever possible (Department of Health 1989). For situations where this was not possible or appropriate, the National Health Service (NHS) and Community Care Act (Department of Health 1990) introduced a contracting system whereby social services departments were given the responsibility of purchasing packages of care from a range of providers that included private, voluntary and statutory services. In effect, these changes reduced the state's involvement in the management of long-term care services and diverted responsibility for funding and capital investment to the private and voluntary sectors (Stanley & Reed 1999). Furthermore, the funding arrangements that developed as a result of the Act introduced eligibility criteria based on dependency measurement

scores. As a result, the decision to enter long-term care became inextricably linked to advanced physical and/or mental frailty and older people in care homes are significantly more frail and vulnerable than had been the situation before the Act. Several commentators have observed that an indirect consequence of these changes is that admission to long-term care is, for many older people, precipitated by crisis when family and statutory services are unable to sustain support in the community (Reed & Payton 1996, Victor 1997). Research too has identified admission to long-term care as a stressful event for an older person's family and carers, accompanied by feelings of regret and ambivalence (Nolan & Dellasega 1999). This set of circumstances militates against the decision to enter long-term care ever being seen as a positive and life-affirming choice for the older person.

A recent development that has sought to prolong the ability of older people to stay in their homes or to be discharged from hospital with intensive time-limited support to ensure they are then able to regain their independence at home is intermediate care.

INTERMEDIATE CARE

The policy interest in intermediate care highlights two areas of concern. First, that schemes that enable older people to remain or return to being independent and active in their own homes are preferable to institutional alternatives and secondly, that access to hospital services is delayed because of avoidable admission and delayed discharge of older people. It is delayed discharge, often termed 'bed-blocking' – a derogatory label that blames the older person, not the service – that most commentators agree has been the impetus for the recent initiatives in intermediate care (Pollock 2000, Thomas & MacMahon 2001). Despite the ageing population in the UK, combined with older people being the main users of hospital services, there has been a steady and dramatic reduction in the number of hospital beds. One report states that two-thirds of hospital beds are occupied by people over 65 and suggests that, of these, at least 20% could be provided with alternative care, in other words, care that is closer to home and based within the local community (Department of Health 2001a). This Department of Health circular promoting intermediate care, coupled with publication of the *National Service Framework for Older People* in 2001 (Department of Health 2001b), has brought intermediate care into mainstream health policy (Gentles & Potter 2001).

As many writers have observed, intermediate care is not a new concept (Steiner & Vaughan 1996, Cornes & Clough 2000). However, central government (Department of Health 2001a) has attempted to introduce a clear and consistent approach for health and local-authority services by establishing five criteria for defining intermediate care. These criteria expand the description of intermediate care provided in *The NHS Plan* (Department of Health 2000b) and the *National Service Framework for Older People* (Department of Health 2001b) that emphasize promotion of independence, prevention of hospital or care-home admission and intermediate care as a targeted and intervention-based service. When reporting investment and activity in this area of work, only those services that meet *all* the criteria will be regarded as providing intermediate care. The five criteria for services are those that:

1. are targeted at people who would otherwise face unnecessarily prolonged hospital admission or inappropriate admission to acute inpatient care, long-term residential care or continuing NHS inpatient care
2. are provided on the basis of a comprehensive assessment, resulting in a structured individual care plan that involves active therapy, treatment or opportunity for recovery
3. have a planned outcome of maximizing independence and typically enabling patients/ users to resume living at home
4. are time-limited, normally no longer than 6 weeks and frequently as little as 1 or 2 weeks or less
5. involve cross-professional working, with a single assessment framework, single professional records and shared-care protocols.

Within this guidance is an explicit statement about the voluntary sector's contribution to intermediate care, an indication of increasing policy recognition that statutory services alone cannot provide continuing care for older people. The suggested input for voluntary services includes acting as a support to statutory services in helping older people regain confidence as part of their rehabilitation, providing social support or taking up a residual care role as an intermediate care episode ends.

Intermediate care: negotiating the health and social care divide

Lewis (2001), in a review of health and social care policy over the last 50 years, highlights how the particularly sharp divide between health and social care provision that exists in the UK has affected older people with non-acute or intermediate care needs. Their needs, she suggests, have consistently been

rationed, ignored or treated inappropriately by both sides of the 'boundary'. Even with the greater emphasis on partnership and increased funding for intermediate care services within government policy (Department of Health 1998, 2000b), Lewis suggests there are still many issues to resolve, not least what kind of care should be provided for this group of older people. It is not clear whether intermediate care, as described in policy documents, fully recognizes the needs of a group which does not easily fit with the existing health and social care services, or whether intermediate care is a compensation and replacement strategy for diminished and inadequate hospital and residential provision as well as community nursing services, and so is a relocation of services rather than a new development. Similarly, MacMahon (2001) considers whether intermediate care represents a reduction of access to assessment and relevant expertise for older people, and so is, in fact, a euphemism for indeterminate care. Pollock (2000) expresses concern that some aspects of intermediate care policy, including the increasing involvement of the private sector, reduce rather than enhance individuals' access to appropriate health care. It is acknowledged that there are unmet needs for older people and that attempts to address this through intermediate care strategies are necessary, but questions persist as to whether what is offered is sufficient. Are intermediate care services patient- or organization-focused and is intermediate care rehabilitation by another name? It is not clear which services are best for which patient, which professionals should be involved or how known differences in assessment and care should be resolved (Twigg 1997, Griffiths 1998, Worth 2001). A recent review of the literature highlights the lack of detailed knowledge on the value of intermediate care for residents of care homes and refers to a scathing attack of the concept of intermediate care by two leading geriatricians in the UK (Thompson & Crome 2001).

Approaches to intermediate care

Steiner (2001), in an overview of intermediate care services, suggests that most are supportive rather than directive, that care is emphasized more than cure and that nursing predominates. There are several distinctive approaches to intermediate care, some of which have been well documented in the literature. These include projects designed to provide extra social support to avoid admission to institutional care (Challis 1994) or rapid-response teams that aim to give intensive nursing support at home to avert an acute hospital admission

(Thomas 1999) or teams that provide extra support for a time-limited period for older people recently discharged from hospital (Townsend 1994). Hyde et al.'s (2000) review of research into supporting discharge of people from hospital to home argues that there is sufficient evidence to suggest that the approach is valid but they also recommend further research.

Intermediate care can also encompass those services provided between home and hospital that offer rehabilitation for older people. The *National Service Framework for Older People* identifies care homes that offer residential care as important providers in the development of intermediate care services to reduce hospital admissions and facilitate discharge from acute services (Department of Health 2000b, 2001b). Nursing-led units are another example of care provided between acute hospital care and care at home. Evaluation of nursing-led care against conventional services suggests that, whilst there are some measurable benefits, the cost benefits and how the service is integrated within the wider health service need further research (Richardson et al. 2001, Wiles et al. 2001). Richardson's group conducted a randomized controlled trial to compare a nursing-led inpatient intermediate care unit for older people with matched patients who received usual hospital care (Griffiths et al. 2000). They found no difference between the groups in functional dependence at discharge, though there was a significant difference in length of stay: the patients in the usual-care group stayed in hospital for a shorter time than the experimental group but the same number in both groups were in hospital 90 days after recruitment to the study because of readmissions. The nursing-led unit's strategy of longer patient stays may have been effective, therefore, in avoiding the need for readmission. As the authors conclude, the nursing-led inpatient unit provides a potentially viable alternative to acute hospital care for patients in the recovery phase of illness, and it may also substitute for a period of primary care.

There does not appear to be significant literature that examines the older person and carers' experiences of being recipients of intermediate care services, its process and perceived outcomes. Within a policy culture of collaborative and public, private and voluntary alliances, little is known as to how the different services interpret their roles and responsibilities within intermediate care and what this kind of care means for the recipients. There is, though, recognition that the need to engage older people in developing both services for them and research about them is key and that their experiences, perspectives and priorities should be the knowledge base that informs service delivery and the focus of studies into their needs

(Hope and Older People & Help the Aged 2000, Owen & Harding 2000).

LONG-TERM CARE FOR OLDER PEOPLE

Concerns over the costs of long-term care and that some care homes might not be fit to cater for very frail and highly dependent people led to the establishment in 1997 of a Royal Commission on long-term care chaired by Sir Stuart Sutherland (Royal Commission on the Funding of Long-Term Care 1999). The aim of the Commission was to examine the short-term and long-term options for a sustainable system of funding of long-term care for older people both in their own homes and in other settings. The Commission's principal recommendation was that nursing and personal care should be centrally funded for anyone needing long-term support but that accommodation and food costs should continue to be means-tested. It was also recommended that nurses should be more involved than in the past in assessments for entry to care homes. The Commission's report was well received but the key message that care should be centrally funded was diminished by a minority report from two dissenters who argued that central funding for personal care would do little to improve the quality of care in the majority of care homes and that resources would be better spent on developing intermediate care services. The government's response in England was to accept the minority proposal that only nursing care supervised by a registered nurse should be free at the point of delivery and that charges for personal care should continue to be means-tested along with accommodation costs. Older people in long-term care settings in England now have their need for nursing care assessed by a nurse within three predetermined funding bands that reflect the level of demand on nursing time. In England, the NHS pays a contribution towards the nursing care that assessors determine needs to be provided by a registered nurse in a nursing home. From April 2005 the payment was set at £40.00, £80.00, or £129.00 per week, according to nursing need assessed as low, medium or high, respectively. This contribution applies whether care is funded privately or by the local authority. The Registered Nursing Care Contribution (RNCC) tool, that was partly derived from an instrument developed by the Royal College of Nursing as a standardized assessment tool for older people, has as its assessment criteria the level of complexity of care required, the predictability of care, the stability of the older person and the degree of risk (Department of Health 2001c). By contrast, the Scottish parliament has not opted for a banding system of payment. The Scottish Executive announced its intention to provide free personal and nursing care for older people from April 2002. It has proposed a flat rate of £145 per week for personal care, plus £65 per week for those assessed as needing nursing care, and the Welsh National Assembly has introduced a flat-rate contribution of £100 per week (at 2003 prices).

Changes in care-homes regulation

In April 2002, the Care Standards Act (Department of Health 2001c) replaced the Registered Homes Act 1984 as the legal framework for the regulation of care services in care homes in England and Wales. The Act makes no distinction in registration between residential and nursing homes, stating under section 3 that an establishment is a care home if it provides accommodation together with nursing and/or personal care. Laing & Buisson (2000) argue that this creates a more flexible regulatory regime in which it is possible to vary regulatory requirements (in particular (registered) nurse staffing levels) according to residents' assessed needs. The National Care Standards Commission (NCSC) was also established within the Care Standards Act as an independent regulatory body for social care and private and voluntary health care agencies, so replacing local councils and health authorities as the former regulators (Department of Health 2001c). Section 23 (1) of the Act has paved the way for the development of national minimum standards in care homes for older people. Standard 8 is of particular relevance to nursing, stating that 'the registered person promotes and maintains service users' health and ensures access to health care services to meet assessed needs', the outcome of the standard being that service users' health care needs are fully met (Department of Health 2001b: p. 9). It is hoped that these changes will encourage the development of outcome measures that are specific to the health needs of older people in long-term care settings (Hartley 1999, Royal College of Physicians, Royal College of Nursing, British Geriatrics Society 2001). Such is the rate of policy change in this sector of health and social care regulation that in April 2004 the Care Standards Commission merged with the Social Services Inspectorate to form the Commission for Social Care Inspection (CSCI). The Commission carries out local inspections of all social care organizations, public, private and voluntary, against national standards. The review and inspection of the independent health care sector for which the NCSC took responsibility has been absorbed by the Health Care Commission that also came into being in April 2004 (formerly known as the Commission for Health Care, Audit and Inspection, CHAI).

A legacy of suspicion

A significant and influential literature highlights the negative, controlling and often dehumanizing consequences of institutional care that can be traced back to the work of Goffman (1961). Many studies have detailed the loss of privacy and enforced dependency and routinized care characteristic of long-term settings for older people that reflect decades of concern about dysfunctional care (for example: Wilkins & Hughes 1987, Willcocks et al. 1987, Victor 1994, Koch & Webb 1996, Black & Bowman 1997). However, Stanley & Reed (1999) challenge what they see as an oversimplified view that institutional care exercises a uniform and inevitably debilitating power on residents. They argue that much of the research into institutional care has isolated care from its wider social context. Particularly for older people, it is not institutional or long-term care itself that causes poor care but rather the prevailing social and professional beliefs and attitudes about older people who happen to need extra support that shapes the care received. Stanley & Reed demonstrate the therapeutic and life-affirming contribution that care in these settings can and should achieve and provide an understanding of why it is that care workers and nurses perpetuate practices that do not enable nor empower the older person. Some nurses have, however, responded to this perplexing question by developing new practices in nursing development units and nurse-led units and new roles in nursing (see section below on changes in nursing). Others have introduced new practices into existing settings for older people, such as incorporating a biographical approach to care in which care workers use individuals' life stories as a basis for planning their care (Clarke et al. 2003). Kitwood's (1997) work and research with people who suffer from dementia who often require long-term care has demonstrated persuasively what can be achieved when the culture and approach to care alter and the person becomes the focus of care (see Chapter 24 for more information on dementia and its care, including Kitwood's contribution).

It is important to look at quality of care for older people in continuing care settings alongside the quality of working life for the staff working in them. Research in the early 1990s demonstrated the value of small-scale NHS-managed residential units, known as domus units, for continuing care of mentally frail older people who had been living in hospital psychogeriatric wards (Lindesay et al. 1991). The authors found that by paying attention to the needs of front-line care staff, care was of good quality and the well-being of residents as well as staff was high. However, a more recent review of the literature found very little research in continuing care settings for older people (nursing homes, residential homes and long-stay wards) that links perceptions of workers with the quality of care and outcome for residents (Hannan et al. 2001). Research that has been done shows equivocal results: some studies found that worker satisfaction is positively related and worker stress is negatively related to quality of care and well-being of residents, but other studies did not. A subsequent empirical study in one nursing home in London, by the same research group, found that the more satisfied and committed and the less stressed the care staff were, the higher was the quality of care and well-being for residents (Redfern et al. 2002). This was just one small study, however, and more research that uses multimethods and that triangulates data from many sources is needed.

LONG-TERM CARE PROVISION FOR OLDER PEOPLE

In England, the majority of care homes for older people offer only residential and personal care and, of these, 90% are provided by the independent sector (i.e. voluntary, private and small homes; Department of Health 2000a). In 2001 there were 341 200 places in homes offering residential care (Office of National Statistics 2001). The total number of residential homes and residential home places for all client groups stood at 24 800 homes and 346 000 places in England at 31 March 2000, although geographical variation is wide (Department of Health 2000a). A total of 12 200 homes were for older people (excluding older mentally infirm people), for whom there were 240 300 places.

In addition to these mainstream kinds of long-term care provision are sheltered and warden-controlled housing that provide a degree of on-site support and protection for older residents but ensure that they are able to maintain their independence within their own home. Multilevel care facilities are also becoming more popular where older people can remain in the same locality as their needs increase.

Sheltered housing

Research done in the 1980s found that older people prefer sheltered housing to residential care if they cannot look after themselves at home (Sinclair 1988). More recently, it has been confirmed that poor health is the most commonly reported reason for moving to sheltered housing followed by the related reason of their

home no longer being suitable (e.g. stairs), and because they want access to a warden or alarm system should the need arise (Field et al. 2002). A study in Quebec, Canada confirmed the positive effect of an alarm system on feelings of security by tenants (Proulx 1999). However, a UK study in the 1990s into life in sheltered housing from the tenants' point of view revealed some perceptions to be as negative as those expressed by residents in care homes (Percival 1996). Percival found that most of the tenants living in a local-authority sheltered-housing scheme in London had little choice about the move to sheltered housing and its timing. When they got there they found that social mores existed with respect to perceived invasion of one's privacy and socializing with other tenants, and disapproval was apparent if these were transgressed. The warden's role was crucial in influencing the atmosphere in which social contacts took place. Even then – in the 1990s – the 'workhouse' was a term quite often used to describe sheltered housing because the 'warden' title seemed to suggest a controlled, institutional environment, and living with other people conjured up a workhouse image. Percival notes how important it is to keep long-standing friendships with older people living outside the sheltered-housing scheme. Morale was high when social contacts in the surrounding locality were numerous. This finding has been supported by Field et al.'s (2002) more recent work which reported that residents with locally integrated social networks were less likely than those with a private network to be physically inactive or to report often being lonely. Field's group revealed that most tenants said they were happy living in sheltered housing and only a minority expressed unhappiness or loneliness.

Autonomy is important to tenants. Percival's tenants wanted freedom to be independent and to make their own choices without fear of recrimination, whereas the warden, they felt, tended to overemphasize the need for a safe, secure and protected environment. It is not always easy to strike the right balance between tenants respecting another's need for privacy and being friendly and offering help. The would-be helper may be accused of prying into personal affairs. Yet, at times, tenants complained that other tenants who could have helped did not.

Very little research has been found on older people from ethnic minorities living in sheltered housing. A study of black British, Afro-Caribbean and Chinese older people who were diagnosed as suffering from dementia or depression and were living in sheltered housing in Liverpool reported evidence of violence by tenants towards wardens, wandering and neglect of rooms (Boneham et al. 1997). Implications for service providers were reported to be considerable, especially the need to work closely with ethnic-minority groups in order to reduce feelings of mistrust and increase cultural sensitivity in the services provided.

There has been a long-running debate over the last 25 years on the value of sheltered housing. Proponents see it as the answer to the accommodation needs of people who need some support. Opponents think the scheme was badly thought-out and overprovided, with the result that there are now many 'difficult-to-let' sheltered-housing flats (Clapham 1997). Clapham refers to Tinker et al.'s (1995) finding that 8% of local authorities and 14% of housing associations in England and Wales have difficulty letting half their sheltered-housing stock. Reasons include overprovision, poorly maintained schemes, concentration in areas of deprivation and poverty, and lack of what are deemed these days to be essential amenities (e.g. lift access, personal bathrooms). The community care reforms of the 1990s have also had an impact in that older people can choose to stay at home and have their housing and care needs met there.

Some housing agencies now allocate sheltered flats to people with needs other than older people, such as young homeless people or people with mental health problems. This practice may not suit older tenants. Other agencies have converted their schemes into 'very sheltered' or 'extra-care' housing, so bringing care provision closer to the concept of the residential care home with independent living units. Some schemes have extended the services offered to the community: for example, by extending the warden service, running preventive health care programmes such as music and movement classes, or basing the home-care team in a sheltered-housing location (Clapham 1997). Others have not, with tenants objecting to community use of 'their' facilities, just as residents object to extension of services offered by their residential homes to the wider community (Wright 1994).

The Tinker report (Tinker et al. 1995) recommends that, to be successful, sheltered-housing schemes should be audited regularly, should assess the needs of tenants and others, and should consult tenants. A fundamental weakness of the sheltered-housing model is that it is not necessarily the most cost-effective way of meeting needs. Critics want a radical change that ensures more flexible links between housing, support and care to meet people's changing needs. This would require housing agencies to become full partners with social services departments in the strategic planning process as well as in implementation.

Multilevel care settings

Increasingly, policy-makers have begun to engage with the need to develop a range of housing initiatives that can cater for an ageing population, can address both health and social care needs and can ensure stability for residents and continuity of care. Many initiatives have drawn on North American models of care (provision of retirement villages and multilevel care facilities that cover all levels of dependency in one setting) and are designed to ensure that, once the older person has moved to live within one of these schemes, there is no need to move again if their needs for care and support increase with advancing years. Thus, the older person is able to own a home and have guaranteed access to services on site, such as help with personal care and domestic tasks, podiatry and social activities. There is also access to 24-h nursing support that is either provided by a visiting nursing team or in a nursing home that is on the same site as the independent-living units. The UK government has provided funding for initiatives such as these under its supported housing scheme and 'extra-care' initiative that encourages local government authorities and housing associations to work together to achieve integrated provision. In 2003 the Department of Health committed £87 million to increase the development of extra-care housing so enabling older people to stay in specialist forms of housing that include 24-h support from health and social care teams as well as other communal amenities. It is envisaged that the extra care could be achieved through a remodelling of sheltered housing and residential care homes and through partnership funding with the voluntary and private sectors (Department of Health 2003). Charities such as the Joseph Rowntree Foundation have also pioneered the development of villages for older people that ensure that the residents can retire independent and healthy to their own homes, confident that should they need further help and support in the future there will be no need to move, or be separated from their partners or experience unexpected financial costs for care and support (Joseph Rowntree Foundation 2003). These initiatives reflect a move towards an integration of health and social care, and public and private funding for older people. Nevertheless, current provision for the very old still relies on care-home settings.

This first half of the chapter has discussed the kind of provision that is available to older people in need of extra support. The second half considers the literature on older people's experience of the move into care, the range of health needs that older people in long-term care have and their access to health care. Assessment of older people in long-term care is mentioned only briefly because it is the subject of another chapter (Chapter 28). This chapter ends with a discussion of changes in nursing, specifically developments in nurse-led units and nursing roles (Figs 9.1 and 9.2).

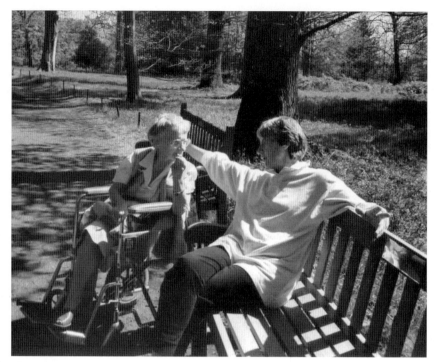

Fig. 9.1   Enjoying the spring.

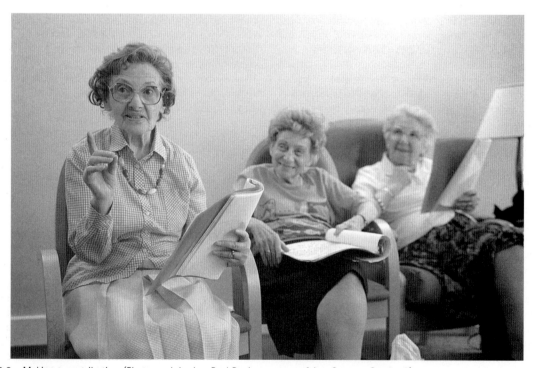

Fig. 9.2   Making a contribution. (Photograph by Jon-Paul Davis, courtesy of Age Concern Scotland.)

The move into residential care

Considerable evidence confirms that admission to residential care is often precipitated by a sudden crisis or psychological factors such as loneliness, grief or the lack of companionship that might follow bereavement (Allen et al. 1992, Warburton 1994, Burholt 1998, Lee et al. 2002). In particular, the fear of moving into an 'institution' or the lack of involvement older people have had in the decision-making process can constitute a threat to an older person's sense of individuality (Peace et al. 1997). Morgan et al. (1997) suggest that older people who perceive the process of relocation to a care home as stressful are at risk of developing either physical illness or negative psychosocial states. The focus of nursing research in this area, therefore, has been on the importance of involving and providing continuity of care for the older person and carer(s) during the transition period and on the maintenance of a sense of self. Hunter et al. (1993) suggested that district nurses and community psychiatric nurses might be best placed to engage older people and their carers in discussions about their care options. Reed & Morgan (1999) interviewed 20 older people and 17 of their family members following discharge from hospital to a care home. They found that few people had been offered opportunities to discuss their move with nurses and that older people tended to adopt a stoical attitude. Nolan et al. (1996), Reed & Payton (1996) and Reed & Morgan (1999) suggest how nurses might facilitate such discussion as well as support older people and their carers through the process of adapting to their new environment. Lee et al. (2002) reviewed 30 years of research into older people's experiences of residential care placement and concluded that, although there is information on the transition to care, little is known about how older people, and particularly those from different ethnic backgrounds, come to terms with residential life. This area of research draws attention to the issues that might face older people prior to, during or following a move to residential care and suggests that nurses are appropriately placed to undertake sensitive interventions.

A Department of Health-funded longitudinal study of residential and nursing-home care followed 2544 people from 18 authorities admitted to a home between October 1995 and January 1996. At 30 months they found that 67% had died and 8% of the original sample had left the care-home setting. Nursing-home residents (46%) were generally more dependent on admission than those admitted to residential care. The average survival times from the time of admission were 10.5 months for those in nursing-home care, and 25 months for those in residential care. A third of nursing-home residents died in the first 3 months after admission. Factors affecting subsequent mortality, in order of size of effect, were: a cancer diagnosis; high dependency score (measured on the Barthel index); male gender; admission to a nursing-home bed; admission from hospital as opposed to a private residence; and respiratory disease. Interestingly, dementia, cardiovascular disease, stroke illness and incontinence had little impact on the mortality rate (Bebbington et al. 1999).

A review by Smith & Crome (2000) examined the possible psychosocial factors that affect subsequent health of older people following admission to long-term care. They reviewed 40 years of resettlement literature, and focused on the debate surrounding mortality of residents post-relocation, variously termed 'relocation stress', 'transplantation shock', 'transfer trauma' and 'pure relocation'. They found that evidence for a causative link between relocation and mortality is equivocal and contradictory partly because of methodological and measurement limitations in the research studies reviewed. They concluded that mortality after relocation depends on the transfer process, specifically preparation for it and the degree of environmental change, as well as the health of the person transferred. People with physical or mental impairment who receive no preparation for the transfer before being relocated are at risk of death or decline in their mental health status after transfer to a care home. It follows that, the more people are involved in the relocation decision and perceive the transfer process and new environment to be within their control, the better the outcome post-relocation. Smith & Crome also highlight the lack of knowledge of how families, carers and staff cope with relocation of older people, particularly when their location experience is a negative one and the person declines in health or dies. These authors point to the need for more research and analysis into these questions and also into ethnic and class differences in the relocation experience. As we concluded earlier, nurses are well placed to take the lead in improving the relocation experience for older people and their families.

HEALTH NEEDS OF OLDER PEOPLE IN LONG-TERM CARE SETTINGS

Physical health needs

Older people resident in care homes have a range of systemic health problems, including non-stroke cardiovascular disorder, rheumatological diseases, dementia, stroke illness and neurodegenerative disease (Challis et al. 2000, Royal College of Physicians, Royal College of Nursing, British Geriatrics Society 2001). However most research has focused on the prevalence and management of specific health needs such as continence (Peet et al. 1995, 1996), infection (Yates et al. 1999), pressure sores (Shiels & Roe 1999), hip fracture (Butler et al. 1996, Norton et al. 1999), dental health (Lall 1999), diabetes (Taylor & Hendra 2000), visual problems (Sturgess et al 1994), hearing impairment (Stumer et al. 1996) and terminal care (Komaromy et al. 2000). All these conditions are responsive to good nursing, as demonstrated in other chapters of this book (for example: Chapter 11 on hearing, Chapter 12 on sight, Chapter 17 on elimination, Chapter 19 on maintaining healthy skin and Chapter 26 on terminal care). It is difficult to generalize from the few research studies done because they have been based on small samples, have not all been carried out in the UK or do not distinguish between residential—and nursing-home populations. Nevertheless, they indicate that prevailing health needs are inconsistently managed and could be improved by nurses supporting and collaborating with care assistants who provide most of the direct care. For example, two separate surveys by Peet et al. (1995) ($n = 6079$) and Roe & Shiels (2000) ($n = 652$) found that about a third of residents from residential homes had a problem with urinary and/or faecal incontinence. Eighty-seven per cent of homes in the Peet survey (Peet et al. 1996) reported using continence aids and appliances. Both studies claimed that in only two-thirds of the homes was promotion or management of continence adequate.

A study in nursing homes in the Netherlands found that health professionals do not do enough to encourage autonomy (self-determination, independence and self-care) in stroke patients to promote recovery (Proot et al. 2000).

Mental health needs

High levels and comorbidity of cognitive impairment, depression, dementia and behavioural problems have been identified by several care-home-based studies (Jagger & Lindesay 1997, Medical Research Council Cognitive Function and Ageing Study 1999, Godlove Mozley et al. 2000). Jagger & Lindesay (1997) found that, in a population of 6079 people living in different types of residential facilities, 38% were moderately or severely cognitively impaired and behavioural problems were present in 12%. The research conducted by Challis and colleagues (Godlove Mozley et al. 2000) identified clinically significant cognitive impairment in 61% of new admissions to the 18 residential homes in their sample, and nearly 45% were classified as 'depression cases'. Comorbidity of cognitive impairment and depression was found in 24% of the residents

and a correlation was found between cognitive impairment and increased dependency, depression and reduced mobility, and between depression and lower social class. Depression, in particular, has been identified as a major health threat for older people in residential homes (Ames 1990). However, it has been argued that an awareness of depressive disorders in this population is poor and symptoms of depression often go unrecognized by care staff (Bagley et al. 2000). The evidence suggests that mental health conditions are common, that they may mask other physical problems such as pain, are a challenge for assessment and indicate a need for specialist expertise for this population (Godlove Mozley et al. 2000, Royal College of Physicians, Royal College of Nursing, British Geriatrics Society 2001). Chapters 24 and 25 provide further information on care of older people with dementia and depression respectively.

Palliative-care needs

Long-term care settings are places where many older people die. Although less than 15% of older people in care homes die of a terminal disease such as cancer, many more die following a period of slow deterioration and, although it cannot be assumed that all people who die in care homes have the same care needs, there is a growing need to develop and support palliative care in these settings (Katz et al. 2000, Froggatt & Hoult 2002). Demands for care-home places for older people who are dying will continue to increase as health and care policy discourages long-stay hospital provision and hospices begin to refer patients to care homes as their focus shifts to short-term crisis intervention and the provision of care in the last days of life (Field & Froggatt 2003). However, unlike hospices, the philosophy of many care homes does not necessarily incorporate preparing residents for death, training staff in palliative-care skills or even how to manage older people with chronic conditions (Katz & Peace 2003).

As has already been shown, the need for palliative care and support in this population is compounded by the presence of other conditions. This has implications for palliative care. Studies of dying patients (not in care-home settings) with dementia have identified the following symptoms as common: pain, dyspnoea, urinary incontinence, low mood, constipation and loss of appetite. In particular, the management of pain for people with dementia is often inadequately assessed and managed even when individuals are suffering from illnesses that are potentially painful (Cooke et al. 1999). Cooke's group reported that dementia patients saw their general practitioners (family doctors) less often than cancer patients did, even though those dying from dementia had comparable symptoms and health care needs (Lloyd-Williams 1996, McCarthy et al. 1997, Lefebvre-Chapiro 2001, Albinsson & Strang 2002). Care homes which do not have on-site nursing support but are looking after older people who are dying are therefore likely to encounter a complex range of resident needs that could benefit from palliative-care nursing support. Exploratory work on district nursing experiences of providing palliative-care support to residential care homes indicates that, despite a strong professional commitment to providing this kind of care, actual provision is erratic and constrained by confusion over what constitutes nursing and personal care and when care-home managers identify the need for nursing support (Goodman et al. 2003b).

Empirical studies on palliative care and older people in care homes have concentrated on nursing homes or studied both types of care homes without distinguishing clearly between the two. They discuss the process of care within the homes, the constraints to care that arise from the physical environment, limited resources, care staff's need for continuing educational support and the contribution of specialist intervention to enhance care for older people (Patterson et al. 1997, Avis et al. 1999, Katz et al. 2000, Komaromy et al. 2000, Casarett et al. 2001, Froggatt et al. 2002). The particular care needs of older people, such as pain management, staff attitudes to palliative care and how staff and older people in these settings engage with end-of-life decisions, have also been discussed (Gibbs 1995, Cohen et al. 2002, Travis et al. 2002). There is a consensus that palliative care in care-home settings needs more recognition, investment and practice development that is organized within the care-home setting. Komaromy et al. (2000) found that, although care-home staff were committed to providing high-quality terminal care for residents, barriers to good practice included staff shortage, a lack of knowledge of palliative care and the restricted physical layout of the home.

Intervention–based studies

A few intervention studies have targeted the specific needs of older people living in long-term care settings with varying degrees of success. These have included evaluation of specialist outreach teams introduced into care homes to improve the quality of resident–staff interaction and residents' mental health (Proctor et al. 1999). Two randomized controlled trials in residential care homes that had introduced exercise promotion and falls prevention interventions showed improvement in their intervention groups in the short term (McMurdo & Rennie 1994, McMurdo et al. 2000). One study however, described the introduction of an oral health training programme for care staff and concluded that, despite evidence of need and an increase in care staff knowledge, actual oral care did not improve 1 week or 1 year after the intervention (Simons et al. 2000). In contrast to experimental and before-and-after evaluation designs, other intervention studies have focused on specific conditions such as depression or behavioural difficulties and have aimed to raise staff awareness. For example, Ames (1990) attempted to evaluate treatment of depression among older residents of 12 residential homes. Psychiatric interventions proved to be difficult to implement and there was no evidence to suggest efficacy of the interventions at 3 months or after 1 year. Llewellyn-Jones et al.'s (1999) randomized controlled trial evaluated the effectiveness of a population-based multifaceted shared-care intervention for late-life depression in residential care. Although their methods have been criticized (Cameron 2000, Hawe 2000), they claim a significantly greater movement to 'less depressed' levels of depression at follow-up in the intervention group than in the control group.

It is likely that many intervention studies have underestimated the effects of the culture of a care home on the uptake of innovation or have not addressed the challenges care homes face when seeking to develop the skills of their staff (Bland 1999). It is unusual for care homes to have a training budget and care-home staff, as an underpaid, often transient and undervalued workforce, do not necessarily find intrinsic value in training (Goodman et al. 2003c, Sidell 2003). It is also difficult for care-home staff to attend training and education programmes when limited staff numbers, particularly of nursing staff in nursing homes, mean that there are few opportunities for paid absences from work (Field & Froggatt 2003).

One study that aimed to work with care-home staff describes the preliminary findings of a partnership project where a project nurse using an action research approach was able to work with care-home staff to review training and development needs and inform the commissioning of education and services (Meehan et al. 2002). The authors describe a range of new initiatives that arose because of the partnership approach but did not discuss the implications of the changes for the older people. All the intervention studies reviewed relied on extra researchers or specialists to implement the intervention, and follow up the interventions for a year or less, and they did not consider how existing health care services (and primary care nursing services in particular) could be used to sustain change in these settings. To be able to address the health needs of older people in long-term care settings that are outside hospital, it is important to understand how older people gain access to their health care and how primary health care services support this population.

Assessment of older people in long-term care settings

Chapter 28 of this volume contains a comprehensive discussion of assessment and care planning for older people, including reference to policy guidance on assessment in the *National Service Framework for Older People* (Department of Health 2001b). We recommend that chapter to readers and here, we confine ourselves to a few points about research on the benefits of assessment for long-term care of older people.

The benefits of systematic comprehensive assessment of older people is reasonably well established, with systematic reviews and meta-analysis demonstrating that it is effective in combination with long-term management in improving survival and function and avoiding hospital admissions (Stuck et al. 2002, Wells et al. 2003). However, there is little research on the assessment of older people in long-term care settings that considers the benefits of assessment on long-term outcomes for this population. What research there has been has tended to focus on assessing older people's levels of dependency and function at time of admission to long-term care rather than as the means by which care is planned, monitored and evaluated (Challis et al. 2000). Stewart et al. (1999) reviewed assessment documentation for social care and found that activities of daily living were covered to some extent in the majority of documents. However, very few documents were designed to elicit information on the potential for rehabilitation. In the UK, the introduction of the single assessment process (Department of Health 2001b) has been designed to encourage collaborative working between health and social care practitioners and ensure that older people are not subjected to multiple assessments that duplicate information. The care-home setting is one that would be likely to benefit from such an approach.

Access to health care from long-term settings

The move to shorter hospital stays has led to an increase in availability of health care services to care homes in many western countries (Välimäki et al. 2001, Goodman & Woolley 2004). A national survey of access to NHS services by older people living in care homes in England found that as a condition of their registration all care homes have medical cover from general practitioners and almost all care homes have access to district nursing services (Jacobs et al. 2001). However, access to specialist nursing support and therapy services was reported to be limited and the frequency of contact care homes have with all these services is highly variable. This variability and apparent confusion surrounding what services are available to older people in care homes caused Jacobs' group to conclude that there are real concerns about how services are funded and the resultant inequities for older people in care homes.

Since 1992, the number of district nursing contacts in care homes offering residential care has risen by 13%, even though actual numbers of older people in residential care are not increasing at an equivalent rate. Older people in care homes consistently account for about 7% of all district nurse contacts, and the proportion of this population being seen by district nurses is rising as the average age of the resident rises (Audit Commission 1999). Little is known about the kind of nursing support that residential care homes receive from generalist and specialist community-based nursing services (Crosby et al. 2000). Cope & Roberts (2002) undertook a census, in one county of England, of district nursing involvement in care homes and suggest that their work is primarily concerned with wound care and the management of continence. However, the census was based on care-home managers' responses to a range of six predetermined nursing interventions. This may have meant that only a partial account was given of the range of district nursing work in care homes.

In a series of studies that considered district nursing involvement in residential care homes, district nurses reported it to occupy a significant part of their workload and often to be shaped by factors unrelated to patient need, such as organization of work through general practitioner-attachment, availability of resources and confusion about their role and responsibilities. The nurses believed they were frequently dealing with health care problems that arise not from the frailty of the older person but from a lack of anticipatory care. Also, they were often involved in undocumented support and training work with care assistants in the homes (Goodman et al. 2003a, 2003b). The only other recent study that has considered nursing involvement surveyed 730 palliative-care nursing specialists' work in residential and nursing homes (Froggatt et al. 2002). The authors conclude that the work was reactive, intermittent and task-specific. There were only a few reported examples of nurses having adopted a more proactive approach in these settings.

To round off this discussion of long-term care provision, we describe the case of an older person (Case study 9.1) to illustrate the complexity of a life as it moves from one of independence and activity to a process of withdrawal that was to be the prelude to final illness and death. This case illustrates many of

Case study 9.1:   Margaret Elliott

Margaret Elliott was 83 years old and lived by herself in a second-floor flat that had been her home for the last 30 years. She had been a widow for 15 years and had one son who lived with his family in Canada. She had a wide network of friends through her church, working as a volunteer one day a week in a local charity shop and through frequent contact with her immediate neighbours in the block of flats. She was a supporter of the local hospice and was a committee member of two local charities. She made every effort to keep active and had just acquired a second-hand computer and begun to learn how to use e-mail to keep in touch with her son and grandchildren. She still drove her car but only for short journeys and she avoided driving at night. She had been diagnosed with mild heart failure and high blood pressure. She also experienced quite severe arthritic pain in her knees from osteoarthritis and was finding the stairs to her flat increasingly difficult to manage.

She had a very real fear of having to go into a care home, partly based on her experiences of having visited church friends in the local residential care home. She had made her good friend and neighbour Wilma (who was also an executor of her will) promise never to let her go into a home.

One morning Wilma discovered Margaret comatose in bed having had a severe stroke. She was admitted to the stroke unit of the local hospital and, after 2 days and contrary to expectations, she regained consciousness. She had right-sided weakness and dysphasia. After 2 weeks of intensive rehabilitation she was transferred to a ward in the elderly-care unit, able to walk very slowly with a frame with someone walking by her side and with her speech gradually improving. She was able to eat and drink but her sense of taste had been affected by the stroke and she had little interest in food.

Margaret did not like the ward and felt that very little was being done to help her compared with the care and the attention she had received in the stroke unit. She complained to her visitors and repeatedly asked staff when she could return to her flat. A case conference with the ward nurses, the geriatrician, occupational therapist and social worker agreed that Margaret could be discharged home to her flat with support from social services. A package of care was established that involved care workers visiting three times a day to help Margaret get up and dressed and have her breakfast, have her lunch and finally have her supper at night and be helped to bed. She was also provided with an alarm to wear round her neck that was linked to a call centre and the district nurse was asked to call to make an assessment visit once Margaret had been home for a few weeks and a routine had been established. Wilma agreed to be the contact person for carers if there were any problems with access and she and other friends would pop in at the times when no carers were visiting.

For the first few weeks Margaret was delighted to be home and had a steady stream of visitors who brought her shopping and were happy to spend time talking with her. She told the district nurse that she was fine and accepted the nurse's suggestion that she would pop in to see how she was progressing in a few weeks' time. However, as the weeks passed Margaret became discouraged that her walking was not improving and that she felt weak and tired all the time. One attempt to go out with the help of friends to a church social event had been disastrous when, even with help, she had been unable to manage the stairs from her flat. If no one was with her she was not confident walking in the flat with her frame. There had been several occasions when she had been unable to reach the toilet in time and she had found this very distressing. Friends still visited, but less regularly, which meant that Margaret had to ask Wilma for help more often. She increasingly stayed in bed, refusing to walk to her chair in the living room; reading was impossible and she disliked television. Her general practitioner thought she might be depressed but Margaret was adamant she would not take any more medication. The district nurse visited again, they talked through some of the problems Margaret was having and the nurse arranged for her to have a commode in her bedroom and incontinence pads as a precaution against accidents.

Margaret found it difficult having so many different carers visiting each day and they always seemed to be in a rush. She also found the night times the most difficult as she felt very vulnerable and alone. Wilma was finding it difficult too, as she had not realized how often Margaret would call her to come and help her; she was 70 years old herself and was feeling stressed by the responsibility. In desperation she contacted Margaret's son who had been over when his mother was first admitted to hospital but had returned to Canada before she was discharged home. He agreed to come over for 2 weeks and it was he who raised the question of whether Margaret might feel happier in a care home. Wilma had been worried about suggesting this and expected Margaret to reject the idea. She was surprised when she did not. It emerged that Margaret and the district nurse had discussed whether her current situation was working and what the options might be. Margaret did not think that sheltered accommodation or any intermediate care option would help as she could see she was not improving and could not bear the thought of having to move again if she became more debilitated. Privately, the district nurse did not think she was eligible for sheltered accommodation. Margaret realized that her greatest need was to feel safe and free from worry; she had come to see her flat as a prison where she had little control over what happened to her. Her reluctance to go into a residential home was based on her observation that many of the residents 'were not with it' and that she would have to sell her flat to finance the move.

Continued

Case study 9.1: Cont'd

It was agreed that her son would visit some local care homes and identify those he thought might be suitable and then take Margaret to visit them. He found two that were close to the flat and her church and so easy for friends to visit. She visited both and decided on one that was run by a private company and had been purpose-built. She liked it because it was very bright and clean, her room had a large en-suite bathroom and she knew Lucy, the senior care assistant who worked there. Her son returned home and her solicitor arranged the sale of the flat and her possessions, something she later told Wilma was like a bereavement, losing part of her life.

Margaret stayed in her room for most of the day, and the care-home staff were happy to bring meals to her. She would go to the dining room each day for lunch and had identified three other women to sit and chat to over the meal. However, she was reluctant to take these friendships any further and still relied on Wilma's visits as the person she was closest to and could confide in. Margaret frequently told visitors she felt like a burden had been taken from her since she had come into the care home. She felt safe. She liked the continuity of the care-home staff and the fact that they learnt what she liked to eat, what she preferred to wear and how she liked her hair done. It was important to her too, that only Lucy, the senior care assistant, called her Margaret. There was a residents' forum in the care home that met once a month to discuss any matters that had arisen to do with the care home, plan social events and raise any issues of concern with the staff that the residents may have. Margaret participated in this and felt that her opinions were valued and listened to, although she would confide in Wilma her frustration with particular residents who always seemed to say the same thing at every meeting. She also found it distressing to see other residents who were confused and this was one of the reasons why she preferred her own room to the care home's sitting room.

The care home had well-tended gardens with specially raised flowerbeds that on fine days saw Margaret weeding and planting from a wheelchair. Residents could attend concerts once a month and go on short outings into town, both of which she enjoyed, and occasionally friends took her out in a wheelchair, but a lot of the time she found the days long and often felt bored and tired. As the months went by, she gradually withdrew into herself, she did not participate as much and told staff that the outings were too much of an upheaval. When visitors came, she would listen and respond but not offer any conversation. Staff wondered if she had had another stroke as she found it very difficult to stand on her own and needed help to transfer between her bed and chair and to go to the bathroom. Gradually the incontinence pads Margaret had insisted on wearing as a precaution needed changing regularly. The district nurse kept in touch and visited the care home. She reassessed Margaret and checked she did not have a urinary tract infection. The district nurse discussed with staff how to help Margaret keep active, trying chair-based exercises, and she also encouraged them to check that Margaret was having enough fluids each day. After 10 months in the care home Margaret was having all her meals in her room, was eating very little and was hardly speaking, although she was always more animated when Wilma visited. The care-home staff were concerned about what they saw as Margaret's gradual deterioration and the general practitioner prescribed antidepressant medication; this time Margaret did not refuse. In fact she took very little interest in what was happening and was very passive. The district nurse visited and suggested that they give her supplement drinks and organized a pressure-relieving mattress and cushion as she had lost weight and had become increasingly sedentary. When asked, Margaret did not report any pain and appeared comfortable.

After a year in the care home, Margaret had another stroke, she was unresponsive to touch or sound and unable to coordinate her movements. The care-home staff were keen to carry on looking after her, even though this was very difficult to manage with the other demands on their time. They discussed how they would provide the care with the general practitioner and district nursing team. For 2 weeks they cared for Margaret with the district nursing team and twilight nursing service between them visiting three times a day. Even with this support the care-home staff found it difficult to spend time with Margaret and were growing increasingly concerned about how long this level of care could be sustained. In the last 3 days, as Margaret's breathing became more laboured, the district nurse was able to organize a night sitter to be with her and Margaret died in her sleep with Wilma and Lucy present.

This case study has several learning points and shows how some aspects of care and services for older people as they move from home to a care-home setting are easier to organize than others. Margaret was fully independent and self-caring until her first stroke. Although the different health and social care professionals were 'successful' in helping her regain mobility and achieve a degree of independence in her own home, Margaret's need to feel safe was not met.

The continuity of contact that she had with the district nurse meant she was able to discuss her concerns and consider moving to a care home although it was the lack of satisfaction with her informal care that precipitated her decision to move. For many older people, entry to a care home occurs as a response to a crisis of care or breakdown in support at home.

Case study 9.1:   Cont'd

The care home was a refuge for Margaret and it allowed her to engage socially as much or as little as she wanted and, initially, still participate in activities in and outside the care home that she enjoyed. The care-home staff achieved a degree of person-centred care and this meant they were able to review and assess her needs and, when her condition deteriorated, collaborate with the general practitioner and district nurse to maintain her health.

They were able to establish a close relationship with her, so much so that it was important to them to carry on caring for her when she was dying. Without the close relationship that the care-home staff had with the district nurse and her continuing involvement in the assessment and reviewing of Margaret's health, it is possible that the last year of Margaret's life would not have been so comfortable and settled.

Although the move into the care home was not her first or even preferred choice in this last period of Margaret's life, the carers, the district nurse and care-home staff recognized and respected her need for choice and time to make decisions. When she was living at home after the first stroke, the large number of carers who came and went in such a rush distressed her. In contrast, the district nurse and care-home staff discussed various options with Margaret and gave her the time she needed to decide what she wanted to do; for example, with the district nurse over whether and when to move into a care home, and with the care-home staff over where to eat her meals and how much to participate in activities. These carers also acknowledged Margaret's family and friends and involved them when it was appropriate to do so; for example, involving her distant son in the decision to move into the care home, and ensuring that her closest friend and favourite carer were present when she died.

the issues raised earlier, such as admission to acute hospital care, wanting to return home, the fear of moving into a care home and the need for health, social and palliative care.

CHANGES IN NURSING: NEW UNITS AND ROLES

The need for health care organizations to have strong leaders to respond effectively to the political, economic, social and cultural forces influencing health and social care has been articulated in research carried out in the USA as well as the UK. In Seattle, USA, Bond & Fiedler (1998) identified organizational culture as a framework for implementing change. They highlighted the 'inefficient, rigid and resistant' bureaucratic culture of the traditional health care organization and developed a resident-centred model of care that would create a long-term residential care environment which encourages values such as choice, dignity, independence, privacy and security – values that are similar to those of the UK's *National Service Framework for Older People* (Department of Health 2001b). Bond & Fiedler describe the following as characteristics of the resident-centred culture:

- staff are treated with dignity and respect
- leaders are effective in promoting resident-centred values
- performance of staff reflects the core values of dignity, choice, privacy and independence for residents

- the organization demonstrates an effective interface with its environment
- care meets residents' health, psychosocial and safety needs.

In a subsequent empirical study, Bond & Fiedler (1999) investigated the effects of perceptions by staff of the culture of three units in a long-term care facility before and after specified interventions (physical modification, social intervention or no change). One unit operated as the control unit where no changes were made. The unit given the physical intervention was modified architecturally to create a more relaxed and home-like atmosphere which encouraged closer interaction between residents and staff. The social intervention in the third unit consisted of cultural change through modification of the management style (through goal-setting and role-modelling) and this encouraged residents to lose their passivity and become more self-directed and self-sufficient. The authors conclude that the study demonstrates the value of effective unit leadership and architectural renovation in improving staff performance and resident outcome but first, staff resistance to change has to be successfully overcome through education about the organization's new values.

Recent research in the UK on achieving change in nursing practice confirms the need for a supportive organizational culture, a credible leader or change agent, and a staff group committed to the need for change and actively involved in it (Ross et al. 2001, Redfern & Christian 2003). This work confirms the importance of understanding the complex interplay between the context, process, content and outcome of change in the real world if health care practice is to be successfully implemented and sustained. The huge and complex literature on organizational change is beyond the scope of this chapter but the reader interested in research on achieving change and leadership for change in health care organizations is referred to Ferlie et al. (2000) and Dopson & Mark (2003) respectively. In the two sections that follow, we summarize some of the developments implemented in the UK on new units and new roles in nursing.

Nurse–led units

There will always be a minority of older people who require continuing nursing care which cannot realistically be provided in their own homes, in sheltered housing or in residential homes. The case for nurse-managed NHS nursing homes was advocated in the 1980s (Baker 1983, Wade et al. 1983) and 1990s (Thomas 1996), though this development did not continue beyond a few pioneering units because, as we have seen, the NHS relinquished responsibility for long-term residential and nursing-home care to the independent sector. In this section, we provide a brief overview of developments in nurse-led units which, far from being consigned to the dustbin of history, have helped shape later developments in care, most notably, intermediate care units and new roles in nursing.

Research in the 1980s, sponsored by the then Department of Health and Social Security (DHSS), into the provision of care for older people in long-stay hospital wards, residential homes and private-sector nursing homes confirmed the inappropriateness of providing continuing care in 'geriatric' wards, and recommended that most long-stay beds should be phased out except for a few for medical assessment and short-term treatment, and for respite care to give families a rest (Wade et al. 1983). The authors recommended that alternative provision should be in state-run nursing homes in which care is organized along 'supportive model' lines as distinct from 'protective', 'controlled' or 'restrained' models. The supportive model removes the organizational control, lack of resident choice and subordination to the care regime characteristic of the more restrictive models.

The DHSS followed the Wade study by funding another major piece of research (Bond 1984, Atkinson et al. 1986, Bond & Bond 1987, Bond et al. 1989a, 1989b). Three NHS nursing homes headed by nurses were established in different areas of England to cater for the same kind of older person then found in long-stay wards in hospitals. The research compared the provision, effectiveness and costs of care and the experiences of the residents in these nursing homes with those provided in the wards. On the whole the results favoured the NHS nursing homes. Personal well-being was greater for residents of two of the nursing homes compared with their counterparts in wards, although the results were inconclusive in the third home. User satisfaction was higher in all three homes. There were differences between the nursing homes but they all provided a more positive environment than the wards. The physical environment of the homes was of higher quality, especially in the provision of single rooms for most residents. The homes had more staff than the wards, particularly care assistants. Relatives favoured nursing-home care which was found to be no more expensive than hospital care.

Nurse-led units question the need for a medically dominated setting for people who have progressed beyond the acute stage of illness but who continue to require skilled nursing care. Nursing development units (NDUs) proliferated in the UK in the 1990s and were based on the influential work by Lydia Hall and her colleagues at the Loeb Center in New York, USA (Hall 1969, Hall et al. 1975). The first NDUs were set up in England and evaluated favourably (Pearson 1983, Wright 1989, Black 1993). The success of these pioneering units led the Department of Health to pump-prime four more NDUs and to fund an external evaluation of them (Turner Shaw & Bosanquet 1993).

These 'first-wave' NDUs were soon followed by a Department of Health grant of £3.2 million to develop 30 'second-wave' NDUs and to evaluate their 'added value' to nursing practice (Redfern et al. 1997). Many of the 30 NDUs catered for older people and a few were based in continuing care settings. The evaluation focused on leadership, research, audit and dissemination activity, staff development, job satisfaction, support from the host organization, development of nursing practice, and resources and costs. The findings show how complex are the mechanisms by which the NDUs may have contributed to improvements in nursing practice. The NDUs were significantly more active than non-NDU comparison units in research and dissemination (Redfern & Murrells 1998) but long-term staff sickness absence (episodes longer than 3 days) was significantly greater in the NDUs (Redfern et al. 1997). Further research is needed to see whether this higher level of sickness is characteristic of working under constant scrutiny in a pioneering and stressful environment. Development of a culture to promote changes in practice depends on strong leadership: the ability of clinical leaders in the NDUs to get the balance right between strategic leadership and day-to-day management, and the influence of organizational context on leadership style were important (Christian

& Norman 1998). The study also looked at job satis-faction of staff working in the NDUs and compared community NDUs with hospital NDUs. Levels of sat-isfaction were not high for either group but commu-nity staff were significantly less satisfied than hospital staff. Many reasons were given, such as reported poor staffing level and mix, resource inadequacy, and insuf-ficient continuing education and professional devel-opment opportunities (Redfern et al. 1999).

A more recent evaluation of six NDUs and their progeny, practice development units, which were developed under an accreditation programme pro-vided by the University of Leeds, UK, supported many of the findings of the earlier evaluation by Redfern's group (Gerrish 2001). Gerrish found that all six units were actively involved in innovative practice and evaluation, dissemination and networking activi-ties. The authors also identified factors influencing the success of the units to be the clinical leadership role, motivation and commitment of unit staff, financial resources and support from managers, medical staff and education institutions. Success of the units was judged according to seven criteria, described as: (1) achieving optimum practice; (2) providing a patient-/ client-oriented service; (3) disseminating innovative practice; (4) team-working; (5) enabling staff to reach their full potential; (6) taking a strategic approach to change; and (7) autonomous functioning.

This last criterion of autonomous functioning is supported by a recent study of 14 'magnet hospitals' (hospitals with a strong nursing culture and a rich skill-mix in terms of registered nurses) in Arizona, USA, which found a high correlation between degree of nursing autonomy and nurses' job satisfaction and quality of care. The authors underline the importance of managers rewarding and sanctioning nurses' autonomy (Kramer & Schmalenberg 2003). This study was based in hospitals rather than the continuing care sector, but research in nursing homes in the USA has also found that high nurse-to-resident ratios are asso-ciated with better health outcomes for residents (Harrington 2001).

In the UK, NDUs and practice development units have given nurses a tremendous opportunity to expand the scope of their practice and to enhance quality of care. However, the impact of the units on patient/client/res-ident outcomes has not been confirmed through rigor-ous research and there is very little discussion in the UK literature of the nurse-to-resident ratio needed and the nature of skills required to achieve the best health out-comes for older people in long-term care.

One attempt to measure the impact of a nursing-led unit for older patients in the post-acute stage of their ill-ness, using a randomized controlled trial, is the work by Griffiths' group (Griffiths & Wilson-Barnett 1998, 2000; Griffiths et al. 2000). This nursing-led unit had evolved from its orginal status as an NDU to one in which the nurse is the designated leader of the clinical team and nurses have authority to admit and discharge patients. A review of the literature by this group shows that the impact of such units on patient outcomes is generally favourable, with improved patient independ-ence, fewer readmissions, lower mortality and cost sav-ings in some or all of the studies when compared to usual-care controls. As we have seen, the Griffiths study found that length of patient stay was significantly longer in the nursing-led unit, though the readmission rate was higher for the control patients, suggesting that the experimental unit may have provided more com-prehensive and enduring care to promote patient recovery and avoid readmission.

New roles in nursing

Developing nursing leadership within health and social care settings is seen by policy-makers in the UK as central to improving the organization and delivery of services to achieve safe optimal care for patients (Department of Health 1999, 2000b). The implementa-tion of the NHS modernization programme into serv-ices for older people requires effective clinical leadership (Department of Health 2001b), which nurs-ing is in a key position to provide. Leadership in nurs-ing through the development of new clinical roles has become commonplace in the UK over the last 20 years (Wilson-Barnett et al. 2000, Spilsbury & Meyer 2001), though similar roles were introduced much earlier in the USA. Clinical nurse specialists and nurse practi-tioners, and more recently, consultant nurses and 'modern matrons' were introduced in the UK to increase clinical nursing leadership, implement evi-dence-based practice, include extended technical and medical skills and lead practice developments that improve the quality of health care provision for serv-ice users (Wilson-Barnett & Beech 1994, Read et al. 1999, Wilson-Barnett et al. 2000, Roberts-Davies & Read 2001, Carnwell & Daly 2003, Redfern et al. 2003). Evaluations show that most of the post-holders assess their roles positively but pressures associated with high expectations, work overload, role confusion and lack of support from managers, peers or medical staff are considerable (Read et al. 1999, Wilson-Barnett et al. 2000, Guest et al. 2001, 2004, Redfern et al. 2003).

There is a growing body of literature demonstrat-ing positive findings in terms of the impact of clinical nurse specialists and advanced nursing practitioners on outcomes for patients when compared to medical practitioners doing similar work (Wilson-Barnett

& Beech 1994, Shewan & Read 1999, Reynolds et al. 2000), although service enhancement by nurse practitioners and specialists is apparent rather than mere substitution for doctors (Spilsbury & Meyer 2001). There is also evidence that patients who have access to specialist nurses are more knowledgeable, more proficient in caring for themselves and more satisfied with their care than those who do not have access to specialist nurses (Maslin-Prothero & Masterson 1998). Many of these specialist nursing roles focus on services for older people, including those with stroke illness, rheumatoid arthritis and Parkinson's disease. Carnwell & Daly's (2003) study explored the advanced nursing practitioner role in primary care settings and they consider the role to be the penultimate step in the clinical career pathway to consultant nurse.

A study in long-term care institutions in Finland discusses the importance of promoting autonomy for residents, arguing that older people who are hard of hearing, or are unable to assimilate information quickly and need time to answer questions, have not necessarily lost their capacity to make decisions about their care (Välimäki et al. 2001). This study demonstrates the ways in which clinical nurse specialists working in care homes can promote the autonomy of the residents.

More research on the impact of new roles in nursing in long-stay settings has been found in the USA compared with the UK. 'Gerontologic advanced practice nurses' working with nursing-home staff to integrate care protocols into routine care achieved good outcomes for residents with pressure ulcers, incontinence, depression and aggressive behaviour (Krichbaum et al. 2000). Nurse practitioners working in long-stay settings have been reported as improving adherence to treatments as a result of more effective communication strategies (Kaakinen et al. 2001) and as having a major role in identifying and managing depression of residents together with staff of the homes (Bell & Gross 2001). Melillo (1990) found that substituting nurse practitioners for traditional medical care improves functional impairment of older residents in nursing homes and may improve recruitment and retention of nurses in long-term care.

Proliferation of nurse practitioners, clinical nurse specialists and consultant nurses may fulfil the need for what Pearson (2003) describes as a generic worker who has multidisciplinary skills, who acts therapeutically with a 'warm-blooded' personal touch with residents, who is a competent leader and can successfully cross professional and organizational boundaries. Evaluating the impact of the nursing contribution on quality of care and outcomes for service users is always going to be a problem when the nature of nurs-

ing changes with the introduction of new roles, when the contexts in which nurses work are never static, and when nurses work as part of a multiprofessional team, so making it neither possible nor advantageous to disentangle their contribution from that of others. It follows that, as Spilsbury & Meyer (2001) argue, rigorous methodological research strategies that go beyond the randomized controlled trial and that investigate processes as well as outcomes from the service users' point of view are needed if the nature of nursing and its impact on practice and patients are to be fully understood.

CONCLUSION

This chapter, on intermediate and long-term care, has focused on what it is like for older people and their families when they need support from health and social services that is likely to increase and may become a permanent feature of the final period of their lives. We have looked at changes in policies and provision in intermediate and long-term care and at recent developments in nurse-led care and new roles in nursing. We need to understand much more than we do about the impact of care provision on the recipients of intermediate care as well as long-term care and on their families. What is beyond doubt is that long-term care in residential settings will continue to be part of a mixed economy of care. More research and evaluation is needed which can take account of care environments that have to keep up with constant demands by central government policy-makers to change their practices.

Rapid change in policies and practices has advantages too. Nurses are taking the initiative: they are uniquely placed to evolve into independent but collaborative practitioners in this area of long-term care. They are in an ideal position to take a leadership role in providing care that is anticipatory, holistic and continuous rather than reactive, task-specific and intermittent. They can be instrumental in reducing the causative link between relocation and mortality in older people who move into care homes. That is to say, nurses can take steps to involve older people in the relocation decision and give them choice over the new environment and control over the transfer process. Many nurses work in this way as a matter of course but their contribution is frequently overlooked and underestimated.

Many care homes are thriving nurse-led units in which residents, their families and care staff work together to create the environment they want. Staff can be forgiven, though, for feeling that they have continually to swim against the tide in the struggle to improve practice. Resources are scarce, nurses with adequate qualifications and experience are thin on the ground and most of the direct care is left to care assistants who do not have the support and supervision they need. But where the ratio of nurses to care assistants is high, where there is regular clinical supervision of all direct-care workers and where resources are available to enable nurses and care assistants to keep up to date with continuing education, then quality of working life, quality of care and quality of life for residents are high.

Recommended reading

Clarke A, Hanson EJ, Ross H 2003 Seeing the person behind the patient: enhancing the care of older people using a biographical approach. Journal of Clinical Nursing 12: 697–706.

A biographical approach that encourages person-centred care.

Davies S 2003 Creating community: the basis for caring partnerships in nursing homes. In: Nolan M, Lundh U, Grant G, Keady J (eds) Partnerships in family care: understanding the caregiver career. Open University Press, Maidenhead, pp 218–237.

Discusses the different cultures and particular approaches to care in care homes and how this can shape the older person's experience of care.

Katz J, Peace S (eds) 2003 End of life in care homes: a palliative care approach. Oxford University Press, Oxford.

and

Clark D, Hockley J (eds) 2003 Palliative care for older people in care homes. Open University Press, Buckingham.

These two edited books include contributions by authors who are acknowledged experts on palliative care in long-term settings. The texts explore in detail the issues that arise in providing palliative care in care homes in particular.

Stanley D, Reed J 1999 Opening up care: achieving principled practice in health and social care institutions. Arnold, London.

An exceptional book that challenges prevailing thinking, provides an excellent critique of the issues and discusses care homes from health and social care perspectives.

References

Albinsson L, Strang PA 2002 A palliative approach to existential issues and death in end-stage dementia care. Journal of Palliative Care 18: 168–174

Allen I, Hogg D, Peace S 1992 Elderly people: choice, participation and satisfaction. Policy Studies Institute, London

Ames D 1990 Depression among elderly residents of local-authority residential homes: its nature and the efficacy of intervention. British Journal of Psychiatry 156: 667–675

Atkinson DA, Bond J, Gregson BA 1986 The dependency characteristics of older people in long-term institutional care. In: Phillipson C, Bernard M, Strang P (eds) Dependency and interdependency in old age. Croom Helm, London, pp 257–269

Audit Commission 1999 First assessment: a review of district nursing work. Stationery Office, London

Avis M, Jackson JG, Cox K, Miskella C 1999 Evaluation of a project providing community palliative care support to nursing homes. Health and Social Care in the Community 1: 32–38

Bagley H, Cordingley L, Burns A et al. 2000 Recognition of depression by staff in nursing and residential homes. Journal of Clinical Nursing 9: 445–450

Baker DE 1983 'Care' in the geriatric ward: an account of two styles of nursing. In: Wilson-Barnett J (ed) Nursing research: ten studies in patient care. Wiley, Chichester, pp 101–117

Bebbington A, Brown P, Darton R, Miles K, Netten A 1999 Longitudinal study of elderly people admitted to residential and nursing homes: 30 months on. Report P42. PSSRU, Canterbury, pp 1–2

Bell M, Gross AJ 2001 Recognition, assessment and treatment of depression in geriatric nursing home residents. Clinical Excellence for Nurse Practitioners 5: 26–36

Black M 1993 The growth of the Tameside Nursing Development Unit: an exploration of perceived changes in nursing practice over a ten year period. King's Fund Centre, London

Black D, Bowman C 1997 Community institutional care for frail elderly people. British Medical Journal 315: 441–442

Bland R 1999 Independence, privacy and risk: two contrasting approaches to residential care for older people. Ageing and Society 18: 539–560

Boaz A, Hayden C, Bernard M 1999 Attitudes and aspirations of older people: a review of the literature. Department of Social Security report 101. Corporate Document Services, Leeds

Bond J 1984 Evaluation of long-stay accommodation for elderly people. In: Bromley DB (ed) Gerontology: social and behavioural perspectives. Croom Helm, London, pp 88–101

Bond J, Bond S 1987 Developments in the provision and evaluation of long-term care for dependent old people. In: Fielding P (ed) Research in the nursing care of elderly people. Wiley, Chichester

Bond G, Fiedler F 1998 The visibility of organizational culture in a long-term care facility. Journal of Nursing Administration 28: 7–9

Bond G, Fiedler F 1999 A comparison of leadership vs. renovation in changing staff values. Nursing Economics 17: 37–43

Bond J, Bond S, Donaldson C, Gregson B, Atkinson A 1989a Evaluation of continuing-care accommodation for elderly people. Report no. 38, vol 7. Health Care Research Unit, School of Health Care Sciences, University of Newcastle upon Tyne, Newcastle

Bond J, Bond S, Donaldson C, Gregson B, Atkinson A 1989b Evaluation of an innovation in the continuing care of very frail elderly people. Ageing and Society 9: 347–381

Boneham MA, Williams KE, Copeland JRM et al. 1997 Elderly people from ethnic minorities in Liverpool: mental illness, unmet needs and barriers to service use. Health and Social Care in the Community 5: 173–180

Burholt V 1998 Pathways into residential care: service use, health, help and health prior to admission. Health Care in Later Life 3: 1358–7390

Butler M, Norton R, Lee-Joe T, Campbell AJ 1996 The risks of hip fractures of older people from private homes and institutions. Age and Ageing 25: 381–385

Cameron I 2000 Intervention for late life depression in residential care: being old, depressed and disabled is to be in triple jeopardy. British Medical Journal 320: 119–120

Carnwell R, Daly WM 2003 Advanced nursing practitioners in primary care settings: an exploration of developing roles. Journal of Clinical Nursing 12: 630–642

Casarett DJ, Hirschman KB, Henry MR 2001 Does hospice have a role in nursing home care at the end of life? Journal of the American Geriatric Society 49: 1493–1498

Challis D 1994 Case management: a review of UK developments and issues. In: Titterton M (ed) Caring for people in the community: the new welfare. Jessica Kingsley, London

Challis D, Mozley CG, Sutcliffe C et al. 2000 Dependency in older people recently admitted to care homes. Age and Ageing 29: 255–260

Christian SL, Norman IJ 1998 Clinical leadership in nursing development units. Journal of Advanced Nursing 27: 108–116

Clapham D 1997 Problems and potentials of sheltered housing. Ageing and Society 17: 209–214

Clarke A, Hanson EJ, Ross H 2003 Seeing the person behind the patient: enhancing the care of older people using a biographical approach. Journal of Clinical Nursing 12: 697–706

Cohen L, O'Connor M, Blackmore AM 2002 Nurses' attitudes to palliative care in nursing homes in Western Australia. International Journal of Palliative Care Nursing 8: 88–98

Cooke KR, Niven C, Downs M 1999 Assessing the pain of people with cognitive impairment. International Journal of Geriatric Psychiatry 14: 421–425

Cope BS, Roberts DI 2002 Nursing and care homes: a census view. Journal of Community Nursing 16: 14–18

Cornes M, Clough R 2000 Assessment in community care: disputed territory. Executive summary of a comparative operational analysis across three northern localities, Department of Applied Social Science, Lancaster University, Lancaster

Crosby C, Evans KE, Prendergast LA 2000 Factors affecting demand for primary health care services by residents in nursing homes and residential care homes. Edwin Mellen Press, Ceredigion

Department of Health 1989 Caring for people: community care in the next decade. HMSO, London

Department of Health 1990 National Health Service and community care act. HMSO, London

Department of Health 1998 Partnership in action: new opportunities for joint working between health and social services. Department of Health, London

Department of Health 1999 Making a difference: strengthening the nursing, midwifery and health visiting contribution to health and healthcare. HMSO, London

Department of Health 2000a Shaping the future NHS: long term planning for hospitals and related services. Consultation document on the findings of the national beds inquiry and supporting analysis, Stationery Office, London

Department of Health 2000b The NHS plan: a plan for reform. London, Department of Health

Department of Health 2001a Intermediate care. HSC 2001/01: LAC (2001)1. Department of Health, London

Department of Health 2001b National service framework for older people. Department of Health, London. Available online at: www.doh.gov.uk/nsf/olderpeople.htm

Department of Health 2001c Care homes for older people: national minimal standards. C80/077240. Department of Health, London

Department of Health 2003 Government announces funding for extra care housing. Available online at: www.wired-gov.net/WGArticle.asp?WCI=htm, 03.07.03

Dopson S, Mark A L 2003 Leading health care organizations. Palgrave, Basingstoke

Ferlie E, Fitzgerald L, Wood M 2000 Getting evidence into clinical practice? An organisational behaviour perspective. Journal of Health Services Research and Policy 5: 92–102

Field D, Froggatt K 2003 Factors affecting provision of palliative care. In: Katz JS, Peace S (eds) End of life in care homes. Oxford University Press, Oxford, pp 175–193

Field EM, Walker MH, Orrell MW 2002 Social networks and health of older people living in sheltered housing. Aging and Mental Health 6: 372–386

Froggatt K, Hoult L 2002 Developing palliative care practice in nursing and residential care homes: role of the clinical nurse specialist. Journal of Clinical Nursing 11: 802–808

Froggatt KA, Poole K, Hoult L 2002 The provision of palliative care in nursing and residential homes: a survey of clinical nurse specialist work. Palliative Medicine 16: 481–487

Gentles H, Potter J 2001 Alternatives to acute hospital care. Reviews in Clinical Gerontology 11: 373–378

Gerrish K 2001 A pluralistic evaluation of nursing/practice development units. Journal of Clinical Nursing 10: 109–118

Gibbs G 1995 Nurses in private nursing homes: a study of their knowledge and attitudes to pain management in palliative care. Palliative Medicine 9: 245–253

Godlove Mozley C, Challis D, Sutcliffe C et al. 2000 Psychiatric symptomatology in elderly people admitted to nursing and residential homes. Aging and Mental Health 4: 136–141

Goffman E 1961 Asylums. Anchor Books, New York

Goodman C, Woolley R 2004 Older people in care homes and the primary care nursing contribution: a review of relevant research. Primary Health Care Research and Development 5: 179–187

Goodman C, Woolley R, Knight D 2003a District nurses' experiences of providing care in residential care home settings. Journal of Clinical Nursing 12: 67–76

Goodman C, Woolley R, Knight D 2003b District nurse involvement in providing palliative care to older people in residential care homes. International Journal of Palliative Care Nursing 12: 521–527

Goodman C, Robb N, Drennan V 2003c Training and development needs of care staff, nurses and therapists working in care homes for older people. Unpublished report. North Central London Workforce Confederation, London

Griffiths J 1998 Meeting personal hygiene needs in the community: a district nursing perspective on the health and social care divide. Health and Social Care in the Community 6: 234–240

Griffiths P, Wilson-Barnett J 1998 The effectiveness of 'nursing beds': a review of the literature. Journal of Advanced Nursing 27: 1184–1192

Griffiths P, Wilson-Barnett J 2000 Influences on length of stay in intermediate care: lessons from nursing-led inpatient unit studies. International Journal of Nursing Studies 37: 245–255

Griffiths P, Wilson-Barnett J, Richardson G et al. 2000 The effectiveness of nursing care in a nursing-led in-patient unit. International Journal of Nursing Studies 37: 153–161

Guest D, Redfern S, Wilson-Barnett J et al. 2001 A preliminary evaluation of the establishment of nurse, midwife and health visitor consultants. Report to the Department of Health by a team from King's College London and Birkbeck College. Management Centre, King's College, London. Available online at: www.kcl.ac.uk/nursing nru/nru

Guest D, Peccei R, Rosenthal P et al. 2004 An evaluation of the impact of nurse, midwife and health visitor consultants. King's College, London. Available online at: www.kcl.ac.uk/nursing/nru/nru.html

Hall LE 1969 The Loeb Center for nursing and rehabilitation, Montefiori Hospital and Medical Center, Bronx, New York. International Journal of Nursing Studies 6: 81

Hall LE, Alfano GJ, Rifkin E, Devine HS 1975 Longitudinal effects of an experimental nursing process. Loeb Centre for Nursing, New York

Hannan S, Norman I, Redfern S 2001 Care work and quality of care for older people: a review of the research literature. Reviews in Clinical Gerontology 11: 189–203

Harrington C 2001 Strengthening the care giving workforce: improving the quality of long term care. American Journal of Nursing 101: 55–56

Hartley BL 1999 Government misses the point on residential care. British Journal of Nursing 8: 1124

Hawe P 2000 Intervention for late life depression in residential care: how much trial and error should we tolerate in community trials? British Medical Journal 320: 120

Hope and Older People and Help the Aged 2000 Our future health: older people's priorities for health and social care. Help the Aged, London

Hunter S, Brace S, Buckley G 1993 The interdisciplinary assessment of older people at entry into long term institutional care: lessons for the new community care arrangements. Research, Policy and Planning 11: 2–9

Hyde C, Robert IE, Sinclair AJ 2000 The effects of supporting discharge from hospital to home in older people. Age and Ageing 29: 271–279

Jacobs S, Alborz A, Glendinning C, Hann M 2001 Health services for homes: a survey of access to NHS services in nursing and residential homes for older people in England. National Primary Care Research and Development Centre, University of Manchester, Manchester

Jagger C, Lindesay J 1997 Residential care for elderly people: the prevalence of cognitive and behavioural problems. Age and Ageing 26: 475–480

Joseph Rowntree Foundation 2003 Hartrigg Oaks housing. Available online at: www.jrf.org.uk/housingandcare/hartriggoaks/care.asp (accessed on 17 July 2003)

Kaakinen J, Shapiro E, Gayle BM 2001 Stategies for working with elderly clients: a qualitative analysis of elderly client/nurse practitioner communication. Journal of the Academy of Nurse Practitioners 13: 325–329

Katz J, Peace S (eds) 2003 End of life in care homes: a palliative care approach. Oxford University Press, Oxford

Katz J, Sidell M, Komoromy C et al. 2000 Death in homes: bereavement needs of residents, relatives and staff. International Journal of Palliative Care Nursing 6: 274–279

Kitwood T 1997 Dementia reconsidered: the person comes first. Open University Press, Buckingham

Koch T, Webb C 1996 The biomedical construction of ageing: implications for nursing care of older people. Journal of Advanced Nursing 23: 954–959

Komaromy C, Sidell M, Katz JT 2000 The quality of terminal care in nursing and residential homes. International Journal of Palliative Nursing 6: 192–201

Kramer M, Schmalenberg CE 2003 Magnet hospital staff nurses describe clinical autonomy. Nursing Outlook 51: 13–19

Krichbaum KE, Pearson V, Hanscomb J 2000 Better care in nursing homes: advanced practice nurses' strategies for improving staff use of protocols. Clinical Nurse Specialist 14: 40–46

Laing W, Buisson E 2000 Laing's healthcare market review 2000–2001. Laing & Buisson, London

Lall B 1999 A pilot screening programme to assess the dental treatment needs of older people in residential and nursing care. Journal of BASE (British Association for Service to the Elderly) 68: 19–23

Lee D, Woo J, Mackenzie AE 2002 A review of older people's experiences with residential care placement. Journal of Advanced Nursing 37: 19–27

Lefebvre-Chapiro S 2001 The DoloPlus scale 2 – evaluating pain in the elderly. European Journal of Palliative Care 8: 191–194

Lewis J 2001 Older people and the health and social care boundary: half a century of hidden policy conflict. Social Policy and Administration 35: 343–359

Lindesay J, Briggs K, Lawes M, Macdonald A, Herzberg J 1991 The domus philosophy: a comparative evaluation of a new approach to residential care for the demented elderly. International Journal of Geriatric Psychiatry 6: 727–736

Llewellyn-Jones RH, Baikie KA, Smithers H et al. 1999 Multifaceted shared care intervention for late life depression in residential care: randomized controlled trial. British Medical Journal 319: 676–682

Lloyd-Williams M 1996 An audit of palliative care in dementia. European Journal of Cancer Care 5: 53–55

McCarthy M, Addington-Hall J, Altmann D 1997 The experience of dying with dementia: a retrospective study. International Journal of Geriatric Psychiatry 12: 404–409

MacMahon D 2001 Intermediate care: a challenge to the specialty of geriatric medicine or its renaissance? Age and Ageing (suppl.) 3: 19–23

McMurdo ME, Rennie LM 1994 Improvements in quadriceps strength with regular seated exercise in the institutionalized elderly. Archives of Physical Medicine and Rehabilitation 75: 600–603

McMurdo MET, Millar AM, Daly F 2000 A randomised controlled trial of fall prevention strategies in old peoples' homes. Gerontology 46: 83–87

Maslin-Prothero S, Masterson A 1998 Continuing care: developing a policy analysis for nursing. Journal of Advanced Nursing 28: 548–553

Medical Research Council Cognitive Function and Ageing Study (MRC CFAS) and Resource Implications Study (RIS MRC CFAS) 1999 Profile of disability in elderly people: estimates from a longitudinal population study. British Medical Journal 318: 1108–1111

Meehan L, Meyer J, Winter J et al. 2002 Partnership with care homes. Nursing Times Research 7: 348–359

Meijer A, van Campen C, Kerkstra A 2000 A comparative study of the financing, provision and quality of care in nursing homes. The approach of four European countries: Belgium, Denmark, Germany and the Netherlands. Journal of Advanced Nursing 32: 554–561

Melillo KD 1990 Evaluation of nursing process and outcomes of care utilizing nurse practitioners to provide health care for elderly patients in Massachusetts nursing homes. Unpublished PhD thesis. Brandeis University, Waltham, MA

Morgan D, Reed J, Palmer A 1997 Moving from hospital into a care home: the nurse's role in supporting older people. Journal of Clinical Nursing 6: 463–471

Nolan M, Dellasega C 1999 'It's not the same as him being at home': creating caring partnerships following nursing home placement. Journal of Clinical Nursing 8: 723–730

Nolan M, Walker G, Nolan J et al. 1996 Entry to care: positive choice or fait accompli? Developing a more proactive nursing response to the needs of older people and their carers. Journal of Advanced Nursing 24: 265–274

Norton R, Campbell AJ, Reid IR et al. 1999 Residential status and risk of hip fracture. Age and Ageing 28: 135–139

Office of National Statistics 2001 Community care statistics 2000. Stationery Office, London

Owen T, Harding T 2000 Involvement of older people in primary care groups. Help the Aged, London

Patterson C, Molloy W, Jubelius R, Guyatt GH, Bedard M 1997 Provisional educational needs of health care providers in palliative care in three nursing homes in Ontario. Journal of Palliative Care 13: 13–17

Peace SM, Kellaher L, Willcocks D 1997 Re-evaluating residential care. Open University Press, Buckingham

Pearson A 1983 The clinical nursing unit. Heinemann, London

Pearson A 2003 Multidisciplinary nursing: re-thinking role boundaries. Journal of Clinical Nursing 12: 625–629

Peet SM, Castleden CM, McGrother CW 1995 Prevalence of urinary and faecal incontinence in hospital and residential and nursing homes for older people. British Medical Journal 311: 1063–1064

Peet SM, Castleden CM, McGrother CW, Duffin HM 1996 The management of urinary incontinence in residential and nursing homes for older people. Age and Ageing 25: 139–143

Percival J 1996 Behind closed doors: inside views of sheltered housing. Journal of the British Society of Gerontology 6: 5–7

Pollock A 2000 Will intermediate care be the undoing of the NHS? British Medical Journal 321: 393–394

Proctor R, Burns A, Stratton Powell H et al. 1999 Behavioural management in nursing and residential homes: a randomised controlled trial. Lancet 354: 26–29

Proot IM, Abu-Saad HH, de Esch-Janssen WP, Crebolder HFJM, ter Meulen RHJ 2000 Patient autonomy during rehabilitation: the experiences of stroke patients in nursing homes. International Journal of Nursing Studies 37: 267–276

Proulx M 1999 Evaluation of the project "vie autonome chez soi" – alternative for reconciling aging, loneliness and feeling of security among the elderly. Canadian Journal on Aging 18: 64–83

Read S, Lloyd Jones S, Collins K, McDonnell A, Jones R 1999 Exploring new roles in practice: implications of developments within the clinical team (ENRIP). Report for the Department of Health by a team from Sheffield University, England. School of Nursing and Midwifery, University of Sheffield, Sheffield

Redfern S, Christian S 2003 Achieving change in health care practice. Journal of Evaluation in Clinical Practice 9: 225–238

Redfern SJ, Murrells T 1998 Research, audit and networking in nursing development units. Nursing Times Research 3: 275–288

Redfern S, Normand C, Christian S et al. 1997 An evaluation of nursing development units. Nursing Times Research 2: 292–303

Redfern S, Murrells T, Christian S 1999 Job satisfaction in community and hospital nursing development units. British Journal of Community Nursing 4: 349–358

Redfern S, Hannan S, Norman I, Martin F 2002 Work satisfaction, stress, quality of care and morale of older people in a nursing home. Health and Social Care in the Community 10: 512–517

Redfern S, Guest D, Wilson-Barnett J et al. 2003 Role innovation in the NHS: a preliminary evaluation of the new role of nurse, midwife and health visitor consultant. In: Dopson S, Mark A (eds) Leading health care organizations. Palgrave Macmillan, Basingstoke, Hampshire, pp 153–172

Reed J, Morgan D 1999 Discharging older people from hospital to care homes: implications for nursing. Journal of Advanced Nursing 29, 819–825

Reed J, Payton V 1996 Working to create continuity: older people managing the move to the care home setting. Report no. 76. University of Newcastle upon Tyne Health Services Research, Newcastle

Reynolds H, Wilson-Barnett J, Richardson G 2000 Evaluation of the role of the Parkinson's disease nurse specialist. International Journal of Nursing Studies 37: 337–346

Richardson G, Griffiths P, Wilson Barnett J, Spilsbury K, Batehup L 2001 Economic evaluation of nurse led intermediate care unit. International Journal of Technology Assessment in Health Care 17: 442–450

Roberts-Davies M, Read S 2001 Clinical role clarification using the Delphi method to establish similarities and differences between nurse practitioners and clinical nurse specialists. Journal of Clinical Nursing 10: 33–43

Roe B, Shiels C 2000 Focus on continence: surveys of care policies. Elderly Care 12: 34–38

Ross F, McLaren S, Redfern S, Warwick C 2001 Partnership for changing practice: lessons from South Thames Evidence-Based Practice project (STEP). Nursing Times Research 6: 817–828

Royal College of Physicians, Royal College of Nursing, British Geriatrics Society 2001 The health and care of older people in care homes: a comprehensive interdisciplinary approach. Royal College of Physicians, London

Royal Commission on the Funding of Long-Term Care 1999 With respect to old age: long-term care – rights and responsibilities. HMSO, London

Shewan JA, Read SM 1999 Changing roles in nursing: a literature review of influences and innovations. Clinical Effectiveness in Nursing 3: 75–82

Shiels C, Roe B 1999 Pressure sore care. Nursing Standard 14: 41–44

Sidell M 2003 The training needs of carers. In: Katz J, Peace S (eds) End of life in care homes: a palliative approach. Oxford University Press, Oxford

Simons D, Baker P, Jones B, Kidd EA, Beighton D 2000 An evaluation of an oral health training programme for carers of the elderly in residential homes. British Dental Journal 188: 206–210

Sinclair I 1988 Residential care for elderly people. In: Sinclair I (ed) Residential care: the research reviewed (the Wagner report). HMSO, London

Smith AE, Crome P 2000 Relocation mosaic – a review of 40 years of resettlement literature. Reviews in Clinical Gerontology 10: 81–95

Spilsbury K, Meyer J 2001 Defining the nursing contribution to patient outcome: lessons from a review of the literature examining nursing outcomes, skill mix and changing roles. Journal of Clinical Nursing 10: 3–14

Stanley D, Reed J 1999 Opening up care: achieving principled practice in health and social care institutions. Arnold, London

Steiner A 2001 Intermediate care: a good thing? Age and Ageing 30 (suppl. 3): 33–39

Steiner A, Vaughan B 1996 Intermediate care: a discussion paper arising from the Kings Fund seminar 30th October 1996. Kings Fund, London

Stewart K, Challis D, Carpenter I, Dickinson E 1999 Assessment approaches for older people receiving social care: content and coverage. International Journal of Geriatric Psychiatry 14: 147–156

Stuck AE, Egger M, Hammer A, Minder CE, Beck JC 2002 Home visits to prevent nursing home admission and functional decline in elderly perople: systematic review and meta regression analyses. Journal of the American Medical Association 287: 1022–1028

Stumer J, Hickson L, Worrall L 1996 Hearing impairment, disability and handicap in elderly people living in residential care and in the community. Disability and Rehabilitation 18: 76–82

Sturgess I, Rudd AG, Shilling J 1994 Unrecognised visual problems amongst residents of part III homes. Age and Ageing 23: 54–56

Taylor C, Hendra T 2000 The prevalence of diabetes mellitus and quality of diabetic care in residential and nursing homes: a postal survey. Age and Ageing 29: 447–450

Thomas L 1996 Editorial. Nursing Standard 10: 1

Thomas S 1999 Rapid response: a look at Bolton. Primary Health Care 8: 8–10

Thomas S, MacMahon D 2001 Elderly: intermediate care. Journal of Community Nursing 15: 1–11

Thompson S, Crome P 2001 Intermediate care. Reviews in Clinical Gerontology 11: 205–207

Tinker A, Wright F, Zeilig H 1995 Difficult to let sheltered housing. HMSO, London

Townsend J 1994 Early and supported hospital discharge: the hospital and community interface. Journal of the Royal Society of Medicine 87: 348–351

Travis SS, Bernard M, Dixon S et al. 2002 Obstacles to palliation and end-of-life care in a long-term care facility. Gerontologist 42: 342–349

Turner Shaw J, Bosanquet N 1993 A way to develop nurses and nursing. King's Fund, London

Twigg J 1997 Deconstructing the 'social bath': help with bathing at home for older and disabled people. Journal of Social Policy 26: 211–232

Twigg J, Atkins K 1994 Carers perceived: policy and practice in informal care. Open University Press, Buckingham

Välimäki M, Leino-Kilpi H, Scott P A et al. 2001 The role of CNSs in promoting elderly patients' autonomy in long-term institutions: problems and implications for nursing practice and research. Clinical Nurse Specialist 15: 7–14

Vetter NJ 1999 Long-term care for elderly people in the UK. Reviews in Clinical Gerontology 9: 383–393

Victor C 1994 Old age in modern society. Chapman and Hall, London

Victor C 1997 Community care and older people. Stanley Thorne, Cheltenham

Wade B, Sawyer L, Bell J 1983 Dependency with dignity: different care provision for the elderly. Occasional Papers on Social Administration, no. 68. Bedford Square Press, London

Wanless D 2001 Securing our future health: taking a long-term view. Interim report. HM Treasury, London. Available online at: www.hm-treasury.gov.uk

Warburton R 1994 Home and away: a review of recent research to explain why some elderly people enter residential care homes while others stay at home. Department of Health, London

Wells JL, Seabrook JA, Stolee P, Borrie MJ Knoefel F 2003 State of the art in geriatric medicine and rehabilitation, part one: review of frailty and comprehensive geriatric assessment. Archives of Physical Medicine and Rehabilitation 84: 890–897

Wiles R, Postle K, Steiner A, Walsh B 2001 Nurse led intermediate care: an opportunity to develop enhanced roles for nurses? Journal of Advanced Nursing 34: 813–821

Wilkins D, Hughes B 1987 Residential care of the elderly: the consumer's view Ageing and Society 7: 175–201

Willcocks D, Peace S, Kellaher L 1987 Private lives in public places. Tavistock, London

Wilson-Barnett J, Beech S 1994 Evaluating the clinical nursing specialist: a review. International Journal of Nursing Studies 31: 561–571

Wilson-Barnett J, Barriball L, Reynolds H, Jowett S, Ryrie I 2000 Recognising advancing nursing practice: evidence from two observational studies. International Journal of Nursing Studies 37: 389–400

Worth A 2001 Assessment of the needs of older people by district nurses and social workers: a changing culture? Journal of Interprofessional Care 15: 257–266

Wright S 1989 Defining the nursing development unit. Nursing Standard 4: 29–31

Wright F 1994 Multi-purpose residential homes: a fair deal for residents? Ageing and Society 14: 383–404

Yates M, Horan MA, Clague JE et al. 1999 A study of infection in elderly nursing/residential home and community-based residents. Journal of Hospital Infection 43: 123–129

SECTION 3

Nursing older people: independence, autonomy and self-fulfilment

SECTION CONTENTS

Chapter 10

Communication challenges and skills

Andrée C. le May

SUMMARY

This chapter starts by defining communication and discussing its continuing importance in older age. The chapter then goes on to highlight reasons for communicating and discuss some of the factors that shape and influence communication between older people and the nurses who care for them in either acute or longer-term care facilities. The central part of the chapter focuses on some of the most commonly occurring communication challenges that older people face. These challenges to communication include those associated with the natural course of ageing (for example, altered hearing and seeing), illness (for example, stroke or dementia), sensory deprivation and challenging behaviours. Communication strategies and pointers for good communication are detailed in relation to each of these challenges; these are usually targeted towards the nurse though, in many instances, they may also be useful for informal carers, relatives and friends. The chapter concludes by reminding readers of the therapeutic value of communication with older people.

INTRODUCTION

Communication is often described as a two-way process, involving the transmission and comprehension of a message. This complex interaction is so well integrated into our daily lives that most of us take it for granted and it is only when the effectiveness of the process is challenged that its importance becomes clear. In some instances growing older may present such challenges by limiting our ability to communicate as a result of natural ageing (for instance, through its effects on hearing or vision), illness or its treatment, or a reduction in opportunities available for communication. Alternatively, growing older may provide great opportunities for people to communicate with each other through the greater availability of time they may have to talk to one another or undertake activities with others.

WHAT IS COMMUNICATION?

Communication is a complex process that involves passing a message intentionally, or unintentionally, between two or more people. This process is often explained using a simple model that suggests four essential features required for communication:

1. a source from which the message is communicated
2. a message to be sent
3. a channel for communicating the message
4. a receiver of the message.

Once the message has been received another message (feedback/a response) is usually sent to the source, creating a dynamic and ongoing process between the interactors (Monaghan 1995).

In order to convey a message the source (or sender) needs to determine the content and purpose of the message as well as targeting a recipient for the message. The message will usually have arisen from stimulation of a sensory or cognitive nature. Therefore an interruption in the usual functioning of these processes, for instance a cognitive impairment, will lead to the disruption of communication at an early stage. Any alteration in the ability to recognize the transmission or content of messages will also have an impact on the effectiveness of the communication, as will the receptiveness of the receiver of the message.

Although this model forms a useful basis for understanding the theory underlying communication, it does not acknowledge the complexity of the process or show how impairment of the communication channels has an impact on the effective transmission of messages. To understand how growing older may challenge communication it is necessary to consider the mechanisms for conveying and recognizing messages more closely.

Each message is transmitted in a unique way through a series of sensory, motor and cognitive channels. The meaning of each message is shaped by each interactor's psychological and social status and experiences (Fig 10.1). In unimpaired communication the complexity of this process may make messages hard to decipher and lead to misinterpretation; this may be compounded when ageing or illness compromises sensory, motor or cognitive functioning or a person's psychological or social condition. Alteration in any of these five key areas will impinge on communication, with the neurological

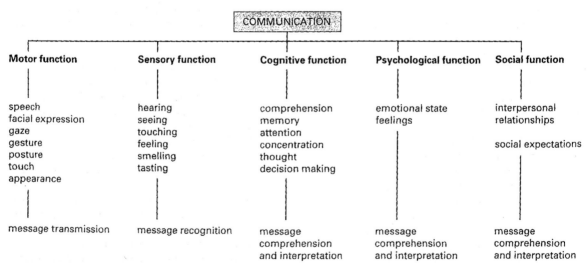

Fig. 10.1   Conveying and receiving messages.

site of damage or underlying illness/deficit determining the effect(s) on communication.

Message transmission, recognition, comprehension and interpretation are primarily learnt behaviours that incorporate a variety of coordinated activities in relation to achieving a goal. Any alteration to these activities will result in a challenge to communication. Message transmission occurs through the use of verbal and non-verbal cues. The use of each of these cues is situation-specific, individually determined, socially constructed and used as a basis for judging the interpersonal effectiveness of the communicator(s) (Hargie 1993). Verbal and non-verbal cues are complementary to each other. Recognition, comprehension and interpretation of messages are primarily associated with the sensory and cognitive processes of sight, hearing, touch, smell, taste and cognition. Any impairment to these may result in ineffective communication through misunderstanding the message and/or giving inappropriate feedback to the sender of the message. These processes are closely linked to the use of verbal and non-verbal cues.

REASONS FOR COMMUNICATING

Argyle (1994) suggests that most people spend most of their time communicating with others with whom they live, work or socialize. They communicate to 'be approved of and to make friends, to dominate or to depend on others, to be admired, to be helped or given social support, [and] to provide help to others' (Argyle 1994: p. 1). Communicating is one of our principal pastimes, and so to be deprived of it, or for it to be inhibited in any way, will have a major impact on our lives, regardless of age.

Worrall & Hickson (2003) emphasize the 'everydayness' and pervasiveness of communication for older people, reminding their readers that communication, in some form, occurs in almost everything – whether it is taking money out of the bank or playing bingo. Worrall & Hickson (2003: p. 12) also highlight several reasons why effective communication is important for older people who use it as a means of:

1. 'Exerting influence and power
2. Relieving loneliness, depression and anxiety
3. Receiving high-quality care
4. Establishing and maintaining friendships
5. Participation in activities of living
6. Facilitating adaptation to change
7. Involvement in decision-making
8. Stimulating thinking
9. Maintaining social networks
10. Enhancing well-being'

Worrall & Hickson (2003) quote Shaddon's (1998) unpublished study of older people's communication partners; the study reported that the most frequently occurring communications were between older peers (50%) and the next most common were with family members (25%). Typical topics of communication included discussions of past life experiences (the most commonly reported), family matters, health, politics and financial concerns (one of the least commonly reported).

Communicating becomes increasingly important for older people if they are dependent on others for care. Isolation may make older people feel vulnerable and increase their need to maintain social interaction and gain support through communication networks. Communication possibilities may be actively sought and maximized through, for example, interactions with friends and family, seeking advice from health care professionals, or attending day centres or clubs. Conversely, with the increased likelihood of very old people experiencing communal living within nursing and /or residential homes, opportunities that minimize communication with others may be welcomed in order to promote privacy and solitude. In these situations nurses are in a key position to facilitate a more equal balance of social interaction with opportunities for privacy and solitude which meet each resident's needs.

Within the nursing context communication is of vital importance, helping nurses to establish, define and maintain relationships between themselves and older people. This has most recently been emphasized in the minimum standards for *Care Homes for Older People* (Department of Health 2003a) and the *Essence of Care* benchmarks (Department of Health 2003b), as well as being implicit in the *National Service Framework for Older People* (Department of Health 2001).

Nurses can, through the use of skilled communication:

- obtain information about the older person's physical, social and psychological well-being
- assess any deficits in communication skills
- assess any opportunities for communication which may increase feelings of support and the development of rapport
- assess an older person's requirements for increased privacy/solitude or increased involvement
- determine how communication deficits may be overcome (e.g. by using glasses, hearing aids or interpreters)
- monitor and explain change in relation to altered communication skills or general health status

- provide appropriate information through the most effective communication channels
- evaluate progress and the impact of care on the person's general condition and ability to communicate
- make referrals to other relevant health care professionals (e.g. speech and language therapists) if necessary.

It is also essential, particularly when older people experience long hospital stays or need continuing care, that nurses consider ways in which they might facilitate communication between older patients/residents. They may consider, for instance, encouraging storytelling between individuals or more formally in designated groups or instigate a peer mentoring system amongst older patients/residents.

SHAPING THE MEANING OF COMMUNICATION

Several mediating factors may be associated with message interpretation and feedback. Hargie & Marshall (1993: p. 31) defined these mediating factors as 'internal states, activities or processes within [each] individual which mediate between the feedback which is perceived, the goal which is being pursued and the responses that are made'. These variables affect the ways in which all messages are interpreted and include age, gender, sociocultural background, the context of the communication, the way we think and feel and the roles we play. These are all important within the context of nursing older people, as communicators bring with them, to every interaction, a unique set of variables that will influence the transmission and interpretation of each message. Older people are not a homogeneous group and, while it is acknowledged that age-related changes are variable and cannot be generalized, the following summary of the likely impact of ageing and its effects on communication may help readers to identify some of the actual or potential communication challenges which some older people will face.

Dowd (1986: p. 183) reminds us that older people have 'been socialized at a different time and to a different set of cultural imperatives' compared with those in younger age groups, and this influences their communication abilities and strategies. In line with this, Biggs (1993) suggests that people of different ages have different hopes, fears and activities to perform, leading to intergenerational differences which may affect communication.

These differences raise several issues that nurses, being naturally of a different generation to older patients, should be aware of:

- The undertakings of the young and the old may be different and have differing associated societal values
- The organization of people into age-specific groups may reduce opportunities for intergenerational communication. Generally people prefer interacting with those whom they see as equals in some way, which may result in, as Dowd (1986: p. 152) puts it, 'an eventual outcome [of] disinclination toward cross-age social interaction'
- The need for care may throw people together who would not usually interact
- Younger people may find it hard to concur with older people's views and feelings because they have not had the same experience of ageing. Conversely, older people have had the experience of being younger but within a different culture, thereby minimizing the potential for shared experiences. This may make the establishment of an empathic rapport difficult, as the mismatch of experiences may also result in misinterpretation of messages between people
- Generations may fail to share the same 'language' athough the same words may be used, they may hold different meanings and conversations may take on different structures and functions between generations.

Biggs (1993) and Armstrong & McKechnie (2003) maintain that all these factors influence the quality of interaction and the development of a relationship between the younger and the older person. Biggs also suggests that, owing to age-related changes, communication becomes increasingly reliant on the sensitivity and good will of others who will need to adjust their communication styles and channels to meet the needs of older people who have deficits in communication.

The idea of intergenerational communication differences became prominent in the 1980s. Nussbaum et al. (1989), though acknowledging that people of all ages generally communicate in the same way, proposed some characteristics that were unique to older people. They suggested that older people might be more cautious in their willingness to communicate with younger people, be more reluctant to suggest specific courses of action or ask for information and take longer to react during interactions. All of these have important repercussions for nurses and other health care professionals when skilled communication is a contributor to high-quality care.

Older people may place more value on talk, particularly 'small talk', seeing it as a more vital component of relationship-building than younger people, who may be sceptical about the value of this type of verbal interchange (Giles & Coupland 1991). These dissimilar values may limit social interactions between people of different generations. Nurses need to consider these factors so that they are able to distinguish between normal age-related changes and those associated with illness, such as the early stages of dementia.

There are, however, many examples in the literature of positive intergenerational communication. For example, Armstrong & McKechnie (2003) studied intergenerational communication by interviewing schoolchildren, care home staff and older women about what it meant to grow old and the value of communication with older people. They concluded that all three groups held generally positive views about old age and older people, although some gender stereotyping (older men were perceived as being grumpy whereas older women spoilt children) was evident in the children's views. Ford & Sinclair (1987) in their study of older women found that one woman reported an enhanced quality of life when a group of young women lived next to her and offered her considerable companionship. The older woman's life changed: 'For a while my life was so different ... We helped each other quite a lot' (p. 9). Old age does not have to be a time of communicative isolation from those of younger years, despite intergenerational differences.

Ryan et al. (1995) proposed a model of 'communication predicament' in relation to older people receiving health care from younger carers. They suggested that the predicament is linked to the older person's communication skills changing alongside certain barriers (maybe linked to intergenerational issues) associated with their communication partners. These altered skills and barriers and led to compromised communication. Ryan et al. (1995) also suggested the existence of a 'communication enhancement' model that focuses on the promotion of health through communication. Both models emphasize the importance of the conversational partner(s) of the older person, suggesting that any 'problem may not lie with the older person's communication, but rather with the interaction between the two, based on the appropriateness of the accommodation that occurs' (Worrall & Hickson 2003: p. 36).

Old age can also be a time when illness and age-related functional changes – such as impaired sight, hearing, speech or cognition – present extra challenges to communication and the maintenance of communication skills. These are covered in detail below.

CHALLENGES TO COMMUNICATION IN OLDER AGE

Worrall & Hickson (2003: p. 93) describe five areas of communication in which impairments can occur as a result of the natural course of ageing or illness (language, conversational discourse, speech, voice and hearing). Deficits in these areas are likely to have the following effects:

1. Language: decreased speed and ability to retrieve words; decreased ability to understand increasingly complicated messages
2. Conversational discourse: difficulty in understanding long and complicated conversations; lessened efficiency and increased ambiguity in conversing; decreased cohesion within conversations
3. Speech: decreased respiratory support for speech output; imprecise articulation; slower rate of speech
4. Voice: increase in pitch for men; decrease in pitch for women; decreased voice quality
5. Hearing: diminished sensitivity to pure tones; difficulty in discriminating speech when it's hard to hear

In addition to these, any deficit in seeing will also have an impact on communication as will alterations in cognition, sensory awareness and behaviour. The main communication challenges associated with each of these areas are discussed below.

Visual impairment

Many older people experience some reduction in vision. Visual impairment significantly affects individuals' ability to collect information about their surroundings and therefore can have a marked impact on an older person's ability to communicate.

The most common problems likely to affect visual acuity are:

- presbyopia
- cataracts
- glaucoma
- senile macular degeneration
- diabetic retinopathy.

Regardless of the cause of visual impairment, it is likely to have some effect on communication leading to:

- reduced orientation to the environment
- reduced ability to discriminate between non-verbal cues

- reduced ability to read or write
- reduced ability to interact with others.

Assessing vision

Obtaining an accurate history of visual impairment and determining how an older person deals with reduced vision is clearly within the remit of the nurse. In order to determine this, nurses should consider, together with the older person and relatives/friends:

- the nature and duration of the visual impairment
- its impact on daily living
- the anticipated impact on sight of hospitalization or admission to a residential nursing home
- mechanisms for reducing the visual impairment
- the cause of the impairment, if known to the older person.

This type of general assessment will help the nurse to recognize signs and symptoms that require referral to a specialist. However, as Gravell (1988) warns, the accuracy of any assessment may be compromised if the older person has any memory loss, or is suffering from a mental or physical illness.

Communicating with an older person with a visual impairment

Helping a person with a visual impairment involves skilled communication, using both verbal and non-verbal cues sensitively. The following pointers may be useful in facilitating this:

- Ensure that spectacles are appropriate, clean and within easy reach
- If a magnifier is used, ensure it is held close to the eye and the object being magnified is moved closer until it is in focus
- Ensure appropriate glare-free lighting and that bedside lights work and are within easy reach
- Avoid glare from windows; draw curtains or blinds accordingly
- Ensure some lighting at night to avoid disorientation or accidents
- Facilitate orientation to the environment through colour-coded doors with large clear labels
- Ensure that call-bells or alarm systems are within easy reach
- If writing information down, use a black felt-tip pen, after checking that the patient can read the size and style of your writing
- Encourage regular eye tests
- Stand or sit within the older person's visual field so that he or she is aware of your presence

– this is particularly important when visual impairment minimizes peripheral vision
- Suggest the use of large-print books/papers or talking books.

Ebersole & Hess (1994) suggest the following strategies which will complement those listed above and help to enhance communication with older people who have a visual impairment:

- Identify yourself clearly
- Make it clear when you are leaving, as well as entering the room
- Make sure you have the person's attention before you speak; you may find touch useful in gaining or holding attention.

Since people with a visual impairment find it hard to become oriented to a new environment, particular care is required to help familiarize them to anything unfamiliar. This will be particularly acute when older people are admitted to a hospital or nursing care from the familiar surroundings of their own home. For more information on sight and older people, see Chapter 12.

Auditory impairment

A third of people aged over 55 years report that they have a problem with their hearing (Royal National Institute for the Deaf 1998). Gravell (1988) suggests that hearing loss is the greatest age-related barrier to communication and disruptive influence on everyday life. Deafness in old age can result from:

- blockage of the ear canal by wax or narrowing, closure or hardening due to ageing
- infection of the middle ear with subsequent auditory damage
- tinnitus (ringing in the ears)

and is generally categorized into conductive or sensorineural hearing loss, although a combination of the two is possible.

Effects of auditory impairment on communication

Hull (1989) describes the frustrations of older people with hearing impairments, emphasizing the consequences of not being able to understand the sounds of a previously familiar world. Hearing impairment may be associated with misinterpretation, embarrassment, fear, making inappropriate responses and withdrawal. These are likely to lead to isolation and diminished well-being. Hull suggests that hearing loss may also result in an older person feeling that control of the senses is being lost, particularly if others confirm this.

Hearing Concern (1996: p. 5) described the effects of hearing loss as 'exclusion from conversation, exclusion from day to day interaction, exclusion from information, exclusion from leisure activities, exclusion from family and friends [and] exclusion from mainstream life'. These exclusions clearly show the challenge of auditory impairment to an older person's well-being and opportunities for communication.

Deafness has an impact on the sender and receiver of the message in a variety of ways:

- The ability to listen will be diminished
- As hearing levels decrease, the older person may suggest that others are not speaking clearly, thereby creating strained relationships
- Hearing loss may affect the person's speech as auditory monitoring of speech is compromised
- Non-verbal communication may also be affected, for example gaze or eye contact may be minimized as the hearing-impaired person focuses attention on the speaker's lips, trying to lip-read
- Responses may be slower because of the need to seek clarity through several communication channels, rather than through listening alone.

All of these will have an impact on the relationship which the nurse establishes with a person with compromised hearing and the degree to which the older person feels able to re-establish independence and autonomy (Fig. 10.2).

Assessing hearing

Once again, assessment plays a vital part in establishing a therapeutic partnership with the person who has an auditory impairment. Nurses need to be able to determine if hearing difficulties are present in order to provide appropriate care and to make rapid referrals for treatment or monitoring by other skilled health care workers. The following steps may be used to guide initial assessments:

- Establish details of the hearing loss, its duration and if any compensatory mechanisms (e.g. hearing aid, lip-reading) are used
- Establish how the hearing loss affects the person's life
- Establish when hearing was last checked
- Check current drug therapy to rule out ototoxicity
- Discuss the anticipated impact of hospitalization or moving into an unfamiliar environment
- Observe the person's behaviour to determine signs of auditory impairment.

Communicating with an older person with an auditory impairment

Hull (1989) suggests that health care professionals can help older people with hearing impairments in a number of ways. First, he proposes amplification using hearing aids. In relation to this the nurse can ensure that if a hearing aid is used it is working, set at the appropriate level and is worn. The nurse may also be able to monitor the effectiveness of the hearing aid in enhancing communication. Second, Hull draws attention to the environment in which the interaction occurs: nurses should, whenever possible, seek to ensure that interactions occur in noise-free environments. Third, he suggests the use of alternative communication strategies,

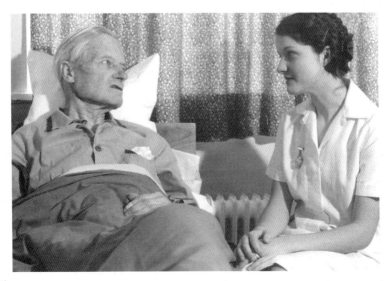

Fig. 10.2 Eye contact.

such as using written information, ensuring that lip-reading is facilitated by careful positioning during interactions and using a variety of communication skills. In addition, Andersson et al. (1994) highlight the positive effects of counselling older people with hearing loss. The use of specialist social workers who can make individual assessments of a person's auditory needs and recommend supportive equipment to help people to adapt and live with hearing loss is becoming increasingly common and is likely to reduce the effects of isolation experienced by older people with hearing deficits.

The following may be useful ways to improve communication techniques when caring for someone with an auditory impairment:

- Make sure that your mouth can be seen to facilitate lip-reading
- Use non-verbal cues, such as facial expressions and gesture, to enhance speech
- Articulate words carefully
- Face the person with whom you are interacting, sitting or standing at the same level
- Make sure there is sufficient light on your face
- Gain the person's attention before speaking: touching may be a useful way of doing this
- Speak at a normal volume; do not shout
- Pause between sentences and confirm if you have been understood
- If you are misunderstood repeat the sentence using different words
- Supplement spoken information with written information
- Reduce background noise such as radios or televisions or find a quiet area
- Make sure that hearing aids, if used, are switched on and work

More information on hearing loss can be found in Chapter 11.

Speech and language impairment

Several types of speech disorder are associated with illness-related changes during old age and may, in some way, impinge on verbal communication. The three most commonly occurring speech disorders are:

- disorders of reception (exacerbated by, for example, hearing impairment, anxiety or altered consciousness)
- disorders of perception (exacerbated by, for example, strokes, dementia or delirium)
- disorders of articulation (exacerbated by, for example, compromised respiratory function or stroke illness).

These disorders may be categorized into four groups:

1. anomia: difficulties in retrieving words during conversation
2. aphasia (or dysphasia): impaired language through disruption in the understanding and expression of language. This affects listening, speaking, calculating, reading and writing
3. apraxia: difficulties in carrying out voluntary movements associated with speech
4. dysarthria: difficulties due to muscle weakness or uncoordinated speech production.

For older people, speech impairment is most commonly associated with aphasia and dysarthria and these are discussed further below.

Aphasia

The most common cause of speech impairment in older people is likely to fall within the category of aphasia and be a consequence of a stroke. The extent of the impairment will depend on the severity and location of the stroke. Damage to the right hemisphere of the brain can result in alteration in attention, orientation, perception, retention and integration. Damage to the left hemisphere is likely to result in damage to centres associated with language.

The complexity of aphasia is emphasized by Groher (1989), who discusses several types of aphasia. He categorizes them into fluent and non-fluent aphasias, due to their impact on speech. Fluent aphasias include:

- Wernicke's aphasia, in which speech is usually fluent but the content of the message is impaired; for instance, incorrect words may be used or words mispronounced. Older people with this type of aphasia may find it hard to find the correct word or syllables and often speak in repetitive jargon. Comprehension of the spoken language may also be impaired. These difficulties will result in compromised speech, reading and writing
- Conduction aphasia, typified by difficulties in repeating words despite sound auditory comprehension. Speech may remain intact
- Anomic aphasia – difficulties occur in recalling specific words. People with this disorder may learn to substitute alternative words for the intended one, thus keeping the content of the message intact. Speech and understanding remain intact
- Transcortical sensory aphasia – less common than the other forms of fluent aphasia. The symptoms are similar to those found in Wernicke's aphasia but more severe. Speech may still be fluent but incomprehensible and words may be replaced by sounds that mimic the intended word but have

no meaning. People with this aphasia may accurately echo sounds that they hear.

The non-fluent aphasias include:

- Broca's aphasia – characterized by problems of verbal production. Grammatical structure goes awry and increased length of time is taken to produce words, resulting in slow speech that uses a minimum of words. In this aphasia comprehension may remain intact
- Transcortical motor aphasia – people with this disorder exhibit problems finding words during conversations and their auditory abilities range from poor to good. As with those with transcortical sensory aphasia, people with this disorder are able to echo sounds which they hear, although initiation may be difficult
- Global aphasia is characterized by severe problems with language, reception and expression, linked with unintelligible speech and compromised understanding.

These communication-linked disorders have far-reaching effects, ranging from an inability to speak coherently to difficulties interpreting and comprehending messages conveyed orally or in writing. Clearly any of these will have a profound effect on an older person's social and psychological well-being and may ultimately impinge on physical status as well.

Communicating with an older person with aphasia

Ebersole & Hess (1994) provide a series of pointers which nurses may find useful when communicating with older people with aphasia:

- Explain interventions in an accessible way
- Avoid child-like or patronizing language
- Keep calm and patient, and allow enough time for responses
- Speak slowly and clearly
- Ask one question at a time and wait for an answer before moving on to the next
- Speak about things that will interest the person
- Augment verbal communication with visual cues (pictures, objects) and non-verbal cues
- Encourage speech, even if it is hard to understand
- Show interest in the person.

Groher (1989) reminds us to stand on the unaffected side of the person with stroke illness, thereby maximizing the likelihood of non-verbal cues being seen. He offers useful advice in relation to word-finding problems, suggesting that if you know the word being searched for that you could consider helping with sentence completion by saying, for instance, 'I want a

drink of . . .' (and then pause); the patient may then find it easier to fill in the missing word (p. 35).

Aphasia often has an isolating effect on older people and several clubs and groups have been established to try to help people with aphasia to communicate more effectively. Recently Rayner & Marshall (2003) trained six volunteers from one such group as 'conversation partners' for other people with aphasia. The training aimed to extend the volunteers' knowledge of aphasia and provide them with a selection of communication strategies that would help them to talk with people with aphasia (and also enhance their own communication skills). The initiative was evaluated positively and highlights the benefits that innovations designed specifically to address older people's communication needs could have on older people's well-being. Case study 10.1 illustrates a nurse's awareness of how to communicate with a patient who had suffered a stroke.

Case study 10.1: Communicating with a stroke patient: a nurse's story

Mr Jenkins lay motionless in bed – he had just been admitted to my ward from the Medical Assessment Unit after having had a stroke. Although he was unable to talk or move, his eyes followed every movement that I made as I tried to make him comfortable and adjust his intravenous infusion. I was to work with him for the rest of the shift.

After about 10 minutes, I realized that it felt rather eerie being watched so closely – I wasn't used to that. I went to fetch another pillow and thought about it and then I realized that this was his way of communicating with me, that I'd been so busy adjusting the intravenous infusion and trying to make him comfortable that I'd said very little. Recognizing this absence of verbal communication took me by surprise. I was usually aware of the importance of talking with people even when they weren't able to respond in words. After that I started to talk more about what I was doing. His eyes continued to follow me and my conversation more attentively, as if they were listening themselves to what I was saying. He began to relax as I continued to talk about what was going to happen to him during the rest of the shift, who I was and who the rest of the team were who would be looking after him and how long he might expect to have the intravenous infusion up.

Recognizing his need for explanation and the degree of normality conferred by my talking was an important way to settle Mr Jenkins into the ward and to reassure him about his care.

Dysarthria

Dysarthria is the second most common disorder related to speech impairment to affect older people (Ebersole & Hess 1994). Dysarthria compromises the intelligibility of speech by poor muscle coordination and can be associated with respiratory function, difficulties in articulation, phonation (the ability to produce sounds) and resonance (the quality of the sounds, e.g. loudness, depth; Groher 1989). These problems can cause distortions of all sounds. Dysarthria is therefore classified as an expressive disorder affecting the structural mechanisms of speech. The consequences can range from voice tremors to slow, uncertain speech. Sensitive communication, which uses the principles suggested by Ebersole & Hess (1994) for older people with aphasia (outlined above) and takes into account the treatment prescribed by a speech and language therapist, will be necessary to establish therapeutic communication.

Assessment

Nurses may be among the first people to identify a speech impairment, which should be accurately noted and referred for specialist intervention early on to facilitate an appropriate plan of action. Assessment may be facilitated through the use of the skilled communication and enhanced, in the case of aphasia, by using the Frenchay Aphasia Screening Test (FAST) (Enderby et al. 1987).

Coping with a speech impairment may be an all-consuming task for an older person, taking up a large amount of energy and concentration. For many people speech impairment causes considerable frustration as speech is generally regarded as the mainstay of communication and effective alternatives are hard to find. Nurses caring for people with a speech disorder need to be aware of the far-reaching effects of this impairment on an older person's social, psychological and physical well-being.

Communication and dementia

Bollinger & Hardiman (1989) described the principal characteristics of dementia as:

- memory impairment
- intellectual impairment
- personality deterioration
- disorientation and confusion
- emotional change
- disorders of communication.

All of these characteristics will, either individually or collectively, have marked effects on communication. Despite this it is important to remember, as Goldsmith (1996) suggests, that communication, although altered to suit each person with dementia, is still possible.

Effects of dementia on communication

Dementia can have a far-reaching impact on the ways in which people communicate. When these alterations to communication are combined with other difficult behaviours linked to dementia (e.g. wandering or forgetfulness) they may result in frustration, anger and isolation for both the person with dementia and/or those providing care (Goldsmith 1996). Some of the most common effects of dementia on communication are outlined below:

- Speech and language disruption will vary with the stage of dementia. This disruption is likely to include, during the course of the disease, poor comprehension, reduced vocabulary resulting in the need to search for appropriate words, difficulty in naming objects, fragmentation of sentences, digression from the topic of conversation, echoing sounds or, in the extreme, the older person may become mute. As the dementia progresses the person's insight will diminish and it will become harder to cover up these speech and language deficits. This will have a significant effect on both the older person's communication skills and the quality of interactions
- Written skills will also deteriorate, with difficulty in choosing correct words or constructing sentences
- Difficulty in following conversations will result from poor comprehension and diminished attention span. Conversations may be easier when long-term memory is used.

Assessing communication impairments associated with dementia

This is a complicated process in which all members of the multidisciplinary team have a role. Nurses will find it useful to consider Jacques' (1992) advice that listening to the older person speaking provides important information on the use of the right words, appropriate sentence structures, difficulties in articulation and naming objects. Consideration of each of these will help the nurse to determine the effect of dementia on communicative abilities and how these will impact on the care planned for the person. Assessment at an early stage helps nurses to recognize progressive deterioration in communication skills and alerts them to the need to modify their own skills to suit the older person's needs (see Chapter 24 for more information on assessment in dementia).

Communicating with an older person with dementia

As the disease progresses it is unlikely that significant improvements can be made in the older person's communicative ability. Therefore efforts need to be directed towards modifying the communication skills of all those interacting with the person. This will naturally be time-consuming, as the abilities and needs of the person with dementia may vary from day to day and person to person. The goal of successful communication, in this instance, is to create an environment that facilitates flexible communication by all carers (lay and professional) and is guided by the older person's changing needs. Carers will need to adapt their communication styles to suit the ways in which the dementia is experienced by the older person. Goldsmith (1996) suggests some useful general strategies for communicating with someone who has dementia:

1. Make the environment conducive to communication. For instance, make sure that the TV or radio is switched off
2. Leave enough time for the interaction
3. Approach the older person slowly and from within his or her line of vision
4. Reinforce your verbal communication with touch if this is appropriate
5. Listen
6. Use short sentences
7. Allow enough time for responses and do not immediately decide that the older person hasn't understood the conversation if he or she doesn't respond
8. Try to illustrate what you are saying with photos or objects
9. Don't feel that it is necessary to correct mistakes in conversations
10. Do not be embarrassed by the expression of emotions in the interaction.

In addition to these strategies, Tanner & Daniels (1990) highlighted a series of behaviours which carers could use to enhance communication. These are based on their observations of interactions between eight carers and their relatives with dementia, and may be useful for nurses to consider in relation to their own practice or to give as advice to relatives of people with dementia.

Behaviours that enhance communication (Tanner & Daniels 1990)

To gain attention:

- using non-verbal cues – touch, eye contact, gesture
- being in close proximity during the interaction
- turning to face the older person
- saying the person's name
- using a focus such as an object or photograph.

During the conversation:

- using a warm and encouraging tone of voice
- speaking slightly louder
- saying the person's name
- making the content clear and simple by using short sentences
- repeating and rephrasing statements
- checking understanding by asking for clarification
- using non-verbal cues – eye contact, gesture, facial expression
- using an object as a focus
- interpreting the older person's behaviour or communication.

In response to communication from the older person:

- using non-verbal communication – touch, eye contact, gesture, facial expression, laughter
- using an appropriate tone of voice
- using short sentences with simple content
- giving confirmation
- asking for clarification.

Behaviours that inhibit communication (Tanner & Daniels 1990)

- addressing older people while they are doing something else and not getting their attention
- speaking too quickly and too quietly
- not checking understanding
- using a frustrated/exasperated tone of voice
- using complicated sentences
- having unrealistic expectations
- giving insufficient explanation
- using patronizing language
- excluding the older person from communication
- not listening
- using minimal non-verbal communication.

Communicating with a person with dementia is an extremely time-consuming and complex undertaking but one that, if done successfully, has the potential to increase physical, social and psychological well-being (see Chapter 24 for further details).

Sensory deprivation

Sensory deprivation may be associated with any of the communication challenges discussed above. It may also occur as a result of diminished social contact, isolation or living in an unstimulating environment. Within care settings nurses have a key role to play in keeping sensory deprivation to a minimum. Skilled communication, using both verbal and non-verbal cues, is particularly valuable in overcoming sensory deprivation, whether it is associated with age- or illness-related changes to communication. The information given earlier in this chapter will help nurses minimize the likelihood of older people experiencing sensory deprivation.

Sensory deprivation may have far-reaching effects on older people:

- exaggerate personality traits
- cause emotional changes – boredom, restlessness, irritability, anxiety
- cause perceptual disorganization – alterations in perceptions of colour, shapes, movements
- lead to an inability to think and solve problems
- in extreme cases result in hallucinations
- increase somatic complaints
- contribute to fluctuating emotional states
- disturb usual routines, e.g. sleeping
- cause disorientation due to an unusual environment.

These may be exacerbated when combined with illness.

Nurses need to create a stimulating environment for those who are not acutely ill. Increasingly nurses work alongside other health care professionals, particularly occupational therapists, to facilitate this. The nurse's communication skills and knowledge of the older person are central to establishing a partnership so that each person feels involved in decisions regarding activities designed to meet individual interests. The net result of this partnership will be to offer a choice of activities that will minimize boredom and restlessness.

Sensory deprivation may also be minimized by helping older people to maintain their own identity by bringing special items from their homes when they need to move into long-term care settings or their hospital stay becomes lengthy. For people requiring acute care, a stay in hospital will detach them from the pace of life outside the hospital so that they may feel deprived of their everyday routines or fearful of returning to their previous lifestyle. Nurses will find it useful to discuss this issue with patients and their friends or relatives so that readjustment following discharge from hospital can be optimized.

Challenging behaviour

Sometimes older people exhibit what is often referred to as 'challenging behaviour', either physically or through their style of communication. With reference to the latter this may include:

- expressions of frustration with one's physical, social or psychological status
- expressions of anger
- misunderstandings
- having insufficient information on which to base decisions.

Alternatively, it may be part of a person's natural character. In these situations nurses will find it useful to determine the source of the problem and discuss how the problem can be resolved. The following strategies may be useful:

- keeping calm
- allowing the person to express strong feelings
- acknowledging that these have been heard
- using assertive statements (clear, honest and direct) or assertive techniques in reply (such as the 'broken-record technique' – repeating, in a relaxed way, what you think is important, or want from the situation, with the aim of getting the other person to begin negotiating the way forward with you)
- listening to what is being said
- negotiating a way forward
- if the interaction becomes too heated, leaving and saying you will return later – and returning later.

THE THERAPEUTIC VALUE OF COMMUNICATION BETWEEN OLDER PEOPLE AND NURSES

Nursing is an interactive process where the quality of the relationship between nurse and patient can have marked effects on the physical, social and psychological well-being of patients and their quality of life. For many years nursing has been described as therapeutic through its ability to help people make positive movements towards health (Ersser 1997). The use of highly developed communication skills may be one way of facilitating this movement.

This interpersonal relationship may start by the negotiation of partnerships between nurses and patients. For nurses, Christensen (1993) suggests, this involves attending, enabling, interpreting, responding and anticipating with patients. For patients, negotiation means managing one's self, surviving the ordeal, affiliating with experts and interpreting the experience. Each of these activities is intrinsically associated with communication and thus provides a link between the notion of therapeutic nursing and communication with the nurse during the process of care, and becoming 'a companion through the ordeal' as a result (Christensen 1993: p. 34). Once the partnership is negotiated the work of the nurse and patient centres on maintaining the therapeutic nature of the partnership, again relying on the use of sensitive communication skills. There remains continued emphasis on partnership development during the care, either acute or continuing, of older people within hospital and/or community-based settings; therefore this would seem to be an underlying principle of nursing older people

Ford (1994), in semistructured interviews, asked four older people living in continuing care wards what they valued in nurses. In relation to communication the ideal nurse was 'organized, calm and professional ... intuitive ... A nurse who really cares does things differently and they are greatly valued by patients' (p. 45). Patients know what they want from nurses and what sets the 'good' nurse apart. Expert nurses were able to show understanding, caring and friendship or, perhaps, as Christensen (1993: p. 34) suggests, become 'a companion through the ordeal'. Christensen identified several elements that were central to the relationship between nurses and patients, such as sociability (civility, humour and socializing), reciprocity (friendship, sharing and solving problems) and the idea of 'being my nurse' (showing involvement, partnership, being a confidante and caring individually for each person). These elements clearly show what older people expect of nurses and emphasize the centrality of communication to this process.

Communication may be affected by the underpinning values of the nurse or the unit where the nurse works. This is illustrated by Thomas (1994) who found that the nursing values espoused by the nurses in elderly-care wards influenced the amount of time qualified nurses and auxiliaries spent talking to older people. Nurses and auxiliaries in wards using primary nursing spent significantly more time talking with patients than those in wards using team or functional approaches to care. These differences were particularly marked when making choices and providing patients with explanations about their care. The primary nursing staff felt positively about communicating with older people and transmitted this to their practice.

Communication is affected by the professional and personal characteristics of the nurse, patient and family or friends who may accompany the elderly person during the interaction (Cook et al. 1990). This triad can often complicate interactions, as well as facilitate them, as the nurse may find conflicting opinions being presented by the older person and the carer(s). Careful negotiation between all involved is required to retain the focus of the interaction and enhance its therapeutic nature.

Communication allows nurses to gather information from older people and their carers that will facilitate sensitive assessment, planning, delivery and evaluation of care. Coupled with the potential to develop a rapport between the nurse and the older person, this kind of communication builds up trust, support and understanding, so enabling a partnership to be established which facilitates collaborative decision-making (Fig. 10.3).

SUCCESSFUL COMMUNICATION

Although there is no foolproof recipe for successful communication, the following general pointers will help nurses to consider how their communication

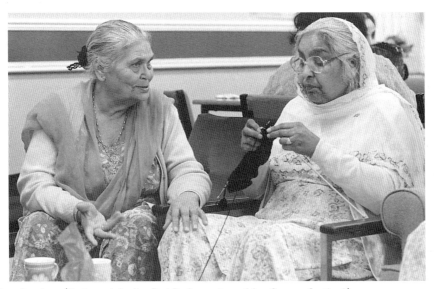

Fig. 10.3   Touch and gesture. (Photograph by Jon-Paul Davis, courtesy of Age Concern Scotland.)

skills could be enhanced when working with older people:

- create an open atmosphere between interactors
- be available
- listen
- watch
- consider alternative forms of communication (signing, simple preset movements, e.g. 'nod your head if the answer is yes')
- acknowledge an older person's reality. Nussbaum et al. (1989) warn us against the use of disconfirming statements which do not acknowledge the older person's reality (e.g. ignoring comments or using child-like language in response to comments). Disconfirming statements can make people doubt themselves and their understanding of their own situation. This is particularly important as many older people fear exactly that, in their fear of dementia and confusion. Older people may be seen as disconfirming to the young too through, for example, forgetfulness
- avoid oversimplification of language and thinking that older people lack intelligence if they do not understand. Child-like or patronizing language is never appropriate
- check out interpretations
- avoid ritualistic or unrewarding conversations
- consider alternative communication media, for example music, art or literature
- create an environment which is conducive to communication or facilitates welcome solitude.

This list can be augmented by Holden's (1988) guidelines for helping older people who have verbal and non-verbal deficits. In relation to verbal challenges she proposes the following strategies. First, recognize that communication impairments do not go hand-in-hand with older age. Second, talk with and do not ignore the person. If the patient is unable to speak to you, try alternatives such as writing notes or using gestures. Talk normally using simple language. Keep to one topic to avoid confusion and choose a topic that is relevant. Do not fill in the blanks and complete sentences for the other person. Remember to check for communication aids – the correct dentures, working hearing aids, clean spectacles. Always retain your patience and understanding.

Holden (1988) addresses non-verbal challenges related to memory loss and movement disorder. In relation to memory loss she advises certain games (e.g. Scrabble, I spy, Kim's game and Monopoly) and quizzes, together with reminder notes, lists, written directions and large-face clocks and calendars to facilitate everyday activities. Movement disorders are likely to affect communication through clumsiness, the inappropriate use of gestures or difficulty with daily living activities, such as dressing, which will alter appearance and affect interactors' perceptions. Holden suggests hand exercises to increase dexterity and formal relearning of other movements. Where older people have difficulty in recognizing objects through one channel (e.g. sight), Holden advises the use of other channels – touching, smelling or listening – to enhance information and therefore provide a more complete picture of the object.

These approaches can be enhanced through the use of reminiscence or story-telling to promote intergenerational understanding by:

- sharing attitudes, histories, backgrounds and experiences
- increasing the nurse's awareness of life events
- allowing the nurse to assess psychological and social feelings of well-being
- allowing the nurse to gather information about the older person's physical, psychological and social function
- allowing the nurse to identify deficits in communication skills
- facilitating rapport.

Successful communication between nurses and older people can be enhanced and evaluated through an assessment of the older person's communication ability, ranging from language comprehension and expression through to the use of non-verbal skills. Sweeney et al. (1993) proposed, in their study of communication disorders in older people in hospital, some possible approaches using standardized tests administered by a research nurse. The most useful test was the FAST (Enderby et al. 1987), which can be used to identify language deficits (language comprehension, expression, reading and writing) and problems associated with articulation. This test is particularly useful because it is designed for use by non-specialists. It may be used with other tests of sight, hearing and cognition to provide a useful starting point for formal assessment by nurses of communication skills, although the informal collection of information through everyday interactions should not be overlooked. Nurses must be able to highlight problems with communication so that their care can be sensitively tailored to meet individual need and they can make prompt referrals for specialist help when problems are apparent. Case study 10.2 demonstrates a nurse's awareness of how to improve her communication with a patient with Parkinson's disease who had a history of falling.

Case study 10.2: Communicating with a patient with Parkinson's disease and a history of falls: a nurse's reflections

For once I was early . . . I walked slowly into the day hospital. It was my first day back from holiday and I felt refreshed and ready to tackle some of the challenges that I'd left behind. I was thinking about how to solve some of those problems when, as I walked past the sitting room, my attention was drawn to a new patient. She was sitting by herself next to the window. She was smartly dressed and didn't seem distressed but she had a distant look – her face strangely stiff and mask-like. I carried on walking, thinking that I would find out more about her at the handover report, especially as I was the primary nurse for that half of the unit.

Mrs Jackson had just been referred to the day hospital. Her general practitioner had been worried by the increased number of falls that she had experienced over the last fortnight and referred her for assessment by the rehabilitation team. She had had Parkinson's disease for the last 10 years. She lived on her own and until recently had been very independent. Now, however, she was becoming more and more depressed because of her increased immobility and fear of falling.

The handover report ended and I went straight to talk to Mrs Jackson. We spoke generally about her falls and tried to identify reasons for them. We thought about the layout of her home and the sort of activities that she liked to do and tried to work out a plan of how she might do things which she could talk through with the occupational therapist when he visited her later that morning. All the time we were together I was aware of how slowly and carefully Mrs Jackson spoke to me – conversation took a lot of effort because of this and I was aware that I was constantly thinking of finishing her sentences to hurry things along. I didn't though because that wouldn't really have helped.

When I handed over my patients at lunchtime to the afternoon staff, I talked through my concerns about communicating with Mrs Jackson – how I had had to listen very carefully to her because she spoke slowly and quietly, how I had had to be careful not to finish her sentences for her because I wanted to get on and how when she wrote down some of the things that she needed to talk about with the occupational therapist I noticed how her hand had a slight tremor. I realized as I passed this information on how important it was for other people to know these things so that they would encourage her to talk rather than leave her in isolation at her next visit, and also recognize that, although her speech seemed slow and laborious, she was able to direct what was going on around her and was very enthusiastic about reducing the falls that she had been experiencing.

As I went home I thought more about Mrs Jackson. I reflected on how some chronic illnesses affect the ways in which people communicate and how, although the person with the illness is used to these changes, sometimes carers (either professional or lay) find the effects of this alteration difficult to deal with. I was pleased that I'd had time to spend talking with Mrs Jackson and that I hadn't felt rushed in the ways through which I communicated with her.

CONCLUSION

Many older people requiring nursing care, either in the community or in hospital, have problems associated with communication. This chapter has focused on the most common challenges to communication presented in older age and has highlighted ways in which nurses can enhance their communication skills in order to help older people and their friends and relatives cope with these challenges. Each of these challenges requires skilled therapeutic intervention to maintain or enhance every older person's physical, social and psychological well-being and therefore quality of life.

All nurses, regardless of their speciality, need to be constantly aware of the changes associated with ageing and illness that might affect communication and also of the intergenerational differences between themselves and older people. Knowledge of these factors and the development of sensitive styles of communication will facilitate therapeutic communication that provides information, support and social interaction to older people and their carers.

Recommended reading

Argyle M 1994 The psychology of interpersonal behaviour, 5th edn. Penguin, London.
This classic book is an easy-to-read, informative work on social behaviour. It addresses verbal and non-verbal communication in detail and provides useful information on how people interact either individually or in groups. Discussions also centre on social skills in relation to different professional groups including nurses and different types of interactions (e.g. interviews, supervision, public speaking).

Hargie O (ed) 1993 A handbook of communication skills. Routledge, London.
This edited text is, as the title suggests, a handbook detailing a variety of communication skills ranging from questioning to

negotiating and bargaining. Hargie's book is a useful companion to this chapter and several relevant chapters will help readers to refine their communication skills.

Rau M 1993 Coping with communication challenges in Alzheimer's disease. Singular Publishing, San Diego.

This book is written for people who have friends or relatives with Alzheimer's disease. It covers the progress of Alzheimer's disease and portrays a vivid picture of what can be expected, in relation to communication, for someone at each stage of the disease. Nurses might recommend this book for friends and relatives of people with Alzheimer's disease.

Worrall L, Hickson L 2003 Communication disability in aging: from prevention to intervention. Thomson, Clifton Park, NY.

This book, although primarily written for speech and language therapists, is an informative text that sensitively discusses communication changes in older age. It provides an overview of communication disability and a host of assessment scales which nurses may find useful.

References

Andersson G, Melin L, Scott B et al. 1994 Behavioural counselling for subjects with acquired hearing loss. A new approach to hearing tactics. Scandinavian Audiology 23: 249–256

Argyle M 1994 The psychology of interpersonal behaviour, 5th edn. Penguin, London

Armstrong L, McKechnie K 2003 Intergenerational communication: fundamental but under-exploited theory for speech and language therapy with older people. International Journal of Language and Communication Disorders 38: 13–29

Biggs S 1993 Understanding ageing. Open University Press, Buckingham

Bollinger R, Hardiman C 1989 Dementia: the confused-disorientated communicatively disturbed elderly. In: Hull R, Griffin K (eds) Communication disorders in aging. Sage, Newbury Park, pp; 61–77

Christensen J 1993 Nursing partnership. A model for nursing practice. Churchill Livingstone, Edinburgh

Cook M, Coe R, Hanson K 1990 Physician–elderly patient communication: processes and outcomes of medical encounters. In: Stahl S (ed) The legacy of longevity. Sage, Newbury Park, pp 291–309

Department of Health 2001 National service framework for older people. Department of Health, London

Department of Health 2003a Care homes for older people. National minimum standards. Stationery Office, London

Department of Health 2003b Essence of care: patient focused benchmarks for clinical governance. NHS Modernisation Agency, London

Dowd J 1986 The old person as stranger. In: Marshall V (ed) Later life. The social psychology of aging. Sage, Beverly Hills, pp 147–189

Ebersole P, Hess P 1994 Toward healthy aging: human needs and nursing response. Mosby, St Louis

Enderby P, Wood V, Wade D, Langton Hewer R 1987 The Frenchay aphasia screening test: a short simple test for aphasia appropriate for non specialists. International Rehabilitative Medicine 8: 11–13

Ersser S 1997 Nursing as a therapeutic activity: an ethnography. Avebury, Aldershot

Ford P 1994 What older people, as patients in continuing care, value in nurses. MSc thesis. Keele University, Keele

Ford J, Sinclair R 1987 Sixty years on: women talk about old age. Women's Press, London

Giles H, Coupland N 1991 Language: contexts and consequences. Open University Press, Milton Keynes

Goldsmith M 1996 Hearing the voice of people with dementia: opportunities and obstacles. Jessica Kingsley, London

Gravell R 1988 Communication problems in elderly people: practical approaches to management. Croom Helm, Beckenham

Groher M 1989 Neurologically based disorders of speech and language among older adults. In: Hull R, Griffin K (eds) Communication disorders in aging. Sage, Newbury Park, pp 23–37

Hargie O 1993 Communication as skilled behaviour. In: Hargie O (ed) A handbook of communication skills. Routledge, London, pp 7–21

Hargie O, Marshall P 1993 Interpersonal communication: a theoretical framework. In: Hargie O (ed) A handbook of communication skills. Routledge, London, pp 22–56

Hearing Concern 1996 Understanding deafness. Hearing Concern (British Association of the Hard of Hearing), London

Holden U 1988 Recognizing the problems. In: Holden U (ed) Neuropsychology and ageing. Croom Helm, London, pp 1–22

Hull R 1989 The hearing-impaired older adult. In: Hull R, Griffin K (eds) Communication disorders in aging. Sage, Newbury Park, pp 91–102

Jacques A 1992 Understanding dementia. Churchill Livingstone, Edinburgh

Monaghan A 1995 Communication. In: Heath H (ed) Foundations in nursing theory and practice. Mosby, London, pp 275–298

Nussbaum J, Thompson T, Robinson J 1989 Communication and aging. Harper & Row, New York

Rayner H, Marshall J 2003 Training volunteers as conversation partners for people with aphasia. International Journal of Language and Communication Disorders 38: 149–164

Royal National Institute for the Deaf 1998 It's time for a hearing test – a report on hearing tests, ear health and public attitudes. Royal National Institute for the Deaf, London

Ryan E, Meredith S, MacLean M, Orange J 1995 Changing the way we talk with elders: promoting health using the communication enhancement model. International Journal of Aging and Human Development 41: 89–107

Sweeney T, Sheahan N, Rice I et al. 1993 Communication disorders in a hospital elderly population. Clinical Rehabilitation 7: 113–117

Tanner B, Daniels K 1990 An observation study of communication between carers and their relatives with dementia. Care of the Elderly 2: 247–250

Thomas L 1994 A comparison of the verbal interactions of qualified nurses and nursing auxiliaries in primary, team and functional nursing wards. International Journal of Nursing Studies 31: 231–244

Worrall L, Hickson L 2003 Communication disability in aging: from prevention to intervention. Thomson, Clifton Park, NY

Chapter 11

Hearing

Debbie Tolson and Iain R.C. Swan

INTRODUCTION

Communication is an important part of all social life and hearing difficulties in all age groups can present many challenges for individuals, their families and their contacts. Difficulty with hearing is not an inevitable consequence of growing old, but epidemiological data demonstrate an increasing prevalence of hearing impairment in people over the age of 60 years (Davis 1995). Hearing impairment in older people may cause greater disability than in younger people because of the impact of other disabilities, especially visual impairments, on their everyday life. There is enormous potential for nurses to support people who are affected by age-related hearing problems providing that they know how to recognize problems and understand the ways in which individuals and their families can be supported. This chapter explores the evidence which should inform the practice of all nurses who work with older people across all care settings.

We start with an overview of the function of the ear and hearing mechanisms and move on to the activities of hearing and listening. Prevalence and aetiology of hearing impairment are discussed, as are ear wax and the concepts of disability, handicap and participation. From this foundation we focus on the knowledge essential to understanding and caring for older people with hearing disability and those who choose to use hearing aids. Advice is given on ways that nurses can contribute to enabling care for both individuals and their regular communication partners. Finally we look at tinnitus to complete our exploration of common problems that older people may experience with their auditory functioning.

THE FUNCTION OF THE EAR

The function of the ear is to convert sound waves in the air around us to electrical impulses in the auditory nerve. The ear is divided into the external, middle and inner ears. The external ear comprises the pinna and the external auditory canal which collect sound and direct it to the tympanic membrane which divides the external and middle ears. The middle ear is an air-filled cavity which contains the ossicular chain: the malleus, incus and stapes. This chain of tiny bones converts sound waves in air to sound waves in the fluid filling the inner ear, or cochlea. The sound waves in the fluid of the inner ear bend the hairs on the hair cells. As the hairs bend chemicals are released which generate an electrical impulse in the auditory nerve.

A basic understanding of how the normal ear works enables nurses to appreciate normal function and the principles of auditory rehabilitation. It will also facilitate information-giving to older people and in particular making sense of hearing aids and other assistive listening devices. A useful overview of age-related changes in the auditory system is provided by Brant (1999).

Abnormalities of the external or middle ear, such as impacted wax or a perforation of the tympanic membrane, cause a conductive hearing impairment. The conduction of sound to the inner ear is impaired so that loudness is reduced, similar to turning down the volume on a TV or radio. A sensorineural hearing impairment is due to pathology in the inner ear or the auditory nerve, most commonly loss of hair cells in the cochlea. In addition to reduced loudness there is commonly loss of frequency and temporal resolution so that, even though sounds may be heard, discrimination of individual sounds is poor. Thus, in addition to the reduced perception of sound, the way sounds of different pitches or frequencies are heard is affected. This is similar to a radio where the volume is too low and, in addition, it is not tuned properly. So while some sounds may be audible, they are distorted and difficult to recognize and word recognition can become difficult.

HEARING AND LISTENING

Hearing and listening are integral to communication that involves speech or other sounds. Hearing is a passive activity in that an individual's ability to hear is a given; listening on the other hand is an active and dynamic process. A person's capacity to listen and motivation to engage in the act of listening depend on a number of factors. To begin with we need to be alert to sounds and, in effect, tune in and focus on interesting ones. Lack of interest in the topic, tiredness, distractions and low mood make us disinclined to listen. Similarly if a conversation does not include us, while

we may be aware that people are talking, we may to some extent ignore them and exercise a degree of choice over intentional listening. In difficult listening circumstances such as in the presence of background noise or when hearing ability is poor it requires a greater effort to understand what is being said and the work of listening becomes harder. A common complaint of older people is that sometimes people, including nurses, exclude them from conversations or expect them to communicate in a disabling listening environment (Tolson & McIntosh 1997). It is important for nurses to recognize and make distinctions between hearing and listening and consider interventions that enable older people to maximize their communication potential.

PREVALENCE OF HEARING IMPAIRMENT

Hearing impairment is defined as a mean hearing level of 25 dB or greater (Fig. 11.1). It is common. About 20% of the UK adult population have a hearing impairment in their better hearing ear (Davis 1989, 1995). These data are from the National Study of Hearing carried out in several centres in the UK by the Medical Research Council Institute of Hearing Research. The proportion of the population with hearing impairment rises significantly in older people (Table 11.1). Those with thresholds of 25 decibels hearing level (dBHL) or worse have at least a mild hearing impairment. Those with thresholds of 45 dBHL or more have at least a moderate impairment and should have audiological rehabilitation. Of those people in the UK with a hear-

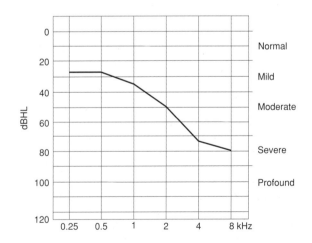

Fig. 11.1 Typical pure-tone audiogram of sensorineural hearing impairment with normal descriptors for hearing thresholds. dBHL, decibels hearing level.

Table 11.1   Prevalence of hearing impairment in the better-hearing ear in age bands

Age group (years)	Hearing ≥ 25 dBHL (%)	Hearing ≥ 45 dBHL (%)
61–70	36.8	7.4
71–	60.3	17.6
81+	93.4	63.6

dBHL, decibel hearing level.

ing impairment in their better hearing ear, about three-quarters are over 60 years of age and one-quarter are over 80 years of age. In the great majority of cases it is a sensorineural hearing impairment.

AETIOLOGY OF HEARING IMPAIRMENT

Sensorineural hearing impairment becomes increasingly common with advancing years. This does not mean that it is caused by age, and indeed it is unfair to older people to blame it on their age. The only significant cause of sensorineural hearing loss that can be readily identified is noise exposure, most commonly industrial noise. People who have worked in shipyards, steelworks and similar heavy industries commonly have sensorineural hearing impairment, hence the old terms such as 'boilermaker's deafness'. However, the majority of older patients with hearing impairment have not worked in noisy occupations. There are probably many factors involved, some related to lifestyle and some to the environment. In the great majority of people we cannot identify specific causes.

Sensorineural hearing impairment is usually more marked at high frequencies (Wiley et al. 1998). These are the frequencies at which vocal sounds such as 'd', 't', 's', 'sh' and 'f' occur. This is part of the reason why older people often say that they can hear people speaking but have difficulty in making out what is said. They can hear vowels and laryngeal tones – commonly the middle of words – but cannot hear the beginning or the end. Shouting at such a person usually does not help and may make things more difficult.

Older people can also have a conductive hearing impairment, though this only affects a small proportion of the hearing-impaired in this age group. This can be caused by simple obstruction of the external auditory canal by wax, or diseases of the middle ear. The most easily identified is chronic otitis media where there is usually a perforation of the tympanic membrane, sometimes with discharge. The ossicles

may also be damaged, either eroded by infection or fixed by scar tissue.

EAR WAX

Ear wax is produced in the lateral third of the external auditory canal. It keeps the lining of the ear canal moist and serves a protective function. Ear wax or cerumen is continuously moved outwards by the natural migration of the skin in the ear canal and can be removed by normal washing with soapy water and a flannel. Repeated use of cotton buds is not recommended as this can push the ear wax into a compact clump deep in the canal, and if used with force can cause damage to the delicate lining of the canal (Somerville 2002). Ear wax tends be less copious but harder in older adults due to increased amounts of keratin.

Where wax has become impacted there are three options. The most desirable is to use softening ear drops which may be purchased over the counter or prescribed by a physician or nurse prescriber. It is preferable to use gentle preparations such as docusate sodium or simple oil-based solutions rather than solvents, which, if used incorrectly, can lead to irritation and inflammation. An informative review of the evidence on the most effective products is offered by Somerville (2002), and this reveals that some frequently prescribed preparations are not as effective as practitioners may believe. If ear drops fail, ear syringing can be performed by a skilled nurse or doctor (Aung & Mulley 2002); however the evidence base for mechanical methods of removing ear wax is limited (Browning 2001). In the community, practice nurses or general practitioners undertake ear syringing; in hospital services physicians and nurses working within specialist services or who have demonstrated competence may undertake ear syringing. Although a relatively safe procedure in skilled hands (Browning 2001), some patients dislike it, particularly if they experience the unpleasant sensation of vertigo, but more usually due to the water being too cold or too hot.

It has been estimated that one-third of older adults experience cerumen impaction (Stone 1999). If wax is impacted against the tympanic membrane or if it totally occludes the ear canal, it may cause a conductive hearing impairment. Where impaction has occurred removal can improve a person's perception of ability to hear. However, many older people incorrectly assume that wax removal will significantly improve their hearing and are left disappointed. Wax obstruction can feel uncomfortable and interferes with hearing-aid fitting and for these reasons its removal is often indicated (Somerville 2002). It is important that older people understand that they are unlikely to notice a marked improvement in their ability to hear given the high prevalence of acquired sensorineural hearing impairment.

HEARING DISABILITY AND HANDICAP

A useful way to begin thinking about the scope for nursing interventions is to reflect on the international classifications of impairment, disability and handicap (World Health Organization 1980) and the recent revision of terminology which helpfully focuses on activity and participation (World Health Organization 1999). In other words, nursing interventions should be striving to minimize the impact of a hearing problem on an older person's activity not just in conversation with others but in all forms of participation.

Impairment is the abnormal function of the hearing mechanism that can be measured, for example by audiometry. Disability is about the hearing difficulties a person experiences in daily life, for example hearing in a noisy place. Handicap is the effect of hearing loss on the individual's life. Disability and handicap can be estimated by questionnaire and interview (Stephens & Hetu 1991) and a variety of tools exist.

Measurement of impairment and disability are recognized to be important for assessment and follow-up, for although it is not possible to reduce the impairment, the goal of auditory rehabilitation is disability reduction and improved participation. The most effective models of rehabilitation embrace the physical and social environment (Hetu & Noble 1994, Tolson & Stephens 1997) and reflect understanding of psychological aspects including motivation (Stephens 1996).

ASSESSMENT OF HEARING

Self-report

Optimal understanding of the nature of a person's hearing problem and the benefits or limitations one might anticipate from interventions require an appreciation of the individual's perception of the problem and others in the immediate environment. Studies have shown that older people tend to underreport hearing difficulties and often ask for help by saying that a member of their family thinks they have a problem (Chmiel & Jerger 1993). The usual admission query 'do you have problems with your hearing?' is totally inadequate as most will answer 'no'. More useful questions to ask include whether they need the television or radio volume

louder than others do and to explore their experience and ability to participate in conversation within noisy situations such as social gatherings, when in shops and church. As telephones are efficient transmitters of sound, people with mild to moderate hearing impairment do not usually report difficulties hearing on the telephone (Tolson & Swan 1991). An older person who reports a difficulty should be referred for specialist assessment. Unfortunately some nurses and doctors continue to dismiss this as an expected part of growing old. This type of complacent response reflects ignorance and ageism (Tolson 1997). For older people who are ambivalent about their hearing problem or find it difficult to acknowledge, it can be helpful to raise their awareness and offer referral based on informal testing using the whispered-voice test.

Whispered-voice test

Free-field, live-voice tests offer an inexpensive form of screening that can be undertaken by nurses with a little training and supervised practice. The whispered-voice test involves whispering as loudly as you can combinations of three numbers such as five, three, seven, or letters, for example 'a', 's', 'm', and asking the patient to repeat. The task should be explained carefully and practised prior to completion. Each ear should be tested and the non-test ear should be masked so that you know in which ear the sound is being heard. The best way to mask the non-test ear is to press on the tragus (the flap of cartilage immediately in front of the ear canal) with your finger so as to occlude the ear canal and then rub gently. With one hand masking the non-test ear, you should stand to the side of the test ear as far away from the ear as your arm will allow and without the patient seeing your lips. It is not necessary for patients to hear every number or letter but if they can correctly repeat at least 50% of the numbers then they pass the test (Tolson & Swan 1991). Over 90% of individuals with a pure-tone hearing average over 30 dBHL will be unable to repeat more than 50% of the numbers and letters whispered at arms-length from the test ear (Browning et al. 1989). The individuals who fail the whispered-voice test in both ears should be considered as candidates for a hearing aid or other form of hearing management and specialist advice should be sought (Swan & Browning 1985). Live-voice testing by competent examiners has been demonstrated to be reliable (Browning et al. 1989); however, poorly trained assessors who fail to perform voice tests in quiet environments render the test meaningless and unreliable (Philp et al. 2002). It is therefore important for nurses who wish to use this method to receive appropriate brief training and clinical supervision from experts.

Audiometry

Pure-tone audiometry is the basic test that assesses hearing thresholds over a range of frequencies for each ear (Fig. 11.1). The approved methodology for testing has been written by the British Society of Audiology (1981). Testing is carried out in sound-proofed rooms or booths. Tones through a range of frequencies are played into each ear and the patient reports when he or she hears them. The scale is designed so that normal hearing thresholds are between 0 and 20 dB. Rather than reporting audiometry as numerical thresholds that mean relatively little to the non-specialist, it is usually reported in terms that convey the hearing disability the individual with those thresholds is likely to suffer. The terms in Figure 11.1 are those that are widely used.

Measuring hearing disability

The aim of understanding a person's hearing disability is to facilitate care planning to focus on promoting participation in the activities which are most important to that person. A number of person-centred questionnaires exist, some of which combine scales with open-ended questions. Stephens et al. (2001) offers a concise overview of key instruments in terms of their focus on activity restriction and participation. A common purpose of these instruments is to allow the clinician insight into how the hearing deficit restricts day-to-day life and agree priorities for auditory rehabilitation.

The Glasgow Hearing Aid Benefit Profile (GHABP) is a client-centred outcome measure designed to evaluate the effectiveness of hearing-aid provision (Gatehouse 1999). It is a valid, easy self-completion questionnaire that is popular in the UK as a tool for the clinician to use to assess hearing-aid benefit over time. If no benefit is evident or an individual is dissatisfied this may indicate that a different aid is required, that the existing aid is not working properly or requires fine adjustments, or perhaps that other aspects of auditory rehabilitation require attention, such as the listening environment. Nurses can facilitate completion of the GHABP to problem-solve in collaboration with experts and offer advice. For nurses who support older people over an extended period of time, such as district nurses and those in long-term care settings, it is important to review progress at agreed intervals to ensure that the reduction in disability is maintained or improved. Being alert to increasing hearing disability

facilitates early referral and, where appropriate, corrective interventions.

THE EXPERIENCE OF AGE-RELATED HEARING DISABILITY

The overall effect of age-related hearing disability for the individual is that communication is incomplete and frustrating. Misunderstandings are embarrassing and, particularly if individuals do not openly acknowledge their difficulties but attempt to hide them, others may misinterpret incorrect or unexpected responses as a sign of confusion. The association with senility has fuelled stigma which makes some people who realize that they have a problem reluctant to admit it and others who would benefit from amplification refuse a hearing aid (Bridgewood 2000).

The impact of hearing loss on a person's life varies but can include threats to self-esteem, a reduced sense of security and loneliness (Chen 1994). Such reduced feelings of well-being can contribute to the risk of depression and an increased dependence on others (Gilhome Herbst et al. 1991, Tolson et al. 2002). The consensus view in the literature is that hearing difficulties reduce the quality of life of older people by interfering with communication and the social and emotional domains of their lives. Successive studies have shown this to be true for people living independently and those who are classified as dependent, such as residents within care homes (Tsuruoka et al. 2001).

To understand the impact on an individual's life is an essential step in audiological rehabilitation. Some studies suggest that the restrictions people experience in their ability to participate (hearing handicap) will influence their decision to seek help (Stephens et al. 2001). Using a new Life Effects Questionnaire which asks individuals to list the effects of their hearing problems on life, Stephens et al. (2001) have categorized the experiences of older people under five headings: (1) functional impairment; (2) activity limitation; (3) participation restriction; (4) environmental factors; and (5) personal factors. The main functional problem was the inability to hear. Some people report sleep disturbance due to tinnitus. Inability to hear the television, doorbell, telephone bell or radio were identified as important activity limitations. Participation restrictions included reports that individuals no longer watched television with family and other shared recreation and leisure activities were reduced. Using transport and moving around was limited, as were shopping, caring for others, participation in community life and going to church. Environmental factors that impact on people's experience include physical and non-physical attributes of their worlds. Important factors include communication skills of the person's immediate family members and their ability to create an enabling listening environment within the home. Although personal factors are specific to an individual, common experiences include frustration, embarrassment, irritability, anxiety and feeling upset. These experiences commonly culminate in a developing sense of isolation, becoming unsociable and feeling awkward in company. There is evidence that hearing-impaired older people show more symptoms of depression than their counterparts with good hearing (Tolson et al. 2002).

Age-related hearing impairment tends to develop slowly and people may be unaware until it restricts their daily lives. In one of the few phenomenological studies of older individuals' experience of hearing problems, Karlsson Espmark & Scherman (2003) highlight that individuals may consider that it is other people's fault that they cannot hear, blaming others for mumbling or talking too quietly. Such complaints are usually indicative of impaired hearing. Importantly, Karlsson Espmark & Scherman's study illuminates the dilemma that on the one hand being with others is desirable but on the other hand it brings hearing difficulty to the fore, thus creating distress. In terms of personal identity their work also explores the association of hearing problems with the state of being old, and the discomfort of realizing that you must be old because you have a problem hearing and yet otherwise do not feel old.

This issue of 'spoiled identity' affects how people cope with the problem. For example, they might mask difficulties by guessing and using a range of techniques to give the impression that they can hear. Hetu (1996) links the threat to social identity and associated stigma with shame and argues that these feelings interfere with an individual's search for the most effective solutions. This often manifests as a reluctance to acknowledge the problem, and in part explains why hearing aids may sit hidden in drawers as an unwelcome symbol of personal failure.

The existential value of hearing (Karlsson Espmark & Scherman 2003), that is to say, the sense of hearing promoting a feeling of existing and being alive, provides a compelling reason to maximize a person's opportunity to hear. To support older people who are living with hearing difficulties effectively the nurse needs to understand the role of hearing in personal identity, its contribution to well-being and the day-to-day experience. In addition, for nurses who have the opportunity to support families, it is important to consider the impact of the hearing problem on significant others.

THE IMPACT OF HEARING DEFICIT ON FAMILIES AND ACQUAINTANCES

As communication is a shared experience it is inevitable that a hearing deficit has an impact on those around the older person. For some this may result in restricting conversations to the essential and for others the distress may reduce their own health and fuel family tension. Several studies suggest that the impact on spouses and significant others is a reflection of the experience of the person with the impaired hearing (Stephens et al. 1995, Brooks et al. 2001). So there is mutual frustration at having to repeat things and annoyance at the different volumes desired for comfortable television and radio-listening. For partners intimate interactions are restricted and there is a tendency for tension to build in relationships (Hetu et al. 1993).

Caring families also suffer and in particular the well-being of the main carer is threatened due to increasing levels of stress (Tolson et al. 2002). Nurses concerned with the alleviation of caregiver stress may find that unmanaged hearing disability is adding an intolerable burden which can be alleviated with appropriate audiological management and nursing interventions, whereas solutions to other problems can be more elusive. The provision of a hearing aid, provided it is used, has been shown to reduce the main family carer's perception of the hassles associated with the hearing problem significantly (Tolson et al. 2002).

MANAGEMENT OF HEARING DISABILITY

Some cases of conductive hearing impairment can be managed surgically. However, the principal management of sensorineural hearing impairment is provision of a hearing aid or aids. It is estimated that only about one-third of the UK population who would potentially benefit from a hearing aid has one (Haggard & Gatehouse 1993). There are probably many reasons for this low take-up but one of the main ones is that hearing impairment is often seen as a sign of ageing and people therefore do not wish to be seen with an aid. Anyone with a hearing disability and who is motivated has the potential to benefit from a hearing aid. Motivation is essential because it takes some time and effort on the part of the patient to learn how to use an aid. Patients who are persuaded by relatives to get a hearing aid often do not use it.

Hearing aids are chosen and appropriately adjusted so that the amount of amplification varies across frequencies to match the hearing thresholds of the individual ear. They are like spectacles – a hearing aid will probably not suit another person and may not even suit the opposite ear of its owner.

People who have a hearing aid but still have significant hearing disability should be reassessed as they probably require their hearing-aid prescription to be updated. Those with a more severe hearing impairment often benefit significantly by using hearing aids in both ears.

Provision of hearing aids is only one part of audiological rehabilitation. Patients require instruction in operating their hearing aid and advice on its use in different listening situations. They should be reviewed a few weeks after fitting to confirm that the aid is providing adequate reduction in disability and that they understand how to use it. Advice should also be given on hearing tactics and environmental aids (see below).

What happens in the hearing–aid clinic?

Patients visiting a hearing-aid clinic for the first time will be reassured if they know what to expect (Swan & Tolson 1991) and may find it easier to attend with the support of a companion or, for those in care, with a social carer or nurse. Prior to the visit it is desirable that obstructive wax is removed as this will interfere with hearing-aid fitting. The visit to the audiology clinic normally starts with seeing the audiologist who will take a brief history and then examine the ears to check for obstructive wax or middle-ear disease. Tests for hearing often begin with voice tests followed by pure-tone audiometry and an assessment of disability. Further tests may also be undertaken.

Pure-tone audiometry is carried out by an audiologist in a room with special sound-deadening to keep ambient noise levels low. The patient wears earphones so that tones can be presented to one ear at a time. The hearing assessment will take 10–15 min and is used to determine how powerful a hearing aid is required and what sort of specific adjustments will be needed to maximize benefit.

Patients prescribed with behind-the-ear (BTE) or in-the-ear (ITE) aids will require a tailor-made transparent acrylic ear mould to connect the aid to the ear. An impression is taken of the ear using soft silicon. This is not a difficult or painful procedure, although it may feel a little strange and the silicon will feel warm. It is similar to the experience of getting dentures or teeth crowns fitted. When the patient returns to have the hearing aid fitted at the next appointment, the fit of the mould will be checked to ensure that it fits snugly so that amplified sound from the aid is kept in the ear canal. Ill-fitting moulds allow escaping amplified sound to re-enter the microphone and a whistle will be heard due to acoustic feedback.

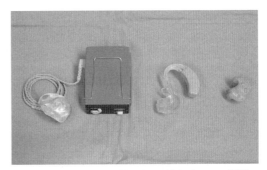

Fig. 11.2   Different types of hearing aid: body-worn (BW), behind-the-ear (BTE) and in-the-ear (ITE).

Types of hearing aid

There are many types of hearing aid (Fig. 11.2). The first hearing aids were large body-worn devices that were attached to clothing and were connected by wire to an ear mould. Such devices are rarely used nowadays except for individuals with profound hearing impairment or those requiring aids with large controls. These aids were replaced in the 1970s by BTE hearing aids: a small aid is placed behind the ear and sound is transmitted to an ear mould by tubing. The ear mould is custom-made for the patient. Now many hearing aids are ITE aids which fit in the concha: the electronics are within an ear mould. The aid itself is custom-made for the patient. There are also even smaller aids that fit in the ear canal (ITC): the power of ITC aids is limited so they are only of use for patients with a relatively mild impairment.

Basically all hearing aids consist of a microphone, an amplifier and a loudspeaker, and are powered by a battery. They have an on/off switch, a volume control and a battery compartment. Everyone dealing with patients, particularly elderly patients, should be able to manipulate a hearing aid, as some patients have difficulty doing it themselves. In body-worn and BTE aids, the on/off switch is usually labelled O for off, T for telecoil and M for microphone on (Fig. 11.3). At the telecoil position, the aid only picks up sound by electromagnetic induction from a loop system. Loop systems are found in some public places such as railway ticket offices, some churches, cinemas and theatres, and sometimes in telephones. This has the advantage of not picking up extraneous, unwanted sound. The appearance of the volume control varies but it is easy to identify, and sometimes it has helpful numbers. The battery compartment is obvious on inspection. The batteries are similar to those used in other small electronic devices such as watches and cameras.

Hearing aids should not usually whistle. This is acoustic feedback where sound coming out of the

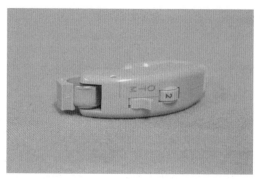

Fig. 11.3   Controls on a behind-the-ear hearing aid with open battery compartment.

speaker re-enters the microphone. If the hand is placed over the ear when the aid is worn then some feedback is to be expected, for example when brushing hair. If hearing aids whistle at other times, a common reason is that the mould has not been inserted properly in the ear. Other causes are a poorly fitting ear mould, broken tubing and the mould being blocked by wax.

A simple and effective way to tell if a hearing aid is working – that it has a charged battery – is to hold it in your hand, switch it on, turn up the volume and listen for the whistle when you put your other hand over it.

There are factors other than hearing that influence the choice of hearing aid. A reasonable degree of manual dexterity is required, so very small hearing aids may not be practical. In addition, the smaller the aid, the easier it is to lose; it may be inadvertently sent to the laundry or dropped unseen into pockets or down the side of chairs.

Supporting new hearing-aid users

Evidence demonstrates that new hearing-aid users require a period of time to adapt before they can derive maximum benefit in listening with amplified sound. For the more independent older person, limiting use to 15–30 min daily at first and stepping up use is recommended by Le May (1999). For frail and dependent older people more intensive support is recommended by Tolson & McIntosh (1997), who offer a flexible person-centred care plan that may take 7–28 days or longer before maximum gain is experienced. Regardless of the age and ability of the individual, all new hearing-aid users are advised to begin using the aid within quiet situations before they attempt to listen in situations of competing noise or near traffic. They may have little influence over noise levels where they live and, where opportunity exists, nurses should promote opportunities for older people to begin using

their hearing aid for one-to-one conversations in an environment with minimal distractions.

Hearing aids are designed to amplify speech but they do not restore normal hearing, so patients are sometimes disappointed at first by their new hearing aid. A period of acclimatization is needed for hearing sound differently that takes at least 3 months (Gatehouse 1992). The brain has become used to hearing sounds at low volume, particularly at frequencies where the impairment is most marked. As hearing aids, if well fitted to the patient's impairment, amplify differently across different frequencies, everyday sounds, particularly speech, sound different. Many patients at first describe the sound as 'tinny', because it is different to the sound to which they have become accustomed.

Nurses can also support older people by reinforcing information about how hearing aids work, how to insert the aid and use the controls and on maintenance, including battery replacement and cleaning. An equally important role is to develop the skills of communication partners who are unfamiliar with talking to people who use hearing aids.

Cochlear implants

Some patients with a profound hearing impairment do not benefit from hearing aids because they have so little residual hearing. Such patients can sometimes be helped by a cochlear implant. This is a management option for some older people. A cochlear implant is a speech processor connected to a row of electrodes that are fed directly into the cochlea. The device sends an electrical signal that stimulates the auditory nerve directly. Inserting a cochlear implant is a straightforward surgical procedure but the patient requires a lot of training over a period of many months to learn how to use the implant. This may not be a feasible option for some people and careful consideration must be given to an individual's capacity to adapt. Cochlear implants are very expensive and so there must be a reasonable prospect of patient benefit to make them worthwhile. However, several studies have shown that patients over 65 years of age obtain significant benefit from cochlear implantation, similar to that obtained by younger adults (Pasanisi et al. 2003).

Environmental aids

Environmental aids to hearing are also referred to as assistive listening devices and are designed to promote independence and safety. Older people with hearing impairment may have difficulty hearing the doorbell or the telephone ring. This can lead to increased isolation as carers have difficulty in making contact. Simple measures such as moving the doorbell and the telephone to a more appropriate area of the house can be helpful. Doorbells and telephone bells can be amplified or, for the more severely hearing-impaired, can be linked to a light. Simple measures like these can have a significant effect on the person's quality of life and can also reduce stress levels in relatives who are concerned when the door or telephone is not answered.

Telephones with amplified handsets are readily available. Telephones can also be purchased with built-in inductive couplers which allow hearing-aid users to select the 'T' setting which is designed for listening when using any loop induction system.

Loop systems enhance clarity as there is no background noise. Loop systems can be used by people without a personal hearing aid by using a device called a loop listener which can be a small device worn behind the ear or as a headset. A loop is a length of wire laid around the edge of a room connected to a loop amplifier which is attached to the equipment you wish to listen to. This can be, for example, a television set in a shared lounge or a microphone in a church. Several people can listen simultaneously within a loop providing that they have a hearing aid with 'T' function or a loop listener. Alternatively, individuals may prefer a personal loop system, a neck or ear loop which they plug into the equipment to which they are listening. Some of the most popular devices are those designed specifically for television and radio listening which allow volumes to be raised for people with hearing disability without disturbing others.

Communicators are devices that amplify sound and are designed to assist with one-to-one conversation (Fig. 11.4). There are several designs on the market with the basic features of a microphone for the speaker to use and an ear piece for the listener. Unlike personal hearing aids there is no scope for fine adjustments, simply a choice of volume setting. The ear piece is standard and, provided the ear piece is wiped clean between users,

the communicator can be used as required by anyone. Although communicators can be very useful they have a tendency to be forgotten resources rather than pieces of enabling equipment which should be readily available to older people (Tolson & McIntosh 1997).

It is important that older people and their families/carers are made aware of the choices available to them and a good source of information is the Royal National Institute for Deaf People helpline at www.rnid.org.uk. Local social service departments, social workers, occupational therapists and, where available, hearing therapists and specialist sensory impairment nurses will be able to provide advice and referral and assist in the selection and provision of appropriate environmental aids.

Listening environment

The environment in which we exist and communicate has important implications for both our ability to hear and desire to listen. From Nightingale's early reference to the benefits of a quiet healing environment (Nightingale 1859), a more comprehensive appreciation of the factors within the environment of care has emerged. Tolson & McIntosh (1997), for example, in their exploration of the complexity of the listening environment highlight the following as important considerations for an enabling environmental approach to nursing people with age-related hearing problems:

- intentional sounds (specifically directed to the individual) and unintentional sounds (background noise)
- the array of social, psychological and physical factors that promote or encourage an individual to engage in the act of listening or meaningful communication
- the hearing disability, auditory rehabilitation and personal factors
- the skill, knowledge and attitude of people, including professionals, who shape enabling communication opportunities or limit an individual's opportunity to participate in communication
- the availability of enabling listening devices.

Background noise is particularly disabling and effort should be made to provide quiet environments that promote opportunity for conversation. Families that appreciate the impact of noise and take steps to reduce it during social gatherings such as family meals can facilitate the impaired listener's ability to participate and feel included. Nurses in hospital wards and care homes who turn off radios and televisions during visits from families and health professionals are promoting an enabling listening environment.

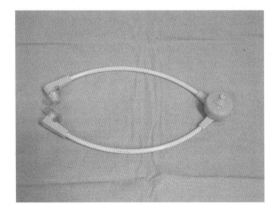

Fig. 11.4   Communicator.

A balance is required between quiet times and access to sounds that provide stimulation and an enjoyment such as music. However, rather than simply providing background music for entertainment, attention should be paid to enabling a person to hear the music with clarity such as may be achieved using induction loops and personal earphones. There is some evidence to suggest that, if people can control the noise level and type of noise to which they are exposed, this will facilitate a positive listening experience.

Physical environments with hard sound-reflective surfaces give rise to high levels of reverberation. Reverberation increases difficulties with word discrimination and the ability to understand speech. Clinical areas such as outpatient departments can present challenges as background noise combines with reverberation from hard surfaces. The provision of soft furnishings and wall coverings to dampen room reverberation is particularly helpful and desirable in areas where an older person's stay may be lengthy, such as in wards and care homes.

Hearing tactics

The behaviours that hearing-impaired individuals develop to improve their communication in various listening situations are collectively described as hearing tactics. Popular hearing tactics used by older people include:

- reinforcing messages with visual cues such as speech or lip-reading
- taking cues from facial expression and gestures
- keeping background noise to a minimum
- positioning themselves as close to the speaker as possible
- turning the better-hearing ear towards the person who is talking
- asking questions or indicating to the speaker if they have not heard, and developing conversational skills
- telling strangers what they can do to make it easier, for example speaking up but not shouting or exaggerating their lip movements
- showing appreciation when people adapt to help as this reinforcement is likely to encourage them to do it again
- adjusting the balance of treble to bass when listening to radio; some people find it easier to understand speech when there is more treble than bass
- keeping calm and trying not to worry if they miss some things (www.brighton-healthcare.nhs.uk/audiology/tactics; accessed 17 June 2003).

Understanding how people use or could develop their use of hearing tactics is an important part of auditory rehabilitation. The formal assessment of hearing tactics may be undertaken by specialists and, where available, hearing and speech therapists. Nurses can contribute to this process by observing behaviours; a brief observational checklist designed for nurse use is described by Newman (1990). Experienced nurses and nurses who have the opportunity to get to know an individual over time will find it relatively easy to identify such adaptive behaviours. An interesting exercise is casually to observe an older person during communication from a distance and watch for such tactics. By understanding, raising awareness, reinforcing successful strategies and skill-building, a nurse can help the listener and speaker to maximize communication potential (Fig. 11.5).

Nursing interventions

There is evidence that older people benefit from nursing interventions which seek to enable them to maximize their ability to communicate with others, enjoy entertainments and be independent (Schofield 2002). For some people who do not have the capacity or energy to adapt to a hearing aid or choose not to try one, interventions will be limited to improvements in the listening environment and developing the communication skills of family, friends and other caregivers (Tolson & McIntosh 1997). For the majority of older people, however, rehabilitation will focus on the issue of a hearing aid, the benefits of which can be augmented through skilled nursing care (Tolson & Nolan 2000).

Nurses can offer initial support by providing information and reassurance and helping individuals to understand that hearing impairment does not signify senility. Hearing disability is a problem that is easier to adapt to and less devastating if it is managed early. Once a hearing problem has been recognized and the older person decides what action to pursue there are a number of ways that nurses can help. These include referral to audiological services, preparation for the visit (e.g. information-giving, removal of ear wax, organizing transport) and supporting the person throughout the agreed auditory rehabilitation pathway.

For new hearing-aid users who may find adjustments hard work, a planned approach to encourage them to persevere as they adjust to amplified sound is essential; otherwise the aid will be discarded. A critical factor will be whether their early experience of hearing-aid use is undertaken within a disabling or enabling listening environment (Tolson & McIntosh 1997). When no improvement is observed or reported,

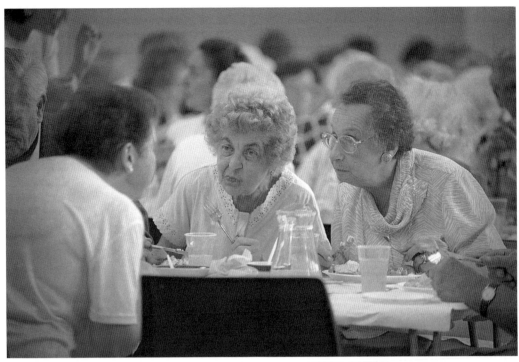

Fig. 11.5   Intense listening. (Photograph by Jon-Paul Davis, courtesy of Age Concern Scotland.)

rather than give up the nurse should encourage a return visit to the hearing-aid clinic where the situation will be reviewed and, if considered helpful, a new prescription for a different hearing aid can be offered.

An important issue for hearing-aid users is a problem known as 'recruitment'. This may be explained as functionally restricted auditory space; there is a fine distinction between the level of sound amplification that allows sound to be heard and the volume that results in discomfort and, in the extreme, pain. This is why expert assessment and prescription of the fine adjustments to each aid are crucial, and why hearing-aid users may flinch when people shout or there is sudden excess noise.

By developing the skills of older people and their usual communication partners through provision of information and instruction, nurses can promote independence and effective communication. Sometimes, as in the case of someone who is extremely weak or confused, it will be impossible to quantify the gain that is experienced, which may be modest. However, for the majority of older people who can use hearing aids, the improved communication will make a difference to their daily lives and should at the very least promote the opportunity for them to participate in decisions about their own care. As confidence grows, opportunities for greater forms of participation will increase, the

negative impact of unmanaged hearing loss should gradually decline and this improvement should be sustainable. Age-related hearing difficulties increase slowly over time and when a sudden onset of difficulty arises it is wise to check first that the hearing aid and battery are functioning properly and that wax obstruction has not developed. If in doubt, a referral to the hearing-aid clinic for reassessment is indicated. It is worth reminding people that a faulty aid, or an aid that is switched off, acts as an ear plug. Enabling communication involves ensuring that listening devices are working properly and are used in the most advantageous listening environment.

Enabling communication

Communication models abound in the literature and Chapter 10 has covered this topic in more detail than will be offered here. In terms of supporting older people with hearing disability we find one of the most useful representations for practitioners is that presented by Gravell (1988: p. 4). Gravell's chain of communication starts with the desire to communicate and reminds us that we need the capacity to receive and understand messages and to formulate and give a response, that is, if we choose to reply. In considering the best approach to communication we need to acknowledge that the cycle of communication can be limited by a range of factors including the individual's hearing, listening, cognitive abilities, vision, mood, well-being and motivation. The listening environment must be considered along with the skills and attitudes of those in regular contact with the person.

Interestingly, some nurses describe older people as being able to hear when they want to and being deaf when it suits. This apparent fluctuation is nothing to do with fluctuating levels of hearing impairment, but so-called patchy auditory performance is a product of changes in the listening environment. Knowing this helps us to understand why a ward patient, for example, can hear parts of the nurses' handover report when all else is quiet, but cannot hear when they are asked to do something during mealtime clatter. This phenomenon can be an unfortunate source of misunderstanding.

The principles of enabling communication when speaking to older people with impaired hearing embrace strategies that are general good practice and some more specific aspects concerned with use of amplified sound systems.

Always pause and consider the listening environment and timing if the communication is to involve important and complex messages rather than being an opportunistic and brief episode of social contact. Try to reduce levels of background noise by closing doors/windows and turning off radios, or alternatively arrange a quieter place for the conversation.

Attract the person's attention and encourage use of glasses if worn and check that the hearing aid is switched on and is working or use a communicator if preferred. Tapping a person on the arm may be appropriate in some situations, but you can also cause alarm if such contact is unexpected. If you enter a room and the person does not turn when spoken to, it may be useful to flick the light on and off, and most people will look around. Attention should be paid to the distance between the speaker and listener, which should be less than 1 m. According to a study by Erber et al. (1998), the ideal distance for some older hearing-aid users may be as close as 30 cm.

Ensure that there is adequate light for the person to see your face and try to talk at eye level. Standing with your back to a window in bright daylight can cast a shadow on your face and the visual cues that enhance understanding will be masked. Always face the person you are talking to and try to keep relatively still. If you need to pick up something or turn away, stop talking and resume when you are facing forward.

Speak clearly and do not shout as this will distort the shape of your mouth and hinder speech-reading and may also give rise to discomfort. It might be helpful to talk slightly more slowly than normal but not overly so, as this will distort mouth patterns. Get to the point quickly to avoid fatigue.

If you can, indicate the topic you want to discuss and again when you change topic, this allows people to anticipate the vocabulary you may use. Use straightforward language, short sentences and reinforce with natural gestures, adjusting the pace of your conversation in response to the person. Check understanding, by sensitively asking the recipient to tell you what you have said; if you ask 'do you understand?' people tend to say 'yes', but they may not have received the message you thought you had delivered. This is partly because they may be speech-reading to supplement what they hear and many of the mouth shapes made by different words are similar. For example, the words mother and meal, taught and saucer involve the same mouth patterns but have very different meanings.

If a person does not understand correctly, rephrase rather than repeat the same words, particularly single words, again and again. If helpful write the message down and don't give up. Be alert to the person becoming tired and losing interest and remember that, if you are finding the conversation difficult or frustrating, the older person will share your irritation and will find the experience demeaning. Sometimes when communication is particularly challenging, it may be possible to locate someone else whom the older person finds easier to understand. When communication has been particularly successful make a record of the enabling factors which you believe contributed to success so that others may learn from your experience.

Nurses' knowledge and skills

There are many ways in which nurses can support older people and contribute to the process of auditory rehabilitation and enabling communication. However, despite compelling evidence that nurses should be proactive in therapeutic approaches to age-related hearing loss, it is often a neglected aspect of care (Tolson 1997). Studies in hospital wards (Heron & Wharrad 2000, Tolson 1997) and care homes (Norwood-Chapman & Burchfield 1999) consistently highlight that, in general, nurses' knowledge, skills and attitude towards hearing loss and hearing aids are relatively poor. Few registered nurses understand how hearing aids work or how to maintain them and even fewer know how to screen older people or are familiar with referral criteria. Given that communication is at the heart of nurse–patient relationships and a prerequisite to person-centred care, it is curious that many nurses are failing to address one of the most common problems that limit an older person's ability to communicate and participate. Case study 11.1 demonstrates

---

Case study 11.1:   Harry Donaldson's experience

Mr Donaldson attended his local health centre for a routine health check, accompanied by his daughter. The assessment results were similar to the previous year. Mr Donaldson considered himself fit of a man of his age. His daughter mentioned that he seemed a bit low. The practice nurse noticed that his daughter occasionally answered for him and he tended to joke and tease, avoiding direct answers to some of her questions.

Although he stated that his hearing was fine, the practice nurse was not convinced and carried out a whispered-voice test, which he failed in both ears. He explained this was due to wax and said he did not want a hearing aid. At this point his daughter argued with him, complaining bitterly about how bad his hearing had become and how difficult it was for everyone else. He denied any problem with his hearing. The nurse gently encouraged him to allow her to look in his ears for wax and to repeat the whispered-voice test once any wax had been removed.

When he returned to the health centre his daughter was asked to wait outside while ear syringing was completed. The practice nurse took the opportunity to spend time discussing how hearing may change with age and the impact that this can have on people's lives. She explained the results of the repeat whispered-voice test, which were identical to the first test. She also persuaded him to try a communicator, to see if it helped him to follow what she was saying. His relief was visible, admitting that he would far rather be deaf than daft. He told her how he had become known by family and friends as the 'really man', as he said 'really' so much in an attempt to answer appropriately when he did not follow what others were saying. He agreed to be referred for a proper hearing test (audiometry) and was reassured that if prescribed a hearing aid he could decide when, where and how often he used it.

Recognition of the hearing problem and the provision of reassuring information were crucial steps for both Mr Donaldson and his daughter. Mr Donaldson's daughter can now help her father to learn how to use his hearing aid and maximize the benefit from it.

---

successful management by a nurse of an older man who was reluctant to admit to his hearing loss.

TINNITUS

Tinnitus is the perception of sound in the ear or in the head that does not arise from the external environment. Sounds such as vascular bruits are not tinnitus and neither are auditory hallucinations such as hearing voices. Sounds are most often described as ringing (38% of patients), buzzing (11%), like a cricket (9%), hissing (8%), whistling (7%) and humming (5%) (Stouffer & Tyler 1990). The nature of the perceived sound is of little relevance in management. Around 20% of older people have tinnitus (Davis 1989).

In a small proportion of tinnitus sufferers it is severe enough to affect their everyday life. Some people find it very distressing. Many tinnitus sufferers also have depression, though it is unclear which comes first (Sullivan et al. 1988).

Management of tinnitus

The most important aspect of management of tinnitus is reassurance. It is important to teach patients that tinnitus is a symptom, not a disease. Patients with tinnitus are often worried that they have some serious condition, most often a brain tumour. They need reassurance that this is not likely to be the case.

Tinnitus is usually associated with hearing impairment and is uncommon in people with normal hearing. Most people with significant tinnitus should have their hearing tested. Other investigations are rarely indicated.

Tinnitus seems worse in quiet surroundings. Patients often say it is louder when they go to bed at night – the world is quieter. They need an explanation of the helpful role of background noise; radio or television provides other noise that masks the tinnitus. Those who have significant hearing impairment should be fitted with a hearing aid. This helps their hearing but also increases the level of background noise, so making the tinnitus less obvious. Patients should be given information about local self-help groups and national organizations that provide advice to tinnitus sufferers.

Many medications have been tried for tinnitus. None has been shown to be effective (Waddell & Canter 2001). People who also suffer from depression should have appropriate antidepressant treatment. This helps their depression and general quality of life but does not affect the severity of their tinnitus (Dobie et al. 1993).

Tinnitus maskers are sometimes provided. These are small devices similar to hearing aids that create a high-frequency noise in the ear to conceal the tinnitus. Some patients find these helpful on occasion, probably mainly because it is a noise that they can control, unlike the noise in their ear, but the overall benefit is minimal (Stephens & Corcoran 1985).

Recently, tinnitus retraining therapy has been increasingly used. This combines directive counselling and sound therapy over a period of 1–2 years (Jastreboff & Hazell 1993). Some practitioners have found this beneficial for their patients (Bartnik et al. 2001). However, others are dubious because of the lack of good evidence for its efficacy (Kroener-Herwig et al. 2000).

At present, the scope for intervention for people with tinnitus is limited and for nurses perhaps the most useful strategy is to take the problem seriously and facilitate problem-solving, particularly when sleep is disturbed. This can be challenging as remedies such as playing a radio or positioning a loud ticking clock next to the bed can disturb partners. An increase in reports of the distress associated with the experience of tinnitus may be indicative of an underlying problem and nurses should be alert for other signs of low mood and take steps to detect and prevent depression.

CONCLUSION

Nurses are ideally placed to contribute to selected aspects of auditory rehabilitation and to help the large number of older people who acquire hearing disability. One of the most difficult challenges is to promote a positive attitude towards intervention and challenge the passive acceptance of hearing disability as an unalterable feature of growing old. As people grow older other opportunities for self-actualization may diminish and the importance of promoting communication increases. Hearing disability is but one example of a chronic problem that may limit individuals' opportunities to communicate and participate as they would like, but thankfully with skilled intervention it can be effectively managed and the negative impact on individuals and those around them can be reduced. Unfortunately, many nurses have limited knowledge and skills in this aspect of care and, like many other people in society who are well-meaning but badly informed, do little to promote communication opportunities for the hearing-impaired older listener.

Recommended reading

Le May A 1999 Sensory and perceptual issues of ageing. In: Schofield I, Heath H (eds) Health ageing; nursing older people. Mosby, London, pp 273–295.
A well-referenced chapter which explores sensory and perceptual issues related to ageing. It highlights the complexity of nursing older people and the need to understand the connections between the sense of safety and well-being and a range of sensory disabilities, including hearing, vision and disorders of speech.
Schofield I 2002 Caring for older people who have hearing disability. Nursing Older People 13: 20–25.

This practical article is a must for nurses interested in developing their role in supporting older people with hearing disability. It teases out key skills and the role of the registered nurse. Ideal for the novice or experienced practitioner who is not confident in this aspect of care.
Stephens D, France L, Lormore K 1995 Effects of hearing impairment on the patient's family and friends. Acta Otolaryngologica (Stockholm) 115: 165–167.
An accessible, albeit specialist paper which provides important background to understanding the impact of hearing disability on close contacts.
Tolson D 1997 Age-related hearing loss: a case for nursing intervention. Journal of Advanced Nursing. 26: 1150–1157
This piece reviews and makes accessible key literature from the field of audiology and builds an argument for nursing intervention based on an intervention study. The literature review provides a useful introduction to nurses who wish to make a case for change or who are beginning a scholarly piece or to justify research in this area.
Tolson D, Nolan M 2000 Gerontological nursing 4: age-related hearing explored. British Journal of Nursing 9:205–208.
Building on the emerging evidence base, this article uses the management of hearing disability to illustrate how gerontological nursing can be advanced. It argues that hearing disability is one of the most prevalent but neglected health issues affecting older people and is highly critical of our current laissez-faire approach.

Useful addresses

British Tinnitus Association, Room 6, 14–18 West Bar Green, Sheffield S1 2DA
Royal National Institute for Deaf People (RNID), 19–23 Featherstone Street, London EC1Y 8SL
Tel: 0808 808 0123; textphone 0808 808 9000; informationline@rnid.org.uk; www.rnid.org .uk; RNID tinnitus helpline 0345 090210

References

Aung T, Mulley G 2002 Removal of ear wax. British Journal of Medicine 325: 27
Bartnik G, Fabijanska A, Rogowski M 2001 Effects of tinnitus retraining therapy (TRT) for patients with tinnitus and subjective hearing loss versus tinnitus only. Scandinavian Audiology (Suppl.) 52: 206–208.
Brant BA 1999 Sensory disorders. In: Stone JT, Wyman JF, Salisbury SA (eds) Clinical gerontological nursing: a guide to advanced practice, 2nd edn. WB Saunders, Philadelphia, pp 527–530
Bridgewood A 2000 People aged 65 and over. General household survey. Office of National Statistics, London
British Society of Audiology 1981 Recommended procedures for pure-tone audiometry using a manually operated instrument. British Journal of Audiology 15: 213–216

Brooks DN, Hallam RS, Mellor PA 2001 The effects on significant others of providing a hearing aid to the hearing-impaired partner. British Journal of Audiology 35: 165–171

Browning G 2001 Wax in ear. Clinical Evidence 6: 420–427

Browning GG, Swan IRC, Chew KK 1989 Clinical role of informal tests of hearing. Journal of Laryngology and Otology 103: 7–11

Chen HL 1994 Hearing in the elderly: relation of hearing loss, loneliness and self esteem. Journal of Gerontological Nursing 6: 22–28

Chmiel R, Jerger J 1993 Some factors affecting assessment of hearing handicap in the elderly. Journal of the American Academy of Audiology 4: 249–257

Davis AC 1989 The prevalence of hearing impairment and reported hearing disability among adults in Great Britain. International Journal of Epidemiology 18: 911–917

Davis AC 1995 Hearing in adults. Whurr, London

Dobie RA, Sakai CS, Sullivan MD, Katon WJ, Russo J 1993 Antidepressant treatment of tinnitus patients: report of a randomized clinical trial and clinical prediction of benefit. American Journal of Otology 14: 18–23

Erber NP, Holland J, Osborn RR 1998 Communicating with elder: effects on speaker–listener distance. British Journal of Audiology 32: 135–138

Gatehouse S 1992 The time course and magnitude of perceptual acclimatization to frequency response: evidence from monaural fitting of hearing aids. Journal of the Acoustic Society of America 92: 1258–1268

Gatehouse S 1999 Glasgow hearing aid benefit profile: derivation and validation of a client centred outcome measure for hearing aid services. Journal of the American Academy of Audiology 10: 80–103

Gilhome Herbst KR, Meredith R, Stephens SDG 1991 Implications of hearing impairment for elderly people in London and Wales. Acta Otolaryngologica (Suppl.) (Stockholm) 476: 209–214

Gravell R 1988 Communication problems in elderly people: practical approaches to management. Croom Helm, Beckenham

Haggard MP, Gatehouse S 1993 Candidature for hearing aids: justification for the concept and a two-part audiometric criterion. British Journal of Audiology 27: 303–318

Heron R, Wharrad H 2000 Prevalence and nursing staff awareness of hearing impairment in older hospital patients. Journal of Clinical Nursing 9: 834–841

Hetu R 1996 The stigma attached to hearing impairment. Scandinavian Audiology 25 (suppl. 43):12–24

Hetu W, Noble W 1994 An ecological approach to disability and handicap in relation to impaired hearing. Audiology 33: 117–126

Hetu R, Jones L, Getty L 1993 The impact of acquired hearing impairment on intimate relationships: implications for rehabilitation. Audiology 32: 363–381

Jastreboff PJ, Hazell JW 1993 A neurophysiological approach to tinnitus: clinical implications. British Journal of Audiology 27: 7–17

Karlsson Espmark AK, Scherman MH 2003 Hearing confirms existence and identity – experiences from persons with presbyacusis. International Journal of Audiology 42: 106–115

Kroener-Herwig B, Biesinger E, Gerhards F et al. 2000 Retraining therapy for chronic tinnitus: a critical analysis of its status. Scandinavian Audiology 29: 67–78

Le May A 1999 Sensory and perceptual issues of ageing. In: Schofield I, Heath H (eds) Health ageing; nursing older people. Mosby, London, pp 273–295

Newman D 1990 Assessment of hearing loss in elderly people: the feasibility of a nurse administered screening test. Journal of Advanced Nursing 15: 400–409

Nightingale F 1859 Notes on nursing. What it is and what it is not (reprinted 1969). Dover Publications, New York

Norwood-Chapman L, Burchfield SB 1999 Nursing home personnel knowledge and attitudes about hearing loss and hearing aids. Gerontology and Geriatics Education 20: 37–47

Pasanisi E, Bacciu A, Vincenti V et al. 2003 Speech recognition in elderly cochlear implant recipients. Clinical Otolaryngology 28: 154–157

Philp I, Lowles RV, Armstrong GK, Whitehead C 2002 Repeatability of standardized tests of functional impairment and well-being in older people in a rehabilitation setting. Disability and Rehabilitation. 24: 243–249

Schofield I 2002 Caring for older people who have hearing disability. Nursing Older People 13: 20–25

Somerville G 2002 The most effective products available to facilitate ear syringing. British Journal of Community Nursing 7: 94–101

Stephens D 1996 Hearing rehabilitation in a psychological framework. Scandinavian Audiology 25 (suppl. 43): 57–66

Stephens SD, Corcoran AL 1985 A controlled study of tinnitus masking. British Journal of Audiology 19: 159–167

Stephens D, Hetu R 1991 Impairment, disability and handicap in audiology: towards consensus. Audiology 30: 185–200

Stephens D, France L, Lormore K 1995 Effects of hearing impairment on the patient's family and friends. Acta Otolaryngologica (Stockholm) 115: 165–167

Stephens D, Gianopoulos I, Kerr P 2001 Determination and classification of the problems experienced by hearing-impaired elderly people. Audiology 40: 294–300

Stone CM 1999 Preventing cerumen impaction in nursing facility residents. Journal of Gerontological Nursing 25: 43–45

Stouffer JL, Tyler RS 1990 Characterization of tinnitus by tinnitus patients. Journal of Speech and Hearing Disorders 55: 439–453

Sullivan MD, Katon W, Dobie R et al. 1988 Disabling tinnitus. Association with affective disorder. General Hospital Psychiatry 10: 285–291

Swan IRC, Browning GG 1985 The whispered voice as a screening test for hearing impairment. Journal of the Royal College of General Practitioners 35: 197

Swan IRC, Tolson D 1991 Hearing aid clinics. Nursing Times 87: 46–47

Tolson D 1997 Age-related hearing loss: a case for nursing intervention. Journal of Advanced Nursing 26: 1150–1157

Tolson D, McIntosh J 1997 Listening: the care environment – chaos or clarity for the hearing impaired elderly person. International Journal of Nursing Studies 34: 173–182

Tolson D, Nolan M 2000 Gerontological nursing 4: age-related hearing explored. British Journal of Nursing 9: 205–208

Tolson D, Stephens D 1997 Age-related hearing loss in the dependent elderly population: a model for nursing care. International Journal of Nursing Practice 3: 224–230

Tolson D, Swan IRC 1991 Gentle persuasion. Nursing Times 87: 29–31

Tolson D, Swan IRC, Knussen C 2002 Hearing disability: a source of distress for older people and carers. British Journal of Nursing 11: 1021–1025

Tsuruoka H, Masuda S, Ukai K et al. 2001 Hearing impairment and quality of life for the elderly in nursing homes. Auris Nasus Larynx 28: 45–54

Waddell A, Canter R 2001 Tinnitus. Clinical Evidence 6: 412–419

Wiley TL, Cruickshanks KJ, Nondahl DM et al. 1998 Ageing and high frequency hearing sensitivity. Journal of Speech and Language and Hearing Research 41: 44–45

World Health Organization 1980 International classification of impairments, disabilities and handicap. World Health Organization, Geneva

World Health Organization 1999 International classification of impairments, disabilities and handicap. World Health Organization, Geneva

Chapter 12

Eyesight and older people

Avril Charnock

INTRODUCTION

Visual impairment, low vision and partial sight are terms used to describe the state of reduced visual acuity which, despite the best optical correction, results in below-average visual performance. These terms are clearly defined in the *International Classification of Impairments, Disabilities and Handicaps* (first proposed by the World Health Organization in 1980) and, when applied to ocular disease, indicate the relationship between disease, impairment, disability and handicap for ocular pathology.

Visual impairment is thought to be the fifth main disability in the community in the UK. There is 5.6% prevalence for people aged 60–74, increasing to 26.2% in those aged 75 years and over (Department of Health 1991). It is estimated that over one million people in the UK are registered as blind or partially sighted, the majority of whom are over 65 years of age. This is in addition to a significant number who are not registered, either from choice or because the impairment has not been identified in full (Bruce et al. 1991). There is thought to be an underregistration of at least 50% within the community (Robinson et al. 1994).

Visual impairment or loss is often combined with other illnesses or disabilities such as deafness, and in some cases may be overlooked since many organizations providing services for disabled people tend to follow a single-disability approach. This is a particular problem for people with learning disabilities, many of whom do not have other needs assessed or catered for (Levy 1997).

The incidence of eye disease increases considerably over the age of 75 years. A recent study by Evans et al. (2002) looked at the prevalence of visual impairment in people aged 75 years and older in the UK, in the Medical Research Council trial of assessment and management of older people in the community. A visual acuity screening test was conducted by trained nurses in a group of almost 15 000 people aged 75 years and older, recruited from general practitioner practices. The results confirmed that vision impairment is common in this age group. The risk of low vision and blindness increases rapidly with advancing age, especially for women: approximately 37% of those over 90 years old were visually impaired. The prevalence of eye disease will affect the ability of older people to perform daily activities and remain independent. A large number of older people do not have regular eye examinations, possibly due to acceptance or unawareness of reduced vision, anxiety about the possible outcome or the cost implications (Salford Eye Care Project 1993).

Work in progress shows that there is a high prevalence of visual disability in older people presenting with falls. Scuffham (2002) has estimated the incidence and cost of accidental falls for the UK population with visual impairment. In 1999 there were 2.35 million accidental falls that required hospital treatment. There were 189 000 falls which occurred in people with visual impairment; 89 500 of these falls were attributed directly to the visual impairment itself and the majority of these occurred in individuals aged 75 years and over.

VISION

Perception of an object occurs when light from that object passes through the various structures of the eye, focusing on the retina at the macula, where specialist cells transform the light into nervous impulses. These impulses are then transmitted via the optic nerve and visual pathways to the occipital cortex. Problems may arise at any of these structures, and such problems may result in reduced visual function (the structure of the eye is shown in Fig. 12.1).

The components of sight or visual function can be divided into light sense, form sense and colour vision.

Light sense

Light sense is the ability to perceive light/dark and the variable intensities between the two. It is possible to measure it by finding the minimum visible stimulus, but this will vary according to the area of retina stimulated. A seminal study by Hecht et al. (1942) answered the basic question about human vision regarding the minimum amount of light required to produce the perceptual response of seeing light. The researchers presented a subject with a series of flashes of light with various intensities to a preselected position on the retina in a dark-adapted eye and asked whether the light was seen. The absolute threshold for detecting light is usually referred to as the 'absolute threshold of vision' and is usually only recorded when form sense cannot be demonstrated.

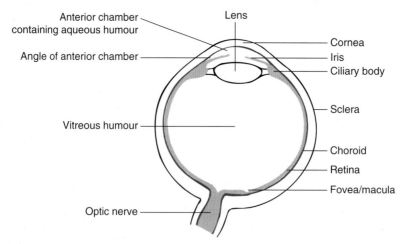

Fig. 12.1 Structure of the eye.

Form sense

Form sense depends on the ability of the eye to distinguish between two spatially separate but adjacent stimuli and to perceive the nature of the object from its size, shape, position and orientation. Visual thresholds are the most common psychophysical measurement. To determine whether a subject can see something would require a detection task to find the absolute threshold for detecting a stimulus, e.g. a light. A discrimination task would determine whether one or two objects were visible to a subject. A recognition task, in which the object is already visible, requires the subject to name the object. Visual acuity tests, in which letters are identified, fall into this category (Corliss et al. 2002). Form sense comprises visual acuity and contrast sensitivity.

Visual acuity

Visual acuity can be subdivided into central and peripheral vision.

Central vision is the capacity of the central retina to distinguish fine detail. This depends on the ability of the fovea to resolve two points or lines that are 0.5 min of arc apart. This is the minimum angle of resolution (MAR). Resolution acuity for letter targets is easily degraded by optical defocus due to a mild refractive error. Identification acuity relies on the ability of a subject to identify individual letters by resolving their details.

The focusing power of the eye decreases after 45 years of age with the onset of presbyopia. This is a refractive condition in which the accommodative ability of the eye is insufficient for close work, which occurs as a natural consequence of ageing. It is due to a hardening of the lens and a reduction of the elasticity of the lens capsule. It is corrected by wearing spherical (plus) lenses for reading. People living in hot climates tend to become presbyopic earlier than those living in European and North American countries.

Numerous physical changes occur in the eye and visual system over time. As the lens thickens and hardens it prevents accommodation and the change in absorption of certain wavelengths produces progressive yellowing and in time lens opacities may develop.

Increased light scatter, increased absorption by the ocular media and senile miosis of the pupil reduce contrast and retinal illuminance. By the age of 60, retinal illuminance is approximately one-third of what it is in a 20-year-old. At the retinal level, foveal cone density decreases; there is a gradual loss of photoreceptors, which become less responsive to light. There may also be cell loss and changes in the neurotransmitters in the visual pathway and cortex leading to a decline in numerous visual functions. The visual fields also become smaller with age.

Regular eye examinations by an optometrist should be encouraged so that the correct glasses are prescribed and to enable the early detection of conditions associated with the ageing eye, which can be treated and monitored effectively. Such conditions include: primary open-angle glaucoma; cataract; diabetic retinopathy; degenerative retinal diseases; vascular disease; and optic atrophy.

The peripheral field of vision is that portion of space in which peripheral objects are visible at the same time as the object of central fixation. A reduced awareness or depression of the field of vision can be of any shape, size or depth depending on the condition present. The horizontal visual field measures approximately 180°, of which 120° forms the binocular visual field (Fig. 12.2). The vertical field extends 55° upward from the midline and 65° below the midline.

There are three types of visual field deficit: scotoma, sectional field loss and peripheral constriction.

Scotoma

A scotoma is an area of partial or complete blindness surrounded by normal or relatively normal visual field. An absolute scotoma is one in which vision is entirely absent in the affected area. It can occur at the centre of fixation, as in age-related macular degeneration (ARMD), optic neuritis or optic atrophy, or as an arcuate defect resulting from retinal nerve fibre branch defects, as in primary open-angle glaucoma. These conditions may start in one eye and later affect the other eye.

Sectional field loss

Sectional field loss occurs when a section of the visual field is defective. This can affect the same half or quadrant of the visual field in both eyes, termed homonymous hemianopia, as occurs in cerebrovascular lesions, or the lateral side of each visual field, bitemporal hemianopia, as in chiasmal lesions, or an altitudinal field defect, as in retinal vascular lesions or glaucoma where it does not cross the horizontal midline.

Peripheral constriction

Peripheral constriction occurs when the visual field of one or both eyes is generally restricted and reduced to the central area of visual function, as in advanced primary open-angle glaucoma, optic neuropathy or retinitis pigmentosa.

A visual field test will give information about the location and degree of disturbance at the retina and visual pathways and helps monitor the progress of the disease. A central field test assessing the central 30° of the field is usually carried out on patients with glaucoma using a computerized perimeter such as the

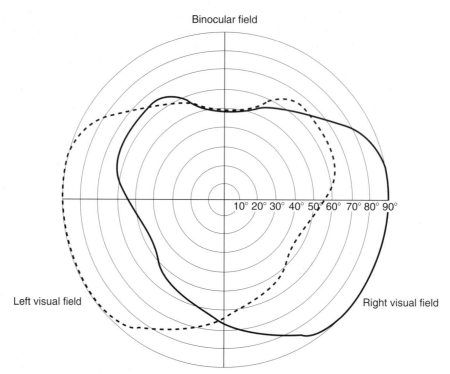

Fig. 12.2 Binocular field, Dashed line, left visual field; continuous line, right visual field.

Humphrey Field Analyzer (first developed in 1985), Octopus, Dicon or Henson CFA 3000. The presentation of the light stimuli and the recording are carried out electronically under the control of an integral computer. The advantages of computerized perimeters are: that the examination strategy is reproducible; the testing routine can be altered by modifying the program; and each instrument contains several examination routines aimed at detecting a number of ocular/neurological conditions. The Humphrey Field Analyzer II is wheelchair-accessible and provides the latest technology for early diagnosis and management of diseases resulting in visual field loss.

The Goldmann perimeter consists of a hemispherical bowl and targets of varying intensity and size are projected manually on to the white interior surface. The practitioner monitors the patient's fixation through the telescope at the back of the bowl. It is used for kinetic perimetry (using a moving target of fixed luminance) of patients with neurological disorders resulting in field defects such as hemianopia, or inherited genetic conditions such as retinitis pigmentosa which results in constricted visual fields and also for plotting the field of binocular single vision in patients with diplopia due to a muscle palsy.

Contrast sensitivity

Contrast sensitivity is the ability to detect differences between a light and dark pattern at varying spatial frequencies. Contrast is defined as the luminance difference between an object and its background, e.g. the luminance of black letters on a white page. This ability decreases when the contrast between the text and the background decreases. A person with reduced contrast may have good visual acuity and visual fields but still complain of blurred vision, as if looking through a mist.

A lower than optimal illumination level results in a loss of visual acuity and contrast sensitivity and it becomes more difficult to carry out tasks which require high acuity and adequate contrast. Visual acuity and contrast sensitivity are optimal at illuminance levels of 100 lux in normally sighted people. There is no significant improvement at higher levels of illuminance; however, over 50 years of age the required level of illumination is higher and this may be significantly higher for people in their 70s and 80s.

Measurement of the contrast sensitivity threshold can assist in the early detection of visual loss and the diagnosis of certain conditions, for example, cataract. Clinically, the contrast sensitivity threshold can be measured using gratings to detect the contrast level at which they are first discernible, or low-contrast letter charts can be used, such as the Pelli–Robson, in which the letters are of equal size but provide decreasing contrast. The contrast threshold is recorded as the contrast of the letters on the last line where characters can be recognized (Whittaker & Lovie-Kitchin 1994).

Sudden changes in lighting conditions can be disabling and give rise to visual discomfort due to glare. Disability glare, which impairs the ability to see detail, can be caused by strong lights illuminating the eyes which cause stray light within the eye. The degree of disability will depend on the extent of stray light and the type of ocular abnormality such as cataract or corneal abnormalities that cause light dispersal within the eye.

Colour vision

Colour vision, or perception, is the ability to distinguish different colours and occurs when light impulses of varying wavelengths are perceived by the retina as a range of hues within the visible spectrum. Hundreds of thousands of different colour sensations are possible due to the presence of three types of retinal cones. The cone types differ in the light-absorbing pigment they contain, creating short-wavelength, middle-wavelength and long-wavelength sensitive receptors. Three photopigments are needed to distinguish the full spectrum of colours. Measurement of colour vision can be done uniocularly and binocularly and can contribute to the diagnosis of certain ocular conditions where acquired colour deficits are prevalent, for example, optic nerve lesions and optic neuritis. Loss of short-wavelength sensitivity due to increased absorption by the lens can have a dramatic impact on colour vision. Vivid blue-green and green colours may be confused, which suggests that reliance on colour coding, e.g. for medicines, can be confusing for an older person.

The presence of good colour discrimination indicates functional cones in the macular area, whereas poor discrimination may suggest that these photoreceptors are not functioning due to the presence of a central scotoma. The reduced ability to discriminate colours may also occur in some cerebral lesions. Cerebral achromatopsia is a condition that presents as a loss of colour vision and is often permanent. The most frequent cause of cerebral achromatopsia is a stroke, which damages two local areas of cortex in the inferior regions of both hemispheres. Most cerebral achromats also suffer from propagnosia, a failure to recognize familiar faces, suggesting that the cortical mechanisms involved in colour vision and facial recognition lie in close proximity (Zeki 1990).

Few colour vision tests are available for acquired colour vision defects, associated with eye disease. The association of retinal and visual pathway disease with colour vision defects is characterized by Kollner's rule, that lesions at the level of the photoreceptors, or outer retinal layers, are more commonly associated with blue-yellow disorders of colour vision, e.g. ARMD. Lesions in the inner retinal layers and ganglion cells are more likely to exhibit red-green colour deficiencies, e.g. optic neuritis.

VISUAL DISORDERS ENCOUNTERED IN OLDER PEOPLE

There are five main conditions where visual function is particularly affected: (1) ARMD; (2) glaucoma; (3) cataract; (4) diabetic retinopathy; and (5) cerebrovascular accident (CVA, stroke).

Age-related macular degeneration (ARMD)

ARMD accounts for almost one-third of registerable visually impaired people in the 65–74 age group and approximately 50% of the 75+ age group. It is a major cause of visual disability in the community (Evans & Wormald 1996), and is the most significant cause of blindness in older people. ARMD may be caused by a late-onset genetic disease or be the result of high-risk environmental factors such as smoking, light and diet. The most significant risk factor is age (Marshall 2002).

There is currently no fully accepted definition of ARMD. The International Epidemiological Study Group (1995) defines age-related maculopathy (ARM) as a disorder of the macular area, most often clinically apparent after 50 years of age. The signs are:

- discrete whitish-yellow spots identified as drusen
- increased pigment or hyper-pigmentation associated with drusen
- sharply demarcated areas of de-pigmentation or hypo-pigmentation of the retinal pigment epithelium and associated drusen.

These age-related changes with progressive accumulation of debris under the retina are predisposing factors in late-stage ARM, which is identified as Age Related Macular Degeneration (ARMD), and which may be wet or dry. The most common type in over 85% of cases is dry ARMD, which causes drusen to be deposited in the macular region with subsequent cellular degenerative changes. This may also be accompanied by the growth of new blood vessels into, or under, the retina in wet ARMD, causing more rapid progression of the disease. The drusen rarely present before the age of 45 years, are relatively uncommon between 45 and 60 years, but steadily increase after this. It is a binocular disease but it may appear in one eye some time before it appears in the other eye.

The main symptom of macular disease is the impairment of central vision (a normal peripheral field with central field loss is shown in Fig. 12.3). This may present as difficulty with close-work activities, straight lines may appear wavy or distorted and dark patches may occur in the central field of vision. Read-ing and other activities will be difficult due to blurring or distortion of the print; some letters or parts of words may keep disappearing, thus reducing the flu-ency of reading. Difficulties with face recognition and change of lighting also occur. A dark patch that rap-idly fades may also occur on waking. Outdoor activi-ties will also be affected, although peripheral vision remains intact (Figs 12.4 and 12.5).

General practitioners, nurses and optometrists need to be aware of the urgent nature of referral for patients with recent onset of distortion and visual loss. Such patients may still have treatable disease and should be referred urgently to their local hospital eye service (Royal College of Ophthalmologists Guidelines).

The Amsler grid test (Fig. 12.6) may be used in an eye clinic by an ophthalmologist or can be done by a nurse with a patient at home and helps to detect and locate early visual problems related to macular dis-ease. The grid should be held at 30 cm from the eye, reading glasses must be worn and each eye should be tested in turn. While looking at the central dot, patients should be asked if they can see all four cor-ners of the grid and if any of the lines are missing or appear to be blurry, bent or wavy.

The aim of management is to minimize visual loss and disability in order to maintain independence. Figure 12.7 shows a 90-year-old woman preparing broccoli with a magnifying glass at her side. However, despite a growing interest in AMD, the options for treatment are limited. Argon laser photocoagulation may be used in

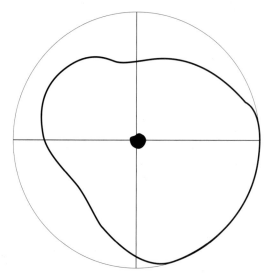

Fig. 12.3 Normal peripheral field with central loss (scotoma) typical of macular degeneration.

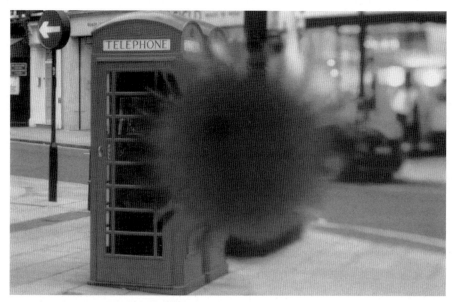

Fig. 12.4 Photograph showing the effect of central field loss with intact peripheral vision. (Reproduced with permission of Novartis Ophthalmics.)

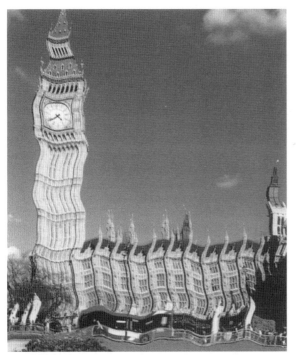

Fig. 12.5   Visual distortion caused by macular degeneration. (Reproduced with permission of Novartis Ophthalmics.)

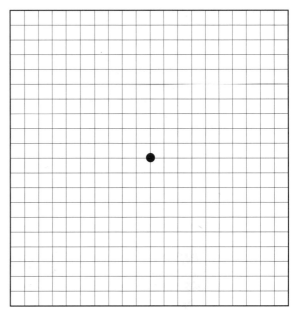

Fig. 12.6   The Amsler grid chart.

cases where the visual acuity is still good (6/12 or better) and the duration of symptoms short (less than a month). Following the onset of reduced visual acuity and changes in the Amsler grid chart, which can detect slight abnormalities, normally undetected by usual methods of perimetry, the diagnosis of AMD is made by fluorescein angiography and colour photography. Intravenous fluorescein is administered to the patient and photographs of the central 30° of the retina are taken.

More recently, a number of alternative managements have been proposed or are the subject of clinical trials. These include photodynamic therapy using a photosensitizing dye that works in the eye by binding the photosensitizer to liposomes and low-density lipoproteins to produce reactive oxygen intermediates (Harding 2001). The efficacy of this treatment is still being evaluated, as it is costly and only available to relatively few patients. The role of nutritional supplements and vitamins in delaying the progression of AMD and vision loss has been the subject of a number of clinical trials in the USA where scientists have established a link between lutein (a carotenoid found in leafy green vegetables, corn on the cob, orange peppers, egg yolk and zeaxanthin, also a carotenoid) and a reduced occurrence of the disease (Bernstein 2002).

A carotenoid is a powerful antioxidant responsible for yellow and red pigments in fruits and vegetables and is a precursor of vitamin A. Antioxidants are a group of nutrients that neutralize dangerous free radicals, molecules charged with oxygen, that can damage healthy cells. It is theorized that lutein protects by blocking harmful blue light from reaching the retina. Researchers Bartlett and Eperjesi at Aston University, Birmingham, UK are currently investigating the role of nutritional supplements on the progression of AMD in an 18-month randomized controlled trial to determine the effect of a normal-dose supplement, including lutein, on ARM/ARMD. Tests will include visual acuity, contrast sensitivity, colour vision, central visual field function, glare recovery and fundus photography.

In older people with AMD, concurrent ophthalmic disease, such as cataract and glaucoma, may also occur and needs to be identified and treated appropriately. Macular degeneration accounts for one of the most significant causes of visual impairment in older people. With the increase in population of over-60-year-olds set to increase by 45% in the next 20–25 years, the increased load on both health and social services is likely to be considerable.

Glaucoma

Glaucoma is a group of disorders in which the optic nerve fibres are susceptible to progressive loss. The

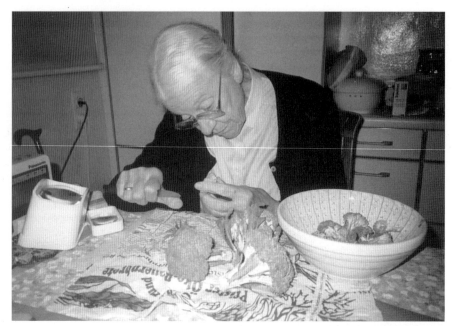

Fig. 12.7 Keeping going: a 90-year-old woman with macular degeneration preparing vegetables.

intraocular pressure may be elevated, causing damage to the nerve fibres at the optic nerve head. This results in impairment of visual acuity and visual fields, with reduced visual function increasing considerably after 75 years of age. There has been a shift in thinking about the disease over the last 5–10 years and the definition of glaucoma no longer includes intraocular pressure since there are many patients with low-tension or normal-tension glaucoma (Barneby 2002).

There are two main types of glaucoma: primary open-angle glaucoma, which is the most common form found in the older population, and primary angle-closure glaucoma. Approximately 13% of individuals who are registered blind and almost 9% of those who are registered partially sighted are as a result of primary open-angle glaucoma (Balatsoukas et al. 1995). This is the second most common cause of blindness in the 65+ age group. Risk factors for glaucoma include age, familial tendency, Afro-Caribbean origin, myopia and diabetes. It is thought to affect 1% of the population over 40 years of age. Studies have suggested that as many as 30–60% may go undetected within the community. Late detection may lead to poor prognosis and a high risk of being registered as visually impaired (Salford Eye Care Project 1993). Figure 12.8 illustrates glaucomatous loss and peripheral constriction.

The principal factors determining the level of intraocular pressure are the rate of production of aqueous humour, the resistance encountered in the outflow channels and the equilibrium of the arterial and venous blood pressure. In primary open-angle glaucoma, the elevation of the intraocular pressure is related to the resistance in the outflow channel of the eye, whereas in primary angle-closure glaucoma, the rise in pressure is due to the mechanical obstruction at the angle of the anterior chamber by the iris, which prevents aqueous humour reaching the outflow channels.

Primary open-angle glaucoma

This is a long-standing, chronic disease that requires continual monitoring. Early detection through regular eye examination is essential to ensure treatment in the early stages of the disease, so that its progress can be arrested or controlled. The threat of progressive damage remains, however, as the sensitivity of the optic nerve to a particular level of intraocular pressure may change with time, and damage may occur at a level not previously associated with it. The changes are insidious, causing nerve fibre bundle damage. The visual fields become patchy and, as the loss of field progresses, it follows the nerve fibres, producing an arcuate scotoma which may appear in the upper or lower midfield. Continued loss in both the mid- and peripheral field will eventually join, resulting in a grossly restricted field, with only a small central field of vision remaining. It is often symptom-free at the onset, usually affecting peripheral vision. Extensive visual loss may occur in one eye before there is any awareness of a problem. Distance visual acuity is initially good, with near vision only becoming problematic if there is defective visual field close to the area of central fixation, especially if it occupies the lower field. For example, a person may not be aware of objects on a table near by, but can see birds in a tree at the end of the garden. As the visual field becomes more constricted, navigating inside and outside the home will prove increasingly difficult. Driving will also be compromised and advice concerning the person's continued eligibility to drive should be sought from the medical division of the Driver's Vehicle Licensing Authority (DVLA). If necessary, the DVLA may request a binocular driving field (Esterman program on the Humphrey Field Analyzer) to be carried out.

The initial treatment for primary open-angle glaucoma may be medical. Depending upon the stage of the disease on examination, and in the absence of systemic contraindications, treatment is usually the lowest dosage of beta-blockers required to achieve the desired effect. Beta-blockers reduce intraocular pressure by decreasing aqueous secretion. In the USA the medical treatment of glaucoma has shifted away from beta-blockers towards prostaglandin analogues. These help to regulate the diurnal fluctuation of intraocular pressure and have been found to be particularly effective in treating African-American patients (Schachnow

2002). Miotics are also used to reduce intraocular pressure by inducing contraction of the longitudinal muscle of the ciliary body to enhance aqueous outflow; they have no effect on aqueous secretion.

A study in the USA by Glynn et al. (1991), analysing the number of falls in 489 older patients with glaucoma, found the greatest single risk factor for falls was the use of non-miotic topical eye medication. Additional risk factors for falls were female sex, the use of cardiac medication, the use of miotic eyedrops, visual field loss of 40% or more and the use of sedatives. This has implications for falls prevention programmes.

Primary angle-closure glaucoma

This condition occurs in anatomically predisposed eyes and, like primary open-angle glaucoma, it has a genetic basis. There can be a number of severe symptoms: a painful red eye which may be accompanied by frontal headaches; eye-ache; blurred vision; visual loss; and nausea. Attacks of this disease may be intermittent and precipitated by physiological mydriasis, for example watching television in a dark room, thus causing the pupils to dilate (physiological mydriasis is the normal dilation of the pupil in dim (mesopic) conditions). When attacks occur, the intraocular pressure may rise considerably and impairment of vision may be associated with seeing haloes around lights due to corneal

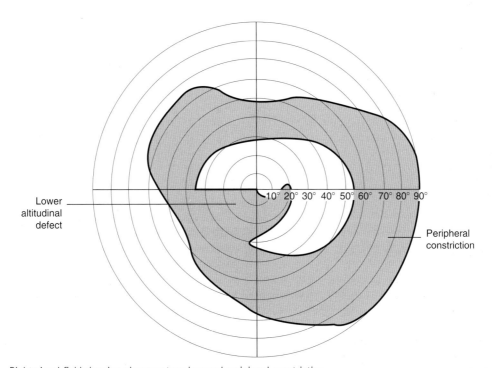

Fig. 12.8   Right visual field showing glaucomatous loss and peripheral constriction.

oedema resulting from raised intraocular pressure. Exposure to bright light or sleep may relieve the symptoms. This disease should be treated as a medical emergency due to its sight-threatening nature. Management is surgical, although intensive miotic therapy (drugs that constrict the pupil) may be used initially. Once the intraocular pressure has been reduced, peripheral iridectomy, laser iridotomy or filtration surgery is carried out to prevent further attack. It may be that for some frail older people and/or those in poor general health, medical treatment only may be advocated.

Cataract

Age-related cataract is the main cause of eye-disease pathology in the community (Webb 1994). However, with modern surgical intervention, it is not the main cause of permanent visual loss in older people. It is prevalent in up to 20% of the 65+ age group, and in over 46% in the 75+ age group. It is a considerable public health problem worldwide and the subject of research on identifying the contributory risk factors (Hodge et al. 1995).

Cataract is generally a bilateral disease but can affect one eye at a time. It is an opacity of the lens following lens fibre degeneration due to physical and chemical factors. The terminology of different types of cataract depends on the area of lens affected, and the degree to which it has developed. Cataract can be cortical, nuclear or subcapsular. Discolouration of the lens occurs for no other reason than the general deterioration of tissue, increased pigmentation and lack of elasticity without any hereditary or systemic influences.

Nuclear sclerosis is usually the first stage, in which the lens nucleus becomes progressively inelastic and hardens, producing some difficulty with distance vision but improvement in near vision (myopic effect). The sclerosis generally progresses into a nuclear cataract, in which the central part of the nucleus becomes opaque. As the opacity increases, preventing light from reaching the macular area of the retina, objects become blurred and colours dull.

In cortical cataract, the cloudiness of the lens is initially caused by excess fluid between the lens fibres, leading to small white opacities within the periphery of the cortex. Opacities of the posterior capsule of the lens cause scattering of light, and disability glare becomes a problem. Thus car headlights when night-driving or low winter sun can often reduce visual function considerably (Anderson & Holliday 1995). Shading the eyes with a visor or hat with a brim is often helpful in daylight conditions.

An additional source of uniform retinal illumination in the presence of cataract is the lens fluorescence, which occurs when short-wavelength light is absorbed by the lens, and re-emitted as radiations of a longer wavelength. Fluorescence is the production of visible light from the absorption of ultraviolet radiation. Crystalline lens fluorescence increases with age. A spectacle lens which absorbs the lower wavelength would prevent this. Driving is not advisable by patients whose visual acuity is less than 6/12 as tested on a Snellen chart.

Treatment for cataract is usually surgical and can be done by either removing the entire lens (intracapsular extraction) or leaving the posterior capsule (extracapsular extraction), followed by inserting a small Perspex or silicone lens implant (intraocular lens). Laser treatment may be necessary after extracapsular extraction if the remaining posterior capsule develops opacities. After surgery the eye is allowed to settle for about 4–6 weeks before a refraction check is carried out and any glasses prescribed to bring the vision up to normal standards. The presence of certain ocular conditions, such as advanced glaucoma, may be a contraindication to surgery.

Cataract surgery is often done as a day case. The shift towards community care and the increased use of local anaesthesia have led to same-day discharge. The advent of improved surgical techniques such as phacoemulsification, followed by insertion of an intraocular lens, coupled with the increasing demand caused by an ageing population, have provided further impetus for day-case cataract surgery. It is interesting to note that 30 years ago patients were in hospital for 10 days following cataract surgery. Today, they are discharged a few hours after the operation. This dramatic change has significant implications for the role of nurses in ophthalmic and community settings who must challenge and develop current practices to meet changing patient and service needs (Stuckey 1999).

The need for visual improvement is the most common indication for cataract extraction, although requirements vary from person to person. Medical indications for surgery are those in which the presence of a cataract is seriously affecting the health of the eye, and cosmetic indications are those in which a mature cataract in an otherwise blind eye is removed to restore a black pupil.

Nursing care of an older person with a cataract
Preoperative assessment by an ophthalmic nurse usually takes place within the month before admission for surgery. It is the first opportunity for the nurse to discuss and inform the patient about the operation and postoperative care. The preoperative assessment will include the following procedures as part of an integrated care pathway (ICP):

1. general health check and visual acuity test using the Snellen letter chart
2. nursing history – to include screening for disease/disability that could prevent the patient from remaining still and supine for approximately half an hour
3. calculation of a suitable power for the intraocular lens using a special formula which incorporates keratometry readings – a non-contact method of measuring corneal curvature, and biometry – an A-scan ultrasound procedure that measures the axial length of the eye
4. applanation tonometry, which is a contact method of measuring intraocular pressure
5. information is given about the operation and postoperative management.

It is helpful if one nurse is able to perform all aspects of the preoperative assessment as this develops a more supportive relationship, and it can be a valuable experience for both patient and nurse in terms of exchange of information. It is also important for nurses to provide a contact telephone number for the patient to use pre- and postoperatively if queries arise. Preoperative patient education may also include written information and, in some cases, use of a video to describe the day-surgery experience (Rose 1997).

Aftercare following surgery
One of the disadvantages of removing the lens in cataract surgery is that it takes away the best yellow filter that the eye has and the retina is confronted with higher levels of hazardous radiation (Marshall 2002). This has resulted in the incorporation of ultraviolet-A blockers into intraocular lenses. However, this can still leave the vulnerable ageing retina exposed to high levels of potentially damaging blue light. To overcome this, new polymer technology is under development to incorporate an artificial yellow pigment into a foldable intraocular lens. This may improve visual acuity by reducing chromatic aberrations and could prove a significant advance in cataract surgery.

About 10% of patients experience posterior capsule opacification. This is caused by the growth of a layer of cells over the posterior capsule, resulting in worsening vision. It may not become apparent for several months and can be successfully treated by YAG laser in an outpatient clinic. After surgery, the eye is allowed to settle for about 4–6 weeks before a refraction check is carried out and glasses prescribed if necessary to bring the vision up to normal standards. The prognosis for a successful outcome after surgery may however be compromised if other ocular conditions, such as glaucoma or ARMD, coexist with a cataract.

A rise in day surgery and the empowerment of patients have increased the need for preoperative patient education. The benefits of reduction of anxiety, promotion of recovery, successful self-medication and patient satisfaction have all been recognized. This will increase the need for ophthalmic nurses to promote learning by preparing a teaching programme, supported by written explanations, thereby enabling patients to assume more responsibility for their care (Cooper 1999).

Postoperative management of patients who have undergone cataract surgery
Most patients will be ready to leave hospital about 2 h after cataract surgery. After the operation patients will have the operated eye protected by an eye shield (cartella) which is left in place for 24 h. This is removed the day after surgery and the eye may be cleaned with normal saline solution or boiled water which has cooled. The eye should be wiped gently from the inner to the outer canthus using a clean cotton-wool swab. It is important to advise the patient or relative who will be doing this that their hands should be washed before and afterwards to reduce the risk of infection.

In order to reduce the risk of accidental trauma to the operated eye, the eye shield must be worn at night for 2 weeks after the first postoperative day. The eye shield must be washed daily with mild detergent, and dried and stored carefully. Postoperatively most patients will be prescribed eyedrops by their ophthalmic surgeon. These are usually antibiotics and will usually need to be instilled for up to four times a day for about 2 weeks.

A study by Rendell (1998a) examined the relevance of written and verbal advice given on discharge from hospital after cataract surgery. It was found that patients given written instructions were more compliant with the advice regarding the instillation of eyedrops and instructions about postoperative eye-care methods than those who were not given this information.

It was recommended that written discharge information should be concise and easily understood by patients and carers. Patients generally prefer this text to be in large bold print (font size 20). Rendell (1998b) also investigated discharge instructions after cataract surgery and professional factors. One of the factors was the ophthalmic surgeon's advice regarding the restriction of daily living activities following cataract surgery. The most usual restrictions recommended for a period of 4–6 weeks are: lifting heavy objects; playing contact sports and swimming.

Two to three postoperative visits to the eye clinic will be necessary and patients are usually discharged 6–8 weeks after surgery. They will be advised to go to an optometrist for an eye-test to determine whether any spectacle correction is necessary. A few patients may experience complications and anyone who complains of worsening vision, severe pain (including headache), an increase in inflammation or a cloudy cornea should return to the ophthalmic department immediately (Rose 1997).

Cataract integrated care pathways

ICPs are now in common use for patients undergoing cataract surgery. These are task-oriented care plans that clearly define the steps to be taken for the management of a specific clinical condition such as cataract, and that describe the patient's expected clinical progress.

The aim of ICPs is to introduce clinical guidelines and continuing audit into clinical practice. They also give patients access to a written summary of their expected clinical course and plan of care. The ICP describes the timing and sequence of the tasks to be carried out for a patient who is to have cataract surgery. This will include: the preoperative outpatient visit; preassessment clinic; day of admission for surgery; the record of cataract surgery; the postoperative care and discharge checklist. It will also specify the professional discipline involved in completing the task and requires signatures of these personnel (Campbell et al. 1998).

Diabetic retinopathy

Diabetic retinopathy is a disease where microvascular changes have developed in the retina over a number of years as a result of diabetes mellitus. It is a bilateral disease that may affect each eye at differing rates. The disease is the major cause of new blindness in working-age people and accounts for 4–6% of newly registered blind people, with the majority of cases over 60 years of age and approximately three-quarters of these being female.

Studies suggest that there are a large number of older diabetic people with undiagnosed retinopathy (Gonzales-Villalpando et al. 1994). Considerably more diabetics are likely to have registerable blindness than non-diabetics and the incidence increases with the duration of the disease. Late-onset diabetics may often present with diabetic retinopathy at the initial assessment and 50% will have developed the disease within 10 years. Studies suggest that diabetics over 80 years of age are also more likely to develop cortical lens opacities (Klein et al. 1995). Degenerative changes in other areas of the eye may also be present.

There are four main stages of diabetic retinopathy, which are important indicators for the prognosis of this disease and possibly the outcome of diabetes mellitus in general: (1) background retinopathy; (2) pre-proliferative retinopathy; (3) proliferative retinopathy; and (4) end-stage retinopathy. The disease may continue from background retinopathy through to the other stages, with the resulting degree of visual impairment having variable effects on the independence of the person involved. Between 10% and 40% of patients with pre-proliferative disease will develop proliferative disease within 1 year. In mature-onset diabetes, 70% with proliferative disease will be blind within 5 years.

The retina is fed by a network of blood vessels, the walls of which become fragile and start to break, causing small haemorrhages and, over time, fatty exudates. The amount of blood may be small and the only symptom may be a few areas of blurring as the patient sees floating spots in front of the eye. If the haemorrhages occur on the macula, however, loss of central vision will be an early symptom. If they are restricted to the peripheral retina, visual loss may not be experienced for some time. Other blood vessels also become constricted and may stop carrying blood permanently and the retinal cells die from lack of nourishment, producing a gradual loss of sight. When old blood vessels close down, new abnormal ones grow in their place, but are unable to nourish the retina adequately and vision may be affected. Vitreous haemorrhage and fibrosis may occur and scar tissue may form which pulls at the retina, causing a detachment. Rubeotic glaucoma, which is secondary glaucoma due to new blood vessels growing into the iris, is a late complication prior to blindness found in diabetes. These later complications may not always respond to surgical treatment.

Recommendations for a national risk reduction programme to preserve the sight of those with diabetes were produced by an advisory panel convened by the British Diabetic Association at the request of the UK National Screening Committee in 1999–2000 (Advisory Panel Final Report to the UK National Screening Committee 1999–2000). The aims of the programme are to reduce the rate of avoidable visual loss by:

- detection of sight-threatening retinopathy so that it can be treated
- detection of any retinopathy, so that diabetic patients can be made aware that changes have begun to occur in their eyes
- improvement of glycaemic and blood pressure controls.

An annual eye surveillance programme of all people with diabetes has been recommended by the BDA Advisory Panel to bring about a reduction in the risk of sight loss from diabetic retinopathy. This should be accessible to all those with diabetes, whether they are cared for in the community or in secondary care. There are two main approaches to screening for diabetic retinopathy, ophthalmoscopy and retinal photography with subsequent grading. Digital fundus photography has replaced slide and Polaroid photography as the photographic medium of choice and it provides ease of image acquisition and storage, and may also be transmitted electronically.

Fundus photographs may be taken by dedicated staff such as ophthalmic nurses, orthoptists or medical photographers, in a health or community service; or by optometrists in their own premises. The digital images may then be read by specially trained non-medical graders supported by second opinions from ophthalmologists. Patients attending digital camera-based screening clinics for diabetic retinopathy monitoring should be advised that they still need to attend their optometrist for their regular eye-tests.

Laser photocoagulation treatment is very effective at saving sight in the early stages of sight-threatening diabetic retinopathy. Hart & Harding (1999) found that for proliferative retinopathy with high-risk characteristics there is a relative risk reduction in severe visual loss of 52% and that early treatment of clinically significant macular oedema reduces moderate visual loss at 3 years with a relative risk reduction of 50%.

Severe visual loss compromises independent living and moderate loss has an impact on quality of life (Ferris 1993). Data from epidemiological studies indicates that each successful treatment will give at least 5 years of preserved sight (Klein et al. 1999).

In some cases, vitreous haemorrhages may resolve spontaneously, restoring vision, although at times surgery may be indicated. The later complications of rubeotic glaucoma and retinal detachments do not always respond to surgical treatment.

Cerebrovascular accident (stroke)

CVA causes considerable neurological dysfunction, the consequences of which produce varying degrees of disability for the survivors. Two-thirds of those with CVA are over 65 years of age. The incidence of reduced visual function associated with CVA is thought to be more prevalent than had previously been demonstrated. Studies by orthoptists working with stroke patients have indicated that a high proportion have some form of visual disturbance (Freeman & Rudge 1988). Clisby (1995) found that 70% of patients with CVA in older care wards exhibited a variety of visual dysfunctions. These can have a considerable impact on the rehabilitation process if not identified.

Reduced vision, manifest squint, ptosis, cranial nerve defects, binocular gaze dysfunction, reduced depth perception and binocular convergence, nystagmus and visual field defects produce a variety of symptoms that can cause confusion and disorientation. Symptoms include: blurred vision; double vision (diplopia); the inability to read easily or for any length of time; jumbled letters or words; poor hand–eye coordination; difficulty judging distances; difficulty in discriminating between objects; and blocking out part of the visual field, either centrally or peripherally as for example in homonymous hemianopia.

Visual perception disorders and visual inattention or neglect can also be evident but these are not produced by anomalies of visual function. Assessment by an orthoptist may take place initially in the stroke unit. The *National Service Framework for Older People* (Department of Health 2001) recommends that all those who are thought to have had a stroke should have access to diagnostic services, be treated appropriately by a specialist stroke service, and subsequently, with their carers, participate in a multidisciplinary programme of secondary prevention and rehabilitation.

For patients with diplopia, an eye-patch or some form of occlusion of their spectacle lens may be given initially when seen by the orthoptist in the ward. A full outpatient orthoptic assessment, including a Hess chart to plot any abnormality of the extraocular muscles, should be carried out as soon as the patient is well enough and, if appropriate, a plastic Fresnel prism can be applied to the patient's glasses to correct diplopia. The diplopia may be present for near and/or distance fixation and may be due to defective nerve function supplying the extraocular muscles, e.g. third, fourth or sixth nerves.

The principle of the Fresnel optic was developed by French engineer Augustin Fresnel in the 1820s, and was first applied to the lens in a lighthouse in order to refract and concentrate the light coming from the source into a narrow horizontal beam. Fresnel's principle was that the thickness and the weight of the lenses could be considerably reduced by using a series of stepped concentric rings. This principle was later applied to prisms and, in the twentieth century with the development of high-quality plastics, it was possible to produce plastic Fresnel prisms. The power of a conventional plastic prism is incorporated in a thin plastic membrane in which a series of small plastic prisms lie adjacent to each other. By the end of the 1970s the Fresnel prism had become an essential aid in the orthoptic management of diplopia (Henderson & Wylie 1997). Fresnel prisms are available in strengths ranging from 1 prism dioptre to 30 prism dioptres. Once the correct power has been determined, they are cut to the size of the patient's spectacle lens. They can be used as horizontal or vertical prisms and in some cases are tilted to incorporate both features. They are applied under running water, can be cleaned easily in situ and can be removed at any time when no longer required. They are an inexpensive and effective way of relieving the symptom of diplopia.

Patients with homonymous hemianopia that does not resolve spontaneously should be referred to an ophthalmologist who can advise patients on their eligibility for registration as partially sighted.

FUNCTIONAL VISION ASSESSMENT

To assess functional vision it is necessary to establish the needs of older people and what they can achieve in their everyday tasks with the visual acuity they have. In order to do this the nurse (hospital and community) or other eye-care professional must take the time to listen and observe how well they are able to cope in their environment. Listening to information concerning their ability to perform various activities or questioning patients about how they are coping will inform the observer about any difficulties.

Questions to be asked include: does the patient have any difficulty reading books or newspapers? How much reading is possible? Or has reading been abandoned because of poor vision, or poor memory?

Observing the patient will help to establish whether problems with mobility are due to reduced visual acuity or visual field defects. A nurse may observe whether the patient is consistently bumping into things on the right or left side, or trips over things on the floor, and whether a compensatory head posture is adopted to overcome any visual difficulties.

In order to assess a patient's visual performance, it is necessary to measure visual acuity. Snellen letter charts are most commonly used clinically to measure recognition acuity and are scored using the Snellen fraction. The test distance is the numerator, and the standard distance of the smallest letter correctly identified is the denominator. The usual test distance is 6 m and normal visual acuity is considered to be 6/6. The patient should be seated comfortably with good overhead lighting. The correct glasses for distance viewing should be worn and each eye tested separately with the other eye adequately occluded. More recently, researchers and clinicians have found that the log of the minimum angle of resolution (logMAR) is the preferred scale for representing visual acuity. Unlike the Snellen letter chart, an equal number of letters is presented on each line with equal spacing between lines. Each row contains five letters and each letter has a value of 0.02 log units. An acuity change of 0.10 log unit is equally significant whether the acuity is 0.0 (6/6 Snellen equivalent), or 1.0 (6/60 Snellen equivalent).

The logMAR chart can be used at a number of viewing distances from 4 m to 1 m, each one representing progressive 0.1 log unit steps which magnify the letters on each row by a factor of 1.26.

If a portable visual acuity test is required for assessing a person at home or in the ward, then Keeler crowded acuity cards are both accurate and practical. The test is performed at 3 m. This test was originally developed for use in assessing children, but has been shown to give equivalent measurements to the logMAR chart used at 4 m in adult eye clinics.

If the visual acuity is reduced in either eye, it is necessary to repeat the test using a pinhole occluder. If the vision improves, an optometric referral should be recommended for an eye-test. If the visual acuity does not improve with a pinhole then referral to an ophthalmologist is advised.

The near visual acuity tests based on print size and the 'N' notations are interchangeable and must be recorded with the viewing distance. This is 40 cm for the normally sighted and 25 cm for the visually impaired. Reading glasses should be worn and each eye tested separately, followed by both eyes together. In general, anyone reading N5–N8 has good functional vision and can read a book with normal-sized print or a newspaper with good contrast. Fluent reading of print (threshold print size) is generally considered to be three times the near visual acuity, e.g. N8 × 3 = N24 (Johnston 1991). To establish to what extent the reading task can be enhanced, it is necessary to increase the size of print and record the point at which the fluency and speed of reading can improve no further. This is known as the critical reading print size and is used to calculate the magnification required for fluent reading of newsprint.

Another aspect of functional vision is the continued ability to drive. The DVLA standard for driving is a visual acuity of 6/12 with both eyes open and a horizontal visual field of 120°, with no field loss 20° above or below fixation throughout the 120°. If there are any doubts about a patient's field of vision and eligibility to drive, the medical division of the DVLA should be contacted and a binocular driving field performed by an orthoptist or an optometrist.

For an immobile or house-bound person, the visual fields can be assessed by the 'confrontation' method. One eye is covered and the subject is asked to fixate on the opposite eye of the examiner. The test object is moved in a plane midway between the examiner and the patient starting in the periphery, and moving it towards the patient in various meridians until it is seen. Visual fields become smaller and peripheral sensitivity decreases with age. By the age of 70 years, the binocular field declines from approximately 180° to

140°. Visual field sensitivity has also been evaluated as a possible basis for poor driving amongst older adults. It is thought that peripheral field loss is more difficult to compensate for than a central field defect, particularly when navigating around the home or outdoors. The level of illumination plays an important role in minimizing the effects of field loss. People with modest levels of visual impairment have fewer difficulties with mobility tasks in high illuminance conditions. People with low vision have more difficulties when performing tasks at low light levels.

When an older person is admitted to hospital for acute, respite or rehabilitation care, careful note should be taken of any ophthalmic history and any comments made by the patient and carer about visual problems. Patients with glaucoma, for example, should continue with their normal routine of eyedrops and any other regular medication.

STRATEGIES TO ENHANCE LOW VISION

Non-optical strategies

Specific visual tasks such as reading become more difficult under conditions of low luminance. Strategies such as improved contrast, colour, light and size can all be used to improve visual performance. It has been noted above that older people are more likely to benefit from improved task illumination as it is suggested that the decrease in the amount of light reaching the retina is the cause of poorer performance.

However, increasing the illuminance cannot compensate completely for the small size and low contrast of a visual task, thus changing the size of the task detail may be effective. Increases in reading performance may follow by improving the contrast of the material. However, if excessive illumination is used this may further reduce performance because of glare. Light rays falling on a surface are partly reflected and if the surface is glossy paper, this could cause reflection glare when reading. This can be minimized by changing the position of the lighting or by changing to matt paper (C Dickinson 1998).

Everyday tasks such as preparing food, eating and drinking can be hazardous, but by making more use of colour and contrast in the home, such tasks can be made easier. For example, non-white crockery on a contrasting tablecloth or using a sheet of dark paper on a desk to make the edges of a sheet of paper or a book more visible may be helpful. The use of light décor on walls with contrasting (darker) floors and doors/door frames and door handles will assist the visually impaired user, and all surfaces should be matt so that there is no specular reflection to create a glare source.

Lighting should be uniform throughout and light switches must contrast clearly with the wall, or have a dark surround. As a rule, a coloured object on a white surface is preferable to a white object on a dark surface as a bright surface reflects up to 70–80% of light falling on it, while a dark one reflects less than 20%.

A survey carried out by the Royal National Institute for the Blind (RNIB) in 1991 suggested that about one million people in the UK suffer from some form of visual deficit involving part of the visual field (Bruce et al. 1991). Impairments such as macular degeneration cause loss of central vision and, in glaucoma, central vision is relatively unimpaired but peripheral sensitivity to coarse moving patterns is reduced. In both cases, colour discrimination is also impaired.

A research group for inclusive environments at Reading University, UK, has looked at the selection of colour and contrast and the impact on the ability of visually impaired users of buildings. The researchers published a booklet giving design guidance for domestic interiors which are attractive to the normally sighted and provide sufficient contrast to help those with low vision (Bright et al. 1997).

General lighting, that is, the global level of illumination in an internal environment, can be improved cheaply and effectively. In the majority of homes there is inadequate lighting for the ageing eye; this increases the incidence of poor visual functioning. Studies have shown that improved lighting can improve a person's visual acuity in the home environment (Cullinan et al. 1979). Clients are advised to make optimum use of natural daylight by drawing back curtains, cleaning windows and positioning chairs near to the window so that light falls over the shoulder.

To assess an individual's lighting needs in the home, where the level of illuminance is likely to be very different from a clinical setting, a visibility indicator devised by Grundy (1989) can be given to the patient to show whether the lighting levels at home are adequate. The visibility indicator consists of three rows of squares of different contrasts printed on a card. Each square is made up of dots which decrease in size going down each column of squares. Holding the card in the reading position, and viewed through reading spectacles, the patient identifies the squares containing the smallest dots visible. This test is first carried out in a low-vision clinic and is then repeated in the patient's home with the instruction to increase the lighting level until the same size of detail can be seen.

Light levels between each room may vary and, when the eye is unable to react quickly to a change in illumination, moving from a bright to a dim level may cause glare. Discomfort glare can result in visual discomfort, eyestrain and fatigue. The positioning of a light source is important and, for a visually impaired person, a higher illumination level may be required for reading. The light source chosen will depend partly on the internal lighting conditions. Desk lamps are ideal 'task lights' and come fitted with different types of bulbs, e.g. incandescent, halogen, fluorescent and compact fluorescent bulbs. The lamps should be positioned so that light falls directly on the work and not into the user's face, causing glare. It is important to remember that, while the bulbs of incandescent and halogen bulbs are small, they create a higher temperature than fluorescent and compact fluorescent lamps. Decreasing the distance between the light source and the work surface can also be effective: halving the distance between the two will result in a fourfold increase in illumination.

Glare and dazzle can be a problem for people with cataract and also after lens implant. This can be remedied by wearing a cap or wide-brimmed hat outdoors. Plano ultraviolet and short-wavelength absorbing tinted overspectacles with additional overhead and side shielding can be worn alone, or over prescription glasses. The tint is designed to minimize light scatter, and can easily be removed when going indoors.

Coloured tints can be incorporated into prescription lenses and a number of research groups have investigated the potential of these tints to improve vision by increasing retinal image contrast. Unfortunately these experiments have produced very mixed results. Disability glare may be caused by strong lights illuminating the eyes, causing stray light within the eye. Complaints that a person's vision varies on a daily basis are mostly related to the brightness outdoors compared with the illumination within the home.

The size of objects can be enlarged to enhance functional vision. Distance vision can be improved by moving closer to the object, for example, a person with a distance visual acuity of 6/36 on the Snellen chart can improve this to 3/18 by positioning the chart at 3 m. Instead of only reading two lines, the individual can now read four lines on the chart, therefore bringing the letters to half the distance doubles the viewing angle.

Magnification of text can be achieved in several ways. Print can be enlarged on a photocopier or printer up to 1.5–2 times. Real image magnification over a wide range of sizes is possible with a closed-circuit TV connected to a monitor screen which displays the magnified text. The size of characters, the contrast and colour of the text and background can be adjusted to suit the needs of the client. The advantage for clients is that they can be the same distance from the image on the screen as from the original object and therefore their existing refractive correction will be appropriate.

A whole range of everyday objects are produced in enlarged sizes specifically for the visually impaired,

e.g. telephone dials, clocks, large-print books and heavy-lined stationery, and are available from voluntary agencies such as the RNIB.

For older people with impaired vision, the ability to cope with sight loss may be due to a number of factors such as fear of the consequences of having a fall and unsteadiness when walking rather than solely due to a visual inability to navigate safely. Visual field defects can cause difficulty with reading and close work as the text may disappear on the side of field loss, especially if the macular area is involved. Reading may be easier if the text is placed in a seeing area, or techniques such as eccentric viewing (deliberate fixation to the side of the object of interest) may be taught. Patients with hemianopia may be helped to read by using a typoscope, a device invented in the nineteenth century. It consists of a rectangle of matt, black card with a window cut out. It is placed over a page of text revealing two or three lines of print. The aim is to enable the client to read along the text and when the end of the line is reached, the typoscope is moved down to the next line. It increases contrast by preventing scattering of light from the white background.

Placement of objects on the side of the still functional field is very helpful and carers should endeavour to place themselves on the side of the patient that is in the 'seeing' area of vision. Patients with central scotomas due to macular degeneration can be taught eccentric viewing by a low-vision therapist. This technique allows the person to use an area of retina, other than the fovea, for fixation; this is called the 'preferred retinal location' and should be as near as possible to the fovea on the edge of the scotoma.

The RNIB's survey (Bruce et al. 1991) found that about one million people in the UK suffer from visual field loss, involving central or peripheral vision.

Gross field defects in the lower field of vision can cause difficulties when going downstairs or stepping off kerbs. Depressing the chin when looking down will bring the object of regard into the upper field of vision. Grossly restricted visual fields of less than 20° in total may occur in advanced glaucoma and can cause great difficulty as the only visible field is around the central area of fixation, and so the patient will find it difficult to gather enough information from the environment for effective orientation and mobility. Care should be taken to ensure that food, utensils and reading texts are placed within the area of restricted field. The only optical aid that may help in this situation is one that minifies the object of regard by expanding the field of view by using a Galilean telescope the wrong way round. This may be helpful in some cases but field expanders are generally considered to be difficult to use and the results disappointing. 'Minifies' is a technical term from the word 'minification' meaning a reduction in the apparent size of an object, which occurs when viewing a distant object through a Galilean telescope (Millodot 2000).

Optical strategies

Most older people require spectacles for close work and also distance viewing, worn as bifocals, varifocals or as two separate pairs of glasses. These should be kept clean by washing with a mild washing-up detergent or using an impregnated cleaning cloth or special cleaning liquid that can be purchased from an optician. It may be helpful to label the spectacle cases if two pairs are worn.

A routine eye-test should be carried out by an optometrist approximately every 2 years. The optometrist will: test the vision and prescribe the appropriate corrective lenses; check for eye disease by examining the fundus (retina) and media by ophthalmoscopy; carry out a screening visual field test and also check the intraocular pressure by non-contact tonometry. The tonometer sends a puff of air towards the cornea with sufficient strength to estimate the intraocular pressure. Binocular function is also assessed using diagnostic equipment.

If any ocular abnormality or general health problem is detected, the patient will be referred to an ophthalmologist via the patient's general practitioner. If an urgent sight-threatening condition is suspected then the patient is directly referred to the local ophthalmic accident and emergency department for immediate investigation.

If patients have an ocular condition which results in permanently reduced vision, or restricted visual field such as ARMD, diabetic retinopathy or glaucoma, they should be referred to a low-vision clinic. Assessment of visual acuity, contrast sensitivity and visual fields will give a clear indication of patients' needs and the tasks with which they have most difficulty. This may be close work or reading, face recognition or mobility.

If required, low-vision aids such as high-plus spectacle lenses, hand-held or stand magnifiers, with or without internal illumination, may be prescribed for close work, or hand-held and spectacle-mounted telescopes for near or distance. These are provided on loan to the patient through the hospital eye service. It must be clear for which activity the low-vision aid is needed and adequate training in the correct use of the aid must be given. In addition to this advice on lighting, use of contrast and enlarged material should also be available.

The internally illuminated magnifiers are powered by batteries or by the mains power supply. The optician must ensure that the patient is able to change the batteries in the appliance, as failure to do so may result in the magnifier being discarded. For patients who are not helped by magnifiers or cannot manage them, there are ways of magnifying text using a closed-circuit TV. The magnified text is displayed on a monitor screen that can be connected to a video camera, a closed-circuit TV magnifier, television screen or a computer. There are also computer programs such as zoom text which can be incorporated into the computer enabling the user to adjust the size, colour and contrast of text and background. Additional magnification can be produced by using a very close viewing distance.

Low-vision services are provided in many eye outpatient departments by dispensing opticians, optometrists, orthoptists, low-vision therapists and rehabilitation workers. There are also low-vision clinics run by voluntary organizations such as the Partially Sighted Society, RNIB and other local agencies. The aim of any low-vision service is to enable a person to maximize the potential use of residual vision, by providing low-vision aids, vision training, advice and emotional support.

IDENTIFICATION AND REGISTRATION OF BLIND AND PARTIALLY SIGHTED PEOPLE

Statutory support

The current process of registration in the UK as blind or partially sighted is based on the BD8 form, a certificate signed by an ophthalmologist and by the patient to indicate a certain level of visual impairment. Copies of the BD8 form are sent to the patient, the patient's general practitioner, social services and the Office of Population Censuses and Surveys.

Following receipt of the BD8 the patient is invited by the local social services to be put on the register of blind or partially sighted people in the borough. This process is voluntary and the patient can withdraw from the register at any time. The register is used to give visually impaired people access to specialist support and financial benefits and concessions to which they are entitled.

The current standards for registration are conditional on the level of distance visual acuity and visual fields. The definition of blind is 'so blind as to be unable to perform any work for which eyesight is essential', and the definition of partially sighted is 'substantially and permanently handicapped by defective vision caused by congenital defect, illness or injury'.

Standards for blind registration are:

- visual acuity 3/60 with good visual field
- visual acuity > 3/60 with grossly constricted visual field.

In some cases the visual acuity could be as good as 6/6 but with a constricted field to within a few degrees of fixation. There is currently no provision for consideration of sight loss in one eye only.

Standards for partially sighted registration are:

- visual acuity 6/60–6/24 with a good visual field
- visual acuity 6/18 with a constricted visual field
- visual acuity of 6/6 with homonymous hemianopia.

Once registered, a person will be visited by a rehabilitation worker from the local social services department, who will carry out an assessment of the person's needs, the aim of which is to help the visually impaired person to be as independent and confident as possible in spite of visual difficulties (Westminster Social and Community Services 2002). The emphasis is on rehabilitation and training. An action plan will be drawn up, which will outline the daily living skills training, help with communication and lighting, mobility skills, equipment, information and advice required by the individual.

A revision by the Department of Health and Social Care in England of the process by which blind and partially sighted people are identified is currently taking place. One of the aims is to recognize the needs of the current older population. It is suggested that three separate forms would be used to enable early identification of those people with visual impairment requiring low-vision services and/or social care and to increase the take-up of registration.

The RNIB survey published by Bruce et al. (1991) revealed a considerable underregistration of those eligible, mostly amongst the older population. It was found by Robinson et al. (1994) that, of those patients routinely attending ophthalmic clinics, less than 50% of those eligible were in fact registered.

Voluntary agencies

Most areas in the UK have local associations for the visually impaired; help is extended to all who are in need even if they are not registered. National organizations such as the RNIB, Partially Sighted Society and Action for Blind People all provide extensive information on eye conditions, financial benefits and concessions, publications on research, campaigns aimed at improving services as well as special equipment for

daily living and specialist services such as talking books and newspapers, and large-print books.

The RNIB has set up a number of hospital-based information desks staffed by volunteers who give patients literature on eye conditions and advice on the range of services and equipment available from their organization. In London, the Metropolitan Society for the Blind has a network of 'visitors' who visit older, blind people who live alone, in order to provide companionship, to help with their correspondence and to accompany them outdoors if required.

A significant number of older people with visual impairment have additional disabilities and some also have significant learning disabilities. These people are usually cared for by local community services for the learning disabled, or by organizations such as See-Ability, and who provide facilities such as workshops, education in daily living skills, crafts, recreation and computer skills, as well as residential accommodation.

LOW-VISION SERVICES

Recommendations for service delivery

In 1998 a Low Vision Services Consensus group was formed by representatives from a cross-section of organizations concerned with helping people with sight loss. A number of problems were identified: a lack of multidisciplinary and multiprofessional working; a wide disparity in quality and quantity of services between different parts of the country; and a lack of information for those who would benefit from a low-vision service.

To address these issues the group prepared a national framework document for the provision of low-vision services which should not be considered in isolation from other services, but should be part of a comprehensive service for people with visual impairment. The Low Vision Services Consensus Group document (1999) was followed by the establishment of a Low Vision Implementation Group Committee and the appointment of a Low Vision Implementation Group officer, and a network of local low-vision services committees have been established around the UK. These groups bring together representatives from local optical, social, health and voluntary care providers and service users to discuss ways of implementing the recommendations in the *Low Vision Services* document in order to improve low-vision service provision in their local areas.

Acknowledgement

I would like to acknowledge the contribution made by Chris Clisby and Christine Cox in the chapter they wrote for the third edition of this book.

Recommended reading

Association of Directors of Social Services (ADSS) 2002 Progress in sight. Available online at: www.adss.org. uk/eyes.shtml.
National standards of social care for visually impaired adults.
Department of Health 2001 National service framework for older people (NSF). Available online at: www.doh.gov. uk/nsf/olderpeople.htm.
Government document outlining eight national service framework standards for the care of older people in the UK, aimed at improving services, and improving co-operation between the NHS and social services.
Dickinson C 1998 Low vision – principles and practice. Butterworth-Heinemann, Oxford.
This book for optometrists gives a comprehensive review of their role in working with the visually impaired. It will also be of interest to all health care professionals involved in the care of patients with low vision.
Hawker M, Davies M (eds) 1991 Distance learning pack on visual handicap. Disabled Living Foundation, London.
Resource for nurses and therapists working with visually impaired patients. It is an easy-to-read guide to problems encountered by this group of people.
Kanski J 1994 Clinical ophthalmology – a systematic approach, 3rd edn. Butterworth-Heinemann, Glasgow.
Clear, concise text for those requiring an indepth knowledge of ophthalmology.
Lomas G 1998 Low vision in the UK. The Partially Sighted Society, Doncaster.
Discussion papers exploring key issues in developing a post-qualifying scheme of staff training as part of continuing professional development.
McBride S 2000 Patients talking one. Royal National Institute for the Blind, London.
McBride S 2002 Patients talking two. Royal National Institute for the Blind, London.
Experiences of visually impaired users of hospital eye services.
Pitts-Crick R, Trimble RB 1986 Clinical opthalmology. Hodder & Stoughton, London.
Excellent, concise text on all aspects of clinical ophthalmology.
Ryan B, Culham L 1999 Fragmented vision. Royal National Institute for the Blind, and Moorfields Eye Hospital, NHS Trust, London.
National quantitative research on the nature, extent and geographical distribution of low vision services.
Ryan B, McCloughan L 1999 Our better vision. Royal National Institute for the Blind, and Heriot-Watt University, Edinburgh.
Qualitative and quantitative research into the experience and needs of service users with regards to low vision services.

Useful addresses

Action for Blind People, London Office, 14–16, Verney Road, London SE16 3DZ
Diabetes UK Central Office, 10 Parkway, London NW1 7AA
International Glaucoma Association (IGA), 108c Warner Road, London SE5 9HQ
Macular Disease Society, Darwin House, 13A Bridge Street, Andover, Hants SP10 1BE
Partially Sighted Society. Queen's Road, Doncaster, South Yorkshire DN1 2NX
Royal National Institute for the Blind (RNIB), 105 Judd Street, London WC1H 9NE
Talking Newspaper Association of the UK, National Recording Centre, Heathfield, East Sussex TN21 8D13

References

Advisory Panel Final Report to the UK National Screening Committee 1999–2000. Available online at: http://www.diabetic-retinopathy.screening.nhs.uk/ recommendations.html
Anderson SJ, Holliday IE 1995 Night driving, effects of glare from vehicle headlights on motion perception. Ophthalmic and Physiological Optics 15: 545–551
Balatsoukas DD, Sioulis C, Parisi A et al. 1995 Visual handicap in south-east Scotland. Journal of the Royal College of Surgeons 40: 49–51
Barneby H 2002 Safety of prostaglandin analogues and the hyperaemia debate. Protecting Vision. 2nd Alcon Scientific Symposium, Monte Carlo. Alcon Laboratories, Hemel Hempstead, pp 14–15
Bernstein PS 2002 New insights into the role of the macular carotenoids in age-related macular degeneration. Resonance Raman studies. Pure Applied Chemistry 74: 1419–1425
Bright K, Cook G, Harris J 1997 Colour, contrast and perception. Design guidance for internal built environments. Project rainbow. University of Reading, Reading
British Diabetic Association 1999–2000 Advisory panel final report to the UK. National screening committee 1999–2000. Available online at: www.diabeticretinopathy. screening.nhs.uk/recommendations
Bruce I, McKennell A, Walker E 1991 Blind and partially sighted adults in Britain: the RNIB needs survey, vol 1. HMSO, London
Campbell H, Hotchkiss R, Bradshaw N, Porteous M 1998 Integrated care pathways. British Medical Journal 316: 133–137
Clisby C 1995 Visual assessment of patients with cerebrovascular accident on the older care wards. British Orthoptic Journal 52: 38–40
Cooper J 1999 Teaching patients in post-operative eye care: the demands of day surgery. Nursing Standard 13: 42–46
Corliss DA, Norton TT, Bailey JE 2002 The psychophysical measurement of visual function. Butterworth-Heinemann, Woburn, MA, USA
Cullinan TR, Gould ES, Irvine D, Silver JH 1979 Visual disability and home lighting. Lancet 1: 642–644
Department of Health 1991 On the state of the public health. HMSO, London

Department of Health 2001 National service framework for older people. Available online at: www.doh.gov.uk/nsf/olderpeople.htm.

Dickinson C 1998 Low vision – principles and practice. Butterworth-Heinemann, Oxford

Evans JR, Wormald RPL 1996 Is the incidence of registerable age-related macular degeneration increasing? British Journal of Ophthalmology 80: 9–14

Evans JR, Fletcher AE, Wormald RPL et al. 2002 Prevalence of visual impairment in people aged 75 years and older in Britain: results from the MRC trial of assessment and management of older people in the community. British Journal of Ophthalmology 86: 795–800

Ferris L 1993 How efficient are treatments for diabetic retinopathy? Journal of the American Medical Association.269: 1290–1291

Freeman CF, Rudge NB 1988 Cerebrovascular accident and the orthoptist. British Orthoptic Journal 45: 8–17

Glynn RJ, Seddon JM, Krug JH et al. 1991 Falls in older patients with glaucoma. Archives of Ophthalmology 109: 205–210

Gonzalez-Villalpando ME, Gonzalez-Villaalpando C, Arredondo Perez B et al. 1994 Diabetic retinopathy: prevalence and clinical characteristics. Archives of Medical Research 25: 355–360

Grundy JW 1989 A visibility indicator. Optometry Today 20: 6–10

Harding S 2001 Treatment of AMD (excluding surgery): past, present and future. Royal College of Ophthalmologists congress 2001, Elizabeth Thomas seminar. Available online at: rcophth.ac.uk/congress/eliz_thomas_treatment/html

Hart PM, Harding S 1999 Is it time for a national screening programme for sight threatening retinopathy? Eye 13: 129–130

Hecht S, Shlaer S, Pirenne MH 1942 Energy, quanta and vision. Journal of General Physiology 25: 819–840

Henderson M, Wylie J 1997 An historical look at Fresnel. British Orthoptic Journal 54: 24–28

Hodge WG, Witcher JP, Satariano W 1995 Risk factor for age-related cataracts. Epidemiology Review 17: 336–346

International ARM Epidemiological Study Group 1995 An international classification and grading system for age-related maculopathy and age-related macular degeneration. Survey of Ophthalmology 39: 367–374

Johnston AW 1991 Making sense of the M, N and logMAR systems of specifying visual acuity. Problems in Optometry 3: 394–407

Klein BE, Klein R, Wong Q, Moss SE 1995 Older onset diabetes and lens opacities. The Beaver Dam study. Ophthalmic Epidemiology 2: 49–55

Klein R, Klein BEK, Moss SE, Cruickshanks KJ 1999 Association of ocular disease and mortality in a diabetic population. Archives of Ophthalmology 117: 1487–1494

Levy G 1997 Access to eye care for adults with learning difficulties. Royal National Institute for the Blind, London

Low Vision Services Consensus Group 1999 Low vision services – recommendations for future service delivery in the UK. Royal National Institute for the Blind, London

Marshall J 2002 The blue light hazard and cataract surgery. Protecting vision. 2nd Alcon Scientific Symposium, Monte Carlo. Alcon Laboratories, Hemel Hempstead, pp 4–5

Millodot M 2000 Dictionary of optometry and visual science, 5th edn. Butterworth-Heinemann, Oxford

Rendell J 1998a Discharge instructions after cataract surgery: the patient's perspective. Ophthalmic Nursing 2: 4–9, 10–16.

Rendell J 1998b Discharge instructions after cataract surgery: professional factors. Ophthalmic Nursing 2: 4–9

Robinson R, Deutsch J, Jones JS et al. 1994 Unrecognised and unregistered visual impairment. British Journal of Ophthalmology 78: 736–740

Rose KE 1997 Caring for patients with cataract. Nursing Standard 11: 49–55

Royal College of Ophthalmologists Guidelines (undated) The management of age related macular disease. Available online at: www.site4sight.org.uk/quality/RGov/Guidelines/ARMD.htm 1-18

Salford Eye Care Project 1993 Henshaws Society for the Blind in partnership with Salford family health services authority. Salford Social Services Department, Salford

Schachnow P 2002 The importance of diurnal IOP variation in glaucoma and the role of prostaglandin analogues. Protecting vision. 2nd Alcon Scientific Symposium, Monte Carlo. Alcon Laboratories, Hemel Hempstead, pp 12–13

Scuffham PA 2002 Falls associated with visual impairment. Visual Impairment Research 4: 1–14

Stuckey S 1999 Health Promotion for cataract day-case patients. Professional Nurse. June 1999 14(9): 638–341.

Webb J 1994 A framework for the care of older people. Vision and older people. Support paper 1. South Thames Regional Health Authority, London

Westminster Social and Community Services 2002 Visual impairment rehabilitation service. City of Westminster, London

Whittaker SG, Lovie-Kitchin JE 1994 The assessment of contrast sensitivity and contrast reserve for reading rehabilitation. In: Kooijman AC, Looijestijn PL, Welling JA et al. (eds) Low vision – research and new developments in rehabilitation. IOS Press, Amsterdam, pp 47–50

World Health Organization 1980 International classification of impairments, disabilities and handicap. World Health Organization, Geneva

Zeki S 1990 A century of cerebral achromatopsia. Brain 113: 1721–1777

Chapter 13

Promoting safe mobility

Janet M. Simpson and Elaine New

IMPORTANCE OF MOBILITY

The skilled guidance and encouragement that nurses and health care assistants give are crucial to helping older people regain, maintain and improve their mobility in both health and social care settings. According to the Royal College of Nursing (RCN), mobility is one of the aspects of care that requires special consideration among older people (Royal College of Nursing 1993: p. 3). Furthermore, although the RCN acknowledges physiotherapists' and occupational therapists' responsibility for developing an outline treatment plan with respect to mobility, it emphasizes nurses' particular responsibility for carrying it through (Royal College of Nursing 1991). Thus a good relationship between nursing staff and rehabilitation staff is essential for success. Our view is that nurses approach their contribution to mobility promotion as supporting and facilitating the work of physiotherapists and occupational therapists and in encouraging patients to take responsibility for following their rehabilitation programme. (Chapter 34 develops this theme.) Moreover, we consider that facilitating clients to return to previous levels of mobility after an illness is an integral part of gerontological nursing. After an acute illness entailing no threat to mobility status, e.g. urinary tract or chest infection, specialist therapy input is not necessarily indicated as encouragement and practice alone will usually help older people back on to their feet. The importance of team work is also stressed repeatedly in the *National Service Framework for Older People* (Department of Health 2001). Henceforth we shall refer to this important document as the NSFOP.

In this chapter we summarize some common major intrinsic and extrinsic challenges to older people's mobility, and make suggestions for combating them.

The World Health Organization defines mobility as 'the individual's ability to move about effectively in his surroundings' (World Health Organization 1980: p. 192). In practice this means the ability to transfer safely from one position to another (lying to standing, sitting to standing, etc.), walk in the home and outside over rough ground, manage steps and climb stairs. When necessary it may be augmented by extrinsic factors such as an artificial limb, walking stick, wheelchair or an electric buggy, and it may be facilitated by slopes, handrails and other environmental adaptations. In practice, nurses need to know how much help a person requires to transfer from one position to another. This information is central to the European regulations on moving and handling and we shall pay particular attention to this important issue.

Loss of mobility leads to loss of independence. People with mobility problems may be more or less dependent on other people for help which, in turn, restricts their ability to do what they want to do and their participation in social life. For example, pathological change associated with osteoarthritis in a knee joint can lead to pain and joint stiffness. In turn these impairments might cause activity limitations such as inability to walk far enough to reach the lavatory or inability to climb on and off a bus in order to visit friends or relatives. Among frail older people in particular, however, it is often inability to get up from a chair or from the toilet or otherwise transfer position, rather than inability to walk, that most affects their level of independence. Activity limitations that restrict participation in social activity or lead to a person becoming house-bound can have detrimental consequences for mood and life satisfaction. The relationship between these three function-related concepts is detailed in the *International Classification of Functioning, Disability and Health*, commonly known as the ICF (World Health Organization 2001). In this classification 'disability' is used as an umbrella term to cover impairments, activity limitation and participation restrictions. Disability and functioning are viewed as outcomes of interactions between health conditions (diseases, disorders and injuries) and contextual factors, such as environmental factors (social attitudes, architectural characteristics, terrain) and personal factors (gender, age, coping styles, social background).

Rehabilitation of mobility takes account of all these factors. In the early stages of management, professionals direct their efforts at helping the person to recover from or overcome impairments associated with the initial pathology, such as fractured neck of femur or acute stroke. But as the person progresses toward greater independence the professionals reduce or change any environmental support and foster the person's confidence in their ability to do what they want to do within any limitations set by chronic impairments or progressive deterioration.

It is important to remember that the majority of people over 65 years of age are fit and able to look after themselves. Mobility problems, however, do tend to increase in very old age as is shown in the *Health Survey for England 2001: Disability* (Bajekal & Prescott 2003). Over 23 000 people were interviewed in all age groups from age 16 upwards, including 2172 older people aged over 74. Mobility difficulties were identified by presence of locomotor problems, inability to walk 200 m independently, climb 12 steps or retrieve a shoe from the ground. The proportion of men and women in a range of age groups who reported being *free* of any locomotor problems is shown in Table 13.1. Although the likelihood of having such problems increases with age, it is only amongst people over 85 years of age that they are common. The participants in the *Health Survey for England 2001* (Bajekal & Prescott 2003) were all living in their own homes. But the previous one, *Health Survey for England 2000* (Hirani & Malbut 2002) dealt with people in care homes, and, not surprisingly, showed the prevalence of locomotor problems to be greater amongst this client group.

In the title to this chapter, we emphasize *safe* mobility. Postural instability (related terms: imbalance, disequilibrium, unsteadiness) is difficulty in correcting displacements of the centre of gravity while standing or walking. This problem and concomitant anxiety about falling are common among the older people in touch with the health and social care services. So it is understandable that nurses and rehabilitation professionals may come to regard their client's reluctance to move about without holding on to something as normal in old age. As the survey data show, this is not so. We regard the promotion of postural stability as a key component of safe mobility and confidence in the ability to move about safely as the key outcome of

Table 13.1 The proportion of men and women in a range of age groups who were *free* of mobility problems

Age group (years)	Men (%)	Women (%)
16–24	99	97
35–44	95	94
65–74	75	76
75–84	67	57
85+	45	31

Adapted from Bajekal & Prescott 2003: Table 3, p. 39.

rehabilitation. Equally important is the safety of the person giving assistance when it is required.

MOVING AND HANDLING REGULATIONS

Under European Union regulations it is a legal requirement to assess patients' handling needs. These regulations, together with a wealth of useful information and guidance, are set out in a series of essential guides. We shall frequently cite the two most recent editions, referring to the 4th edition (Guide to the Handling of Patients, Royal College of Nursing 1997) as The 'Guide 1997' and to the 5th edition as The 'Guide 2005' (Smith J 2005). Of course, the regulations apply to all patients who need to be moved or helped to move. But, as we have noted above, many older patients have mobility problems so familiarity with these guides is particularly relevant to nursing and rehabilitation of this client group.

The patient handling assessment must be completed and documented, preferably as part of a patient care plan, as soon as possible after admission or referral. Its main purpose is to work out how to give patients more control over their daily activities and to improve the chances of successful rehabilitation.

Introducing this law in health care practices has promoted a much-needed philosophical change in both the attitude to, and application of, patient handling techniques. Above all, the need for nurses to *lift* patients manually is challenged. The law sets new standards for moving and handling to be achieved in all patient care circumstances, and emphasizes the safety and comfort of both patient and carers. It has led to a fundamental change in nurse education and requires commitment from employers to provide safe work systems, including adjustable-height beds, couches, trolleys, hoists and bathing equipment and to set up staff training and supervision in all aspects of patient handling as part of an overall safe handling policy. Qualified coordinators are appointed to ensure that standards of handling are achieved in accordance with guidelines laid down by the Health and Safety Executive and the appropriate professional body, i.e. the RCN. Nurses also have obligations. Following training, they are obliged to adhere to safe handling practices and to use equipment when the patient handling assessment indicates this to be necessary.

Applying the law in practice

Historically nurses have lifted, or otherwise moved and handled patients, using techniques that have now been proved to be biomechanically unsafe, e.g. the so-called 'bear hug' stand and the underarm 'drag-lift'

(Stubbs et al. 1983). The quantity and frequency of these manoeuvres, particularly in care of older people, have undoubtedly contributed to the huge numbers of nurses suffering from serious musculoskeletal problems, especially low-back pain.

The law is clear on how this problem must be tackled and on the consequences of failing to do so. Each element of a patient handling task must be brought together and assessed to determine whether there is any risk of injury to either patient or helper. Any hazards are identified and the level of risk associated with them is calculated and formally documented. It has been shown that a comprehensive nurse training programme and systematic risk assessment reduce the rate of injury and sickness absence in the workplace. *The Guide* 1997, Chapter 2, gives several examples of how improvement has been brought about. A notable tale tells about the ward sister in Glasgow who, more than 10 years ago, took the initiative and successfully introduced a no-handling policy in her own ward, which was then extended to the whole hospital.

Introducing hoists and other small handling aids has an added bonus. Since patients can be moved more easily and comfortably, they are likely to be moved more often, for example back on to the bed after lunch for a nap and back into the chair for tea. These position changes reduce the risk of complications associated with lack of movement, such as chest infections, and enhance successful rehabilitation.

Good training, regularly updated, ensures that nurses and other staff are confident and competent to develop appropriate handling strategies and to advise patients, relatives and other carers in their use. But insufficient practice and incomplete understanding of assessing patients' handling needs may lead to rigid or extreme views: 'This patient needs to be hoisted at all times' is misleading and denies people the chance to practise helping themselves. Given clear instructions and light assistance, they may be able get out of bed to a chair or commode at the side of the bed. It may just be necessary for their legs to be lowered over the side of the bed, for example. However, they may *not* be able to perform this procedure in reverse, so using a hoist is the safest and most comfortable way for getting back into bed.

As with all good nursing care, clear communication is crucial while handling patients. The term 'therapeutic handling' emphasizes that manually handling a patient could be considered an 'art', in contrast to the techniques used to handle large, heavy, inanimate loads. Simple explanation of the handling procedure in non-technical language delivered in an encouraging tone of voice, coupled with calm, gentle but purposeful touch, eye contact and a friendly facial expression, distinguishes good from poor handling. Particularly in the care of older people it fosters a relationship of trust and confidence.

There are few rules concerning patient handling. The clear underlying principle, however, is that any manoeuvre should be accomplished while allowing patients to do as much as possible for themselves and with minimal physical strain on the nurses. The law, when correctly applied, encourages rehabilitation of functional mobility. In summary, good handling practice:

- facilitates independent movement within the patient's capability
- reduces the likelihood of injury to the carer.

FACTORS ASSOCIATED WITH DECLINING MOBILITY: 'WHAT DO YOU EXPECT AT YOUR AGE?'

Getting older increases our chance of accumulating health problems due to, for example, disease, trauma and environmental pollutants, and it allows the effects of chronic disease to become more obvious. Among these intrinsic health problems are several that can profoundly restrict activity and social participation: impairments of sight and hearing reduce awareness of the environment and any potential hazards nearby. (For further discussion of hearing and sight, see Chapters 11 and 12.) Joint and soft-tissue diseases can give

rise to pain and stiffness; diseases affecting the nervous system can lead to impairments in the control of movement; respiratory and cardiovascular disease can reduce endurance and the ability to sustain activity. A metabolic problem, such as diabetic neuropathy, may lead to gangrene in one or both lower limbs and eventually to amputation; apparently minor disorders affecting a person's hands or feet can also severely restrict activity. In addition, anxiety can affect mobility if people lose confidence in their ability to move about.

Age-related physiological changes mean we can all expect to get physically slower and weaker, although changes may not start to become apparent until we are in our mid-60s (see Chapter 5 on the biology of ageing). However, it is difficult to disentangle the inevitable effects of ageing on the locomotor system from changes that may equally well be attributable to the adoption of a more sedentary way of life. Weakness and slowness will be exacerbated by lack of fitness, lack of use and, on top of that, by fatigue, poor general health and acute illnesses. The NSFOP (standard 8) stresses the need to extend the healthy life expectancy of older people. The very least we can all do is to try to remain physically as fit as possible as we age by taking plenty of exercise. As health professionals we should encourage all older people to take brisk walks (i.e. brisk for them), go swimming and dancing, play golf and to take up other enjoyable physical activities (Figs 13.1). Even very old

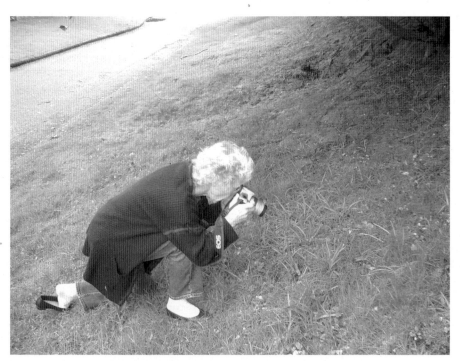

Fig. 13.1   Example of enjoyable physical activity – photographing flowers.

people who have been leading sedentary lives can show remarkable improvements in muscle strength and walking speed once given the opportunity to exercise (Fiatarone et al. 1994).

Abnormal joint pain and stiffness

The *Health Survey for England 2001*: Disability (Bajekal & Prescott 2003) showed that, among adults, 40% of all disabilities are attributable to musculoskeletal problems. So, not surprisingly, these disorders are very common among older people, often giving rise to their most bothersome complaints. Pain and joint stiffness present intrinsic barriers to mobility and the main causes include osteoarthritis, inflammatory arthropathies such as rheumatoid arthritis, and bone disorders such as osteoporosis. Most of these chronic disease processes are thought to arise from a mixture of genetic predisposition and environmental factors, including trauma and infection. Especially when they affect the lower limb, these processes can seriously impede a person's mobility. The very high rate of disability has a huge impact on the health and social services. People with these diseases need help to adjust to a life restricted by pain, discomfort and disability. We shall focus on the two most common joint problems afflicting older people: osteoarthritis and rheumatoid arthritis.

Generalized osteoarthritis describes a widespread pattern of synovial joint involvement, not only in hips and knees but also in terminal interphalangeal joints and thumb bases, with ankles and shoulders usually spared. However, the characteristic focal loss of articular cartilage occurs most commonly in the knees, hips, hands and apophyseal joints of the spine, either unilaterally or bilaterally. It is accompanied by a hypertrophic reaction in the subchondral bone and margins of the joint. The joint space narrows, subchondral bone thickens and within it cysts develop. Bony outgrowths, termed osteophytes, form at the joint margins.

Dieppe (1995) describes the clinical features familiar to nurses working with older people. Use-related aching and pain are the most commonly reported symptoms. Pain may start soon after activity begins and may last for hours after it has ceased. About 50% of sufferers report rest pain and 30% pain at night. Sensations of tenderness around the affected joint often accompany the pain and the area may be extremely painful if knocked or handled roughly. Long-term sufferers often find the unsightly deformities embarrassing.

Most patients also report joint stiffness. This can mean difficulty in starting a movement, a limitation of available range, and pain or aching while moving. Problems with getting the joint to move after a period of rest, called 'gelling', are characteristic of osteoarthri-tis joint stiffness. 'Getting going' after rest may be severe initially but usually only lasts a few minutes and is particularly noticeable first thing in the morning. If preventive exercise is not performed regularly, serious loss of joint range can ensue. People with knee osteoarthritis, in particular, often describe a feeling of insecurity or instability. They feel as if the joint is going to 'give way'. This sensation is probably due to weak and wasted muscles failing to give support.

Like osteoarthritis, rheumatoid arthritis is a disease of synovial joints but it is also a systemic condition, being one of the most common autoimmune diseases, affecting about 1% of the UK population (Dieppe & Klippel 1995). In autoimmune disease the immune system, which normally acts to protect the host from infectious agents, reacts against some of the host tissues, the autoantigens, leading to disease by generating local inflammation and tissue damage. At least three or more joint areas are usually involved. Usually initial signs of joint inflammation, tenderness and swelling appear in the proximal interphalangeal joints of the hands but these can extend to the metacarpophalangeal joints, wrist, knee, ankle, and metatarsophalangeal joints. Patients may feel generally unwell. Within the joints the synovial membrane becomes inflamed and proliferates; then, as the disease progresses, the articular cartilage is destroyed and the bone surfaces are eroded. In the later stages definite joint damage and accompanying deformity are evident, such as ulnar deviation of the fingers. Bone damage can affect tendons passing over joints which, in the hands, can lead to weak grip strength. Patients complain of morning stiffness but, unlike that associated with osteoarthritis, it lasts longer than 30 min, usually up to 1 h at least before maximal improvement is achieved. Rheumatoid arthritis affects the patient's body as a whole, not just the articular system, and it invariably impacts on every aspect of the patient's physical and psychosocial life.

With some exceptions, the inflammatory disease will no longer be active by the time a person reaches old age. It is then said to be 'burnt out'. Nevertheless, deformities and loss of normal joint movement remain so that, in common with osteoarthritis sufferers, the most serious effects for an individual's mobility arise from problems in the main weight-bearing joints, i.e. the hips and knees.

As yet, there is no totally effective way of halting or controlling the progress of either form of arthritis. Instead, interdisciplinary management programmes encourage patients to take charge of their problem, cope with the unpleasant symptoms and, as far as possible, maintain their level of functioning.

Physiotherapy for patients with rheumatic conditions aims to help them maintain and if possible improve functioning, although improvement may be limited in older people with advanced and poorly managed disease. Physiotherapy interventions include methods to reduce pain, flexibility exercises to maintain range of movement and muscle-strengthening exercises to improve the ability of muscles acting over the joints to maintain stability (Riley 1998).

Special considerations apply when the disease moves into an active phase and, especially in rheumatoid arthritis, periods of rest may be advised for the affected joints to alleviate the symptoms of inflammation. Special resting splints may need to be applied to support affected joints or to keep them comfortable at night. With good management, soft-tissue contractures around joints, which are very difficult to correct, should be prevented by regular careful, assisted active movement and good positioning. If a contracture becomes established – fixed flexion of the knee, for example – taking weight through the abnormal joint can be extremely painful and severely limit activity. Depending on the joint affected, contractures can also interfere with dressing and self-care. Methods to prevent them will form elements of the care plan.

Nurses play a key part in patient education (Hill 1998, le Gallez 1998). They work closely with physiotherapists and, appreciating the positive benefits of regular exercise, give patients confidence in their ability to carry out the daily regime and reinforce their understanding of the value to themselves of doing so. The goal is to achieve patient self-management. Working with patients in this way is proving to be very successful in managing chronic conditions (Bodenheimer et al. 2002).

Abnormal motor control: Parkinson's disease

Motor control is the ability to regulate and direct the mechanisms essential for movement (Shumway-Cook & Woollacott 2001). Loss of normal motor control means loss of the ability to adapt responses to changing tasks and environmental demands. 'Parkinsonism' describes the abnormal movement that characterizes Parkinson's disease (PD) but is also seen in other conditions. At present there is no cure for PD. Drugs can help mobility but, as with other chronic diseases, the nurse's goal, as a member of the care team, is to help patients understand and come to terms with PD and to help them and their carers learn how to manage the symptoms as well as possible.

This chronic progressive neuropsychiatric disorder affects between 1 in 1000 and 1 in 600 people in the UK (Mutch & Lien 2001). The signs and symptoms of PD, once known as the shaking palsy, originate in degeneration of the nigrostriatal tract which projects from

the substantia nigra, in the midbrain, to the basal ganglia, deep within the forebrain. These organs contribute to the planning and control of complex motor behaviour, so abnormal output from the basal ganglia leads to disordered function in the motor cortex and therefore impaired movement (Stewart 2001). Movement impairments are:

- akinesia – lack of movement
- hypokinesia – poverty of voluntary and spontaneous movement
- bradykinesia – failure to initiate movements, slowness of movement, difficulty with sequential or complex movements
- rigidity – increased resistance in the muscles to passive stretching but not dependent on the speed of muscle stretch. It is described as 'lead-pipe' rigidity when smooth, or 'cog-wheel' when jerky
- tremor – an involuntary, oscillatory rhythmic movement of a limb or the head, most commonly when it is at rest. It does not occur in all patients, and is not a great functional problem but can be socially embarrassing, e.g. when the knife and fork rattle against the plate.

Given these impairments, people with PD commonly develop balance and mobility limitations of varying severity. They may also exhibit slow mental information-processing, slow speech and depressive symptoms.

Early in the course of the disease they may have difficulty in turning over in bed or in rising from a low chair; they may walk slowly and even fall over. Eventually these problems increase. People with established disease have a stooped posture, tending to stand with their knees, hips, trunk, neck and elbows all slightly flexed and with their hips adducted, giving a narrow base of support between their feet. It is a great effort for them to try to correct this posture voluntarily and they resent being commanded brusquely to 'straighten up'. Patients may sit much more motionless than other people, showing little in the way of spontaneous weight-shifting, head-turning or other small movements. The patient's face seems expressionless, which can lead uninformed carers to assume some mental impairment.

Getting about becomes increasingly difficult. At first people may shuffle their feet as they walk, but, with time, they may lean forward more and more so that their centre of gravity gets pushed ahead of their narrow base of support. They may be forced to walk on tiptoes, which further increases their tendency to topple forwards and fall.

Bradykinesia means that quick compensatory movements, e.g. to regain balance and prevent a fall, become almost impossible, especially on turning around. Noticeably, their trunk and arms are moved as one unit, with reduced arm swing and shoulder rotation. Complex sequential movements such as getting out of a car, even rising from a chair or bed, may become difficult or impossible. Gait initiation can be frustratingly slow. It becomes difficult to shift body weight on to one foot in order to step with the other. This leads to 'freezing', when a person seems stuck to the spot. It can happen when a hazard is encountered, such as a narrow doorway, or a change of direction is required. Then the individual needs help to break out of the 'frozen' thought and movement pattern. Many patients learn tricks to help themselves. Simple instructions given authoritatively but kindly can also help. Some ideas for unfreezing are listed in Box 13.1. Robertson et al. (2001) and Edwards (2002) discuss these issues in further detail. Patients find it extremely frustrating if other people do not understand their problem and blame them for not getting going.

People with PD must work hard at retaining physical fitness and as much independent mobility as possible. 'Working hard' means 'hard for them' at whatever level of fitness they are starting from. Climbing stairs is relatively easy for PD patients: the visual cueing helps, and it should be encouraged as a fitness exercise (Case study 13.1). But in general it becomes so difficult to initiate movement that they readily succumb to being helped and eventually come to rely on others to do everything. On the other hand, people with PD should

---

Case study 13.1

Mrs A suffered from Parkinson's disease. She lived in a small, three-storey terrace house. There were one or two small rooms on each floor, all connected by flights of stairs. Mrs A was resisting her social worker's encouragement to move into residential care. 'It would all be on the flat there and I would not be able to manage as well as I do now. I can go up and down my stairs at home better than I can walk on the flat.'

---

not be left to struggle in vain at a task when patience and just the correct amount of help at a crucial moment can help them to succeed. To enable concentration on a task it is best to avoid talking unnecessarily or otherwise dividing their attention.

Drug therapy can facilitate mobility, especially in the early stages, though in due course it may become less effective. Depending on the length of time they have been on treatment, patients vary in how long it takes for the drug effect to 'come on' and start to 'go off'. It is important, therefore to know when a particular patient will be getting maximum benefit and plan important activities such as bathing, toileting, dressing and feeding for this interval. Likewise, when the effect is wearing off, people begin to slow down mentally and physically and should not be pushed to undertake demanding tasks. For this reason, people may have great difficulty during the night in turning in bed or getting out of it to go to the toilet and may need extra help. It is important to understand that the same drugs that can facilitate movement may also bring on feelings of tiredness.

Extreme emotion can affect a patient's mobility, overriding the beneficial effects of medication. For example, anxiety about something or excitement at going home can trigger exaggerated symptoms. Patients themselves are aware that they have good days and bad days and their judgement should be accepted and activities planned accordingly.

Abnormal motor control: stroke

In contrast to chronic progressive disorders such as PD, stroke, as its name implies, is of very sudden onset. The person exhibits 'rapidly developing signs of focal or global disturbance of cerebral functions lasting more than 24 hours or leading to death'. Strokes are caused by cerebral haemorrhage, thromboembolic occlusion or cerebral infarct, any of which compromises the normal blood flow and supply of oxygen to a part of the brain. Interruption of the oxygen supply

---

Box 13.1   Strategies to 'unfreeze'

When Parkinson's disease patients' feet seem stuck to the floor and they seem unable to move, try:

Sequence of instructions
1. Stand as straight as you can
2. Press your heels down on the floor
3. Lean back with the weight of your body over your heels
4. Now rock your body weight over (e.g.) your right foot
5. With your left foot, forward *step!*

Alternative strategies
- Patient marches on the spot, observer counts: 'one, two, three, four, forward *step!*'
- Patient slides one foot back, or steps back with it, in preparation to bring it forward briskly to step
- To keep themselves walking rhythmically, patients often count or sing

for more than 3–4 min leads to widespread damage and death to nerve cells

Although the *Health Survey for England 2001* recorded very little disability attributable to stroke in their sample, stroke care accounts for 4% of the total annual National Health Service budget. In the UK and other developed countries stroke is among the four most common causes of death, especially among people over 65 years of age (McGovern & Rudd 2003). Many people who survive experience severe disability with concomitant devastating impact on their family. Nevertheless, by the end of a year, with good team management, about half of those who survive can live independently and many continue to recover for several more years.

The NSFOP (standard 5) requires that all people with stroke are treated by a specialist stroke service. Evidence shows that stroke patients are best admitted to specialized hospital stroke units, i.e. a designated ward, run by a team of experienced nursing, rehabilitation and medical staff (McGovern & Rudd 2003). During the acute phase skilled nursing is essential. Without it patients may suffer considerable discomfort and complications may develop that seriously inhibit recovery of mobility. In the first 24 h after the initial damage, many patients will be unconscious or semiconscious. Subsequently the sufferers may have difficulty in moving and controlling their head, trunk and the limbs on one side of the body (hemiplegia). They may experience disturbances of speech, swallowing, skin sensation, vision, balance and mental function as well as impaired control of their bladder and bowels. Once the patient's medical condition has stabilized the next phase of recovery begins when the focus turns from survival to rehabilitation.

There has been controversy over the precise nature of the impairments arising from the neural lesions which interfere with motor performance. According to Carr & Shepherd (2003: Chapter 6) it is now generally recognized that these are: (1) paralysis and weakness, i.e. decreased muscle force, and (2) loss of the ability to carry out any motor task precisely, quickly, rationally and deftly, i.e. loss of coordination, also termed loss of dexterity. This term is used to encompass all skilled motor activity, not just hand movements.

At present, although research is underway, these impairments cannot be prevented. What can be prevented, to some extent, are the complications that arise when people are unable, or only partially able, to move their limbs voluntarily. During movement muscles are stretched, thereby maintaining their length. If they are not stretched they, and other soft tissues surrounding joints, contract and become stiff. Furthermore, muscles that are already weak because the lesion blocks descending commands become even weaker due to inactivity. Good nursing is essential in trying to prevent these maladaptations to disuse from developing.

For some time the difficulty with voluntary movement has been attributed to 'spasticity', a term which is probably often used inappropriately. Narrowly it means overactive stretch reflexes but it is often used interchangeably with 'hypertonus' or 'hypertonia'. These terms should be reserved to label increased resistance to passive movement, i.e. to stretching. These differences in nomenclature reflect underlying differences in neurophysiology but the properties may be less easily distinguishable in clinical practice.

In contrast to muscle stiffness, only a limited number of stroke patients develop spasticity. A feature of spasticity, when it does occur, and which can be particularly difficult to control, is clonus. It happens when a single quick movement, e.g. dorsiflexion of the foot, leads to rapidly alternating bursts of activity in the flexor and extensor muscles acting over the corresponding joint (Latash 1998). To stop clonus the responsible muscle group has to be subjected to sustained stretch. When it occurs at the ankle and the person is seated in a chair the trick is to get the foot flat on the floor and press down firmly on top of the bent knee to exert pressure directly down through the lower leg to the heel. Then maintain this stretch on the calf muscles until clonus subsides.

There does not appear be any evidence that spasticity is related to functional performance. In contrast, hypertonus may contribute significantly to functional limitation. Carr & Shepherd (2003: Chapter 6) and Latash (1998) discuss the issue of terminology and the research underpinning these arguments. In clinical practice carers need to focus on their goal of maintaining muscle length and joint flexibility regardless of the precise name given to the underlying phenomenon.

Immediately after a stroke, the muscles of the affected side may show decreased resistance to passive stretching, so that the limbs feel floppy. Subsequently, over days or weeks there is mounting resistance to stretch and muscle stiffness builds up. The extent to which these features develop depends not only upon the severity of neural damage but also on external influences. These include the person's posture in bed or in a chair and in particular, the overflow of tension into the affected limbs when the person feels uncomfortable and makes efforts to change position. So, not surprisingly, Wade (2000, 2002), in the *National Clinical Guidelines for Stroke*, emphasizes the importance of team work and the prevention of complications. Wade states that:

All staff should be trained to place patients in positions to reduce the risk of complications such as contractures, respiratory complications, shoulder pain and pressure sores (sections 4.2 and 8.3.1).

Contractures cause pain, restrict movement and impede recovery of function. It is essential therefore that patients who cannot change their position themselves are helped to do so regularly and that muscles and joints in weak limbs are placed in the optimal positions for regaining function. In addition, to ensure that muscles and soft tissues around joints in paralysed limbs maintain their length as much as possible, specialist physiotherapists assess the state of the limbs and if appropriate, move them carefully through their full range of movement regularly. Soft inflatable splints are also used to keep limbs in functional positions.

On the whole nurses and physiotherapists have reached agreement on the most advantageous functional positions for the trunk and limbs of the affected side while the person is sitting out in a chair or is lying horizontally in bed, usually on each side alternatively. Nevertheless some variation in practice remains. Carr & Kenney (1992) found agreement for:

- protraction of the shoulder when lying on the affected side
- alignment of the spine
- avoidance of external rotation of the hip
- extension of the fingers on the affected side
- avoidance of pressure against the soles of the feet.

There is less consensus regarding positioning of the unaffected limbs and whether the elbow of the affected side should be flexed or extended. It is useful to display diagrams of the recommended positions close to the patient's bed and chair so that relatives can also be involved in preventing complications. Chatterton et al. (2001), Rowat (2001) and Booth et al. (1996) examine these issues in detail. Usefully, Booth et al. give examples of positioning diagrams.

Routine position changes ensure patient comfort and are made safe and easy with correct handling systems and techniques. A point to remember is that physiotherapists have to deal with the consequences of poor positioning when pressure sores and contractures get in the way of functional retraining so they appreciate the benefits of good staff training in this skill.

Irwin (Booth et al. 1996) identifies the nurse's role in the acute phase of stroke as follows:

- to maintain hygiene, in particular the integrity of the skin, bowels and bladder
- to organize and coordinate care on a 24-h day-to-day basis
- to support, educate and counsel patients and their carers
- to promote continuation of therapy.

During the rehabilitation phase however, it may be that the contribution of nursing appears less focused. Always in line with clinical guidelines (Wade 2002), patients should be given as much opportunity to practise as possible and Irwin highlighted the importance of nurses in enabling patients to practise their exercises, thereby ensuring that therapy becomes a 24-h process rather than a sessional one with therapy staff. Especially in the early stages, nurses can control the physical environment of the ward. It should offer possibilities for intensive and meaningful exercise and social interaction and promote physical activity. Improvement in motor skill depends on the amount and type of practice the patient carries out (Carr & Shepherd 2003: Chapter 1).

From admission and throughout rehabilitation, nurses and all team members will be aware of the need for careful handling of the limbs on the affected side. Paralysed muscles are unable to react to protect themselves and surrounding soft tissue from being overstretched. It is essential, therefore, to avoid trauma to joints lacking such protection, especially the shoulder on the affected side. Many stroke patients suffer considerable pain and discomfort in this unstable joint so the arm should be moved with great care. In particular it is crucial that care staff avoid pulling the vulnerable arm. When the person is sitting up or standing upright the aim is to support the heavy limb and stop it dragging on the lax soft tissues around the joint. In sitting this is achieved by supporting the arm on a lapboard or pillow. Previously, strapping techniques and devices to approximate the joint were recommended but research has shown these to be of little benefit so the advice has been withdrawn (Wade 2000, 2002). The distress caused by painful shoulders and other joints inhibits people from cooperating in rehabilitation, as well as complicating nursing care.

The introduction and use of joint patient handling assessments, referred to earlier, facilitate good team work so that the person with a stroke is handled consistently. The care team aims to encourage the patient to utilize all currently available movement and balance ability in order to cooperate in moving and doing as much as possible independently. At the same time, to ensure confidence and safety, the person receives the agreed amount of physical support. As the law demands, handling assessments are jointly revised as often as indicated by the patient's rate of progress. For example, as a person regains ability, using the hoist for transfers from bed to chair can be replaced by using a turntable for a guided pivot transfer with one or two staff assisting as appropriate. Naturally, more experienced and therefore more confident staff will be able to make these progressions sooner than novices.

We are not suggesting that nurses should be required to give physiotherapy but we are emphasizing the value of consistent good handling. *The Guide 1997*, Chapter 18, makes the point that certain techniques, which may be acceptable when used by a specialized neurological physiotherapist, can become unsafe if attempted by a novice lacking specialist skills.

The role of the nurse in promoting safe mobility among stroke patients continues in the community when patients return to their own homes: enabling them to practise their functional tasks and ensuring they do not sit for long periods in a poor position and that vulnerable joints remain painfree through careful handling.

Hand, wrist and foot problems

Besides interfering with washing, dressing and other self-care activities, deformity of the hands can impede mobility in frail older people. The very old with postural instability and multiple pathology may need to support themselves by holding on to furniture or fixtures or by using a walking aid of some sort. If they are unable to use their hands, either to place them flat on a surface for support or to grip a rail or walking stick or frame, the ability to move may be impeded and disability exacerbated. Arthritic conditions such as rheumatoid arthritis can result in severe hand deformities but nevertheless sufferers often retain a surprising range of functional ability. Suitably adapted and specially shaped handles may be needed for walking aids and sticks as well as cutlery.

Contracture of the palmar fascia, Dupuytren's contracture, can leave individuals unable to grasp any sort of walking aid or to feed themselves independently. Some people have surgery to correct the contractures but the condition frequently goes unrecognized until the deformity is beyond correction. It causes permanent flexion of the metacarpal phalangeal joints and, eventually, of the wrist. It becomes impossible for people to stretch out their hands, to support themselves on furniture, to get their fingers around the hand grip on a walking aid, to grasp a banister rail, or to pull up underclothes. It can be very disabling when it occurs bilaterally.

Following a Colles fracture of the wrist, not only will the person be severely handicapped by having the forearm in plaster but, once it is off, will be left with restricted wrist movement and inability to take weight through that arm for several months until rehabilitation is complete. Similar problems usually arise after other fractures of the upper limb, all of which can restrict mobility if the person is dependent on using a walking aid. Various specially adapted alternatives may have to be considered, such as gutter crutches or frames.

Safe walking depends on safe footwear (see the section on clothing and footwear, below). If the person is unable to put on safe shoes the risk of falling increases and the ability to get about decreases. Swollen feet or pressure sores on the heels prevent people getting their shoes on. These are avoidable barriers to mobility. Painful, uncared-for feet with calluses, bunions and claw-like toenails commonly have the same effect. See Chapter 14 for more information on care of the foot.

Anxiety about falling and postural instability

The intrinsic barriers to mobility considered so far arise predominantly from physical impairments. Now we turn to a barrier arising from anxiety – a psychological impairment. When students are asked whether they are ever afraid of falling, they give answers such as: 'When I am drunk and wearing very high heels' or 'When I am on a narrow ridge high in the mountains with a gale blowing'. But most older people are familiar with this concept in daily life and either say that are not afraid of falling or admit to being concerned about hazards such as 'kids on bikes', 'catching my foot on a paving stone', or what the consequences could be, 'I might break a bone', or, especially if they live alone, 'I might not be able to get up again', 'who would help me?'

For many older people, taking measures to avoid falling can be an everyday activity (Simpson et al. 2003). They often talk about 'taking care', which may involve always holding on to something or always looking out for hazards on the ground. Some older people become so worried about falling that they lose their confidence in their ability to move about and do what they want to do. They may restrict their activities and social participation considerably, even to the extent of threatening their health (Case study 13.2). Thus anxiety about falling can be a barrier to mobility.

Case study 13.2

Mrs Y was very old and lived at home on her own. She did not go outside and could only walk short distances with her wheeled frame. She also became very afraid indeed of falling over. To reduce her risk of falling while getting up from her chair and walking to the lavatory she drank less and less so that she did not need to pass urine so often. She became very dehydrated and her urine became thick and dark.

It is related to feeling unsteady, being unsteady and fearing the consequences (Simpson et al. 1997, Simpson 2001). In turn postural instability, being unsteady, as indicated by taking more than five steps to turn through 180°, is itself an important risk factor for falling (Nevitt et al. 1989).

In the *Health Survey for England 2001*, non-fatal accidents are classed as major or minor (Malbutt & Falaschetti 2003). Major accidents are those severe enough for the person to consult a doctor or to receive hospital treatment afterwards. The survey collected data from a systematically drawn sample of community-dwelling adults aged over 65. Falls were found to be the most common major accident in this age group, although the percentage of the sample reporting a major fall in the last 6 months was low: men 2%, women 4%. The major fall rate increases with age in both men and women but is higher in women: at 85 years or older the rate reaches 7 per 100 in men and 17 per 100 in women. But many older people experience so-called minor falls. The usual figure given is that one in three people over 65 years old fall each year, but some people fall many times.

Lord et al. (2001: Chapter 1) report that about 50% of all falls among independently living older people occur during everyday activities in the home or nearby. In institutional settings, where the people are older and frailer, transferring positions seems to carry risk, both for the residents and for the staff who are helping, for example, getting in and out of bed, up or down from a chair or the toilet. Considering just major falls, however, the *Health Survey for England 2001* (Bajekal & Prescott 2003) found no difference between the community sample and a separate sample of older people in care homes, nor did it find any difference in the fracture rates between the two locations. But, when minor falls are also taken into account, several studies show that many more occur in care homes, and that people with old stroke or PD are particularly susceptible (Lord et al. 200: Chapter 1). Even though the overall rate of major falls may be low, their cost to health and social care services is very high in terms of admissions to hospitals and to care homes. The greatest cost, however, is the threat to older people's well-being.

The NSFOP recognizes the problem. Standard 6 states that action is to be taken 'to prevent falls and reduce resultant fractures or other injuries' and that 'older people who have fallen receive effective treatment and rehabilitation and, with their carers, receive advice on prevention through a specialised falls service'.

Furthermore, it acknowledges the detrimental effect that fear of falling can have on older people's well-being and lists 'being very afraid of falling' as an indicator to refer to the falls service. Together with physiotherapists and occupational therapists, nurses are usually key members of falls service teams.

Younger people's and fit older people's falls are usually the result of a single event such as a trip or a fit. But frail older people fall following the interaction of long-term and short-term predisposing factors and short-term precipitating factors in the environment, i.e. their falls are multifactorial in origin (Tinetti 2003). A person whose postural stability and mobility are already compromised by chronic disease or lack of fitness presents a background of long-term risk predisposing to loss of balance when additional short-term predisposing factors, such as an acute infection, and one or more situational factors further threaten balance and stability. Precipitating factors can be environmental, such as a wet, slippery floor, an item of furniture temporarily out of its usual place, or a sudden impulse to pick up a fallen object. Several prospective studies, summarized by a group of American and British experts (American Geriatrics Society, British Geriatrics Society, American Academy of Orthopaedic Surgeons Panel on Falls Prevention 2001) have identified risk factors for falling. Some of these factors are not amenable to intervention, such as being aged over 80 years or having a history of falls, but many of the rest can be grouped as threats to postural stability such as muscle weakness, gait deficit, balance deficit and impaired vision. Drugs are often implicated. Their action is probably due to the effect they have on postural stability, centrally sedating or blood-pressure-lowering medications in particular. People aged over 74 who have bladder problems at least once per week have higher fall rates than those without such problems, especially women (Malbutt & Falaschetti 2003). This is probably associated with hurrying to the lavatory. Diuretics may be implicated because they can make people, who may already be unsteady on their feet, feel an urgent need to void.

The onset of falling may indicate an underlying medical condition. Cotty (1999) gives guidance about when to refer an older person for medical examination. This will establish whether or not there is a medical explanation, perhaps cardiac, neurological or an infection, that can be addressed and maybe reduce the likelihood of more falls (see also Lord et al. 2001: Chapters 4 and 5). But people who turn out to have a medical explanation for their falls may still be afraid of falling and may need help to overcome it even after their problem has been resolved (Simpson & Hawke 1998).

Most adults are unaware that keeping one's balance requires little attention except, for example, negotiating an ice-covered steep slope. But some older people find just walking about so attention-demanding that they have to stop if they also want to talk to someone. Lundin-Olsson et al. (1997) found that those people who stopped walking regularly tended to have poor gait patterns and were more likely to fall over compared with those who could walk and talk at the same time. So, this and similar findings show that distraction can be a precipitating factor for falling. It is safer therefore to let some older people concentrate on one task at a time and to avoid distractions, especially while they are moving about.

Sadly the only 'treatment' offered to some frail, unsteady older people is to provide a walking frame and then teach the person how to manoeuvre it. This can be unwise. Inappropriately prescribed frames can lead to loss of balance confidence (Case study 13.3). The risk is that, once having started to hold on all the time, people may never again stand unsupported to test their balance mechanisms, which then deteriorate to the point they cannot let go any more (Simpson & Richardson 2002). Several times each day, people who use frames should practise standing unsupported, but with a sturdy support in front of them, should they feel unsteady.

In fact there is very good evidence, summarized by Tinetti (2003) and Lord et al. (2001: part 2), that the likelihood of falling can be reduced among older people. Multifactorial assessment followed by interventions to target the person's particular predisposing and precipitating risk factors is most likely to be effective. The first programme to reduce falls statistically significantly followed this model and involved nurses and physiotherapists (Koch et al. 1994, Tinetti et al. 1994). But addressing just the dominant risk factor, postural instability, by a programme of tailored progressive exercise is also successful in reducing falls (Robertson et al. 2002). The programme, supervised by a specialist physiotherapist, was followed by older people at home.

Gardner et al. (2001) describe it in detail. Furthermore, when nurses, who had been trained by a physiotherapist, delivered the programme, it was also very effective (Gardner et al. 2002).

Addressing environmental risk can also reduce falls. Cumming et al. (1999) showed that safety checks made by an experienced occupational therapist visiting people at home reduced their likelihood of falling. But the therapist also gave advice on safe behaviour in the home so the falls reduction may have been due to either intervention (Gill 1999). The potential danger posed by clothing and other garments is often overlooked, whether in hospital or at home. Ill-fitting slippers or down-at-heel shoes increase postural instability and should be discouraged; likewise trousers that are too long or likely to fall down and poorly fitting incontinence pads (Case study 13.4). Lord et al. (2001) devote a whole chapter (Chapter 10) to the role of footwear in falls prevention.

In line with the NSFOP, specialist services for people who have fallen or are afraid of doing so are being developed throughout the UK. These services address all aspects of the problem, starting with a multifactorial assessment which usually involves specialist nurses.

Practice guidelines have been developed (American Geriatric Society, British Geriatrics Society, American Academy of Orthopaedic Surgeons Panel on Falls Prevention 2001, Feder et al. 2000). When any underlying medical reasons have been addressed then rehabilitation guidelines are available (Simpson et al. 1998, NSFOP standard 6: Department of Health 2001).

Case study 13.3

Eighty-year-old Mrs B was independently mobile and enjoying life when she experienced sudden onset of falling. She reported this to her general practitioner who asked the community nurse to visit her. The nurse provided Mrs B with a walking frame. Some time later the falls were recognized as being caused by syncope associated with a cardiac problem. A pacemaker was inserted. In the meantime no one thought to 'wean' Mrs B off the walking frame, which she continued to use. A year later she admitted to a physiotherapist that she could no longer do without the frame as she had lost her confidence.

Case study 13.4

Mrs C was in an acute elderly-care unit recovering from a chest infection. She was getting used to walking again with her frame, which she needed because of her painful osteoarthritic knees. In the afternoon, her visitor was shocked to see Mrs C's face covered with bruises. Mrs C explained that the previous evening when she walked out of the lavatory into the corridor she had fallen down, got entangled in her walking frame and hit her face on the floor. Close questioning revealed that she had stooped down to pick up her incontinence pad which had suddenly, embarrassingly, dropped to the floor. It transpired that the ward had run out of the elastic mesh knickers that Mrs C should have been wearing and instead the assistant who had helped her had fitted her with a pair of ordinary, rather baggy knickers. The pad had been stuffed inside them.

The intervention that older people themselves may welcome most is the chance to talk about any anxiety they have about falling and concomitant loss of confidence in moving about and doing the things they want to do. In particular they may be concerned about how they would cope with a fall; we address this topic later in this chapter. Theoretically, people should become less anxious about falling and more confident in safe movement as they feel stronger, more posturally stable and confident that they could cope after a fall. Some support for this theory emerged from a study in which a subgroup of participants performed balance exercises and showed a significant improvement in balance confidence (Tinetti et al. 1994). But more research is needed in this area.

SETTING MOBILITY GOALS

In this and the following sections we consider assessment of the person's current mobility level compared with a premorbid level in order to set realistic mobility goals. We consider problems in relation to current moving and handling needs and how mobility goals are set in consultation with the patient, family and community care staff, and with other members of the team. We shall stress the patient's contribution to this process as, in the end, they must feel confident that they can do what they need to do without fear of losing their balance or falling (Simpson & Jones 2004). People preparing to be discharged from hospital may wish to regain confidence in walking to the toilet, negotiating stairs, or in making themselves a hot drink. People already at home may wish to become confident enough to go into the garden or to the shops.

Many older people, especially those over 75, present with more than one health problem. Following illness or surgery, together with even brief periods of enforced bedrest, they are in danger of becoming even less able to cope at home than they may have been prior to their current episode of care. Inexperienced doctors, nurses and rehabilitation staff can find it difficult to know where to start when planning management and eventual discharge. They are in danger of being distracted by the numerous diagnoses people may have collected, some long-standing, rather than focusing in the first place on pinpointing the patient's functional needs: these are the activities an older person or the person's carer identifies as being those which she or he needs to be able to perform with confidence in order to be ready for discharge from care.

These needs vary, depending not only on the person's physical abilities but also on the amount of carer support or social service support available. Therefore the discharge mobility goal should be that, given whatever support is on offer, the person feels confident that he or she will be able to cope at home, wherever that is. Often a goal may be that the patient or the patient plus carer feel confident in getting to and using the lavatory or going up and down stairs or getting in and out of bed.

Once the main functional limitation to be addressed has been agreed, the underlying impairment is identified. Only by treating at the impairment level can a mobility problem be resolved by alleviating the cause of the disability rather than by compensating for it. Take, for example, the limitation of being unable to rise from the toilet without carer assistance. If the underlying impairment is weakness in the extensor muscles of knees and hips, the problem may be resolved by increasing the power in these muscles by progressive resistance exercise, which matches the movement required. If this strategy proves only partially successful, then installing a higher toilet seat compensates for the remaining weakness.

How much could the person do recently?

For mobility goals to be set all members of the team need an accurate mental picture of each person's home surroundings and usual daily routine. Initially, nurses and medical staff gather at least some of this information during the admission procedure: whether the person lives in a house or flat, has to negotiate steps and receives social service support. Nurses' contribution to gathering this information is crucial. Not only do they assess patients very soon after admission but they are most likely to see visiting relatives and neighbours. These people are valuable sources of detailed information about the patient's home circumstances, especially when the patient, because of illness or mental state, is unable to supply it. Similarly, home care assistants or other professionals who can be contacted by telephone can describe the person's usual daily surroundings and level of ability. Further details are added by other staff who may need to be clear about a particular set of circumstances. Occupational therapists, for example, often conduct a 24-h interview in which they carefully lead people through an account of their daily activities. Starting with 'tell me how you get out of bed in the morning', and moving on to personal hygiene, preparing breakfast and so on, they listen for details of activities that present difficulties or have been solved, prompting sensitively to elicit more detail as necessary. They aim to build up a picture of the person's usual daily routine and the points at which occupational therapy interventions seem indicated. Key points from this information are shared with nurses and the rest of the team so that problems may be tackled jointly while the person is still in care.

If team-working is not well established, with clear routines and well-planned documentation, patients and/or their relatives may become irritated by finding themselves questioned repeatedly about their home circumstances by various professionals: nurse, doctor, occupational therapist, physiotherapist, social worker.

Apart from recording any diagnosis as a clue to the type of care the patient will require, a useful question to ask is: 'Why has the person become a patient?' If he or she was middle-aged rather than older, would the person have been admitted for the same problem? If the answer is no, a younger person would have been looked after at home, then a clue to the care problem is revealed. Either there is no one at home to care for the person who was managing well enough previously, or the person has become too difficult for the carer to manage. Old people's carers are often quite old themselves. Sometimes 'not coping at home', or the rather insulting term 'acopia' may be given as a diagnosis by someone who has not taken the trouble to find out why the person has lost the ability to manage. In these circumstances careful questioning reveals whether difficulties have extended to many functions or, as is often the case when a carer is involved, to one main problem. The carer may have been managing quite awkward transfers using appropriate handling aids but, due to deterioration in the patient's condition, these manoeuvres are no longer possible (Case study 13.5).

Only a minority of patients are admitted to hospital or nursed at home for problems that pose a dramatic threat to their mobility status. Such threats arise from stroke, lower-limb fracture, amputation or sudden severe deterioration in a chronic condition. Most patients, however, are suffering infections or other acute illnesses that, once resolved, should allow them to regain previous levels of mobility. But, as we have noted above, a period of bedrest associated with an acute medical problem or surgical intervention can result in older people feeling weak and lacking energy. Patients often express the need to 'test' themselves before they can feel confident in managing at home. By this they mean finding out if they can still do the things for themselves that they were able to do prior to the current episode.

In these circumstances the long-term mobility goal is that people return to their premorbid levels of mobility, which they should be able to regain given the opportunity and encouragement as well as attention that no intrinsic barriers to mobility are allowed to develop (e.g. contractures, pressure sores, swollen feet) and that no extrinsic, environmental barriers to safe mobility are in place (e.g. unsafe clothing and footwear, chairs from which egress is difficult). Good team work ensures that sufficient opportunities to practise moving about safely, to regain mobility and confidence, are built into the patient's day as soon as he or she is well enough to cooperate.

Ideally, however, the opportunity should be grasped to help people recover the physical fitness they had before the acute episode in order to increase margins of safe functional mobility. In old age even healthy people's maximum oxygen uptake has declined to the extent that energy expenditure on a functional task may be double that in earlier years. As Harridge & Young (2000) point out, this brings them perilously close to the point where even a small further decline in aerobic power, as might follow a period in bed, may render some essential daily activities, such as rising from a toilet seat, extremely stressful to perform. Thus a discharge mobility goal should be that the person can walk more than the required distance, climb more than the necessary number of steps, get up from the toilet and in and out of bed with ease given the adaptations and help deemed necessary.

How much can the person do now?

Among older people, as among younger people with temporary or long-standing mobility problems, assessing present mobility status is combined with assessing the amount of physical help they need to be able to move. During the process information from the person or carer is augmented by direct observation of what the patient can do, or is willing to do. Managers must ensure that nurses acting as assessors are trained in risk assessment and able to identify all aspects of the problem and to record all relevant details.

After recording the history of the present condition, and social and home circumstances, the person's ability to perform essential functional, physical tasks is observed to identify current mobility problems, while at the same time decisions can be reached about the

---

Case study 13.5

Mrs D was short, while her husband, Mr D, was very large. Although he had suffered a stroke several years ago, Mrs D had been managing to transfer Mr D on and off the toilet quite satisfactorily with the help of a transfer belt. But he had to be admitted to an elderly care ward because he suffered an acute infection which left him unable to muster the small effort he contributed to the success of the transfer, thus leaving Mrs D unable to help him. Until he had recovered from the illness and been retrained in toilet transfers so that Mrs D could cope again, he could not return home.

best way to solve them. Also, short-term goals must be set around safe ways of handling people in their present state of health, but ones that can be reset progressively as people regain muscle strength and joint flexibility. This process may be guided by a checklist of tasks which ensures nothing is forgotten. An example is given in Box 13.2.

Assessment is most economical and successful when the person's nurse works together with the physiotherapist or occupational therapist. In this way all rehabilitation staff learn how much an older person can do and the way to do it. By observing and analysing the separate components of the activity (e.g. getting out of bed) and listening to the patient's views, they can establish which element is preventing the total, combined effort from being successful and agree the best way to solve the problem now and plan steps to resolve it further in the future. For example, a female patient wants to get out of bed and use the commode rather than continue using the bedpan. The assessors (i.e. nurse and physiotherapist or occupational therapist) will want to find out how much of each stage in the manoeuvre she can perform herself:

- Can she raise herself from lying (or half-lying) to unsupported sitting?
- Can she progress to bringing her legs over the edge of the bed and manoeuvre her upper body around?
- What height must the bed be at for her to be able to put her feet on the floor prior to standing?
- How should the commode be placed strategically so that she can utilize the arm rest to support some body weight during the standing phase?

Box 13.2   Checklist of tasks for patient handling assessment

Patient care plan – moving and handling section
Can the patient manage the following mobility tasks completely independently, not even requiring verbal prompts?
- Sitting/standing   yes/no
- Walking   yes/no
- Toileting   yes/no
- Bathing   yes/no
- Transfer to/from bed   yes/no
- Movement in bed up/down   yes/no
- Rolling and turning in bed   yes/no

If the answer to any question is 'no' then the details of how the problem is solved are recorded in the patient handling section of the care plan.

- Can she turn her body safely to position herself accurately ready for sitting down?
- Will she need help to adjust her clothing?

The crucial components therefore are the ability to:

- sit unsupported
- use arms to support body weight
- weight-bear through the legs
- turn the body in preparation for sitting
- lower the body on to the seat.

It follows that this sequence must be performed in reverse order when getting into bed. A deficit in just one component or more of this sequence means she will need help. Before proceeding with the next step at any stage of the manoeuvre, the assessors must quantify the extent to which her ability is compromised and judge the amount of help to be given. If they do not, the patient could collapse on the floor, injuring both parties. Nurses who have been trained and are competent in using handling aids know how to select the appropriate device to overcome the problem posed by the missing component or know how to give assistance without undue strain on themselves.

We all become slower at processing information as we grow older (see Chapter 4); therefore, even if the person does not have overt dementia, it helps assessment to keep language clear and simple and enhance requests with appropriate gestures and avoidance of confusion-inducing terms. 'Bend in the middle' is probably meaningless to someone without any concept of where the 'middle' of the body is. Moreover, difficult movements, especially ones that require balance maintenance or that generate pain, are attention-demanding. It is best to concentrate on the task in hand and avoid anything that diverts attention (see the section on anxiety about falling and postural instability, above).

When older people are confused because of acute infections, after anaesthetic or because they have dementia, even greater care is required when encouraging functional movement during day-to-day care. Eye contact, a look of friendly expectancy and simple, unambiguous requests to move, augmented by visual cues and clear gestures, are most likely to elicit a response. (For further information on communication methods, see Chapter 10.) For example, smacking the seat of a chair to attract a person's attention reinforces the request to 'please sit down here'; tapping the hips of a person practising chair-to-chair transfers indicates the direction of the turn which the hips must make (Oddy 1998). *The Guide* 1997, Chapter 18 has advice for handling patients who are reluctant to cooperate or who may be aggressive.

Checklists may act as memory aids during the handling assessment but the outcome is recorded in the moving and handling section of the patient care plan. This information forewarns other team members of the tasks that the person cannot perform independently. It then informs the team members how to assist that person, and which handling devices to use, thereby reducing the risk of injury to themselves. In *The Guide* 2005, Chapters 11 to 17 focus on risk assessment and giving a summary of the scientific evidence for managing functional tasks e.g. lying-to-sitting, sitting-to-standing, assisted walking, dealing with falling and a fallen person. The help required with a task might be recorded as follows:

- getting in and out of the bath – needs bathing hoist or needs bath with bathing seat
- walking from chair to toilet – needs one assistant using a handling belt.

A rating or coded system may be used and an example is given in Box 13.3.

Using this code, a patient at home requiring help from the community nurse may score 3˙C which indicates the level of help required in relation to the circumstances and the skills of the nurse. Using such a system depends on all assessors and those using the assessment being fully conversant with the rules for assigning and interpreting codes; otherwise it will not yield reliable information. This issue is discussed further in the section below on using standardized assessment tests and tools.

USING PATIENT HANDLING SYSTEMS AND PROMOTING INDEPENDENCE

Given the array of patient handling systems, it is now unnecessary to lift all or part of a patient's weight. As noted earlier in the chapter, the law puts the onus on the handler to utilize, as appropriate, all the patient handling devices that have been designed and are available for use. It also places a vicarious responsibility on health care providers to ensure that staff are trained to a sufficiently high level of expertise to assess, prescribe and use any appropriate pieces of equipment. The necessary moving and handing techniques must be perfected, in the first instance, in the classroom and not on patients. It is a very serious misconception that such equipment can be used without any or only minimal previous experience. Some of the most commonly used systems are described in Box 13.4 and information about the whole range of patient handling devices can be obtained from disabled living centres throughout the UK. Addresses can be found in *The Guide* (National Back Pain Association, Royal College of Nursing 1997).

Assessing an older person's current moving and handling needs at the beginning of an episode of care is not the end of this process. Reassessment may indicate that the person is ready to cope with less physical support or to use a small handling aid with less help. For example, the person may be keen and ready to learn to

---

Box 13.3   A patient handling assessment using codes

Patient's ability rating
- – Independent
- 1 Needs minimal assistance/supervision
- 2 Cooperative but needs assistance for several tasks
- 3 Limited ability to assist during most tasks
- 4 Limited ability + unpredictable/uncooperative behaviour
- 5 Conscious but totally unable to assist
- 7 Unconscious/totally dependent

Environment rating
- *   No attachments but limited space/non-adjustable bed
- **   Constraints present, e.g. catheter/oxygen/intravenous infusion/cardiac leads/other (please state)
- *** Multiple attachments/severely restricted space

Handling task rating
- – No assistance required
- A Moves under supervision + walking aid
- B Needs support when walking or transferring
- C Manual handling technique required to move in bed/light assistance
- D Manual handling technique + handling aids + two (or more) nurses
- E Hoist required for transfers/bed manoeuvres/bathing

Box 13.4 Patient handling systems

Sliding sheets
These are very-low-friction sheets, two flat ones or one roller type, that are placed directly under the patient, or under the bed sheet. The sheet can then be used as a means of moving the patient in whichever direction is desired. This technique is particularly useful for highly dependent patients or people who are unable to sit up and must be nursed flat, prone or on alternate sides. Sliding sheets are used to:

- assist patients to sit up
- move patients up or down the bed
- move patients across the bed
- sit patients further up the bed
- rotate patients in bed or towards the edge of the bed
- move patients out of bed into a chair
- transfer patients across on to the toilet or commode
- transfer patients from bed to bed or trolley or couch
- transfer patients from a wheelchair into a car.

In some situations a 'bridging' device may also be necessary, such as a transfer board (straight or angled) or full-length Pat Slide in order to bridge gaps between surfaces.

Not only do sliding sheets eliminate all previous lifting techniques but they have the added bonus of permitting transfer and rotation of the patient's body weight without the risk of friction shear and tear on the skin. However, they should:

- never be used if patients can perform the task themselves
- only be used in accordance with the manufacturer's instructions
- only be used after training and practice as they can be dangerous if overenthusiastic force is applied.

Transfer boards
These devices (often used in conjunction with sliding sheets) facilitate easy assisted or independent seated transfers, especially bed to chair, or chair to toilet. Several designs are available, either straight or curved (which allows transfers even if the chair or commode has a fixed arm rest). Boards should be light, very smooth and made of a material that is strong and durable.

Handling belts
Using a handling belt allows the handler to support a patient without actually having to 'grasp' the person or his or her clothing. Patients are therefore free to use their arms to assist or use a walking aid. Soft, wide handling belts are particularly useful to assist patients with poor sitting or standing balance. The extra support can be used to assist control in positioning in a chair, getting up or down and walking short distances. The belt must always be firmly fastened and grasped by the handler.

Turntables/turning discs
Two types are available, soft or rigid, depending on the application. For use on the floor, the rigid type can be used to assist patients who cannot lift their feet to transfer, i.e. stroke patients or those suffering from PD. The soft disc is used for seat transfers, i.e. when a patient needs to swivel the lower body in a car seat or on to a bed.

Handling blocks
These are designed for patients to use themselves. By raising the elbow angle, patients with reasonable upper-body but poor lower-body strength (or unilateral impairment) can move themselves in and around the bed, or use them on the floor in the event of a fall. They are especially useful for patients learning to cope with a lower-limb amputation, or during stroke recovery or any disability preventing the use of the lower body.

Jacob's ladder or pull-strap
This is a self-help device. Patients pull themselves up from lying to sitting. It is attached to the foot of the bed and must extend far enough for the patient to grasp the rungs to bring the upper body forwards. Older people often have weak abdominal muscles but surprisingly strong arm strength. It helps individuals to move forward independently to reach the over-bed table or reposition themselves comfortably in the bed, so they do not need to call a nurse for assistance.

use a sliding sheet or transfer board independently. Already, as this skill is mastered, patients may be planning ahead to becoming independent in manoeuvres that, until then, they believed they would always need help to complete. Eventually, for example, it may be possible to transfer from bed to chair, chair to toilet and back, or wheelchair to car seat with surprising ease.

When people are going to need assistance at home, then carers should have the chance to learn how to use such devices well before discharge. It is essential that all agencies involved with future care are consulted, and any equipment needed at home is in place and checked before the person returns.

Using standardized assessment tests and tools

Standard 2 of the NSFOP requires the National Health Service and social care services to develop a single assessment process for older people in order to avoid overlap and duplication. Mobility is to be assessed as part of personal care and physical well-being. This can be done by practical performance tests, by an observer's report or by self-report. Whichever method is used care must be taken that accurate ratings and scores are assigned. A standardized measure is one that has been carefully developed to achieve this.

Standardization implies that, for a given measuring instrument, such as a functional assessment scale or a performance test, there is a recommended procedure for it to be administered and scored. The term also implies that, when these recommendations are followed, the scores are consistent. This means that when the same person administers the same test or procedure to the same patient, or patient and carer, under the same circumstances but over a brief interval, the results will be the same. Similarly, different observers scoring the test at the same time should get results which are the same or very close.

Patient handling assessment records can, under certain circumstances, be used to monitor change over time. By repeating the assessment regularly and by using a numerical scoring system, for example using higher numbers to indicate more of a problem (i.e. higher levels of dependency), changes in people's ability over time towards or away from independence can be monitored easily. To be used in this way, however, complete and unambiguous criteria for the assignment of scores must be available and the extent to which different observers assign the same score to the same activities should be examined and any ambiguities ironed out.

A scheme for recording the amount of help people need, not only for getting about but for all key activities of daily living, is the modified Barthel index (Collin et al. 1988). It has been recommended for routine use with older patients in community settings (Ross & Bower 1995) and is used frequently as a measure of outcome in research. However, it is important to note that scoring of the item relating to transfers, e.g. bed to chair, now contravenes the moving and handling regulations. It describes the situation where a patient has no sitting balance and requires 'two people to lift or use a hoist'. However, the law is clear. No two nurses should ever take the weight of a person weighing more than 50 kg (*The Guide* 1997: p. 16). In fact, two people should always be present when a hoist is used. There is considerable overlap between the transfer items of the Barthel index and the corresponding items on a handling assessment. But the latter emphasizes patient and staff safety rather than patient dependency. We suggest that staff focus on completing a detailed moving and handling assessment and regularly reassess to monitor progress.

The are many standardized assessments of mobility designed for use with older people or for people with specific pathology such as stroke patients (Wade 1992, Lennon 1995). Whereas most of the procedures familiar to nurses require ratings to be made, there are several performance tests familiar to physiotherapists and occupational therapists that measure physical ability directly. A quick, standardized test of balance while moving is TURN180 (Simpson et al. 2002, Fitzpatrick et al. 2005). The score is the number of steps taken to complete a 180° turn, which indicates whether they are at risk of falling. Also it can be used in people's homes as well as in health centres.

Aids to mobility

Appropriate walking aids allow people to walk further in safety than they can without them, and thereby considerably improve their quality of life. But inappropriate use of aids may prolong dependency and reduce balance ability (Simpson & Richardson 2002). The aids to mobility most commonly used by older people are walking sticks and walking frames, wheeled or unwheeled. The most common aid to stability is the grab bar.

Reasons for the use of walking aids are:

- to take weight off a lower limb that is still healing and might be damaged, e.g. after a fracture or joint replacement
- to take weight off a painful joint, e.g. osteoarthritis
- to provide support when a person feels at risk of losing balance

- to signal to others that users have a problem, i.e. avoid jostling the user and allow them time, e.g. to get on or off a bus
- any combination of the above.

The height of the hand grip from the ground of both sticks and frames is adjusted to match the height of the person's wrist crease from the ground with the arm hanging straight by the side of the body, but with the elbow very slightly bent. Wooden sticks are sawn to the correct length; metal ones and frames have adjustable legs. All metal adjustable walking aids must be inspected regularly to ensure that pressure is not distorting the holes, making the device unsafe. Ferrules on all walking aids need regular checking and replacement before they become dangerously worn.

Choice of walking aid has tended to be unsystematic but clearly has to relate to the environment in which the aid is to be used and the reason for needing one in the first place. Holliday & Fernie (1995) suggest the model with two wheels at the front is probably most suitable for posturally unstable elders. It allows a more normal walking pattern. The disadvantage of non-wheeled walkers is that they break up the natural rhythm of walking as they have to be picked up in advance; this action also creates a moment of instability when the person is not being supported by the device. However, one of the greatest problems with any very supportive device such as a walking frame is that older people become too attached to them (Simpson & Richardson 2002). A very simple test of standing balance is described below.

Promoting balance skills and confidence

A person may have enough physical ability in terms of motor control, joint flexibility and muscle strength to perform a task independently but, lacking confidence, may be unwilling to try. A fit young person may be wary of walking across a narrow mountain ridge; an older person may be equally wary of walking across a room without having something to hold on to.

Being able to stand confidently without holding on, let alone walk, is a prerequisite for most functional activities, but many frail older people are reluctant to let go. Among 52 people consecutively admitted to an acute older people's care unit (mean age 83 years, SD 6.4, 61% women), only 29 (56%) could stand up without holding on to the table in front of them for 3 min or longer. None of the remaining 23 (44%) could stand steadily without holding on for more than 40 s (Simpson et al. 1996). Without the table in front of them, more would have given up sooner.

People who are reluctant to discard their walking frames are in danger of their balance reactions deteriorating and of entering a cycle of loss of confidence, loss of balance skill and further loss of confidence. To reduce this risk, team members should encourage older people, particularly those who depend on a walking frame, to practise balance exercise regularly. People who are worried or afraid of falling are much more likely to cooperate if they see that there is something nearby that they can hold on to. Box 13.5 contains some suggestions.

Just as people are more likely to risk letting go of the support as long as it remains within reach, so they are more likely to agree to walk independently, apart from any walking aid, if a seat is clearly in view at an agreed distance. The distance is gradually increased, by agreement, as the person gains confidence, until it matches the distances the person needs to manage before discharge (see above, under Setting mobility goals).

When the person is out of practice, the initial distance may be negligible, perhaps just a transfer between two chairs, maybe with a sliding board and some sturdy support to hold on to. Team members provide as many opportunities for practice as possible to ensure steady progress. A well-defined rehabilitation task is one that, once it has been set up, e.g. sturdy furniture arranged as supports, the person is able to perform with confidence and without close supervision. But the task should also be sufficiently taxing to bring about strength and balance gains.

Other people's behaviour can either facilitate older people's confidence and mobility or hinder it. The person in hospital who is soon to return home may be encouraged to walk about the ward when confident to

---

Box 13.5   Simple balance-retraining exercises

Standing at the sink or other firm support, with a sturdy chair behind ready to sit in:
- Let go with one hand
- Let go with both hands
- Stand unsupported

Goal: to stand steadily unsupported for at least 60 s and preferably for 3 min

Progression while standing:
- Turn head from side to side
- Arrange flowers in a vase without leaning against the table
- Stand further away from the support
- Fix trousers or skirt with both hands after using the toilet
- Walk around a table without holding on to it

do so safely and independently. Encouragement may have to be quite positive as many older people in hospital feel obliged to sit still by their beds and it is all too easy for staff to tell them to sit down when they could easily be more active. Suggestions about places to go (to see the television in the day room) or people to visit ('the lady in the next room who went to the same school as you') can 'give permission' to walk about or just 'do feel free to walk about the ward' may be enough. However, people at home rarely have to manage the long distances presented by many hospital wards, which may be very tiring if walking is still a struggle. So, to promote confidence and encourage walking, chairs are placed about wards, where space permits, so that rehabilitation patients can always keep a seat-goal in view.

Elderly-care medical wards, which tend to be geared toward rehabilitation, are at an advantage in this respect compared with general medical wards, where patients who are not yet fully confident in their own balance may be inhibited from walking because 'there are so many people and trolleys rushing about, I might get knocked over'. Moreover, people admitted to elderly-care rehabilitation units are usually encouraged to wear their own clothes. This is rarely the case in general medical wards. Not only is normal clothing more dignified but probably it makes a positive contribution to rehabilitation and to promoting mobility.

Older people who are recovering from an acute episode such as an operation or infection, whether in general medical wards or elderly-care units, often express a need to 'test' themselves. By this they mean reassuring themselves that they are still capable of the tasks they were able to carry out safely prior to admission. As soon as the acute episode is under control they should be able to do this by deciding, with their nurse, on an achievable goal and then having the chance to reach it.

Coping with a fall

One of the four goals addressed in the guidelines for the collaborative rehabilitative management of older people who have fallen (Simpson et al. 1998) is that older people learn to cope with a fall and to prevent a 'long lie' and its possible consequences. The other aspect of this problem is how nurses cope should a person fall in hospital, nursing home or at home during one of the nurse's domiciliary visits.

After a fall in hospital or in a care-home, older people must have an opportunity to recount what happened after any previous fall, especially how they managed afterwards, and then to discuss how they will cope after the next fall. It can be very reassuring for

them to learn that, although falls are common in old age, only a few result in serious injuries (see above under Anxiety about falling and postural instability). The aim is to ensure that people are equipped with strategies for summoning help should they fall again, and that they know how to avoid the complications of spending a long time on the floor waiting for help to arrive. No older faller should be discharged from hospital or community care without this problem having been sorted out. Whether the person's primary nurse, physiotherapist, occupational therapist or a trained volunteer takes responsibility is a matter for local negotiation but someone, or maybe two people, must develop the expertise and knowledge to take on this task.

Physiotherapists have techniques for training people in how to get up from the floor (Reece & Simpson 1996). If this is not feasible then people should practise moving about the floor to reach an alarm cord or a telephone that has been placed on a low table where it is accessible from the floor. They should also have to hand the telephone numbers of people willing to come in to help them. However, lifting someone up from the floor is not an easy task and moving and handling regulations must be heeded. Some people contact the ambulance service.

On being asked about the dangers of spending a long time on the floor, most older people answer 'hypothermia'. Few of them will think of thirst and dehydration, pressure sores or even about the difficulty of passing urine with dignity. Encouraging people to work out their own solutions to these problems, especially if they are participating in small discussion groups, can be extremely rewarding:

- What can be used to keep warm and where can it be kept so that it is also accessible from the floor?
- Where can drinks be kept so that they can be reached from the floor?
- How can you pass urine without spoiling the carpet if you are sitting on the floor (see Case study 13.6)?

The team should build up a store of tips and anecdotes to help people develop strategies for coping. Of course, many people will have or will acquire alarm buttons. Nevertheless, discussing strategies for survival on the floor helps to foster a sense of control and self-efficacy and may reduce worries and fears about falling. Safety groups, often run by occupational therapists and nurses, discuss these matters and ways of improving safety at home in order to avoid trips and promote hazard-free mobility.

Immediately after a fall, it is advisable for the nurse and other professionals to avoid fanning panic in the

Case study 13.6

In a safety group Mrs P talked with pride about how she had coped after her last fall. She knew her daughter would be visiting within the next couple of hours so she did not exhaust herself trying to heave herself up from the floor. She made herself comfortable and waited. Soon, however she needed to pass urine. She was proud of her neat, clean flat and did not want to spoil her carpet. She worked out what to do. She shuffled on her bottom into the bathroom and pulled her bath-towel down from the rail. She pulled her underpants down, rolled the towel into a 'sausage' and pushed it high up between her legs. She passed urine on to it, without a drop finding its way on to the carpet. Then she threw the damp towel into the bath.

Hearing this, Mrs W said that she had used a similar method. In her house, the bathroom and towels were upstairs so when she found herself on the floor downstairs and wanted to pass urine, she pulled her oldest cushion off its chair and used it in the same way.

faller and any carers, so a calm authoritative manner should be adopted. All too often well-meaning carers fail to recognize the floor as the safest place to be and attempt to get the person off the floor as quickly as possible, with little regard as to how this may be achieved in safety. Once it is established that no injury has been sustained, the person should be given pillows and otherwise made comfortable and kept warm while the next move is planned.

In due course the person may be able to get up or into a chair if given clear and confident instructions and possibly a little physical assistance, especially if the individual has had prior training in the technique or has coped successfully with a fall in the past. Reece & Simpson (1996) set out the usual steps followed in getting up. If a person falls frequently and has a carer at home, an inflatable lifting cushion may be kept to hand. In care settings a hoist or lifting cushion must be used if the person cannot make a substantial contribution to the manoeuvre. No attempt should be made to raise the greater part of the patient's weight, especially from a low level, as the likelihood of injury is very high. The problem is also discussed in depth in *The Guide* 1997, Chapter 20 and *The Guide* 2005 Chapter 17.

REMOVING EXTRINSIC BARRIERS TO MOBILITY

Clothing and footwear

In contrast to the intrinsic barriers to mobility considered so far, extrinsic barriers are aspects of the environment immediately surrounding people, as well as more distant from them, that limit or hinder their ability to move about and exercise choices. During domiciliary visits community nurses and health visitors are alert to the extrinsic barriers presented by furniture arrangements or unsuitable clothing. In the hospital nurses are similarly alert to barriers to patients' mobility and act to reduce their effect to a minimum, often working with the team occupational therapist or physiotherapist.

Safe walking is commonly hindered by unsuitable footwear, especially ill-fitting slippers (Lord et al. 2001: Chapter 10). All rehabilitation-conscious staff are alert to this problem. If possible, people who are being admitted to hospital are encouraged to bring with them their usual footwear, comfortable shoes and well-fitting slippers. Otherwise relatives and friends are asked to bring them in before patients recover from an acute episode or start their rehabilitation programme. Sometimes elderly-care units have stocks of footwear to lend to patients, or run a scheme that allows then to buy suitable slippers while still in hospital. Having personal footwear is particularly important when the person has been using an orthopaedic shoe or appliance, perhaps to compensate for difference in leg length or a deformed foot. Older people may still be using, and be quite content with, 'old-fashioned' models of bespoke shoes or appliances supplied when they were much younger, even seemingly ancient artificial limbs. Needless to say, without these items restoration of mobility will be seriously impeded. Every effort has to be made to have them brought into hospital (Case study 13.7).

Furthermore, although it seems obvious, it is necessary to remind students and assistants to ensure that people are not wearing dangerous clothes. Not only may unsteady people be tripped up by long trousers, or loose skirts that threaten to fall down, but awareness of this danger inhibits their walking. Similarly, incontinence pads that are not held firmly in place by the correct type of pants are very uncomfortable and restrict safe walking, and gowns that flap open at the back, risking loss of dignity, are not conducive to confident mobility.

Chairs and rising from sitting

The key ability with respect to mobility, at least in western societies, is the ability to transfer from sitting to standing. Wheelchairs may compensate for inability to walk. Unsuitable seating, therefore, is a major barrier to mobility among older people, especially for those already burdened with intrinsic mobility impairments. The wide range of human shapes and sizes

---

Case study 13.7

Mrs R had been admitted as an emergency to an acute medical ward and had not brought in any of her usual clothes or footwear. Once recovered, the rehabilitation team were puzzled at the difficulty she had trying to walk. On examination it was found that her right ankle dorsiflexion was very limited. On careful questioning Mrs R recalled that as a young girl she had jumped off a fence and that her foot had never been quite right after that. Increasingly, she had found that she could only walk in shoes with a fairly high heel. Mrs R, who was from a modest background, had probably ruptured her Achilles tendon, but in her youth, before the National Health Service was founded, one did not go to the doctor other than in life-threatening situations. She had become so adapted to the problem that it had not occurred to her to point out to the staff that, in order to be able to walk, she needed her usual shoes.

---

further complicates the issue. An adjustable-height chair is the obvious solution, but these are rarely to be found in hospitals. However, providing a variety of chairs allows the right chair to be selected for the right user, although this is usually an approximation or compromise.

Here we concentrate on rising from a seat rather than on comfort while sitting. Chapter 15 of *The Guide* 1997 and Chapter 12 of *The Guide* 2005 examine this critical issue in detail. But, as a great deal of time may be spent in sitting, a contradiction arises: higher seats allow easier egress, and lower seats are more comfortable for prolonged sitting. But fixed flexion deformities of the hips and knees, which make nursing very difficult, are often the result of prolonged sitting in a low chair.

Most chairs are too low for older people who need assistance, but for an independent user of very small stature, a lower chair may be ideal. A raised chair seat will be more comfortable, as well as facilitating early ambulation for people with hip problems or in the early stages following hip surgery when flexion is definitely contraindicated.

Besides chair height, other features, such as seat depth and slope, back angle or rake, are important for easy egress. Most tall people have long legs, so the seat depth must be adequate to support the thigh length but will require the patient to lean much further forward to get up from the chair. This sort of problem may be reduced by inserting a wedge-shaped cushion with the thin edge of the wedge to the front; the forward slope makes rising easier, although it may not be tolerated for prolonged sitting. Conversely, a seat that

slopes back is comfortable but makes egress much more difficult. The height, slope and forward projection of chair arms can facilitate or hinder ease of egress or safe sitting-down. People with limited wrist extension may prefer a chair arm which is rounded toward the front. Once a person has got the hips to the front of the seat, standing up comprises three overlapping phases: trunk flexion, hip and knee extension and trunk extension. It is important to encourage the person to concentrate on pushing the knees straight before starting to lift the head and extend the back – 'push your knees straight', 'keep your head down'. This is to prevent the individual tipping backwards.

Given that the hips are to the front of the seat, the usual chair drill follows this routine:

1. feet apart and back, close to or under the chair
2. hands on the arms of the chair
3. 'lean forward' or 'get your nose over your knees'
4. (if applicable) encourage rocking forward and backward to give momentum to the movement
5. 'push up to standing'.

Usually the person is discouraged from holding the walking frame or stick until upright. The critical manoeuvre in sitting down is that people do not start to turn around to get their back to the chair while still at some distance from the chair (or lavatory). Once close enough, they must turn right round in order to ensure they will land on the seat and not on the chair arm. Older people should not be expected to walk so far before sitting down that they get exhausted. Then they are at risk of rushing and missing the seat.

Besides paying attention to the design of the actual seat, standing up may be easier if people feel confident that their feet will not slide forwards. This may happen if they are not far enough forward in the chair or if they cannot get their feet back far enough because, for example, of stiff knees. Feelings of insecurity are exacerbated if the soles of the shoes are very slippery. Sometimes carers wedge the person's feet with their own. This is not advised as it can be very uncomfortable for the older person. However, a 30-cm square of non-slip material placed under the feet will help to overcome this problem. Suitable material can be found in carpet shops and is easily carried in a pocket. It is helpful if several pieces are available in wards and rehabilitation areas.

Immediate surroundings and ergonomic assessment

Assessment of the ergonomic implications of any handling situation is largely a matter of careful observation to make sure that what has to be done can be done in the safest and least stressful way for all concerned.

Problems can often be solved by simple means. In a residential or hospital setting, for example, a bed, as long as it has good working brakes, can be moved away from the wall to provide greater space to move a patient without the locker or chair getting in the way. Sometimes radical solutions are indicated, such as changing a swing-style door to a sliding model or replacing a bath with a seated shower unit. Especially in a community setting, there are many ways in which nurses can influence or change unsatisfactory situations. They may be the first to notice obstructions, problem furniture, unsatisfactory flooring, insufficient lighting, inadequate temperature control, poor ventilation or disturbing noise. Once having noticed problems they are well placed to report them and suggest solutions.

CONCLUSION

The ability to move about and exercise choices is key to quality of life. In old age, however, many intrinsic and extrinsic barriers to mobility may become apparent. But a great deal can be done to help older people restore functional movement following an acute threat and to help them compensate for losses that cannot be corrected with the onset of chronic disorders. Promoting safe functional mobility is a central rehabilitation task for the interdisciplinary team. However, neither patients nor staff need to take risks during the rehabilitation period that might put themselves in danger of injury.

In the first chapters of both recent editions of *The Guide* it is pointed out that: 'The law as it relates to lifting and handling of patients has two principal objectives, accident prevention and compensation for the injured lifter.' Based on expert opinion, the guidance on moving and handling patients has been drawn up with a view to fulfilling these objectives. However, if the other aspect of the guidance is ignored, older people with mobility problems could be in danger of losing what mobility they do have as they are hoisted from one seat to another and pushed around in wheelchairs. Sensible interpretation of the guidance, however, should promote rather than impede older people regaining or improving their mobility. Both recent editions of *The Guide* stress the contribution that patients should be allowed to make. In fact many patients benefit from contributing to a move during rehabilitation once assessed as safe to do so.

Acknowledgements

Our thanks to colleagues who have kindly advised us during the revision of this chapter: Professor Valerie Pomeroy, Rebecca Impson, Fiona Jones, Elizabeth Reilly, Stella Smith, Helen Mann, Jill Phipps and Catherine Donaldson.

Recommended reading

Coene EH, Griffiths KK 2000 (eds) Parkinson's disease self care manual. September Foundation, Amsterdam.
Hignett S, Crumpton C, Ruszala E et al. 2003 Evidence-based patient handling. Tasks, equipment and interventions. Routledge, Taylor and Francis, London.
A systematic review of the research evidence relating to patient handling. It provides a source of reference and the foundation for future practice for a range of professionals.
Pickles B, Compton A, Cott C et al. (eds) 2000 Physiotherapy with older adults. WB Saunders, London.
Not just physiotherapists but all health care professionals working with older people will find this book useful. Besides the chapters referenced, others deal with pain, ageing with a disability, interdisciplinary assessment, osteoporosis and fractures.
Royal College of Nursing 2003 Safer staff, better care. RCN manual: handling training guidance and competencies. Royal College of Nursing, London.
Part of the Working Well Initiative, this pamphlet puts manual handling guidance in the context of a fully integrated management system that meets all the legal requirements.
Sassoon R 2002 Understanding stroke. Pardoe Blacker, Felbridge.
The author suffered a stroke and wrote this book for patients, carers and health professionals. The information ranges from personal experiences to research in progress.
Steed R 1999 Safer handling of people in the community. National Back Care Association, 16 Elmtree Road, Teddington, Middx TW11 8ST.
For professional carers and their managers, to reduce the risk of back injuries when working in someone's home or in a residential care home.

Useful websites

Arthritis Care: www.arthritiscare.org.uk
Disabled Living Foundation: www.dlf.org.uk
Parkinson's Disease Society: www.parkinsons.org.uk
Stroke Association: www.stroke.org.uk

References

American Geriatrics Society, British Geriatrics Society, American Academy of Orthopaedic Surgeons Panel on Falls Prevention 2001 Guideline for the prevention of falls in older people. Journal of the American Geriatrics Society 49: 664–672
Bajekal M, Prescott A 2003 Disability. In: Bajekal M, Primatesta P, Prior G (eds) Health survey for England 2001. Stationery Office, London

Bodenheimer T, Lorig K, Holman H et al. 2002 Patient self-management of chronic disease in primary care. Journal of the American Medical Association 288: 469–475

Booth B, Warren A, Garbett R 1996 Professional development unit 30. Stroke. Nursing Times 92: 27–29

Carr EK, Kenney FD 1992 Positioning of the stroke patient: a review of the literature. International Journal of Nursing Studies 29: 355–369

Carr JH, Shepherd RB 2003 Stroke rehabilitation. Butterworth-Heinemann, Edinburgh

Chatterton HJ, Pomeroy VM, Gratton J 2001 Positioning for stroke patients: a survey of physiotherapists' aims and practices. Disability and Rehabilitation 23: 413–421

Collin C, Wade DT, Davies S et al. 1988 The Barthel ADL index: a reliability study. International Disability Studies 19: 61–63

Cotty MA 1999 Recognising medical reasons for falling. Physiotherapy Theory and Practice 15: 135–140

Cumming RG, Thomas M, Szonyi G et al. 1999 Home visits by an occupational therapist for assessment and modification of environmental hazards: a randomised trial of falls prevention. Journal of the American Geriatrics Society 47: 1397–1402

Department of Health 2001 National service framework for older people. Standard 5 Stroke, standard 6 Falls, standard 8 Promotion of health and active life in older age. Stationery Office, London

Dieppe PA 1995 Clinical features and diagnostic problems in osteoarthritis. In: Klippel JH, Dieppe PA (eds) Practical rheumatology. Times Mirror International, London, pp 141–156

Dieppe PA, Klippel JH 1995 Disorders of the musculoskeletal system. In: Klippel JH, Dieppe PA (eds) Practical rheumatology. Times Mirror International, London, pp 1–20

Edwards S 2002 (ed) Neurological physiotherapy: a problem solving approach. Churchill Livingstone, London

Feder G, Cryer C, Donovan D et al. 2000 Guidelines for the prevention of falls in people over 65. British Medical Journal 321: 1007–1011

Fiatarone MA, O'Neill EF, Ryan ND et al. 1994 Exercise training and nutritional supplementation for physical frailty in very older people. New England Journal of Medicine 330: 1769–1775

Fitzpatrick C, Simpson JM, Valentine JD et al. 2005 The measurement properties and performance characteristics among older people of TURN 180: a test of dynamic, postural stability. Clinical Rehabilitation 19: in press

Gardner M, Buchner M, Robertson M et al. 2001 Practical implementation of an exercise based falls prevention programme. Age and Ageing 30: 77–83

Gardner M, Robertson M, McGee R et al. 2002 Application of a falls prevention program for older people to primary health care practice. Preventive Medicine 34: 546–553

Gill TH 1999 Preventing falls: to modify the environment or the individual? Journal of the American Geriatrics Society 47: 1471–1472

Harridge S, Young A 2000 Strength and power. In: Grimley Evans J, Williams TF, Beatie BL et al. (eds) Oxford textbook of geriatric medicine. Oxford University Press, Oxford, pp 963–968

Hill J 1998 Rheumatology nursing. Churchill Livingstone, Edinburgh

Hirani V, Malbut M 2002 Health survey for England 2000: disability among older people. Stationery Office, London

Holliday PJ, Fernie GR 1995 Assistive devices: aids to independence. In: Pickles B, Compton A, Cott C et al. (eds) Physiotherapy with older people. WB Saunders, London, pp 360–381

Irwin P 1996 The role of the nurse in stroke. In: Wolf C, Rudd T, Beech R (eds) Stroke services and research. Stroke Association, London

Koch M, Gottschalk M, Baker D et al. 1994 An impairment and disability assessment and treatment protocol for community-living older persons. Physical Therapy 74: 286–295

Latash ML 1998 Neurophysiological basis of movement. Human Kinetics, Champaign, IL

le Gallez P 1998 Patient education and self-management. In: le Gallez P (ed) Rheumatology for nurses. Whurr, London, pp 98–123

Lennon SM 1995 Using standardised scales to document outcome in stroke rehabilitation. Physiotherapy 81: 200–202

Lord SR, Sherrington C, Menz HB 2001 Falls in older people. Cambridge University Press, Cambridge

Lundin-Olsson L, Nyberg L, Gustafson Y 1997 'Stops walking when talking' as a predictor of falls in older people. Lancet 349: 617

Malbutt K, Falaschetti E 2003 Non-fatal accidents. In: Bajekal M, Primatests P, Prior G (eds) Health survey for England 2001. Stationery Office, London

McGovern R, Rudd A 2003 Management of stroke. Postgraduate Medical Journal 79: 87–92

Mutch WJ, Lien C 2001 Epidemiology. In: Playfer JR, Hindle JV (eds) Parkinson's disease in the older patient. Arnold, London, pp 30–40

National Back Pain Association, Royal College of Nursing 1997 Guide to the handling of patients, 4th edn. National Back Pain Association and Royal College of Nursing, London

Nevitt MC, Cummings SR, Kidd S et al. 1989 Risk factors for non-syncopal falls. Journal of the American Medical Association 261: 2663–2668

Oddy R 1998 Mobility in dementia care: a problem solving approach for carers. Age Concern, London

Reece A, Simpson JM 1996 Preparing older people to cope after a fall. Physiotherapy 82: 227–235

Riley HS 1998 Role of physiotherapy in rheumatology. In: le Gallez P (ed) Rheumatology for nurses. Whurr, London, pp 186–222

Robertson D, Aragon A, Moore G et al. 2001 Rehabilitation and the multidisciplinary team. In: Playfer JR, Hindle JV (eds) Parkinson's disease in the older patient. Arnold, London, pp 250–272

Robertson MC, Campbell AJ, Gardner MM et al. 2002 Preventing injuries in older people by preventing falls: a metaanalysis of individual level data. Journal of the American Geriatrics Society 50: 905–911

Ross FM, Bower P 1995 Standardised Assessment For Older People (SAFE): feasibility study in district nursing. Journal of Clinical Nursing 4: 303–310

Rowat AM 2001 What do nurses and physiotherapists think about the positioning of stroke patients? Journal of Advanced Nursing 34: 795–803

Royal College of Nursing 1991 The role of the nurse in rehabilitation of older people. Scutari Press, London

Royal College of Nursing 1993 The value and skills of nurses working with older people. Royal College of Nursing, London

Shumway-Cook A, Woollacott M 2001 Motor control: theory and practical applications, 2nd edn. Lippincott, Williams & Wilkins, Baltimore

Simpson JM 2001 Having fallen does not fully explain fear of falling. Proceedings of the British Psychological Society 9: 146 (abstract)

Simpson JM, Hawke J 1998 Self-esteem after syncope and falls: a qualitative study. Age and Ageing 27 (suppl. 2): 19 (abstract)

Simpson JM, Jones F 2004 Physical or psychological change? Which is the most important rehabilitation outcome for older people who fall? Age and Ageing 33: 204–211

Simpson JM, Richardson B 2002 Why do older people use walking aids? Physiotherapy 88: 174–175 (abstract)

Simpson JM, Worsfold C, Hunter I 1996 A simple test of balance for frail old people. Clinical Rehabilitation 10: 354 (abstract)

Simpson JM, Worsfold C, Hastie I. 1997 Is fear of falling really fear of the consequences? Age and Ageing 26 (suppl. 3): 12 (abstract)

Simpson JM, Harrington R, Marsh N 1998 Managing falls among older people. Physiotherapy 84 (4) 173–177

Simpson JM, Worsfold C, Reilly E et al. 2002 A standard procedure for using TURN180 to test dynamic postural stability among older people. Physiotherapy 88: 342–351

Simpson JM, Darwin C, Marsh N 2003 What are older people prepared to do to avoid falling? A qualitative study in London. British Journal of Community Nursing 8: 133–141

Smith J (ed) 2005 The Guide to the Handling of People. Backcare. Teddinghton, Middlesex

Stewart DA 2001 Pathology, aetiology and pathogenesis. In: Playfer JR, Hindle JV (eds) Parkinson's disease in the older patient. Arnold, London, pp 12–29, 30–40

Stubbs DA, Buckle PW, Rivers PM et al. 1983 Back pain in the nursing profession. Part 1: Epidemiology and pilot methodology. Ergonomics 26: 755–765

Tinetti ME 2003 Preventing falls in elderly persons. New England Journal of Medicine 348: 42–49

Tinetti ME, Baker DI, McAvay G et al. 1994 A multifactorial intervention to reduce falling among older people living in the community. New England Journal of Medicine 331: 821–827

Wade D 1992 Measurement in neurological rehabilitation. Oxford University Press, Oxford

Wade D 2000 Intercollegiate working party for stroke. National clinical guidelines for stroke. Royal College of Physicians, London. Available online at: www.rcplondon.ac.uk/pubs/

Wade D 2002 Intercollegiate working party for stroke. Updated guidelines for stroke. Royal College of Physicians, London. Available online at: http://www.rcplondon.ac.uk/pubs/

World Health Organization 1980 International classification of impairment, disability and handicap. World Health Organization, Geneva

World Health Organization 2001 International Classification of Functioning, Disability and Health. World Health Organization, Geneva. Available online at http://www.who.int/classification/icf

Chapter 14

Care of the foot

Christine Hanks and Margaret Bruce

INTRODUCTION

The effect of hurting feet is legendary: they make us irritable and reduce our concentration and the desire to be mobile.

Foot problems in older people (65 years +) are common. The effect of foot problems in older people is significant, as they can result in instability (leading to falls), reduced mobility and social isolation (Menz & Lord 2001a, 2001b). Many foot problems can be avoided by taking care of the feet. This care may be undertaken by the individual, a family or informal carer, or a care professional who is not a foot specialist, such as a health care assistant or nurse. The role of the nurse in relation to the client's feet involves:

- health education
- assessment
- non-specialist foot care
- referral to a foot-care specialist (podiatrist).

Benvenuti et al. (1995) found that 86% of a sample of 459 'community dwelling older people' had 'at least one foot symptom or sign', many of which would reduce mobility. For older people, a decrease in mobility can leave them unable to participate in their regular normal activities. Consequences can range from loss of independence to severe alterations in lifestyle.

Our feet consist of skin, bones, muscles, tendons, ligaments, nerves and blood vessels. Healthy feet enable us to balance our body effectively in walking, running, dancing and in many other daily activities. Our feet are vulnerable to repetitive mechanical stress and skin irritation due to heavy daily usage but, like the rest of the body, the foot succumbs to changes that occur with age and older patients with foot problems exhibit degenerative changes of the soft tissues of the foot and lower limb.

Feet may be misused and abused throughout life, as the person follows shoe fashion, ignorant of the problems being established for the future. Consider the ancient cultural tradition of binding the feet in China and the effect on women of wearing high-heeled shoes or shoes with pointed toes. Most shoes are not the shape of a healthy foot. Not surprisingly, it is women who have statistically more problems with their feet than men as they get older (Munroe & Steele 1998, Menz & Lord 2001b, Dawson et al. 2002).

COMMON CHANGES IN THE FOOT WITH AGE

Ageing causes a thinning of epithelial and subcutaneous fatty layers (see Chapter 5 for more information on the biology of ageing). The number of fibroblasts, which are responsible for the synthesis of protein and collagen, are reduced. The resulting reduction in collagen and elastic fibres in connective tissue causes the tissue to become denser and the fragile skin loses elasticity and resilience and becomes prone to injury (Edelstein 1988). There is a decrease in both active sweat glands and sebaceous glands, leaving the skin at risk of becoming dry, flaky and scaly. The older skin, which is easily damaged, repairs at a slower rate than in younger individuals (Weg 1973) and is at greater risk of infection. The fat pads under the feet (plantar surface) are important as a shock absorber and the reduction in fat makes the foot prone to injury.

Toenails grow more slowly with age, due to the decreased vascular supply to the nailbed, and there is a thickening of the nail plate, resulting in brittle, thick and dull nails, which are prone to infection. Improper shoe wear can cause persistent trauma to the nail matrix and lead to further thickening. As in bone in other parts of the body, osteoporosis can affect the bones of the feet, predisposing feet to fractures even during normal, everyday activities. There is a reduction of elastic fibres in the ligaments which increases the rigidity of the foot. The reduction in muscle fibre in old age leads to thinner feet, and loss of integrity of the arches. There is often a reduced blood supply to the feet with age, as arteriosclerosis increases peripheral resistance to blood flow. The delivery of oxygen and nutrients is reduced, resulting in an increase in healing time after injury.

With ageing, sensory acuity diminishes, which may be exacerbated by pathological conditions. This reduced capacity for sensation may mean that the older individual is unaware of uncomfortable shoes. Foreign objects can, for example, get into shoes and cause significant damage to persons with diminished sensation. In addition, a decrease in temperature sensitivity may increase susceptibility to thermal trauma, and so the individual should guard against burns from hot-water bottles or when sitting near to a fire.

As people get older, the impact of loss of visual acuity and loss of strength and suppleness can interfere with self-care of the feet, which in turn increases pain and further reduces mobility. Loss of mobility may lead to loss of contact with family and friends who used to help with foot care. Lack of interest and neglect may ensue.

PREVALENCE OF FOOT PROBLEMS

Foot pain and deformity are very common problems for older people and they can have a serious impact on quality of life. When these problems are successfully managed the relief from pain can facilitate the older person's rehabilitation from chronic disorders and other disabilities (Bruno & Helfand 1990).

Several studies have found a high prevalence of foot disorders in the older population and, although the numbers of older people assessed as having foot pathology vary, they consistently form a large proportion. Harvey et al. (1997) found that a total of 53% of people in a population aged 60 and over had three or more foot problems. Another study stated that more than half of those aged 75 years or more obtained care from podiatry services (Crawford et al. 1996). Over 70% of a population aged 65 and over reported that they were suffering from foot problems and also a higher incidence of foot disorders was reported by women (Munroe & Steele 1998). In another study it was estimated that 40% of people over 65 years of age need podiatry treatment but only half of this number received it (Pushpangadan & Burns, 1996). This was supported by Harvey et al. (1997), who found that 20% of people whose feet had been assessed had sufficient pathology to be in need of care from a podiatrist but they were not receiving it. The group least likely to receive treatment for their foot conditions were older people living alone (Harvey et al. 1997). The most prevalent problems that affect older people are toenails that are difficult to cut, pain from corns and calluses and toe deformities (White & Mulley 1989). The podiatry services may not be being targeted towards those with greatest need, and where podiatric services are available, not all older people with painful feet consult practitioners for treatment or guidance (Munro & Steele 1998).

There is a clear relationship between painful feet and impaired balance. It has been found that older people with multiple foot problems are at a higher risk of falling than those with fewer problems, or those with normal feet (Hylton et al. 2001). Painful and deformed feet can impair the mobility of the individual to such a degree that they can become house-bound.

COMMON FOOT PROBLEMS

Common foot problems in older people include dry skin, calluses, corns, toenail pathologies, fungal infection and chilblains. The normal changes of ageing are often aggravated by inadequate foot care, mechanical causes and infection, in addition to systemic disease such as diabetes, vascular disease and arthritis.

Corn and callus

These common skin pathologies arise when excessive mechanical stresses are affecting the foot. These hyperkeratotic lesions are produced when the outermost layer of the skin, the stratum corneum, becomes thickened as a result of the epidermis being stimulated by the stresses to produce more cells. A callus can be described as a diffuse area of hyperkeratosis of a regular depth while a corn is a denser area of hyperkeratosis, which forms a nucleus and indicates that the pressure is concentrated in that area. These lesions are found typically on the plantar surface of the foot and the apex and the dorsum of the prominent joints of the toes. They are not always painful and serve to protect the underlying tissues from excessive stresses. However, corns and calluses may produce pain on walking.

Podiatric treatment of corn and callus usually consists of debridement with a scalpel followed by relief of pressure. This is usually in the form of an individually made cushioning insole for the older person or sometimes an orthotic, which is a custom-made insole designed to compensate for mild degrees of abnormality in the functioning of the feet or lower limbs.

Bunions

'Bunion' is a lay term associated with a deformity of the hallux (first or big toe) – hallux abducto valgus – and is one of the most common forefoot problems, especially affecting women (Fig. 14.1). Hallux abducto valgus refers to the lateral deviation of the hallux and the splaying of the first metatarsal medially. The bunion is the prominence on the inside of the foot around the big toe joint and usually consists of a chronically inflamed adventitious bursa (a bursa not present at birth), which arises on the medial side of the head of the first metatarsal and serves to protect the deeper tissues from injury when the area is traumatized by shoe pressure. The movement of the big toe towards the other four toes commonly produces various toe deformities of these lesser toes, i.e. hammer, mallet or claw toes.

The symptoms of bunions include inflammation, swelling and sometimes acute pain in the affected area. The discomfort may affect the patient's gait. A similar deformity can arise on the outside (lateral) side of the foot over the joint at the base of the little toe and this is sometimes known as a 'tailor's bunion'; in times gone by, tailors would sit cross-legged and so this area, on the lateral side of the foot, was susceptible to constant trauma. These deformities develop from an abnormality in foot function but may be exacerbated by wearing ill-fitting footwear. It is important for the patient to wear shoes that can accommodate the extra width of the foot caused by the deformity and so avoid trauma to the exposed bony prominences.

Toenails

The most common soft-tissue problem is related to the nail (Karpman 1995) and many older people are particularly affected by nail deformities. Patients may present with very long, neglected nails. This often painful and potentially problematic condition may arise from an inability to bend to reach the feet as a consequence of arthritic conditions of the knees or hips. Difficulty in manipulating nail nippers or scissors because of stiffness in the hands and fingers or visual impairment also makes this simple task impossible for many older people to carry out (Helfand et al. 1998).

Simple thickening of the nails may cause lesions on the toes and affect walking. Onychauxis is simple thickening of the nail plate without any associated deformity and is often caused by impaired nutrition to the nailbed and matrix in the older person.

Onychogryphosis usually occurs as a result of trauma to the nailbed or matrix and results in a deformity, which is often referred to as a 'ram's horn nail'. The nail plate is very distorted and deviates to one side as it grows. When neglected, this nail type can curve under or over the adjacent toes, frequently causing painful lesions and ulceration.

Onychomycosis is the term given to a nail that has become infected by fungal organisms. The nail will appear thickened, discoloured and crumbly with a characteristic odour. Occasionally the nail plate is only partially affected and the infection may be evident by white discolouration from the free edge of the nail.

Insufficient arterial supply may cause dystrophic thinning and sometimes absence of the nail plate.

Skin fungal infections

Chronic skin fungal (mycotic) infections are relatively common foot problems in older people and often accompany onychomycosis (fungal infection of the

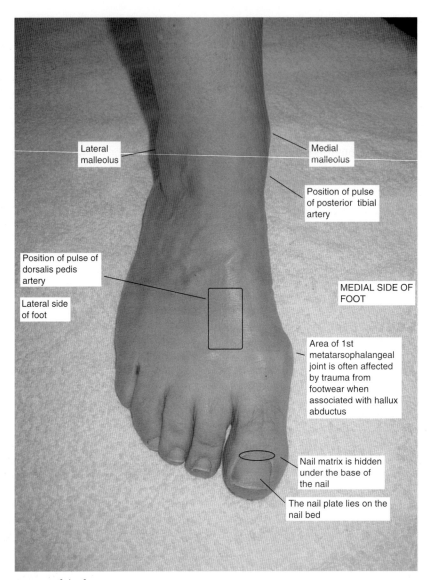

Fig. 14.1 Surface anatomy of the foot.

nail plate). The condition is referred to as 'tinea pedis' – the lay term is 'athlete's foot'. Tinea refers to the organism causing the infection (tinea rubrum, tinea mentagrophytes). Pedis refers to the foot. Clinical features include excessive desquamation, skin fissures and vesicles and itching is often a troublesome symptom. Fungal infections are common interdigitally and often present with moist inflamed skin between the toes with vesicles extending on to the surrounding skin. There is sometimes a characteristic 'cheesy' odour. Fissuring, or splitting, of the skin can occur, which can be very painful. The patient should be encouraged to dry carefully and gently between the

toes and then apply an antifungal preparation as described below.

These fungal infections can often become chronic (or tend to keep recurring) and nurses can play a useful role in preventing this by advising the patient to carry out some simple practical measures. To identify the fungal organism, a scraping of the affected skin can be sent to the local microbiology laboratories for microscopy and culture. The infected skin can be treated by using one of the over-the-counter antifungal preparations: clotrimazole 1% or miconazole nitrate 2% is effective against a range of organisms. Occasionally a more widespread or particularly pertistent infection may require a more potent preparation (for example, terbinafine hydrochloride 1%), which can be obtained on medical prescription from the patient's general practitioner. It is sensible to encourage prompt treatment of these infections to prevent development of a skin fissure (crack) and secondary bacterial infection. These problems can lead to more serious complications, especially if the patient has impaired arterial flow to the feet or a disorder such as diabetes, when ulceration may result.

To prevent reinfection, the patient's socks, towels and bed linen should be washed at 60°C to destroy any fungal elements and shoes and slippers should be sprayed with any of the above preparations that are available in aerosol form. The patient should be encouraged to wear different shoes on alternate days and then leave them to dry out, preferably in sunshine, which helps to eradicate any remaining fungal spores from the shoes.

Chilblains

Chilblains develop in older people who experience an abnormal response to cold in the blood vessels of the skin of the extremities. The cold temperature damages areas of the skin and as a result localized inflammation occurs (Case study 14.1). The blood supply is diverted away from the skin when entering a cold atmosphere in order to help to conserve the body's core temperature. Normally, when returning into the warmth, the blood supply is restored almost immediately but, when a person is susceptible to chilblains, the blood supply is not immediately restored, although the tissues of the skin warm up and metabolism returns to normal. The metabolites build up, the sluggish blood flow becomes deoxygenated and the area appears cyanosed. This is described as the congestive phase of chilblains. The arterial supply is eventually restored to normal and the area becomes inflamed, with the classic features of chilblains becoming evident as the area becomes locally hot, red and swollen and intensely itchy. Common sites for chilblains are the apices of toes, over the exposed medial border of the foot associated with hallux abducto valgus and at the back of the heel. The susceptible individual can avoid chilblains by wearing warm footwear and take care to avoid exposing the feet to direct heat after coming in from the cold. Proprietary chilblain preparations can also be very helpful.

Metatarsalgia

Loss of subcutaneous fat and thinning of the skin result in a loss of shock absorption and pain, particularly over the plantar metatarsal heads. Chronic inflammation of the soft tissues causes pain in this area. Hyperkeratosis may result as the skin thickens in a response to the extra stress and sometimes corns arise over the metatarsal heads.

Ulceration

Several types of ulcer may be found on the feet of older people. Amongst these are: (1) ischaemic; (2) venous; (3) neuropathic; (4) pressure; and (5) diabetic ulcers.

Case study 14.1

Mrs Dunn, a fit and active woman of 85 years of age, lives with her husband in a flat in an area of town that is being renovated. They are hoping to be rehoused in the near future. Mrs Dunn is visiting the practice nurse, Michelle, at her general practitioner's practice for her annual flu vaccination. The weather is unusually cold and she has to remove layers of clothing, which takes some time, during which she chats with Michelle. Mrs Dunn sits down with relief and complains about how sore her feet have been recently, and so Michelle takes the opportunity to examine her feet. She finds small dark cyanosed patches on her toes and on the ball of her feet and Mrs Dunn's feet feel very cold. Michelle suspects that these lesions are typical of the congestive stage of chilblains and advises Mrs Dunn to buy a proprietary preparation to treat chilblains, which acts as a vasodilator and may help to relieve the symptoms. She also advises her to keep her feet warm by wearing a thin pair of socks over her stockings and to find some insulating insoles to wear in her boots. Michelle also says it is a good idea to keep outdoor shoes on when returning home until her feet warm up. Rubbing the feet gently with the towel after washing them in comfortably warm water may also help to improve the blood flow in her feet. Avoiding standing in the cold and getting exercise walking is also sensible advice. Mrs Dunn reveals that her flat is very cold and draughty and she admits to toasting her feet in front of the electric fire, which Michelle warns against. She reassures Mrs Dunn that, when she and her husband move into their new well-insulated, centrally heated home, her chilblains will probably be less of a problem. Keeping warm and preventing chilblains from forming is the best form of management in susceptible people.

Ischaemic ulcers

These are ulcers caused by insufficient arterial supply to the area of the lesion, resulting in the tissues of the skin becoming devitalized and necrosed. These patients will present with signs and, often, symptoms, which are characteristic of arterial insufficiency usually caused by arteriosclerosis. Signs include an abnormally cool foot with a temperature gradient increasing proximally, the leg being warmer than the foot. The foot appears pale unless there is also venous insufficiency, when the pallor may be masked by cyanosis. There may be thin atrophic skin and a lessening of hair growth. The nails may be small and thickened.

Symptoms include pain in the calf on walking which disappears when the person rests for a few minutes (intermittent claudication). Pain in the foot can also waken the person at night; this may be 'rest pain', which is a sign of serious arterial insufficiency. The dorsalis pedis and posterior pulses (locations indicated on Fig. 14.1) may not be palpable and, if they are audible when using Doppler ultrasound, will be monophasic. A monophasic pulse is one in which only one sound can be heard, indicating reduced flow in the diseased artery. The pulse normally has three sounds, otherwise known as triphasic, which indicates a healthy elastic artery, and therefore a good blood flow to the area it supplies. The ischaemic ulcer is often shallow and located over bony prominences on the margins of the feet. These ulcers are less common on the dorsum, due to better perfusion of blood to this part of the foot, which is subjected to less pressure (Sumpio 2000). The ulcer may have a 'punched-out' appearance and have well-demarcated borders. This sort of ulcer often causes the patient a great deal of pain.

Venous ulcers

This type of ulcer is commonly present in the area of the medial malleolus or occasionally the lateral malleolus (Fig 14.1). Varicosities will probably be evident and other clinical findings will include oedema and venous dermatitis. Venous stasis ulcers can vary in size from a few centimetres to many centimetres in diameter and they occasionally extend round the entire circumference of the leg above the ankle.

Neuropathic ulcers

These ulcers are most frequently caused by diabetes in the western world, but can be associated with other neurological disorders in which a sensory deficit exists, such as spina bifida and leprosy, or as the result of injury to the peripheral nerves. Neuropathic ulcers are often deep and complicated by infection.

The neuropathy not only affects the sensory nervous system, preventing the person from feeling pressure or pain: it can also affect the autonomic nervous system, through innervation of the sweat glands, which results in a marked diminution in the production of sweat in the lower limb, often leading to the development of dry cracked skin on the foot.

The motor nervous system can also be affected by neuropathy, with the result that the impulses of the peripheral nerves to various groups of muscles are reduced. This can lead to muscle imbalance in the foot and lower limb and often deformity.

Neuropathic ulceration usually occurs over the areas of the foot that receive the greatest pressure, such as the metatarsal heads, medial aspect of the first toe, the heel and any other areas which, because of deformity, may receive excessive load. In a patient with neuropathy, any callosity may increase the likelihood of ulceration because the callus traumatizes the tissues of the foot by acting like a foreign body in the shoe whilst the patient is walking. A person with neuropathic ulceration should be encouraged to rest to relieve pressure on the ulcer. The podiatrist can remove pressure from the ulcer by applying a contact cast or supplying an air-cast boot, rocker-soled shoe or arranging for other specialist footwear to be made.

Osteomyelitis may be present in 68% of neuropathic foot ulcers (Crerand et al. 1996). This may be suspected if the ulcer is deep and bone may be visible at the base of the ulcer. If a toe is involved it may be enlarged and 'sausage-shaped'. The patient's blood sugar may be elevated and poorly controlled. A patient with suspected osteomyelitis should be referred urgently to the diabetes specialist podiatrist or the patient's general practitioner.

Pressure ulcers

These are found located over bony prominences in patients with reduced mobility. Tissue necrosis is caused by prolonged tissue pressure, capillary occlusion and subsequent local necrosis of tissue. The reader is referred to Chapter 19 for information on the causes and treatment of pressure ulcers.

Diabetic ulcers

Common complications of diabetes mellitus include not only peripheral neuropathy, as discussed above, but also microangiopathy (abnormality of small blood vessels) and arteriosclerosis (disease of the large blood vessels), making the feet extremely vulnerable to ulceration. Enabling patients to maintain their blood glucose levels as close as possible to normal can reduce these complications of diabetes.

Diabetic ulcers are most commonly described as 'neuroischaemic', that is, they are produced by a mixed aetiology of ischaemia and neuropathy (Case study 14.2). They are therefore more difficult to manage because the impaired blood supply may result in rapid deterioration in the ulcer, increased tissue loss and gangrene. These ulcers are best treated by team work between the tissue-viability nurse, diabetes specialist nurse and podiatrist. Patients with diabetes are also likely to develop deep infection in any ulceration. Hyperglycaemia affects the body's ability to fight infections because it lessens the effectiveness of the white blood cells (Pecoraro et al. 1991).

MANAGEMENT OF FOOT PROBLEMS

It may be necessary for the older person with painful feet to be referred to a podiatrist for management. However, as already indicated, nurses can provide the everyday foot care that older people are unable to provide for themselves. This includes cutting toenails unless they have become too thickened to shorten using normal nail nippers. Some nurses are not confident in providing this basic level of care (Turner & Quire 1996), even though it has been shown to be a very useful service (Wesley & Glick 1997). This lack of confidence indicates a need for podiatrists to become involved in nurse training and professional development. Nurses can also advise people how best to reduce their discomfort.

Self-care

It is easy to neglect one's feet until discomfort draws attention to a problem. In order to prevent foot problems, a regular regime of foot care and surveillance should be established. Older people should be encouraged to inspect their feet regularly, looking for cracks or cuts in the skin or peeling or scaling of the skin on the plantar aspect of the feet or between the toes, which could indicate fungal infection. Moist sodden skin is often seen between the toes of older people as the joints of the toes are stiff, making separation of the toes difficult. Sweat does not evaporate in these circumstances and the area is also difficult to dry properly. The skin loses its elasticity and can split or fissure, which can be very painful and allow the entry of microorganisms.

Feet should be washed regularly and dried carefully, especially between the toes. Moisturizing cream

---

Case study 14.2

Mr White is a retired farm worker who lives alone in an isolated cottage in a rural area. He is suffering from type 2 diabetes, which was diagnosed 10 years ago by routine screening of his blood chemistry before he underwent a minor surgical procedure at the local hospital. His diabetes is controlled by diet and by metformin (oral medication that helps to lower the blood glucose levels). He finds it difficult to maintain his blood glucose levels at a low level and they have been found to vary between 10 and 18 mmol/l (normal fasting blood glucose levels are 3.0–6.5 mmol/l; World Health Organization guidelines (1999) for diagnosing diabetes mellitus specify a fasting blood glucose level of more than 6.9 mmol/l). He is also overweight and has a body mass index of 30 (normal range 18.5–25.0).

The district nurse, Julie, visits Mr White to have a chat about how he can improve his blood glucose levels. He shows her a 'blister' on his big toe, which has been present for about a week but which does not cause him any pain. Julie examines the lesion and discovers that he has a 2-cm-diameter ulcer on the dorsum of the hallux of his left foot. She uses a 10g Semmes–Weinstein monofilament to detect the presence of any neuropathy (see section on Assessment undertaken by the podiatrist) and finds that he is unable to feel the filament at all on that foot, and also cannot feel the pain of the ulcer. These findings indicate that he has severe peripheral neuropathy. Julie is concerned and arranges an urgent appointment for him with the local diabetes specialist podiatrist who finds that only one pulse is palpable in this foot, indicating that the ulcer is neuroischaemic in origin. The specialist podiatrist discusses this with the district nurse and advises Mr White to start taking aspirin 75 mg per day. A referral to the vascular team is arranged. Lifestyle changes are discussed with Mr White by Julie and reinforced by the podiatrist. Mr White is encouraged to take some gentle exercise and adopt a healthier diet. The general practitioner is also involved and he agrees that the patient's dose of metformin should be increased. A plan of care is discussed by the podiatrist, the district nurse and Mr White to facilitate healing of the ulcer. The podiatrist persuades Mr White to buy a larger pair of shoes, as those that he had been wearing were too small for his feet and were traumatizing the toe.

Mr White's blood glucose levels came down to 8–9 mmol/l and, with suitable dressings and the change in footwear, the ulcer healed in 6 weeks. He is now waiting for his appointment with the vascular team to assess for the presence of arterial disease in the affected leg. If this can be treated, the likelihood of further tissue loss in that limb may be avoided. In future, the podiatrist will monitor Mr White's condition regularly and the district nurse will continue to visit him to keep an eye on his medication and diabetes control.

applied to the feet will help to keep the skin in good condition but should be avoided interdigitally. Excess moisture between the toes can be managed by the use of an antiperspirant spray several times a week or surgical spirit can be applied with cotton wool. If the skin is allowed to become too sodden in this area it can split or fissure. Toenails should be cut straight across and not too short, and sharp corners or edges should be smoothed out with a nail file. Cutting down the sides of the nails is inadvisable as this can lead to the development of an ingrowing toenail.

It is always advisable that older people do not walk barefoot, as this can increase the risk of injury, and wearing any form of footwear will provide protection.

Home remedies for foot pain are best avoided. The use of 'corn cures', the contents of which often contain acids, can cause damage to the skin around the area. It may be tempting but is unwise to treat one's own painful corns or callus using a razor blade or a pair of scissors.

Nurses can help with these problems by advising the patient to soak the feet for no more than 5–10 min and then, after drying carefully, especially between the toes, applying a moisturizing cream; not especially a 'foot cream', which can be expensive, but any moisturizing cream will help. A thin layer of petroleum jelly can also be applied to the most painful areas after bathing and before retiring to bed, and a sock worn to protect bed linen. This will prevent the moisture from escaping in the area of callosity and will help the area to soften and so become less painful. As many older patients have trouble reaching their feet, a partner, other relative or friend may be willing to help them with this beneficial routine.

The most helpful advice can be to encourage the wearing of adequate and well-fitting footwear, as described below. A change in footwear often brings about a tremendous improvement in pressure lesions and a much more comfortable pair of feet. This may enable the older person to enjoy walking.

Footwear

The choice of footwear is important in order to prevent (or exacerbate existing) foot problems and to reduce the risk of falls (Menz & Lord 1999, Burns et al. 2002, Sherrington & Menz 2003). Nurses are in a good position to advise patients (and their informal carers) on their choice of footwear. Style is commonly seen as being more important than comfort in every age group but the older person, particularly with foot pain, should ideally choose shoes for comfort and support rather than fashion. Drawing around the patient's foot when standing on a piece of paper and then compar-

ing this to a similar drawing made around the patient's shoe can reveal a mismatch which may persuade the patient to discard ill-fitting shoes.

A correct fit is important and length of shoe may be inadequate. Width and depth of the toe box of the shoe should be roomy enough to allow for natural spread of the toes. It can be difficult to find well-fitting shoes when there is gross toe deformity. Ideally the shoe should have a fastening in the form of a lace, bar or Velcro strap which will enable the shoe to be held snugly to the foot while the foot moves through the gait cycle and adapts to uneven walking surfaces. A thick sole to absorb the stresses that pass through the foot during walking is also desirable. It is beneficial if the upper of the shoe is made of leather as it will conform more easily to the foot shape but sometimes cheaper shoes with synthetic uppers are acceptable. Shopping for shoes late in the day when feet tend to be at their largest is a good idea to ensure a good fit and avoid wasting money on inadequate, unsuitable and uncomfortable shoes.

Some people have such difficult foot deformities or gross oedema around their feet and ankles that it is almost impossible for them to buy shoes that they can wear. These people can be referred to the local National Health Service disablement services centre for footwear to be made for them.

People with mobility difficulties can get equipment to assist with fastening shoes (see address for Disabled Living Centres, below). Replacing ordinary shoelaces with elastic ones, or shoes with a zip fastener may be easier to manage than a lace. Long-handled shoehorns can also assist people who cannot bend to put on their shoes.

If slippers are worn indoors they should provide support and fit properly, with firm non-slip soles, so that there is no need to shuffle to keep them on, which increases the risk of falls.

Loose-fitting socks and stockings will avoid restriction to the superficial circulation over the toes and heels. Cotton socks, which absorb sweat, are useful for people who are prone to developing fungal infections where the skin is moist.

Surgery

Surgery is sometimes an excellent option to relieve foot pain. Particularly successful procedures can be carried out on deformed toes, which rub against the shoe when walking and cause dorsal or apical corns and callus to develop. Surgical interventions such as digital arthroplasty (which restores function in an abnormal joint or the joint is replaced with a prosthetic joint) or arthrodesis (correction of the joint with fusion so no movement occurs) straighten toes and prevent further trauma from the shoe. If a lesser toe is excessively dorsiflexed (pushed upwards and out of normal alignment with the other toes) it may be simpler to amputate it and keep a cosmetically acceptable result. Extreme dorsiflexion can occur in the second toe from pressure from a medially deviated first toe (hallux abductus), which comes to lie under the second toe and forces the second toe into this position.

Assessment undertaken by the podiatrist

When a nurse finds patients have painless lesions or wounds on their feet it is advisable to refer them to a podiatrist, as there may be an undiagnosed underlying sensory neuropathy. Any patient who has signs and symptoms of arterial insufficiency to the feet (see above) may also benefit from the specialist assessment and advice of a podiatrist.

The podiatrist will question the patient and note any relevant surgical or medical history, including drug regimes. A detailed examination of the lower limb will be made to reveal any minor deformities that may hinder the normal mechanics of the leg and foot, which can cause tissue stress and therefore pain. A non-invasive assessment may be performed, including determining the ankle brachial pressure index (ABPI) to determine the presence and degree of any arterial disease. The patient will also be carefully questioned to identify any symptoms of arterial disease by asking, for example, 'when you are walking, do you get cramps in your legs which make you stop?' If the the answer is 'yes' this may indicate intermittent claudication (muscle cramping due to an insufficiency of oxygen to the muscle group caused by reduced flow in the artery supplying the muscles). The patient will stop walking because of the pain and this allows the oxygen supply to increase in the resting muscles. After a few minutes the pain passes and the patient continues to walk. The advice to a patient with this symptom should be to 'walk through the pain' as this will encourage the development of an alternative blood supply (collateral circulation) to the area.

A brief physical examination is then carried out to detect any signs of arterial disease in the limbs. This includes assessing for reduction in temperature in the limbs, pallor of the tissues and hair loss, which is especially significant if it occurs in one limb and not the other, suggesting that the limb may be ischaemic. The skin may be fragile and atrophic and the nails brittle and slow to grow on an affected limb. The pulses are examined to determine their strength and palpability. The ABPI may be recorded; this allows the severity of any ischaemia to be determined.

Using a sphygmomanometer and Doppler ultrasound, the systolic pressures of the brachial artery in the arm and the dorsalis pedis artery and posterior tibial arteries in both legs are determined. The higher systolic reading in each leg is used as this indicates the highest flow to that leg. The ABPI is calculated for each leg from the ratio of ankle systolic pressure to the brachial systolic pressure. This ratio is a sensitive indicator of the presence of the arterial insufficiency in the lower limb. Table 14.1 shows ABPI values indicating normal, moderate and severe arterial insufficiency. The results help to determine whether a patient is at risk of tissue loss and gangrene and indicates when a referral to a vascular team for further investigations may be appropriate.

An example of a patient with arterial insufficiency is Mrs Drew, who was examined for ischaemia because she complained of pain in her right calf when walking, which caused her to stop.

- The brachial pressures were both 130 mmHg (always take both and use the highest reading)
- Right foot systolic pressures: dorsalis pedis 100 mmHg, posterior tibial 80 mmHg
- Left foot systolic pressures: dorsalis pedis 125 mmHg, posterior tibial 135 mmHg
- ABPI right side = 100/130 = 0.76
- ABPI left side = 135/130 = 1.03

This indicates that Mrs Drew had a normal blood flow in her left foot (1.03) but a moderate amount of ischaemia in the right leg (0.76). The right-leg symptoms suggest intermittent claudication and so the podiatrist referred her to her general practitioner with a letter containing the results so that onward referral to the vascular team could be made for further investigations.

Neurological assessments can also be carried out, if the patient history indicates that this may be necessary. These take the form of quantifiable tests, such as the Semmes–Weinstein monofilament test to determine pressure perception. The Semmes–Weinstein monofilament was developed to detect patients who are at risk of neuropathic ulceration. Assessment of pressure

Table 14.1 Significance of ankle brachial pressure index	
Ratio value*	Indicates
1.0 and above	Normal
0.5–0.9	Moderate ischaemia
Below 0.5	Severe ischaemia

*See text for method of calculating ratio.
Source: Donnelly and London (2000)

threshold in the insensitive foot is reported as being the ideal method for testing patients at risk of ulceration. Unrecognized pressure can cause injury to the foot (Hall & Brand 1979). Semmes–Weinstein monofilaments are a set of 20 graded nylon filaments of standardized lengths and thickness. They increase in calibre and buckle at reproducible stresses identified by the manufacturer, ranging from 1.65 to 6.65. The 10g monofilament (5.07) is now commonly used in clinical assessment, as failure to feel the monofilament has been associated with an increased risk of developing foot ulcers (Bell-Krotoski & Tomancik 1987, Armstrong et al. 1998). If the patient cannot feel a 5.07 monofilament, about 98% of the ability to feel pressure has been lost in this area (Jeng et al. 2000). It has been recommended that clinical examination, to determine if the patient has any deformity of the feet, together with testing with the 10g monofilament, is the most sensitive method of identifying patients who are at risk of foot ulceration (Pham et al. 2000). There are many different methods of use of monofilaments described in the literature but no universally accepted guidelines. However it has been recognized that one of the most accurate methods of using the monofilaments is as follows: (Young et al. 1994).

- Patients should be in a comfortable warm atmosphere with shoes and socks removed and they must be able to understand the procedure when it is carefully explained
- Ask patients to close their eyes and indicate by saying, for instance, 'now' whenever they feel the monofilament touching an area of the foot
- The monofilament should be applied to the palm of the tester several times before applying it to the skin of the patient to remove any stiffness
- Apply the monofilament to the skin surface of the patient perpendicular to the test site
- Apply pressure until the filament bends by about 1 cm
- Remove the filament
- Allow several seconds before applying to the next site.

The plantar aspects of the foot's metatarsal heads should be used as test areas (these are zones of the foot that are subject to particularly high pressure and so most likely to develop ulceration). Any area that has developed callus should be avoided because sensation will be impaired by the presence of hard, thickened skin and a false diagnosis of neuropathy may be made. Armstrong et al. (1998) have determined that, out of 10 sites tested using the 10g monofilament on various areas of the foot, a score of 4 out of 10 is indicative of a loss of protective sensation (Armstrong et al. 1998). The monofilament is a widely used tool for the identification of diabetic neuropathy as it is cheap, practical, easily transported and easy to use. The International Diabetes Federation and the World Health Organization have recommended the use of the 10g Semmes–Weinstein monofilament (Kumar et al. 1991) to simplify and standardize detection of neuropathy by using a tool that can be applied by all health professionals. Birke & Rolfson (1998) considered that the monofilament was probably the tool most easily applied to the 'entire diabetic population' to detect neuropathy when considering cost, portability and ease of use, and Olaleye et al. (2001) recommended its use for annual screening. The monofilament has been used in the Exeter Integrated Diabetes Foot Project to establish the presence of neuropathy in a community setting (Donohoe et al. 2000). The effects of using different testing sites and buckling strengths on the sensitivity and specificity of using monofilaments to detect diabetic neuropathy have been examined and results revealed a sensitivity of 80% and a specificity of 86% (McGill et al. 1999).

Neuropathy in diabetes can also produce pain in the feet and legs which often coexists with a lack of sensation. Painful neuropathy can be severe and common, affecting up to 10% of patients (Chan et al. 1990), and can also cause uncomfortable sensations such as pins and needles. Clinical examination may reveal sensory loss, muscle weakness and depressed reflexes. Neuropathy can have a profound effect on the quality of a patient's life (Rajbhandari & Wilson 1998) and the symptoms are often described as becoming much worse or unbearable at night (Archer et al. 1983). Patients who are worst affected are confined to home, unable to carry out basic tasks, and often become depressed (Tesfaye et al. 1996). Allodynia (pain due to a stimulus that does not normally provoke pain) may be suffered, which can make the simple task of toenail cutting unbearably painful. This condition can often be managed effectively by prescribing antidepressant drugs such as amitriptyline.

Vibration perception testing is the most widely studied quantitative sensory test and is well established as a predictor for ulceration (Young et al. 1994). The test reflects disturbances in the function of mechanoreceptors and thick myelinated sensory nerve fibres. Various types of equipment can be used to assess the perception of vibration clinically, including the 128 Hz tuning fork, and the neurothesiometer.

Studies have found the tuning fork to be a poor indicator of the degree of vibration perception (Claus et al. 1988). The neurothesiometer, a more accurate reflector of peripheral nerve function than other methods (Bril et al. 1997), contains a linear scale, which displays the applied voltage (0–50 V). A vibration perception threshold (VPT) is the threshold of intensity of vibration at which the patient becomes aware of the sensation. Most healthy people would have a threshold below 5 V. A higher score may indicate a degree of neuropathy. A score greater than 25 V is associated with foot ulceration (Edmonds et al. 1982, Kastenbauer et al. 2001). Patients with a VPT greater than 25 V have a sevenfold increased risk of ulceration over 4 years, compared with those with a VPT less than 15 V (Young et al. 1994). Armstrong et al. (1998) point out that the hallux VPT is the only site tested for sensitivity and specificity for ulceration. Cassella et al. (2000) demonstrated the importance of the correct use of the hand-held neurothesiometer, as the vibrating head must be perpendicular to the site without any extra pressure being applied.

Cold perception is often impaired and may develop without any other signs or symptoms of sensory abnormality. Although it would seem sensible to assess for the patient's ability to detect changes in temperature, as this may help to identify abnormal sensory nerve function and prevent trauma from cold in those at risk (Claus et al. 1987), there is at present no accurate method of estimating temperature-sensitivity in a normal clinical situation.

Neuropathy associated with diabetes is the primary or contributory cause of 90% of diabetic foot ulceration (Pham et al. 2000), which unfortunately has the common sequel of lower-limb amputation (Young et al. 1992, Armstrong et al. 1997). As neuropathy is commonly asymptomatic and therefore the patient has no awareness of a loss of sensation, accurate assessment of neuropathic status is essential. Patients with neuropathy can be targeted with care and given advice to prevent them developing ulceration. Nurses can ensure that patients with neuropathy take simple but important steps to prevent the skin being damaged without them being aware of it, or to find small lesions which can be dealt with before they become major problems, for example:

- Look inside shoes or slippers before putting them on – a small stone, for instance, can cause tremendous damage
- Examine feet every day for wounds or areas that are inflamed, especially on the soles of the feet and between the toes.

If they discover a problem, patients should seek professional help from the district nurse, practice nurse, podiatrist or general practitioner as soon as possible. If they are unable to see or cannot get down to examine their feet it would be helpful if a relative, neighbour or friend could assist them with this extremely important task. A mirror on the floor may allow the arthritic but normally sighted person to examine the soles of the feet.

This assessment will help the podiatrist, nurse and patient to understand the cause of the patient's problems and enable a suitable management plan to be derived, which takes into account the patient's wishes. Management may take the form of the debridement of corns or callus, or manufacture of special insoles, which will help to relieve mechanical stresses and so lessen pain. Referrals can be made where appropriate, for instance to the vascular team if a patient presents with a critical vascular status. Liaison will be made and discussions will take place between district or practice nurses or hospital nurses and podiatrists if extended wound care is required.

The nurse has an extremely important role to play in discovering foot pathology in older patients, in advising the older patient about self-care and in carrying out practical interventions and assessments when appropriate. Nurses and podiatrists working together can do much to lessen discomfort from foot problems and enable older people to carry out their day-to-day activities by helping to lessen their disability.

Recommended reading

Boulton AJ, Connor H, Cavanagh PR (eds) 2000 The foot in diabetes, 3rd edn. Wiley, Chichester.
This book looks widely at the epidemiology of the diabetic foot and explores in some depth the provision of foot care services. It also comprehensively examines the complications of diabetes, their effects on the lower limb and their management.

Donnelly R, London N (eds) 2000 ABC of arterial and venous disease. BMJ Books, London.
This book presents a clear overview of the presentation, investigation and management of vascular disease in the lower limb. This would be a very comprehensive source of referral for a nurse who wishes to find out further information about vascular problems.

Edmonds ME, Foster AVM 2000 Managing the diabetic foot. Blackwell Science, London.
This excellently illustrated book covers all aspects of diabetic foot care with a practical and succinct approach. It is published as a pocket-sized paperback which is easily portable for straightforward access for rapid reference.

Neale D (ed) 1997 Common foot disorders. Churchill Livingstone, Edinburgh.

Merriman LM, Tollafield DR (eds) 1995 Assessment of the lower limb. Churchill Livingstone, Edinburgh.
These two books are directed at students of podiatry but much of the contents will be useful to all health professionals who are concerned about lower-limb pathology.

Sinclair AJ, Finucane P (eds) 2001 Diabetes in old age, 2nd edn. Wiley, Chichester.

This comprehensive book details how diabetes can affect the older person and includes epidemiology, pathophysiology and methods of diagnosis as well as covering the general complications of diabetes and those that are particularly relevant to the lower limb, and how they may be prevented and managed.

Useful addresses

British Diabetic Association, 10 Queen Anne Street, London W1M OBD.
Tel: 020 7323 1531; fax: 020 8742 2396; textphone: 020 7462 2757; helpline: 020 7636 6112; e-mail: bda@diabetes.org.uk.

British Footwear Association, 3 Burystead Place, Wellingborough, Northants NN8 1AH.
Tel: 01933 229 005; fax: 01933 225 009.

Clothing and Footwear Advisory Service, Disabled Living Foundation, 380–384 Harrow Road, London W9 2HU.

Disabled Living Centres, Council for the Regional Disabled Living Centre, Redbank House, 4 St Chads Street, Manchester M8 8QA.
Tel: 0161 834 1044; fax: 0161 835 3591; e-mail: dlcc@dlcc.demon.co.uk; website: www.dlcc.org.uk.

Society of Shoe Fitters, The Anchorage, 28 Admirals Walk, Hingham, Norwich, Norfolk NR9 4JL.
Tel: 01953 851171.

References

Archer AG, Watkins PJ, Thomas PK, Sharma AK, Payan J 1983 The natural history of acute painful neuropathy in diabetes mellitus. Journal of Neurology, Neurosurgery and Psychiatry 46: 491–499

Armstrong DG, Lavery LA, Harkless LB, Van Houtum WH 1997 Amputation and reamputation of the diabetic foot. Journal of the American Podiatric Medicine Association 87: 255–259

Armstrong DG, Lavery LA, Vela SA 1998 Choosing a practical screening instrument to identify patients at risk for diabetic ulceration. Archives of Internal Medicine 158: 289–292

Bell-Krotoski J, Tomancik E 1987 The repeatability of testing with Semmes–Weinstein monofilaments. Journal of Hand Surgery 12: 155–161

Benvenuti F, Ferrucci L, Guralnik JM, Baroni A 1995 Foot pain and disability in older persons: an epidemiologic survey. Journal of the American Geriatrics Society 43: 479–484

Birke JA, Rolfson RJ 1998 Evaluation of a self administered sensory testing tool to identify patients at risk of diabetes related foot problems. Diabetes Care 21: 23

Bril V, Kojic J, Ngo M, Clark K 1997 Comparison of a Neurothesiometer and Vibratron in measuring vibration perception thresholds and relationship to nerve conduction studies. Diabetes Care 20: 1360

Bruno J, Helfand AE 1990 Physical medicine considerations in managing the older patient. Journal of the American Podiatric Medical Association 80: 364–369

Burns SL, Leese GP, McMurdo ME 2002 Older people and ill fitting shoes. Post Graduate Medical Journal 78: 344–346

Cassella JP, Ashford RL, Meakin J 2000 The effect of caffeine on Neurothesiometer readings. Diabetic Foot 3: 18–20

Chan AW, MacFarlane IA, Bowsher D 1990 Short term fluctuations in blood glucose concentrations do not alter pain perception in diabetic-patients with and without painful peripheral neuropathy. Diabetes Research 14: 15–19

Claus D, Hilz MJ, Hummer I, Neundorfer B 1987 Methods of measurement of thermal thresholds. Acta Neurologica Scandinavica 76: 288–296

Claus D, Caervalho VP, Neundorfer B, Blaise JF 1988 Perception of vibration. Normal findings and methodologic aspects. Nervenarzt 59: 138–142

Crawford VLS, Ashford RL, McPeake B, Stout RW 1996 Palliative podiatric care: service provision and treatment in an elderly population. The Foot 6: 10–12

Crerand S, Dolan M, Laing P et al. 1996 Diagnosis of osteomyelitis in neuropathic foot ulcers. Journal of Bone and Joint Surgery 1: 51–55

Dawson J, Thorogood M, Marks S-A et al. 2002 The prevalence of foot problems in older women: a cause for concern. Journal of Public Health Medicine 24: 77–84

Donnelly R, London N (eds) 2000 ABC of arterial and venous disease. BMJ Books, London

Donohoe ME, Fletton JA, Hook A et al. 2000 Improving foot care for people with diabetes mellitus – a randomized controlled trial of an integrated care approach. Diabetic Medicine 17: 581–587

Edelstein JE 1988 Foot care for the aging. Physical Therapy 68: 1882–1886

Edmonds ME, Blundell MP, Morris M et al. 1982 The combined diabetic foot clinic: a major development in diabetic foot care. Diabetologia 23: 468A

Hall DC, Brand PW 1979 The etiology of the neuropathic ulcer. Journal of American Podiatry 69: 173

Harvey I, Frankel S, Marks R, Shalom D, Morgan M 1997 Foot morbidity and exposure to chiropody: population based study. British Medical Journal 315: 1054–1055

Helfand AE, Cooke HL, Walinsky MD, Demp PH 1998 Foot problems associated with older patients. Journal of the American Podiatry Association 88: 237–241

Hylton B, Menz B, Lord SR 2001 The contribution of foot problems to mobility impairment and falls in community-dwelling older people. Journal of the American Geriatrics Society 49: 1651

Jeng C, Michelson J, Mizel M (2000) Sensory thresholds of normal human feet. Foot and Ankle International 21: 501–504

Karpman RR 1995 Foot problems in the geriatric patient. Clinical Orthopaedics and Related Research 316: 59–62

Kastenbauer T, Sauseng S, Sokol G, Auinger M, Irsigler K 2001 A prospective study of predictors for foot ulceration in type 2 diabetes. Journal of the American Podiatric Medical Association 91: 343–350

Kumar S, Fernando DJ, Veves A et al. 1991 Semmes–Weinstein monofilaments: a simple, effective and inexpensive screening device for identifying diabetic patients at risk of foot ulceration. Diabetes Research and Clinical Practice 13: 63–67

McGill M, Molyneaux L, Spencer R et al. 1999 Possible sources of discrepancies in the use of the Semmes–Weinstein monofilament. Impact on prevalence of insensate foot and workload requirements. Diabetes Care 22: 598–602

Menz HB, Lord SR 1999 Footwear and postural stability in older people. Journal of the American Podiatric Medical Association 89: 222–229

Menz HB, Lord SR 2001a The contribution of foot problems to mobility impairment and falls in community dwelling older people. Journal of the American Geriatrics Society 49: 1651–1656

Menz HB, Lord SR 2001b Foot pain impairs balance and functional ability in community dwelling older people. Journal of the American Podiatric Medical Association 91: 222–229

Munroe BJ, Steele JR 1998 Foot-care awareness: a survey of persons aged 65 years and older. Journal of the American Podiatry Association 88: 242–248

Olaleye D, Perkins BA, Bril V 2001 Evaluation of three screening tests and a risk assessment model for diagnosing peripheral neuropathy in the diabetes clinic. Diabetes Research and Clinical Practice 54: 115–128

Pecoraro RE, Ahroni JH, Boyko EJ, Stensel VL 1991 Chronology and determinants of tissue repair in diabetics lower extremity ulcers. Diabetes 40: 1305–1313

Pham H, Armstrong DG, Harvey C et al. 2000 Screening techniques to identify people at high risk for diabetic foot ulceration: a prospective multicenter trial. Diabetes Care 23: 606–611

Pushpangadan M, Burns E 1996 Caring for older people: community health services: British Medical Journal 313: 805–808

Rajbhandari SM, Wilson RM 1998 Unusual infections in diabetes. Diabetes Research in Clinical Practice 39: 123–128

Sherrington C, Menz HB 2003 An evaluation of footwear worn at the time of fall-related hip fracture. Age and Ageing 32: 310–314

Sumpio BE 2000 Foot ulcers. New England Journal of Medicine 14: 787–793

Tesfaye S, Stevens LK, Stephenson JM et al. 1996 Prevalence of diabetic neuropathy and its relation to glycaemic control and potential risk factors: the EURODIAB IDDM complications study. Diabetologia 39: 1377–1384

Turner C, Quire S 1996 Nurses' knowledge, assessment skills, experience and confidence in toenail management of older people. Geriatric Nursing 17: 273–277

Weg RB 1973 Aging and the aged in contemporary society. Physical Therapy 53: 749–756

Wesley CJ, Glick DF 1997 Foot care: an innovative nursing service in a community nursing centre. Journal of Community Health Nursing 14: 15–21

White EG, Mulley GP 1989 Foot care for very old people: a community survey. Age and Ageing 18: 276–278

World Health Organization 1999 Definition, diagnosis and classification of diabetes mellitus and its complications. Report of a WHO consultation, Part 1: diagnosis and classification of diabetes mellitus. World Health Organization, Department of Noncommunicable Disease Surveillance, Geneva

Young MJ, Manes C, Boulton AJM 1992 Vibration perception threshold predicts foot ulceration Diabetes Medicine 9 (suppl. 2): 542

Young MJ, Breddy JL, Veves A, Boulton AJM 1994 The prediction of diabetic foot ulceration using vibration perception thresholds; a prospective study. Diabetes Care 117: 557–560

Chapter 15

Breathing

Tina Day and Suzanne Bench

This chapter focuses on aspects of breathing in the older person. There are well-documented physiological changes associated with ageing. Respiratory conditions can be debilitating and have an impact on physical and emotional well-being, resulting in feelings of helplessness and depression. The chapter builds on issues raised in Chapter 5 and emphasizes the importance of a thorough respiratory assessment. A range of therapeutic interventions intended to maximize breathing in the older person is explored (a useful list of abbreviations used and their definitions can be found in Table 15.1).

OVERVIEW OF THE RESPIRATORY SYSTEM

The main function of the respiratory system is gas exchange. Oxygen is required at cellular level for the production of energy, which the cells use for metabolism. If oxygen is not readily available to the tissues, the cells will cease to function and may ultimately die. Elimination of carbon dioxide occurs by an elegant transport mechanism, which begins when atmospheric oxygen is drawn into the lungs via the respiratory tract, and comes into contact with the alveolar membrane. Oxygenation occurs through three main processes: ventilation, external respiration and internal respiration.

Ventilation refers to the mechanism by which atmospheric gases are delivered to the alveolar membrane and alveolar gases are expelled. This is a mechanical process that is dependent on volume changes within the thoracic cavity (Bassett & Makin 2000). When there is a change in volume, there is a corresponding change in pressure, which leads to an increased flow of gases to equalize the pressure. This is explained by Boyle's law, which forms the basis of inspiration and expiration (Carola et al. 1992). Ventilation is affected by the action of the muscles of the thorax and controlled by the respiratory centre in the brainstem via the phrenic

Table 15.1 Abbreviations used in Chapter 15

Abbreviation	Definition
ABG	arterial blood-gas analysis
BiPAP	biphasic positive-pressure ventilation
BTS	British Thoracic Society
CAL	chronic airways limitation
COPD	chronic obstructive pulmonary disease
CPAP	continuous positive airway pressure
CVA	cerebrovascular accident
CXR	chest X-ray
EPAP	expiratory positive airway pressure
FEV_1	forced expiratory volume in 1 s
FRC	functional residual capacity
FVC	forced vital capacity
GOLD	Global Initiative on Chronic Obstructive Lung Disease
Hb	haemoglobin
HbO_2	oxyhaemoglobin
HME	heat moisture exchanger
IPAP	inspiratory positive airway pressure
LTOT	long-term oxygen therapy
MDI	metered-dose inhaler
NIPPV	non-invasive positive-pressure ventilation
NIV	non-invasive ventilation
$Paco_2$	partial pressure of carbon dioxide in arterial blood
Pao_2	partial pressure of oxygen in arterial blood
PCP	*Pneumocystis carinii* pneumonia
PEEP	positive end-expiratory pressure
PEFR	peak expiratory flow rate
RV	residual volume
Spo_2	saturation of peripheral haemoglobin
TB	tuberculosis
TLC	total lung capacity
V/Q	ventilation–perfusion

and intercostal nerves. The respiratory centre is mainly stimulated by raised levels of arterial carbon dioxide and also by low levels of oxygen. Breathing is not normally under conscious control, although it can be stopped for a few seconds at will.

A number of gases make up the atmosphere, including oxygen, carbon dioxide, nitrogen and water. Each of these gases has its own molecular weight and each is pulled to earth by gravitational forces. The term used for the collective pressure of all these gases is atmospheric pressure, which equates to 760 mmHg (101 kPa) at sea level (Hinchcliff et al. 1996). Inspiration occurs when atmospheric pressure is greater than the pressure within the lungs and expiration when pressure inside the lungs exceeds the atmospheric pressure. However,

each gas also exerts its own pressure independently (Dalton and Henry's laws). These are referred to as partial pressures and can be measured in clinical practice by arterial blood-gas (ABG) analysis.

Once inspiration is complete, oxygen is able to move from the alveoli to the pulmonary blood capillary by a process of diffusion. Similarly, carbon dioxide diffuses from the pulmonary blood capillary to the alveolus for elimination during expiration. This process is referred to as *external respiration*. Once oxygen has moved across the alveolar membrane, 97% combines with haemoglobin (Hb) to form oxyhaemoglobin (HbO_2). The remaining 3% is dissolved in the plasma. Each molecule of Hb can carry four molecules of oxygen.

The final stage of respiration involves the exchange of gases at tissue level, between the capillaries and tissue cells. This is known as *internal respiration*. Gas exchange occurs as a result of changes in pressure gradients by the same process of diffusion. Carbon dioxide is then carried as a waste product of metabolism. The majority (70%) of carbon dioxide is carried as bicarbonate, via the carbonic acid bicarbonate buffer system. The remaining carbon dioxide is carried as either carbaminohaemoglobin (23%) or dissolved in the plasma (3%). Carbon dioxide is then expelled from the lungs during expiration. In health, the amount of carbon dioxide produced should be equal to the amount exhaled, and this forms the basis of acid–base balance. For a more detailed discussion, please refer to Hinchcliffe et al. (1996) or any general physiology text.

ACUTE AND CHRONIC BREATHING PROBLEMS ASSOCIATED WITH THE OLDER PERSON

There are many acute or chronic respiratory conditions that may affect the older person. Chronic respiratory problems develop throughout life, many of which may be associated with smoking or environmental factors. The disabling effects tend to increase with age, leaving some individuals house-bound. Chronic obstructive pulmonary disease (COPD) and chronic airways limitation (CAL) are terms used to encompass conditions such as chronic bronchitis, emphysema and asthma (British Thoracic Society 1997). The most recent guidelines from the Global Initiative on Chronic Obstructive Lung Disease (GOLD) acknowledge that there are deranged inflammatory processes associated with noxious particles or gases in the lungs of a patient with COPD (Gross 2001, MacNee & Calverley 2003). A diagnosis of chronic bronchitis is usually made by the presence of a productive cough for most days of the week for a minimum of 3 months over a 2-year period. Asthma is associated with symptoms of wheezing and breathlessness rather than sputum production. Patients with emphysema have enlarged air sacs distal to the terminal bronchioles, accompanied by destruction of the alveolar walls. Acute problems such as influenza and pneumonia may affect any age, but in the older person this may have more serious consequences. COPD is a major cause of global morbidity and mortality. Figures indicate that in 1990 more than 44 million people worldwide were affected, and in 2000 almost 3 million died from this condition (Lomas 2002).

Recently, there has been an increase in cases of tuberculosis (TB) in the UK, especially in the older population. For all ages, the incidence increased by 6% between 1987 and 1989. In 2001 this had risen to 10% (World Health Organization 2003). In view of the fact that people are living longer, these figures are likely to rise. Couser & Glassroth (1993) believe that the increased risk to the older person may be due to the fact that many may have been infected by TB in their youth. However, diagnosis is often difficult in this age group, as the classic signs of chronic cough, weight loss and clear evidence on chest X-ray (CXR) may be absent. Furthermore, even in the presence of active disease, the results of tuberculin tests may be negative, as older people do not necessarily show an appropriate inflammatory response. It is clear, therefore, that an increased awareness is essential for the prompt recognition, diagnosis and treatment of TB in this population.

FACTORS AFFECTING BREATHING IN THE OLDER PERSON

Factors affecting breathing in the older person may be physiological, psychosocial and/or environmental. It is difficult to assess physiological ageing processes, as few lungs are free from some pathophysiological or environmental changes. However, older lungs are known to have lost much of the protein elastin, which is necessary for maintaining airway patency. As a consequence lungs become less compliant, which increases airway resistance. Loss of elasticity may result in alveolar hypoventilation, resulting in a ventilation–perfusion mismatch (Camhi & Enright 2000).

Changes also occur in the composition of collagen. Cross-links form between the subunits of the collagen, resulting in increased rigidity, which is thought to be responsible for the alterations of respiratory mechanics (Camhi & Enright 2000). General musculoskeletal changes associated with ageing may also affect the mechanics of breathing. For example, osteoporosis affecting the ribcage and vertebra can result in kyphosis. Kyphosis is observed as a stooped posture, which compromises respiratory effort and impairs inspiration.

Epithelial mucus production is increased and macrophages become less efficient, which impairs the immunological processes that protect an individual against infection. Loss of muscle tone and strength in the diaphragm, intercostal and accessory muscles, together with an increase in sensitivity of the upper respiratory tract may lead to a reduced and less effective cough reflex.

In younger people, the respiratory system is able to respond to challenges, such as an infection or heavy exercise, by compensatory mechanisms (for example, increased respiratory rate and depth, strong cough reflex). However, where changes have occurred due to age, that option is reduced. Weak respiratory muscles are thought to contribute to reduced lung volumes. These effects are confounded by inactivity and lack of stamina.

Environmental conditions, both at home and at work, also affect the overall respiratory status of the individual. Dunn et al. (1995) established clear links between factory emissions and cases of asthma. The older person may have had a longer period of exposure to such unfavourable conditions. Some may even have been exposed without protection to environmental pollutants, including asbestos dust or mustard gas, conditions which would not be tolerated today. Housing conditions may also contribute to respiratory problems. A cold, damp home environment will reduce resistance to infection, thus predisposing the occupant to bronchitis and TB. Dietary deficiencies will also have an adverse effect. For example, iron-deficiency anaemia will reduce the oxygen-carrying capacity of the blood, which will result in breathlessness and lethargy.

Whilst it is acknowledged that maintaining a healthy lifestyle from an early age will give the best chance later on, few individuals reach old age without some compromise to health. However, it is never too late to benefit from positive changes to lifestyle and environment. Cigarette smoking is the chief initiating agent in the development of COPD. It causes hypertrophy of the mucus-secreting glands and increases the risk of infection by reducing the number and efficiency of the epithelial cilia. Tobacco has been shown to play a major role in the development of emphysema, due to an imbalance between protease and antiprotease activity in the lung. Excess protease activity damages and dissolves alveolar walls and the small airways. Cigarette smoke induces the proliferation of alveolar macrophages, which contain proteases. On the death of the macrophages, the proteases released exceed the neutralizing capacity of the antiprotease system (Higgins et al. 1993). This allows tissue damage to occur. Cigarette smoke is also carcinogenic.

The most important intervention in modifying the course of COPD and, indeed, many other respiratory disorders is to encourage smoking cessation (Parrott et al. 1998). However, alternative strategies must be considered, as nicotine dependency is a relapsing condition that may require multiple interventions (The Tobacco Use and Clinical Practice Guideline Panel 2000). Despite the overwhelming evidence for the adverse effects of cigarettes, consideration should also be given to the individual who cannot or does not wish to stop smoking. The habit may have started when it was not only acceptable to smoke, but was also considered chic and sophisticated.

Physiological and social/environmental factors will also have an impact on the psychological status of the older person. Chronic respiratory conditions can be debilitating, which may affect psychological well-being, resulting in feelings of helplessness and depression. Community nurses and general practitioners are ideally placed to note all these factors and to assist in obtaining the appropriate help and advice. There is also evidence that increased levels of physical activity may help to reduce the likelihood of hospital admission. In a prospective study of 340 patients with COPD, Garcia-Aymerich et al. (2003) reported a 46% reduction in hospital admission for those patients with higher levels of physical activity.

Patterns of hospital readmission may also be affected by health care delivery factors, and a general practitioner may prefer to admit an older person with chronic breathing problems to hospital than to deal with an exacerbation at home (Morgan 2003). Nevertheless, there is evidence to suggest that the risk of readmission can be greatly reduced by improving domestic activity and breaking the cycle of hospital dependency (Garcia-Aymerich et al. 2000).

RESPIRATORY ASSESSMENT

A thorough respiratory assessment is key to planning effective care to prevent, manage or treat respiratory conditions. This process is not very different in the older person than it is in the younger person. However, it may be complicated by difficulties such as unreliable historians and complex multiple pathologies and therapeutic regimes which affect the clinical symptoms seen (Camhi & Enright 2000). These issues, although more common in the older adult, are not exclusive to this population (Epstein et al. 2000).

It is of vital importance to gain an accurate patient history. Memory and concentration loss may however be apparent. Similarly, the older person may have sensory deficits such as hearing or vision loss, which may impede the process. Other sources of information should therefore be used to validate information where necessary. These might include family and significant others, and previous medical or nursing documentation, although it should be remembered that retrospective documentation has the potential for inaccuracies. When considering history, it is prudent to enquire about social circumstances. A number of older people live alone, and may be financially less secure following retirement. This could have repercussions on their lifestyle and diet and may contribute to respiratory problems. Questions relating to smoking habits, exercise regimes, living arrangements, heating and pastimes should be asked in a sensitive manner. It is also important not to forget occupational history just because a person has retired. Conditions such as asbestosis, for example, can occur years after initial exposure (Epstein et al. 2000).

All clinical assessments should follow a logical systematic approach such as that outlined by Epstein et al. (2000). This involves utilizing the skills of inspection, palpation, percussion and auscultation to obtain primary data, and then supporting these findings using secondary data such as CXRs. Table 15.2 outlines and discusses the primary data that might be ascertained during a clinical respiratory assessment. Assessment is best performed with the person sitting upright and forward. However, this may be difficult for some older clients and support may be required to sustain such a position (Kwaiser Khun & McGovern 1992). Adaptations will need to be made to the assessment technique depending on individual needs.

A number of older clients will rely on long-term therapies for chronic respiratory conditions. Assessment of their respiratory status must be undertaken in relation to these therapies. The amount of respiratory support the person is receiving at the time of assessment should be noted. This should include treatments such as oxygen, drugs and fluids. It is important also to understand the effects of these therapies, for example an increased fluid input may lead to cardiac failure and subsequent pulmonary oedema which may present as dyspnoea. Furthermore, Weilitz & Lueckenotte (1995b) note that this is a useful time in which to get patients to demonstrate the use of metered-dose inhalers (MDI), and to discuss competence issues in relation to equipment being used, such as home oxygen therapy. Exercise tolerance should also be noted so that it can be used to evaluate any improvement or deterioration in the condition of the patient over time. This is especially important when the patient has been diagnosed with a chronic condition such as COPD (British Thoracic Society 1997).

Table 15.2 Clinical respiratory assessment: primary data

Assessment	Data obtained	Assessment issues
Inspection	Respiratory rate, pattern and depth Signs of dyspnoea, e.g. sitting forward, use of accessory muscles Conscious level/mental acuity Signs of pain Colour Chest movement/structure/spinal deformities Patient position Ability to speak/move Finger-clubbing/nicotine staining/evidence of tremor Jugular venous pressure Presence of cough Colour, consistency and culture of sputum	Inspection may increase respiratory rate Older persons have increased respiratory rate (16–25 beats/min) (Weilitz & Lueckenotte 1995a) Trend of respiratory rate most sensitive indicator of deterioration. Rate should be accurately counted and documented (Goldhill et al. 1999) Mental status changes most sensitive indicator of hypoxia and hypercapnia in older adults (Weilitz & Lueckenotte 1995a) Colour changes may be indicative of common respiratory pathologies (Eliopoulos 2001) Older persons can have a larger anterior posterior chest diameter, especially in the presence of chronic obstructive pulmonary disease (Eliopoulos 2001) Barrel chest can indicate chronic airflow limitation (Epstein et al. 2000) Abnormal spinal curvatures may impede adequate ventilation Decreased chest expansion may be caused by pain, poor position and reduced mobility Older persons may have decreased effectiveness of cough mechanism and reduced ciliary action (Weilitz & Lueckenotte 1995a) Alterations in sputum colour and consistency may indicate tuberculosis, malignancy or infection
Palpation	Pulse Blood pressure Skin temperature/skin turgor Tracheal position Chest-wall tenderness/movement Abnormal lesions Presence of systemic oedema Presence of lymph nodes Tactile fremitus	Environmental factors may alter findings, e.g. fan therapy/blankets Systemic oedema may indicate cardiac or hepatic dysfunction causing secondary respiratory difficulties May reveal presence of masses (Eliopoulos 2001) Older person would be expected to have reduced skin turgor (Weilitz & Lueckenotte 1995b) Vibrations over chest wall during expiration may indicate retained secretions (Weilitz & Lueckenotte 1995b, Epstein et al. 2000)
Percussion	Areas of density/consolidation Presence of air Hyperresonance	Percussion not often performed by nurses Chronic obstructive pulmonary disease patients may have hyperresonant chest, whereas those with pneumonia, consolidation or fluid-filled areas would have areas of dullness (Weilitz & Lueckenotte 1995b)
Auscultation	Normal bilateral air entry to all zones Added breath sounds (e.g. crackles, wheeze, stridor)	Should be performed from the back over each lobe of lung Commence auscultation at bases as most pathologic conditions occur here in an older person (Kwaiser Khun & McGovern 1992) Do not to continue for too long as patient may become dizzy and exhausted (Kwaiser Khun & McGovern 1992) Older person may have decreased basal breath sounds due to spinal changes, poor position, reduced mobility and decreased ability to take deep breaths (Weilitz & Lueckenotte 1995b) Crackles can indicate fluid or secretions Older clients can have increased retention of mucus due to age-related decreased pulmonary function (Kwaiser Khun & McGovern 1992) Wheeze can indicate airflow restriction

Secondary data

Pulmonary function tests

Pulmonary function testing is a useful adjunct to clinical assessment. Static lung volumes such as total lung capacity (TLC), residual volume (RV) and functional residual capacity (FRC), and dynamic lung volumes such as forced vital capacity (FVC) and forced expiratory volume in 1 s (FEV_1) can be measured. However, these require specialist equipment, which may not always be readily available in the acute setting. Changes in pulmonary function in the older person are related to musculoskeletal changes of the chest wall and changes in elastic recoil (Camhi & Enright 2000). Baseline assessment of these data may be useful to determine changes in any chronic condition over time.

Although TLC remains essentially unchanged in the older person, some of its components alter, for example, FRC increases as elastic recoil decreases (Camhi & Enright 2000). They may also present with increased RV, particularly if diagnosed with emphysema and/or chronic bronchitis (Camhi & Enright 2000, Epstein et al. 2000). In both restrictive and obstructive diseases, FVC and FEV_1 are reduced, the difference lying in the amount of RV, and the ratio between FVC and FEV_1, described as $FEV_1\%$ (Epstein et al. 2000).

Peak expiratory flow rate

The measurement of peak flow is a useful guide to dynamic lung function in the more acute setting, and serial measurements are used to diagnose and monitor asthma (Epstein et al. 2000), and to evaluate the effect of therapies such as nebulized salbutamol. The British Thoracic Society (BTS) guidelines insist its use on all asthmatics, and it may also be indicated for other patient groups (British Thoracic Society 2003). Peak expiratory flow rate (PEFR) or peak flow, as it is commonly termed, is the flow generated in the first 0.1 s of a forced expiration; the resulting figure is then extrapolated over a minute. Results indicate the degree of airway resistance, with reducing volumes being achieved as the condition deteriorates. Three readings should be taken, with the patient standing or sitting well upright where possible as this increases inspiratory capacity, and the same device should be used for successive readings as different peak flow meters can give different readings (British Thoracic Society 2003).

Pulse oximetry

The use of the pulse oximeter in clinical practice has become widespread over recent years, providing a useful non-invasive method of estimating peripheral oxygen delivery. Normal readings are cited by most authors to be > 95% (Hough 1996, Hogsten & Switzer 2001). However, patients with chronic respiratory conditions such as COPD may have a lower normal baseline due to changes in chemoreceptor activity. Cyanosis is not normally visible unless oxygen saturation drops below 75% (Hanning & Alexander-Williams 1995). The main function of the pulse oximeter is to facilitate the early detection of hypoxaemia before it can be seen clinically (Lowton 1999). The pulse oximeter estimates oxygen delivery by measuring the saturation of peripheral Hb with oxygen and expressing this as a percentage (SpO_2). It is important therefore to ensure that the person has an adequate Hb before accepting the result as being valid. The probe should be applied to a warm, well-perfused digit or to the nose or earlobe, and the area should not be under direct sunlight as this may affect readings. Heavy nail varnish will also obscure the light penetrating through the nailbed. It is sensible to avoid using the dominant hand, which is more likely to be moved, as motion has been shown to affect readings (Barker & Shah 1997). Roffe et al. (2001) provided reassurance in their study that oximeters can be applied to either side in a patient with hemiparetic stroke. However, a hand with a tremor will affect readings, and so patients with problems including Parkinson's disease or muscle tremor may be better with the probe placed upon the earlobe, which is less likely to be affected by motion artefact or vasoconstrictive effects (Awad et al. 2001).

Most studies have demonstrated earlier detection of hypoxaemia in patients with whom a pulse oximeter was used (Moller et al. 1993), but there remains little evidence that this translates into improved outcome (Hess & Medoff 1999). However, the pulse oximeter has been shown to be a useful adjunct to clinical respiratory assessment when used properly. Kaye et al. (2002), for example, performed a case-control study in a group of nursing-home residents. Their study suggested that in this population a decrease in oxygen saturation of > 3% from the baseline or a saturation of < 94% suggested the presence of pneumonia (Kaye et al. 2002). However, the accuracy of the pulse oximeter is also dependent on a skilled user. For example, a survey of house officers and nurses in 1993 revealed that many lacked knowledge of the basic principles, and made serious errors in interpreting the data (Stoneham et al. 1994). The SpO_2 should always be interpreted in light of the clinical picture, and the degree of oxygen therapy being received.

The most important thing to remember about pulse oximeters is that they do not measure the adequacy of ventilation or lung performance, only peripheral oxygenation (Lowton 1999). Therefore, it is not possible to assess carbon dioxide elimination with a pulse oximeter. An increase in carbon dioxide may be present in a patient with a chest infection, for example, when the metabolic rate and thus production of carbon dioxide is increased, but the patient is unable to increase the rate and depth of breathing to exhale the increased production. In such a patient, capnography or an ABG would be necessary to evaluate the patient's condition fully.

Arterial blood gases

ABG analysis is considered to be the gold standard for evaluating gas exchange (Hess & Medoff 1999), and its use is indicated in any patient with severely deteriorating respiratory or haemodynamic function. It may also be used in order to obtain a baseline for patients prior to surgery where a chronic condition might indicate potentially varied values from normal. Blood gas analysis provides information regarding the partial pressure of oxygen (Pao_2), carbon dioxide ($Paco_2$), and the presence of acid–base disturbances by evaluating the blood pH (normal range 7.36–7.44). The normal Pao_2 is considered to be > 12 kPa and $Paco_2$ 4.7–6.0 kPa on room air (Driscoll et al. 1997). Patients with chronic conditions such as COPD may need to have ABG analysis performed frequently in order to evaluate their condition, and thus the use of capillary sampling from the earlobe is becoming increasingly common in some areas. This method is preferred to sampling from an artery due to the reduction in risk factors associated with the procedure and the fact that specialist nursing staff may therefore be able to undertake this procedure, ensuring that patients receive effective treatment as quickly as possible. Murphy (2001) undertook a review of the use of this method in COPD patients from 1996 to 2000 and found only four pieces of research (Langlands & Wallace 1965, Begin et al. 1975, Pitkin et al. 1994, Dar et al. 1995). From this review it was concluded that properly taken capillary samples accurately reflect ABG measures of Pao_2, $Paco_2$ and pH (Murphy 2001).

If a patient has a blood-gas sample taken, it is important to ensure that a heparinized syringe is used, all air bubbles are expelled from the syringe, the sample is processed as quickly as possible, and that the site (if arterial) has firm pressure applied for at least 5 min after sampling. This is particularly important if a large artery, such as the femoral artery, is used or if the patient has known blood-clotting problems. As with any other method, it is again important to evaluate results in light of any therapy, such as oxygen, being received by the patient, and the patient's normal baseline.

Radiography

Many older patients will need to have a CXR taken at some point, perhaps as part of a preoperative respira-

tory assessment or to evaluate the progress of an ongoing or acute condition. A CXR can offer information regarding both local and diffuse problems, for example, local consolidation due to a tumour or infection, or diffuse shadowing due to the presence of fluid in the lungs (pulmonary oedema). A CXR can also provide information regarding rib fractures, position of the diaphragm, size of the thoracic cage and the amount of functioning lung present (Epstein et al. 2000). In most cases, patients will have CXRs performed in the radiography department of a hospital, but in some circumstances, mobile equipment can be used to go to the patient. All CXRs should be reviewed and reported upon by a radiologist who has specialist training in the technique. Some patients may also have other radiographic investigations (e.g. ventilation–perfusion (V/Q) scans, ultrasounds) for certain conditions, which may require specific preparation and aftercare. It is always important therefore to explain to the patient fully what to expect, and to be aware of any particular side-effects, such as allergic reactions to dyes, that will need to be looked for following the procedure.

NURSING INTERVENTIONS FOR THE OLDER PERSON WITH BREATHING DIFFICULTIES

Airway management

In some cases breathing difficulties may be due to a partial or complete obstruction of the airway. This could be caused by unconsciousness due to a cerebrovascular accident (CVA), post anaesthetic or to airway obstruction from foreign objects or the presence of a tumour. In such circumstances, airway manoeuvres and/or adjuncts may be required.

The most basic method of opening the airway is to ensure proper positioning of the head and neck. Often, a simple chin lift may be adequate to remove signs of obstruction such as snoring, and ease any dyspnoea that may have been evident. Such patients should also be nursed in a lateral position to prevent the tongue from falling back and to protect the airway from aspiration in the case of vomiting.

Positioning may need to be combined with the use of an oropharyngeal airway in some patients where no gag reflex is present to maintain an open airway and to provide a route for oropharyngeal suction. This device (sometimes referred to as a Guedel airway) prevents the tongue from falling back and obstructing the airway, but does not protect from gastric aspiration, and thus again the patient should be positioned laterally. Oropharyngeal airways come in sizes 2, 3 and 4 and before insertion should be sized to correspond to the vertical distance between the patient's incisors and the angle of the jaw (Jevon & Pooni 2001, Resuscitation Council UK 2002). Care should be undertaken to avoid damage to the hard palate, and the airway should be inserted in an upside-down position, before rotating 180° when the soft palate is reached. It should then be further inserted until it lies in the oropharnynx. This reduces the risk of the tongue being pushed back, causing further obstruction. The flat portion of the airway should fit snugly against the patient's teeth (or gums if edentulous), and following insertion, patency of the airway should be rechecked (Resuscitation Council UK 2002).

Nasopharyngeal airways may be used to facilitate the removal of secretions from the patient who has an inadequate cough, and are better tolerated by the semiconscious or awake patient. They are also useful as an airway adjunct for patients with trismus (lock jaw) or maxillofacial injuries, although they are contraindicated in any patient with a suspected basal skull fracture (Resuscitation Council UK 2002), and should be used with caution in a patient with any history of bleeding or epistaxis (nose bleeds). Adult sizes are 6–7 mm in diameter and are often measured by the diameter of the patient's little finger. Before insertion the tube should be lubricated and the right nostril should be checked for patency; this is the nostril recommended by the Resuscitation Council UK (2002). Some makes of airway also have a safety pin, which needs to be placed at the flange end before insertion to prevent the airway disappearing beyond the nasal flares (Resuscitation Council UK 2002). The airway should be directed towards the patient's feet, with the bevelled end inserted first, using a slight twisting action (Resuscitation Council UK 2002). If it is not possible to pass the airway through the right nostril, the left nostril may be used. As with the oropharyngeal airway, patency should be checked following insertion. In addition, consideration needs to be given to discomfort, which might be experienced by the more awake patient.

A *tracheostomy* is an opening in the wall of the trachea, below the cricoid cartilage. With the increase in critical care facilities and the growing population of older persons, many older patients may be found with either permanent or temporary tracheostomy tubes in place, either in the hospital or community environment. Most tracheostomies are temporary following respiratory failure and weaning from mechanical ventilation or following trauma when there has been a potential risk to the airway (Docherty & Bench 2002). Nursing a patient with a tracheosotomy requires vigilance and a good level of knowledge and skill to prevent complications such as obstruction, which could lead to a respiratory arrest. For a full discussion of the care required by such patients, please refer to review articles such as Docherty & Bench (2002) or Woodrow (2002a). The key aspects of management are based on the maintenance of adequate tube patency, with the use of humidification, suctioning and cleaning of the inner tube on a regular basis. Vigilance for signs of respiratory distress is required and should be reported immediately. Any patient with a tracheostomy should have emergency equipment available nearby, including spare tracheostomy tubes, tracheal dilators and equipment for manual ventilation (ambu-bag) and suctioning. It should also be remembered that such patients may be highly anxious about the presence of a tracheostomy tube, which can also hinder their ability to speak, and so psychological support and reassurance are vital parts of care.

In an emergency situation (e.g. cardiac arrest), the use of an endotracheal tube may be required to provide a secure airway for ventilation. Such patients will then usually be transferred to a critical care unit. Insertion of such devices is the responsibility of a trained anaesthetist, but nurses may be required to assist with the procedure. Familiarity with the equipment required for such a procedure is important to facilitate a smooth intubation process. Nurses should check the equipment found on the emergency trolley with this in mind. Following extubation, close monitoring of respiratory status is required.

Removal of secretions

In the older person, the cough reflex may not be very effective, making the removal of secretions difficult. Patients with COPD may have copious secretions, which may prove difficult to expectorate. Nurses should work with the physiotherapist, assisting the patient with coughing and deep breathing. The patient should be shown how to inspire deeply, pause, and then cough forcibly to expel secretions. This manoeuvre may be too exhausting, in which case the patient is encouraged to take deep breaths on inspiration and long exhalations. This may move secretions sufficiently to stimulate a cough reflex. The patient may also be taught how to breathe through pursed lips, which increases pressure in the lungs during expiration and prolongs the period for gas exchange. This increases intrinsic positive end-expiratory pressure (PEEP) and arterial oxygen tension (Pa_{O_2}).

Expectoration may be perceived as an antisocial activity. The patient can be given assistance by providing sputum pots and tissues and by recognizing the importance of clearing secretions. An upright posture, either in bed or chair, can be achieved by careful positioning of pillows to allow support and full chest expansion, thus permitting maximum ventilation. Positioning may be especially important when osteoporosis has resulted in kyphosis. The patient may find it easier to manage lung expansion by leaning over a cushioned table (the orthopnoeic position). Careful attention should be paid to the patient's hydration status, as dehydration will make the secretions more sticky, tenacious and difficult to expectorate. Caution should also be taken to prevent cross-infection through expectoration, in view of the increasing incidence of TB and other respiratory pathogens.

If secretions cannot be expectorated, it may be necessary to use oropharyngeal or nasopharyngeal suction. However, the procedure has been identified as potentially hazardous, with many associated risks and complications. These range from hypoxaemia (Adlkofer & Powaser 1978) to cardiac dysrhythmias (Stone et al. 1991a), trauma (Czarnik et al. 1991) and even cardiac arrest and death (Fiorentini 1992, Raymond 1995).

In view of such hazards, there is an increasing body of evidence to suggest how and when suctioning should be performed (Table 15.3). However, in spite of the available evidence, clear guidelines and protocols are often lacking in the practice setting. Moreover, suctioning appears to be performed on an individual basis with varying techniques and with little reference to research (Day et al. 2001, 2002). If the patient requires suctioning to remove secretions, a full explanation, together with possible pain relief, should be given in order to minimize the potential traumatic effects. This is especially important, as suctioning has been associated with feelings of choking and loss of breath (Bergbom-Engberg & Haljamae 1989). Case study 15.1 describes a patient who required suctioning.

An alternative way to help with the removal of secretions is the use of mucolytic agents. Until recently, the effectiveness of these drugs had been questioned, and some clinicians have suggested that nebulized saline or water is equally effective. However, research by Gallon (1996) demonstrated that sputum viscosity was reduced and expectoration increased by the administration of nebulized N-acetylcysteine. There were also associated improvements in oxygen saturation levels. Nebulized normal saline,

Table 15.3 Summary of recommended practice for tracheal suctioning

Action	Recommended practice
Assessment	Undertake a respiratory assessment, including auscultation (Glass & Grap 1995, Griggs 1998)
Patient preparation	Provide an appropriate explanation, sedation and pain relief in order to reduce pain and anxiety (Peruzzi & Smith 1995, Wood 1998a)
Preoxygenation	Preoxygenate with 100% oxygen to reduce risk of cardiac dysrhythmias (Stone at al. 1991b) and hypotension (Wood 1998a). Preoxygenate with 20% above baseline in patients with chronic obstructive pulmonary disease (Rogge et al. 1989)
Infection control	Wash hands before and after suctioning; wear gloves and goggles during suctioning (Wood 1998a, Parker 1999a, 1999b, Pratt et al. 2001)
Catheter selection	Use the correct size of suction catheters to prevent trauma (Young 1984). Calculate using the formula: size of tracheostomy tube − 2 × 2 (Odell et al. 1993)
Depth of catheter insertion	Insert the catheter to the carina and then withdraw 1 cm before applying suction (Dean 1997, Wood 1998a)
Negative pressure	Negative pressure should be between 80 and 150 mmHg or 10.6–20 kPa (Boggs 1993, Luce et al. 1993). Suction should only be applied during withdrawal and should be continuous (Glass & Grap 1995)
Duration of suction	Take no longer than 10–15 s to suction to minimize the risk of hypoxaemia and trauma (Boggs 1993)
Number of passes	Limit the number of suction passes to three during one episode (Wood 1998a)
Reconnection to oxygen therapy	Reconnect the patient to oxygen within 10 s post-suctioning to minimize the risk of hypoxaemia (Adam & Osbourne 1997, Day 2000)
Assessment	Undertake an assessment (including auscultation) post-suctioning (Glass & Grap 1995, Day 2000)
Reduction of stress and anxiety	Provide reassurance to the patient after suctioning to minimize stress and anxiety
Reduction of oxygen	Ensure that the level of inspired oxygen is returned to presuctioning parameters to prevent oxygen toxicity (Pierce 1995)

Case study 15.1

Mrs Lillian Harvey, a 72-year-old woman, is in the ward following a laryngectomy. She has a tracheostomy tube in place and has been reluctant to mobilize since her operation 3 days ago. Upon assessment, the following was noted:
- respiratory rate increased from 26 to 34 breaths/min
- an increased use of accessory muscles
- restlessness and sweaty appearance
- Spo_2 reduced from 96% to 91% on 40% oxygen
- noisy breath sounds upon auscultation.

This picture indicated the need for tracheal suctioning, which was performed using a clean technique (Table 15.2). Ignoring such assessment findings could result in tracheostomy tube occlusion, deteriorating respiratory status and possible respiratory arrest. Prior to and during suctioning, the nurse explains and reassures Mrs Harvey about the procedure to ensure compliance and limit the possibility of distress and further complications. During the procedure, the nurse evaluates its effectiveness and considers whether further intervention is required.

When the suctioning is finished, the nurse reapplies Mrs Harvey's oxygen therapy at the prescribed level and helps her into an upright position to enhance chest expansion. The nurse and physiotherapist encourage her to do deep breathing exercises and to mobilize. The nurse documents all events precisely and discusses with her nursing and physiotherapy colleagues any concerns she has about Mrs Harvey's ability to manage her secretions. If Mrs Harvey's condition does not improve following suction, her oxygen therapy may need to be increased and further investigations undertaken, such as an arterial blood-gas analysis and chest X-ray, under the direction of her medical team.

---

however, had no such effects. Nebulized N-acetylcysteine is now commonly used in patients with cystic fibrosis to aid secretion removal.

The effectiveness of mucolytic agents has recently been reviewed in a meta-analysis by the Cochrane Collaboration and shown to produce a statistically significant reduction in the number of acute exacerbations of chronic bronchitis (Grandjean et al. 2000, Poole & Black 2000). However, whilst these results are indeed encouraging, the studies are of a short duration (2–6 months) and in patients with mild COPD. Mac-Nee & Calverley (2003) argue that the routine use of mucolytic agents in COPD is not yet recommended.

Humidification

The humidification of inspired gases may be necessary if any part of the patient's airway has been bypassed (for example, in a patient with a tracheostomy) or in conjunction with respiratory support. Humidification will assist with clearing thick tenacious secretions and prevent drying of mucosa and cilia (Adam & Osborne 2001). Hot-water humidification provides a greater level of humidity than cold-water systems. However, this method is not without complications, as it has been associated with higher levels of infection and has the potential to overheat and overhydrate (Thomacot et al. 1998). Heat moisture exchangers (HME) are an alternative method. HMEs function by transferring heat and moisture from the patient's exhaled breath to a filter. Heat and moisture are then transferred to the

inhaled gas during inspiration (Adam & Osborne 2001). HMEs can also be used with non-invasive ventilation (NIV).

Administration of nebulizers

Prevention and relief of symptoms are central to managing the patient with breathlessness, and bronchodilators are the key agents. The major benefit of bronchodilator therapy is to improve lung-emptying during expiration and to reduce hyperinflation (Belman et al. 1996). However, the degree to which this occurs is not easy to predict (Hay et al. 1992). MacNee & Calverley (2003) argue that the best way to assess the effectiveness of bronchodilators is to ask patients simple questions about their symptoms.

For the older person, nebulizers may be used both in hospital and also at home. A nebulizer converts a drug in solution to a fine mist for inhalation, and can be driven by either air or oxygen via a mask or mouthpiece. The choice of beta-agonists, anticholinergic drugs, theophylline or combination therapy will depend on the individual response. However, improvements are often found by combining agents (MacNee & Calverley 2003). Moreover, the availability of longer-acting inhaled beta-agonists, such as salmeterol and formoterol, may be of particular benefit to the older person, as they have a duration of action of up to 12 h and can significantly improve symptoms, exercise capacity and health status (Ulrik 1995, Boyd et al. 1997).

Corticosteroid therapy may also be given through nebulizers, as an anti-inflammatory agent. However, their effects in asthma and COPD remain controversial (Keatings et al. 1997, Confalonieri et al. 1998). The bronchodilator should always be given first and time allowed for it to take effect (5–10 min) so that when the corticosteroid is inhaled it is delivered to the bronchioles, where its anti-inflammatory effects are required. After using the nebulizer it is advisable to wash the patient's face to prevent skin irritation. It is also advisable to rinse the mouth after steroid inhalation to avoid the risk of oral candidiasis (Cowan 1996).

If patients are going to be discharged home with a nebulizer it is essential that they are given specific information regarding the number of inhalations per day, instructions on how to prepare the nebulizer and how to clean and care for the equipment. Written instructions should also be provided and help should be available through community nurses and general practitioners, who are ideally placed to provide appropriate advice and assistance.

Alternatively, patients may be discharged home with an MDI. Unlike nebulizers, these require a greater level of coordination for effective use. Jarrett's study (1988) demonstrated that up to 89% of people of all ages were unable to use MDIs correctly, and that even after appropriate teaching 30% were still unable to coordinate their use. In the older person with chronic respiratory weakness and/or arthritis, this may make MDIs impossible to use. To make this as easy as possible, time should be taken to teach them how to use the inhaler. For some patients, the use of a device attached to the MDI which allows the medication to be held in the chamber long enough for inhalation over a number of breaths (spacer device) may be more appropriate. This eliminates the need to coordinate triggering the MDI with inspiration and so may be the best option (Connolly 1995).

RESPIRATORY THERAPIES

Oxygen therapy

Oxygen is probably one of the most common drugs given to patients both within the hospital and in the community setting. The indications for its use are to treat or prevent hypoxaemia. Although the administration of oxygen may be life-saving, it is not without risks and these should be considered at all times (Howell 2001). Guidance on the short- and long-term administration of oxygen is available in the *British National Formulary* (British Medical Association/Royal Pharmaceutical Society of Great Britain 2003). Particular attention should be paid to the risks associated with

smoking, and the need for the amount of oxygen therapy to be prescribed. (Case study 15.2 gives details of a patient with COPD.) Patients who have COPD with carbon dioxide retention should not normally be administered high percentages of oxygen (> 24–28%) as this may cause their respiratory drive to be affected (British Medical Association/Royal Pharmaceutical Society of Great Britain 2003), although this traditional approach to oxygen therapy in such patients has recently been challenged (Gomershall et al. 2002). Similarly, high flow rates of administered oxygen are said to cause hypercarbia to become worse (Chien et al. 2000). Oxygen at higher concentrations given over prolonged periods of time can also be toxic to the cells of the respiratory tract and alveoli, causing possible irreversible damage. Thus, the smallest amount of oxygen necessary to maintain an adequate PaO_2 should be given for the shortest period of time possible (Howell 2001). This means that the patient on oxygen therapy needs to be regularly evaluated using clinical assessment, SpO_2, ABG analysis and other available tools.

Oxygen may be administered using a variety of different devices of both fixed and variable rate. Nasal cannulae are suitable for low-flow oxygen rates (up to approximately 6 l/min), or for short-term use to enable a dyspnoeic patient to remove the facemask whilst eating or talking. Nasal cannulae may also be useful for the confused patient who is unable to tolerate a facemask. However, caution should be applied if the patient breathes through the mouth as nasal cannulae will be of limited benefit. Simple facemasks may be more useful in the acute situation. Both nasal cannulae and simple facemasks are termed low-flow devices or variable-performance devices as the amount of oxygen delivered to the patient may be variable because it is affected by the patient's own breathing depth and rate. Documentation should state the flow in l/min but the percentage of oxygen cannot be accurately calculated. Fixed performance systems such as the Venturi system or high-humidity device are not dependent on the minute volume of the patient and thus the percentage of oxygen delivered to the patient using these systems can be determined accurately so long as the correct flow of oxygen is set at the oxygen flowmeter. There are also some devices that allow up to 100% oxygen to be delivered by a system of rebreathing expired gas, which is housed in a reservoir bag beneath the mask. These systems are commonly referred to as 100% masks or reservoir masks, and are useful in the acute setting.

The patient who is receiving oxygen therapy for long periods of time may find masks claustrophobic. Alternatively, feeling unable to breathe may make the patient highly anxious and dependent on the mask, and then unwilling to remove it for any reason. Close

---

Case study 15.2

Mr Patrick O'Reilly, a retired 87-year-old builder, is admitted from a residential home with an acute onset of respiratory distress. He was diagnosed with chronic obstructive pulmonary disease 15 years ago and continues to smoke 30 cigarettes a day. He is normally unable to walk more than 20 m without becoming breathless and has required hospital admission three times over the past year. He is prescribed 24% oxygen, 4-hourly Salbutamol and Atrovent nebulizers, and steroid therapy. A sputum pot is provided and a specimen is collected for microbiological assay. He is also referred for chest physiotherapy. Following nursing assessment, the following priorities are identified:

- psychological support and reassurance to alleviate fears regarding his condition and inability to breathe, and an awareness of the effects of a change in environment to the older person
- positioning to enhance chest expansion and the ability to cough and clear secretions
- assistance with activities of daily living (e.g. hygiene, mobilization, nutrition, sleep) taking account of his level of dyspnoea and oxygen therapy
- ensuring nebulizers and oxygen therapy are delivered according to the prescription, assembled correctly and appropriately humidified. Mr O'Reilly must be informed of the dangers of smoking whilst receiving oxygen and steps taken to ensure that the therapy is tolerable (e.g. mouth and eye care)
- ongoing assessment and monitoring of clinical observations, noting the importance of an increase in respiratory rate over time and ensuring data are interpreted according to Mr O'Reilly's normal parameters.

Two weeks later, Mr O'Reilly's condition has improved sufficiently for him to be discharged back to the residential home. Before this, the following issues are considered:

- rehabilitation programme to increase respiratory muscle strength and level of mobility
- assessment of most appropriate inhaler device for Mr O'Reilly and teaching him how to use it correctly
- follow-up appointment at chest clinic and associated transport arrangements
- future medical management of Mr O'Reilly's condition
- discussion of potential lifestyle changes that might reduce recurrence of acute illness (e.g. nutritional advice to enhance immune function and smoking reduction).

---

attention needs to be paid to good psychological care, ensuring effective communication between the nurse and the patient, and the development of a trusting and supportive relationship. Negotiation may be necessary to achieve an optimal outcome in such situations. Oxygen is also a dry gas, which is likely to dry the mucous membranes of the oro/nasopharynx, and thus attention needs to be given to adequate humidification and frequent oral hygiene or drinks. Eyes too are at risk of drying, particularly if masks are incorrectly fitting, and so attention should be given to ophthalmic care. Oxygen equipment should be changed regularly, labelled with the patient's details, and kept clean and dry to prevent infection and discomfort. This may be a particular problem with humidification systems fitted into the circuit, which can cause accumulation of water in the tubing, thus making it more difficult for the patient to breathe through.

Long-term oxygen therapy (LTOT)

LTOT improves pulmonary function in patients with COPD and lengthens survival in patients with COPD and other chronic respiratory conditions (Tarrega et al. 2002).

It is advisable for all patients to be assessed by a respiratory physician prior to its use. Guidelines from the British Thoracic Society (1997) suggest that patients with COPD who have a PaO_2 of <7.3kPa, with or without hypercapnia, and an FEV_1 of < 1.5 l should receive LTOT, and that it should be administered for at least 15 h/day to achieve maximum benefit (British Thoracic Society 1997). When home oxygen is arranged, the type of facility (concentrator and/or portable oxygen) and the recommended flow rate should be recorded. Three systems are currently available (gas cylinders, liquid oxygen systems and oxygen concentrators; Kacmarek 2000). A concentrator with nasal prongs is recommended as the best method of delivery, with the flow rate set at 2–4 l/min (British Thoracic Society 1997). With these systems air is drawn into the unit through a filter and compressed. Room air is then separated into oxygen and nitrogen plus trace gases. The concentrated oxygen is stored in a small cylinder for delivery to a flow meter. Oxygen concentrators are able to deliver oxygen concentrations of up to 95% depending on the flow rate set (Kacmarek 2000).

LTOT can be very restricting for patients, which in turn can further affect both their physiological and psychological state. Portable systems may be considered for some patients, and development of technology which allows systems that are both light-weight and compact, and capable of providing oxygen for extended periods, is ongoing (Kacmarek 2000). Some patients may use extension tubing to increase mobility. Tubing up to 15 m (50 ft) can maintain accurate flow rates, but a second unit may be required in some cases (McInturff & Dunne 1998). Nursing considerations with LTOT are similar to those with in-hospital oxygen administration. It is generally recommended however, that humidification is unnecessary with nasal cannulae if the flow rate is < 5 l/min (American Association for Respiratory Care 1992). If humidifiers are used they should be washed in soapy water and dried twice weekly (Findeisen 2001). The use of cannulae may cause soreness around the nasal cavity. Patients should be advised to use only water-based lubricants, as petroleum can increase the risk of combustion in the presence of oxygen (Findeisen 2001). Education regarding fire hazards when using oxygen in the home is important, and smoking must cease before LTOT is offered. Patients must understand why they are having the therapy, how the equipment functions, how to care for it and what to do if there are problems. Follow-up and reassessment for all patients on LTOT at regular periods are vital, as studies have highlighted a number of problems associated with the use of LTOT (British Thoracic Society 1997). Assessment should involve regular ABG analysis (British Thoracic Society 1997). However, if a patient is receiving nocturnal therapy, daytime ABGs have been shown not to correlate with nighttime gas exchange (Tarrega et al. 2002). ABG analysis should therefore be performed at 07.00 h in order to determine appropriate settings for night-time therapy (Tarrega et al. 2002).

Non-invasive ventilation

Over the past decade, NIV has become an important treatment option for patients with severe breathing difficulties (British Thoracic Society 1997, Bach et al. 2001, Jolliet et al. 2001). For the older person with COPD, who may not previously have been considered suitable for invasive ventilation, this has been shown to improve survival significantly (Plant et al. 2001). NIV is a global term that encompasses a number of respiratory therapies, including continuous positive airway pressure (CPAP) and non-invasive positive-pressure ventilation (NIPPV).

Continuous positive airway pressure

For some patients, oxygenation is not improved through oxygen therapy alone, and the use of CPAP can be of great benefit. CPAP increases the volume of

Table 15.4 Continuous positive airway pressure (CPAP)

Indications for CPAP	Possible applications
Hypoxic respiratory failure (type 1)	Acute left ventricular failure
Atelectasis/low lung volumes	*Pneumocystis carinii* pneumonia (PCP)
Increased work of breathing	Acute lung injury
	Pulmonary oedema
	Asthma
	Obstructive sleep apnoea

gas in the lungs at the end of quiet respiration (i.e. the FRC). This will increase compliance and help to correct any ventilation–perfusion mismatch (Bassett & Makin 2000). The indications for CPAP are outlined in Table 15.4.

The application of CPAP involves using a tightly fitting mask, which some patients find claustrophobic and uncomfortable (Fig. 15.1). In addition, the constant high-flow gas can be difficult to tolerate, and CPAP is therefore only suitable for patients who are alert and able to maintain their own airway and clear their own secretions (Bassett & Makin 2000). Setting up CPAP requires skill and expertise. CPAP can either be delivered by continuous or demand flow systems:

- *Continuous flow* systems use a continuous flow of gas throughout the respiratory cycle and are very noisy, which can interfere with the sleep and rest of all other patients in close proximity.
- *Demand flow* systems are only triggered at the start of inspiration. However, whilst these systems are indeed quieter and more economical, they do create additional respiratory effort and may therefore be unsuitable for many patients.

The type of valve attached determines the amount of CPAP delivered. Many patients are started on a fairly low level of CPAP, such as 2.5 or 5.0 cm H_2O. These are easier to tolerate but may not increase the FRC sufficiently to improve oxygenation. Higher levels of CPAP can be used, such as 7.5 or 10.0 cm H_2O, although this can in itself cause problems and increases the risk of barotrauma (pressure damage). Attention needs to be paid to the risks of circuit blockage, which would be recognized by an increase in airway pressure and obvious distress in the patient. This should be rectified immediately to prevent the occurrence of barotrauma.

Non-invasive positive-pressure ventilation

NIPPV can be used as an alternative to intubation and mechanical ventilation in patients with type 2

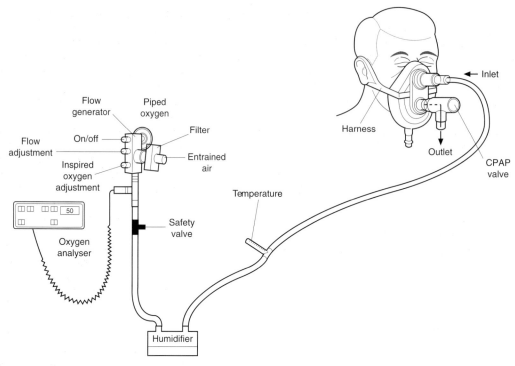

Fig. 15.1   Patient with continuous positive airway pressure (CPAP) circuit.

(ventilatory) respiratory failure (Doherty & Green-stone 2000). NIPPV augments alveolar ventilation by positive-pressure ventilation without the need for an endotracheal tube. Biphasic positive-pressure ventila-tion (BiPAP) is one type of NIPPV, and is now so widely used it is becoming the main mode of NIV in the acute-care setting (British Thoracic Society 2002, Woodrow 2002b). Woodrow (2002b) describes BiPAP as being similar to two alternating pressures of CPAP: a higher one is set during inspiration (inspiratory pos-itive airway pressure, IPAP) and a lower pressure dur-ing expiration (expired positive airway pressure, EPAP). Levels of IPAP and EPAP should be set accord-ing to prescribed parameters based upon the patient's condition and assessment data. The indications for NIPPV/BiPAP as identified by the British Thoracic Society (2002) are outlined in Box 15.1.

The British Thoracic Society (2002) also recom-mends that NIPPV should be used as a holding meas-ure, with a view to intubation if unsuccessful, and as a maximum level of treatment for patients who are not candidates for intubation and invasive ventilation. For the older person, the latter may indeed apply, as it may not always be appropriate to admit the patient to an intensive care unit.

Setting up NIPPV also requires skill and expertise, and there are potential problems. The British Thoracic

***

Box 15.1   Indications for non-invasive positive-pressure ventilation and biphasic positive-pressure ventilation

Patients with chronic obstructive pulmonary disease
Hypercapnoea: $Paco_2 > 6.5$ kPa
Hypoxaemia: $Pao_2 < 8$ kPa
Respiratory acidosis: pH < 7.30

***

Society (2002) recommends that a 24-h service should be available for NIV. However, it is not clear who should lead this service. Physiotherapists are often the experts in this field and commonly initiate treatment.

Nasal or full-face masks can be used. A nasal mask may be more comfortable and easier to tolerate, and can facilitate communication. However, they cannot be used if the patient is mouth-breathing. Another advantage of NIPPV is that the ventilator is able to deliver additional predetermined breaths should the patient become hypoxic or apnoeic. Because of the sys-tem back-up and the comfortable masks, this method of treatment is often well tolerated for relatively long periods of time. Patients can also be discharged home with NIPPV as long as there is appropriate support in the community.

Both CPAP and NIPPV can be extremely frightening for the patient, and it should not be forgotten that many patients are also confused as a result of the associated hypoxia. It can take up to 20 or 30 min for the physiological effects of CPAP and NIPPV to take place at an alveolar level. It is therefore important that treatment, once started, is not stopped abruptly and that care is grouped together to accommodate these factors. An ABG should be taken 1 h after starting treatment to assess and monitor the effects on oxygenation and acid–base balance.

In view of the complex issues associated with caring for the older person receiving NIV, it is essential that nurses have a good understanding of the key issues and nursing interventions required. Frequently, it is more appropriate for the patient to be nursed in a high-dependency unit for closer assessment and monitoring. A more detailed discussion of NIV can be found in Woodrow (2002b).

Monitoring and evaluating the effectiveness of respiratory therapies

Place (1997) suggests that the success of CPAP can be assessed by observing improvements in oxygenation (i.e. through ABG analysis or pulse oximetry), a reduction in respiratory rate, an increase in tidal volume and reduced work of breathing. This also applies to patients receiving oxygen therapy and/or NIV. The need for high levels of vigilance when caring for these patients cannot be overemphasized, as deterioration can be rapid, particularly in the older person who has less compensatory capacity. Patients receiving high levels of oxygen (greater than 50%) or NIV should not be left unattended. Observations of respiratory rate, depth and rhythm, level of consciousness and vital signs should be documented at frequent intervals and any deterioration should be reported immediately.

ASSOCIATED CARE ISSUES

Nutrition

Breathing difficulties may lead to insufficient intake of fluid and/or nutrition due to oxygen administration, open-mouth-breathing, an increased insensible loss with pyrexia, and the inability to eat and drink due to the level of dyspnoea experienced. All these factors will lead to secretions becoming more tenacious and difficult to expectorate, and thus may exacerbate any difficulties that might already be present. Adequate systemic hydration is therefore a priority and nurses should be vigilant in monitoring input and output. However, with conditions such as pulmonary oedema, fluid restriction may be required. Some patients, for example those with a tracheostomy in place, may also be `nil by mouth', and so strict attention should be given to ensuring the mouth remains moist by the provision of mouthwashes and toothbrushing. Those patients who have an irritating cough or unpleasant-tasting mouth may also obtain some relief from sipping warm drinks or sucking ice cubes, sweets or lozenges if appropriate. Referral or discussion with a speech and language therapist may be required before starting oral intake for some patients.

Nutritional requirements of the older person are different to those of younger people, with specific requirements for increased protein, some vitamins and calcium (Hegney 1997). These requirements may be further altered in the presence of breathing difficulties, thus requiring an appreciation of the special needs of the older person (Coutts 2001). For example, medical conditions and/or drug therapies can affect the absorption of nutrients (Hegney 1997). Malnutrition can increase the risk of pulmonary infection due to a decrease in respiratory muscle function (Holmes 1998). This may be compounded by the presence of foul-tasting sputum and hypoxia, which can also lead to anorexia and a disinclination to eat or drink. Weight loss has been shown to be a particularly important predictor of poor prognosis in COPD, and so attention should be given to its avoidance (Chapman-Novakofski 2001). Supplementary nutrition via either the enteral or parenteral route may be necessary as part of acute care requirements, and the importance of ensuring that the mouth, teeth and any dentures are kept in good condition cannot be overemphasized if malnutrition is to be avoided, thus helping to prevent the occurrence of chest infections, which could cause breathing difficulties. Small meals may be better tolerated by the patient with dyspnoea, and will help to prevent any abdominal distension, which could impede adequate lung expansion. Similarly, obesity needs to be addressed as this will increase the work of breathing and make any breathing difficulties worse. Therefore, health promotion plays an important part in the ongoing plan of care. More information on eating and drinking can be found in Chapter 16.

Sleep, rest and activity

The older person with breathing problems may find it increasingly difficult to maintain a balance between activity and rest. Lack of energy to perform even the simplest activity is often experienced. Rest is disturbed by dyspnoea, which is aggravated if the patient falls into an unsuitable position. Coughing can also disrupt sleep and rest. Regular position changes, to aid ventilation, prevent consolidation in the dependent areas of the lung, and for pressure area care will also disturb sleep.

There is little doubt that being unable to breathe, or fighting for breath, is one of the most frightening experiences for people of all ages. For the older person with chronic breathing difficulties, the fear of falling asleep and not waking is very real. This anxiety can turn a restful night into a time of terror. Hypnotics can rarely be used as they may cause respiratory depression. Alternative strategies need to be considered to aid patient comfort and provide reassurance. In the hospital setting, consideration should be given to the position of the patient within the ward. Some patients may find reassurance by being placed close to the nurse's station. Others may prefer a quieter place in the ward to allow them to sleep without disturbance. If sleep during the night is broken, patients may be encouraged to sleep and rest during the day. More information on sleep and rest in older people is available in Chapter 20.

In addition to ensuring sufficient sleep and rest, it is also essential to consider the importance of activity. The position of the patient is important, as a recumbent position will reduce the capacity for gas exchange and exacerbate any hypoxia, which could result in an acute confusional state and increase the risks to the patient. It is therefore important that early mobilization is achieved. Movement and exercise should be increased each day and planned with each individual patient.

An association between physical activity levels and hospital admission rates has also been demonstrated (Garcia-Aymerich et al. 2003). Furthermore, progression to a more comprehensive rehabilitation programme has been found to be beneficial for older patients with COPD (Couser et al. 1995).

SUMMARY

This chapter has highlighted the normal pathophysiological changes associated with breathing in the older person, and has discussed the process of respiratory assessment and management. The importance of treating each person individually and holistically is emphasized. In order to meet the needs of this patient group, nurses should ensure that they develop the knowledge and skills necessary to work with patients to achieve optimal goals for each individual.

Recommended reading

Bassett C, Makin L 2000 Caring for the seriously ill patient. Arnold, London

A good introductory text which focuses on acute respiratory management for all adult patients.

British Thoracic Society 1997 BTS guidelines for the management of chronic obstructive pulmonary disease. Thorax 52 (suppl. 5): S1–S28 and British Thoracic Society 2003 British guideline on the management of asthma. Thorax 58 (suppl. I).

These two guidelines produced by the British Thoracic Society provide useful information to practitioners caring for patients with chronic obstructive pulmonary disease and asthma.

Weilitz PB, Lueckenotte A 1995 Respiratory assessment of older adults: part I. Perspectives in Respiratory Nursing 6: 3–4

and

Weilitz PB, Lueckenotte A 1995 Respiratory assessment of older adults: part II. Perspectives in Respiratory Nursing 6: 1, 3–4

These papers focus on respiratory assessment in the older person. They cover anatomical and physiological changes and the process of undertaking a systematic assessment.

Woodrow P 2002 Managing patients with a tracheostomy in acute care. Nursing Standard 16: 39–48.

A comprehensive article which describes and discusses the care required by patients with a tracheostomy. The paper also addresses issues associated with humidification and suctioning and includes a useful self-assessment tool.

References

Adam S, Osborne S 1997 Critical care nursing: science and practice. Oxford University Press, Oxford

Adam SK, Osborne S 2001 Critical care nursing – science and practice. Oxford University Press, Oxford

Adlkofer R, Powaser M 1978 The effect of endotracheal suctioning on arterial blood gases in patients after cardiac surgery. Heart and Lung 7: 1011–1014

American Association for Respiratory Care (AARC) 1992 AARC clinical practice guideline. Oxygen therapy in the home or extended care facility. Respiratory Care 37: 918–922

Awad A, Ghobashy M, Ashraf M et al. 2001 Different responses of ear and finger pulse oximeter wave form to cold pressor test. Anesthesia and Analgesia 92: 1483–1486

Bach PBX, Brown C, Gelfand SE, McCrory DC 2001 Management of acute exacerbations of chronic obstructive pulmonary disease: a summary and appraisal of published evidence. Annals of Internal Medicine 134: 600–620

Barker S, Shah N 1997 The effects of motion on the performance of pulse oximeters in volunteers. Anesthesiology 86: 101–108

Bassett C, Makin L 2000 Caring for the seriously ill patient. Arnold, London

Begin R, Racine T, Roy JC 1975 Value of capillary blood gas analysis in the management of acute respiratory distress. American Review of Respiratory Diseases 112: 879–881

Belman M, Bornick W, Shin J 1996 Inhaled bronchodilators reduce dynamic hyperinflation during exercise in patient with chronic obstructive pulmonary disease. American Journal of Respiratory Critical Care Medicine 153: 967–975

Bergbom-Engberg I, Haljamae H 1989 A retrospective study of patients' recall of respiratory treatment: nursing care factors and feelings of security/insecurity. Intensive Care Nursing 4: 95–101

Boggs RL 1993 Airway management. In: Boggs RL, Woodridge-King M (eds) AACN procedure manual for critical care, 3rd edn. Philadelphia: WB Saunders

Boyd G, Morice A, Pounsford J 1997 An evaluation of salmeterol in the treatment of chronic obstructive pulmonary disease (COPD). European Respiratory Journal 10: 815–821

British Medical Association/Royal Pharmaceutical Society of Great Britain 2003 British national formulary 48. September 2004. British Medical Association/Royal Pharmaceutical Society of Great Britain. Available online at: www.bnf.org (accesssed 2 February 2005)

British Thoracic Society 1997 BTS guidelines for the management of chronic obstructive pulmonary disease. Thorax 52 (suppl. 5): S1–S28

British Thoracic Society 2002 Non-invasive ventilation in acute respiratory failure. Thorax 57: 192–211

British Thoracic Society 2003 British guideline on the management of asthma. Thorax 58 (2): (suppl. I): 95–188

Camhi SL, Enright PL 2000 How to assess pulmonary function in older persons. Journal of Respiratory Diseases 21: 395–399

Carola R, Harley J, Noback C 1992 Human anatomy and physiology. McGraw-Hill, New York

Chapman-Novakofski K 2001 Nutrition management in long-term care and home health: nutrition management of chronic obstructive pulmonary disease in older adults. Journal of Nutrition for the Elderly 20: 45–46

Chien JW, Ciufo R, Novak R et al. 2000 Uncontrolled oxygen administration and respiratory failure in acute asthma. Chest 117: 3

Confalonieri M, Mainardi E, Della P 1998 Inhaled corticosteroids reduce neutrophilic bronchial inflammation in patients with chronic obstructive pulmonary disease. Thorax 53: 583–585

Connolly M 1995 Inhaler technique of elderly patients: comparison of metered dose inhalers and large volume spacer devices. Age and Aging 24: 190–192

Couser J Jr, Glassroth J 1993 Tuberculosis: an epidemic in older adults. Clinics in Chest Medicine 14: 491–499

Couser J Jr, Guthmann R, Hamadeh MA, Kane CS 1995 Pulmonary rehabilitation improves exercise capacity in older elderly patients with COPD. Chest 107: 730–734

Coutts A 2001 Nutrition and the life cycle 5: nutritional needs of older adults. British Journal of Nursing 10: 603, 605–607

Cowan T 1996 Nebulisors for use in the community. Professional Nurse 12: 215–216, 218–220

Czarnik RE, Stone KS, Everhart CC Jr et al. 1991 Different effects of continuous versus intermittent suction on tracheal tissue. Heart and Lung 20: 144–151

Dar K, Williams T, Aitken R et al. 1995 Arterial versus capillary sampling for analysing blood gas pressures. British Medical Journal 310: 24–25

Day T (2000) Tracheal suctioning: when, why and how? Nursing Times 96: 13–15

Day TL, Wainwright S, Wilson-Barnett J 2001 An evaluation of a teaching intervention to improve the practice of endotracheal suctioning in intensive care units. Journal of Clinical Nursing 10: 682–696

Day TL, Farnell S, Haynes S et al. 2002 Tracheal suctioning: an exploration of nurses' knowledge and competence in acute and high dependency ward areas. Journal of Advanced Nursing 39: 35–45

Dean B 1997 Evidence based suction management in accident and emergency: a vital component of airway care. Accident and Emergency Nursing 5: 92–98

Docherty B, Bench S 2002 Tracheostomy management for patients in general ward settings. Professional Nurse 18: 100–104

Doherty M, Greenstone MA 2000 Non-invasive ventilation in acute exacerbations of chronic obstructive pulmonary disease (COPD): who is eligible? Care of the Critically Ill 16: 126–130

Driscoll P, Brown T, Gwinnutt C et al. 1997 A simple guide to blood gas analysis. British Medical Journal publishing group, London

Dunn C, Woodhouse J, Bhopal R et al. 1995 Asthma and factory emissions in northern England; addressing public concern by combining geographical and epidemiological methods. Journal of Epidemiology and Community Health 49: 395–400

Eliopoulos C 2001 Gerontological nursing, 5th edn. Lippincott, New York

Epstein O, Perkin G, de Bono D et al. 2000 Clinical examination, 2nd edn. Mosby, London

Findeisen M 2001 Long term oxygen therapy in the home. Home Healthcare Nurse 19: 692–699

Fiorentini A 1992 Potential hazards of tracheo-bronchial suctioning. Intensive and Critical Care Nursing 8: 217–226

Gallon AM 1996 Evaluation of nebulised acetylcysteine and normal saline in the treatment of sputum retention following a tracheostomy. Thorax 51: 429–432

Garcia-Aymerich J, Barreiro E, Farrero E 2000 Patients hospitalised for COPD have a higher prevalence of modifiable risk factors for exacerbation (EFRAM study). European Respiratory Journal 16: 1037–1042

Garcia-Aymerich J, Farrero E, Felez MA 2003 Risk factors of readmission to hospital for a COPD exacerbation: a prospective study. Thorax 58: 100–105

Glass C, Grap M 1995 Ten tips for safe suctioning. American Journal of Nursing 5: 51–53

Goldhill D, Worthington L, Mulcahy A et al. 1999 The patient at risk team: identifying and managing seriously ill ward patients. Anaesthesia 54: 853–860

Gomershall C, Joynt G, Freebairn R et al. 2002 Oxygen therapy for hypercapnic patients with chronic obstructive pulmonary disease and acute respiratory failure: a randomised, controlled pilot study. Critical Care Medicine 30: 113–116

Grandjean E, Berthet P, Ruffmann R 2000 Efficacy of oral long-term N-acetylcysteine in chronic bronchopulmonary disease: a meta-analysis of published double-blind, placebo controlled clinical trials. Clinical Therapy 22: 209–221

Griggs A 1998 Tracheostomy: suctioning and humidification. Nursing Standard 13: 49–53

Gross N 2001 The GOLD standard for chronic obstructive pulmonary disease. American Journal of Respiratory Critical Care Medicine 163: 1047–1048

Hanning CD, Alexander-Williams JM 1995 Pulse oximetry: a practical review. British Medical Journal 311: 367–370

Hay J, Stone P, Carter J, 1992 Bronchodilator reversibility, exercise performance and breathlessness in stable chronic obstructive pulmonary disease. European Respiratory Journal 5: 659–664

Hegney T 1997 Know how; vitamins and minerals. Nursing Times 49 (suppl.): 60–61

Hess D, Medoff B 1999 Respiratory monitoring. Current Opinion in Critical Care 5: 52

Higgins MW, Enwright PL, Kronmal RA et al. 1993 Smoking and lung function in elderly men and women. Journal of the American Medical Association 21: 2741–2748

Hinchcliff S, Montague S, Watson R 1996 Physiology for nursing practice 2nd edn. Baillière Tindall, London

Hogsten P, Switzer M 2001 Hemodynamic monitoring. In: Kidd PS, Wagner KD (eds) High acuity nursing, 3rd edn. Prentice Hall, Upper Saddle River, NJ, p 315

Holmes S 1998 The aetiology of malnutrition in hospital. Professional Nurse Study 13 (suppl.): S5–S8

Hough A 1996 Physiotherapy in respiratory care, 2nd edn. Chapman & Hall, London

Howell M 2001 An audit of oxygen prescribing in acute general medical wards. Professional Nurse 17: 221–224

Jarrett DRJ 1988 Differential diagnosis: asthma and its mimics. Geriatric Medicine 18: 31–36

Jevon P, Pooni JS 2001 Practical procedures for nurses. Cardiopulmonary resuscitation: insertion of an oropharyngeal airway. Nursing Times 97: 39–40

Jolliet P, Abajo B, Pasquina P et al. 2001 Non-invasive pressure support ventilation in severe community-acquired pneumonia. Intensive Care Medicine 27: 812–821

Kacmarek R 2000 Delivery systems for long-term oxygen therapy. Respiratory Care 45: 84–92

Kaye K, Stalam M, Shershen W et al. 2002 Utility of pulse oximetry in diagnosing pneumonia in nursing home residents. American Journal of Medical Science 324: 237–242

Keatings V, Jatakanon A, Worsdell Y 1997 Effects of inhaled and oral glucocorticoids on inflammatory indices in asthma and COPD. American Journal of Respiratory Critical Care Medicine 155: 542–548

Kwaiser Khun J, McGovern M 1992 Respiratory assessment of the elderly. Journal of Gerontological Nursing 18(5): 40–43

Langlands JH, Wallace WF 1965 Small blood samples from ear-lobe puncture. Lancet ii: 315–317

Lomas DA 2002 Chronic obstructive pulmonary disease: introduction. Thorax 57: 735

Lowton K 1999 Pulse oximeters for the detection of hypoxaemia. Professional Nurse 14: 343–350

Luce JM, Pierson DJ, Tyler ML 1993 Intensive respiratory care, 2nd edn. Philadelphia, WB Saunders

MacNee W, Calverley P 2003 Chronic obstructive pulmonary disease. 7: Management of COPD. Thorax 58: 261–265

McInturff S, Dunne PJ 1998 Home care equipment. In: Dunne PJ, McInturff SL (eds) Respiratory home care: the essentials. FA Davies, Philadelphia, pp 43–83

Moller JT, Pederson T, Rasmussen LS et al. 1993 Randomized evaluation of pulse oximetry in 20 802 patients: I. Anesthesiology 78: 436–444

Morgan MDL 2003 Preventing hospital admissions for COPD: role of physical activity. Thorax 58: 95–96

Murphy R 2001 Capillary blood gases in COPD. Emergency Medicine Journal 18: 117

Odell A, Allder A, Bayne R et al. 1993 Endotracheal suction for adult non-head injured patients. A review of the literature. Intensive and Critical Care Nursing 9: 274–278

Parker LJ 1999a Infection control 1: a practical guide to glove usage. British Journal of Nursing 8: 420–424

Parker LJ 1999b Importance of handwashing in the prevention of cross-infection. British Journal of Nursing 8: 716–720

Parrott S, Godfrey C, Raw M 1998 Guidance for commissioners on the cost effectiveness of smoking cessation interventions. Health Education Authority. Thorax 53 (suppl. 5): 31–38

Peruzzi WT, Smith B 1995 Bronchial hygiene therapy. Critical Care Clinics 11: 79–93

Pierce L 1995 Guide to mechanical ventilation and respiratory care. WB Saunders, Philadephia, pp 92–143

Pitkin AD, Roberts CM, Wedzicha JA 1994 Arterialised earlobe blood gas analysis: an underused technique. Thorax 49: 364–366

Place B 1997 Using airway pressure. Nursing Times 93: 42–44

Plant PK, Owen JL, Elliott MW 2001 Non-invasive ventilation in acute exacerbation of chronic obstructive pulmonary disease: long term survival and predictors of in-hospital outcome. Thorax 56: 708–712

Poole P, Black P 2000 Mucolytic agents for chronic bronchitis or chronic obstructive pulmonary disease. Cochrane Database Systematic Review 2: CD001287

Pratt RJ, Pellowe C, Loveday HP, Robinson N, Smith GW 2001 The epic project: developing national evidence-based guidelines for preventing healthcare associated infections. Phase 1: Guidelines for preventing hospital-acquired infections. Journal of Hospital Infection 47 (suppl.): S1–S82

Raymond S 1995 Normal saline instillation before suctioning: helpful or harmful? A review of the literature. American Journal of Critical Care 4: 267–271

Resuscitation Council UK 2002 Advanced life support course: provide manual. Resuscitation Council UK, London. Available online at: www. resus.org.uk (accessed 29 May 2003)

Roffe C, Sills S, Wilde K et al. 2001 Effect of hemiparetic stroke on pulse oximetry readings on the affected side. Stroke 32: 1808–1810

Rogge J, Bunde L, Baun M 1989 Effectiveness of oxygen concentrations of less than 100% before and after endotracheal suction in patients with chronic obstructive pulmonary disease. Heart and Lung 18: 64–71

Stone KS, Bell SD and Preusser BA. 1991a The effect of a repeated endotracheal suction on arterial blood pressure. Applied Nursing Research 4: 152–158

Stone KS, Preusser BA, Groch KF et al. 1991b The effect of lung hyperinflation and endotracheal suctioning on cardiopulmonary haemodynamics. Nursing Research 40: 76–80

Stoneham MD, Saville GM, Wilson IH 1994 Knowledge about pulse oximetry among medical and nursing staff. Lancet 344: 1339–1342

Tarrega J, Guell R, Anton A et al. 2002 Are daytime arterial blood gases a good reflection of nighttime gas exchange in patients on long term oxygen therapy? Respiratory Care 47: 882–886

The Tobacco Use and Dependence Clinical Practice Guideline Panel 2000 A clinical practice guideline for treating tobacco use and dependence. Journal of the American Medical Association 283: 244–254

Thomacot L, Vialet R, Viguier JM 1998 Efficacy of heat and moisture exchangers after changing every 48 hours rather than 24 hours. Critical Care Medicine 26: 477–481

Ulrik C 1995 Efficacy of inhaled salmeterol in the management of smokers with chronic obstructive pulmonary disease: a single centre randomised, double blind, placebo controlled, cross over study. Thorax 50: 750–754

Weilitz PB, Lueckenotte A 1995a Respiratory assessment of older adults: part I. Perspectives in Respiratory Nursing 6: 3–4

Weilitz PB, Lueckenotte A 1995b Respiratory assessment of older adults: part II. Perspectives in Respiratory Nursing 6: 1, 3–4

Wood C 1998 Endotracheal suctioning: a literature review. Intensive and Critical Care Nursing. 14: 124–136

Woodrow P 2002a Managing patients with a tracheostomy in acute care. Nursing Standard 16: 39–48

Woodrow P 2002b Measuring respiratory function to wean patients from non-invasive ventilation in a ward environment. Nursing in Critical Care 7: 136–143

World Health Organization 2003 Global tuberculosis report: surveillance, planning, finance. Available online at: www.who.int/gtb/publications/globrep/pdf/region/europe.pdf (accessed 28 May 2003)

Young C 1984 Recommended guidelines for suction. Physiotherapy 70: 106–108

Chapter 16

Eating and drinking

Susan M. McLaren

CHAPTER CONTENTS

INTRODUCTION

Eating and drinking are pleasurable activities which meet vital biological, social, psychological and cultural needs. In this chapter, the diverse variables that can affect intakes of food and fluids in older persons are examined, encompassing the effects of ageing on appetite regulation, social, economic and psychological factors, the impact of diseases, and unpleasant symptoms. The fact that disease can affect dietary intake and nutritional status adversely, and that diet may exert a positive or negative effect on risk factors for disease, is a conundrum that continues to fascinate. Attempts to modify risk by dietary change are the mainstay of health promotion, disease prevention and nutrition education initiatives. For these reasons examples of relationships between diet, risk factors and disease are considered in the following pages, with specific reference to dietary fats, cholesterol and coronary heart disease (CHD), salt and hypertension. The extent to which dietary guidelines targeted at young to middle-aged adults in the context of primary prevention are appropriate for older populations is a continuing source of debate.

A particular emphasis has been placed in this chapter on the prevention and management of malnutrition associated with either low or excessive body weight, since surveys have shown this to be a common finding in older persons in both community and institutional settings (Finch et al. 1998, Griep et al. 2000, Saletti et al. 2000, Kyle et al. 2003). This is a matter for concern, as indicators of disease-related undernutrition, predominantly in institutionalized populations, have been associated with increased risks of developing an infection, a major life-threatening complication, increased duration of hospitalization and costs, together with an increased risk of dying in hospital or following discharge home (Green 1999, Isabel et al. 2003). In overweight obese older people, reduced functional abilities and decreased quality of life accompany the development of complications such as diabetes and vascular disorders (Kennedy et al. 2004).

An urgent need exists to identify individuals who are significantly at risk of malnutrition, in order to implement appropriate nutritional and lifestyle interventions in the hope of improving outcomes.

Assisting older patients with eating and drinking is acknowledged to be a fundamental aspect of nursing care, requiring knowledge and skills to identify a range of physical, emotional, cognitive and social problems which can impair eating, and to plan appropriate interventions. At one extreme this may involve reading a menu to a visually impaired patient, at the other utilizing a range of knowledge and skills to feed a demented older person who cannot lift a cup, retain food in the mouth, chew or communicate. Whatever nursing support is given to enable older persons to eat and drink, it is performed in the context of the professional relationship and, as with other aspects of caring, should be endowed with trust, dignity and respect for the patient's autonomy in relation to dietary practice. More broadly, within the scope of professional practice, nurses need to work collaboratively with other health professionals to ensure that nutritional standards for screening, assessment and support are of the highest quality. This chapter aims to provide constructive, practical information for nurses who assist patients in a range of health care settings to eat and drink. Above all, it aims to provide food for thought.

AGEING: NUTRITIONAL PERSPECTIVES

During the normal process of ageing, consumption of food and fluids may be affected by physical changes and altered appetite. Alterations in dietary energy and protein requirements also occur, reflecting the effects of ageing on body metabolism. Despite these changes, many older people remain healthy; however, the imposition of ill health on reduced consumption of food and fluids may lead to loss of body weight, resulting in protein-energy malnutrition (PEM). The amount of energy consumed is controlled by central and peripheral mechanisms regulating appetite which adjust intake to balance energy expended in metabolism and physical activity. The autonomic nervous system provides another control system for energy expenditure. If the control systems malfunction, at one extreme body weight can fall, at the other it may rise, causing obesity. In ageing adults, great individual variation is evident in energy balance, but the two distinct phases summarized below can be identified (Glick 1995, Morley 2001):

1. a phase of positive energy balance most marked between the ages of 40 and 65 years by a rise in body weight and fat stores ('middle-age spread'), attributable to a decline in physical

activity and resting metabolic rate, rather than an increase in food intake

2. a second phase of negative energy balance in persons over 65 years, marked by weight loss, reduced food intake, a decline in muscle mass (sarcopenia) and increased risk of malnutrition.

Possible reasons for the second phase are discussed below.

Appetite regulation: taste and smell

It has been suggested that the decrease in appetite associated with old age, 'the anorexia of ageing', is in part attributable to altered homeostatic regulation (Morley 2001). Specifically, impairment in the ability to control energy intake and regulate energy balance occurs. This is manifest in lower levels of hunger and increased levels of fullness (satiety) observed in older people at mealtimes, and may explain the reduced consumption of dietary energy and fewer between-meal snacks in this age group. Early satiety is caused by a reduction in adaptive relaxation of the fundus of the stomach, resulting in more rapid filling of the antrum and slower rates of gastric emptying (Glick 1995, Morley & Thomas 1999). An array of endocrine and neurochemical changes underlies the pathogenesis of the anorexia of ageing (Glick 1995; Morley 2001). These include increased basal levels of cholecystokinin secretion, together with an increased production of anorectic peptides and reduced production of orexigenic peptides in the central nervous system. In men, a decline in testosterone secretion leading to elevated leptin levels may account for most of the reduction in food intake (Morley 2001).

The extent to which sensory changes consequent on ageing affect appetite has not been investigated extensively in humans. However, although a decline in taste and olfactory acuity occurs, a recent study has shown that this does not result in weight loss (Griep et al. 2000). Murphy (1993) found that flavour preference changes with ageing and that high concentrations of sugar and salt are rated more pleasant by older than by younger persons. Such taste alterations may lead to an increased use of salt as a contributory factor to hypertension in older people. This is addressed in more detail in the section on cardiovascular disease, below. Rolls et al. (1995) also noted that 'sensory specific satiety' is altered in old age. In younger groups, people tire of the taste of a specific food, which leads to reduced consumption and a requirement for variety in dietary tastes. In contrast, older people tend to lose this satiety mechanism and continue to eat the same food without tiring of its taste, a factor which could contribute to the consumption of a monotonous diet. Side-effects of a number of drugs may also diminish appetite in older people.

Oral food ingestion and transport

The processes of ingesting food into the oral cavity, forming a bolus and transporting this to the oropharynx for swallowing, can be impaired by the physiological changes associated with ageing, summarized below (Hudson et al. 2000):

- loss of teeth
- reduced mass of the tongue and masseter muscles in the jaw
- increased chewing strokes required per mouthful
- reduced salivary volume, enzyme content, increased viscosity
- diminished tongue sensation resulting in slightly delayed pharyngeal swallowing
- decreased sensory capacity in the laryngopharynx
- shorter duration of pharyngeal reflex swallow
- minor slowing of oesophageal peristalsis.

Metabolism

Analysis of cross-sectional and longitudinal survey data reveals that food intake gradually declines with age; the magnitude of decreases in total daily energy intake varies considerably, by 1000–1200 kcal in men and 600–800 kcal in women (Wakimoto & Block 2001). As food and therefore energy intake declines, energy expenditure also falls in both men and women due to a decrease in the basal metabolic rate (BMR) and levels of physical activity (Glick 1995). BMR is the energy needed each day to maintain vital physiological functions and is influenced by body size, and particularly, lean body mass. Reasons for the decline in BMR associated with ageing include reduction in the skeletal muscle mass, activity of thyroid hormones and responsiveness to hormones such as noradrenaline (norepinephrine). In young adults skeletal muscle mass accounts for about 45% of body weight, declining to less than 27% at 70 years and above. In contrast, the non-muscle protein mass remains unchanged and an increase in body fat occurs. The fall in muscle mass is largely due to loss of the trophic effects of growth hormone, testosterone and the autonomic nervous system, in conjunction with a decrease in the capacity for muscle fibre regeneration. The magnitude of decline in skeletal muscle mass is reflected in the change in BMR, from a median of 7.40 mJ/day at 25 years to 5.78 mJ/day at >70 years in men. Corresponding values in women are 6.49 mJ/day declining to 4.99 mJ/day. The impact of these changes in basal metabolism and activity is to reduce energy requirements in healthy older people.

DIETARY RISKS: AN OVERVIEW

Obesity

Definition

Obesity can be defined as 'an excess of adipose tissue for a given weight', but there is no consensus as to what constitutes 'an excess' (Morley & Glick 1995). Body mass index (BMI) provides a simple measure of the spectrum of underweight–obesity, and is calculated by dividing body weight in kilograms by the square of height in metres. As a general approach, the following ranges are used to indicate degree of fatness:

- < 20: underweight; long-term hazard to health
- 20–25: desirable range
- 25–35: overweight
- > 30: severely obese.

In the UK National Diet and Nutrition Survey in people aged > 65 years, about two-thirds of free-living participants and a little under half of those in institutions were classified as overweight or obese, on the basis of a BMI of > 25 (Finch et al. 1998). However, in free-living men, the proportion who were overweight decreased by 18% between the age groups of 65–74 years and > 85 years. What are the causes, risks and advantages associated with weight gain in older people and at what point is weight reduction advisable? What approaches to weight reduction can be safely used? These questions are addressed in the following sections.

Aetiology

With increasing age a decline in the rate of metabolism (BMR) occurs due to a reduction in muscle mass, hormone secretion and responsiveness. This is accompanied in many individuals by a decline in physical activity, such that energy intake exceeds output and weight gain results from this. Side-effects of drugs and pathological endocrine disorders can also contribute to the development of obesity or play a substantive role in its aetiology (Box 16.1).

Risks

Obesity has been associated with many diseases affecting older age groups, including diabetes mellitus, CHD, hypertension, specific cancers, osteoarthritis and psychological morbidity (Masaki et al. 1997, Defay et al. 2001, Visscher et al. 2001, Kennedy et al. 2004).

Box 16.1   Obesity: aetiology in older people

- Decline in basal metabolic rate
- Reduction in level of physical activity
- Hypothyroidism (5% > 60 years)
- Hypothalamic tumours (uncommon)
- ? Growth hormone, somatomedin C deficiency
- Drug side-effects: corticosteroids, monoamine oxidase inhibitors, tricyclic antidepressants

---

Moreover, a longitudinal investigation conducted over 3 years in a community-dwelling population of older adults has confirmed that obesity was an important determinant of functional ability and predicted decline in functional status (Jensen & Friedman 2002).

However, in relation to mortality, a prospective longitudinal study conducted over a 14-year period in a free-living population of 1 million (mean age of 57 years at study commencement), found only relatively modest relationships between BMI and risk of death, which became less marked with increasing age (Calle et al. 1999). In marked contrast, underweight resulting from non-intentional weight loss has been associated with underlying disease states and is thought by many to constitute by far the greater risk to health and mortality in older people (Lehman 1991; Ho et al. 1994). Findings of an early survey by Campbell et al. (1990) illustrate this contrast between overweight, obesity and mortality in older people > 70 years. Anthropometric indicators of malnourishment were significant prospective predictors of mortality, in contrast to a high BMI and other indicators of substantive subcutaneous fat, which were not predictive over the same time period.

Importance of body fat

Body fat constitutes an important means of survival, offering protection to body organs and a vital store of energy in situations of metabolic stress. Obesity also offers some protection from fracture of the hip, an effect which has been attributed to physical absorbance of the impact of falling, together with beneficial effects on bone mineral density produced by increased weight-loading of bone and secretion of oestrogenic steroids by adipose tissue (Vellas et al. 1995).

Management

Given that moderate overweight in older people is not associated with significant increase in mortality, who needs treatment for obesity? Opinions vary, but the selective dietary management of obese individuals requires consideration of the morbidity which may be attributed to specific levels of obesity, the presence of medical conditions such as diabetes mellitus which may be exacerbated by obesity, the impact of weight reduction on quality of life and nutritional adequacy of the diet. Morley & Glick (1995) suggest weight reduction is mandatory for individuals over 65 years of age who are morbidly obese (> 130–140% of average body weight). Individuals suffering from diabetes mellitus with > 110% average body weight should be advised to reduce their body weight.

In overweight older people, increasing energy expenditure by taking regular gentle to moderate exercise can be a useful weight-reducing strategy. Walking, swimming and t'ai chi can form part of effective and enjoyable weight-reduction programmes. Specific exercises under supervision can be recommended for disabled individuals with restricted mobility, e.g. upper-body exercises for individuals immobilized by arthritis affecting the hip, knee and feet. Others may benefit from a home-based exercise programme. For example, a randomized controlled trial of a home-based, 12-month exercise programme of moderate intensity in older women resulted in decreased weight together with reduced total and intra-abdominal fat in the intervention group (Irwin et al. 2003). Excessive dieting should not be attempted by any individual without medical consultation and professional supervision. Practical approaches to the promotion of safe weight loss are outlined in Box 16.2. It is important to include the patient/client's partner in discussions about diet and

---

Box 16.2 Achieving safe weight loss: practical considerations

- Seek expert advice; set realistic goals for slow, steady weight loss of 0.25–0.5 kg/week on a diet which is within financial budget
- Eat three meals daily; avoid snacking; put down fork between bites
- Avoid fried food: grill, poach and bake instead
- Increase dietary intakes of fibre, wholemeal bread, wholegrain cereals, vegetables, fruit
- Trim visible fat from food; drink semiskimmed milk, reduce intake of butter, spreads, sweets
- Use artificial sweeteners in tea or coffee; consume sugar-free soft drinks; drink alcohol in moderation; ensure total fluid intake is adequate
- Gradually increase levels of physical activity; i.e. benefits from walking, swimming, t'ai chi
- Low-calorie or crash diets should not be used; do not reduce energy intake to < 1000 kcal/day, which could result in inadequate micronutrient intakes

---

lifestyle changes. Increasing knowledge and understanding of the energy and nutrient content of foods is important, as are learning to recognize and avoid cravings and coping positively with days when the diet degenerates. The social benefits and positive aspects of peer support to be gained by joining a slimming club may be helpful for some people. In contrast, fad diets and very-low-calorie diets are not recommended, neither is dieting during periods of acute illness, when a deterioration in nutritional status could have harmful effects. Prospective trials relating to the use of antiobesity drugs (e.g. sibutramine) have not included older adults; potential dangers associated with side-effects may limit their use (Kennedy et al. 2004). In relation to surgical interventions, laparoscopic adjustable silicone gastric banding has been shown in one evaluation to be a safe technique for the treatment of morbid obesity in older people (Abu-Abeid et al. 2001).

Malnutrition

Definition
Malnutrition is a term which can be applied very broadly to describe a number of states indicative of nutrient depletion or overrepletion. These include overnutrition due to excessive food consumption; undernutrition due to deficient food consumption; and various types of specific dietary deficiencies or imbalances due to inadequate or disproportionate consumption (Keller 1993).

In the context of this chapter, which is concerned principally with the nutritional care of older people in the community and in hospital, a major concern is that of undernutrition due to inadequate food provision or consumption. A more specific definition to describe PEM is 'a change in body composition and physiology resulting from an absolute or relative deficiency of dietary energy and protein'. 'Absolute' refers to the fact that the intake of nutrients does not meet normal requirements for the individual; 'relative' describes the deficiency state when intake meets normal requirements, but these have increased due to defective utilization of nutrients, catabolism or losses (Taylor & Goodinson-McLaren 1992: p. 13). PEM is usually accompanied by deficiencies of micronutrients, i.e. vitamins, minerals and trace elements.

In recent years, a number of surveys of older populations in the community and in hospital or nursing-home settings have suggested a significant prevalence of PEM. In the UK a national survey of older people found that 16% of men and 15% of women living in residential or nursing homes had a BMI < 20 kg/m^2 indicative of underweight, in comparison with 3% and 5% respectively of free-living older people (Finch et al.

1998). More recent comparative figures from a Scandinavian survey revealed that PEM indicated by a mini-nutritional assessment risk score of < 17 was present in 21% of older people living in service flats, 33% in old people's homes, 38% living in group dwellings for those suffering from dementia and 71% in nursing homes. Dependency on assistance at mealtimes was highest in the nursing-home population where 37% of residents needed some help and 36% needed to be fed (Saletti et al. 2000). Comprehensive reviews of research reports emanating from surveys in nursing homes in the USA report that 10–85% of older residents suffer from varying degrees of malnutrition (Green 1999). Prevalence figures for undernutrition in adults admitted to hospital, which incorporate data on older age groups, suggest about 40% are at least mildly malnourished and many undergo further deterioration in nutritional status during hospitalization (McWhirter & Pennington 1994, Allison 2002). Given these findings, a number of questions arise. What factors can place older populations at risk of developing malnutrition? How can individuals at risk be identified? What preventive measures are indicated? Finally, what are the most appropriate and effective therapeutic interventions and support services for older, malnourished individuals?

Community risk factors

A number of socioeconomic, psychological, pathological and drug-related factors, alone or in combination, can predispose to or cause malnutrition in older people. Such effects are superimposed on the effects of ageing, which result in changes in nutritional status.

Socioeconomic factors   Social isolation, poverty and poor levels of education predispose to PEM. Living alone poses a significant risk, notably after a bereavement. Older men appear to be particularly vulnerable, as those living with a spouse have better dietary habits than those living alone. Those with adequate social networks, outside interests and support fare better from a dietary perspective than those who have poorer social anchorage. Eating alone is associated with eating less regularly, increased use of convenience foods and reduced amounts, quality and variety of nutrients consumed (McLaren et al. 1997).

Poor nutritional status in older people has also been associated with poverty. Low income can restrict food purchase and limit facilities for storing and preparing food. Consequences of this are the consumption of a diet which is dull, monotonous and limited in variety, in which the intake of selected nutrients is low, notably in energy. For example, in studies comparing dietary intakes in impoverished and affluent older

groups, the former were found to have lower intakes of energy, calcium, vitamin D, iron and B-complex vitamins. Low income particularly affected the purchase of milk, cheese and fruit. In contrast, affluent groups consumed greater quantities of fibre and vitamin C, fewer high-fat foods and less salt. Poor dietary habits and failure to comply with dietary regimens may also result from inadequate levels of education and illiteracy, which frequently accompany low socioeconomic status (Chandra et al. 1991).

Psychological factors   Anxiety and depression may have extrinsic or intrinsic causes, resulting in anorexia and weight loss. Admission to a hospital or nursing home, or relocation to another ward or unit within the same institution, are common causes of anxiety and depression in older people. Reactions to an unpleasant or devastating illness and bereavement have also been associated with anorexia, weight loss and malnutrition. A positive approach to screening for depression in individuals who have lost significant amounts of body weight together with antidepressant treatment may result in an improvement in appetite (Morley 1997). The benefits of antidepressants were illustrated by investigations in a nursing home which found that 36% of malnourished patients resident for > 3 months had depression and that pharmacological treatment of the depression reversed their weight loss (Morley & Kraenzle 1994; Morley 2001).

Pathological factors   A number of disease-related factors can result in, or contribute to, the development of PEM (Green 1999). Nutrient intakes can be reduced due to disability and handicap associated with chronic illnesses such as rheumatoid arthritis, osteoarthritis, Parkinson's disease and stroke. Here, loss of motor skills and mobility impairs the ability to shop for food, prepare a meal, cut food, load cutlery and ingest food. Stroke and dementia can also result in cognitive and sensory deficits which make it extremely difficult to concentrate on eating a meal, recognize items of food, chew and swallow safely. Food intakes can also be reduced in the cachexia of cancer, or due to gut obstruction, nausea and vomiting associated with cancer treatment. Anorexia can result from renal and liver diseases, uncontrolled pain and sepsis. Providing effective support for patients suffering from these factors, which reduce food intake, involves treating the underlying cause and providing symptomatic relief in a variety of ways, using both physical and psychological approaches. For further discussion of these, see the section on the impact of distressing symptoms on eating and drinking, below.

Pathological factors may also cause malnutrition by decreasing the digestion and/or absorption of nutrients (in inflammatory, neoplastic and infective conditions affecting the gastrointestinal tract and liver disease). Pernicious anaemia can impair vitamin B_{12} absorption. Impaired absorption and loss of nutrients may also follow surgery to the gastrointestinal tract, notably if a cutaneous-enteral fistula forms as a complication. Pathological factors may also increase the metabolic requirement for nutrients and their disposal, thereby contributing to the development of a malnourished state. Neurohumoral responses to injury, trauma, sepsis and the presence of severe chronic wounds such as grade IV pressure sores can significantly elevate requirements for energy, protein, micronutrients and fluids. Cancer cachexia features a rise in metabolic rate and increasing nutrient requirements, as does hyperthyroidism and the presence of chronic pulmonary disease associated with sepsis and hyperventilation.

Drug effects

Older people consume high quantities of drugs as a consequence of the degenerative diseases which are increasingly prevalent in old age. In older adults, undetected food–drug interactions may lead to serious morbidity and mortality and be misdiagnosed as chronic disease progression (McCabe 2004). Polypharmacy, with its associated risk of drug–drug and drug–food interactions, is the result of multiple prescribing and increased use of some non-prescription drugs, including herbal remedies and dietary supplements (see Chapter 27 for more information on drugs and older people). What are the implications of drug treatment for older people in relation to impact on nutritional status? Drugs can affect nutritional status by altering food consumption, nutrient absorption, metabolism, utilization and excretion (Hamilton-Smith 1995). Such effects are superimposed on those of ageing, which may increase vulnerability to drug side-effects or toxicity. For example, in old age significant loss of nephrons reduces the ability to excrete drugs, while a reduction in lean body mass and increase in body fat may alter the duration and onset of action and distribution of fat-soluble drugs respectively. Reductions in liver mass and hepatic blood flow may reduce transformation of some drugs (limited evidence). Some potential side-effects of common drugs in impairing nutritional status are summarized in Table 16.1.

Acute hospital admission

Following admission to hospital, many older people are known to lose weight and sustain a further deterioration in their nutritional status, with its associated risks of an increased morbidity and mortality (King's

Table 16.1 Common drugs: potential side-effects in older people

Drug	Effect
Cholestyramine	Malabsorption of lipids, carotene, calcium, iron, vitamins A, D and K. Anorexia, nausea, vomiting
Furosemide	Increased excretion of Na^+, K^+, Ca^{2+}, water diarrhoea, anorexia, dry mouth, thirst
Aspirin	Increased excretion of ascorbic acid, iron-deficiency anaemia, nausea, vomiting, gastric pain, ulceration, anorexia
Corticosteroids	Increased catabolism
Methotrexate, anticonvulsants, alcohol	Altered folate metabolism, folate-deficiency anaemia

Fund Report 1992). Findings of a study by McWhirter & Pennington (1994) exemplify the problem. In this survey of 500 patients, 40% were found to be malnourished on admission to hospital. However, the majority lost weight following hospitalization, with the most extensive weight loss occurring in those who were malnourished at the time of admission. Since catering and nutrition support services are available, what are the contributory problems? Undoubtedly, effects of disease, unpleasant symptoms, treatment effects and drugs continue to play a part. However, a number of organizational and environmental problems are also known to influence various aspects of food selection, delivery and consumption (Table 16.2), all of which can be remedied.

Effects of hospitalization on established food habits in older people raise both organizational and environmental issues which cannot be overestimated. Culture and tradition are powerful determinants of dietary habits, and religious beliefs are an important determinant of food acceptability (Holmes 1986). Adherence to habits is important in creating feelings of familiarity, security, stability and a sense of belonging. Familiarity in particular is one of the most important factors underlying food choices (Steptoe et al. 1995). Following hospitalization it is vital that catering and nutrition support services provide a range of diets which will meet the spectrum of cultural, religious and individual requirements of the older population. It is known that individuals who receive a 'familiar diet' which is comparable to that consumed at home eat better and with greater enjoyment. Consultation with patients to ascertain their needs will avoid problems

Table 16.2   Organizational and environmental influences on eating: acute hospital settings

Problems	Solutions
Sterile decor, poor lighting, temperature extremes	Provide designated eating area, bright cheerful decor, good lighting, warm ambient temperature, varied table settings
Solitary eating, lack of socialization	Ask patients their preferences of eating alone or in company; socialization enhanced by providing small, square tables, group size 4–6.
	Consistent seating arrangement may help older people with memory problems
	Encourage staff to socialize with patients at mealtimes; use mealtime 'buddy' system
Noise, interruptions for medical investigations, ward rounds	Turn off sources of noise at mealtimes (television sets, cleaning equipment)
	Prioritize mealtimes; reschedule ward rounds, special investigations not to coincide with meals
Untrained personnel responsible for meal selection, delivery, removal of meal trays, meals delivered in inappropriate portion size, texture	Patients to have choice in meal selection with appropriate assistance; request patient's permission before removing meal trays
	Supervision of mealtimes by nurses; referral and involvement of dieticians, speech therapists, medical staff in meal selection, as appropriate
Meal timing too close (3–4 meals in 8 h followed by 16 h starvation)	Swallowing/chewing problems to be rapidly assessed following admission; videofluoroscopy may be necessary to ascertain safe swallowing capacity; speech therapist assessment also vital
	Review timing of meals; provide bedtime snacks; individual habits and preferences should be considered
Staff not trained to identify patients at risk of protein-energy malnutrition	Ensure high-quality standards and training operationalized in nutritional screening and assessment
Lack of nursing skills in feeding disabled patients, particularly those needed to compensate for dysphagia and visual/perceptual problems	Provide education/training in assessment of disabilities which impair eating and appropriate, safe, compensatory skills for all nursing personnel
Inadequate mealtime supervision of patients; ward handovers and reports occurring at lunch and supper; rapid turnover of staff feeding patients in long-stay wards	Ensure sufficient staff available to meet level of patient dependency and assign to patients on a consistent basis to ensure continuity of care
	Reschedule handovers/reports so they do not coincide with meals
Inadequate documentation of nutritional problems, dietary management, nutritional assessment/screening data	Review/develop audit standards for recording systems which support effective decision-making
	Record dietary information/nutritional screening/assessment data on admission, during hospitalization at recommended monitoring intervals and prior to discharge
Inadequate provision of aids to posture and eating	Referral of patients requiring aids to physiotherapist/occupational therapist
	Review of aid resources in relation to demand
Lack of foods appropriately presented to help patients with lack of manual dexterity to eat	Involvement/presence of physiotherapists and occupational therapists at mealtimes to assess/supervise patients
	Provision of some finger foods which are easier for disabled patients to eat

arising in relation to inadequate choices and delivery of meals of an unsuitable texture or portion size which are frequently the focus of dissatisfaction (Association of Community Health Councils 1997).

Nursing responsibilities in assisting patients to eat have recently been emphasized by the United Kingdom Central Council for Nursing, Midwifery and Health Visiting (1997). Respect for autonomy requires that individuals who are able to select their own meals do so with appropriate help and guidance if specific dietary problems (e.g. dysphagia) are present. Support may be needed for those suffering from auditory and visual field deficits, perceptual problems, dysphasia and lack of manual dexterity which make verbal expression of meal preferences, responses to instructions and selection from a menu very difficult. Plated meal serving systems with prior menu selection have become increasingly popular, yet for older people selecting from a visible choice of dishes, stimulated by the sight and smell of food, may result in improved food consumption (Elmstahl 1987). Many older patients are disabled as a consequence of chronic diseases and require sensitive help to eat and drink. Providing assistance which is appropriate to their level of dependency is vital, not only to ensure an adequate food intake of a safe volume and texture, but also to maintain dignity and maximize whatever degree of independence is possible during rehabilitation. Failure to identify patients at risk of PEM and to provide an appropriate level of support have been identified as problems (King's Fund Report 1992, United Kingdom Central Council for Nursing, Midwifery and Health Visiting 1997). Approaches to nutritional screening, assessment and management of symptom distress, including that arising from disability, are discussed later in this chapter.

Effects of malnutrition

A vast plethora of literature is now available documenting the adverse effects which PEM can exert on body function and in delaying recovery from illness. For older people, effects of malnutrition are superimposed on the effects of ageing on physiological systems. When effects of disease, malnutrition and ageing are considered together, the apparent significant negative impact on morbidity and mortality can be appreciated only too well. Preventive measures which seek to improve nutritional status by modifying risk factors in conjunction with dietary health promotion strategies are essential. In addition, commitment and action are needed to raise the profile of nutritional support in the context of both organization and environment. Hopefully this will result in more effective screening and assessment of 'at-risk' patients, with efficient and effective systems to ensure appropriate meal selection, delivery and consumption.

EFFECTS OF DISEASE: DIETARY FACTORS

Nutrition–related anaemias

Anaemia is a general term used to describe a diminution in the oxygen-carrying capacity of blood, below the normal limit. Table 16.3 summarizes the characteristic haematological profile and symptoms of different types of anaemia. During human ageing, few changes occur in basal erythropoiesis, yet a number of surveys have suggested a higher prevalence of mild anaemia with advancing age in apparently healthy individuals (Yip et al. 1984). It has been suggested that nutritional deficiencies may contribute to this, as anaemia is very rare in affluent communities but has a higher prevalence in low socioeconomic populations where other nutritional problems are significant (Lipschitz 1995).

Iron deficiency

Older people may be affected by a number of complex factors which either enhance iron losses or reduce absorption from the gut. These include:

Table 16.3 Anaemias: haematological profile and symptoms

Common name	Type of anaemia	Haematological profile	Symptoms
Iron-deficiency	Microcytic hypochromic	Serum ferritin < 13 mg/l (normal ranges: males 40–340 mg/l; females 14–148 mg/l)	Brittle spoon-shaped nails, tiredness, shortage of breath, fatigue, palpitations
Folate-deficiency	Macrocytosis	Red-cell folate < 140 mg/l packed cells (normal range: 150–600 mg/l packed cells)	Peripheral neuropathy, ataxia, mental changes
	Megaloblastic anaemia	Serum folate < 3 mg/l (normal range: 3–25 mg/l)	
Vitamin B_{12}-deficiency	Macrocytosis	Serum vitamin B_{12} < 100 pg/ml	Peripheral neuropathy; mental changes; subacute combined degeneration of the cord; paraesthesiae; glossitis
	Megaloblastic anaemia	(normal range > 150 pg/ml)*	

*Varies with biochemical method used. A picogram (pg) is 10^{-12} of a gram; a microgram (mg) is 10^{-6} of a gram. These are weights of compounds dissolved in a given volume of liquid.

- chronic loss of blood from the gut, attributed to use of aspirin, presence of neoplasms, ulceration, haemorrhoids, diverticular disease
- reduced gastric acid secretion in atrophic gastritis, neoplasms
- low vitamin C intake which can adversely affect iron absorption from the gut, as can the presence of fibre, tetracyclines, phosphates and antacids.

Inadequate intake of dietary iron is rarely the sole cause of anaemia in older individuals, despite the prevalence of other nutritional deficiencies, but it may contribute to development. Treatment consists of eradicating the underlying cause and taking oral ferrous sulphate or gluconate. If the condition is severe, blood transfusion may be necessary. Dietary recommendations (RNI, reference nutrient intake; Department of Health 1991) for iron intakes for older people are 8.7 mg daily. Foods rich in iron include red meats, offal, eggs, wholemeal bread, cereals and green vegetables.

Vitamin B_{12} deficiency

This type of anaemia has four principal causes:

1. reduced absorption of vitamin B_{12} due to antibodies produced against gastric parietal cells and intrinsic factor leading to atrophic gastritis and decreased secretion of intrinsic factor (pernicious anaemia)
2. vegan diets deficient in vitamin B_{12}
3. disorders of the terminal ileum which result in failure to absorb vitamin B_{12}–intrinsic factor complex, e.g. gluten-sensitive enteropathy, blind-loop syndrome and postileal resection
4. long-term complications of gastrectomy; the treatment of this type of anaemia consists of intramuscular injections of vitamin B_{12}, e.g. 100 mg weekly until repletion occurs followed by a monthly to 3-monthly maintenance dose of 1000 mg.

Folate deficiency

A folate deficiency severe enough to cause anaemia in older people can usually be attributed to deficient diets, PEM or drugs that interfere with the absorption or metabolism of folate (anticonvulsants, alcohol, methotrexate). Increased requirements for folate may increase the vulnerability of older people to deficiency, e.g. inflammation, cancer. Treatment of folate-deficiency anaemia comprises folic acid tablets and dietary attention together with correction of the underlying cause of malnutrition. Folate requirements are 200 mg daily for individuals over 50 years. Prime sources of dietary folate are vegetables and offal. The vitamin is destroyed by prolonged cooking.

In recent years the protective role of folate in the prevention of CHD has generated considerable interest. Both folate and vitamin B_{12} are substrates or cofactors for the metabolism of homocysteine, elevated levels of which are a risk factor for CHD. As elevated plasma homocysteine levels are inversely related to those of folate and vitamin B_{12}, the effectiveness of improving folate and vitamin B_{12} status as an intervention to reduce CHD has been under investigation (Tice et al. 2001, Stanger 2002).

Osteoporosis

Osteoporosis is defined as 'a progressive systemic skeletal disorder, characterized by low bone mass and microarchitectural deterioration of bone tissue with a consequent increase in bone fragility and risk of fracture' (World Health Organization 1994). Features of bone loss are greatest in areas of cancellous bone, which forms the centre of vertebral bodies and the femoral neck. It is therefore not surprising to find that crush fractures of the spine and fractures of the hip are frequent concomitants to osteoporosis. In England and Wales it has been estimated that 180 000 osteoporosis-related symptomatic fractures occur annually and that costs of treating osteoporosis in postmenopausal women alone are about £1.5–1.8 billion (National Institute of Clinical Excellence 2003). The principal risk factors are well known, as are their mechanisms of action, which are prevention of the attainment of peak bone mass (PBM), acceleration of bone loss after PBM has been reached, or both operating together (Pachucki-Hyde 2001). Risk factors encompass genetic predisposition, ageing, nutrition, lifestyle and medical conditions as summarized below:

- Caucasian and Asian racial groups, family history of osteoporosis
- ageing (> 35 years) associated with gradually decreasing bone mineral density
- postmenopausal oestrogen deficiency in women
- inadequate dietary intakes of calcium, vitamin D and a low BMI < 19 kg/m^2
- vitamin D deficiency caused by lack of exposure to sunlight
- excessive use of alcohol, smoking, immobilization, a sedentary lifestyle
- Cushing's disease, malabsorptive syndromes, hyperparathyroidism, renal and liver disease
- use of glucocorticoid and cytotoxic drug therapy.

Guidance issued by expert committees, in conjunction with the systematic reviews and meta-analyses derived through the Cochrane Collaboration summarized below, can be helpful in preventing osteoporosis through risk-factor modification (Department of Health 1998, Royal College of Physicians 1999, National Institutes of Health 2001, Bonaiuti et al. 2004, Homik et al. 2004):

- lifestyle modification at all ages, encompassing increased exercise, smoking cessation, avoidance of excessive alcohol consumption
- maintenance of body weight in older adults
- maintaining dietary intakes of calcium and vitamin D which meet RNIs
- hormone replacement therapy in postmenopausal women can protect against bone loss and risk of fragility fractures; aerobics, weight-bearing and resistance exercises can also benefit bone mineral density
- prophylaxis of steroid-induced osteoporosis using calcium and vitamin D treatment.

A number of interventions can be used in the management of osteoporosis. Calcium supplementation can exert small, positive improvements in bone density in postmenopausal women and decreases bone loss in women with osteoporosis (Royal College of Physicians 1999, Shea et al. 2004). Use of vitamin D with calcium has been recommended in older osteoporotic women and in frail older people these supplements can exert beneficial effects on bone density and tooth retention (Royal College of Physicians 1999, De Jong et al. 2000, Krall et al. 2001). In considering therapeutic interventions utilizing vitamin D in older adults, Sahota & Hosking (2001) draw attention to the need to consider, in relation to the underlying deficiency state, which form of vitamin D is likely to be most effective, i.e. either the parent form 25-OHD or an analogue of the active form, 1-25 (OH)2D. Continuing benefits of hormone replacement therapy, alone or in combination with exercise and exercise alone, have demonstrated benefits on bone mass in postmenopausal women (Cheng et al. 2002). Exercise alone was also found to be helpful in the treatment of osteoporosis in postmenopausal women in a recent Cochrane review of randomized controlled clinical trials (Bonaiuti et al. 2004).

Cardiovascular disease

A number of risk factors for CHD have been identified over the last 40 years: smoking, high intakes of saturated fats, raised plasma cholesterol concentrations and hypertension. A major aim of primary prevention has been to modify risk factors in order to reduce the morbidity and mortality associated with CHD (Ezzati et al. 2002). Over the same timescale, the 'dietary lipid-heart' hypothesis gained significant credence, i.e. a high saturated fat intake increasing low-density

lipoprotein (LDL) cholesterol concentrations in plasma, leading to the deposition of atheroma in arterial plaques and to the development of CHD. This hypothesis had a number of weaknesses, notably that plasma cholesterol concentrations are affected by a number of variables with diet exerting relatively minor effects. The question then arose: what implications does this have for older people?

- The high relative risk of CHD associated with any concentration of plasma cholesterol declines with age, but cholesterol remains a predictor of CHD up to 70 years (Gordon & Rifkind 1989)
- Plasma cholesterol concentrations rise with age, most markedly in postmenopausal women, where 22% aged over 65 years have plasma cholesterol concentrations > 7.8 mmol/l (cf. 2% in males), and its relationship to morbidity is unclear (White et al. 1993).

Despite some of the unanswered questions regarding cholesterol-lowering interventions, the expert working group Committee on Medical Aspects of Food Policy (1992) encouraged older people to adopt diets that 'moderated their plasma cholesterol levels'. Furthermore, the researchers specially recommended consumption of oily fish to reduce the risk of coronary thrombosis. The latter recommendation followed investigations demonstrating a low CHD risk in populations consuming a relatively high $n3$ fatty acid intake and reduced rates of reinfarction in subjects consuming a diet enriched with these fatty acids in oily fish or as a supplement (Burr et al. 1991, British Nutrition Foundation 1992). Specifically, the consumption of $n3$ fatty acids appears to affect haemostasis, reducing thrombogenicity by decreasing platelet adhesiveness, lowering plasma triglycerides and LDL cholesterol.

It is not recommended that supplements containing high concentrations of fish oil are routinely consumed by older people. Instead their use has been reserved for specific types of hyperlipidaemia and other high-risk groups. However, consuming 2–4 portions of oily fish weekly may offer potential benefits to those who are at low risk of CHD (Committee on Medical Aspects of Food Policy 1992, Department of Health 1992b, Morley 1995). Box 16.3 summarizes some of the key recommendations of a number of expert groups aimed at the reduction of CHD and its associated dietary risk factors (United States Drug Administration 1985, Paffenbarger et al. 1986, Committee on Medical Aspects of Food Policy 1992, Macnair 1994).

Recently guidelines have become available relating to diet in the secondary prevention of cardiovascular disease (British Dietetic Association 2004). General recommendations are to increase $n3$ fatty acid intake

---

Box 16.3 Recommendations aimed at the reduction of coronary heart disease and its associated dietary risk factors

- Maintain a desirable body weight
- Increase/maintain physical activity
- Eat a variety of foods
- Increase consumption of fruit and vegetables
- Reduce saturated fat intake to 15% or 10% of total dietary kilocalories
- Consume oily fish regularly (herring, mackerel, salmon)
- Moderate excessive alcohol consumption

---

from dietary or supplemental fish oils, but with caution in men suffering from angina where such an increase might elevate the risk of death. A reduction in saturated fats, with total or partial replacement by unsaturated fats (rapeseed or olive oil) is also advised. Adoption of a Mediterranean type of diet, encompassing increased $n3$ fats, fruit, vegetables and fresh foods, together with a reduction in saturated fats and processed foods, is protective. In the interpretation of guidelines, attention is drawn to the fact that some dietary interventions may be unsuitable at an individual level, for example the ingestion of a low-saturated-fat diet in an older, frail person suffering from angina. Sih & Morley (1995) also drew attention to the fact that aggressive use of unappetizing low-fat diets might increase the risk of PEM in older people and furthermore, changing long-established eating habits might be unrealistic.

The advent of statin therapy to reduce LDL cholesterol has revolutionized the treatment of individuals at high risk of cardiovascular disease. Findings of the UK MRC/BHF Heart Protection Study (2002a), conducted in 20 536 adults in the age ranges 40–80 years with evidence of coronary disease, occlusive vascular disease or diabetes, demonstrated that the use of simvastin in comparison with placebo significantly reduced all-cause mortality. Significant reductions in the coronary death rate and also in non-vascular deaths were found. Conclusions were that adding simvastin to existing treatments conferred added benefits for high-risk patients, irrespective of initial cholesterol concentrations.

The role of antioxidant vitamin supplements in reducing the incidence of vascular disease has also been extensively investigated over a 5-year period in high-risk individuals in the MRC/BHF Heart Protection Study (2002b). Ingestion of supplements of vitamins E, C and beta-carotene in the intervention group did not produce any significant benefits in comparison

with controls across a range of outcomes, including deaths due to vascular or non-vascular causes and incidence of vascular disease.

Hypertension

Over many years a number of investigations have shown that blood pressure rises with age, as does the prevalence of hypertension (Freis 1976, White et al. 1993). Extensive use of antihypertensive drugs in older populations reflects the latter and, as these are associated with a 30% incidence rate of adverse effects, the use of non-pharmacological approaches to control hypertension is important (Tschamm et al. 1988).

Dietary salt consumption appears to contribute significantly to the rise in blood pressure which occurs with age. A positive correlation between average dietary sodium intake and the rate of rise in blood pressure with age has been shown (Intersalt Cooperative Research Group 1988). This study also found:

- a negative correlation between dietary potassium intake and blood pressure
- a significant association between the combined effects of obesity and high sodium and alcohol intakes.

To what extent can manipulation of dietary sodium intake bring about beneficial therapeutic effects in control of hypertension? Early studies by Myers & Morgan (1983) investigated the effects of both low and high sodium intakes in normotensive and hypertensive subjects in relation to age. Key findings to emerge were that older normotensive and hypertensive subjects greatly increased their blood pressure with sodium loading, but they also achieved greater reduction in blood pressure with sodium restriction. The underlying rationale for these observations seems to be the decline in glomerular filtration rate which occurs with age, inability to conserve sodium during deprivation and loss of functioning nephrons. More recently, a Cochrane review of the literature has assessed the effect of long-term modest salt reduction on blood pressure (He & MacGregor 2004). Conclusions following analysis of data extracted from randomized trials were that a modest reduction in salt intake for a duration of > 4 weeks or more significantly reduces normal and elevated blood pressures. Within a range of daily salt intakes from 3 to 12 g/day, reductions in intake paralleled reductions in blood pressure.

It has been estimated that the average daily salt intake in the UK is 9 g (James et al. 1987). Reductions in average dietary salt intakes to < 6 g/day were recommended by the World Health Organization (1998). In comparison, for adults > 50 years RNIs of sodium are 1.6 g/day (Department of Health 1991, 2001). In practice, this means changing the type and frequency of foods consumed, in addition to reducing salt added during or after cooking. Approximately 75% of dietary salt intake is derived from that added during manufacture and preparation, notably to cheese, bacon, bread, canned foods and preserved meats.

Dietary potassium intakes are also vital in the maintenance of blood pressure. Krishna et al. (1989) found that mean arterial blood pressure levels were higher in subjects consuming a low-potassium diet. Currently the RNI for potassium in adults over 50 years is 3.5 g daily (Department of Health 1991, 2001). Potassium is found in abundance in fruit and vegetables, notably bananas and potatoes.

Calcium intakes and hypertension

McCarron et al. (1982) found that a low dietary calcium intake and alterations in calcium metabolism predisposed to hypertension in some populations. The precise role of calcium deficiency in the genesis of hypertension in older populations is not clear, nor are the potential benefits of increasing dietary calcium intakes on blood pressure. Since the risk of hypertension appears to increase at intakes lower than 400–600 mg daily, the maintenance of intakes at the current RNI of 700 mg daily is supported.

Alcohol and vascular disease

Low-to-moderate alcohol consumption has been consistently associated with a reduced total mortality, and that attributed to heart disease, in comparison with complete abstinence. Age does not change this relationship between alcohol consumption and mortality. In contrast, excessive alcohol consumption is associated with increased risks of cancer, hypertension, liver disease, stroke and accidental injury. Current safe levels of consumption (maximum) are 21 units weekly for females and 28 for males; where 1 unit equates with a single glass of wine, measure of spirits, and half a pint of beer (Department of Health 1997).

There is no evidence to suggest that excessive alcohol consumption is a particular problem in the older population, since a survey by the Ministry of Agriculture, Fisheries and Food (1993) has shown that in pensioners' households per-capita expenditure on alcohol is only 40–45% of that found in other age groups. In older males aged over 75 years 17% consumed fairly high to high intakes of alcohol, in comparison with 20% in the 65–74-year age group and 28% in the 16-years-plus group. In females only 3% over 75 years consumed fairly high levels of alcohol.

Non-insulin-dependent diabetes mellitus (NIDDM)

Non-insulin-dependent, type 2 diabetes mellitus is notably prevalent in countries where the food supply is plentiful. Although the disorder has a genetic basis, it can be precipitated by risk factors such as obesity, inactivity and smoking. The principal feature is a relative decrease in insulin secretion, resulting in changes in glucose, fat and protein metabolism. The prevalence of NIDDM increases with age and has been estimated to affect up to 30% of individuals aged over 75 years (Department of Health 1991). Glucose homeostasis is impaired with age and is manifest as impaired glucose tolerance in response to an oral glucose load, i.e. an elevation in blood glucose concentration evident 2–3 h following loading, when insulin secretion in healthy subjects has returned the blood glucose concentration to resting levels of 4–5 mmol/l. The impairment in glucose tolerance has been attributed to a relative decrease in insulin production by pancreatic beta cells, and a reduced sensitivity of insulin-sensitive tissue to the hormone, known as 'insulin resistance' (Kaiser 1995). Possible mechanisms underlying the development of age-related hyperglycaemia or NIDDM include postreceptor defects in beta cells, and deposition of amylin in the pancreatic islets. Insulin resistance as a phenomenon appears to be associated with obesity, specifically the distribution of body fat, as shown in a high hip-to-waist ratio (Kohrt et al. 1993).

NIDDM is associated with a reduced life expectancy and a morality ratio 2.3 times higher than that recorded for non-diabetics (Morley & Kaiser 1990). This is not surprising, considering the wide range and variable severity of complications associated with the disorder. These include nephropathy, retinopathy, cataract, neuropathic changes, myopathy, impaired cognitive function and vascular problems caused by autonomic dysfunction, such as arrhythmias and hypotension. People with diabetes also have an increased risk of atherosclerosis and associated cardiovascular disease. However, recent findings of a multicentre randomized controlled clinical trial in the UK have demonstrated that atorvastin, a statin with lipid-lowering effects, is highly effective in the primary prevention of cardiovascular disease in patients suffering from type 2 diabetes mellitus, without high concentrations of LDL cholesterol (Colhoun et al. 2004).

The cornerstone of managing NIDDM in older individuals is based on a reduced fat/sugar diet, high in complex carbohydrates and fibre (Department of Health 1991, 2001). Specific features are as follows:

- Maintain a desirable body weight and pattern of physical activity
- In obesity, achieve a slow, steady weight loss of 0.25–0.50 kg per week
- 50–55% of dietary energy should be obtained from carbohydrate (complex carbohydrate rich in fibre raises peripheral insulin sensitivity)
- 30–35% of dietary energy should be provided by fat, of which no more than one-third is derived from saturated fats
- 10–15% of the dietary energy should be provided by protein
- Non-soluble polysaccharide (NSP) derived from the plant cell wall, which is not digested or absorbed in the colon, is essential to slow glucose absorption from the gut and reduce absorption of cholesterol
- A diet rich in NSP is also fibre-abundant and low in energy density, which enhances weight control and slows gastric emptying – all beneficial to diabetic control.

Although it has been acknowledged that initial dietary management is a vital aspect of treatment following the diagnosis of type 2 diabetes mellitus, evidence concerning dietary efficacy has not been critically appraised. However, a recent systematic review by Moore et al. (2004) evaluated the impact of dietary advice provided to adults on measures of diabetic control in randomized controlled clinical trials of 6 months' duration, in which diet constituted the major intervention. The dietary approaches investigated included low-fat/high-carbohydrate, high-fat/low-carbohydrate, low-calorie (1000 kcal/day) and very-low-calorie (500 kcal/day) regimens. Conclusions were that there was no high-quality evidence on the efficacy of dietary treatment, although exercise may have exerted beneficial effects on glycosylated haemoglobin levels, a measure of glycaemic control. Further longitudinal comparative research trials are urgently needed to provide evidence for dietary interventions.

A number of proprietary brand foods are manufactured for use in diabetic diets; they contain fructose or sorbitol, or other types of sweetening agents (aspartame). In general, these are relatively expensive to purchase, which may preclude or limit their use for the older population. In some individuals NIDDM may be controlled by diet alone; in others, oral hypoglycaemic drugs may be used in combination with diet.

Eye disorders

In older persons, disorders which contribute markedly to visual loss are glaucoma, diabetic retinopathy, cataracts (opacity of the lens) and age-related macular degeneration (ARMD) in which the macula of the eye used to visualize fine detail degenerates. In recent years, both cataracts and ARMD, which are the most common disorders, have generated a great deal of interest in relation to the possible role of nutrition in their prevention and treatment. Eye disorders are discussed in Chapter 12, therefore the focus here is on nutritional uses.

Cataracts have been attributed to the damaging effects of ultraviolet radiation, degenerative changes associated with diabetes mellitus and a low dietary intake of the antioxidant vitamins A, C and E. A number of early surveys suggested the following:

- vitamin E intake might decrease the development of cataracts in older people
- older persons consuming fewer than 3.5 portions of fruit or vegetables each day increased the risk of cataract (Jacques & Chylack 1991)
- consumption of multivitamin supplements reduced the risk of cataract (Leske et al. 1991).

However, more recent findings of a double-masked clinical trial conducted over a 7-year period in 4629 well-nourished adults of 55–80 years, with at least one natural lens present, did not find any significant reduction in the risk of developing age-related lens opacities, or loss of visual acuity resulting from the consumption of supplements of antioxidant vitamins C, E and beta-carotene (Age Related Eye Disease Study Research Group 2001).

Megadoses of vitamins can have toxic visual and other physiological effects, therefore unsupervised use of supplements is not recommended. Further research is necessary to clarify optimal doses of specific vitamins.

Neurological disorders

Dementias

A survey of carers, health professionals and people suffering from dementia reported by the Alzheimers Society (2000) revealed that inadequate intakes of food and fluids, swallowing problems, weight loss and anorexia were cause for concern in hospitals and care homes. Prior to institutional care in the early stages of dementia, forgetting to eat and difficulties with shopping and preparing food can be experienced. Later phases may be marked by severe agitation, an inability to self-feed, hoarding of food in the cheek pouch due to impaired chewing and dysphagia. Food may not be recognized and aversion behaviour, marked by a refusal to cooperate with feeders, can occur, manifest in spitting food out and turning the head away when carers attempt to insert food in the mouth (Watson 1996). This creates a number of challenges for carers in the ethical, practical and emotional dimensions of care. A number of strategies have attempted to increase food intake and prevent a deterioration in nutritional status, for example using supplements, finger foods, modified food textures and modifying the environment using animal-assisted therapy (Edwards & Beck 2002, Faxen-Irving et al. 2002). However, although results of these interventions show that it is possible to increase energy intakes and promote weight gain, practical solutions to the complex, aversive eating behaviours resulting from dementia remain elusive. Barratt (2004) recommends that researchers investigating these problems need to consider the broader social, environmental and cultural aspects of eating, together with the views of carers and patients as a basis for finding solutions. In the interim, the Voluntary Organizations Involved in Caring in the Older Sector (VOICES 1998) report suggests a number of constructive standards of care to assist carers feeding older people suffering from dementia, covering planning and organization, giving choice and resolving practical issues. Identification of eating difficulties by nurses can be enabled using the EdFED assessment scale (Watson 1996) which provides a helpful basis for care-planning and monitoring progress (McLaren & Crawley 2000). For more information on care of people with dementia, see Chapter 24.

Stroke

The neurological deficits that result from stroke can lead to a formidable array and combination of eating problems constituting 'eating disability'. These include arm dysfunction caused by paralysis or paresis, which can be either unilateral or bilateral and result in an inability to cut food, load cutlery, lift a cup, unwrap food items or lift heavy plate covers. Visual field deficits can impair the ability to see food items on a meal tray, or select items from a menu unaided, problems enhanced by the presence of aphasia or dysphasia which impair communication. Paralysis affecting the circumoral muscles can lead to impaired lip closure and repulsion of food or liquids from the mouth, and chewing impairment can lead to impaction of food in the cheek sulcus.

One of the most serious eating problems resulting from stroke is dysphagia, which may vary in severity but carries with it the risk of aspirating food or fluid into the respiratory tract. Visual neglect, i.e. lack of attention to half the visual space, may result in a bizarre problem of failing to eat food on one side of the plate. A reduced attention span and short-term memory loss may result in an inability to follow through the sequence of activities necessary to eat; food consumption following stroke may also be adversely affected by anorexia resulting from depression. Any one of these problems may constitute a serious difficulty to inde-pendent eating; in combination they are formidable, and frequently difficult to assess. The presence of severe poststroke eating problems has been associated with reduced food intake, a decline in nutritional status and mortality (Axelsson et al. 1984, McLaren & Dickerson 2000). Such problems pose a significant challenge for the nurse to manage. Development, implementation and evaluation of evidence-based guidelines for nutritional support following acute stroke have shown that improvements in documented nursing practice that result can reduce infective complications experienced by patients (Perry & McLaren 2003).

Cancer

Malignant disease is a major cause of mortality in the ageing population and it has been suggested that dietary factors are implicated in the aetiology of 50% of all cancers in women and 30% in men (Dickerson & Williams 1988, Havlick 1992). Reasons for this are that a number of natural carcinogens or contaminants in food may act as initiators of cancer, and that specific dietary components and food additives may be cancer promoters. Examples of specific cancers and their dietary risk factors include:

- oesophageal cancer (high alcohol intakes, pickles, moulds)
- stomach cancer (smoked, salted, spiced foods)
- colon cancer (low-fibre diet)
- breast cancer (high fat intake).

It is important to bear in mind that dietary factors may not act independently, but are only carcinogenic in combination with other factors. For example, cancers affecting the mouth and oesophagus are associated with the combination of smoking and high alcohol consumption. The contribution of dietary factors to overall risk should feature in health promotion strategies aimed at reducing the incidence of malignant disease in all age groups.

In individuals suffering from malignant disease, alterations in the consumption of food and fluids can be caused by a combination of disease and treatment-related factors. In the main, these can lead to severe weight loss and the development of a malnourished state, in which disease and treatment-related effects worsen in a vicious cycle. Specific examples of these include:

- dysgeusia, cachexia, depression arising from the pathophysiological and psychological impact of disease (dysgeusia is alteration in taste; cachexia in cancer is a syndrome marked by anorexia, profound weight loss and abnormal metabolism)

- mucositis, ageusia, xerostomia caused by side-effects of chemotherapy and radiotherapy (mucositis induced by radiation treatment is an inflammatory condition of the mucous membrane of the mouth marked by xerostomia, erythema, ulceration and pseudomembrane formation; ageusia is loss of taste; xerostomia is a feeling of mouth dryness not always associated with a decrease in salivation).

Both disease and treatment can lead to the development of other distressing symptoms, such as nausea, vomiting, anorexia, wasting, diarrhoea, fatigue, altered sensation and increased vulnerability to sepsis due to depressed immunity. Alone, or in combination, these symptoms can exert a significant negative effect on food intake and quality of life. Motivating and assisting patients to eat and drink in these circumstances pose an enormous challenge in which respect for autonomous choice is paramount.

Surgery, trauma, sepsis

Surgery, trauma and sepsis can produce significant changes in the direction and magnitude of body metabolism, increasing requirements for energy, protein and micronutrients. Older patients are at risk of increased perioperative morbidity and mortality; it is likely that poor nutritional status may be a contributory factor (Hirsch 1995). Malnourished patients undergoing surgery have been shown to sustain a higher incidence of wound-related and other complications, for example episodes of sepsis that hinder recovery and lengthen periods of hospitalization. It has been previously noted that, unfortunately, 10–40% of older patients admitted to hospital are already malnourished as a consequence of socioeconomic, psychological and disease-related factors. Effects of trauma, sepsis and surgery superimposed on this can lead to further depletion of nutrient stores (fat, glycogen) and reserves (muscle) as a consequence of metabolic responses which are catabolic. It is vital that individuals who are malnourished, or likely to become so following surgical treatment, are identified at an early stage so that appropriate nutritional support can be given to improve clinical outcome. Minimizing periods of nil-by-mouth for diagnostic tests and pre- and postoperative fasting are vital considerations here.

Why do the direction and magnitude of body metabolism change following surgery, trauma and severe sepsis? The reason is that a metabolic neuro-humoral response is evoked which is designed to ensure survival and promote healing. This is accomplished by mobilizing nutrient stores and reserves through neural and humoral mechanisms. The magnitude of the meta-bolic response is proportional to injury severity and is influenced by many factors, which include pre-existing nutritional status (diminished in depletion) and the presence of sepsis (increased) in older people. The response has been shown to occur following burns, femoral fracture, head injury and stroke. Readers are referred to Elia (1990) and Bastow et al. (1983) for details of metabolic responses to these catastrophes.

IMPACT OF DISTRESSING SYMPTOMS ON EATING AND DRINKING

Many of the medical conditions discussed above can result in the development of unpleasant, distressing symptoms that impair food consumption and can contribute to the development of PEM and impaired quality of life in older people. High-risk distressing symptoms (e.g. dysphagia) may be identified during nutritional screening. More comprehensive assessment, which includes taking a dietary history, can identify other symptoms of dietary relevance. During the assessment, management and monitoring of symptom distress, the following should be determined:

- symptom severity and duration
- factors triggering or exacerbating symptom distress
- aetiology of symptoms, diagnostic information from special investigations
- impact of symptom distress on food and fluid intake, nutritional status, general clinical condition
- effectiveness of specific interventions in symptom palliation for the individual patient/client
- need for interdisciplinary team work at all stages.

Some approaches to symptom distress management in the context of nutritional status, eating and drinking are discussed below.

Alteration in taste and smell

In older people deficits in taste and smell appear to be associated with ageing (see Chapter 5). Smell appears to decline more markedly than taste. However, alteration in taste (dysgeusia), diminished taste (hypogeusia) or complete loss of taste (ageusia) may also be caused by a number of diseases and as side-effects of drug or other forms of therapy. Such changes can diminish pleasure in eating and drinking or contribute to a reduced food intake.

Dysgeusia is reported to affect 25–50% of patients suffering from cancer, who may report a raised taste threshold for some foods (tastes appear weaker) or a lower threshold where the reverse is experienced

(Twycross & Lack 1986). Taste changes may also occur as a consequence of chemotherapy or radiotherapy to the head and neck. The latter is usually a temporary effect, since taste is restored in most cases between 20 and 60 days following radiotherapy (Mossman 1986).

Altered, diminished or complete absence of taste may also occur in vitamin and mineral-deficiency states, notably of vitamins A, B and zinc. Taste changes have also been reported in response to metronidazole and lithium carbonate therapy, the latter causing an unpleasant metallic taste. Hypogeusia or dysgeusia may also result from neurological damage associated with stroke or cerebral surgery. Approaches which may help in the management of taste alteration or impairment include the following:

- dietetic manipulation to select foods that maximize acceptable taste sensation, or use of condiments to enhance particular flavours
- use of spices or herbs during food preparation which maximize aroma detectable by smell
- vitamin and mineral replacement in established deficiency states
- attention to oral hygiene and giving up smoking.

The benefits of adding flavour enhancers selected according to the protein component of the meal and the cooking process have been evaluated in older nursing-home residents with stable health status (Mathey et al. 2001). Over a 16-week period, increased hunger feelings, improvements in smell perception, and average body weight were reported in a flavour intervention group in comparison with controls.

Nausea and vomiting

Diverse factors may lead to nausea and vomiting, ranging from relatively innocuous constipation or transient gastrointestinal infection to drug side-effects and serious underlying neurological, renal and liver disease, cancer and its treatment. Effective treatment is aimed at alleviating or palliating the underlying cause, replacing lost fluids and electrolytes and removing any environmental contributory factors. Some general interventions that can be helpful include:

- pre-emptive use of antiemetic drugs (Table 16.4) appropriate to the underlying disorder
- eating small amounts of food slowly in an upright posture, maintained for 30 min after a meal to prevent regurgitation
- avoidance of fatty and/or fried food
- sipping cool, clear fluids through a straw; use of nutritious food supplements in small quantities

- reducing or reviewing the dosage of drugs with emetic side-effects, e.g. antibiotics, opioid analgesics
- removing unpleasant smells or other trigger factors.

For patients suffering from nausea and vomiting associated with the use of cytotoxic drugs, use of complementary therapies such as acupuncture has proved helpful. Behavioural techniques based on guided imagery, relaxation and deep breathing can also be of benefit (Morrow & Morrell 1982, Dundee & Yang 1991). For further information on complementary therapies, see Chapter 31.

Constipation

It has been estimated that constipation affects about 20% of the population over 65 years old and that women are more severely affected than men. Although difficult to define due to the great variation in normal healthy people, in individuals constipation is infrequency in bowel habit marked by fewer than three occasions per week, a gut transit time of more than 5 days and stool weight of less than 50 g/day (Department of Health 1991, 2001). In healthy older individuals, constipation can be prevented by maintaining physical activity, ensuring an adequate fluid intake of 2–3 l/day and consuming fibre-rich, NSP in natural foods. The latter non-digestible components of food are found in leafy vegetables, peas and beans (cellulose) and in fruit, vegetables, cereals and fungi (non-cellulose); the recommended average daily intake of NSP is 18 g (range 12–24 g). More information on constipation can be found in Chapter 17.

Anorexia

In older people anorexia may be due in part to the process of ageing, but specific medical conditions, drugs and environmental factors may initiate the problem. Anorexia has been closely linked with the presence of apathy, anxiety, depression and weight loss; treating the underlying cause of depression or anxiety is vital in resolving the problem (Morley & Kraenzle 1994). Cachexic syndrome resulting from malignant disease is associated with anorexia, alterations in taste and smell, catabolism and severe wasting. It is initiated by tumour metabolites and mediators of the host response, notably by cytokines, including tumour necrosis factor and the chemicals known as interleukins (Argiles et al. 2003). Arresting cachexia has proved a difficult challenge, but use of progestational drugs such as megestrol acetate and

Table 16.4 Nausea and vomiting: antiemetic use

Feature	Rationale	Antiemetic
Anticipatory nausea and vomiting	Fear, anxiety	Benzodiazepine Haloperidol
Precipitated or worse on movement	Infection of middle ear Ménière's disease Tumour; side-effects of drugs	Cyclizine
Stimulation of medullary vomiting centre directly	Metastases in brainstem	Dexamethasone
	Traumatic/vascular causes of raised intracranial pressure Radiotherapy to head/neck	Cyclizine
Stimulation of peripheral autonomic afferent nerves	Metastatic distension of the liver capsule Constipation Irritation of the pharynx (infection, sputum)	Cyclizine
Distension of the stomach	Gastric atony	Nasogastric suction to remove fluid, air
Stimulation of the chemoreceptor zone	Morphine/cytotoxic drugs Uraemia Hypercalcaemia	Haloperidol
Regurgitation of food and fluids, saliva	Obstruction of the oesophagus by tumour Impaired swallowing reflex in stroke Oesophagitis	High-dose corticosteroids/radiotherapy to decrease obstruction Reduce pharyngeal secretions with hyoscine Antifungal treatment for infection
Gastric stasis	Morphine/anticholinergic drugs Outflow obstruction (partial) due to tumours, ascites, liver distension	Metoclopramide Domperidone
Gastritis	Non-steroidal anti-inflammatory drugs or corticosteroid oral drug treatment Alcohol Biliary reflux	Metoclopramide Domperidone

Modifed from Allan (1995).

medroxyprogesterone acetate have proved to be of benefit and are widely prescribed, except when tumours are hormone-dependent. Improved appetite, weight gain and enhanced feelings of well-being have been reported (Loprinzi 1990; Alexander & Norton 1995). These drugs exert their effects by down-regulating the production of cytokines. Side-effects including fluid retention and sexual dysfunction may occur (Laviano et al. 2003).

Anorexia may be a symptom of other chronic disorders in older people, including liver and renal disease or gut tumours. Again, treating the underlying medical cause is necessary to alleviate the symptom. Occasionally the problem may be precipitated by factors as diverse as uncontrolled pain, swallowing purulent sputum, unpleasant smells or sights and excessive noise. Removing environmental stimuli and controlling other symptoms effectively are necessary. Opiate analgesics, antibiotics, cardiac glycosides and antineoplastic drugs may also cause loss of appetite as a side-effect. Sometimes this is a transient problem if the treatment period is short, but if the drugs are used for longer periods or indefinitely, adjusting the dose may be necessary to reduce side-effects and serious impairment of nutritional status.

Whatever the underlying cause of anorexia, some general approaches may be helpful in increasing appetite:

- respecting and encouraging autonomous choice in meal selection
- serving small, frequent meals attractively and in a quiet, tranquil setting
- providing an appetite stimulant such as a glass of sherry 20 min before a meal
- prescribing dietary supplements, which are palatable, easily ingested and of significant nutrient value, e.g. Fortical (246 kcal/200 ml supplied in various flavours; glucose polymer); Build-up (106 kcal/38 g; 6.2 g protein made with whole milk, various flavours).

Where anorexia is associated with alterations in taste, use of flavourings which are palatable and aromatic may be helpful.

Diarrhoea

Diarrhoea can be defined as the passage of frequent loose stools on more than 2–3 occasions in a single 24-h period (Sykes 1995). In older persons it can be caused by side-effects of drug therapy, notably with antibiotics, non-steroidal anti-inflammatories (NSAIDs), antineoplastics and laxatives. It may also follow dietary excesses with alcohol, use of bran and spices. Radiotherapy to the gut, the presence of carcinoid tumours, gut infection, inflammatory bowel disease and malabsorption syndromes can also lead to severe diarrhoea and its complications of fluid and electrolyte imbalance (see Chapter 17 for more information).

Initial supportive dietary management of diarrhoea includes:

- rehydration, orally or intravenously, using an appropriate replacement solution
- solely consuming clear fluids for 24 h, following which bland, low-fat foods can be introduced, progressing to solids as the problem resolves
- avoiding milk ingestion if transient lactose deficiency associated with some gut infections is suspected
- review of contributory factors, i.e. drug treatment, diet.

Changes in intestinal microflora have been shown to occur with ageing (Hebuterne 2003). Specifically, a decline in anaerobes and bifidobacteria together with an increase in enterobacteria can occur which, when combined with reduced gut immunity, could favour the development of intestinal infections with organisms such as *Clostridium difficile*, a common nosocomial infection in older adults associated with diarrhoea. The use of probiotics (which incorporate lactobacilli) as a dietary supplement may offer valuable therapeutic effects in *C. difficile*-associated diarrhoea. Further research is necessary to evaluate these therapeutic effects and identify the patients who can benefit most.

Oral repulsion of food and fluids

When food is ingested, the lip muscles are contracted to form an anterior seal which prevents leakage during chewing and swallowing. With increased age, reduced mass of the masseter muscles of the jaw and decreased tone in the circumoral muscles can result in drooling of saliva and repulsion of food and fluids. This is not normally a problem as affected individuals are aware of it, and it usually involves only small volumes of liquid or food which are easily removed. However, more severe problems can occur when motor and sensory loss following cerebral infarction, haemorrhage, trauma, tumours and dementia result in paralysis of facial and circumoral muscles, lack of awareness of food on the lips or in the mouth and loss of effective lip seal. Saliva, food and fluids then leak from the mouth, usually from one side, depending on the location and severity of neurological injury. The problem is compounded by chewing and swallowing impairments, cognitive deficits which reduce awareness of mealtime events and the ingestion of food textures that are difficult to control, i.e. liquids and some semisolids.

Oral repulsion of food and fluids is distressing, causing embarrassment and loss of dignity for the individuals affected. Sensitive assessment is necessary to determine the extent of the problem and identify contributory factors and the awareness of the individual of leakage. Supportive interventions include the provision of mealtime privacy if the problem is severe, and assisting or teaching manual lip-closure techniques. Motor control and sensory awareness can be maximized by positioning food on the unaffected, non-paralysed side of the mouth and tilting the head to this side (Logemann 1997). Provision of food of appropriate volumes and textures is also important, as is ensuring adequate protection of clothing. Referral to a speech therapist can be extremely helpful in identifying exercises that improve mandibular and labial closure and other problems that may be present.

Impaired chewing

With increased age, loss of teeth, reduced salivary output and muscle mass can impair chewing, to the extent that more chewing strokes are needed to reduce a mouthful of test food. Effects of the neurological disorders listed above can also impair chewing and lead to the accumulation of food in the cheek pouch.

Paralysis affecting the muscles of the jaw is not infrequently associated with paralysis of the tongue. The latter impairs localization, separation and formation of a bolus, and its propulsion to the posterior oral cavity prior to reflex swallowing.

Since chewing impairment resulting from neurological disorder is often associated with more complex swallowing problems, assessment by a speech therapist is recommended, and referral to a dietician is necessary for advice on dietary texture, volume and quality. Interventions that can help to resolve chewing impairment include the following:

- dental assessment; correction of problems affecting gums, teeth, dentures and palate
- mild chewing problems can be helped by providing mechanically soft textured foods, prepared without blending or puréeing. Dry, crispy, raw, stringy foods should be avoided, as should nuts and vegetables with tough skins. Meat should be minced and liquids provided as tolerated; medications should be taken in liquid form or as directed by the pharmacist (Martin 1991)
- individuals afflicted with moderate problems which result in reduced tolerance of chewable foods and an inability to swallow thin liquids safely may need a diet based on purées which incorporates some texture, flavour and variety. Liquids require thickening using a commercial agent; water is not taken. No coarse textures are usually permitted, e.g. nuts, raw fruits or vegetables. Creamed rice, scrambled eggs, cottage cheese and puréed meats are included
- where paralysis affects one side of the mouth, positioning food to be chewed on the unaffected side is helpful. Removal of any impacted food from the cheek pouch in conjunction with other oral hygiene measures is necessary after meals
- if sensory impairment is present affecting the gums, mucosa and tongue, localization of a food bolus can be improved by providing cold, thick, non-acid liquids and including foods to which patients are taste-sensitive.

Dysphagia

Dysphagia is an unpleasant, anxiety-evoking symptom that is not uncommon in older people, notably those suffering from a variety of neurological disorders and cancer (Twycross 1995, Finestone & Green-Finestone 2003). Swallowing is a highly complex process, requiring the integration and coordination of sensory and motor activity in the cranial nerves by control centres in the frontal cortex, medulla oblongata, pons and limbic system. The process covers the entire sequence of events following the insertion of food into the mouth to the arrival of a bolus in the stomach. Four stages are involved: (1) oral preparation; (2) oral transport; (3) pharyngeal transport; and (4) oesophageal transport. Manifestations of dysphagia depend on the stage of swallowing affected and can range from leakage of food from the mouth to choking, coughing and regurgitation of food through the nose. Management of some of the symptoms of dysfunctional oral preparation and transport has been discussed earlier.

The presence of dysphagia carries the risk of aspirating saliva, fluids and food into the respiratory tract, leading to bronchopneumonia and airway obstruction. Complications such as this are thought to explain the high morbidity and mortality associated with poststroke dysphagia, which can be difficult to identify (Doggett et al. 2001). For this reason it is vital that rigorous screening followed by more detailed assessment occurs, to identify the presence, type and severity of dysphagia, drawing on evidence gained from the use of validated screening instruments, clinical bedside assessment, videofluoroscopy and fibreoptic endoscopic evaluation. This requires the combined skills of nurse and physician in identifying the problem initially, followed by rapid referrals to speech therapist and radiologist for expert diagnosis. A systematic review by Perry & Love (2001) identified a number of screening instruments for use in neurogenic dysphagia, which varied in meeting criteria for reliability and validity. In content, these included the identification of clinical manifestations of dysphagia with or without an assessment of the patient's ability to swallow a measured amount of water. It is vital that level of consciousness, oromotor and laryngeal function, signs of aspiration and the extent to which the patient can cooperate safely with screening are checked beforehand. Training in the use of screening instruments is mandatory.

Causes of dysphagia can be categorized very broadly as either obstructive or neurogenic, with some mixed types and rare forms. Obstructions of varying degrees affecting the oral cavity, pharynx or oesophagus may be intrinsic or extrinsic in origin. Intrinsic obstructions can arise due to the presence of cancers of the head, neck and oesophagus, specifically those involving the nasopharynx, pharynx, tongue, valleculae and postcricoid area. Severe inflammation and local oedema can also lead to obstruction. Causes include candidiasis affecting the pharynx and oesophagus and postradiation mucositis. Other causes of intrinsic obstruction include oesophageal spasm precipitated by anxiety, achalasia and strictures of benign aetiology (achalasia is the failure of the lower oesophageal segment to relax on swallowing. The achalastic segment causes obstruction and the area above it becomes dilated and hypertrophied). Extrinsic obstruction of the oesophagus can occur due to compression by mediastinal tumours.

In contrast, neurogenic transfer dysphagia may occur following stroke, dementia, cerebral tumours, trauma, motor neurone disease and multiple sclerosis. All these disorders can affect neural control centres, cranial nerves and associated structures coordinating the first three stages of swallowing. Less common neurogenic or neuromuscular causes of dysphagia include dystonic side-effects of drugs, such as metoclopramide, and the hypercalcaemia associated with carcinoma of the bronchus.

Enabling dysphagic patients to eat and drink safely is a vital component of successful management. Some key points relevant in assisting swallowing are summarized in Table 16.5. Assisting or feeding dysphagic individuals is a highly skilled task which should not be delegated to junior nurses, who may have insufficient knowledge and experience to cope. If possible the same nurse should be allocated at mealtimes to assist a patient, to ensure continuity in monitoring progress. Whatever the cause of dysphagia, deteriorating nutritional status, starvation and its associated complications are potential risks that can be prevented by rapid referral to a dietician or nutrition support team, so that nutritional needs can be met by an appropriate method. In relation to nutrition management, Twycross (1995) has emphasized the need to make distinctions between eating for pleasure and nutritional goals for the restoration or maintenance of health, given that some dysphagic individuals are suffering from terminal cancer or irreversible, progressive neurological deterioration, and others have hope of recovery. Where the extent of obstruction or neurological injury renders swallowing unsafe, difficult or impossible, artificial methods of nutritional support may be instituted, either enterally via gastrostomy or jejeunostomy or parenterally.

Dietary advice: obstruction

Tumours causing intrinsic or extrinsic compression usually create difficulties at the outset in swallowing solid textures. Foods to be avoided include nuts, fruit skins, raw or lightly cooked vegetables, pithy segments of orange or grapefruit, fibrous roast meats, hard-boiled eggs and soft doughy bread, which are prone to block the oesophagus (Taylor & Goodinson-McLaren 1992, Penman & Thomson 1998). Food textures of the liquid–soft paste spectrum are usually easier to swallow. Liquidized meals can be highly nutritious and with the use of savoury or sweet garnishes can be made tasty and attractive. To retain nutrient value in small volume, as little liquid as possible should be used in preparation, and care should be taken to use hot liquids and plates to retain an acceptable, palatable temperature. A number of commercial supplements are available which can be sipped between meals to raise energy, protein and fluid consumption. Inflammatory conditions affecting the oesophagus can cause pain on swallowing; to ease swallowing, liquid local anaesthetics such as oxethazaine can be taken 15 min before meals.

Other treatment: obstruction

Inflammatory conditions such as candidal oesophagitis respond well to antifungal drugs, for example nystatin suspension (10^5 units/ml; 1–2 ml as directed) and ketoconazole 200 mg daily. Indometacin can be used to attenuate the extent of radiation mucositis and dexamethasone can be very effective in relieving inflammation associated with external oesophageal compression by tumours (Carter et al. 1982). Insertion of an endo-oesophageal tube, palliative surgery or irradiation can also be used to relieve oesophageal obstruction. Troublesome oral accumulation of saliva as a result of total obstruction can be relieved by treatment with transdermal hyoscine patches.

Dietary advice: neurogenic dysphagia

Patients with neurogenic dysphagia marked by severely impaired oral preparation, oral transport and pharyngeal transport are unable to chew solids or swallow thin liquids safely. Foods to be omitted include those of coarse, hard or brittle textures. Fruits, nuts, raw vegetables, sticky foods requiring bolus formation or thin liquids requiring controlled oral manipulation should not be taken. Thick, homogeneous, smooth, semisolid textures are recommended, with cold, thickened liquids. Poached eggs, soft puddings, custards, thick fruit or vegetable purées are all suitable (Curran & Groher 1990, Martin 1991, Penman & Thomson 1998). Individuals with inadequate fluid bolus control and impaired swallow, cough or gag reflexes require short-term intravenous fluid replacement to prevent dehydration. Artificial methods of feeding may be required subsequently if oral feeding cannot be re-established within a short period of time due to loss of reflex swallow.

Other interventions

Pharyngeal transport or reflex swallowing problems in neurogenic dysphagia can be improved by a range of other therapeutic techniques. Reduced pharyngeal peristalsis may be helped by turning the head to the affected side during eating, which closes the pyriform sinus, directing food down the non-paralysed side. Increasing sensory stimulation to heighten the

Table 16.5 Neurologic swallowing problems: enabling patients to eat and drink safely

Components	Activities
Preliminary screening using validated, reliable method (nurse, doctor)	Dependent on method
	Prescreen checking of conscious level and ability to cooperate safely with screening
	Alertness and attention span checked
Variable depending on method (radiologist)	Swallowing capacity determined from oesophagoscopy, videofluoroscopy, fibreoptic endofluoroscopy and bedside assessment
Assessment of nutrient requirements (dietician) in conjunction with food preferences (patient)	Daily energy, macro- and micronutrient requirements determined, e.g. using predictive formula
	Food and fluids of appropriate volume, quality and texture for safe swallowing provided
Provision of appropriate environment	Quiet and privacy ensured to assist concentration and relaxation
Information exchange	Spectacles, hearing aid checked
	Anxiety diminished, learning facilitated by explaining swallowing techniques using non-technical language
	Patient taught to control a single action, gradually building up a sequence
	Feedback elicited on feelings and difficulties
	Verbal and non-verbal communication used to convey positive praise and support for progress
Posture	Nurse positioned sitting, facing patient
	Patient positioned upright, head stable in midline, slightly flexed forward to protect airway and minimize aspiration risk (depends on nature of swallowing disorder)
	Upright posture maintained for 30 min following meal to prevent regurgitation and aspiration
Ingestion of food and fluids using appropriate aids	Dentures checked in situ
	Small amounts of food or fluids of safe temperature and texture placed in mouth
	Food positioned in mouth on unaffected side using hand mirror to demonstrate correct positioning as appropriate
	Patient taught to inspire, hold breath, swallow, expire, cough on expiration to clear food debris
	Aids to feeding which consider postural problems, impaired arm movement used; a styrofoam mug with cut-out for nose is valuable in assisting drinking without tipping head backwards
Evaluation of swallowing capacity	Detailed assessments of swallowing capacity repeated
	Tolerance, ease of swallowing, time taken to consume meal, exertion required all monitored
	Quantities of food or fluid ingested recorded on chart; dietetic review
	Nutritional status assessed weekly

sensitivity of the swallowing reflex can be achieved by gently touching the faucial area using a cold dental mirror, providing cold, thickened liquids, strongly flavoured foods, or by inserting a palatal training device. The latter consists of a loop of wire attached to a dental plate which projects over the soft palate, stimulating pressure receptors which trigger reflex swallowing. This is well tolerated, effective and reduces aspiration (Selley 1989, Selley et al. 1995). Expert

advice is necessary prior to assisting or implementing these techniques.

Impaired arm movement

Normal eating activities require a formidable range of movement by the arm: using a fork or spoon and drinking from a cup using the dominant hand involve 5–45° of shoulder flexion/abduction, 70–130° elbow flexion, from 40° forearm pronation to 60° supination and 25° wrist extension (Rad 1990). These complex, finely tuned, coordinated movements encompass cutting and spearing food, loading cutlery and transferring food or a cup to the mouth without spillage. Finer movements are needed to remove cling film or food packaging. In older people a number of medical conditions may hinder this, limiting independence in eating. These include spastic or flaccid paralysis of the arm resulting from stroke, cerebral trauma or tumours; muscle tremor, rigidity, and lack of arm coordination in Parkinson's disease; and joint pain, impaired range of motion and deformity caused by acute or chronic arthritic conditions.

A number of aids can be provided by the occupational therapist to compensate limited arm movement. These include modified cutlery with built-up handles, non-slip plate mats, plate guards, light-weight cups and reusable straws. The extent to which arm movement is impaired and individuals are dependent on nursing assistance should be assessed carefully. Individuals suffering from mild degrees of arm impairment may require help at the beginning of a meal to remove plate lids, cling film or packaging. More severe impairment of range of movement may require intermittent or continuous feeding to ensure an adequate food intake. When tremor, spastic paralysis, involuntary movement and pain are major problems, drug therapy may produce some benefits for arm movement. Following neurological injury motor loss affecting a limb may also be accompanied by impaired sensation for temperature. Risks of accidental injury here can be minimized by instructing patients to use the unaffected hand to detect the degree of heat/cold in containers for food and liquids (McLaren 1997).

Impaired vision and perception

With increased age, both elasticity and opacity of the lens of the eye are impaired, in conjunction with loss of photoreceptive cells in the retina. These changes result in far-sightedness and loss of visual acuity which can affect many activities of daily living adversely. In relation to eating, problems can be experienced in reading or selecting from a menu, visualizing food items, preparing or ingesting food, and safety in consuming hot liquids or foods can be compromised. Degenerative visual changes can be compensated in part by corrective lenses, hence 97% of the population aged over 65 years wears glasses. However, frequent monitoring of changes in eye sight is necessary to ensure that the lenses supplied are appropriate (Department of Health 1992a).

Approximately 30–60% of individuals who suffer a stroke develop hemianopia, in which loss of vision is experienced in the right or left halves of both visual fields without affecting the other half-fields (homonymous hemianopia) (Gray et al. 1989). The result of this is that an individual may not be able to locate all the food items on a meal tray and omits to eat them; reading a menu can also be difficult. Risks of accidental injury are increased with this type of impairment. Important nursing interventions include teaching individuals to scan the visual field to compensate areas of loss, using consistent placement of the same items on a meal tray and providing help in selecting from a menu. This type of problem, which can be identified using confrontation testing, is frequently missed by nurses attempting to help patients eat (McLaren 1997).

Quite distinct from visual field impairment are visual perceptual deficits, 'visual neglect', which can follow strokes affecting the visual cortex. This results in lack of attention to half the visual space, causing bizarre manifestations such as ignoring food on one side of the plate or utensils or objects placed in that area. Individuals suffering from this problem require considerable supervision from nurses at mealtimes, a principal aim of care being to enable patients to acknowledge and use the neglected visual space. Approaching patients from the affected side, verbally reminding them of it, placing a bright marker on the side of the plate which is not perceived, and reducing the total number of items on a meal tray to focus attention can all be helpful. Visual neglect is identified using the line bisection test (Wade et al. 1985), but it should be noted that visual field deficits and visual neglect may coexist.

Memory loss: inattention to mealtimes as events

Dementia, stroke and other neurological disorders can result in short-term memory loss and an inability to concentrate on activities of daily living such as eating (Sissons 1988). Observed effects are forgetting to eat, eating courses in the wrong sequence, frequent distraction from eating and slowness in relearning eating skills. Nursing interventions that can be helpful include repeated verbal orientation to time and place and activity engaged, verbal prompts to continue eating, and use of cue cards or alarms to initiate or maintain activity (Johnstone 1991). As far as possible, environmental distractors should be minimized or removed, e.g. noise generated by radios or television sets, ward rounds at mealtimes and moving equipment for diagnostic investigations. In attempting to help older neurologically injured patients to relearn the motor skills necessary for independent eating, activities need to be separated into small sequences and any information given limited in volume and complexity.

Postural problems

The ability to attain and/or maintain an upright posture when eating and drinking is essential for safe swallowing, effective cutting and preparation of food, reaching or lifting utensils and food items and general comfort. A number of acute and chronic medical conditions can impair posture, either directly by affecting postural mechanisms or indirectly by causing profound physical prostration and weakness. Older people recovering from surgical procedures, orthopaedic trauma, chest infections or anaemia may be too weak, immobile and frail to attain an upright posture at mealtimes and can be dependent on nursing assistance for this. In contrast, the neurological deficits that follow acute stroke, head injury and cerebral tumours can affect posture of the head, neck and trunk, causing affected individuals to be unable to support their head and/or to fall towards the paralysed side of the body. Postural techniques to support the head, neck and trunk in the midline after stroke have been described by Carr & Kenney (1992). Other important points to attend to when positioning such patients in an upright sitting posture include protraction of the shoulder with the arm forward and hand pronated. More generally, effective use of postural aids at mealtimes is vital for safety and in ensuring comfort. Examples of such aids which can be provided by the physiotherapist and occupational therapist are backboards for chairs, adjustable-height bed tables, and/or Velcro arm support, and pillow supports of different shapes and sizes.

NUTRITIONAL SCREENING AND ASSESSMENT: MONITORING INDIVIDUALS AT NUTRITIONAL RISK

Preceding sections of this chapter have discussed reasons why older people may be malnourished or at risk of PEM. The use of appropriate methods of screening and assessment is therefore vital for effective management. Currently in the UK, the introduction of the single assessment process for older people as part of *National Service Frameworks* could incorporate nutrition risk screening as part of an overview assessment and more detailed investigation within specialist assessment (Department of Health 2001, 2002a, 2002b). Similarly, in the USA nutritional screening and assessment are incorporated within the process of comprehensive geriatric assessment (Devons 2002). In this section, selective approaches to both processes are reviewed, with an emphasis on the readily available, practically useful and reliable which may be used by nurses. For a broader, more detailed review of screening and assessment methods, readers are referred to the extensive publication by Waitzberg & Correia (2003). Also, Chapter 28 gives more information on the UK's single assessment process and other assessment methods.

Aims and approaches

Distinctions are made between two processes designed to identify individuals who are nutritionally at high risk: screening and assessment. Screening is a first-line filtering process in which a questionnaire, checklist or scaled instrument based on significant prognostic criteria (of PEM) is used to quantify risk (Vellas et al. 2001). Individuals in high-risk categories and/or with high-risk scores can then be referred for more thorough nutritional assessment. Typically a screening instrument could be incorporated into the nursing assessment record for all individuals admitted to an older-care unit or community caseload. Ideally screening instruments should be short, accessible, inexpensive and measure what they are intended to with consistency, i.e. they should have demonstrable validity and reliability. A number of nutritional screening instruments have been developed which are suitable for use with older populations. They vary considerably in content, level of measurement and the extent to which validity and reliability have been tested in different environments and cultures. Two of the three examples in Table 16.6 have been designed for use specifically with older adults and have been tested on some aspects of reliability and validity.

Nutritional assessment is a sequential process intended to pinpoint nutritional status at a given time and to evaluate subsequent changes by repeating measurements. The process can also be used to identify individuals requiring nutritional support and, depending on the method, provide guidelines to quantities of a particular nutrient needed. Any assessment process in human subjects can be affected by extraneous variables and nutritional assessment indicators are no exception. For example, body weight represents the total mass of skeleton, fat, water and protein in the body but the presence of a large, rapidly growing tumour weighing 5 kg can inflate apparent measurements and obscure interpretation of any subsequent changes. In order to compensate for the limitations of any single method of nutritional assessment, it is advisable to use two or three methods together. It is also important to select those that provide the most reliable information, given the potential impact of medical diagnosis and treatment on nutritional indicators. Other important considerations in selecting an appropriate method are patient safety, comfort, availability and cost.

Table 16.6 Examples of nutritional screening instruments

Instrument	Type	Content/components	Author
NURAS (Nutrition risk assessment scale)	12 items Score range: 0–12 >12 high risk for malnutrition Questionnaire	Medical, physical, anthropometric, lifestyle, socioeconomic areas Validated for use with older people	Nikolaus et al. (1995)
MAG (Malnutrition Advisory Group tool plus guidelines for action)	Step 1: 3 items Step 2: establishes overall risk Establishes high-, medium-, low-risk categories based on item combinations	Anthropometric, history of weight loss, decreased food intake, loose clothing, psychological, physical influences on weight loss Validated for use with adults	Elia (2000)
MNA (Mini-nutritional assessment) Stage 1: screening Stage 2: assessment	Stage 1: 6 items Stage 2: 12 items Score range: 0–30 <17 indicates protein-energy malnutrition Well-nourished, at risk of protein-energy malnutrition, malnourished categories based on total scores	Anthropometric measures, dietary and subjective assessment, lifestyle, medication, mobility Validated for use with older people	Vellas et al. 1999; Vellas et al. 2001.

A number of reference tables have been published detailing ranges of specific nutritional indicators (body weight, triceps skinfold thickness, etc.) found in apparently healthy, free-living male and female populations. Important questions are:

- To what extent do such tables represent the ranges of measurements found in older age groups of a specific ethnic origin?
- Is it appropriate to compare values obtained from measurements in a single individual with reference ranges or norms obtained from population surveys?

Given the significant extent of human variation in biological phenomena, it is generally considered more reliable to make serial measurements in an individual and interpret these changes over time, rather than make comparisons with reference norms. Some reference tables contain age cut-off points of 74 years and do not supply values for the 'very old'. Others are not specific for an ethnic group and may therefore be of limited value.

Broadly, nutritional assessment methods can be categorized as anthropometric, biochemical, subjective and functional. A number of methods are accurate but expensive and are not generally available. For this reason, examples given below are confined to those that can be used routinely and may be of particular interest to nurses.

- *Anthropometric methods* relate body dimensions to composition, e.g. triceps skinfold thickness and mid-arm muscle circumference provide information on the volume and changes in energy stores and the protein reserve. Such methods are usually inexpensive, non-invasive and readily available, but are slow to reflect changes and unsuitable for short-term use, i.e. 4 weeks or less
- *Biochemical methods* include serum proteins and nitrogen balance studies. The concentration of specific markers in serum can be affected by non-nutritional variables, notably stress, trauma and sepsis, when their use is not advised. They can be used more reliably in metabolically stable individuals, where the short half-lives of prealbumin and retinol-binding protein ensure rapid sensitivity to PEM

- *Subjective methods* include both a clinical examination and dietary history. The clinical examination is part of the diagnostic medical process and can be useful in the identification of morphological signs of PEM, vitamin and trace-element depletion (Tables 16.7 and 16.8).

The presence of disease can influence the interpretation of specific symptoms. A dietary history can take the form of a checklist or questionnaire intended to provide wide-ranging information about factors that may have affected food intake and nutritional status (Box 16.4). Information can be obtained from the patient or carer directly.

Assessments of food intake can be useful where very detailed information is required on dietary adequacy. A number of approaches can be used:

- dietary recall over periods of 24 h, 3 days, 1 week, 1 month
- food diaries recording actual intakes for 5 days, 7 days, 1 month
- weighed food intakes for 3-day periods
- food-frequency questionnaires designed to cover a range of time periods (day, week, month).

Once records of nutrient intake have been obtained, nutrient composition can be analysed using computer software programs, and average 24-h intakes of energy

Table 16.7 Features of vitamin-deficiency states

Vitamin	Symptoms characteristic of deficiency	Deficiency disease
A	Gradual deterioration in dim vision	Night blindness
	Dryness and scaling of skin (hyperkeratosis)	Xerophthalmia
	Conjunctival dryness	Keratomalacia (corneal softening or liquefaction)
	Bitot's spots	
D	Proximal muscle weakness: 'waddling gait'	Osteomalacia
	Bone pain, exacerbated by weight-bearing	
	Bone deformity with advanced disease state, i.e. bowing of legs, kyphoscoliosis	
E	Individuals with defective fat absorption (rare) may develop deficiency symptoms: ataxic neurological syndromes	Rare spinocerebellar degeneration
C	Weakness, fatigue, lethargy	No characteristic deficiency disease in humans
	Dryness, hyperkeratosis of skin	Scurvy
	Purpura in the lower extremities; muscle, joint haemorrhage	
	Loss of gingival margin, teeth	
	Failed wound healing	
Thiamine (B₁)	Tachycardia, cardiac failure, oedema	Beri-beri (wet)
	Anorexia, nausea, vomiting	Beri-beri (dry)
	Calf-muscle weakness, foot drop	
Riboflavin (B₂)	Angular stomatitis, fissuring at corners of mouth	
	Swelling, redness of mouth or lips (cheilosis)	
	Nasolabial dermatitis	
Niacin	Peripheral neuropathy, dementia, depression, apathy	Pellagra
	Hyperkeratotic, hyperpigmented skin on exposed areas	
	Dermatitis, diarrhoea, atrophic changes in tongue	
Pyridoxine (B₆)	Weakness, irritability, insomnia	
	Depression, confusion	
	Dermatitis (nasolabial, perineal, scrotal), glossitis, stomatitis	

Table 16.8 Features of trace-element depletion

Trace element	Deficiency symptoms
Zinc	Nasolabial dermatitis, diarrhoea, depression
	Disturbances of taste and smell, mouth ulcers
	Anorexia, ataxia, alopecia
	Impaired wound healing
	Low plasma zinc concentration a feature of acute/chronic tissue injury, carcinomas, renal disease, liver disease, acute/chronic infections
Copper	Neutropenia, leucopenia
	Anaemia
	Skeletal demineralization
	Malabsorption, enteropathies, nephropathies associated with deficiency
	Dietary copper requirements are increased if dietary raw bran or phytate intake is high (they bind to copper in an unabsorbable complex)
Iron	Hypochromic, macrocytic anaemia
	Glossitis, cheilosis
	Dyspnoea, paraesthesiae, gastric atrophy
	Blood loss and inadequate iron intakes are main causes of anaemia
Magnesium	Depression, irritability, confusion, restlessness
	Muscle tremor, ataxia, cramps, nystagmus
	Tachycardia, ectopic beats
	Positive Chvostek sign*
	Loss of magnesium a feature of malabsorptive states, chronic diarrhoea
	Renal losses caused by diuretic therapy, renal diseases, untreated diabetic ketoacidosis
Selenium	Reported deficiency states rare
	Low serum concentrations associated with cancers, cirrhosis, renal failure – significance not clear

*Spasm of the facial muscles induced by tapping the skin over the facial nerve. This is a sign of hypocalcaemia, classically associated with parathyroid insufficiency.
(Reproduced with permission from McLaren S, Green S 1998 Nutritional screening and assessment. Professional Nurse 13: S9–S14.)

and nutrients can be compared with recommended intakes to identify any deficiencies present. Although extremely useful, the following problems can arise when using assessments of food intake:

- Recall can be subject to memory error
- Non-compliance or fictitious entries can occur with diary recording
- A variation in foods consumed may be missed
- Reduced palatability can be a problem if food is weighed and allowed to cool.

Westerterp & Goris (2002) have reviewed the issue of misreporting food intake in the interpretation of surveys utilizing dietary recall and dietary record methods by participants. Findings were that physical and psychological characteristics of study participants could influence observed reporting bias. Conclusions were that, as yet, methods for the accurate determination of dietary intake have not been developed. Such limitations need to be borne in mind when analysing and drawing conclusions from survey data.

All nutritional assessment information should be accurately recorded, summarizing baseline and serial measurements, together with actions taken as a consequence of diagnosis. Details of dietary history, dietary regimens, use of supplements and other information should also be recorded. As a means of ensuring effective decision-making on nutritional support, nurses, dieticians, medical personnel and other professional groups may formulate a multidisciplinary recording system for common use on each patient.

USE OF NUTRITIONAL SUPPLEMENTS

Oral feeding: use of supplements

Two types of commercially manufactured supplements can be used to improve nutrient intakes, but not

Box 16.4   Dietary history: key questions

Eating patterns/habits
- What types of food are preferred?
- How frequently is food consumed during the day?
- Quantities of food consumed (portion sizes)?
- Is appetite normally good?
- How has appetite been affected by illness?

Socioeconomic factors
- Living arrangements: alone, with friends, sheltered accommodation, institution or home?
- Assistance needed with food purchase, preparation, delivery?
- Involvement of family, friends in shopping for food?
- Support from social services?
- Mobility, disability in relation to food purchase, preparation and consumption?
- Domestic facilities for heating, cooking food, refrigeration available?
- Bereavement, loneliness, feelings of isolation, extent of social network?
- Adequacy of income, receipt of supplementary benefits?

Distressing symptoms
- Have any unpleasant symptoms affected food intake?
- Severity of symptoms, trigger factors?
- Anorexia, nausea, vomiting?
- Constipation, diarrhoea?
- Dyspnoea?
- Alterations in taste or smell?
- Dysphagia?
- Dental health?
- History of weight gain or loss?
- Postural problems?
- Visual field problems?
- Able to communicate dietary preferences?

Special diets
- Presence of chronic diseases requiring dietary modification, e.g. diabetes mellitus, liver disease, renal disease, inflammatory bowel disease?
- Problems complying with diet?
- Specific nutrient content of diet?
- Any recent change in nutrient requirements?
- Palatability of special diet?
- Use of 'alternative' diets?
- Use of dietary supplements?
- Food allergies, intolerance, aversions
- Reactions to specific foods?
- Types of reaction: skin problems, breathing difficulties, diarrhoea, vomiting?
- Details of food aversions before and after onset of illness?

Drug treatment
- Drugs taken on prescription (name)?
- Details of drug treatment, dose frequency, duration of treatment?
- Side-effects?
- Self-medication: use of over-the-counter drugs?
- Potential for drug–drug and drug–nutrient interactions?

to replace meals, in older people who cannot eat enough to meet their nutritional needs.

- food supplements in the form of nutrient-dense drinks (also called sip feeds), soups and puddings
- vitamin supplements in the form of oral tablets or liquid preparations.

Food supplement beverages are now widely available and are normally prescribed by the dietician. They vary in terms of nutrient composition, hence it is vital that their consumption is carefully considered in the complete picture of assessing dietary requirements and intakes:

- Food supplements should be given at the times and in the quantities prescribed
- Some supplements containing high concentrations of nutrients should not be given in excess due to potential toxicity
- Intake of supplements should be recorded on a food or fluid balance chart
- Unconsumed quantities should be stored or discarded as recommended by dieticians or manufacturers.

Currently, two systematic reviews of research conducted in a range of diagnostic groups have evaluated the effects of ingesting nutrient supplements on indices of nutritional status and other outcomes (Stratton & Elia 2000, Potter 2001). The review by Stratton & Elia included an analysis of studies conducted of older patients, finding evidence of small improvements in body weight when differences between supplemented and unsupplemented groups were examined. Individuals most likely to benefit from supplements in relation to improvements in weight were those with a BMI < 20 kg/m². The review by Potter (2001) was entirely focused on older adults and concluded that use of supplements had been evaluated predominantly in medical patients, in whom improvements to nutritional status had been demonstrated. In contrast, a Cochrane review evaluating use of oral supplements after hip fracture did not find evidence of benefit in five published trials and noted lack of information on compliance data in some that did not help interpretation (Avenall & Handoll 2001).

Vitamin supplements may be prescribed by physicians for people who show evidence of deficiency.

Artificial nutritional support in hospital and community

In order to eat and drink adequate amounts of food and fluids, the gastrointestinal tract must be functional, and an individual must be conscious, motivated and physi-

cally able to eat. Older patients who are unable, for a variety of reasons, to consume food orally may require enteral nutrition if their gut function is adequate. If it is not, then parenteral (intravenous) feeding may be necessary. It is beyond the scope of this chapter to provide a detailed account of the methods of providing artificial nutritional support; readers will find some recommendations in the reading list to further their interest. Rigorous screening and assessment should identify patients who need artificial support either immediately or at a later stage in their treatment. Decision-making should not be delayed in the implementation of support as patients' nutritional status can deteriorate rapidly and contribute to increased morbidity and mortality.

Enteral feeding

Feeding via tube or catheter is indicated for patients in whom an oral intake is contraindicated (coma, stupor, facial injuries, obstructive lesions, dysphagia). Patients suffering from trauma, burns or sepsis may not be physically able to consume sufficient nutrients to meet significantly increased requirements, but can often be successfully nourished via enteral catheter. Enteral feeding is contraindicated in individuals at high risk of pulmonary aspiration and in the presence of peritonitis, gut obstruction, paralytic ileus, gut haemorrhage and intractable diarrhoea and vomiting.

If the upper gastrointestinal tract is accessible and functional, then nasogastric, oesophagostomy or pharyngostomy feeding may be attempted (short-term), or percutaneous endoscopic gastrostomy performed (longer-term feeding). Where the upper gastrointestinal tract is accessible but non-functional or the risk of pulmonary aspiration is high, then naso-duodenal or jejunal feeding may be attempted (short-term) or via gastrostomy (long-term). In cases where upper gastrointestinal tract and upper jejunum are non-functional and/or inaccessible, then jejunostomy feeding is the only option. For further information on this complex area of artificial support, see Jeejeebhoy (2002) and Gopalan & Khanna (2003).

Parenteral feeding

Total parenteral nutrition (TPN) is indicated in acute, temporary and long-term gastrointestinal failure, hypercatabolic states and several conditions where bowel rest is mandatory. Intravenous feeding is costly and carries appreciable risks of infective, metabolic and mechanical complications. For this reason its use should never be routine, but considered carefully. Use of parenteral feeding can lead to disuse atrophy of the gut in 50% of patients after periods as short as 6 weeks; hence, when possible, oral intakes should be maintained while using the intravenous route. Examples where this can be accomplished successfully are in chronic alimentary failure when mechanical integrity of the gut is maintained although efficiency of absorption is extremely low.

Venous access routes for TPN may be either central (via the internal or external jugular and subclavian veins) or via a peripheral vein. Use of the peripheral route is limited by the osmolality and volume of infusate that it is necessary to use, but advantages are a reduction in the septic, thrombotic and mechanical hazards of using a central venous catheter. Further information on central and peripheral TPN can be found in Griffiths (2004) and Culebras et al. (2004).

NUTRITIONAL SUPPORT SERVICES

Older people in hospital and community represent a spectrum of needs for nutritional support services and issues relating to their management require a range of professional expertise. Opinions vary concerning the most appropriate approaches to the management of nutritional support, but in recent years the concept of the nutritional support team has gained credence as evidence has been provided that it can result in more efficient, effective management of nutrition support, with patients suffering fewer complications (Allison 2001, Howard 2001). Despite this, the percentage of hospitals in European countries with teams varies from 2% to 37%.

Nutritional support teams

Although originally conceived as an acute, hospital-located group, the team concept has now broadened to include working across the primary–secondary care interface. It is clear that the aims of a nutritional support team can vary depending on the demand for particular types of nutritional service, in addition to location and remit of operation. Reviews by McLaren & Crawley (2000) and Howard (2001) have suggested that the following may be part of the team function:

- development of evidence-based policies, standards and guidelines for the service
- provision of a high-quality nutrition support service covering screening, assessment, delivery and evaluation which is monitored for cost–benefit outcomes
- education of patients/clients and carers regarding nutritional aspects of treatment, use of specialist aids and equipment, prevention of complications of dietary treatments or diet-induced ill health
- development of education and training programmes for health professionals involved in nutrition support

- initiation of research relating to nutritional interventions and management.

Different approaches to team organization and working have been described (Howard 2001). Possible models include multidisciplinary teams (individual disciplines work to achieve their own targets then meet to review progress), interdisciplinary teams (shared goals, common care plan) and transdisciplinary teams (shared goals and skills), but in reality most nutrition support teams fall into the first two categories. The concept of 'core' and 'extended' teams has also been described; core would include the specialist nurse, dietician, pharmacist and doctor (Cole & Jones 1995). Outside this, the extended team may encompass the speech therapist, occupational therapist, physiotherapist, dentist, catering services manager and clinical psychologist. Roles can and do vary within the team remit, sometimes with overlap; however, within the core team the following are common:

- nurse: nutritional screening or assessment; extended role involving placement or care of enteral/parenteral catheters; liaison with ward or community nurses
- dietician: nutritional assessment; determination of nutrient requirements; formulation of special diets or feeding regimens; use of supplements; cost–benefit calculations
- doctor: nutritional screening or assessment; placement of catheters; monitoring responses to support; prescription of enteral/parenteral feeds, supplements
- pharmacist: preparation of enteral/parenteral solutions; drugs.

Individuals forming part of the extended team normally have a very specific input to make. For example, a speech therapist's role may be confined to the assessment and management of dysphagia; that of the physiotherapist advising on aids to posture at mealtimes. In particular cases it may be necessary to call on the services of an expert consultant to advise on a nutritional support issue. Although team roles may vary, clear accountability, linked to effective communication, referral and monitoring procedures, is essential for effective decision-making. Above all, respect for the autonomy of patients/clients in decision-making on dietary matters should be paramount.

Social services and voluntary organizations

Earlier in this chapter, the risks of malnutrition occurring in frail, older, house-bound people were discussed. How can they be offered support which will attenuate the risk of malnutrition, allow them to cope with disability, retain independence in eating and drinking and maintain nutritional status? A number of community agencies aim to deliver a flexible service to meet such needs. Frail, older, house-bound individuals can benefit from the meals-on-wheels service operated by social services or Women's Royal Voluntary Service. This service delivers a hot mid-day meal, usually of two courses, for a relatively modest cost. Although the precise nature of the service can vary in some areas of the UK, special dietary requirements and cultural needs are considered in meal preparation. The Caroline Walker Trust (1995) has published an extremely valuable summary report of standards and guidelines for the nutritional quality of community meals, including those delivered to the home. The expert working party who devised the standards suggested that a 'meal package' delivered each day to an older person should include a two-course meal and snack for consumption later. The inclusion of a user evaluation of the service was also recommended as a means of providing feedback on the quality of meals provided. The nutritional quality of meals utilized the standards for Department of Health (1992a) reference values. After a community needs assessment, aids to cooking and eating may be provided by social services. In hospital, a domiciliary occupational therapy assessment can establish the nature and range of aids needed to maintain an individual's independence and safety prior to discharge home. Items which can be provided include raised-edge or spiked boards for food preparation, utensils with suction-cup bases, non-slip plate mats, cutlery with built-up handles, kettle or teapot pouring stands and modified can openers. Lever handles can be attached to taps to facilitate turning, split-level hobs installed for wheelchair access to cooking, and food stored in swing-out cupboard baskets. Walking trolleys can be used to move food between rooms. Unsafe steps can be replaced by ramps.

For house-bound individuals unable to shop for food or prepare it, home helps can provide a valuable service. Assistance may be needed from community nurses to interpret a client's needs for the purchase and provision of food which is culturally acceptable. Eating fulfils both social and biological needs, so the informal group interaction provided by attending a luncheon club can be greatly enjoyed by some older people in preference to meals-on-wheels. These clubs are largely supported by voluntary organizations, providing a three-course meal for a modest cost, and in many cases including transport to and from a client's home.

Oral health is vital to pleasurable, adequate eating and drinking. Loss of dentition, with variable effects on chewing and swallowing, can limit both quantities and range of foods consumed. By the ages of 65–74 years just under half the population are edentulous (Department of Health 1992b). Many older people wear dentures, which should be replaced every 5–10 years or following any ailment which can change the shape of the oral cavity (e.g. stroke). In the UK, cost-free dental services are available to older people who are exempt from prescription charges, although National Health Service dentists are increasingly hard to find. Many people view the costs of dental treatment as a significant disincentive to visit a dentist. Health promotion programmes focused on the maintenance of oral health may achieve much in this area.

CONCLUSION

This chapter has reviewed some key issues in the nutritional care of older people, with a particular emphasis on factors affecting eating and drinking. At the time of writing, the problem of malnutrition in both institutionalized and free-living older persons appears to be a significant challenge for all health professional interventions across the spectrum of delivery, encompassing primary, secondary and tertiary care. Are nutritional support teams the key to providing effective prevention and treatment? Time will tell.

Recommended reading

Bond S (ed) 1997 Eating matters. Centre for Health Services Research, University of Newcastle upon Tyne, Newcastle upon Tyne.
This portfolio of documents provides a comprehensive review of a wide range of issues on the nutritional care of older people in hospital and to some extent in the community. Each key document is devoted to a particular aspect of dietary support, the whole covering specific dietary problems and risks, nutritional assessment, organizational aspects of meal preparation and delivery and setting standards or guidelines for audit of nutritional care. The portfolio includes a review of the research literature, policy documents and a set of case studies illustrating best practices in nursing management. The multiprofessional aspects of nutritional support are emphasized.

Devons CAJ (2002) Comprehensive geriatric assessment: making the most of the ageing years. Current Opinion in Clinical Nutrition and Metabolic Care 5: 19–24
This is an excellent review drawing extensively on the international literature. Different components of assessment of older people are appraised, considering the physical, psychosocial and environmental factors which have an impact on the well-being of older individuals. Nutritional assessment is reviewed and helpfully placed in a wider context and experiences in implementing comprehensive assessment are considered. This is recommended to nurses grappling with current policy requirements in the UK to implement

assessment as part of the National Service Framework for Older People.

Holmes S 2002 Wholesome, appealing, balanced: the challenge of food provision and the national minimum standards in residential care for older people. Conference Proceedings, Royal Society of Health, London, October 2002.

This publication of the Royal Society of Health contains full papers presented at an interactive conference to tackle issues relating to the implementation of care standards. Innovative contributions from policy advisers, famous chefs de cuisine, dieticians, academics, food hygiene consultants and catering managers. Highly recommended.

Morley JE, Glick Z, Rubenstein LZ 1995 Geriatric nutrition: a comprehensive review, 2nd edn. Raven Press, New York.

The second edition of this text provides an authoritative review of contemporary research in the field of nutrition of older people, combining pure and applied clinical sciences. The contents cover nutrition and ageing, nutritional-deficient systems, malfunction and nutrition, in addition to a range of special topics. Of the latter, the discussions of drug–drug and drug–food interactions, the roles of nutrition and body composition in falls, gait and balance disorders in older people provide thorough reviews. Readers will find a useful source of practical information in the chapters on dysphagia, pressure ulcers and nutrition, and nutrition and behaviour. The approach is academic, but accessible, written by subject specialists with a real enthusiasm which is communicated to the reader.

References

Abu-Abeid S, Keidar S, Szold A 2001 Resolution of chronic medical conditions after laparoscopic adjustable silicone gastric banding for the treatment of morbid obesity in the older. Surgical Endoscopy 15: 132–134

Age Related Eye Disease Study Research Group 2001 A randomized placebo controlled clinical trial of high dose supplementation with vitamins C and E and betacarotene for age-related cataract and vision loss. AREDS report no 9. Archives of Ophthalmology 119: 1439–1452

Alexander HJ, Norton JA 1995 Pathophysiology of cancer cachexia. In: Doyle D, Hanks GWC, Macdonald N (eds) The Oxford textbook of palliative medicine. Oxford University Press, Oxford, pp 316–329

Allan S 1995 Nausea and vomiting. In: Doyle D, Hanks GWC, MacDonald N (eds) The Oxford textbook of palliative medicine. Oxford University Press, Oxford, pp 282–290

Allison SP 2001 Nutrition support teams: dissociated ions or the yeast in the loaf. Clinical Nutrition 20: 289

Allison S 2002 Institutional feeding of the older. Current Opinion in Clinical Nutrition and Metabolic Care 5: 31–34

Alzheimers Society 2000 Food for thought. Alzheimers Society, London

Argiles JM, Busquets S, Lopez-Soriano FJ et al. 2003 Cytokines in the pathogenesis of cancer cachexia.

Current Opinion in Clinical Nutrition and Metabolic Care 6: 401–406

Association of Community Health Councils 1997 Hungry in hospital. ACHC, London

Avenall A, Handoll HHG 2001 Nutritional supplementation for hip fracture aftercare in the older. Cochrane Review. The Cochrane Library, issue 4. Update Software, Oxford

Axelsson K, Norberg A, Asplund K 1984 Eating after a stroke: towards an integrated view. International Journal of Nursing Studies 21: 93–99

Barratt J 2004 Practical nutritional care of older demented patients. Current Opinion in Clinical Nutrition and Metabolic Care 7: 35–38

Bastow MD, Rawlings J, Allison SP 1983 Benefits of supplementary tube feeding after fractured neck of femur: a randomized controlled trial. British Medical Journal of Clinical Research 287: 1589–1592

Bonaiuti D, Shea B, Iovine R et al. 2004 Exercise for preventing and treating osteoporosis in post menopausal women. Cochrane Review. The Cochrane Library, issue 1. John Wiley, Chichester

British Dietetic Association 2004 Dietetic guidelines: diet in secondary prevention of cardiovascular disease. Journal of Human Nutrition and Dietetics 17: 337–349

British Nutrition Foundation 1992 Unsaturated fatty acids, nutritional and physiological significance. Report of the British Nutrition Foundation's task force. British Nutrition Foundation, London

Burr ML, Fehily AM, Gilbert JF et al. 1991 Effects of changes in fat, fish and fibre intakes on death and myocardial infarction; diet and reinfarction trial (DART). Lancet ii: 757–761

Calle EE, Thun MJ, Petrelli JM 1999 Body-mass index and mortality in a prospective cohort of US adults. New England Journal of Medicine 341: 1097–1105

Campbell AJ, Spears GFS, Brown JS, Busby WJ, Borrie MJ 1990 Anthropometric measurements as predictors of mortality in a community aged 70 years and over. Age and Ageing 19: 131–135

Caroline Walker Trust 1995 Eating well for older people. Caroline Walker Trust, London

Carr EK, Kenney FD 1992 Positioning the stroke patient: a review of the literature. International Journal of Nursing Studies 29: 355–369

Carter RL, Pittam MR, Tanner NSB 1982 Pain and dysphagia in patients with squamous carcinoma of the head and neck: the role of perineural spread. Journal of the Royal Society of Medicine 75: 598–606

Chandra RK, Imbuch A, Moore C, Skelton D, Woolcott D 1991 Nutrition of the older. Canadian Medical Association Journal 145: 1475–1487

Cheng S, Sipila S, Taafe DR et al. 2002 Change in bone mass distribution induced by hormone replacement therapy and high impact physical exercise in post menopausal women. Bone 31: 126–135

Cole KD, Jones FA 1995 Interdisciplinary teams for the solution of nutritional problems. In: Morley JE, Glick Z, Rubenstein LZ (eds) Geriatric nutrition: a comprehensive review, 2nd edn. Raven Press, New York, pp 367–375

Colhoun H, Betteridge DJ, Durrington PN et al. 2004 Primary prevention of cardiovascular disease with atorvastin in type 2 diabetes in the Collaborative Atorvastin Diabetes Study (CARDS) ; multicentre, randomized, placebo-controlled trial. Lancet 364: 685–696

Committee on Medical Aspects of Food Policy 1992 The nutrition of older people. Report on health and social subjects no. 43. HMSO, London

Culebras JM, Martin-Pena G, Garcia de Lorenzo A, Zarazaga A, Rodriguez-Montes JA 2004 Practical aspects of peripheral parenteral nutrition. Current Opinion in Clinical Nutrition and Metabolic Care 7: 303–307

Curran J, Groher ME 1990 Development and dissemination of an aspiration risk reduction diet. Dysphagia 5: 6–12

Defay R, Delcourt C, Ranvier M 2001 Relationships between physical activity, obesity and diabetes mellitus in a French older population: the POLA study (Pathologies Oculaires Liées à l'Age). International Journal of Obesity Relating to Metabolic Disorders 25: 512–518

De Jong N, Paw MJ, de Groot LC 2000 Dietary supplements and physical exercise affecting bone and body composition in frail older persons. American Journal of Public Health 90: 947–954

Department of Health 1991, 2001 (11th impression) Dietary reference values for food energy and nutrients for the United Kingdom. Report on Health and Social Subjects no. 41. HMSO, London

Department of Health 1992a The nutrition of older people. Report on health and social subjects no. 43. HMSO, London

Department of Health 1992b The health of older people: an epidemiological overview. Central Health Monitoring Unit epidemiological overview series, vol 1. HMSO, London

Department of Health 1997 Drinking: adults' behaviour and knowledge. HMSO, London

Department of Health 1998 Nutrition and bone health . Report on health and social subjects 49. HMSO, London

Department of Health 2001 National service plan for older people. HMSO, London

Department of Health 2002a Guidance on the single assessment process. HMSO, London

Department of Health 2002b The single assessment process: tools and scales. HMSO, London

Devons CAJ 2002 Comprehensive geriatric assessment: making the most of the ageing years. Current Opinion in Clinical Nutrition and Metabolic Care 5: 19–24

Dickerson JWT, Williams C 1988 Nutrition and cancer. In: Dickerson JWT, Lee HA (eds) Nutrition in the clinical management of disease. Edward Arnold, London, pp 350–373

Doggett DL, Tappe KA, Mitchell MD et al. 2001 Prevention of pneumonia in older stroke patients by systematic diagnosis and treatment of dysphagia: an evidence-based comprehensive analysis of the literature. Dysphagia 16: 279–295

Dundee JW, Yang J 1991 Prolongation of the anti-emetic action of P6 acupuncture in patients having cancer chemotherapy. Journal of the Royal Society of Medicine 83: 360–362

Edwards NE, Beck AM 2002 Animal assisted therapy and nutrition in Alzheimers disease. Western Journal of Nursing Research 24: 697–712

Elia M 1990 Artificial nutritional support. Medicine International 82: 3392–3396

Elia M 2000 Guidelines for detection and management of malnutrition. British Association for Parenteral and Enteral Nutrition, Maidenhead

Elmstahl S 1987 Hospital nutrition in geriatric long term care medicine: effects of a changed meal environment. Comprehensive Gerontology 1: 29–33

Ezzati M, Lopez AD, Rodgers A, Van der Hoolm S 2002 Selected major risk factors. Lancet 360: 1347–1360

Faxen-Irving G, Andren-Olsson B, Geijerstam A 2002 The effect of nutritional intervention in older subjects residing in group living for the demented. European Journal of Clinical Nutrition 56: 221–227

Finch S, Doyle W, Lowe C et al. 1998 National diet and nutrition survey: people aged 65 years and over. Stationery Office, London

Finestone HM, Greene-Finestone LS 2003 Diagnosis of dysphagia and its nutritional management for stroke patients. Canadian Medical Association Journal 169: 1041–1045

Freis ED 1976 Salt, volume and the prevention of hypertension. Circulation 53: 589–594

Glick Z 1995 Energy balance. In: Morley E, Glick Z, Rubenstein LZ (eds) Geriatric nutrition. Raven Press, New York, pp 15–24

Gopalan S, Khanna S 2003 Enteral nutrition delivery techniques. Current Opinion in Clinical Nutrition and Metabolic Care 6: 313–317

Gordon DJ, Rifkind BM 1989 Treating high blood cholesterol in the older patient. American Journal of Cardiology 63: 43h–52h

Gray CS, French M, Bates J 1989 Recovery of visual fields in acute stroke. Age and Ageing 18: 419–421

Green CJ 1999 Existence, causes and consequences of disease-related malnutrition in the hospital and community and clinical and financial benefits of nutritional intervention. Clinical Nutrition 18: 3–28

Griep MI, Mefs T, Collys K 2000 Risk of malnutrition in retirement homes: older persons measured by mini-nutritional assessment. Journal of Gerontology 55A: M57–M63

Griffiths RD 2004 Is parenteral nutrition really that risky in the intensive care unit? Current Opinion in Clinical Nutrition and Metabolic Care 7: 175–181

Hamilton-Smith C 1995 Drug–food and drug–drug interactions. In: Morley JE, Glick Z, Rubenstein LZ (eds) Geriatric nutrition, 2nd edn. Raven Press, New York, pp 311–328

Havlick RJ 1992 Health statistics on older persons. In: Munro H, Schlierf G (eds) Nutrition of the older. Raven Press, New York, pp 7–16

He FJ, MacGregor GA 2004 Effect of longer term modest salt reduction on blood pressure. Cochrane Review. The Cochrane Library, issue 3. John Wiley, Chichester

Hebuterne X 2003 Gut changes attributed to ageing: effects on intestinal flora. Current Opinion in Clinical Nutrition and Metabolic Care 6: 49–54

Hirsch CH 1995 When your patient needs surgery: how planning can avoid complications. Geriatrics 50: 39–44

Ho SC, Woo J, Sham A 1994 Risk factor change in older persons, a perspective from Hong Kong; weight change and mortality. Journal of Gerontology 49: M269–M272

Holmes S 1986 Determinants of food intake. Nursing 3: 260–264

Homik J, Suarez-Almazor ME, Shea B et al. 2004 Calcium and vitamin D for corticosteroid induced osteoporosis. Cochrane Review. The Cochrane Library, issue 1. John Wiley, Chichester.

Howard P 2001 Organizational aspects of starting and running an effective nutrition support service. Clinical Nutrition 20: 367–374

Hudson H, Daubert CR, Mills R 2000 The interdependency of protein malnutrition, ageing and dysphagia. Dysphagia 15: 31–38

Intersalt Cooperative Research Group 1988 Intersalt: an international study of electrolyte excretion and blood pressure. Results for 24 hour urinary sodium and potassium excretion. British Medical Journal 297: 319–328

Irwin ML, Yasui Y, Ulrich CM 2003 Effect of exercise on total and intra-abdominal fat in post-menopausal women: a randomized controlled trial. Journal of the American Medical Association 289: 323–330

Isabel M, Correia TD, Waitzberg DL 2003 The impact of malnutrition on morbidity, mortality, length of hospital stay and costs evaluated through a multivariate model analysis. Clinical Nutrition 22: 235–239

Jacques PF, Chylack LT 1991 Epidemiological evidence for a role for the antioxidant vitamins and carotenoids in cataract prevention. American Journal of Clinical Nutrition 53 (suppl.): 352s–355s

James WPT, Ralph A, Sanchez-Castillo CP 1987 The dominance of salt in manufactured food in the sodium intake of affluent societies. Lancet i: 426–428

Jeejeebhoy KN 2002 Enteral feeding. Current Opinion in Clinical Nutrition and Metabolic Care 5: 695–698

Jensen GL, Friedman JM 2002 Obesity is associated with functional decline in community-dwelling rural older persons. Journal of the American Geriatric Society 50: 918–923

Johnstone M 1991 Therapy for stroke. Churchill Livingstone, Edinburgh

Kaiser FE 1995 Nutrition and diabetes mellitus in the older. In: Morley E, Glick Z, Rubenstein LZ (eds) Geriatric nutrition. Raven Press, New York, pp 211–218

Keller HH 1993 Malnutrition in institutionalized older: how and why? Journal of the American Geriatrics Society 41: 1212–1218

Kennedy RL, Chokkalingham K, Srinivasan R 2004 Obesity in the older: who should we be treating, and why, and how? Current Opinion in Clinical Nutrition and Metabolic Care 7: 3–9

King's Fund Report 1992 Nutrition: a positive approach to treatment: report of a working party. King's Fund, London

Kohrt WM, Kerwan JP, Staten MA 1993 Insulin resistance in ageing is related to abdominal obesity. Diabetes 42: 273–281

Krall EA, Wehler C, Garcia RI 2001 Calcium and vitamin D supplements reduce tooth loss in the older. American Journal of Medicine 111: 452–456

Krishna CG, Miller E, Kapoor S 1989 Increased blood pressure during potassium depletion in normotensive men. New England Journal of Medicine 320: 1177–1182

Kyle UG, Pirlich M, Schuetz T et al. 2003 Prevalence of malnutrition in 1760 patients at hospital admission: a controlled population study of body composition. Clinical Nutrition 22: 473–481

Laviano A, Meguid MM, Rossi-Fanelli F 2003 Improving food intake in anorectic cancer patients. Current Opinion in Clinical Nutrition and Metabolic Care 6: 421–426

Lehman AB 1991 Nutrition in old age: an update and questions for future research: part 1. Reviews in Clinical Gerontology 1: 135–145

Leske MC, Chylack LT, Suh Yuh W 1991 The lens opacities: case-control study: risk factors for cataract. Archives of Ophthalmology 109: 244–251

Lipschitz DA 1995 Nutrition related anaemias in the older. In: Morley JE, Glick Z, Rubenstein LZ (eds) Geriatric nutrition: a comprehensive review. Raven Press, New York, pp 133–143

Logemann J 1997 Evaluation and treatment of swallowing disorders. College Hill Press, San Diego

Loprinzi CL 1990 A controlled trial of megestrol acetate treatment of cancer anorexia and cachexia. Journal of the National Cancer Institute 82: 1127–1132

Macnair AL 1994 Physical activity not diet should be the focus of measures for the prevention of cardiovascular disease. Nutrition Research Reviews 7: 43–65

Martin AW 1991 Dietary management of swallowing disorders. Dysphagia 6: 129–134

Masaki KH, Curb JD, Chiu D 1997 Association of body mass index with blood pressure in older Japanese American men. The Honolulu Heart Programme. Hypertension 29: 673–677

Mathey M, Siebelink E, de Graaf C, Van Staveren WA 2001 Flavour enhancement of food improves dietary intake and nutritional status of older nursing home residents. Journal of Gerontology 56A: M200–M205

McCabe BJ 2004 Prevention of food–drug interactions with special emphasis on older adults. Current Opinion in Clinical Nutrition and Metabolic Care 7: 21–26

McCarron DA, Morris CD, Cole C 1982 Calcium, magnesium and phosphorous balance in human and experimental hypertension. Hypertension 4: 1127–1133

McLaren S 1997 Eating disabilities following stroke. British Journal of Community Health Nursing 2: 9–18

McLaren S, Crawley H 2000 Managing nutritional risks in older adults. Nursing Times Clinical Monographs no 44. Emap Healthcare, London

McLaren S, Dickerson JWTD 2000 Measurement of eating disability in an acute stroke population. Clinical Effectiveness in Nursing 4: 109–120

McLaren SM, Holmes SH, Green S, Bond S 1997 An overview of nutritional issues relating to the care of older people in hospital. In Bond S (ed) Eating matter. Centre for Health Services Research, University of Newcastle upon Tyne Publications, Newcastle upon Tyne, pp 15–100

McWhirter JP, Pennington CR 1994 Incidence and recognition of malnutrition in hospital. British Medical Journal 308: 945–948

Ministry of Agriculture, Fisheries and Food 1993 National food survey 1992. HMSO, London

Moore H, Summerbell C, Hooper L et al. 2004 Dietary advice for treatment of type 2 diabetes in adults. Cochrane Review. The Cochrane Library, issue 3. John Wiley, Chichester

Morley JE 1995 The role of nutrition in the prevention of age associated diseases. In: Morley JE, Glick Z, Rubenstein LZ (eds) Geriatric nutrition: a comprehensive review. Raven Press, New York, pp 63–73

Morley JE 1997 Anorexia of ageing: physiologic and pathologic. American Journal of Clinical Nutrition 66: 760–773

Morley JE 2001 Anorexia, body composition and ageing. Current Opinion in Clinical Nutrition and Metabolic Care 4: 9–13

Morley JE, Glick Z 1995 Obesity. In: Morley E, Glick Z, Rubenstein LZ (eds) Geriatric nutrition: a comprehensive review. Raven Press, New York, pp 245–256

Morley JE, Kaiser FE 1990 Unique aspects of diabetes mellitus in the older. Clinics in Geriatric Medicine 6: 693–702

Morley JE, Kraenzle D 1994 Causes of weight loss in a community nursing home. Journal of the American Geriatrics Society 42: 583–585

Morley JE, Thomas DR 1999 Anorexia and ageing. Nutrition 15: 499–503

Morrow GR, Morrell C 1982 Behavioural treatment for anticipatory nausea and vomiting induced by cancer chemotherapy. New England Journal of Medicine 307: 1476–1480

Mossman KL 1986 Gustatory tissue injury in man: radiation dose–response relationship and mechanisms of taste loss. British Journal of Cancer 53: 9–11

MRC/BHF Heart Protection Study 2002a Heart protection study of cholesterol lowering with simvastin in 20 536 high risk individuals: a placebo controlled trial. Lancet 360: 7–22

MRC/BHF Heart Protection Study 2002b Heart protection study of antioxidant vitamin supplementation in 20 536 high risk individuals: a randomized placebo controlled trial. Lancet 360: 23–33

Murphy C 1993 Nutrition and chemosensory perception in the elderly. Critical Reviews in Food Science and Nutrition 33: 3–15

Myers J, Morgan T 1983 The effect of sodium intake on blood pressure related to age and sex. Clinical and Experimental Hypertension 5: 99–118

National Institute of Clinical Excellence 2003 Scope: osteoporosis. Available online at: www.nice.org.uk

National Institutes of Health 2001 Osteoporosis and related bone diseases. National Resource Centre. Available online at: http://www.osteo.org/osteolinks

Nikolaus T, Bach M, Siezen S et al. 1995 Assessment of nutritional risk in the older. Annals of Nutrition and Metabolism 39: 340–345

Pachucki-Hyde L 2001 Asssessment of risk factors for osteoporosis and fracture. Nursing Clinics of North America 36: 401–408

Paffenbarger RS, Hyde RT, Wing AL, Hsieh CC 1986 Physical activity, all cause mortality and longevity of college alumni. New England Journal of Medicine 314: 605–613

Penman JP, Thomson M 1998 A review of the textured diets developed for the management of dysphagia. Journal of Human Nutrition and Dietetics 11: 51–60

Perry L, Love C 2001 Screening for dysphagia and aspiration in acute stroke: a systematic review. Dysphagia 16: 7–18

Perry L, McLaren SM 2003 Nutritional support in acute stroke: the impact of evidence-based guidelines. Clinical Nutrition 22: 283–293

Potter JM 2001 Oral supplements in the older. Current Opinion in Clinical Nutrition and Metabolic Care 4: 21–28

Rad RS 1990 Normal functional range of motion of upper limb joints during the performance of 3 feeding activities. Archives of Physical and Medical Rehabilitation 71: 505–509

Rolls BJ, Dimeo K, Shide DJ 1995 Age-related impairments in the regulation of food intake. Journal of Clinical Nutrition 62: 923–931

Royal College of Physicians 1999 Osteoporosis. Clinical guidelines: summary and recommendations. Available online at: www.rcplondon.ac.uk

Sahota O, Hosking D 2001 The contribution of nutritional factors to osteopenia in the older. Current Opinion in Clinical Nutrition and Metabolic Care 4: 15–20

Saletti A, Lindgren EY, Johansson L, Cederholm T 2000 Nutritional status according to mini-nutritional assessment in an institutionalized older population in Sweden. Gerontology 46: 139–145

Selley WG 1989 Respiratory patterns associated with swallowing. Age and Ageing 18: 168–172

Selley WG, Roche MT, Pearce VR, Elhs RE, Flack FC 1995 Dysphagia following stroke: clinical observations of swallowing rehabilitation employing palatal training appliances. Dysphagia 10: 32–35

Shea B, Wells G, Cranney A et al. 2004 Calcium supplementation on bone loss in post menopausal women. Cochrane Review. The Cochrane Library, issue 1. John Wiley, Chichester

Sih R, Morley JE 1995 Lipids. In: Morley JE, Glick Z, Rubenstein LZ (eds) Geriatric nutrition: a comprehensive review. Raven Press, New York, pp 219–233

Sissons R 1988 Alterations in memory. Section 2. In: Mitchell P, Hodges LC, Muwaswes M, Walleck C (eds) Neuroscience nursing. Appleton Lange, CT, pp 171–183

Stanger O 2002 Physiology of folic acid in health and disease. Current Drug Metabolism 3: 211–223

Steptoe A, Pollard JM, Wardle J 1995 Development of a measure of the motives underlying the selection of food: the food choice questionnaire. Appetite 25: 267–283

Stratton RJ, Elia M 2000 Are oral nutritional supplements of benefit to patients in the community? Findings from a systematic review. Current Opinion in Clinical Nutrition and Metabolic Care 3: 311–315

Sykes JE 1995 Constipation and diarrhoea. In: Doyle D, Hanks GWC, MacDonald N (eds) The Oxford textbook of palliative medicine. Oxford University Press, Oxford, pp 299–310

Taylor S, Goodison-McLaren SM 1992 Nutritional support: a team approach. Wolfe, London

Tice JA, Ross E, Coxson PG 2001 Cost-effectiveness of vitamin therapy to lower plasma homocysteine levels for the prevention of coronary heart disease. Journal of the American Medical Association 286: 936–943

Tschamm JM, Adamsen TE, Coates TJ, Gullion DS 1988 Behaviours of treated hypertensive patients and patient demographic characteristics. Journal of Community Health 13: 19–32

Twycross RG 1995 Dysphagia, dyspepsia and hiccup. In: Doyle D, Hanks GNC, Macdonald N (eds) The Oxford textbook of palliative medicine. Oxford University Press, Oxford, pp 291–299

Twycross RG, Lack SA 1986 Taste change. In: Twycross RG, Lack SA (eds) Control of alimentary symptoms in advanced cancer. Churchill Livingstone, Edinburgh, pp 57–65

United Kingdom Central Council for Nursing, Midwifery and Health Visiting 1997 Registrar's letter (20): Nurses are responsible for feeding patients. UKCC, London

United States Drug Administration 1985 Food and nutrient intakes of individuals in one day in the United States, spring 1977. Nationwide food consumption survey 1977–78. Preliminary report no. 2. Department of Agriculture Consumer Nutrition Centre, Hyattsville, MD

Vellas BJ, Baumgartner RN, Garry PJ, Albarede JL 1995 The role of nutrition in falls, gait and balance disorders in the older. In: Morley JE, Glick Z, Rubenstein LZ (eds) Geriatric nutrition: a comprehensive review. Raven Press, New York, pp 343–350

Vellas BJ, Guigoz Y, Garry P et al. 1999 The mini-nutritional assessment (MNA) and its use in grading the nutritional state of elderly patients. Nutrition 15: 116–122

Vellas B, Lauque S, Andrieu S et al. 2001 Nutritional assessment in the older. Current Opinion in Clinical Nutrition and Metabolic Care 4: 5–8

Visscher TL, Seidell JC, Molarius A 2001 A comparison of body mass index, waist–hip ratio and waist circumference as predictors of all-cause mortality among the older: the Rotterdam study. International Journal of Obesity Relating to Metabolic Disorders 25: 1730–1735

Voluntary Organizations Involved in Caring in the Older Sector (VOICES) 1998 Eating well for older people with dementia. VOICES Publications, Potters Bar, Herts

Wade DT, Langton-Hewer R, Skilbeck OE, David RH 1985 Stroke: a critical approach to diagnosis, treatment and management. Chapman & Hall, London, pp 3–40

Waitzberg DL, Correia MI 2003 Nutritional assessment in the hospitalized patient. Current Opinion in Clinical Nutrition and Metabolic Care 6: 531–538

Wakimoto P, Block G 2001 Dietary intake, dietary patterns and changes with age: an epidemiological perspective. Journal of Gerontology 56A: 65–80

Watson R 1996 The Mokken scaling procedure (MSP) applied to the measurement of feeding difficulty in older people with dementia. International Journal of Nursing Studies 33: 385–393

Westerterp KR, Goris AHC 2002 Validity of the assessment of dietary intake: problems of misreporting. Current Opinion in Clinical Nutrition and Metabolic Care 5: 489–493

White A, Nicolaas G, Foster K et al. 1993 Health survey for England (1991). HMSO, London

World Health Organization 1994 Assessment of fracture risk and application to screening for post menopausal osteoporosis. Report of a WHO study group. WHO technical support series 843. World Health Organization, Geneva

World Health Organization 1998 Preparation and use of food-based dietary guidelines. WHO technical report series 880. World Health Organization, Geneva

Yip R, Johnson C, Dallman PR 1984 Age-related changes in laboratory values used in the diagnosis of anemia and iron deficiency. American Journal of Clinical Nutrition 39: 427–436

Glossary of body and arm measures

BMI	body mass index; an estimate of body size obtained from weight (kg) divided by height^2 (m). The range associated with the lowest risk to health is 20–25.
TSF	triceps skinfold thickness; an estimate of subcutaneous fat stores (indirect). The measurement is made at the midpoint of the upper arm using calipers which quantify the thickness of a vertical skinfold in millimetres.
MAMC	midarm muscle circumference; derived from measurements of both the mid upper-arm circumference and triceps skinfold (TSF) thickness. MAMC = midarm circumference − (p × TSF). This measurement provides an index of muscle protein reserves. For this equation to be valid all measurements should be in the same units, preferably millimetres. For further details see Taylor & Goodinson-McLaren (1992).

Chapter 17

Eliminating

Christine Norton

INTRODUCTION

The passage of urine and faeces is, for most people in western society, a very personal and private function, which many are able to take for granted. Continence is one of our first socializations in childhood, and in adult life is a largely subconscious, if still voluntary, function. Considerable control over micturition and defecation is necessary for the commonly accepted criteria of continence to be met. This involves a complex neuromuscular coordination, in conjunction with an awareness of societal norms.

This control may become vulnerable for many older people, most especially at times of illness or disease, amongst disabled older people and those dependent upon the care of others to access toilet facilities at home or in residential or hospital care. The nurse has a key role, in both hospital and community settings, in identifying older people at risk of elimination problems. By a thorough assessment of each individual's needs, appropriate care can be planned to maintain normal function and prevent problems, or to remedy those problems that are already apparent.

Traditionally, nurses approached elimination care in a routinized manner. Most nurses were familiar with bedpan rounds, bottle rounds, bowel books and 4-hourly toileting regimens. Care of bowel and bladder tended to be seen as a low-status task which required little knowledge or expertise, and was often left to the most junior or untrained staff. Working with older people was often identified as synonymous with an endless routine of changing incontinent patients and wet beds. Indeed, this may be partly responsible for the unfavourable image of working with older people held by some nurses. Yet care for elimination needs really is one of the basics of nursing care, and an aspect that nurses do need to take responsibility for.

The majority of old people manage to maintain normal elimination function to the end of their days. Problems are not a necessary or inevitable concomitant of ageing and should never be passively accepted. Problems do not 'just happen'; there must always be a cause or reason for them. If this can be discovered it can often be remedied, or at least the effects upon the individual minimized.

ATTITUDES AND EFFECTS

The patient

Elimination is a difficult subject for most older people to talk about. Many were brought up with Victorian attitudes towards bodily functions – that these are somehow shameful and should never be mentioned in public. Commonly, failure to maintain normal function is thought to reflect adversely on the character of the sufferer. Elimination difficulties are a cause for shame, embarrassment and guilt and are typically kept hidden. Consequently, many people who have problems do not seek help. For example, only a minority of incontinent people seek health care and many delay seeking help for incontinence, often for years.

Younger women with incontinence have been found at interview to find it difficult to focus and think clearly because of the taboo nature of the subject (Ashworth & Hagan 1993). Many were apathetic and never quite got round to taking action. Others felt guilty that incontinence was somehow their own fault (often because of non-compliance with postnatal exercises) or were in a state of defensive denial, struggling to maintain 'normality' and a sense of personal control. The same may well be true of older incontinent women.

It is easy to assume that frail older people are passive recipients of nursing care, with little input themselves to the process. However, Robinson, in a study of nursing-home residents with incontinence using grounded theory methodology, found that people engage in a process she called 'managing urinary incontinence', with a range of strategies used with varying success. Most believed that urinary incontinence is an inevitable part of ageing and within that context sought to protect their own physical, psychological and social integrity (Robinson 2000). Residents invest much more in protecting themselves from the consequences of leakage than in seeking treatment for incontinence, with most expressing the feeling that 'you manage', for example by accepting pads instead of toilet use to reduce the risk of falls, cognitive efforts to preserve dignity and avoiding alienating staff. Six common strategies were identified by Robinson (Table 17.1). For many residents this enabled 'making the best of it' and getting on with other aspects of life. For those who did not employ successful strategies, incontinence caused suffering and physical and/or mental anguish.

Similar beliefs about the inevitability of incontinence are held by community-dwelling older people with symptoms (Branch et al. 1994), with similar strategies employed (Mitteness 1987). These issues

Table 17.1 Nursing-home residents' strategies for managing urinary incontinence

Strategy	Examples
Limiting	Self-imposed restriction on activities
	Avoid taking diuretics
	Restrict fluid intake
	Use pad instead of calling for night staff
	Stay near a toilet, avoid travel
Improvising	Methods to accomplish voiding, e.g. receptacles
	Travel and transfer to the toilet
	Aesthetic and hygienic methods
Learning	Learning how to access toilets in the facility
	Learning how to transfer
	Importance of controlling fluid intake
Monitoring	Environment: routine and other residents
	Checking for evidence of leakage
	Observing staff behaviour
Speaking up	Communicate needs, opinions and ideas
	Express preferences
Letting it go	Accidental, deliberate or negotiated urination outside usual receptacle
	Wait until morning to tell staff when wet at night

were also found to be relevant to older women during indepth interviews with a small sample (seven) of older incontinent women (Dowd 1991). Dowd found that the loss of control associated with urinary incontinence was perceived as a major threat to self-esteem. Those women who had successfully developed methods of managing their incontinence were able to accept it and lead a relatively normal life. To need help was to admit that management was ineffective, that the woman was not in charge, and this was damaging to her self-concept. There was a need to believe that the current situation was the best that can be achieved; then the incontinence could be accepted and minimized. This may explain why so many people fail to seek professional help for incontinence, and why others do not take up offers of assistance, even when these are easily accessible in their own locality.

Many older incontinent women restrict their social activities and will only go out to places where they know the toilet facilities. The degree of incontinence is not always directly related to the degree of restriction. Grimby et al. (1993) have found both emotional disturbance and social isolation in older incontinent women compared with age- and other illness-matched controls. Many avoid social contact. Generally, urge incontinence has more impact than stress leakage, probably because of the unpredictable nature of the symptom (Vinsnes & Hunskaar 1991).

The presence of urinary incontinence may determine where somebody lives, may even rob an individual of the ability to live independently, and is often quoted as a precipitating factor for admission to a nursing home. One year after a stroke people with urinary incontinence are four times more likely to be institutionalized than those who are continent (Kolominsky-Rabas et al. 2003). Even allowing for the consideration that some incontinent people are more disabled than those who are not incontinent, this is a major influence on placement. The same is likely to be true for other conditions.

Unlike urinary incontinence, very little research has been conducted on the effects of faecal incontinence upon the individual, although common sense would suggest that the impact would be even greater.

Elimination problems cause misery and discomfort and can be a burden to carers. Night-time problems, faecal incontinence and the need to have intimate contact with a person of the opposite sex are particularly difficult for relatives to cope with. These problems merit a serious nursing effort to provide a remedy when possible, or optimum management to control symptoms.

Although most older people think that nothing can be done to cure or improve incontinence, it has been found that attitudes can be changed by health education. One randomized study of people in sheltered accommodation in France demonstrated that a 1-h health information meeting not only improved attitudes but also led to increased health-seeking behaviour 3 months later in the intervention group compared with controls who received no intervention. The authors felt that this was a rapid, effective and inexpensive method of improving access to care, with incontinence people more than three times more likely to be receiving help in the intervention group than in those who did not receive the education (Beguin et al. 1997). Another education programme, Dry Expectations, resulted in 80% of older people feeling that they had more control over their bladder (Newman et al. 1996).

The nurse

A nurse needs to approach the subject of elimination difficulties with the utmost sensitivity and tact if a good rapport and trust are to be established, and take the time to find a mutually understood vocabulary. Nurses have unique and privileged access to information and the bodies of their patients (Lawler 1991, 1997). The nurse must also be alert to the possibility of problems with every patient, not just those with overt difficulties. Nurses may be reluctant to bring the subject into the open, either accepting problems as irremediable or pretending nothing is wrong in order to spare the patient's embarrassment. Schwartz (1977) has classically described this as an attitude of 'mutual pretence' between nurses and patients, leading to problems being coped with rather than constructively confronted. Nurses are notoriously good at 'coping' in unsatisfactory circumstances. This is not always in the patient's long-term interest.

Elimination has repeatedly been identified as a major problem for nursing older people. From the time of Norton's study onwards (Norton et al. 1962) it has been known that problems such as incontinence occupy a high proportion of nursing time and energy. Wells (1980) compared several studies which found between 4% and 8% of nursing activity related to elimination. Maybe not surprisingly, she found that the amount of time spent 'promoting continence' was inversely related to the amount of incontinence on a ward. Trained nurses were found to have 'confused, inaccurate' knowledge about the causes of bladder or bowel problems.

Negative attitudes and inadequate knowledge do seem to be becoming less common. Palmer (1995) found that, while the majority of nursing-home nurses had a positive attitude to implementing a continence programme, 20% were resistant, and there was an ingrained belief that incontinence is caused by old age. Up to 10% of nurses were found to believe that wilful behaviour on the part of the patient was a cause of incontinence and changing of pads and clothes was selected as commonly as any toileting programme on a list of possible interventions. Forty-one per cent of nurse respondents reported that incontinent residents in their facilities did not wear undergarments other than pads. Although nurses acknowledged that continence programmes are important, the author felt that more attention needs to be given to organizational support for such programmes. This has been echoed by other authors who describe the difficulty of maintaining behavioural interventions in long-term care (Schnelle et al. 1998).

Attitudes are found to be different among different grades of nursing staff and in different settings. One study has found that, in general, nursing assistants are more positive than registered nurses and those in acute units may be more negative than those working in longer-stay care (Vinsnes 2001). Various continence programmes have been found to reduce incontinence (see below), but compliance with such programmes is often low, even in research settings once the formal study phase is over.

Education alone does not seem to change practice; there need to be organizational changes and communication which support staff in implementing continence programmes (Lekan-Rutledge et al. 1998). There may also be major discrepancies between what staff assume is good practice and how well care is evaluated by independent audit (Peet et al. 1996).

There is a rapidly growing literature on promoting continence (see Wyman 2003 and Lekan-Rutledge & Colling 2003 for comprehensive reviews) and today the motivated nurse has considerable scope for positive management of elimination. However, change in established practice is not always easy to achieve. In a controlled study (Williams et al. 1995), it was found that a clinical handbook and educational focus groups improved knowledge about incontinence amongst nurses working with older people in hospital, but there was poor uptake for the project (only 54% of nurses invited to participate did so, and only 29% completed the study) and improved knowledge did not result in improvements in documented practice on the wards.

DELIVERY OF CONTINENCE SERVICES

It is easy for service providers to make assumptions about those they are supposed to serve. It is only recently that we have seriously asked what people want or need, and with an embarrassing problem like incontinence, the majority of sufferers have been reluctant to tell us, or to complain when things were not good. Most do not seek help and expect little when they do. Simple screening questions have been found to screen effectively for incontinence in primary care (Gunthorpe et al. 2000), but in routine practice such questions are rarely asked. Despite official guidance that service users should be involved in planning and evaluating services (Department of Health 2000), there is little evidence that this is happening in practice.

Multidisciplinary team

For many years incontinence has often been seen as solely a nursing problem, with little interest or input from other members of the multidisciplinary team, either in hospital or community settings. It is still not uncommon for an older person presenting with incontinence to a general practitioner to be told 'it's your age' and referred directly to the district nurse 'for supply of pads and pants', with no physical examination or further investigation considered.

In fact, incontinence is often a complex and multifaceted problem which may need input from a wide variety of disciplines (Norton 1996; Table 17.2). While it is obviously not practical for all of these specialties physically to work together, there needs to be careful consideration of who does what, preferably with protocols to guide appropriate referral and ensure good liaison. It is important to ensure that there are neither gaps nor too many overlaps in the service. It will often be the nurse who is responsible for ensuring this liaison (Department of Health 2000).

Role of the nurse specialist continence adviser

With the recognition of the very positive role of the nurse in managing incontinence, the concept of the nurse specialist has grown. By 2003 there were approaching 500 continence advisers in post in the UK. These nurses have a very diverse role – from clinical casework and running incontinence and urodynamics clinics to

Table 17.2   The multidisciplinary team and incontinence

Community	Hospital
District nurse	Physician
Continence adviser	Urologist
General practitioner	Gynaecologist
Physiotherapist	Geriatrician
Occupational therapist	Neurologist
Social worker	Nurse
	Physiotherapist

teaching, research, acting as a resource and information centre, product development and appraisal, and supplies liaison. It has been found that there is tremendous variation in time allocated to the different elements of the job and that managers don't really understand what the service is about (Rhodes & Parker 1995). Shaw et al., in qualitative interviews with recipients of specialist nursing continence advice, have found that the main themes that emerged were the interpersonal and technical skills of the nurse, which together led to effective treatment (Shaw et al. 2000). An informal friendly approach by nurses with good communication skills relieved patients' embarrassment and anxiety, giving them confidence and trust in the nurse, thus facilitating information exchange and the effectiveness of care. Communication was not too technical, but not patronizing. A friendly rapport was felt to promote compliance, without which treatments cannot be effective. Figure 17.1 shows Shaw et al.'s conceptualization of the effects of interpersonal, technical and communication skills of the nurse on the effectiveness of continence treatment.

ELIMINATION NEEDS

For people who are older or have a disability, the ability to remain continent often depends on a complex interplay of their physical bladder and bowel control and a whole host of other factors. Incontinence may be transient, for example during an acute illness or a urinary tract infection (UTI), and this may be the case for one-third of older people who are incontinent in the community and half of inpatients (Resnick 1995).

Certain basic needs are common to both micturition and defecation if these are to be achieved continently. The individual must be able to identify an acceptable place for elimination; get to that place; hold excreta until that place is reached; empty the bowel or bladder easily, completely and in private once there; and perform a number of toilet-related skills. This may sound obvious, but failure in any one of these abilities makes the individual vulnerable to incontinence and is so common that each is considered in turn, along with possible measures to solve problems.

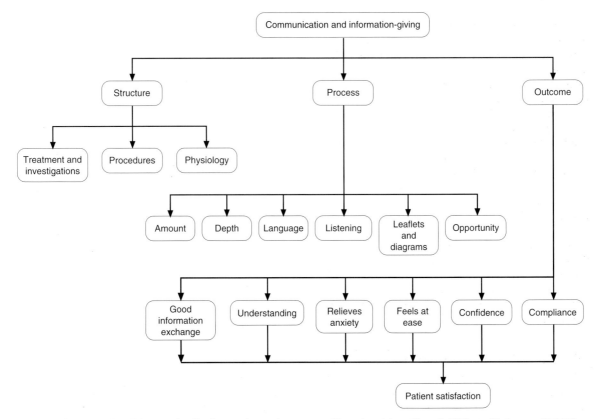

Fig. 17.1 Shaw's model of the nurse's effectiveness in continence care. (Reproduced from Shaw C, Williams KS, Assassa RP 2000 Patients' views of a new nurse-led continence service. Journal of Clinical Nursing 9: 574–584 with permission of Blackwell Publishing.)

Identifying an acceptable place

An older person's ability to identify correctly an acceptable place for elimination may be impaired in several ways. Most people expect to use a lavatory behind a locked door. In unfamiliar surroundings, this presumes an ability to follow signposts and read and correctly interpret labels on doors. Impaired vision, dim lighting or unclear (or absent) signs will create difficulties. Sometimes male and female symbols can be difficult to distinguish. The problem is often compounded by a reluctance or embarrassment to ask for help. In some instances of cerebrovascular disease, the individual loses the ability to recognize the function of common objects (such as a lavatory) by vision alone (agnosia). The confused or demented person may likewise experience difficulty in correctly identifying right and wrong receptacles and may, for instance, use a wastebin or washbasin in error.

In institutional care, expectations are often different from those in general society and people are expected to void into bedpans, bottles, commodes, behind curtains or doors without locks (or even without a door or any privacy), often in close proximity to their peers in shared rooms (Counsel & Care 1991). It is easy to see how a lifetime's conditioned responses only to excrete in private are disrupted and how a disoriented person may not be able to identify which is the 'acceptable' place. The very confused person may lose all 'socially acceptable' behaviour, and the concept of continence or incontinence becomes irrelevant to the individual.

Correct identification can be aided by clear explanations of what is expected, ensuring good lighting, signposting and labelling of facilities (at an appropriate height for older people and using pictures rather than words if patients have lost the ability to read) and, if necessary, improving vision by provision of spectacles.

Ability to get there

It is no good knowing that there is a correct place for elimination unless that place can be reached. The problem may be an unsuitable environment or an individual's physical disabilities. At home, some older people have a lavatory which involves climbing stairs or is outside. If shared with others it may be occupied when needed. Public lavatories are often difficult for anyone with even a slight disability to use and are usually in sparse supply. They may be closed, or vandalized and not repaired (Cunningham & Norton 1995). Many older women have a horror of public lavatories (believing that they risk catching diseases) and would rather avoid their use. Some older-care wards were built in the days when all patients were nursed in bed, and

some nursing homes have been adapted from private residences. Lavatories have been built on as an afterthought, often at the opposite end of the ward to the day room and down a corridor or around a corner. Travers et al. (1992) found that, in a large teaching hospital, none of the toilets met the standards recommended by the British Standards Institution. The worst were on older-care wards, where none of the toilets were suitable for use by disabled people and bedside commodes had to be used instead.

Mobility is essential in getting to the lavatory. Degree of incontinence is closely related to degree of immobility, especially in institutional settings (Ouslander & Schnelle 1995). This may be helped by ensuring that beds and chairs are of the correct height and design to aid rising; that routes to the toilet are uncluttered with obstacles (e.g. loose mats); and that individuals have the optimum mobility aid for their needs. A physiotherapist should be involved in ensuring maximum mobility and in advising carers on safe transfer techniques. Good footcare and well-fitting shoes can make a great difference.

Opening the lavatory door and getting into the compartment may present problems if design is poor. The height of the lavatory and availability of handrails will often determine whether sitting and rising are possible independently. Manual dexterity is crucial in removal of clothing, positioning and cleansing. Appropriate clothing, a raised seat or a dressing aid can facilitate independent toileting.

When physical disabilities are severe, an alternative such as a hand-held urinal (male or female) or a commode may be more appropriate, if privacy in their use can be ensured. However, it has been found that many commodes are supplied without adequate consideration for privacy (120 of 140 commode users felt embarrassed about using their commode and 101 disliked its appearance; Naylor & Mulley 1994). Recent design improvements may improve comfort and safety in future (Nazarko 1995). White (2004) has reviewed the wide range of toilet adaptations and alternatives to suit an individual's disabilities.

Sometimes depression or apathy may result in lack of motivation to attempt to reach the lavatory. The person with an impoverished social environment may simply cease to try. We are all subject to peer pressure and a wish to conform (Stokes 2002). If staff have an attitude that incontinence does not matter, and indeed it can be quicker to change a pad than to toilet someone, they can actively promote incontinence. This is particularly a problem in long-stay care if incontinence has become the norm and no expectation is put upon the individual to attempt to be continent. Occasionally, incontinence seems to be a protest or sign of despair from an individual in an unacceptable personal situation.

Ability to hold excreta

The individual needs to be able to control bladder and bowel contents reliably while getting to the lavatory. This requires competent urethral and anal sphincters and the ability to inhibit detrusor (bladder muscle) and rectal contractions. Any of these may be impaired by disease or ageing (see below). With increasing age, sensation tends to diminish and the individual gets little warning and often experiences increased urgency of micturition or defecation. It is a cruel fact that this urgency may coincide with decreased ability to hurry.

Ability to empty

Constipation and bladder-voiding difficulties are common in old age and have many possible causes (see below). Privacy is an important component in enabling complete evacuation.

Toilet-related skills

Sitting or standing in the correct position for long enough, using lavatory paper, flushing the lavatory, hand-washing and many other incidental skills are all part of independence in toileting. The nurse's assessment will determine which, if any, of these prerequisites for successful elimination are lacking for each individual. Care should be planned that aims to maximize each individual's potential for independent continence.

Drugs

Many different drugs can influence continence (Resnick 1995). The most obvious are diuretics, which will exacerbate urgency and frequency and may contribute to constipation. Sedation in any form can lessen awareness of a full bladder or bowel. Both of these are overused for older people, with 48% of nursing-home patients prescribed diuretics and 33–45% regularly receiving night sedation (Hatton 1990). Only 5% of nursing-home residents have been found to be on no medication at all (Hatton 1990). Many of these drugs would be unnecessary with thoughtful nursing interventions (Nazarko 1994).

Other drugs have unintended side-effects, such as constipation (many analgesics), or difficulty emptying the bladder (Parkinson's drugs, some antipsychotics and antidepressants). Polypharmacy is common in old age and it is essential that all incontinent people have

their drug regimens reviewed to determine if any medication is influencing continence.

Emotions

Many incontinent people appear anxious or depressed. It is very difficult to say whether this is a cause or effect of their problem. Most of us can identify with needing to use the toilet more often when under stress. Unfortunately, worrying about leaking can become a self-fulfilling prophecy, especially for those with urgency.

DEFECATION

Many older people seem obsessed by their bowels. Having lived through an era when the medical profession extolled the virtue of at least one bowel motion per day and weekly purgation, many become distressed if they do not achieve this. In fact, the range of 'normality' is wide and lies between three motions per day and one every 3 days (Connell et al. 1965), and only a minority of adults have the conventionally held 'normal' bowel habit of once per day (Heaton et al. 1992).

Normal defecation

Figure 17.2 shows the normal anatomy of the colon and rectum. The colon receives about 600 ml of faecal matter from the small bowel per day. Normal colonic activity includes propulsion of the faecal matter and absorption of fluid, so that 150–200 ml of faeces finally reaches the rectum each day. Normal defecation usually follows a so-called 'mass movement' of bowel contents. These mass movements are often stimulated by eating or physical activity and usually deliver a substantial proportion of colonic contents to the rectum.

Rectal filling leads to a sensation of needing to defecate and automatic reflex relaxation of the smooth-muscle internal anal sphincter (rectoanal inhibitory reflex). This enables the stool to move into the upper anal canal where sensitive nerve receptors can distinguish different rectal contents (gas, liquid or solid). The external anal sphincter is voluntary skeletal muscle. If passage of stool or flatus is inconvenient at this moment, the person can contract the external sphincter to retain rectal contents. This contraction is maintained for long enough for the internal sphincter to recover its resting tone automatically and the rectum to relax. The stool is propelled backwards into the rectum, and usually the feeling of needing to empty the bowels becomes less acute.

Once at the toilet, the external sphincter and puborectalis muscle are relaxed and this, sometimes coupled with a slight voluntary rise in abdominal pressure,

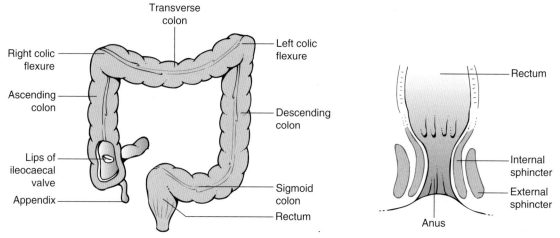

Fig. 17.2 Normal anatomy of the colon and rectum.

stimulates a coordinated rectal contraction and the rectum should empty with minimal effort. If the call to stool is ignored, defecation can be delayed for considerable periods. An increasing amount of fluid is absorbed from the stool, so the longer the delay, the harder the stool tends to become.

CONSTIPATION

There is no universally understood or accepted definition of constipation (Harari 2002). Each of us knows what we mean when we say we are constipated; however, different people mean very different things, depending on past experience and expectations. The most common use of the term refers to difficult and/or infrequent defecation.

Constipation may be associated with a variety of symptoms besides difficulty in evacuating rectal contents. Stools may be hard or pellet-sized and there may be a feeling of incomplete evacuation. Some people can only evacuate by using a finger in the rectum to help. Many constipated people complain of abdominal pain or cramps, bloating and a general malaise or fatigue. In extreme cases nausea, headaches and halitosis may be present.

Of itself, constipation seldom has serious or life-threatening consequences. Minor anorectal conditions such as haemorrhoids, fissure or rectal mucosal prolapse may be precipitated or exacerbated and, in immobile older people, faecal incontinence may result. It may be a factor in confusion in vulnerable individuals. Old wives' tales such as poisoning of the blood have little factual basis, although this does not stop many people still believing in the imperative of a daily bowel motion for inner cleanliness. Constipation does,

however, cause chronic discomfort and distress to very many people. If faecal impact results, then 'overflow' faecal incontinence may occur (Harari 2004).

A large-scale prospective population survey (Heaton et al. 1992) has found that women of child-bearing age are in fact likely to defecate less often than women 60–69 years old, and that younger women have a more irregular bowel habit and firmer stools. A third of women defecate less often than daily, and 1% once per week or less. Women are also more likely to have hard stools than men, and there is no decrease in bowel frequency associated with ageing in those under 70 years. Ageing does not, of itself, appear to decrease colonic motility or transit time, or decrease rectal sensation or bowel frequency (Barrett 1993). It may be that the image of constipation increasing with age has more to do with expectations and attitudes, immobility, frailty and other concomitant conditions rather than age itself (Heaton et al. 1992) as there is no evidence that ageing per se is a cause of constipation, but many more older people take regular laxatives than younger people, often in the absence of symptoms (Harari et al. 1995, 1996).

Constipation results from a failure of colonic propulsion (slow transit) or a failure to evacuate the rectum, or a combination of both. Box 17.1 lists the most common underlying causes of each of these. It is possible to have more than one of these problems contributing to symptoms of constipation and often there is a complex interaction of causes.

Stool consistency affects both transit and evacuation and is to some extent regulated by diet. Dietary fibre is indigestible carbohydrate (non-starch polysaccharides) which is not digested in the small bowel. When it reaches the colon it provides an ideal nutritional

---

Box 17.1   Common causes of constipation

Delay in colonic transit
- Inadequate dietary fibre
- Inadequate fluid intake (dehydration)
- Immobility
- Neuropathy – gut wall (myenteric plexus), or peripheral or central nervous system (e.g. Parkinson's disease, diabetic neuropathy)
- Myopathy
- Megacolon or megarectum
- Hormonal or endocrine disorder (e.g. hypothyroidism)
- Drug-induced (e.g. opiate analgesia, anticholinergics, iron)
- Bowel disorders (e.g. irritable bowel syndrome, diverticular disease, carcinoma)
- Psychiatric disorders (e.g. anorexia nervosa, depression)

Evacuation difficulties
- Hard stools
- Secondarily to painful anorectal conditions (haemorrhoids, fissure, solitary rectal ulcer)
- Descending perineum or rectocoele
- Paradoxical pelvic floor contraction (anismus)
- General debility and ineffective abdominal effort
- Poor toilet facilities (lack of access, privacy or poor posture on toilet)
- Hirschsprung's disease
- Neuropathy
- Confusion or intellectual impairment
- Rectal mucosal prolapse or solitary rectal ulcer syndrome

---

medium for the normal commensal colonic bacteria. Bacterial cell bodies form 40–55% of the bulk of material in the colon, and in addition help to retain fluid in the gut lumen as bacteria contain 80% water. Normally stool weight can vary considerably, despite a constant fibre intake. Although it is commonly believed that low dietary fibre is associated with constipation, and it is known that an increase in fibre improves colonic transit time and increases stool weight, there is little evidence that chronically constipated people eat a different diet from non-constipated people, or that an increase in fibre intake will control the problem if it is severe. Indeed, constipated people seem to respond less well to bran than others (Muller-Lissner 1988).

People who are unwell or generally weak may be unable to generate enough abdominal effort to stimulate a defecation reflex. Poor toilet facilities or lack of privacy may exacerbate this. Confused people may fail to realize what social behaviour is required for toileting and ignore the call to stool.

The physical environment may play a role in constipation for some older people. As physical height declines the toilet may be too high for the feet to touch the floor with ease. This will inhibit effective use of abdominal muscles to aid defecation. Provision of a footstool may enable a better defecation posture. For those in institutional settings, attention to adequate privacy is important.

Each constipated person will need a thorough individual assessment to discover the cause. Rectal examination for stool presence and consistency is an important component of a nursing assessment (Addison & Smith 2000), although digital rectal examination provides an unreliable indicator of colonic loading, particularly when stools are soft and putty-like rather than hard (Barrett 1993). Older people have been found not to find rectal examination distressing (Morgan et al. 1998). Plain abdominal radiography may not be helpful, but a transit study using radiopaque markers will give an accurate picture of the speed of colonic transit (Norton & Barrett 2002).

Treating constipation

Mild constipation may respond to simple dietary manipulation, and this is probably useful in prophylaxis, although the effectiveness of just increasing fibre for someone whose constipation is bad enough to seek medical attention is doubtful (Muller-Lissner 1988). Increased bulk should improve transit time (thus decreasing the opportunity for water absorption and breakdown of bacterial cell bodies) and improve peristalsis, thus delivering a softer stool to the rectum, as well as probably protecting against diverticular disease.

The average UK daily intake of fibre is 12–13 g (Cummings 1994); this can usefully be doubled. However, as noted above, constipated people often derive less benefit from fibre than non-constipated people as the non-starch polysaccharides tend to be broken down more with slow transit. Raw bran may upset mineral balance in vulnerable individuals. Fibre often needs to be combined with minor lifestyle changes, such as allowing adequate time for defecation and not ignoring the call to defecate. Great care should be taken to increase fibre intake gradually as a sudden increase can cause bloating and abdominal discomfort. Fibre supplement should be avoided in immobile older people as it is likely to add to the problem and even result in faecal incontinence (Ardron & Main 1990). A systematic review has not identified strong or consistent evidence for the benefit of fibre in an institutionalized population (Kenny & Skelly 2001). As there are many different types of non-starch polysaccharide, and its content within individual foods can vary, it can be both difficult to estimate intake and to predict response.

The most widely used treatment for constipation is laxatives. Considering how widely used both prescribed and over-the-counter laxatives are, there have been remarkably few comparative trials (Petticrew et al. 1997, Tramonte et al. 1997). It is often a case of trial and error to find a laxative that works for an individual with minimal side-effects (Emmanuel 2002).

Bulking agents may help those who find dietary fibre supplements unpalatable; however, these should always be introduced gradually, after clearance of any impacted faeces and with adequate fluid intake, otherwise there may be a danger of intestinal obstruction or merely adding to the impacted mass. There is no evidence that increasing fluid intake to abnormally high levels helps constipation. While clinically dehydrated individuals may benefit, normal gut secretions far exceed the daily fluid intake, and excess intake is voided by the urinary, not the digestive, system.

Stimulant laxatives should be used with extreme caution if it is suspected that the patient is faecally impacted, especially with those with concurrent disease such as diverticulitis. Osmotic laxatives such as lactulose act by retaining fluid in the stool and thereby softening it. Passmore et al. (1993) have found a senna–fibre combination (Manevac) more effective than lactulose in increasing bowel frequency, improving stool consistency and easing evacuation in non-incontinent long-stay older patients, and at a lower cost. There is a need for many more placebo-controlled studies of this nature before it is possible to make general recommendations on laxative use.

Those resistant to fibre or oral laxatives may find that a rectal stimulant in the form of a suppository or enema has better results. Indeed, the results are often more predictable and so easier to manage (Emmanuel 2002).

As lack of exercise and mobility is widely cited as a cause of constipation in old age, it would seem logical that exercise might improve constipation. The mode of action might be to stimulate colonic motility and mass movements, or that the mobile individual has more opportunity to use the toilet. One pilot study of 12 constipated immobile residents in a long-stay geriatric hospital (Resende et al. 1993) found that an exercise programme with abdominal massage made no difference to intestinal transit time (as measured by radiopaque markers), but significantly decreased faecal incontinence and increased the number of bowel motions compared to a baseline monitoring period. Treatment was a daily 50-min session of relaxation (20 min), abdominal massage (10 min) and exercise (20 min), coupled with cessation of all laxatives unless there has been no bowel action for 5 days. Only one patient needed a laxative on one occasion during the 12-week treatment period. Prior to the study, 11 of the 12 patients had received daily laxatives, suggesting unnecessary use, which may have been the major cause of the faecal incontinence, with withdrawal of laxatives leading to decrease in the proportion of days when incontinence happened.

FAECAL INCONTINENCE

Studies have found widely varying prevalence rates of faecal incontinence, depending on the definition of incontinence used and the population. The largest study to date has found that 6.2% of men and 5.7% of women over 40 years old have some degree of faecal incontinence and for 1.2% of adults this is a significant problem, occurring regularly and limiting activities (Perry et al. 2002). Prevalence increases with advancing age in both sexes, such that more than 11% of people over 80 years old have some faecal incontinence (Perry et al. 2002). Of those reported as anally incontinent in a large telephone survey, 30% were over 65 years old, and 63% were female. Incontinence was particularly associated with poor general health and limited physical capabilities. One-third had restricted their activities as a result of their incontinence and only 36% had consulted a doctor about it (Nelson et al. 1995).

Of older people living in a home or hospital, 21% are faecally incontinent at least weekly (Peet et al. 1995), and for most people in institutional care faecal incontinence is compounded by urinary incontinence. Some homes have been found to have prevalence rates for faecal incontinence of over 90% (Brocklehurst et al. 1999).

There are many different causes of faecal incontinence (Norton & Chelvanayagam 2004; Table 17.3). Childbirth, with consequent sphincter damage, is probably the most common, but chronic diarrhoea, local anorectal pathology and neurological disease are also common. Treatment will depend upon accurate diagnosis and remedy for the underlying cause, and will be the same in old age as for younger folk (Norton & Chelvanayagam 2004). Dependent older people may be incontinent of faeces secondarily to impaction (see below).

Table 17.3 Common causes of faecal incontinence

Primary problem	Common causes
Anal sphincter or pelvic floor damage	Obstetric trauma
	Iatrogenic (e.g. haemorrhoidectomy, anal stretch, lateral sphincterotomy)
	Idiopathic degeneration
	Direct trauma or injury (e.g. impalement)
	Congenital anomaly
Gut motility/stool consistency	Infection
	Inflammatory bowel disease
	Irritable bowel syndrome
	Pelvic irradiation
	Diet
	Emotions/anxiety
Anorectal pathology	Rectal prolapse
	Anal or rectovaginal fistula
	Haemorrhoids or skin tags
Neurological disease	Spinal cord injury
	Multiple sclerosis
	Spina bifida, sacral agenesis
Secondary to degenerative neurological disease	Alzheimer's disease, or environmental (see below)
Impaction with overflow 'spurious diarrhoea'	Institutionalized or immobile older people
Lifestyle and environmental	Poor toilet facilities
	Inadequate care/non-available assistance
	Drugs with gut side-effects
	Frailty and dependence
Idiopathic	Unknown cause

Constipation, impaction and faecal incontinence in old age

There is a well-recognized association between severe constipation with faecal impaction and incontinence of solid or liquid stool, often referred to as 'spurious diarrhoea', particularly amongst the frail older population in institutional care (Harari 2004). However, the mechanism for this incontinence remains somewhat obscure. It has often been suggested that impaction of the rectum causes anal relaxation, but anal resting and squeeze pressures have been found to be similar in impacted individuals compared with pressures in age-matched non-impacted controls. There is, however, a reduction in sensation and in the volume of rectal distension needed to elicit internal sphincter relaxation via the rectoanal inhibitory reflex, and some loss of the anorectal angle in incontinent individuals. It is unclear which of these mechanisms is cause or effect of impaction or subsequent incontinence. It may be that, once impaction is present (possibly caused by a combination of immobility, low fluid and fibre intake, drug side-effects, confusion, lack of privacy and many other factors), lack of sensation makes it difficult to contract the external sphincter appropriately to prevent leakage when the internal sphincter relaxes in response to rectal distension (Harari 2004).

Read et al. (1985) found that 42% of people admitted to an acute geriatric ward were impacted with hard faeces in the rectum and that impacted older people have diminished rectal sensation and so do not experience a normal call to stool. Barrett (1993) has, however, cast doubt on the definition of impaction as the presence of hard stool by finding that 45% of older people with impaction develop massive faecal loading with soft stool. He suggests that laxatives and excess fibre intake are responsible for most of this soft impaction. Treatment of constipation has been found to resolve faecal incontinence in a nursing-home population (Chassagne et al. 2000).

Patients who are generally frail and dependent need to have their bowel care actively planned to attempt to pre-empt problems, particularly impaction with overflow. With meticulous attention to routine, diet, fluid intake, maximizing mobility (with passive movement if necessary), motivation, staff/carer attitudes, defecation posture, drug regimens and the many other factors that can contribute to the problem, many problems can be kept in check. It has, however, often been difficult to implement bowel management programmes in practice because of poor staff compliance (Rands & Malone-Lee 1990).

MICTURITION

Disorders of micturition become increasingly common with age. However, ageing per se does not produce incontinence. It is usually a combination of impairment of bladder function and a variety of precipitating factors that upset an often delicate balance and produce frank incontinence (Resnick 1996). Bladder capacity decreases with age, thereby increasing frequency of micturition. Urethral outlet pressure decreases in women.

Nocturia (rising at night to pass urine) affects most old people, with nocturia 1–2 times at night considered normal. Over the age of 80 years 70–90% of people get up at night to pass urine. There is evidence that many older people experience a disturbed diurnal rhythm of urine production. Instead of producing most urine during waking hours, older people often produce urine evenly throughout the 24 h, or even more at night. This is probably due to changes in the production of antidiuretic hormone, and will be exacerbated by renal or heart disease, worsened if sleep is disturbed for other reasons. Frail older people may additionally spend more hours in bed, increasing the likelihood of needing to empty the bladder while in bed. Simple measures such as elevating the feet or using compression stockings towards the end of the day to encourage venous return, reducing fluid intake for a few hours before bedtime and changing timing of diuretics can be helpful to some people with troublesome nocturia (Fonda et al. 2002).

Many also experience diurnal frequency, urgency and, in community-dwelling adults, about 20% have some degree of urinary incontinence, and this may affect upwards of 50% in nursing homes (Peet et al. 1995, Hunskaar et al. 2002). As age advances, men, who have lower prevalence rates than women in younger age groups, tend to be as incontinent as women. In the very old (85 years+), 43% of women and 24% of men have some urinary incontinence (Hellstrom et al. 1990). Severity of incontinence also increases with advancing age. However, it is important not to assume that everyone reporting incontinence is bothered by it. For some, it is a minor nuisance, and only about 50% of those found to be incontinent find it troublesome (Hunskaar et al. 2002).

Urinary tract infection is present in over 10% of older people and up to 50% of those in institutional care. One in two men is likely to experience symptoms attributable to prostatic hypertrophy by the eighth decade of life. Urge urinary incontinence is associated with a 26% increased risk of falls and a 34% increased risk of fractures (Brown 2000).

Control over bladder function, as with bowels, is likely to face many other insults in addition to physiological dysfunction with increasing age, including other diseases, multiple medications, difficulties with mobility and mental agility. Incontinence is often precipitated by these extra-bladder factors. Resnick (1984) coined the mnemonic 'DIAPPERS' (with two 'p's) to summarize these as follows:

- D – delirium (e.g. confusion)
- I – infection (UTI, symptomatic)
- A – atrophic urethritis or vaginitis (women)
- P – psychological (e.g. severe depression, neurosis)
- P – pharmacologic
- E – excessive fluid intake or output
- R – restricted mobility and environmental
- S – stool impaction (constipation).

It will be most usually necessary to treat both the bladder and these other factors to achieve continence.

Complete urinary continence may not be achievable for all older people. This does not mean that care has 'failed'. A state of 'dependent continence' or 'social continence' may enable the individual to maintain dignity and continue desired activities despite imperfect bladder control (Fonda et al. 2002).

Bladder dysfunction in old age

Most people with urinary symptoms have an underlying bladder dysfunction. Indeed, in old age two or even three separate problems may be present in combination. It is important to obtain an accurate diagnosis, as the treatments are different. Usually a careful history and examination will indicate the cause, but if in doubt urodynamic studies are necessary to distinguish the bladder dysfunctions (Abrams et al. 2002). Figures 17.3 and 17.4 give expert-consensus-derived algorithms for the management of urinary incontinence in old age (Abrams et al. 2002). Assessment should be multidisciplinary and approached in a stepwise logical order, first to identify and treat reversible causes and subsequently to determine the best management option for those with established incontinence. Expert opinion agrees that the fit older person should be treated for incontinence in exactly the same manner as younger people, with the full range of options, including surgery, considered (Fonda et al. 2002).

Lifestyle alteration and education

Box 17.2 gives the suggested components of assessment in frail older adults (Lekan-Rutledge & Colling 2003). Expert opinion is that 'most patients can be managed with non-pharmacologic treatments that nurses can prescribe and implement' (Wyman 2003). Treatment will often involve addressing mobility and

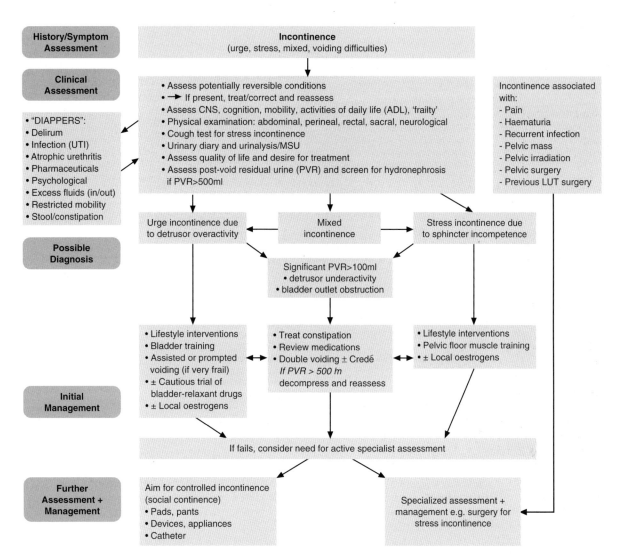

Fig. 17.3 Management of urinary continence in frail and/or disabled older women. UTI, urinary tract infection; CNS, central nervous system; MSU, midstream urine; LUT, lower urinary tract. (Reproduced from Fonda et al. (2002) with permission of Health Books.)

toilet access, diet to avoid constipation, adequate (but not excessive) fluid intake, caffeine reduction and advice on increasing exercise and reducing obesity (Subak 2002). As would be expected, there is evidence that increased fluid intake increases the volume and frequency of voiding. However, increased fluid intake probably does not actually cause frequency or incontinence in the absence of other problems such as an overactive bladder. Ensuring adequate fluid intake does not increase incontinence and helps to protect against UTI and bladder cancer. Excessive fluid intake (over 3 litres in 24 h) may increase incontinence and restricting fluids for 2 h before bed may improve nocturnal voiding (Gray & Krissovich 2003).

Although the evidence base for many suggested 'lifestyle' changes is not strong (Wilson et al. 2002, Wyman 2003), clinically and in combination, they are often found clinically useful. Group learning has been found to be effective in enabling older women to take an active role in tackling their own incontinence (Gerard 1997) as well as encouraging them to seek help from health professionals (Beguin et al. 1997).

Overactive bladder

An unstable or overactive bladder is the most common bladder dysfunction in old age. Overactivity of the detrusor (bladder muscle) is however present in one-third of continent older people, and so cannot

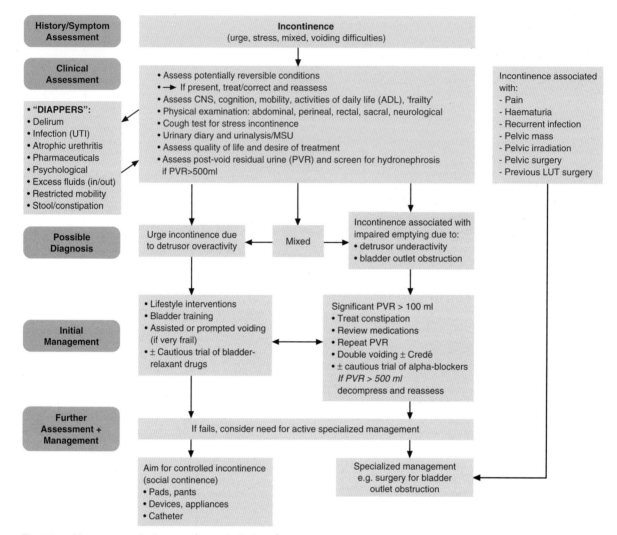

Fig. 17.4   Management of urinary continence in frail and/or disabled older men. UTI, urinary tract infection; CNS, central nervous system; MSU, midstream urine; LUT, lower urinary tract. (Reproduced from Fonda et al. (2002) with permission of Health Books.)

alone be said to be the 'cause' of incontinence (Fonda et al. 2002). The patient loses the ability to inhibit detrusor contractions reliably and so experiences urgency and frequency. If this is severe, or the sufferer is immobile or asleep, or no lavatory is at hand, incontinence may result.

Behavioural interventions are the mainstay of treatment for the overactive bladder. Table 17.4 outlines the various programmes described in the literature (Wyman 2003). However, there are many variations and combinations of therapy described. Bladder training, with or without the help of medication, should be the first option in the treatment for cognitively intact individuals. There is good evidence that bladder retraining reduces urge, stress and mixed urge and stress incontinence in older

women (Wilson et al. 2002, Wyman 2003). While there is no nursing consensus as to what we mean by 'bladder training', most programmes involve keeping a baseline chart for 3–7 days and then working out an individualized pattern of target toilet visits gradually to extend the time between voidings (Norton 1996). With plenty of support and encouragement, many patients can learn to overcome their urgency and establish a normal pattern without urgency. Studies have found cure and improvement rates of 57–87% (Wilson et al. 2002). There is also evidence that there is an incremental benefit from advice on lifestyle and diet (e.g. caffeine reduction), bladder training and pelvic muscle exercise, with a decrease in severity of incontinence of 61% 2 years after behavioural management, compared with an increase of 184% in

---

Box 17.2   Components of assessment in frail older adults

History and symptoms
- Symptoms of stress, urge, mixed or functional incontinence
- Voiding and incontinence pattern
- Fluid intake and type
- Bowel habit
- Smoking
- Functional assessment
    Activities of daily living, mobility and exercise
    Cognition and affect
- Other medical conditions and medication
- Impact of incontinence, quality of life and motivation
- Environment and carers
- Patient's preferences for treatment

Clinical and physical assessment
- Assess for reversible causes and treat if present (DIAPPERS: see text for details)
- Physical examination (abdominal, rectal, vaginal, prostate)
- Bladder diary for 3–5 days (voids, volumes and incontinence)
- Urinalysis
- Postvoid residual urine volume

Environmental assessment
- Distance to toilet
- Accessibility of toilet or alternative (commode or urinal)
- Carer's availability and willingness to help
- Walking aids
- Dexterity and clothing

Formulate diagnosis
- Based on the assessment determine, and where possible address, all factors that may be relevant to each individual patient.
- Consider need for specialist referral

(Adapted from Lekan-Rutledge & Colling 2003.)

---

severity of incontinence in controls (Dougherty et al. 2002). The latter authors found that self-monitoring and bladder training accounted for most of the difference. Timed voiding is also of proven benefit (Wyman 2003). Provision of leaflets and audiotapes suggesting cognitive strategies improve function and increase comfort through 'coaching' but weekly phone calls to reinforce the advice do not add greatly to the effect (Dowd 2003).

Family caregivers have been found able to implement an individualized toileting programme, producing a significant reduction in incontinent episodes compared to controls, especially if the patient is mobile and has only mild to moderate cognitive impairment (Jirovec & Templin 2001, Engberg et al. 2002).

Urge incontinence may also be controlled pharmacologically by inhibiting unstable detrusor muscle contrac-

tions. The antimuscarinics oxybutynin chloride and tolterodine are probably the most successful drugs available at present, although some patients also respond to propantheline or imipramine, and newer preparations such as tropsium chloride are promising (Abrams et al. 2002). Side-effects such as a dry mouth, disturbed vision and constipation are very common with therapeutically effective doses. Postural hypotension is also a possibility in the frail. Oxybutynin has been found superior to placebo in reducing frequency and increasing subjective benefit, but not in reducing incontinence episodes when used in addition to a bladder-training programme in frail older people living at home (Szonyi et al. 1995), suggesting that the benefit of using medication over using bladder training alone may be marginal, but useful if training alone is not successful.

Table 17.4 Bladder-training programmes

	Description	Suitable for
Scheduled voiding	Toileting to a fixed schedule, typically 2-hourly	Patients with physical or cognitive impairments, especially if voiding pattern is erratic
Habit retraining	Scheduled toileting with voiding intervals adjusted to the individual's pattern	Patients with physical or cognitive impairments with predictable incontinence episodes
Patterned urge response toileting	Habit retraining with the use of an electronic monitor	Patients with physical or cognitive impairments
Prompted voiding	Scheduled toileting where carer prompts (asks patient if toilet needed), typically 2-hourly: patient assisted to toileting only if response is positive	Patients who sense the need to void and are able to request assistance, with carer available to assist
Bladder training	Progressive increase in voiding intervals, often combined with urge control and distraction strategies	Cognitively intact, mobile and motivated patient

Electrical stimulation also has a place in alleviating urge incontinence due to detrusor instability (Moore 1994). This is usually administered via vaginal or skin electrodes, at home or in a clinic setting.

Stress incontinence

This complaint is most common in parous women and may be associated with atrophic changes in the vagina and urethra, or vaginal prolapse. The symptom of stress incontinence is leakage upon physical exertion such as cough. If severe, even minimal rises in abdominal pressure, such as during walking or the act of standing from a chair, may provoke leakage. If incontinence is slight to moderate, there is strong evidence that relief can be gained from pelvic muscle exercises (Laycock & Haslam 2002, Wilson et al. 2002) with an average cure rate of 25% from pelvic floor exercises and a cured and improved rate between 47% and 77%. Pelvic floor exercises may also help someone with urgency to hang on a little more effectively, and so avoid urge incontinence.

Simple teaching of techniques such as 'the knack' (intentionally contracting the pelvic floor muscles before and during cough or other rise in intra-abdominal pressure) can dramatically (average of 73% reduction) reduce urine loss within 1 week of teaching (Miller et al. 1998).

Success from pelvic muscle exercises will depend on:

- patient motivation: there is no doubt that these exercises are boring and it is difficult to remember to do them as often as needed. Regular follow-up has an important role to play in keeping the patient motivated and giving feedback on progress
- correct teaching: most people are unaware of the pelvic floor and will not perform the exercises correctly unless properly taught, and reassessed at intervals. A digital vaginal or rectal examination is the best way to teach pelvic floor exercises. Many patients practise them incorrectly, and even counterproductively, without this teaching (Laycock & Haslam 2002)
- a correct initial diagnosis: pelvic floor exercises are not a panacea for all types of incontinence
- sometimes vaginal cones or electrotherapy can be a useful adjunct to pelvic floor exercises alone (Wilson et al. 2002).

Long-term adherence to exercises has sometimes been found to be a problem and long-term benefit probably depends on at least some exercises being performed on an ongoing basis. Various health education techniques have been tried to enhance long-term compliance with exercises, but none has been found more advantageous than good physiotherapy teaching alone (Alewijnse et al. 2003), with women with the highest urine loss initially being the most likely to keep performing the exercises.

Drugs have a limited role in stress incontinence. Oestrogen replacement may improve subjective control for some postmenopausal women, but has not been proven to decrease the actual amount of urine loss (Fantl et al. 1994).

Urinary incontinence in men following prostatectomy has been found to be less severe and resolve more quickly if men practise pelvic muscle exercises (Van Kampen 2000), but long-term results seem to be similar whether or not exercises are performed, suggesting that perhaps it may be most cost-effective to reserve intensive exercise programmes for those who are most symptomatic (Kondo et al. 2002).

More severe stress incontinence, particularly if associated with prolapse, usually requires surgical correction, for which advanced age is no contraindication. Indeed, older women may achieve better results from surgery than younger ones as they are less likely to undertake vigorous exercise which may disrupt the repair. Traditionally, a suprapubic rather than vaginal approach to surgery gives the best results. However, in the past decade a technique for insertion under local or brief general anaesthetic of a 'tension-free vaginal tape' has been developed and is now in widespread use as a minimally invasive technique, usually performed as a day-case without open surgery. Another minimally invasive approach is to inject collagen or similar material around the bladder neck to give added support, and this can be done under local anaesthetic as an outpatient, with improvement rates of 70–80% which last at least in the medium term (Khullar et al. 1997, Stanton & Monga 1997). Sometimes a vaginal ring pessary will produce symptomatic relief (Sasso et al. 2003).

Incomplete voiding

In both sexes postvoid residual urine volume increases with age, often due to a combination of urethral outflow obstruction and impaired detrusor muscle contractility, with 50–100 ml considered normal and volumes above that as potentially significant. Prostatic enlargement in men is the most common cause of outflow obstruction, which may also occur in either gender because of faecal impaction or a pelvic mass. The patient usually experiences frequency and difficulty voiding. Residual urine may accumulate in the bladder, and overflow incontinence usually presents as a continuous non-specific dribbling. Treatment involves relief of the obstruction. Simple mechanical methods such as use of an intravaginal pessary to support genital prolapse are often overlooked but can provide ongoing help to many older women who do not wish for surgical solutions for prolapse (Sasso et al. 2003).

If the detrusor muscle fails to contract for micturition, or if the contraction is not sustained until the bladder is empty, a chronic residual collection of urine may be present. This may become infected and lead to overflow incontinence. It is now recognized that many frail older people have both an overactive unstable bladder, causing frequency, and impaired contractility on micturition, and therefore incomplete emptying,

and that this diagnosis is commonly missed, especially in a nursing-home population (Resnick et al. 1996). An important element of patient assessment is an estimation of postvoid residual urine volume (either using portable ultrasonography or an in–out catheter) as this is very often missed as a cause of incontinence in older people of both genders (Fonda et al. 2002).

The use of intermittent (in–out) catheterization to drain off this residual urine is widespread for younger patients with an underactive detrusor. Its use for older people has not yet been widely reported, but initial results are promising. Some patients can be taught to self-catheterize, in which case a clean, non-sterile technique is taught; for others, a relative or nurse must do the catheterization. Some patients seem to regain detrusor tone with this management and resume voiding; for others, the intermittent catheterization must become long-term management.

Urinary tract infection (UTI)

The presence of 'significant' bacteriuria (commonly accepted as 100 000 organisms/ml of urine) is so high that it must call into question the criterion of significance adopted for younger people. Probably the most useful way to treat UTI is to distinguish between acute and chronic infection. The patient with a sudden onset of the symptoms and cystitis – dysuria, pain, frequency, pyrexia and possibly confusion – should receive the appropriate antibiotic therapy (but it should be noted that symptoms are often a lot less acute than in younger patients). A chronic infection is often asymptomatic, associated with residual urine and will not respond to antibiotics, or will soon return, and should seldom be treated (Wilkie et al. 1992). Routine treatment of UTI, regardless of symptoms or needs, risks the emergence of resistant organisms and should be avoided.

It is wise to remember that symptoms of atrophic urethritis may mimic cystitis in older women. Inspection of the vulva will reveal if atrophic changes, such as dry, inflamed mucosa, are present. Women with recurrent UTI may benefit from low-dose oestrogen therapy (Wilkie et al. 1992)

INCONTINENCE IN INSTITUTIONAL CARE

Prevalence of incontinence in nursing homes varies from 40 to 70%, depending on case mix (Ouslander & Schnelle 1995). An average of over 50% is accepted as usual. It is associated with immobility, reduced ability to perform activities of daily living, use of restraints and cognitive impairment (Brandeis 1997, Lekan-Rutledge & Colling 2003), with dementia and immobility the two factors most strongly associated. It is possible to improve mobility by a structured exercise programme in this group, but the benefits for continence status are unclear, as few who are dependent are capable of becoming independent (Schnelle et al. 1995). Pads are the most commonly used method of management (used by 84%) for urinary incontinence in American nursing homes; 38% of incontinent people are also said to be on scheduled toileting (Brandeis 1997). Some potentially reversible factors include use of trunk restraints and bedrails and prescription of antianxiety/hypnotic medications, with only 22% tested for urinary infection and only 40% examined for faecal impaction (Brandeis et al. 1997). Residents in nursing homes have been found to believe that incontinence is inevitable and to spend more time and energy hiding the problem than in seeking treatment (Robinson 2000). Continence in this patient group has been characterized by four categories (Fig. 17.5; Fonda et al. 2002).

Incontinence in residents in homes or hospitals is often associated with multiple undiagnosed and untreated problems, which, if remedied, may lead to restoration of continence for a proportion of residents. It cannot be overemphasized that an individual assessment is the crucial first step in any nursing intervention. Transient causes may be reversible (e.g. treating an acute UTI or changing medications). However, caregivers have often been found to fail to assess incontinent residents for faecal impaction, vaginal atrophic changes, congestive cardiac failure, diabetes and other potentially reversible causes (Brandeis 1997). If the resident is confused, a behavioural assessment is indicated.

Toileting programmes

Most toileting programmes reported for frail older people achieve an average reduction of 1–2 incontinent episodes per day (Fonda et al. 2002, Lekan-Rutledge & Colling 2003). Few result in total continence in this patient group. Those whose continence resolves have been found to be more ambulant and less

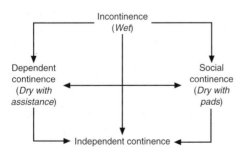

Fig. 17.5 Four possible continence states in frail older people. (Reproduced from Fonda et al. (2002) with permission of Health Books.)

demented than those who remain incontinent despite intervention (Palmer 1991).

Prompted voiding

Prompted voiding provides an opportunity to be assisted to the toilet at regular intervals. Most studies have used a 2-hourly schedule of asking the patient discreetly, up to three times, if they would like help to go to the toilet, and taking them if requested. Social interaction and positive verbal feedback are given when the request is appropriate and the toilet used. It has been found that 20–40% of frail nursing-home residents respond well, with severity of incontinence reduced by approximately half. Success is associated with patients who can accurately recognize the need to void and can successfully do so when taken to the toilet; less successful are those who cannot voluntarily initiate voiding, void low volumes or have high residual urine volumes (Hu et al. 1989, Schnelle 1990). A 3-day trial of prompted voiding is usually sufficient to tell if an individual patient will respond, suggesting that this is not a 'learning' response but a positive response to being provided with the opportunity to be continent. It does not help at night. A 2-hourly programme has been found to maintain 35% of patients at an average of only one incontinent episode per 24 h and take an average of 17 min carer time per patient (Schnelle et al. 1989). Prompted voiding has been found to be more effective than just social contact (Creason et al. 1989). A 3-hourly programme has been found to be as effective as, or even more effective than, a 2-hourly one and possible to implement using normal nursing-home staff if management are supportive (Burgio et al. 1994).

The results of many studies have been found to be statistically significant, but the clinical significance of these results is less clear as few patients become completely continent. Likewise, addition of antimuscarinic medication to a prompted voiding programme may yield results which are statistically significant but probably not large enough an effect to be clinically useful in the nursing-home setting except in occasional individual cases (Ouslander et al. 1995).

Habit training

This is the most complex toileting programme devised for frail older people in nursing homes. It attempts to identify each individual's own natural habit or voiding pattern, and then to implement an individualized prompted voiding schedule. Colling et al. (1992) found a statistically significant reduction in episodes of incontinence in 86% of patients, with one-third showing a 25% or greater improvement.

To achieve an individualized toileting programme is undoubtedly most difficult to implement in an institutional setting using largely untrained staff. Colling et al. (1992) encountered major problems with staff resistance and compliance. The difficulties of introducing innovative programmes and getting staff to comply should not be underestimated. Much depends on the attitude and ethos of care and it should be remembered that elimination care will not be beneficial unless general care is individualized in intent and content. Education of staff alone has been found to be insufficient to sustain improvements once research staff are withdrawn (Schnelle et al. 1998).

MANAGEMENT OF INTRACTABLE INCONTINENCE

Even with the best available management and care, some patients remain incontinent. It is important that this is recognized as inevitable and that nurses do not feel guilty about it. The individual can usually be helped to maintain dignity and comfort in some way. The nurse should teach the patient, or the family, the most suitable management techniques, and has an important supportive role in care (Norton & Kamm 1999).

There is remarkably little research or literature on the practical management of incontinence. The odour and sore skin that can be caused by leakage of faeces are particularly difficult to cope with. Scrupulous attention to personal hygiene, changing and washing (rather than just dry wiping) as soon as possible after an accident seem to prevent soreness for some people. Moist toilet tissue can be a lot more comfortable than dry paper if use is very frequent. But if incontinence is frequent, there is continuous seepage or the faeces are liquid, the perianal skin can become very excoriated. Barrier creams such as Metanium or Sudocrem may be useful in the prevention and treatment of milder cases. Where the skin becomes broken, stoma care products can help healing. The efficacy of these products has not been systematically tested in research studies, and it is often a case of trial and error to find a product that works for an individual.

Smell is an understandable concern of many people with incontinence. In fact, freshly voided urine should not smell unpleasant (and if it does, it may be infected): it is contact with air that leads to breakdown of the constituents of urine and the consequent smell. Prompt changing of soiled pads or clothes and storage of soiled materials in an airtight container, along with the hygiene measures outlined above, is the best option. But this is not always possible and the smell of faeces is hard to disguise. Deodorants developed for use with stoma bags are probably the most useful products to combat smell.

Incontinence products

A good incontinence aid will enable the incontinent person to be socially accepted and to lead a relatively normal life. Despite the huge range and variety of products now available (www.promocon2001.co.uk), some function poorly. An aid must be carefully selected with regard to the individual's degree, type and pattern of incontinence, local anatomy, physical and mental abilities, personal preference, washing or disposal facilities, and cost. No one aid will suit everyone and a range should be provided. The nurse must be the patient's advocate in this and be prepared to make a case for the supply of the most appropriate items.

Body-worn pads and pants

Most incontinent women, and some men, use a disposable, absorbent pad held in place by pants to collect urine or faeces. Sanitary towels are the most commonly used, but will not cope with any but minimal leakage. Plastic pants are undignified, uncomfortable and can cause considerable skin problems and should not be in routine use. Most pads are plastic-backed and held in place with stretch pants. Others have an all-in-one 'diaper'-style design. They vary a lot in the quality of their constituents and design and capacity. The smallest pad that will reliably contain incontinence for an individual should be selected. Many pads now have superabsorbent gel to augment capacity. Most recently, washable, reusable pads and pants with absorbent gussets have become available. Good-quality evidence is available from government-funded sources, such as the Continence Products Evaluation Network (www.medphys.ucl.ac.uk/research-groups/incont/cpe.htm), but unfortunately, product development has often changed the product before evaluations are published.

Male appliances

Some men are able to use a penile sheath or an appliance in preference to a pad. A retracted penis or poor manual dexterity make their use difficult. A penile sheath should be carefully selected for appropriate size and is most satisfactory if a self-adhesive variety is used, or if held in position with a double-sided adhesive strip. It should be connected to a leg-bag. Appliances such as pubic pressure urinals should always be fitted by an experienced appliance fitter.

Bed and chair protection

Bed-pads do have their uses but are often expected, quite unrealistically, to cope with all incontinence needs. Washable bed-sheets with a stay-dry surface have proved to be comfortable, popular and cost-effective, but in some instances laundry provision is inadequate to cope with them. Nurses should consider more carefully the use of bed and chair protection, possibly refocusing care from protection of the environment to protection of the patient.

INDWELLING CATHETERS AND OLDER PEOPLE

Generally, the use of an indwelling catheter should be seen very much as a 'last resort' when all other methods of managing micturition have been tried and failed. Widespread, indiscriminate use of catheters has fallen into disrepute, as has their use solely for nursing convenience. A move away from catheters can be shown to benefit even severely incontinent patients in many instances.

The decision to use a catheter should only be made for clear and valid reasons, with a definite goal that can be evaluated, and in full consultation with all concerned, especially the patient. The individual's quality of life should be the prime consideration – will the use of a catheter significantly improve independence, comfort and dignity? For some patients (e.g. someone with severe incontinence which is poorly controlled by an aid) a catheter can be a great benefit, even enabling community rather than institutional care. Each decision should be made on an individual basis and re-evaluated at intervals.

Managing a catheter

Many long-term catheters are poorly managed (Roe 1996). Confused, ignorant management and a lack of knowledge of the principles of catheter drainage were found to be widespread.

If a patient has to live with a catheter, drainage must be made convenient (Roe 1996). For day use, a leg-bag or a bag attached to a waist-belt, garment holder or in a pocket inside trousers or a skirt will hide the urine from public view. Some systems allow direct connection of night-bags to the bottom of day-bags without breaking the closed system. The outlet tap should be simple to use and to understand, but many fail to meet these criteria.

Patient teaching and individualized care will overcome many problems. The importance of diet, exercise, fluid intake, personal hygiene and avoiding constipation should be emphasized. Sexual function should be discussed, and if the patient is sexually active an alternative to a urethral catheter considered. Sometimes the patient or a partner may be taught to remove and replace the catheter, thus increasing independence; or a catheter can be inserted into the bladder suprapubically via the abdominal wall.

Leaking may be caused by too large a catheter or balloon, or by an overactive bladder (which may respond to anticholinergic medication). Catheter blockage is a recurrent problem in 40–50% of long-term catheters (Getliffe 2003) and is most likely in the presence of alkaline urine, often caused when the bladder is colonized by bacteria which produce the enzyme urease which breaks down urea to release the alkaline ammonia. Routine preventive acidic bladder wash-outs (of 50 ml volume) should only be used when a catheter is found to block persistently, but pre-emptive changing may be a better answer unless blockage regularly occurs in less than 7–14 days (Getliffe 2003). Increasing fluid intake and drinking acidic drinks such as cranberry juice do not seem to prevent blockage in those with the relevant organisms. Infections are inevitable with long-term catheter drainage and should only be treated if the patient is symptomatic (Roe 1996). If a catheter causes repeated problems, its use should be questioned since the patient may be better off without it.

CONCLUSION

Many older people are at risk of less than perfect control over their elimination. It is a nursing responsibility to assess each individual and then to plan care, in collaboration with other members of the multidisciplinary team. That care should attempt to remedy any bladder or bowel problem and to maximize the individual's ability to cope with elimination in a continent manner. In this area nurses can make a significant contribution to the comfort, dignity and well-being of those who come into their care.

Recommended reading

Fonda D, Benvenuti F, Cottenden A et al. 2002 Urinary incontinence and bladder dysfunction in older persons. In: Abrams P, Khoury S, Wein A, Cardozo L (eds) Incontinence. Health Books, Plymouth, 625–695.
Comprehensive review of available evidence by an international multidisciplinary consensus panel, updated every 3 years.
Getliffe K, Dolman M (eds) 2003 Promoting continence: a clinical research resource, 2nd edn. Baillière Tindall, London
Comprehensive reasearch-based textbook.
Newman DK, Palmer MH (eds) 2003 State of the science on urinary incontinence. American Journal of Nursing 103(suppl March): 1–57
Four articles with discussion and commentary which are the proceedings from a symposium held in the USA in 2002, with

recommendations for research, practice, education and policy.
Excellent review of the available nursing evidence.

Norton C, Chelvanayagam S (eds) 2004 Bowel continence nursing. Beaconsfield Publishers, Beaconsfield.

Comprehensive text written for qualified nurses covering all aspects of faecal incontinence assessment and management.

Potter J, Norton C, Cottenden A (eds) 2002 Bowel care in older people. Royal College of Physicians, London.

Edited proceedings of a meeting held in London in 2001 reviewing the state of knowledge about bowel care in older people, including epidemiology, assessment and options for interventions.

References

Abrams P, Khoury S, Wein A, Cardozo L 2002 Incontinence. Health Books, Plymouth

Addison R, Smith M 2000 Digital rectal examination and manual removal of faeces. Royal College of Nursing, London

Alewijnse D, Metsemakers JFM, Mesters IE, van den Borne B 2003 Effectiveness of pelvic floor muscle exercise therapy supplemented with a health education programme to promote long-term adherence among women with urinary incontinence. Neurourology and Urodynamics 22: 284–295

Ardron ME, Main ANH 1990 Management of constipation. British Medical Journal 300: 1400

Ashworth PD, Hagan MT 1993 The meaning of incontinence: a qualitative study of non-geriatric urinary incontinence sufferers. Journal of Advanced Nursing 18: 1415–1423

Barrett JA 1993 Faecal incontinence and related problems in the older adult. Edward Arnold, London

Beguin AM, Combes T, Lutzler P, Laffond G, Belmin J 1997 Health education improves older subjects' attitudes toward urinary incontinence and access to care: a randomised study in sheltered accommodation centres for the aged (letter). Journal of the American Geriatrics Society 45: 391–392

Branch LG, Walker LA, Wetle TT, DuBeau C, Resnick NM 1994 Urinary incontinence knowledge among community-dwelling people of 65 years of age and older. Journal of the American Geriatrics Society 42: 1257–1262

Brandeis GH, Baumann MM, Hossain M, Morris JN, Resnick NM 1997 The prevalence of potentially remediable urinary incontinence in frail older people: a study using the minimum data set. Journal of the American Geriatrics Society 45: 179–184

Brocklehurst JC, Dickinson E, Windsor J 1999 Laxatives and faecal incontinence in long term care. Nursing Standard 13: 32–36

Brown JS 2000 Urinary incontinence: does it increase risk for falls and fractures? Study of osteoporotic fractures research group. Journal of the American Geriatrics Society 48: 721–725

Burgio LD, McCormick KA, Sceve AS et al. 1994 The effects of changing prompted voiding schedules in the treatment of incontinence in nursing home residents. Journal of the American Geriatrics Society 42: 315–320

Chassagne P, Jego A, Gloc P et al. 2000 Does treatment of constipation improve faecal incontinence in institutionalized elderly patients? Age and Ageing 29: 159–164

Colling J, Ouslander J, Hadley BJ, Eisch J, Campbell E 1992 The effects of patterned urge-response toileting (PURT) on urinary incontinence among nursing home residents. Journal of the American Geriatrics Society 39: 135–141

Connell AM, Hilton C, Irvine G, Lennard-Jones JE, Misiewicz JJ 1965 Variation in bowel habit in two population samples. British Medical Journal ii: 1095–1099

Counsel & Care 1991 Not such private places. Counsel and Care for the Elderly, London

Creason NS, Grybowski JA, Burgener S, Whippo SA, Richardson B 1989 Prompted voiding therapy for urinary incontinence in aged female nursing home residents. Journal of Advanced Nursing 14: 120–126

Cummings JH 1994 Non-starch polysaccharides (dietary fibre) including bulk laxatives in constipation. In: Kamm MA, Lennard-Jones JE (eds) Constipation. Wrightson Biomedical, Petersfield, pp 307–314

Cunningham S, Norton C 1995 Public inconveniences: some suggestions for improvement, 2nd edn. Continence Foundation, London

Department of Health 2000 Good practice in continence services. PL/CMO/2000/2. NHS Executive, London

Dougherty MC, Dwyer JW, Pendergast JF et al. 2002 A randomized trial of behavioral management for continence in older rural women. Research into Nursing Health 25: 3–13

Dowd TT 1991 Discovering older women's experience of urinary incontinence. Research into Nursing Health 14: 179–186

Dowd TT 2003 The addition of coaching to cognitive strategies: interventions for persons with compromised urinary bladder syndrome. Journal of Wound Ostomy and Continence Nursing 30: 90–99

Emmanuel AV 2002 The use and abuse of laxatives. In: Potter J, Norton C, Cottenden A (eds) Bowel care in older people. Royal College of Physicians, London, pp 77–88

Engberg S, Sereika S, McDowell J, Weber E, Brodak I 2002 Effectiveness of prompted voiding in treating urinary incontinence in cognitively impaired homebound older adults. Journal of Wound Ostomy and Continence Nursing 29: 252–265

Fantl JA, Cardozo L, McClish D 1994 Estrogen therapy in the management of urinary incontinence in postmenopausal women: a meta-analysis. First report of the hormones and urogenital therapy committee. Obstetrics and Gynecology 83: 12–18

Fonda D, Benvenuti F, Cottenden A et al. 2002 Urinary incontinence and bladder dysfunction in older persons. In: Abrams P, Khoury S, Wein A, Cardozo L (eds) Incontinence. Health Books, Plymouth, pp 625–695

Gerard L 1997 Group learning behavior modification and exercise for women with urinary incontinence. Urologic Nursing 17: 17–22

Getliffe K 2003 Managing recurrent urinary catheter blockage: problems, promises and practicalities. Journal of Wound Ostomy and Continence Nursing 30: 146–151

Gray M, Krissovich M 2003 Does fluid intake influence the risk for urinary incontinence, urinary tract infection and bladder cancer? Journal of Wound Ostomy and Continence Nursing 30: 126–131

Grimby A, Milsom I, Molander U, Wiklund I, Ekelund P 1993 The influence of urinary incontinence on the quality of life of elderly women. Age and Ageing 22: 82–89

Gunthorpe W, Brown W, Redman S 2000 The development and evaluation of an incontinence screening questionnaire for female primary care. Neurourology and Urodynamics 19: 595–607

Harari D 2002 Epidemiology and risk factors for bowel problems in frail older people. In: Potter J, Norton C, Cottenden A (eds) Bowel care in older people, Royal College of Physicians, London, pp 23–45

Harari D 2004 Bowel care in old age. In: Norton C, Chelvanayagam S (eds) Bowel continence nursing. Beaconsfield Publishers, Beaconsfield, pp 132–149

Harari D, Gurwitz JH, Avorn J, Choodnovskiy I, Minaker KL 1995 Correlates of regular laxative use by frail elderly persons. American Journal of Medicine 99: 513–518

Harari D, Gurwitz JH, Avorn J, Bohn R, Minaker KL 1996 Bowel habit in relation to age and gender. Archive of Internal Medicine 156: 315–320

Hatton P 1990 Primum non nocere – an analysis of drugs prescribed to elderly patients in private nursing homes registered with Harrogate HA. Care of the Elderly 2: 166–168

Heaton KW, Radvan J, Cripps H et al. 1992 Defecation frequency and timing, and stool form in the general population: a prospective study. Gut 33: 818–824

Hellstrom L, Ekelund P, Milsom I, Mellstrom D 1990 The prevalence of urinary incontinence and use of incontinence aids in 85-year-old men and women. Age and Ageing 19: 383–389

Hu T, Igou JF, Kaltreider L et al. 1989 A clinical trial of a behavioral therapy to reduce urinary incontinence in nursing homes. Journal of the American Medical Association 261: 2656–2662

Hunskaar S, Burgio KL, Diokno AC et al. 2002 Epidemiology and natural history of urinary incontinence. In: Abrams P, Khoury S, Wein A, Cardozo L (eds) Incontinence. Health Books, Plymouth, pp 165–201

Jirovec MM, Templin T 2001 Predicting success using individualized scheduled toileting for memory-impaired elders at home. Research into Nursing Health 24: 1–8

Kenny KA, Skelly J 2001 Dietary fiber for constipation in older adults: a systematic review, Clinical Effectiveness in Nursing 5: 120–128

Khullar V, Cardozo L, Abbott D, Anders K 1997 GAX collagen in the treatment of urinary incontinence in elderly women: a two year follow up. British Journal of Obstetrics and Gynaecology 104: 96–99

Kolominsky-Rabas PL, Hilz M-J, Neundoerfer B, Heuschmann PU 2003 Impact of urinary incontinence after stroke: results from a prospective population-based stroke register. Neurourology and Urodynamics 22: 322–327

Kondo A, Lin TL, Siroky M, Tammela T 2002 Conservative management in men. In: Abrams P, Khoury S, Wein A, Cardozo L (eds) Incontinence. Health Books, Plymouth, pp 553–569

Lawler J 1991 Behind the screens: nursing, somology and the problem of the body. Churchill Livingstone, Melbourne

Lawler J 1997 The body in nursing. Churchill Livingstone, Melbourne

Laycock J, Haslam J 2002 Therapeutic management of incontinence and pelvic pain. Springer, London

Lekan-Rutledge D, Colling J 2003 Urinary incontinence in the frail elderly. American Journal of Nursing 3 (suppl.): 36–46

Lekan-Rutledge D, Palmer MH, Belyea M 1998 In their own words: nursing assistants' perceptions of barriers to implementation of prompted voiding in long-term care, Gerontologist 38: 370–378

Miller JM, Ashton-Miller JA, DeLancey JO 1998 A pelvic muscle precontraction can reduce cough-related urine loss in selected women with mild SUI. Journal of the American Geriatrics Society 46: 870–874

Mitteness L 1987 So what do you expect when you're 85? Urinary incontinence in late life. Research in the Sociology of Health Care 6: 177–219

Moore KN 1994 Electrical stimulation for the treatment of urinary incontinence: do we know enough to accept it as part of our practice? Journal of Advanced Nursing 20: 1018–1022

Morgan R, Spencer B, King D 1998 Rectal examinations in elderly subjects: attitudes of patients and doctors. Age and Ageing 27: 353–356

Muller-Lissner SA 1988 Effects of wheat bran on weight of stool and gastrointestinal transit time: a meta analysis. British Medical Journal 296: 615–617

Naylor JR, Mulley GP 1993 Commodes: inconvenient conveniences. British Medical Journal 307: 1258–1260

Nazarko L 1994 Drugs, continence, elderly people. Primary Health Care 4: 19–22

Nazarko L 1995 Commode design for frail and disabled people. Professional Nurse 11: 95–97

Nelson R, Norton N, Cautley E, Furner S 1995 Community-based prevalence of anal incontinence. Journal of the American Medical Association 274: 559–561

Newman DK, Wallace J, Blackwood N, Spencer C 1996 Promoting healthy bladder habits for seniors. Ostomy Wound Management 42: 18–28

Norton C 1996 Nursing for continence, 2nd edn. Beaconsfield Publishers, Beaconsfield

Norton C, Barrett JA 2002 Assessing the individual. In: Potter J, Norton C, Cottenden A (eds) Bowel care in older people, Royal College of Physicians, London, pp 47–53

Norton C, Chelvanayagam S 2004 Bowel continence nursing. Beaconsfield Publishers, Beaconsfield

Norton C, Kamm MA 1999 Bowel control – information and practical advice. Beaconsfield Publishers, Beaconsfield

Norton D, McLaren R, Exton-Smith AN 1962 An investigation of geriatric nursing problems in hospital. National Corporation for the Care of Old People, London

Norton C, Baracat F, Gartley CB et al. 1999 Promotion, organisation and education in continence care. In:

Abrams P, Khoury S, Wein A (eds) Incontinence – first international consultation on incontinence (World Health Organization). Health Publications, Monaco, pp 837–868

Ouslander JG, Schnelle JF 1995 Incontinence in the nursing home. Annals of Internal Medicine 122: 438–449

Ouslander JG, Schnelle JF, Uman G et al. 1995 Does oxybutynin add to the effectiveness of prompted voiding for urinary incontinence among nursing home residents? A placebo-controlled trial. Journal of the American Geriatrics Society 43: 610–617

Palmer MH 1991 Risk factors for urinary incontinence one year after nursing home admission. Research into Nursing Health 14: 405–412

Palmer MH 1995 Nurses' knowledge and beliefs about continence interventions in long-term care. Journal of Advanced Nursing 21: 1065–1072

Passmore AP, Wilson-Davies K, Stoker C, Scott ME 1993 Chronic constipation on long-stay elderly patients: a comparison of lactulose and senna-fibre combination. British Medical Journal 307: 769–771

Peet SM, Castleden CM, McGrother CW 1995 Prevalence of urinary and faecal incontinence in hospitals and residential and nursing homes for older people. British Medical Journal 311: 1063–1064

Peet SM, Castleden CM, McGrother C, Duffin HM 1996 The management of urinary incontinence in residential and nursing homes for older people. Age and Ageing 25: 139–143

Perry S, Shaw C, McGrother C et al. 2002 The prevalence of faecal incontinence in adults aged 40 years or more living in the community. Gut 50: 480–484

Petticrew M, Watt I, Sheldon T 1997 Systematic review of the effectiveness of laxatives in the elderly. Health technology assessment 1 (13). NHS Centre for Reviews and Dissemination, York

Rands G, Malone-Lee J 1990 Urinary and faecal incontinence in long-stay wards for the elderly mentally ill: prevalence and difficulties in management. Health Trends 22: 161–163

Read NW, Abouzekry L, Read M et al. 1985 Anorectal function in elderly patients with faecal impaction. Gastroenterology 89: 959–966

Resende TL, Brocklehurst JC, O'Neill PA 1993 A pilot study on the effect of exercise and abdominal massage on bowel habit in continuing care patients. Clinical Rehabilitations 7: 204–209

Resnick NM 1984 Urinary incontinence in the elderly. Medical Grand Rounds 3: 281–290

Resnick NM 1995 Urinary incontinence. Lancet 346: 94–99

Resnick NM 1996 Clinical crossroads: urinary incontinence in an 89 year old woman. Journal of the American Medical Association 276: 1832–1840

Resnick NM, Brandeis GH, Baumann MM, DuBeau C, Yalla SV 1996 Misdiagnosis of urinary incontinence in nursing home women: prevalence and a proposed solution. Neurourology and Urodynamics 15: 599–618

Rhodes P, Parker G 1995 The role of the continence adviser in England and Wales. International Journal of Nursing Studies 32: 423–433

Robinson J 2000 Managing urinary incontinence in the nursing home: residents' perspectives. Journal of Advanced Nursing 31: 68–77

Roe B 1996 Catheterisation. In: Norton C (ed) Nursing for continence. Beaconsfield Publishers, Beaconsfield, pp 194–225

Sasso K, Hanson L, Smith D 2003 Case study: challenges of pessary management. Journal of Wound Ostomy and Continence Nursing 30: 152–158

Schnelle JF 1990 Treatment of urinary incontinence in nursing home patients by prompted voiding. Journal of the American Geriatrics Society 38: 356–360

Schnelle JF, Traighber B, Sowell VA et al. 1989 Prompted voiding treatment of urinary incontinence in nursing home patients. Journal of the American Geriatrics Society 37: 1051–1057

Schnelle JF, MacRae PG, Ouslander JG, Simmons SF, Nitta M 1995 Functional incidental training, mobility performance and incontinence care with nursing home residents. Journal of the American Geriatrics Society 43: 1356–1362

Schnelle J, Cruise PA, Rahman A, Ouslander JG 1998 Developing rehabilitative behavioral interventions for long-term care: technology transfer, acceptance and maintenance issues. Journal of the American Geriatrics Society 46: 771–777

Schwartz DR 1977 Personal point of view – a report of seventeen elderly patients with a persistent problem of urinary incontinence. Health Bulletin 35: 197–204

Shaw C, Williams KS, Assassa RP 2000 Patients' views of a new nurse-led continence service. Journal of Clinical Nursing 9: 574–584

Stanton SL, Monga AK 1997 Incontinence in elderly women: is periurethral collagen an advance? British Journal of Obstetrics & Gynaecology 104: 154–157

Stokes G 2002 Psychological approaches to bowel care in older people with dementia. In: Potter J, Norton C, Cottenden A (eds) Bowel care in older people. Royal College of Physicians, London, pp 97–109

Subak LL 2002 Does weight loss improve incontinence in moderately obese women? International Urogynecology Journal and Pelvic Floor Dysfunction 13: 40–43

Szonyi G, Collas D, Ding YY, Malone-Lee J 1995 Oxybutynin with bladder retraining for detrusor instability in elderly people: a randomized controlled trial. Age and Ageing 24: 287–291

Tramonte SM, Brand MB, Mulrow CD et al. 1997 The treatment of chronic constipation in adults. Journal of General Internal Medicine 12: 15–24

Travers AF, Burns E, Penn ND, Mitchell SC, Mulley GP 1992 A survey of hospital toilet facilities. British Medical Journal 304: 878–879

Van Kampen M 2000 Effect of pelvic floor re-education on duration and degree of incontinence after radical prostatectomy: a randomised controlled trial. Lancet 355: 98–102

Vinsnes AG 2001 Healthcare personnel's attitudes towards patients with urinary incontinence. Journal of Clinical Nursing 10: 455–462

Vinsnes AG, Hunskaar S 1991 Distress associated with urinary incontinence, as measured by a visual analogue scale. Scandinavian Journal of Caring Science 5: 57–61

Wells TJ 1980 Problems in geriatric nursing care. Churchill-Livingstone, Edinburgh

White H 2004 Making toilets more accessible for individuals with a disability. In: Norton C, Chelvanayagam S (eds) Bowel continence nursing, Beaconsfield Publishers, Beaconsfield, pp 267–275

Wilkie ME, Almond MK, Marsh FP 1992 Diagnosis and management of urinary tract infection in adults. British Medical Journal 305: 1137–1141

Williams K, Roe B, Sindhu F 1995 Using a handbook to improve nurses' continence care. Nursing Standard 10: 39–42

Wilson PD, Bo K, Hay-Smith J et al. 2002 Conservative treatment in women. In: Abrams P, Khoury S, Wein A, Cardozo L (eds) Incontinence. Health Books, Plymouth, pp 571–624

Wyman JF 2003 Treatment of urinary incontinence in men and older women. American Journal of Nursing 3 (suppl.): 26–35

Chapter 18

Maintaining body temperature

Joan Adams and Rosamund A. Herbert

INTRODUCTION AND PREVALENCE

The ability of older people to maintain a normal body temperature is one aspect of homeostasis that has been widely discussed over the past few years, not only within the caring professions but also by the general public. Many reports have addressed the issues surrounding hypothermia and excess winter deaths in those aged 55 years and over in the UK (Donaldson & Keatinge 1997, Age Concern 2002, 2004, Pattenden et al. 2003). Reports have also indicated a relationship between hyperthermia, heatwaves and an increase in morbidity and mortality, especially in older people (Rooney et al. 1998, Falcoa & Valente 1997, McMichael & Kovats 1998). However most older people maintain a normal body temperature throughout their lives (to view the biological changes in thermoregulation associated with ageing, see Chapter 5). As always, we must consider the enormous variability of age-related changes from one individual to another. The majority are able to maintain temperature homeostasis under usual conditions; nevertheless, both cold weather and heatwaves do lead to a considerable increase in mortality and morbidity among older people. This increased mortality is not due to a failure in thermoregulation, i.e. the body's ability to maintain a normal body temperature, but rather to other consequences of the heat or cold on the body's physiology. There is reduced efficiency in thermoregulation and a slower ability to adapt to the stressors heat and cold. It is accepted that the number of deaths from all causes provides a more valid measure of the effects of extremes of temperature on older people than simply the number of deaths (as revealed by death certification) due to hypothermia or heat illness.

In the UK more attention has been given to the effects of the cold on older people than to the effects of heat. There was an overall excess winter mortality (December to March) of 21 800 in 2002–2003 in England and Wales among those aged 65 and over (National Statistics 2003) when compared with non-winter months. Figures for 1999–2000 revealed an excess winter mortality of 48 440 in those 65 years and above (Age Concern 2002). The variation in these figures is probably due to winter severity. In the past these excess deaths have been associated with hypothermia, i.e. simple cooling of the body core until death occurs. In reality the actual recorded deaths from hypothermia account for fewer than 1% of these excess deaths; deaths where there is any mention of hypothermia on the death certificate as a contributory factor are approximately 300 per year in the UK (Age Concern 2002, Murphy 2003). Epidemiological studies show that the excess cold-related mortality is predominantly due to myocardial infarctions, cerebrovascular disease (strokes) and respiratory tract infections (Neild et al. 1994, Donaldson & Keatinge 1997, Keatinge et al. 1997). Certainly, hypothermia is a relatively infrequent cause of death in older people.

Although hypothermia is an infrequent cause of death, it has received much publicity and attention because in most circumstances it is considered to be preventable. McAlpine & Dall (1987) undertook a retrospective study and reviewed 81 patients admitted with primary hypothermia (no underlying pathology) and secondary hypothermia. The two groups were compared in a 3-year follow-up study. The results demonstrated that death occurred in 100% of those with primary hypothermia and 24% of those with secondary hypothermia. This report indicates that those who present with primary hypothermia would benefit from a risk assessment and advice on appropriate preventive strategies. When hypothermia does actually occur, it has a potentially poor prognosis. Hislop et al. (1995) reported a 20% death rate in those with mild hypothermia and a 50% death rate in those with moderate to severe hypothermia, although the death rate can be higher if there is concurrent illness. Hypother-

mia is said to exist when the deep body temperature (for example, rectal temperature) falls below an arbitrarily defined limit of 35°C (Royal College of Physicians 1966). However, 35°C is not a physiologically defined lower limit of normality and problems can ensue from body temperatures that are low but do not reach that of the Royal College of Physicians definition.

The prevalence of low body temperatures in older people is difficult to establish with any accuracy. Estimates of the extent of hypothermia have been made from surveys of the temperature of individuals being admitted to hospital, from surveys of body temperature in older people living at home and from mortality statistics. Each of these approaches has given different estimates, and values often differ widely on the prevalence of hypothermia.

Initial estimates of mortality from hypothermia were high. Taylor (1964) estimated that deaths from hypothermia each winter numbered between 20 000 and 100 000 among older people. This estimate was based on oral temperature measurements, which have since been shown to be unreliable indicators in cold conditions (Fox et al. 1973a). Examination of death certificates from before 1979 is unhelpful because hypothermia was not recorded as a separate category in the mortality statistics until 1979.

One study of old people admitted to the University College Hospital group in London found that 3.6% of older patients admitted were hypothermic; this survey assessed the deep body temperature of patients admitted during 3 winter months in selected hospitals (Goldman et al. 1977). In contrast to this, a study undertaken at the London Hospital during January and February, in which the body temperature of all patients entering the hospital as emergencies was measured, found that only three patients (all ages) had body temperatures below 35°C, representing 0.04% of a total 7579 admissions to the emergency department (Coleshaw et al. 1986). This study supports other literature that states that the number of hypothermic patients admitted to hospital is small and patients who are hypothermic are usually cold only because drink or drugs or serious illness caused them to collapse in cold surroundings (Keatinge 1987).

In the winter of 1972, two large-scale surveys of body temperature in older people living at home were carried out (Fox et al. 1973b). This involved a national random sample of 1000 older people aged over 65 living at home. Simultaneously, 1000 older people in the London borough of Camden were assessed and an intensive domiciliary and hospital investigation was conducted on a subgroup of the Camden residents. Only 0.58% of the national sample (0.32% in Camden) were found to have a deep body temperature of 35°C or below. However, a significant number (9.5% of the national sample and 10% in Camden) were found to have a deep body temperature below 35.5°C. So these surveys did not find a high incidence of hypothermia in older people living at home, but a large 'at-risk' group with low body temperatures between 35°C and 35.5°C.

Findings such as these partly account for the large amount of attention that hypothermia received in the 1970s and early 1980s. In 1991, another national survey of older people in cold weather was conducted (Salvage 1993) and many of the findings from Wicks (1978) and others have been supported. However, further work has clarified the relationship between excess winter mortality and older people: first, there have been refinements in the methods used to study hypothermia (some of the earlier methods almost certainly overestimated the occurrence of a low body temperature); secondly, it is now recognized that it is not hypothermia per se that is responsible for the majority of the excess winter deaths. Part of the complexity of investigating and studying the area is that many different factors are involved, including physiological changes with increasing age, superimposed disease conditions and important socioeconomic factors, including poverty.

An analysis of recorded monthly deaths in England and Wales for the years 1962–1967 first showed the fundamental relationship between environmental temperature and death rates (Bull & Morton 1978), although the phenomenon was known about in the nineteenth century. The effect is most clearly seen in the population group older than 60 years. Figures indicate that excess winter mortality is not just a phenomenon in the UK but also in many other countries (Curwen 1991). However, when comparisons are made between various countries with respect to cold-related deaths, the UK, Ireland and southern European countries fare particularly badly when compared with Finland, Germany, the Netherlands and Siberia, where winters are more severe (Healy 2003). Healy examined the variations in excess winter mortality between 14 European countries from 1988 to 1997 to identify potential causal reasons. The UK's seasonal variation rate was 18% (37 000 annual excess deaths). These figures can be further divided: England 19% (31 000 annual excess winter deaths), Wales 17% (1800 annual extra winter deaths), Northern Ireland 17% (800 annual extra deaths) and Scotland 16% (3100 annual extra deaths). Portugal revealed a winter increase of 28%, and Ireland 21%. The reasons proposed by Healy (2003) to explain this disparity between countries included socioeconomic factors, poor housing, poor thermal efficiency, deprivation and poverty. He also cited as important indicators health care spending and hospital bed shortage. Previous studies have questioned deprivation as a causal reason (Lawlor et al. 2002). Shah & Peacock (1999) argue that excess winter mortality is no greater in areas of deprivation, when compared to more affluent areas, and proposed outdoor temperatures and the individual's response to cold indoors as more important determinants. A major finding discussed by the Eurowinter Group (1997) suggested that those countries with the mildest winters (average temperature 5°C) showed higher levels of excess winter deaths. Pattenden et al. (2003) and Healy (2003) reported similar finding. These figures demonstrate clearly the importance of factors other than biological ones in excess winter mortality. Standards of housing, the type and cost of heating, poverty and cultural factors have all been implicated. The 'old and the cold' has become something of a political issue.

Having put the subject of the effect of environmental temperature in perspective, we now consider the factors that influence the ability of older people to maintain a normal body temperature under various conditions. Temperature regulation is an excellent example of homeostasis and, as discussed in Chapter 5, most homeostatic mechanisms function quite adequately in older people. This chapter will first consider the factors normally involved in thermoregulation and then the aspects that change with ageing. Physiological, behavioural and social issues will be examined. The last part of the chapter considers the appropriate nursing care and interventions for older people with abnormal body temperatures.

PHYSIOLOGICAL ASPECTS OF THERMOREGULATION

There are many factors to take into account when considering the possible susceptibility of older people to extremes of environmental temperature. Again, to emphasize a key point, many older people will never have problems with maintaining a normal body temperature. As discussed in Chapter 5, there are many variables that affect an individual's homeostatic capabilities: physiological fitness and training, diet, lifestyle and concurrent illness all have a direct influence on an individual's thermoregulatory capacity.

Normal body temperature

As discussed above, many factors are involved in allowing an individual to maintain a normal body temperature. It is essential to maintain a 'normal' deep body or core temperature for optimum function of the metabolic processes in the cells of the so-called vital organs – brain, heart, lungs and liver. For instance, enzymes in the cells of these organs are very temperature-dependent; in contrast, the cells of the peripheral tissues can function at, and withstand, lower temperatures. So, regardless of the environmental temperature, homeotherms (warm-blooded animals) maintain a constant deep body temperature. This is achieved at the expense of quite wide variations in the temperatures of the peripheral tissues (sometimes referred to as the shell of the body), e.g. hands and feet. Deep body temperature varies with the site of measurement (e.g. rectal, oral) and is different from the skin temperatures recorded at the surface of the body. Thus each part of the body has its own temperature. Core temperature is normally in the range of 36–37°C, while the temperature of the skin and extremities is lower. For instance, oral temperature might be 36.8°C, skin temperature of the back might be 33°C and that of the feet, 27°C.

There has been some debate as to whether the normal core temperature is the same in older people as in, say, younger adults; some authorities initially suggested that core temperature was lower in older people, but the evidence is far from conclusive. A study by Collins et al. (1995) indicated that there is no age-related difference in resting deep body temperature during the daytime and evening. So many factors influence the level of body temperature that it is difficult to attribute any temperature change to ageing per se. So, to all intents and purposes, the normal range for core temperature of 36–37°C should still be used for older people, although it might be expected that an older person would have a temperature nearer the lower limits of normal. Getting a low temperature measurement should not be automatically explained by saying the patient is old.

Normal thermoregulation

In order for the deep body temperature to remain constant in an individual, heat gain must equal heat loss. This is expressed in the first law of thermodynamics:

$$M = E \pm C \pm K \pm R \pm S$$

where: M = heat produced by metabolism; E = heat lost by evaporation; C = heat lost/gained by convection from the air; K = heat lost/gained by conduction from solids/liquids; R = heat lost/gained by radiation; and S = heat storage in the body.

The ideal ambient (surrounding) temperature for comfort and thermal equilibrium for a person sitting down wearing normal indoor clothes is approximately 21°C; the temperature gradients, namely from core to skin and skin to air, under these conditions are just adequate to transfer excess heat from the metabolically active tissues to the surroundings. Heat always flows down temperature gradients. If the ambient temperature is decreased and the temperature difference between the skin and environment increases, heat loss through convection and radiation increases. Thus the body ceases to be in thermal equilibrium. The opposite occurs if the individual is in a hot environment; then the body gains heat from the atmosphere by convection and radiation (and also by conduction if in direct contact with something hot, e.g. a hot-water bottle).

Factors such as clothing and the amount of body fat will also affect heat loss from the body. It is generally believed that fatter individuals are better insulated than their thinner counterparts, but the importance of fat is unclear. It is probably of greater significance in water (e.g. the blubber of marine animals), as water is a better conductor of heat than air. Clothing is the most appropriate insulation for humans.

In order to maintain a constant and normal body temperature, a balance must be maintained between the heat lost and heat gained by the body. The main features of temperature regulation are shown in Figure 18.1. The major source of heat production is the body's metabolic processes: the chemical processes that provide energy for all the metabolic reactions in the body also produce heat. The blood circulating around the body then distributes the heat generated as a byproduct of metabolism around all the tissues. If the metabolic rate increases, for example with exercise or diseases like thyrotoxicosis (the thyroid hormones directly influence the rate of metabolism), more heat will be produced in the body. In order to maintain a normal core temperature under these circumstances, heat loss from the body must be increased – otherwise the body temperature will rise. It is simpler for the body to regulate the amount of heat lost than to alter the metabolic rate.

Thus there is a constant balancing act going on in the body: if the core temperature is elevated, heat loss mechanisms are necessary to restore the equilibrium, whereas if the core temperature falls, a combination of heat conservation and heat gain mechanisms is necessary.

One of the main ways that we regulate heat loss from the body is by varying the blood flow to the surface of the body. If we need to lose heat, vasodilatation occurs, which has the effect of increasing blood flow to the periphery (the skin becomes red and warm) and heat is lost by convection and radiation because the temperature of the surface is higher than the temperature of the surrounding air and objects. If an individual needs to conserve heat within the body, a widespread peripheral vasoconstriction occurs, reducing blood (and hence heat) flow to the limbs especially (the skin appears pale and feels cold to touch); this has the effect of retaining heat in the core of the body as the temperature differential between the surface of the

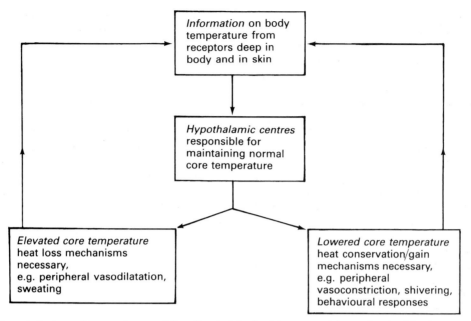

Fig. 18.1   The main features of temperature regulation. Constant feedback is an essential part of maintaining homeostasis.

skin and the atmosphere is reduced. So less heat is lost. This vasoconstrictor/vasodilator response is described as the vasomotor tone and is controlled by the sympathetic nervous system (Fig. 18.2).

The extent of the vasoconstrictor response varies from one region of the skin to another. For example, little change occurs in the cutaneous vessels in the head, whereas in the hands and feet there is considerable nervous control over the calibre of blood vessels. Appreciable quantities of heat can be lost through the head, especially in people who are bald or have thinning hair; hence the reason for wearing a hat in cold environments.

In colder conditions people will need to increase heat production as well as reduce heat loss by vasoconstriction and this is achieved by increasing metabolic heat production. The simple response of clapping hands together or moving generates more heat as a byproduct of muscle metabolism. Shivering is also a way of increasing heat production. Shivering consists of synchronous contractions of small groups of voluntary muscles which contract out of phase with other groups, so that no useful movements of the joints are produced – it simply generates heat. The shivering metabolic response to cold exposure is not great; for short periods a fourfold increase in metabolic rate can be produced and a twofold increase can be maintained over a period of several hours. Ordinary dynamic muscular work is a much more efficient way of increasing metabolic rate, as the rate may increase 10-fold or more.

Babies are unable to shiver (the nerve pathways that control the shivering response have not devel-

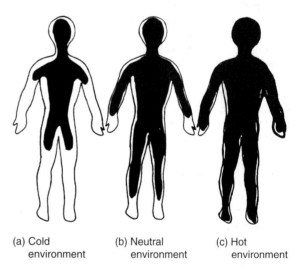

| (a) Cold environment | (b) Neutral environment | (c) Hot environment |

Fig. 18.2   Relationship between vasomotor tone and environmental temperature. The core temperature of the body must be maintained between 36°C and 37°C whatever the external environmental temperature. In cold environments the peripheral vasoconstriction 'reduces' the size of the core of the body (shown in black) and the size of the 'shell' increases (a); in hot environments the peripheral vasodilatation 'expands' the core of deep body temperature and the shell size is reduced (c).

oped fully) and they depend on a process known as non-shivering thermogenesis (NST). NST relies on the high metabolic activity of brown adipose tissue or brown fat. The occurrence of NST due to brown fat in adults remains a contentious issue, although there is some evidence for brown fat in cold-adapted adults (Lean & James 1986), but under usual conditions brown fat is not thought to play a significant role in adult thermoregulation in the cold.

Sweating is an important mechanism in aiding heat loss from the body. The sweat produced in the sweat glands is passed by ducts to the skin surface and then evaporates from the surface of the body. In order to evaporate, the fluid uses heat from the body (the latent heat of vaporization); thus heat is removed and the skin cooled. It is the evaporation of sweat that cools an individual – it is pointless wiping off any sweat from the skin, say after exercise, as this will eliminate any cooling effects.

Of course under normal circumstances we do not rely only on physiological mechanisms to maintain a normal body temperature; behavioural and social aspects are important too. If we are cold we put on additional clothing (which is a good insulator) and this reduces heat loss from the surface of the body. We might also move around more, increase the heat supply to the environment (e.g. put on the fire) and have a hot drink. Eating increases metabolic heat production because the specific dynamic action of food (especially proteins) causes heat to be generated during the absorption and metabolism of the nutrients.

Conversely, if we are too hot we remove items of clothing and manipulate our environment appropriately; we also tend to move around less or move more slowly to minimize heat production, and to have an ice-cold drink.

The environment that we are in as well as our general fitness level affect our ability to thermoregulate. In a very hot environment an individual might gain heat through convection from the air and radiation from the sun. The presence of any air movement and the level of humidity affect our ability to lose or gain heat. If we are in an area with a breeze or draught, convective air loss from the surface of the body will increase as air warmed by heat from the body is constantly replaced by cooler air. If we are in a humid environment, the sweating response is less effective as the air is already partly saturated with water vapour and so less able to accept more water vapour from sweating; an extreme example of this would be in a sauna. Sweat gland activity is more efficient in fit people who take regular exercise, as physical activity demands efficient disposal of heat; thus a fit person has in effect 'trained up' many heat loss mechanisms, e.g. sweating. In general the human body's physiological mechanisms are more efficient at coping with hot environments than cold ones; this is because humans have, it is believed, evolved in tropical climates. Water is a better conductor of heat than is air, and so exposure to hot or cold water in a bath or swimming pool will alter conductive heat loss or gain.

An inherent part of any homeostatic mechanism is the central monitoring and control of the system; receptors to detect the variable being controlled are essential in passing sensory information to the control centre. The hypothalamus is the 'control centre' for thermoregulation and sensory information is passed to the hypothalamus from the temperature sensors in the skin and deeper structures in the body. It is generally accepted that thermal information from the skin surface summates in some manner with that from the body core to stimulate integrated thermoregulatory activity. Information is also fed to the cerebral cortex to give the awareness and perception of body temperature. Temperature perception is important if an individual is to bring into operation the appropriate behavioural responses to aid temperature regulation.

Individual variability

Even in young subjects there is considerable intersubject variation in response to heat or cold stress. For example, in the cold some people exhibit very good vasomotor control while others seem to rely on increased heat production to maintain body temperature. It has also been suggested that females have a greater reliance on vasomotor control and this has been observed in hot environments (Fox 1974). Differences between males and females may also be explained by variations in body fat and in the differences in quantity of metabolically active mass of the body.

CHANGES WITH AGEING

The factors that determine thermoregulation have been discussed in some detail so that the reasons why some older people may be more at risk than younger individuals can be clearly understood. Thermoregulation does not actually fail in older people but the potential for coping with extreme temperatures is diminished. This is in line with the general decline in homeostatic efficiency in older people when the body is stressed. With alterations in environmental temperatures the physiological responses of older individuals are more variable and body temperature oscillates between wider limits of internal temperature.

There are some physiological changes with ageing that may affect thermoregulation. For instance, vasomotor responses to the cold have been shown to be less efficient in minimizing heat loss in some older people, i.e. there is a reduction in the efficiency of the vasoconstrictor response. It has been suggested that some 20% of a normal healthy older group do not constrict significantly on cooling (Collins 1987a). This reduced vasoconstrictor effect does seem to be an age-related phenomenon. One explanation proposed was that cold-induced vasomotor tone changes are dependent on the release of the hormone noradrenaline (norepinephrine) and resultant α-adrenoceptor-mediated vasoconstriction in the cutaneous vessels. Proposed reasons for impaired vasoconstriction are lower levels of released noradrenaline or a reduced vasomotor response for the amount of noradrenaline that is released (Neilsen et al. 1992). Frank et al. (1996) noted that the threshold for triggering noradrenaline release in cold exposure was 1°C lower in older people compared to younger individuals. There is also a noted down-regulation of α-adrenoceptor, which would also impact on thermoregulatory vasoconstriction (Docherty 1990). Compliance of blood vessels might be further exacerbated in those with arteriosclerosis (Collins 1987b).

Some older people also show a reduced metabolic response to cold stress when compared with younger subjects. Many factors interact. There is a smaller proportion of actively functioning cells in older people and so the basal metabolic rate (BMR) is slightly decreased; the BMR decreases significantly until the age of approximately 30 and then there is a gradual decline into old age. Metabolic heat production in older people is generally lower because of reduced activity and a smaller energy intake. Fukagawa et al. (1995) reported a reduced thermic response after the intake of glucose but not protein and fructose. A few older people also suffer a degree of hypothyroidism, which will reduce metabolic heat production.

In some older people the shivering response is altered. Early studies suggested that shivering was reduced or absent in older individuals; however, other work (Collins et al. 1981a) has shown that shivering ability is not lost with ageing, even in those 80 years of age, but changes in the character of shivering do occur. The shivering is often less vigorous and a longer latent period is required to initiate maximum shivering. Detraining is probably a major contributory factor, as well as ageing changes in muscle cell function. Some work has shown that the older people who exhibited the 'best' shivering response were those who showed marked loss of efficiency in their vasomotor response to the cold; this demonstrates the adaptability of human physiology, even in old people.

There is no evidence at present to show changes in the central nervous control of thermoregulation in older people. Some older people may be more susceptible due to the prescription of drugs that interfere with thermoregulation, e.g. phenothiazines, hypnotics and some antidepressants. It has been noted that peripheral blood vessels are less sensitive to vasodilator and vasoconstrictor drugs (Collins 2003). Alcohol has a marked peripheral vasodilator effect, which tends to increase heat loss. Alcohol should never be given to anyone whom you suspect may have a low body temperature; although alcohol gives a general feeling of warmth, it will tend to increase heat loss.

Sensory systems do become less sensitive with age (Chapter 5) and a reduced ability to sense cold or changes in temperature may clearly put some old people at risk. Some older people do appear to have a blunted perception of temperature changes and thus do not experience 'coldness' until environmental temperatures have lowered below those that make younger people feel cold (Watts 1972, Collins et al. 1981b). Collins et al. found deterioration with age in the ability to discriminate between environmental temperatures and this could contribute to the vulnerability of the old. Investigations of behavioural thermoregulation indicate that older people often lack the precision of environmental temperature control shown by younger people (Collins et al. 1981b). If an individual lacks the awareness of 'being cold', he or she might not make use of the important behavioural adaptations to the cold and, for example, may not put on additional clothing or turn up the heating.

However, cultural or economic factors (such as the cost of heating) rather than a blunted temperature sense may cause some older people not to increase the heat supply to the environment. Similarly, it may be more difficult for some old people to increase metabolic heat production by moving around, due perhaps to arthritis or some other health problem. Financial or social factors, e.g. cost and living alone, may also limit food intake, and this in turn will reduce diet-induced thermogenesis. Several studies have shown a link between undernutrition and poor thermoregulation in older people; thus undernutrition may predispose to hypothermia. It has also been suggested that there might be a link between undernutrition, hypothermia and fracture of the femoral neck in the winter months (Bastow et al. 1983, Fellows et al. 1985).

Added to these problems is the fact that many older people in the UK live in a poor standard of housing which stretches physiological responses even further. There is evidence of very low temperatures in the homes of older people and this will particularly put stress on an ageing thermoregulatory system.

In addition to the above factors, clinical or subclinical diseases present in older people, e.g. hypothyroidism and cardiovascular or neurological disorders, may interfere with normal thermoregulation if they decrease an individual's ability to respond to the cold. Prolonged immobility due to conditions such as arthritis, unsteadiness and postural hypotension will reduce heat production. If a person is less active this may lead to a reduced food intake and less diet-induced thermogenesis. Reduced physical fitness will also contribute to this vicious cycle. People with confusional states or dementia are also likely to be at risk.

The importance of these endogenous and exogenous factors is indisputable, but sometimes spontaneous hypothermia occurs that cannot be accounted for by these factors; in such cases, failure of the thermoregulatory processes themselves should be considered.

OTHER EFFECTS OF THE COLD

There are other genuine effects of exposure to the cold that can give rise to concern for older people and also help to explain the increased mortality and morbidity in cold weather. Being in a cold environment has other effects on the body besides challenging temperature homeostasis. For instance, it has a negative effect on dexterity; a low peripheral temperature leads to a loss of sensation which is especially noticeable in the hands and feet. There is a loss of manipulative ability, probably due to an increased viscosity of the synovial fluid in the joints (joints often feel stiffer in the cold) and increased muscle viscosity (Ramsey 1983). So the cold affects neuromuscular and sensory function and this could increase the incidence of falls and fractures.

A seasonal pattern of blood pressure variation has been recognized for some time, with blood pressure being higher in the winter months (in the order of 5 mmHg for both systolic and diastolic pressures; MacMahon et al. 1990). However, experimental work with old people exposed to cold environments for a short period of time has shown that some older people have a greater increase in blood pressure than younger people (Collins et al. 1985, 1995); there was also a strong association between the fall in deep body temperature and increase in systolic blood pressure. The systolic blood pressure is more raised than the diastolic pressure, and the pulse amplitude is increased. This sustained increase in blood pressure and pulse pressure increases the probability of vascular damage (Wilmshurst 1994). Raised blood pressure in the cold may have a long-term effect on the aetiology of arterial thrombosis and this may help to explain winter mortality from coronary and cerebrovascular disease (strokes). Other changes in the blood have been demonstrated: for instance there is an increase in the size and number of platelets in the blood, an increase in the number of red blood cells, a 20% increase in the viscosity of the blood during mild cooling and higher fibrinogen and cholesterol levels (Keatinge et al. 1984,

Stout et al. 1996). These factors together may contribute to the increase in arterial thrombosis in cold conditions, especially in people with atheromatous vessels.

It is known that exposure to cold has other effects on the body's physiology. Cardiovascular reflexes are initiated by cold air on the face and can result in a slowing of the heart rate and changes in blood pressure; these reflexes affect people of all ages but might precipitate illness in older people. Cold also places an additional strain on the heart and circulation by increasing the volume of blood circulating in the core of the body; this may in turn take a significant toll on unfit older people during the winter. Certainly, exercise combined with exposure of the face and extremities to the cold produces a number of cardiovascular responses that increase the strain on the heart and circulation.

As already mentioned at the beginning of this chapter, the high winter mortality is due to deaths from myocardial infarctions, strokes and respiratory disorders (Neild et al. 1994, Donaldson & Keatinge 1997, Keatinge et al. 1997). The 'typical' pattern of illness is an increased incidence of myocardial infarctions occurring 2–3 days after a cold spell, strokes occurring after about a week and an increase in respiratory infections at about 10 days. The changes described above in the blood and the cardiovascular system are thought to account for the raised incidence of cerebral and coronary thrombosis. Exposure to cold air is also known to induce bronchoconstriction and wheezing and it may also alter mucin production and depress ciliary activity. Immunological impairment in older people and the greater risk of exposure to bacterial and viral agents during the winter months, together with these physiological responses, might combine to render some individuals susceptible to respiratory tract infection and explain the trends that are observed in respiratory disease.

Thus the cold does have a potentially damaging effect on old people, even if not by hypothermia. Several studies have highlighted that exposure to cold indoor temperatures may have some influence on excess winter deaths. This association has prompted initiatives to review and improve home standards, heating and insulation. However outdoor exposure is also an important part of the equation. Keatinge (1986) looked at the seasonal mortality in people who lived in homes with unrestricted heating (housing-association homes where the heating bills were paid by the authorities). The continuous high daytime temperatures did not prevent the mortality among the residents from rising in winter by a percentage similar to that among the general population. Extensive outdoor excursions by able-bodied residents and the preference for open windows and no heating at night provided their only substantial exposure to cold. The simplest explanation is that, although the quality of life was higher with heated housing, the beneficial effects on mortality of the high indoor temperatures were balanced by the adverse effects of increased exposure to cold outdoors. These findings were consistent with those of the Eurowinter Group (1998), where the aim was to explore effective measures adopted during the Siberian winter to control excess winter mortality. Conclusions drawn indicated that housing was warm, but what was significant in this group of people was the importance placed on suitable winter clothing when outdoors.

RAISED BODY TEMPERATURE

Less work has been conducted on the effect of heat and hot environments on older people; the adverse effects of high environmental temperatures are not usually a problem in the UK, although recent heatwaves have prompted the UK Department of Health to publish a national plan to alert the public and the National Health Service into taking action to prevent excess deaths during heatwaves (Department of Health 2004). Heatwaves have been observed as a problem more often, of course, in Australia and the USA. Older people are particularly vulnerable to hot weather (Kunst et al. 1993). An estimated excess mortality of 619 deaths in England and Wales was recorded in the 1995 heatwave (Rooney et al. 1998). An analysis of the data during the 1975 and 1995 heatwaves in England and Wales demonstrated that those who were most at risk lived in urban areas and mortality was higher in the more deprived populations (McMichael & Kovats 1998). There is no precise definition of heatwave. Each country identifies its own levels, therefore epidemiological studies have shown varying degrees of environmental temperatures at which heat-related mortality begins. Hajat et al. (2002) analysed London's mortality statistics, daily humidity levels and minimum/maximum temperatures from 1975 to 1996, to determine whether there was a relationship between mortality and heat. The study also set out to identify a temperature threshold where mortality increased. The conclusion drawn suggested that, with average climatic temperatures of 21.5°C, mortality rates increased by 3.34% for every 1°C increase in temperature. Hot days in the early part of the year appeared to have had the greatest impact, suggesting that there is a degree of acclimatization. The excess mortality of older people during heatwaves is mainly attributed to an increased number of deaths from res-

piratory disease, ischaemic heart disease and cerebrovascular disease (Keatinge et al. 1984). The latter two diseases can be explained in the following way: the increase in salt and water loss through sweating reduces plasma volume, and thrombogenic risks are increased with the raised levels of platelets, fibrinogen and red blood cells which influence blood viscosity (Keatinge et al. 1984). While the high incidence of cardiovascular and cerebrovascular disease in older people is probably the primary cause of their enhanced vulnerability, impairment of thermoregulatory function may also be partly responsible. In older people the threshold for sweating is higher and sweat glands atrophy; reduced sweating is more pronounced in women. Other work has demonstrated a diminished sweat response when compared with younger individuals (Collins 2003). With increasing age the core threshold for vasodilatation may increase (Collins 1992), and peripheral vasodilatation may be less efficient. These changes reflect deterioration in sweat gland or blood vessel function, possibly as a consequence of structural changes in the skin and/or changes in autonomic function. Impairment of the skin circulation is a considerable disadvantage since the physical routes of heat loss call for an increased surface temperature. Diminished thermal perception may also contribute to impairment of homeostasis.

An older person who develops hyperthermia or heat illness is at a disadvantage: the frequency of death from hyperthermia increases rapidly after the age of 60 years (Kenney 1989). The effect of high heat loads is cumulative, and the incidence of hyperthermia increases steadily as a hot spell continues. This progressive morbidity is probably due to failure to maintain water and salt balance. The increased demand on the circulation in heat calls for good vascular filling, and sweating requires the availability of large volumes of fluid. The older person may be unaware of the need for, or be incapable of acquiring, the necessary fluid. The course of hyperthermia, once initiated, can be rapid. When the body temperature reaches 41°C, the central control mechanisms become depressed, and at this point the chemical reactions of metabolism take place at an increasing rate so that a positive-feedback situation develops. In this phase the body temperature rises rapidly and death, usually from respiratory depression, ensues when it reaches around 44°C.

There are many risk factors that could predispose an older person to heat-related illness (Vassallo et al. 1995, Kunihiro & Foster 1998, Collins 2003). Table 18.1 illustrates this.

The risk to older people from hot environments can be reduced by:

Table 18.1 Risk factors for heat illness in older people

Risk	Comments
Extreme age	Over 80 years
Degree of dependence	On bedrest, in hospital or nursing-care home
Extrinsic/social conditions	Hot living areas, with increased humidity and no air movement, high-density living area
	Lack of cooling facilities
	Inappropriate clothing
	Social isolation
Intrinsic factors	
Disease processes and iatrogenic factors	
Drugs: examples	Phenothiazines, antidepressants, alcohol, diuretics
	Anticholinergic drugs
Cardiovascular disease	Heart failure, ischaemic heart disease
Neurological disease	Stroke, head injury, autonomic dysfunction, tumours, abscess
Mental health conditions	Confusional states, dementia
Endocrine disorders	Diabetes, hyperthyroidism, hyperpituitarism
Impairment of sweating	Skin disorders
Infections	
Other factors	Obesity
	Dehydration
	Lack of fitness
	Reduced sweating ability

- monitoring the temperature of ill individuals
- monitoring the room temperature and alerting carers of the risk
- ensuring adequate ventilation, the use of fans or air conditioning
- wearing light loose clothing
- cooler food and drinks (fewer drinks containing caffeine, as this has diuretic properties)
- ensuring adequate fluids (the perception of thirst and drugs can alter fluid balance)
- reducing physical activity.

Perhaps more frequent is high body temperature occurring during a fever. Infection is a common problem in older individuals and it is often said that they do not reveal a raised body temperature with an infection. In fever the increase in temperature occurs in response to endogenous pyrogens such as tumour necrosis factor and the increase in synthesis of interleukin-1 and interleukin-6. With the release of prostaglandins the set point of the core temperature level increases (Miller et al. 1991). It has been known for many years that the febrile response is diminished in older people and this may be due in part to ageing changes in the immune system. Part of the problem also stems from the difficulty in defining the upper limit of normal body temperature in the older person and also from difficulties in getting an accurate measurement of core temperature in older people. McAlpine et al. (1986), however, maintain that, with careful and effective monitoring, pyrexia is detectable in the majority of infected older patients. It is obviously important to use, wherever possible, each individual as his or her own control, i.e. 37°C might indicate pyrexia in an individual whose normal temperature was in the range of 36–36.5°C. Certainly the extent of temperature increase may be less marked in older than younger people. It has been proposed that levels of endogenous pyrogens are limited in the ability to exert their physiological effect on the central nervous system. Research undertaken on aged mice demonstrated a reduced synthesis and response to peripheral endogenous pyrogens. When interleukin-1 was injected into the intracerebral region a fever response followed, suggesting an inability of endogenous pyrogens to diffuse from the blood into the central nervous system. This argument could be proposed to account for the blunted febrile response in some older people (Norman et al. 1988). However older people do react like younger ones by developing fever in response to acute and chronic infections, neoplastic growths, deep-vein thromboses, myocardial infarctions and other inflammatory conditions.

MEASUREMENT OF BODY TEMPERATURE

It is obviously important, if we are concerned with temperature homeostasis, to be able to measure core or deep body temperature accurately: measuring body temperature in older people needs careful attention. The most commonly used routes are oral or sublingual measurement, external auditory canal, axilla, rectal and pulmonary artery temperature. Several studies have shown that the oral method can be unreliable in older people, especially if used to assess low body temperatures or in cold environments (Fox et al. 1973a). A study by Sloan & Keatinge (1975) compared sublingual and oesophageal temperatures in subjects in various air temperatures (oesophageal temperature is often used for research purposes, as it gives an excellent measurement of core body temperature). In warm air (25–44°C) Sloan & Keatinge found that sublingual temperature stabilized within 0.45°C of oesophageal temperature, but in air at room temperature (18–24°C) it was sometimes as much as 1.1°C below, and in cold air (5–10°C) the oral temperatures were as much as 4.4°C below oesophageal readings. Thus caution should be exercised in the use of oral temperatures in cold environments. Indeed, it is thought that some of the high incidences of hypothermia reported in early work were due to oral temperatures being taken. For reliable measurements correct positioning of the thermometer is essential and some older people find it difficult to keep a thermometer in the correct place. A study by Nayagam et al. (1986) looked at the best route for recording temperatures in older people by comparing oral, axillary and rectal temperatures. Oral measurements were taken in two ways: once by the nurses using the normal ad hoc timing method and once by the researchers with the thermometer left in situ for 5 min. The results showed that oral temperature was unreliable and would miss over 30% of fevers. In the study axillary temperature was found to be higher and more consistent than ad hoc oral temperature recordings, but still error-prone. The authors recommended that rectal temperature was the best method; they also said that the lack of fever with infection in older people is commonly due to faulty technique rather than the true absence of fever, though the temperature is often only modestly elevated. Darowski et al. (1991) suggested that, in older patients with known infection, rectal measurement was more sensitive than sublingual and axillary measurements. The findings indicated that rectal measurement detected fever in 86% of patients, whereas sublingual detected 66%, and axillary measurements only 32%.

So rectal temperature is still the method of choice if there is particular concern about the level of an individual's temperature, and should certainly be the method used if considering low body temperature. Of course a low-reading thermometer (range 25–40°C) should be used, as the scale of the usual clinical thermometers only starts at 35°C.

The infrared tympanic thermometer (range 25–43°C) correlates more closely with the core temperature due to its close proximity to the hypothalamus and internal carotid artery, though facial cooling can influence the measurement (Shiraki et al. 1988). Several studies have alluded to the inconsistencies of measurements (Schmitz et al. 1995, Giuliano et al. 1999). Gilbert et al. (2002) found no significant difference between oral and tympanic measurements. In a prospective study rectal and tympanic measurements were compared using a sample of 45 older patients. The results suggested a positive correlation between the two methods in detecting fever (Smitz et al. 2000). Weiss et al. (1998) compared the accuracy of three different tympanic thermometers when used in a multi-operator environment. Accuracy was set against pulmonary artery catheter readings. The findings

indicated variation in measurement between thermometers, and inaccuracies in results when incorrect technique was used. Latman et al. (2001) examined the accuracy and reliability of electronic, oral digital, tympanic digital and clinical thermometers and concluded that they were less accurate than mercury thermometers. The results showed significant overestimation at lower temperatures and underestimation at higher temperatures. It would appear that consistency of instrument, correctly calibrated equipment and technique are important for reliable readings.

One method that gives reliable measurements of core temperature and has been shown to be acceptable to older people is the use of urine temperature measurements with a Uritemp bottle (Fig. 18.3). This was used by Fox et al. (1973c) and Salvage (1993) and is simply a plastic container with a funnel in the top and a low-reading thermometer placed inside. The funnel has some small holes in it to allow excess urine to flow through. Provided at least 100 ml of urine is passed, the urine drains slowly through the funnel and the urine temperature is recorded on the thermometer. Since clinical thermometers have a 'kink' in the column of mercury, the maximum temperature is recorded permanently on the thermometer. So, for example, a district nurse could come and read the value at some convenient point later. The early-morning temperatures are likely to be the lowest, as temperature drops during the night due to the circadian rhythm, inactivity and possibly also unheated or cold bedrooms.

There is no easy answer as to the best route of temperature monitoring for older people and so a nurse should use a combination of methods (perhaps also monitoring room temperature) and other clinical skills to assess whether a patient has a normal, high or low body temperature.

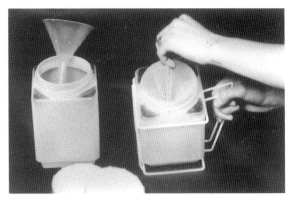

Fig. 18.3 The Uritemp apparatus.

LOW BODY TEMPERATURE

As has been suggested earlier, the development of a low body temperature in an older person results from a complex interaction of physiological, social and behavioural factors. Hypothermia, as defined by the UK Royal College of Physicians (deep body temperature below 35°C), can be divided into primary and secondary hypothermia. Primary hypothermia occurs because of dysfunction of the thermoregulatory system itself. It is most frequently seen during the cold winter months but can happen at any time of the year. Accidental exposure to severe cold alone may also lead to primary hypothermia. Secondary hypothermia occurs as the result of concomitant illness or disability that renders the older person more susceptible to the cold. A survey of 100 consecutive cases of hypothermia conducted by Maclean & Emslie-Smith (1977) found that 85% were over the age of 60 years. Almost half the cases had been found lying on the floor after falling accidentally or as the result of an illness, and few of the older cases had no predisposing illness. The authors concluded that hypothermia is uncommon in older people in the absence of any underlying disease or incapacity. Salvage (1993) estimates that 750 000 older people may be at risk of developing hypothermia during the winter months. The following sections examine in greater detail how social and behavioural factors contribute to the problem of low body temperatures in older people.

Social factors

A large number of older people live alone (currently about 3 million in the UK), often in large houses that were once family homes. Older people tend to live in older properties, which are less thermally efficient and less well maintained. Scandinavian countries and regions of North America where extreme winter conditions are the rule have built housing that incorporates thick walls, window shutters, triple glazing, well-insulated roofs and efficient heating systems. Housing and insulation standards in many of these countries are much higher than our own, although housing built in the UK since 1970 has been found on average to be about 3°C warmer than properties built before 1914. Unfortunately, this has not benefited many older people because they live in much of the poorest housing (Grundy & Holt 2001). A national study undertaken by Shelter (1997) indicated that older people occupied 32% of the worst housing, and 40–60% lived in pre-1919 terraced houses. These houses were in a state of disrepair, and lacking appropriate insulation and heating. Many pensioners occupy privately rented accommodation and may have landlords who have not undertaken renovations and repairs. Others, who are owner-occupiers, may have lost the inclination or physical ability to maintain the property themselves, or have lost their partner who may have been the one responsible for upkeep of their home. Many simply cannot afford the services of builders, plumbers, carpenters and the like.

Housing, fuel and food are the major expenses for older people and the cost of these may account for three-quarters or more of their income. Pensioners spend a larger proportion of their income on fuel relative to the national average but this represents less in absolute terms because of their small pension relative to average earnings. It has been estimated that over 4 million British households are in fuel poverty (Moore et al. 2000). Fuel poverty has been defined as the need to spend 10% of income to maintain an acceptable standard of warmth. Despite the fact that more time is spent at home and that heat is needed throughout the day, it has been estimated that many old people spend less on heating in winter than families do in summer and they live in cold environments. A national survey conducted in 1972 and reported by Wicks (1978) discovered that 90% of pensioners had morning living-room temperatures below the 21°C minimum proposed for old people by the then Ministry of Housing for periods when the outside temperature was −1°C. Seventy-five per cent of pensioners had morning living-room temperatures of less than the 18.3°C minimum recommended by the Parker-Morris report on council housing (Parker-Morris 1961), and 54% had room temperatures below 16°C, the legal minimum established by the Offices, Shops and Railways Act. These findings were confirmed in the 1991 national survey of older people in cold weather (Salvage 1993).

Many pensioners' homes are equipped with obsolete and ineffective heating appliances that are expensive to use. Most fuel costs rose steeply in the late 1970s and early 1980s; this has forced pensioners to economize further on heating in order to make ends meet, at the same time as they have grown older and in some cases become more incapacitated. Bedrooms, bathrooms, lavatories and passages are often left unheated and living rooms may be heated only intermittently. This situation may be very hazardous. Lloyd (1986) suggests that the warmth of the air in a room that is only intermittently heated may be sufficient to abolish vasoconstrictor activity in the skin while radiant heat loss to the cold walls may continue without the individual feeling cold. Falls in unheated parts of the home are then potentially disastrous. Fortunately, during the 1980s there was a considerable rise in the proportion of older people living in households with central heating (Jarvis et al. 1996). The 1991 General Household Survey showed that, whereas in 1980 only half of people aged 60+, and two-thirds in 1985, were living in households with some form of heating, by 1991 the proportion was four out of five. It should be remembered, though, that although people have central heating, they may not necessarily use it, if costs prohibit it.

In addition to shelter and heating in winter, to keep warm people need to eat well, have warm clothing and keep active. The intake of food at regular intervals during the day makes an important contribution to thermogenesis. A diet that is restricted by financial limitations, by the individual's lack of motivation, physical difficulties in obtaining supplies, manipulating cooking and eating utensils or by disorders of the digestive tract, are all factors that will render the vulnerable older person more susceptible to the cold. Weight loss results in a reduction in lean body mass and loss of insulating fat and a relative increase in heat loss from the body surface due to a high ratio of surface area to body mass.

Clothing worn by older people may deteriorate or be neglected for various reasons. There may be a reluctance to spend money on clothes if the budget is tight, and warm winter wear is relatively expensive. There may be a loss of pride in personal appearance, especially after the death of a spouse, and if the spouse was the partner responsible for maintaining and replacing clothing this aspect of self-care may lapse. In addition, it can be hard for older people to obtain items of warm clothing appropriate to their generation. Many have to rely on distant specialist stockists or mail order because high-street stores concentrate on the young fashion market.

Regular exercise is also an important way of keeping warm. To save on their fuel bills many older people may spend longer in bed. This has the unfortunate effect of creating a vicious cycle of muscle weakness, reduced capacity for exercise and immobility.

Social isolation and distance from family aggravate the risk of hypothermia. With rising age, many older people become increasingly isolated. This may be due partly to physical deterioration, but factors such as poor public transport, cost of travel on public transport, fear of being a victim of street crime and death of members of their peer group all contribute to an increasingly isolated existence. Neighbouring families may all be out during the day and social contacts may be few. This can easily lead to situations where the early-warning signs of potential hypothermia may be missed or overlooked.

Behavioural factors

Many older people have attitudes and beliefs which make them reluctant to spend money on heating even when they can afford it. Such attitudes are difficult to change and may be hard for carers of a different generation to understand or respect. The fear of debt is particularly prevalent and the concept of respectable debt relatively new. Many professionals caring for older people will themselves have mortgages, overdrafts and credit cards, but most older people have never owed money, and do not intend to start doing so.

Quarterly bills for gas and electricity may present difficulty to those on a weekly budget and fears about inflation and rising costs may increase levels of anxiety. It was much easier to see how quickly a pile of coal was diminishing than it is to work out how much gas or electricity is being used. In addition, coal was bought and used, whereas modern fuels are used and then bought.

Older people are proud of their independence and were brought up in an era before the welfare state. Many are reluctant to claim state benefits, preferring to live in impoverished situations relying solely on their state pension rather than engage with the bureaucracy of the social security system, which for these people still means the indignity of the means test and the stigma of charity.

Also prevalent amongst the older population are attitudes concerning the healthy qualities of fresh air. In the past, tuberculous patients were nursed in wards open to the outside and many people believe it is healthy to sleep in cold bedrooms and to keep windows open at night whatever the temperature outside. Electric blankets and duvets may be perceived as modern and new-fangled and offers to purchase these by family members may be resisted. Such attitudes and beliefs should be addressed with sensitivity and tact; a sustained and strenuous public education programme targeted at older people is needed in this regard. Salvage (1993) reviewed the behavioural factors possibly linked with hypothermia. The ability to detect falling ambient temperatures and initiate behavioural changes is blunted; studies have indicated that older people are less able to discriminate between close ranges of ambient temperature, and some have difficulty in discriminating temperatures up to 4°C (Collins et al. 1981b).

PREVENTION

The most effective solution to the hypothermia problem is to prevent it, and to relieve the worry and discomfort experienced by many older people each winter. It has been encouraging that since 1982 the number of hypothermia-associated deaths has declined, that is, where hypothermia, either alone or in association with another illness, is stated as the cause of death on the death certificate (Age Concern 2002).

It is important not to become complacent about the problem, especially when the winters are mild. Oliver (1983) reported the findings of a study by the Institute of Consumer Affairs that indicated that 87% of older people had never seen any of the numerous leaflets or pamphlets available, which give advice about keeping warm or about heating problems. There have been subsequent campaigns by government agencies in collaboration with voluntary bodies such as Age Concern and Help the Aged to rectify this at both national and local level, through the use of the mass media and by targeting groups working with and for older people. Winter warmth advice is available and published in many different languages.

There are three main ways of preventing hypothermia:

1. by obtaining as much money as possible for older people
2. by 'burning' that money as efficiently as possible to produce heat
3. by keeping as much as possible of the warmth produced in and around the old person.

Money

It is important that older people are kept aware of all the benefits and grants they may be entitled to and encouraged to apply for these. Age Concern provides a range of services, including individual fact sheets on keeping warm and a freephone helpline (0800 009 966). Help the Aged also provides information and advice on keeping warm in winter; its freephone helpline is 0800 800 6565. The government Warm Front scheme was launched in 2000 and is available to households who qualify for income-related benefit such as pension credit or housing benefit or disability benefit. Scotland, Wales and Northern Ireland have their own funded schemes. Money and grants are available for insulation and heating improvements. Local councils may also offer financial help. Winter fuel payments are paid to households where an occupant is 60 years and over. Those over 80 receive extra payment.

In very cold weather pensioners on income-related benefit may be entitled to cold-weather payments to help with the cost of extra heating, although qualification for this varies according to local average temperatures.

Various budget schemes are operated by the gas regions and electricity boards to assist people paying for fuel. These include weekly, fortnightly, monthly or flexible payment schemes, or, in the case of those on income-related benefit, direct deductions from benefits to clear a debt. All pensioner households are protected from disconnection between October and March by a code of practice operated by the fuel industry. In case of difficulty in meeting payment, it is important that the gas or electricity board is notified as soon as possible.

Grants are also available to assist pensioners with loft insulation, the lagging of water pipes and tanks and the cost of draught-proofing. Local councils may also offer financial help. For further details see *Keep Warm, Keep Well* (Department of Health 2003/2004a).

Heating

The Acheson inquiry accepted the link between cold and damp housing and the effect on health. One of the recommendations was a policy improvement in heating and insulation. A government strategy to end fuel poverty was initiated in 2000. The Warm Front scheme enables those most vulnerable and on income-related benefits to apply for grants to improve heating. However a report from the National Audit Office (2003) stated that one-third of those in fuel poverty were not eligible.

Insulation and draught-proofing are important ways of preventing generated heat from escaping. In addition to the grant aid provided for materials, a number of local community projects provide help with installation. Simple measures such as letterbox covers, heavy curtains over the front door, fabric 'sausage' draught excluders and blocking unused fireplaces can be both cheap and effective. Double glazing is very expensive, but curtains with thermal linings or temporary double glazing with plastic film, combined with aluminium foil behind radiators on outside walls, will all help to conserve heat. However, it is important to remind pensioners that some ventilation is essential when using paraffin, gas, Calor gas or solid-fuel heaters. Economies on water heating can be made by ensuring there is an insulating jacket on the hot-water tank and checking that the thermostat of the immersion heater is not set too high. Dual immersion heaters are useful, but expensive. Dripping taps should be repaired as soon as possible, and the use of a bowl for washing hands and dishes rather than a running hot tap may produce savings.

It is important that older people are familiar and confident with their heating appliances and the controls. Heating systems or appliances with thermostats are a great advantage provided the thermostat is allowed to control the temperature rather than being used as a switch. Equipment should be checked regularly for safety, preferably before the cold weather begins, and all open fires should be guarded. It can be very tempting to sit too close to a source of heat and old people should be warned about the dangers of this, especially if they were to fall asleep. Bedrooms should be heated in cold weather and for at least 1 h before retiring. Electric blankets or hot-water bottles filled with warm rather than scalding water provide useful supplementary heat when going to bed. There are various types of electric blanket commercially available. Certain overblankets can be kept on all night and there is at least one very-low-voltage under-blanket that can be kept on and that has the added advantage of being waterproof if occasional inconti-nence is a problem.

Thermometers can be helpful in monitoring room temperatures in rooms that are regularly used. Rooms should be kept comfortably warm with a temperature of 21°C or thereabouts, according to personal prefer-ence (Department of Health 2003/2004b). In very cold weather some older people choose to live and sleep in the same room to economize on heat. If this is done the bed should be kept away from the outside walls to prevent conductive heat loss. As suggested earlier, leaving parts of the home without heat is not the best solution because the possibility exists of a fall in some unheated area of the home.

Keeping warm

Hot drinks and meals have been identified as impor-tant for keeping warm and healthy in winter and for providing comfort. Meals on wheels is an invaluable service and complete meals and convenience foods, though expensive, are nutritious and useful for those who cannot be bothered, or for those unaccustomed to cooking, provided they are dextrous enough to open tins and packaging. Microwave ovens slow cookers and divided saucepans enable small amounts of food to be heated efficiently. A balanced diet with protein, carbohydrate and fibre will help to prevent under-nourishment and weight loss but food supplements and soups or frequent light snacks can be very helpful for those with small appetites. A hot drink left in a vac-uum flask by the bed is often advisable to provide a warm drink in the night or early in the morning.

Any form of exercise, however leisurely, will gener-ate heat and promote warmth. It is important to encourage older people to keep as mobile as possible and to avoid sitting for long periods (Chapter 13). Even gentle exercise will help and jobs should be spaced out to alternate resting times with periods of activity.

Warm thermal underwear and several layers of thin clothes are more effective insulation against the cold than one thick layer. Natural fibres tend to be warmer than synthetics and an extra loose wool jumper may be as effective as a 2°C rise in room temperature. It is particularly important for old people that they keep all exposed areas, feet, hands and head covered, espe-cially if going outside, and wear non-slip shoes or boots. Even inside, bed socks and a night-cap will help to reduce heat loss in a cold bedroom.

EARLY DETECTION

Vigilance on the part of formal and informal carers, friends, neighbours and anyone who even occasion-ally visits old people is an important part of protecting the older population from the effects of the cold. Hypothermia is notoriously difficult to identify because its symptoms are non-specific and its onset can be insidious and may mimic those of other condi-tions. It is essential that all who come into contact with older people in the community know what to look out for and are alert to cold room temperatures, lack of food in cupboards, heating appliances turned off, inappropriate dress for the ambient temperature, apa-thy and drowsiness, as well as hazards such as trailing flexes and poor lighting that might precipitate an acci-dent in a cold house.

Ideally, it should be possible to construct 'at-risk' registers. These would identify the very aged with multiple pathology, those receiving polypharmacy and those whose social history suggests they are at risk. This might enable better targeting of scarce community resources and enable community nurses, social services staff and workers in the voluntary sector to coordinate their work effectively. For exam-ple, some local authorities, charities and housing associations provide alarm systems for older people, but the criteria for qualifying for these vary from area to area. Some of these emergency alarm systems can be made to work automatically if sensors detect a low room temperature or if there has been an extended period of inactivity. These systems might be a valuable asset to an old person known to be at high risk.

Certain warning signs should alert carers to the possibility of hypothermia. These include:

- no complaints of feeling the cold, even in a very cold room
- drowsiness and apathy
- slurred speech and a husky voice
- skin that is cold to the touch; this applies not just to the extremities but to areas that would nor-mally be warm, such as the abdomen, between the thighs and under the arms
- a puffy face that may appear pale or grey in colour
- apparent confusion and slow responses
- slow and shallow breathing.

Figure 18.4 illustrates the typical facial appearance of a hypothermic patient. This can readily be mistaken for myxoedema.

After summoning help, steps should be taken to warm up the room while avoiding subjecting the older person to any direct source of heat such as a hot-water bottle, a hot bath or a heater. Further heat loss should be prevented by wrapping the person up well, including the head, in light coats, blankets or a duvet. If the victim is conscious and alert, then warm, nourishing drinks can be given, but alcohol, which causes vasodilatation, should not be given, as this would increase heat loss. There are two categories of hypothermia: primary hypothermia due to cold stress without dysfunction in thermoregulation, and secondary hypothermia due to cold stress with abnormal thermoregulation and underlying pathology (Morgan 1997). In the older person hypothermia is more likely to be multifactorial in nature.

As the core temperature drops, the vital organs become progressively functionally defective. There is an increase in the respiratory rate (tachypnoea) and depth, followed by a reduced minute volume, increased bronchial secretions and bronchospasm. As hypothermia progresses the respirations slow (bradypnoea) and breathing becomes shallow. Gaseous exchange becomes increasingly ineffective. Eventually, respiratory arrest develops. The victim becomes confused and unable to respond sensibly and there may be impaired judgement. The level of consciousness reduces and coma follows. There may be a tachycardia initially but, with increasing poor cardiac output, bradycardia develops, with a corresponding fall in blood pressure. Arrhythmias develop, the most serious being asystole or ventricular fibrillation, which cause immediate cardiac arrest. The rationale for cold diuresis is the initial increase in cardiac output and increased peripheral vasoconstriction; this may result in hypervolaemia. Blood pressure is raised with a corresponding increased glomerular filtration rate, resulting in the initial cold diuresis. As hypothermia progresses renal blood flow reduces, with a corresponding reduction of urine (oliguria). Haematological and biochemical changes are observed. In the presence of other disease, such as chronic bronchitis, dementia or ischaemic heart disease, the clinical effects may develop earlier, i.e. with relatively mild hypothermia, cardiorespiratory arrest may be precipitated by cooling in susceptible people even before severe core hypothermia is established. Table 18.2 illustrates the effects of dropping core temperature even in the absence of other pathologies.

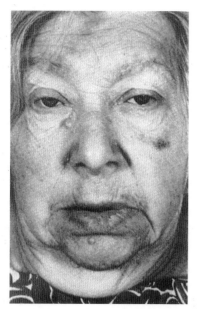

Fig. 18.4 Facial oedema of an elderly hypothermic woman.

Table 18.2 Signs and symptoms of hypothermia

Rectal temperature (°C)	Signs and symptoms
37–35	Cold to touch, pale skin
	Poor muscle coordination
	Shivering
	Hyperpnoea
	Piloerection
	Tachycardia
35–32	No shivering
	Cold skin
	Waxy appearance
	Puffy face
	Confusion
	Bradypnoea
32–30	Rigid muscles
	Dilated pupils
	Poor reflexes
	Low blood pressure
	Bradycardia
	Coma
	Convulsions
30–28	Flaccid muscles
	Bradycardia or tachycardia
	Fixed dilated pupils
	Atrial fibrillation
	Risk of cardiac arrest
28 and below	Cyanosis
	Barely detectable vital signs
	Cardiac arrest

Hypothermia can only be diagnosed accurately by the use of a low-reading thermometer; an older person with an oral temperature of 35°C or less should always have a rectal temperature recorded. Patients whose hypothermia is secondary to underlying disease may present with a mixture of signs and symptoms and it is essential to obtain an accurate core temperature in these individuals. Full diagnosis of their condition may only be possible after rewarming has taken place.

CARE OF AN OLDER PERSON WITH A LOW BODY TEMPERATURE

There is no standard treatment for hypothermia in the older person and careful consideration of each individual case is required, taking into account any known current disease and the degree of hypothermia.

Previously healthy people with a mild degree of hypothermia (core temperature 32–35°C) may not need admission to hospital and may be gently and passively rewarmed at home under careful supervision (Collins 1988). A potential risk of circulatory collapse during rewarming exists and for this reason hospitalization should always be considered. Opinions differ as to whether hypothermic patients can be managed satisfactorily in general wards or whether they should be cared for in intensive care units. Wherever they are, it is important that they can be monitored closely with facilities to hand to institute rapid intervention should complications arise. Initial investigations that are required are shown in Table 18.3.

To end this section, four problems associated with hypothermia are identified, together with their nursing goals and the intervention designed to alleviate or prevent them.

Problem 1

Manifestations of hypothermia caused by low core body temperature (Table 18.2).

Goal

The patient will suffer no further heat loss and rewarming will occur at a rate of approximately 0.5–1°C/h.

Nursing intervention

Rewarming techniques used depend on the degree of hypothermia. Passive rewarming appears to be more generally favoured in the older person rather than aggressive active rewarming used in younger victims of accidental hypothermia. The patient is normally nursed in a room with no draughts, and the room temperature kept between 25 and 30°C. Insulation from further heat

Table 18.3 Common investigations in hypothermia

Investigation	Rationale
Chest X-ray	To detect bronchopneumonia or pulmonary oedema
Abdominal X-ray	To detect severe gastric dilation and risk of aspiration pneumonia
Twelve-lead electrocardiogram	To detect sinus bradycardia and atrial fibrillation. Often shows characteristic J-wave
Arterial blood gases	To indicate degree of hypoxaemia
Blood cultures	To detect underlying septicaemia
Blood	To assess fluid and electrolyte biochemistry requirements and detect blood glucose abnormalities and renal impairment
Haematology	May detect haemoconcentration, raised white cell count, thrombocytopenia and raised red cell count

loss is achieved by the use of light blankets; the head and neck should be covered to reduce heat loss. This technique relies on endogenous thermogenesis. Rewarming should be slow, with observed increases of temperature ranging from 0.5°C/h to 1°C/h.

Active external rewarming is a method that can be introduced if the body temperature is below 32.2°C. Active external rewarming includes using warm baths, radiant heat (Ledingham & Mone 1980) or convection warming therapy (Fritsch 1995). Miles & Thompson (1987) claim successful use of the Clinitron bed for rewarming in two case reports and this may offer useful advantages. The patient needs to be monitored as this method may cause peripheral vasodilatation, decrease in blood pressure and aftershock effect (Morgan 1997).

Active core rewarming includes the administration of humidified oxygen or air at a temperature of 40–45°C and warmed intravenous fluid. Other methods include peritoneal dialysis and warm mediastinal irrigation; these are used in intensive care settings.

Problem 2

Potential complications of rewarming, e.g. hypotension, hypoxia, pulmonary oedema.

Goal

No complications will occur while maintaining spontaneous rewarming.

Nursing intervention

Continuous rectal monitoring of core body temperature is recommended using an electronic probe. Respirations, blood pressure and pulse should be recorded half-hourly to hourly. Pulse oximetry measurements may not be reliable due to vasoconstriction.

If the pulse becomes irregular, if blood pressure falls or if the temperature rises too rapidly then the rate of warming should be slowed and the patient recooled until the vital signs stabilize. This situation occurs when cutaneous vasodilatation reduces the peripheral resistance, blood flows away from the vital organs and cardiac output is unable to compensate. An alternative to recooling is to maintain the blood pressure with administration of dopamine. In addition, cold blood returning to the core from the extremities may produce an 'afterdrop' in core temperature and induce cardiac dysrhythmias.

Warmed oxygen at an appropriate concentration via a mask is frequently administered to correct hypoxaemia. A substantial number of patients require positive-pressure ventilation because lung function deteriorates as a result of pulmonary oedema or because of the development of atelectasis, and it is therefore important to observe respiratory function closely.

The patient's level of consciousness should be assessed regularly and should steadily improve as rewarming occurs. The level of blood glucose should be monitored as hyperglycaemia may be observed in those with temperatures below 30°C because insulin is not effective at this level of temperature. Hypoglycaemia may correct itself during rewarming, although in the case of hypoglycaemic diabetics or the severely malnourished, intravenous glucose may be administered.

Problem 3

Risk of pressure sores as indicated by assessment using Norton or Waterlow scale (Chapter 19).

Goal

No pressure sores will develop.

Nursing intervention

Hypothermic patients may have been immobile and lain or sat in one position for many hours, with poor skin perfusion as a result of cutaneous vasoconstriction. Immediate action should be taken to protect pressure areas. Use of a pressure support system such as a low-air-loss bed, Pegasus bed, ripple bed or Clinitron bed is advocated, as any unnecessary movement of the patient can precipitate ventricular fibrillation

(see Chapter 19 for further information on pressure-sore prevention).

Problem 4

Potential fluid imbalance due to cold-induced fluid shifts.

Goal

Arterial and venous pressures will remain within normal limits and urine output will be adequate.

Nursing intervention

Since blood pressure falls when the body temperature is very low, water moves from the plasma to the interstitial compartments, giving rise to oedema and to the characteristic bloated appearance (Fig. 18.4). These cold-induced fluid shifts often reverse spontaneously on rewarming and intravenous fluids are given based on individual requirements. If given, they should be prewarmed. Oliguria is not uncommon but diuresis should improve as the temperature of hypothermic patients rises. Catheterization is required in moderate to severe hypothermia to monitor urine output. A nasogastric tube to relieve gastric dilation and avoid aspiration of gastric contents has to be balanced against the risk of inducing ventricular fibrillation, and is best avoided while the core temperature remains below 30°C.

Current practice suggests that there are no indications for routine use of thyroxine or steroids, although coexisting disease may need drug therapy (Maclean 1987). A broad-spectrum antibiotic is usually administered prophylactically to treat overt or suspected bronchopneumonia.

If the clinical course of rewarming progresses favourably then recovery is likely. One or more complications indicate a poorer prognosis. Once the patient has been rewarmed, attention must be directed at discharge planning and establishing the home circumstances. Returning an individual who has been hypothermic to the same environment without adequate support or change in the situation will predispose to further attacks.

We end this section with a summary of a patient who experienced hypothermia and include information about the condition, warming interventions, adverse effects and management (Case study 18.1).

CARE OF AN OLDER PERSON WITH A RAISED BODY TEMPERATURE

When an older person develops a fever in response to some infectious agent or inflammatory process, then

Case study 18.1

Mrs Caruthers, aged 80 years, fell after tripping on a mat in the kitchen. Her daughter called an ambulance and she was admitted to the accident and emergency department of the local hospital. Radiological studies revealed she had sustained a fractured neck of femur. Observations on admission revealed the following:

- temperature was 36.2°C (infrared tympanic thermometer)
- pulse 88 beats/min and regular
- respiration 20 breaths/min
- blood pressure 150/70 mmHg
- she was restless and in considerable pain
- she appeared underweight.

Her past medical history revealed that she had been treated for hypertension for the past 40 years and was maintained on atenolol 50 mg/day and bendroflumethiazide 2.5 mg/day. The initial medical intervention consisted of intravenous fluid replacement, pain management and electrocardiogram recording. Biochemical and haematological investigations were undertaken. Mrs Caruthers was admitted to the orthopaedic unit and was to undergo surgery.

She went to the operating theatre at 1600 h on the day of admission. At 1700 h her temperature measurement was 34.8°C. What may have caused this drop in temperature?

Heat loss

Hypothermia is a known consequence of anaesthesia. The definition of hypothermia does vary but perioperative hypothermia is usually defined as a core temperature of less than 36°C (Sessler & Sessler 1998, Enwright & Plowes 1999, Frank et al. 1999). Core temperatures less than 36°C are associated with an increased risk of adverse outcomes in the postoperative period. Both general and regional anaesthesia alter thermoregulation (Matsukawa et al. 1995) and Sessler (1997) has observed that 'anaesthetic drugs inhibit thermoregulation in a dose dependent manner'. The vasoconstriction and shivering response that occur when cold is inhibited is approximately three times greater than the sweating response when hot (Sessler 1997).

Induction of anaesthesia causes vasodilation, which in turn causes a redistribution of heat from the core to peripheral tissues. The core temperature can decrease by 1–1.5°C in the first few hours (Matsukawa et al. 1995). Heat flow depends on the temperature gradient and the rate of decrease in core temperature is determined by the difference between heat loss and heat gain (Sessler 2000). Heat is lost through the mechanisms of:

- radiation: heat flows from the warmer body to the cooler environment; about 50–60% of heat is lost this way
- convection (sometimes called facilitated conduction): heat transfers by movement of air over the body
- conduction: transfer of heat by direct contact with a cooler area (e.g. from skin preparation or surgical instruments)
- evaporation: heat transfers via the respiratory tract, or through loss of skin integrity (Sessler 1997).

Heat loss is also influenced by ambient temperature (Morris 1971, Closs et al. 1986, Frank et al. 1992, El Gamal et al. 2000), skin preparations (Sessler et al. 1993), unwarmed intravenous fluids (Monga et al. 1996), and the surface area exposed (Goldberg & Roe 1966). Other factors that could have influenced Mrs Caruthers' temperature are her low body mass (Roberts et al. 1994) and her age (Morrison 1988, Bynom 1998) as there is an age association with reduced muscle mass, decreased BMR and a reduced vasomotor response when cold. Female gender has also been cited as a risk factor (Sessler 1997).

It is important that the core temperature is monitored during surgery to identify changes and this can be achieved by positioning a temperature probe in the upper oesophagus, or nasopharynx, or by using a tympanic thermometer.

Ambient temperature

Morris (1971) suggested that 100% of anaesthetized patients have temperatures of less than 36°C when the operating theatre temperature is less than 21°C. Studies conducted by Kurz et al. (1996), Frank et al. (1992) and Vaughan et al. (1981) showed an approximately 50% incidence of hypothermia with core temperature less than 36°C when ambient temperatures were between 20°C and 23°C. El-Gamal et al. (2000), in a small comparative study of patients (20 patients aged 20–40 years and 20 patients aged 60–80 years) undergoing orthopaedic surgery, found a 10% incidence of hypothermia postoperatively when ambient temperature was maintained at 26°C. There was no significant difference between the two age groups. Arndt (1999) questioned whether environmental temperatures outside the range of 20–24°C could increase the risk in growth of micro-organisms, and whether higher temperatures would be tolerated by staff.

Case study 18.1—cont'd

Warming interventions
Preoperative and intraoperative warming
Reducing the core-to-peripheral-temperature gradient forms the basis of interventions.

What warming methods could have been considered for Mrs Caruthers and why?

Prewarming using forced air 1–2 h prior to surgery has been shown to reduce redistribution hypothermia (Hynson et al. 1993, Just et al. 1993, Fossum et al. 2001) and patients tend to remain normothermic with a core temperature > 36°C (Sessler 2001).

Intraoperative methods of maintaining the core temperature include warmed cotton blankets, warmed water mattress, forced air warming, warmed intravenous infusion, irrigation fluid and humidified inspired gases. (In neurosurgery mild hypothermia can be of benefit: Todd & Warner 1992.)

Forced air warming works through the mechanisms of radiation replacing cool surfaces of the operating theatre with warm air and convection, when air is warmer than skin. Forced air warming has been shown to be an effective preventive intervention in maintaining perioperative normothermia (Hynson et al. 1993, Kurz et al. 1993). In patients with peripheral vascular disease, a risk assessment should be undertaken prior to its use. There is no empirical literature to support the view that this method increases the risk of infection (Kurz et al. 1996). Two small randomized controlled studies (in a sample of 24 patients aged 20–80) compared three warming methods: circulating water mattress, resistive heat and forced air warming. Conclusions drawn suggest that the circulating water mattress performed less well than the others, with core temperatures continuing to decrease (Matsuzaki et al. 2003, Negishi et al. 2003).

Warming fluids
Sessler (1994) suggested that 1 unit of refrigerated blood decreases the core temperature by 0.25°C. Fluid warmers can be of benefit when large volumes are used.

Airway heating and humidification of gases
Approximately 10% of heat loss occurs through the respiratory tract.

Adverse effects
What are the known and perceived adverse effects of perioperative hypothermia? Areas that need to be considered are as follows:

Increased risk of wound infection
There is an increased risk of wound infection in those whose central core temperature is < 36°C. Flores-Maldonada et al. (1997) concluded that perioperative hypothermia was an independent risk factor for wound infection. Kurz et al. (1996), in a randomized controlled study of patients undergoing colorectal surgery, found that with a mean intraoperative temperature of 34.7°C, 19% of patients developed postoperative wound infections compared with 6% of those actively warmed whose mean intraoperative temperature was 36.6°C. Thus, the incidence of postoperative wound infection tripled in the hypothermic group. It was also noted that the hypothermic group had a longer hospital stay (2.6 days longer). Scott & Buckland (2004) suggested that there is a link between intraoperative hypothermia and tissue viability and a relationship with the formation of pressure ulcers.

Physiological reasoning: perioperative hypothermia is associated with increased levels of noradrenaline, and peripheral vasoconstriction (Frank et al. 1995) and decreased subcutaneous oxygen tension (Kurz et al. 1996, Greif et al. 2000). The immune system of the hypothermic patient is less efficient and neutrophil function is impaired (Sessler 1997).

Blood loss
Schmied et al. (1996) questioned whether perioperative hypothermia influenced blood loss during hip arthroplasty. A randomized controlled trial with a sample of 60 adults aged 40–80 years were allocated to two groups: (1) a normothermic group, for whom the temperature was actively maintained at or near 36.5°C by using warmed intravenous solution (37°C) and warmed forced air cover (Bair hugger); and (2) a hypothermic group who had no active warming and whose temperature was allowed to fall to 35°C. The findings demonstrated that surgical blood loss was significantly greater in the hypothermic patients at the end of surgery and up until 24 h afterwards. A 500 ml loss of blood, 30% more than the normothermic group, was observed.

Case study 18.1—cont'd

Physiological reasoning: hypothermia causes changes in the clotting mechanisms such as impaired platelet function, and an impaired coagulation cascade sequence. Research suggests that the process of fibrinolysis is unchanged and that clot formation is impaired rather than clot (lysis) degeneration (Kettner et al. 1998).

Altered drug metabolism

Hypothermia decreases the metabolism of drugs and alters the pharmacodynamics of volatile anaesthetics. The action of vecuronium, a muscle relaxant, is increased at temperatures 2°C below the core temperature. When the core temperature is 3°C lower, plasma concentration of intravenous propofol is 30% higher. Therefore the effects of anaesthetic medication can be prolonged.

Cardiac arrhythmias and myocardial ischaemia

Frank et al. (1997) suggest that maintenance of normothermia in the perioperative phase (36.7°C versus 35.4°C) can reduce the incidence of cardiac morbidity during surgery and in the early postoperative period. Postoperative shivering has often been cited as leading to myocardial ischaemia and myocardial infarction. Shivering is not common in older people and many studies conclude that shivering does not trigger myocardial ischaemia (Sessler 1997). Laszlo et al. (1990) suggested that potassium levels can alter when a patient is hypothermic.

Physiological reasoning: mild hypothermia can increase levels of noradrenaline, causing vasoconstriction and an increase in blood pressure. This may contribute to arrhythmias and myocardial ischaemia.

Commentary

Mrs Caruthers' temperature in the recovery unit was 35.8°C. How would you assess and manage her care in the initial postoperative period?

Record observations:
- pulse rate: amplitude and rhythm to detect dysrhythmias
- blood pressure: be consistent in method of measurement to ensure reliability; remember she is taking atenolol
- respiratory effort: rate, rhythm and depth, oxygen saturation levels, and presence of cyanosis.

Assess temperature:
- comfort level: shivering, feeling cold (Leinonen et al. 1996), skin cold to touch
- temperature measurement: consistent use of equipment to ensure reliability.

If temperature is in the hypothermic range consider warming methods:
- passive interventions or
- active external rewarming: forced warm air blanket generates the fastest rewarming times when compared with cotton blankets and fluid-filled water-circulating blankets (Grossman et al. 2002). A risk assessment should be undertaken in those patients who have peripheral vascular disease, and skin should be observed for redness, especially in those where skin is fragile. With increasing age, warming is slower (Bush et al. 1995 review the adverse effects; see p. 33).

Evaluate the patient's condition during the warming process:
- vasodilation can cause hypotension; once temperature reaches 36.5°C, remove blanket and observe for afterdrop (see Bush et al. 1995)
- assess for hypokalaemia when rewarming
- neurological assessment: level of consciousness, cognitive awareness, agitation, mental status and confusion
- urine volume, colour and concentration
- hydration state and intravenous fluids
- observe skin for colour and warmth
- comfort: observe for pain
- remember to assess for potential adverse outcomes from intraoperative hypothermia.

Readers may like to analyse their own practice when managing the care of an older person undergoing a surgical intervention and could consider devising a nursing protocol for managing postoperative hypothermia in the older person.

treatment involves management of the underlying cause as it would in a younger person, bearing in mind that the febrile response may be less marked. The principles of treating hyperthermia or heat illness are the same for both older and younger patients.

Problem 1

Dehydration due to water and sodium depletion.

Goal
Rehydration and correction of fluid and electrolyte balance.

Nursing intervention
Whenever the patient's condition permits, oral rehydration with cold drinks (not iced) is the preferred method since this is a more physiologically normal route. Fluid containing caffeine (coffee, some fizzy drinks) has diuretic properties and therefore should be given with caution. When the patient is confused or unable to tolerate frequent drinks, intravenous rehydration will be required. This involves carefully controlled administration to ensure that the cardiovascular system is not further compromised by the rapid infusion of large volumes of fluid. Vital signs should be carefully monitored and the infusion rate varied accordingly. Observation of vital signs to prevent and detect pulmonary oedema is important, especially in patients who have renal or cardiac impairment. Urine output also should be observed as rehydration progresses to establish whether or not renal function has been impaired.

Problem 2

Impaired/ineffective heat loss mechanisms.

Goal
Heat loss will increase and body temperature will drop.

Nursing intervention
The patient should be nursed in a cool room with the minimum of light coverings. Air movement can be created by use of an electric fan, air conditioning or other ventilation systems and this will increase heat loss by convection from the surface of the body. Further heat loss can be promoted by careful use of tepid sponging which will enhance evaporation of moisture from the skin. Vasoconstriction must be avoided. Body temperature should be monitored before and after this procedure and the patient closely observed to ensure that the shivering mechanism is not activated as this would be counterproductive. Cooling units use the methods of evaporation and convection when cooling the body. The procedure is achieved by spraying warm water and air to maintain a skin temperature of 31–32°C (Collins 1996).

We end this section with a summary of a patient who experienced hyperthermia caused by fever following a chest infection and include information about the condition, the negative and positive consequences of hyperthermia, and assessment and management of an older person with pneumonia (Case study 2). Following this is a case study of a patient who suffered from heat exhaustion during a heatwave in England (Case study 3).

Case study 18.2

Mr Connor, aged 82, has been a resident in a nursing home for the past 3 years. He is a sociable man who enjoyed participating in organized activities. He required help with walking, getting in and out of a chair and managing his hygiene needs. In the past few days he has had little appetite and has been feeling unwell. He also appears confused. His aural temperature was 37°C and his respiratory rate 24 breaths/min. The general practitioner saw him and a provisional diagnosis of pneumonia was made. He scored 2 on the (CRB-65; confusion, respiratory rate, blood pressure -age 65 and over) severity score (Lim et al. 2003).

Pneumonia
Pneumonia is an important cause of morbidity and mortality in the older person. Marrie (1994) indicated that, of those aged 75 and over, there is a higher annual incidence of hospital admission, citing 11.6 cases per 1000. It is well documented that older people have a greater risk of developing secondary complication from community-acquired pneumonia such as meningitis, empyema and bacteraemia (Finkelstein et al. 1983, Rajagopalan & Moran 2000). Community-acquired pneumonia is noted to be at its highest during the winter months (Vankatesan et al. 1990).

Case study 18.2—cont'd

Pneumonia-related mortality is associated with comorbid illnesses such as diabetes mellitus, congestive cardiac failure and cancer (Conte et al. 1999, Shua-Haim & Ross 2000), malnutrition (Shua-Haim & Ross 2000), poor socioeconomic status and behavioural changes (Falsey 2003). Also associated are altered functional capacity, including cognitive impairment (Salive et al. 1993) and age (Conte et al. 1999).

With ageing, there is an increased risk of pneumonia due to the biological changes in both the lungs and immune system (see section on changes with ageing, above, for biological changes in the respiratory and immune systems, and Chapter 5 for further information). Specific changes reduce the protective mechanisms: ciliary activity slows, mucociliary clearance decreases (Shua-Haim & Ross 2000) and there is a reduced cough reflex which impairs the older person's ability to clear secretions. Changes in both humoral (antibody response to external antigens) and cell-mediated immunity are associated with increased risk of infection. There may be a diminished fever response (Chan & Fernandez 2001).

The classical signs and symptoms of pneumonia – fever, cough with sputum, pleuritic pain, dyspnoea, tachycardia, leukocytosis – are not always present in the older person (Fein 1999).

Instead, the older person may present with absent or low-grade fever, cognitive impairment, malaise, loss of appetite, decreased functional ability, tachypnoea and tachycardia (Feldman 1999, Chan & Fernandez 2001).

Severity assessment tool
The CRB-65 severity assessment tool identifies specific management pathways for patients who present with community-acquired pneumonia. The tool sets out to identify those at greatest risk, by using a points scheme: 0 points suggests the older person could be cared for in the community setting, and is at the lowest risk of mortality; 1–2 points indicates that assessment and care are needed in hospital, and 3 points suggests a greater risk of death and care is most appropriately provided in an intensive-care setting or high-dependency unit (Lim et al. 2003, BTS guidelines 2004).

Admission to hospital
On admission to the hospital's medical unit, Mr Connor's past medical history revealed that he had a history of mild heart failure and had been prescribed angiotensin-converting enzyme inhibitors. His observations revealed:
- temperature: 37.6°C using an infrared tympanic thermometer
- pulse rate 114 beats/min
- blood pressure 138/88mmHg
- respiration rate of 26 breaths/min with fast, shallow breathing
- pulse oximetry: read 90% on air
- a cough, but he was not expectorating sputum
- he appeared confused.

Fever in older people
It is important to recognize that older people do not always present with a substantial increase in body temperature when challenged with an infection (bacterial, viral or fungal). The evidence confirms that between 20% and 30% of older people have no fever or show a 'blunted response' and this may lead to poorer outcomes (Norman & Yoshikawa 1996, Yoshikawa 1997). As the older person may not present with the classical signs and symptoms of infections, other indicators should be used in the assessment process, such as changes in functional capacity, i.e. cognitive functioning, loss of appetite, falls, fatigue (Norman & Yoshikawa 1996).

In the older person Norman (2000) defines fever as a tympanic membrane temperature or oral temperature of > 37.2°C (rectal > 37.6°C), which is lower than the 38–41°C usually classified as fever (Bernheim et al. 1979, Castle 1979, McCarron 1986). Several studies have reported that older people tend to have a lower baseline temperature when compared to younger individuals (Keatinge et al. 1984, Castle et al. 1991, 1993). An increase of 1.3°C from the baseline would be significant and indicative of fever, and may suggest severe infection. (Norman 2000). Roghmann et al. (2001), in a retrospective study, assessed the effect of age on the febrile response. Temperature measurements were taken on days 1 and 2 and on discharge in 320 patients aged 18–97 with moderate to severe pneumonia. Conclusions drawn from this study showed that the febrile response declined with age. It was noted that the temperature on the first 3 days of infection was lower by 0.15°C with each decade. This study supports the premise that baseline temperatures reduce with age. However, there were acknowledged limitations which could have influenced results: missing data sets of temperature recordings and not all data were available to indicate the use of antipyretics in the first 2 days. Nonetheless,

Case study 18.2—cont'd

the evidence suggests that a lower threshold of 37.2°C (oral or tympanic membrane temperature) or a 1.3°C increase from the baseline should be used as an indicator for infection in older people. Furthermore, changes in functional capacity can be indicators of infection.

Is fever protective?

It is well documented that fever is an important part of the body's defences. It is suggested that fever may inhibit replication of micro-organisms (Roberts 1975). Fever enhances the activity of the immune system (antibody production and cell-mediated immunity, neutrophil and macrophage function and mobility and phagocytic action are more pronounced in temperatures of 38–40°C and interferon levels are enhanced (Holtzclaw 1992)). The other benefits of fever include a fall in plasma iron levels which may inhibit growth of pathogens (Rosenthal & Silverstein 1988, Holtzclaw 1992). It has also been suggested that absorption of sulphonamides is enhanced in fever (Holtzclaw 1992). If older people have blunted fever responses, does lack of this protective element compromise them? In a survey, Ahkee et al. (1997) examined mortality rates of older patients with community-acquired pneumonia. They found that those presenting with temperatures above 37.8°C and a leukocyte count above 10 000cells/mm^3 had a mortality rate of 4% compared with those presenting with no fever or leukocytosis whose mortality rate was 29%. Bender & Scarpace (1997) suggest that, in the older person, lack of fever could indicate a poorer outcome.

Detrimental effects of fever

The increased metabolic demands caused by the febrile response include increase in sympathetic tone, depending on release of noradrenaline, resulting in peripheral vasoconstriction and leading to an increased mean arterial blood pressure (Styrt & Sugarman 1990, Greisman 1997). This response may be compromised in older people because of lower levels of released noradrenaline or reduced vasomotor response (Neilsen et al. 1992). There is an increase in oxygen consumption (Beisel et al. 1980), with a corresponding increase in respiratory rate and heart rate. These changes could compromise a patient who has cardiovascular or pulmonary disease. Insensible fluid loss through respiration can increase, which may lead to dehydration and electrolyte imbalance. Anorexia, weight loss and confusion may also be observed (Davis-Smith 1978, Castle 1979, Bruce & Grove 1992).

There has always been debate concerning the use of interventions that lower fever (i.e. antipyretics and cooling strategies). Mackowiak (2002) argues that there is little empirical evidence to support such therapeutic interventions, and fever of less than 41°C is not harmful (if not persistent). There has been ongoing debate as to whether patients with cardiopulmonary disease are more at risk from the metabolic effects created by fever. Experimental studies have not confirmed the ability of antipyretic medication to reduce fever-induced metabolic demands in older people (Mackowiak 2002).

Investigations

Mr Connor had arterial blood gases taken and oxygen was started at 35% and administered via a facemask (non-invasive ventilation was not required). Further blood tests consisted of blood cultures to identify for bacteraemia, full blood count, electrolytes and urea and liver function tests. Sputum for culture and sensitivity was not obtained, as Mr Connor could not expectorate. Murdoch et al. (2001) and Farina et al. (2002) evaluated the urine antigen test for *Streptococcus pneumoniae* in diagnosing pneumococcus pneumonia, and found a higher sensitivity than sputum cultures and blood tests (BTS guidelines 2004). A chest X-ray revealed consolidation in the left base of the lung.

Assessment

Nutritional screening and assessment were undertaken, as Mr Connor had limited appetite and malnutrition is a risk factor for pneumonia. Assessment was undertaken to detect dehydration as insensible sweating increases with increased respiratory rate and increased core temperature. His confusional state could limit his fluid intake. When older people are challenged by fluid deprivation they exhibit a decreased thirst sensation and reduced fluid intake (Kenney & Chiu 2000). Mr Connor was initially rehydrated with intravenous fluids (he has a history of mild heart failure). His mental status was assessed twice daily.

Management

Mr Connor was prescribed antibiotics, amoxicillin 1 g orally three times daily and clarithromycin 500 mg twice daily (*S. pneumoniae* had been identified). No antipyretics were administered.

Case study 18.2—cont'd

The most important aspects when caring for Mr Connor were:

- to observe for the clinical signs of hypoxia, including altered mental status, assessed twice daily
- detailed observations of respiratory function were continued: respiration rate (observed for tachypnoea) and dyspnoea
- oxygen saturation levels were measured: oxygen therapy was continued whilst pulse oximetry readings read less than 92%
- pulse and blood pressure were monitored, observing for hypotension (< 100 mmHg systolic) and hypertension
- temperature was recorded 4-hourly using the same site and device with an infrared tympanic thermometer to ensure reliability. Accuracy and reliability are important in observing for improvement and deterioration. Devices vary in accuracy, and anatomical differences can affect accuracy of reading as these thermometers measure the heat that radiates from the tympanic membrane. In the older person, the walls of the external auditory canal tend to collapse (Latman 2003), which can affect accuracy. However, with serial measurements, trends can be observed
- nursing activities were clustered to allow Mr Connor time to rest
- he was positioned sitting upright to aid ventilation and to minimize respiratory effort
- physiotherapy was given.

Mr Connor was unable to take adequate fluid or food without prompting and help was offered. Nutritional supplements were introduced. Both fluid and nutritional intake were monitored and reassessment was undertaken daily.

Mr Connor was oriented to his surroundings and interventions specific to his needs were introduced.

His hygiene needs were met: Stein (1990) suggests that colonization of the oropharynx with respiratory pathogens increases the risk of pneumonia in the older person because of potential aspiration. Scannapieco (1999) argues that poor mouth care, reduced salivary flow and malnutrition increase bacterial colonization and, together with aspiration of oropharynx secretions, the risk of pneumonia is increased.

Gentle mobilization was started and gradually increased.

His vaccination status was reviewed.

Mr Connor responded well and was discharged back to the nursing home. On discharge his temperature was 36°C, pulse 88 beats/min, blood pressure 156/86 mmHg and oxygen saturation 95% on air. He was able to maintain his nutritional and oral intake, and his mental status returned to normal.

Case study 18.3

Mrs Bushiza is 84 years old and lives on her own in a small flat on the fourth floor of an apartment block. She has one married daughter who usually visits once a week. Mrs Bushiza has limited mobility due to osteoarthritis and is unable to leave the flat independently. She likes to sit by the window during the day. Social services visit twice weekly to provide help with shopping and housework. Mrs Bushiza has a leg ulcer, which is redressed by the district nurse.

During the last 24 h she has been feeling increasing unwell. When the district nurse visits she finds Mrs Bushiza feeling nauseous and she has been vomiting. The initial assessment reveals that she has a headache and is feeling fatigued and dizzy though, when questioned, she does not display signs of confusion or present with altered behaviour or consciousness levels. She has not been drinking very much during the last 24 h because of her nausea. Her temperature is 37.4°C and she has accompanying tachycardia.

During the past few days there has been a heatwave with daytime temperatures reaching 28°C with a relative humidity of 35–41%. High environmental temperatures and humidity levels can cause heat-related disorders (especially in the older person where the sweating threshold is increased, so increasing the risk of heat-related disorders). The room where she is sitting is hot and Mrs Bushiza had been unable to open the window.

The initial intervention consisted of moving Mrs Bushiza away from the window and to a cooler room in her flat. Her cardigan was removed, she was offered water but could not tolerate it because of her nausea. It was agreed she would be admitted to hospital for assessment.

Case study 18.3—cont'd

On admission, her temperature is 37.8°C and there is a noticeable change in her systolic and diastolic blood pressure from a lying to standing position, indicating orthostasis with an accompanying tachycardia. Her urine appears concentrated, her mouth is dry and observations of her tongue reveal longitudinal furrows. She is still complaining of a headache and feeling dizzy, though she is not disoriented or confused. Her respiratory rate is 18 breaths/min. Blood is taken to evaluate fluid and electrolyte status.

Summary of findings

The assessment data indicate that Mrs Bushiza is in negative fluid balance. She is in fluid volume deficit with both fluid and electrolyte loss due to a decrease in fluid intake, vomiting and loss through perspiration. High environmental temperatures and humidity levels are likely to have contributed to her condition. Blood pressure readings indicate a lying/standing deficit of 20 mmHg systolic and 10 mmHg diastolic with accompanying tachycardia, which could be indicative of intravascular volume deficit.

She presents with reduced urine volume and concentrated urine. The normal urine output should be approximately 1 ml/kg body weight per hour (Pestana 1989). Over a 24-h period with adequate hydration, the output should be approximtely 1000–1500 ml.

She also has a dry mouth and her tongue shows increased longitudinal furrows. In older people this can be a more realistic assessment in reflecting fluid deficit. Skin turgor is less reliable: when lightly pinched, the skin should return to its original position; however this is not only influenced by the interstitial fluid volume but also by skin elasticity and skin elasticity is lost in the ageing process, making this assessment unreliable (for details of fluid homeostasis, see Chapter 5).

Her temperature has increased above the normal range but there are no signs of infection.

From the assessment data, the patient's history and awareness of the recent heatwave, a diagnosis of heat exhaustion is made.

It is important to differentiate heat exhaustion from heat stroke as heat stroke induces multiple organ failure. Heat exhaustion consists of a spectrum of signs and symptoms and can progress to heat stroke if not managed successfully (see Boxes 18.1 and 18.2 for the differences in signs and symptoms, drawn from Ballester & Harchelroad 1999 and Kunihiro & Foster 2002). Patients with heat exhaustion have normal findings on neurological examination.

Interventions

Mrs Bushiza was placed in a cool environment and her clothing was reduced.

An intravenous infusion was started to replace fluid and electrolyte deficit. Initially she was unable to take adequate fluid orally.

Her temperature was taken hourly to observe for any increase or decrease.

Exposed skin can be sprayed with tepid water and a fan used to aid a drop in temperature which may cause shivering and so needs to be monitored closely. Temperature measurement must be undertaken during this process. Peripheral vasoconstriction may reduce blood flow from core to periphery, which will increase pooling of blood in the core and cause subsequent hyperthermia. This cooling method was not necessary for Mrs Bushiza.

The respiratory rate and depth were observed for signs of fluid overload.

All care was explained to Mrs Bushiza.

Mrs Bushiza was positioned comfortably in bed and a pain assessment was undertaken to assess the degree of arthritic pain.

Blood pressure and pulse rate, amplitude and rhythm were taken hourly to assess the effectiveness of the interventions.

Oral hygiene was provided to decrease the risk of mouth infection and provide comfort.

Urinary output was monitored and measured to assess the 24-hourly output. Fluid replacement restores normal urine volumes. Fluid balance charts were used to document all fluid intake and fluid loss.

Capillary refill was measured: pressure is placed on a vein and refill slower than 3 s is indicative of fluid deficit.

Mrs Bushiza's weight was measured.

Oral fluids and diet were introduced when her nausea decreased.

The key messages in reducing heat exhaustion are listed in Box 18.3.

Case study 18.3

Information provided

Mrs Bushiza responded well to both nursing and medical interventions, but prior to discharge it was felt that she would benefit from being aware of various strategies to reduce the risk of heat-related disorders. Her daughter was invited to attend the discussion. There were many influencing factors that could have predisposed Mrs Bushiza to heat exhaustion, including the heatwave, immobility, sitting by the window and taking inadequate fluids. The following information was discussed with Mrs Bushiza and her daughter and they were encouraged to ask any questions.

The information included:

- The importance of maintaining a good fluid intake and increasing amounts during hot weather, even when not thirsty. Recommendations for intake are 2.5 l or eight glasses a day. Drinks should include water, fruit juices and tea. However, reduce drinks containing caffeine as these have a dehydrating effect
- Iced cold water is often less tolerated and only sips are usually taken. Water at room temperature is better tolerated
- If the urine looks more concentrated than usual, increase the amount of fluids taken
- Eat small light meals and more frequently than usual
- Wear clothes that are loose-fitting and light in weight
- Ensure adequate ventilation. It is advisable not to sit by the window on hot days, but in a cooler area of the flat
- Stay inside or in the shade outside
- Use a fan and open windows. Clothing can be moistened (Box 18.4)
- Caregivers should note whether the person is sweating in the hot weather; if not, it could indicate heat illness
- Keep in touch with other people during heatwaves

(Drawn from Keatinge 2003 and McCloskey 2003)

Box 18.1   Heat exhaustion

Signs and symptoms may include:
- Dizziness
- Weakness
- Malaise
- Fatigue
- Myalgias and muscle cramp
- Nausea and vomiting
- Sweating may be present or absent
- Tachycardia and orthostatic changes in blood pressure
- Headache
- Irritability
- Core temperature less than 41°C

Box 18.2   Heat stroke

Signs and symptoms may include:
- Central nervous system dysfunction, including hallucinations, altered mental status, disorientation, confusion and coma
- Anhydrosis
- Nausea and vomiting
- Hyperdynamic circulation, including a tachycardia with an increase in pulse pressure, decreased cardiac output, decreased diastolic blood pressure
- Coagulation disorders
- Oliguria, anuria, haematuria
- Skin is hot and dry
- Increase in respiratory rate and respiratory alkalosis
- Temperature is usually above 41°C

CONCLUSION

This chapter has considered some of the important issues concerning temperature homeostasis in older people. The majority of older people are more than able to maintain a normal body temperature under most circumstances. Our emphasis has been on low body temperatures because this is a particular concern in the UK. However, health professionals should not forget other situations where the thermoregulatory systems can be stressed. For example, low body temperatures are a problem during and after surgery owing to the mode of action of anaesthetic drugs and physical exposure. Even hot or cold baths could be stressors for some vulnerable individuals.

Box 18.3   Key interventions to reduce heat exhaustion

- Cool environment
- Rest
- Replace fluids
- Cooling methods

Box 18.4   Reducing heat in buildings

Keatinge (2003) advises the use of a fan, open windows and moistening clothing as ways of reducing heat-related disorders. These interventions are effective because the moistening of clothing can substitute for sweat and air movement allows for heat loss through evaporation and convection.

Wolfe (2003) argues that fans are only effective when there is low to normal humidity; in high humidity, fans are not an effective cooling method, and cool showers or baths are advised. Air-conditioned buildings are of benefit.

The Centers for Disease Control and Prevention of Heat Related Mortality in Chicago (1995, cited in Wolfe 2003) warn that fans lose their protectiveness in ambient temperatures above 32°C when humidity is greater than 35% because air movement created by the fan is associated with heat-related disorders.

Closing windows helps reduce heat (Pauleau 2003), though Keatinge (2003) would argue that the increased heat production from cooking and people occupancy means that closing the windows can increase indoor heat.

Recommended reading

Collins K 2003 Temperature homeostasis. In: Grimley Evans J, Franklin Williams T, Beattie B, Michel J, Wilcock G (eds) Oxford textbook of geriatric medicine, 2nd edn. Oxford University Press, Oxford.

This book contains a chapter on temperature homeostasis and reviews the mechanisms of heat loss and heat gain. It presents an overview of hyperthermia together with proposed causes, clinical features and management.

Department of Health 2003/2004 Keep warm, keep well: winter guide. Department of Health, London.

An important summary of the important issues, written for the general public, with fact sheets detailing financial help, advice on keeping warm, health issues and where to get help and advice.

Donaldson G, Kovats R, Keatinge W, McMichael D 2001 Overview of climate change: impacts on human health in the UK. In: Health effects of climate change in the UK: an expert review for comment. Department of Health, London, chapter 4.

This chapter reviews the proposed impact of both high and low temperature on the individual, and the significance of climate change on morbidity and heat-related and cold-related deaths. Although not entirely focused on older people, the implications for the older person are stressed throughout.

Rooney C, McMichael J, Kovats R, Coleman M 1998 Excess mortality in England and Wales, and in Greater London, during the 1995 heatwave. Journal of Epidemiology and Community Health 52: 482–486.

This paper reviewed the mortality figures (of England and Wales) during the heatwave of 1995 and compared them with the 1993/94 figures. Examination of the data showed an increase in mortality during the heatwave with an increased incidence of cerebrovascular and respiratory disease. The mortality figures were compared with those of Greater London and the incidence of excess deaths was greatest in this urban population. It is well documented that during cold weather spells there is an excess death rate. This study demonstrates the deleterious effects that heatwaves can have on a population, and how climate changes may influence the nation's health.

Wicks M 1978 Old and cold: hypothermia and social policy. Heinemann, London.

A classic text reporting the national study of hypothermia in older people conducted in 1972, looking at the number suffering in cold homes and low body temperatures during the winter months. This was the first such study and brought to the public's attention the plight of the old in cold weather.

Wilkinson P, Landon M, Armstrong B et al. 2001 Cold comfort: the social and environmental determinants of excess winter deaths in England 1986–1996. Joseph Rowntree Foundation, The Policy Press, London.

A readable and informative report, the objectives set out to review the 'relationship between the housing quality, socio-economic status and excess winter mortality'. The report also examines whether housing conditions modify the relationship between daily mortality and low outdoor temperature. The findings, although not conclusive, lead the authors to propose that indoor temperature and, significantly, the age of the property (those built before 1850 being less thermally efficient than those properties built after 1980) increase the vulnerability of individuals to winter death from cardiovascular disease. The findings lead the authors to focus on the social policy implications, as these, rather than physiological or pathophysiological ones, will deliver greater benefits to public health.

References

Age Concern 2002 Hypothermia and excess winter deaths. Policy unit reference 2501. Age Concern, London

Age Concern 2004 Hypothermia and excess winter deaths. Policy unit reference 0104. Age Concern, London

Ahkee S, Srinath L, Ramirez J 1997 Community acquired pneumonia in the elderly: association of mortality with lack of fever and leucocytosis. Southern Medical Journal 90: 296–298

Arndt K 1999 Inadvertent hypothermia in the OR. AORN 70: 204–218

Ballester J, Harchelroad F 1999 Hyperthermia: how to recognise and prevent heat-related illnesses. Geriatrics 54: 20–24

Bastow M, Rawlings J, Allison S 1983 Undernutrition, hypothermia and injury in older women with fractured femur. Lancet i: 143–146

Beisel WR, Wannemacher RW, Neufeld HA 1980 Relation of fever to energy expenditure assessment of energy metabolism health and disease. Report of the first Ross conference on medical research. Ross Laboratories, Columbus, OH

Bender BS, Scarpace P 1997 Fever in the elderly. In: Mackowiak PA (ed) Fever: basic mechanisms and management, 2nd edn. Lippincott-Raven, Philadelphia, PA, 363–373

Bernheim H, Block LH, Atkins E 1979 Fever, pathogenesis, pathophysiology and purpose. Annals of Internal Medicine 91: 261–270

Bruce JL, Grove SK 1992 Fever: pathology and treatment. Critical Care Nurse 12: 10–49

BTS guidelines for management of community acquired pneumonia in adults – 2004 update. Available online at: www.brit-thoracic.org/docs/ MACAPrevised. april/ 04pdf

Bull GM, Morton J 1978 Environment, temperature and death rates. Age and Ageing 7: 210–224

Bush H, Hydo L, Fisher E 1995 Hypothermia during elective abdominal aortic aneurysm repair: the high price of avoiding mortality. Journal of Vascular Surgery 21: 392–402

Bynom S 1998 Adding OC to old shouldn't read cold. British Journal of Theatre Nursing 8: 9–14

Castle M 1979 Fever: Understanding a sinister sign. Nursing 9: 27–33

Castle SC, Yeh M, Norman DC 1991 Fever response in the elderly: are the older truly colder? Journal of American Geriatric Society 39: 853–857

Castle SC, Yeh M, Toledo S 1993 Lowering the temperature criterion improves detection of infection in nursing home residents. Ageing Immunology Infectious Disease 4: 67–76

Chan E, Fernandez E 2001 The challenge of pneumonia in the elderly. Journal of Respiratory Diseases 22: 139–148

Closs SJ, Macdonald IA, Hawthorn PJ 1986 Factors affecting perioperative body temperature. Journal of Advanced Nursing 11: 739–744

Coleshaw SR, Easton JC, Keatinge WR, Floyer MA, Garrard J 1986 Hypothermia in emergency admissions in cold weather. Clinical Science 70: 93P–94P

Collins KJ 1987a Physiological changes in the older predisposing to hypothermia. In: Maudgal DP (ed) Hypothermia: medical and social aspects. Pergamon, Oxford, pp 7–15

Collins KJ 1987b Effects of cold on old people. British Journal of Hospital Medicine 6: 506–514

Collins KJ 1988 Hypothermia in the older. Health Visitor 61: 50–51

Collins KJ 1992 Temperature homeostasis and thermal stress, In: Grimley Evans J, Williams TF (eds) Oxford textbook of geriatric medicine. Oxford Medical Publications, Oxford, pp 93–100

Collins KJ 1996 Heat stress and associated disorders. In: Cook GC (ed) Manson's tropical diseases, 20th edn. WB Saunders, London, pp 421–432

Collins K 2003 Temperature homeostasis In: Grimley Evans J, Franklin Williams T, Beattie B, Michel J, Wilcock G (eds) Oxford textbook of geriatric medicine. Oxford University Press, Oxford, pp 852–856

Collins KJ, Easton JC, Exton-Smith AN 1981a Shivering thermogenesis and vasomotor responses with convective cooling in the older. Journal of Physiology 320: 76P

Collins KJ, Exton-Smith AN, Dore C 1981b Urban hypothermia: preferred temperature and thermal perception in old age. British Medical Journal 282: 175–177

Collins KJ, Easton JC, Belfield-Smith H, Exton-Smith AN, Pluck RA 1985 Effects of age on body temperature and blood pressure in cold environments. Clinical Science 69: 465–470

Collins KJ, Abdel-Rahman TA, Goodwin J, McTiffin L 1995 Circadian body temperatures and the effects of a cold stress in older and young subjects. Age and Ageing 24: 485–489

Conte HA, Chen Y, Mehal W 1999 A prognostic rule for elderly patients admitted with community acquired pneumonia. American Journal of Medicine 106: 20–28

Curwen M 1991 Excess winter mortality: a British phenomenon? Health Trends 22: 169–175

Darowski A, Najim Z, Weinberg J, Guz A 1991 The febrile response to mild infection in older hospital in-patients. Age and Ageing 20: 193–198

Davis-Smith J 1978 Mechanisms and manifestations of fever. American Journal of Nursing 11: 1874–1877

Department of Health 2003/2004a Keep warm, keep well. Available online at: www.doh.gov.uk/kwkw/booklet-3.htm

Department of Health 2003/2004b Keep warm, keep well. Available online at: www.doh.gov.uk/kwkw/booklet-2.htm

Department of Health 2004 Heatwave – plan for England: protecting health and reducing harm from extreme heat and heatwaves. Available online at: www.dh.gov.uk/ PublicationsAndStatistics/Publications/PublicationsPoli cyAndGuidance/PublicationsPolicyAndGuidanceArticle /fs/en?CONTENT_ID=4086874&chk=opuHhJ

Docherty JR 1990 Cardiovascular responses in aging: a review Pharmacological Review 42: 103–125

Donaldson GC, Keatinge WR 1997 Early increases in ischaemic heart mortality dissociated from, and later associated with, respiratory mortality, cold weather in south east England. Journal of Epidemiology and Community Health 51: 643–648

El Gamal N, El-Kassabany N, Frank S et al. 2000 Age related thermoregulatory differences in a warm operating room environment. Anesthesia and Analgesia 90: 694–698

Enwright A, Plowes D 1999 Inadvertent hypothermia is it just a perioperative problem? Nursing Standard 14: 46–47

Eurowinter Group: Donaldson GC, Keatinge WR 1997 Cold exposure and winter mortality from ischaemic heart disease, cerebrovascular disease, respiratory disease, and all causes in warm and cold regions of Europe. Lancet 349: 1341–1346

Eurowinter Group: Donaldson GC, Ermakov SP, Komarov Y, McDonald CP, Keatinge WR 1998 Cold related mortalities and protection against cold in Yakutsk, eastern Siberia: observational and interview study. British Medical Journal 317: 978–982

Falcoa JM, Valente P 1997 Cerbrovascular disease in Portugal: some epidemiological aspects. Acta Medica Portugesa 10: 537–542

Falsey A 2003 Epidemiology of infectious disease. In: Grimley Evans J, Franklin Williams T, Beattie B, Michel J, Wilcock G (eds) Oxford textbook of geriatric medicine, 2nd edn. Oxford University Press, Oxford, pp 55–63

Farina C, Arosio M, Vailati F, Moioli F, Goglio A 2002 Urinary detection of *Streptococcus pneumoniae* antigen for diagnosis of pneumonia. New Microbiologica 25: 259–263

Fein A 1999 Pneumonia in the elderly: overview of diagnostic and therapeutic approaches. Clinical Infectious Diseases 28: 726–729

Feldman C 1999 Pneumonia in the elderly. Clinics in Chest Medicine 20: 563–573

Fellows IW, MacDonald IA, Bennett T, Allison SP 1985 The effect of undernutrition on thermoregulation in the older. Clinical Science 69: 525–532

Finkelstein M, Petkun W, Metal F 1983 Pneumococcal bacteremia in adults: age dependent differences in presentation and outcome. Journal of the American Geriatrics Society 31: 19–27

Flores-Maldonada A, Guzman-Llanez Y, Castaneda-Zarate S et al. 1997 Risk factors for mild intraoperative hypothermia. Archives of Medical Research 28: 587–590

Fossum S, Hays J, Henson M 2001 A comparison study on the effects of prewarming patients in the outpatient surgery setting. Journal of Peri Anesthesia Nursing 16: 187–194

Fox RH 1974 Temperature regulation with special reference to man. In: Linden RJ (ed) Recent advances in physiology no. 9. Churchill Livingstone, Edinburgh, pp 340–405

Fox RH, MacGibbon R, Davies L, Woodward PM 1973a Problem of the old and the cold. British Medical Journal 1: 21

Fox RH, Woodward PM, Exton-Smith AN et al. 1973b Body temperatures in the older: a national study of physiological, social and environmental conditions. British Medical Journal 1: 200–206

Fox RH, Macdonald IC, Woodward PM 1973c A hypothermia survey kit. Journal of Physiology 228: 4P–6P

Frank SN, Beattie C, Chriopherson T 1992 Epidural versus general anaesthesia, ambient operating room temperature, patient age as predictors of inadvertent hypothermia. Anesthesiology 77: 252–257

Frank SN, Higgins MS, Breslow M et al. 1995 The catecholamine, cortisol and hemodynamic responses to mild perioperative hypothermia. Anesthesiology 82: 83–93

Frank SN, El-Gamal N, Raja SN, Wu PK 1996 Alpha-adrenoceptor mechanisms of thermoregulation during cold challenge in humans Clinical Science 91: 627–631

Frank SN, Fleisher LA, Breslow MJ 1997 Perioperative maintenance of normothermia reduces the incidence of morbid cardiac events: a randomized clinical trial. Journal of the American Medical Association 277: 1127–1134

Frank SN, Raja SN, Bulaco C 1999 Relative contribution of core and cutaneous temperature to thermal comfort and autonomic responses in humans. Journal of Applied Physiology 86: 1588–1598

Fritsch D 1995 Hypothermia in the trauma patient. AACN Clinical Issue 6: 196–211

Fukagawa NK, Viers H, Langeloh G 1995 Acute effects of fructose and glucose ingestion with and without caffeine in young and old humans. Metabolism 44: 630–638

Gilbert M, Barton A, Counsell M 2002 Comparison of oral and tympanic temperatures in adult surgical patients. Applied Nursing Research 15: 42–47

Giuliano K, Scott SS, Elliott S, Guiliano AJ 1999 Temperature measurement in critically ill orally intubated adults: a comparison of pulmonary artery core temperature, tympanic and oral methods. Critical Care Medicine 27: 2188–2193

Goldberg MJ, Roe CF 1966 Temperature changes during anaesthesia and operations. Archives of Surgery 93: 365–369

Goldman A, Exton-Smith AN, Francis G, O'Brien A 1977 A pilot study of low body temperatures in old people admitted to hospital. Journal of the Royal College of Physicians 11: 291–306

Greif R, Akca O, Horn E, Kurz A, Sessler DI 2000 Research group: supplemental perioperative oxygen to reduce the incidence of surgical wound infection. New England Journal of Medicine 342: 161–167

Greisman SE 1997 Cardiovascular alternations during fever. In: Mackowiak PA (ed) Fever: basic mechanisms and management, 2nd edn. Lippincott-Raven, Philadelphia, PA, pp 143–163

Grossman S, Bautista C, Sullivan L 2002 Using evidence based practice to develop a protocol for postoperative surgical intensive care unit patients. Dimensions of Critical Care Nursing 21: 206–213

Grundy E, Holt G 2001 The socioeconomic status of older adults: how should we measure it in studies of health inequalities? Journal of Epidemiology and Community Health 55: 895–904

Hajat A, Kovats R, Atkinson R, Haines A 2002 Impact of hot temperatures on death in London: a time series approach. Journal of Epidemiology and Community Health 56: 367–372

Healy JD 2003 Excess winter mortality in Europe: a cross country analysis identifying key risk factors. Journal of Epidemiology and Community Health 57: 784–789

Hislop L, Wyatt J, McNaughton G et al. 1995 Urban hypothermia in the west of Scotland. British Medical Journal 311: 725

Holtzclaw BJ 1992 The febrile response in critical care: state of the science. Heart and Lung 21: 482–501

Hynson JM, Sessler DI, Moayeri A, McGuire J, Schroeder M 1993 The effects of pre-induction warming on temperature and blood pressure during propofol/nitrous oxide anesthesia. Anesthesiology 79: 219–228

Jarvis C, Hancock R, Askham J, Tinker A 1996 Getting around after 60: a profile of Britain's older population. HMSO, London

Just B, Trevien V, Delva E, Lienhart A 1993 Prevention of intraoperative hypothermia by preoperative skin-surface warming. Anesthesiology 79: 214–218

Keating MJ, Klimek JJ, Leveine DS 1984 Effects of ageing on the clinical significance of fever in ambulatory adult patients. Journal of American Geriatric Society 32: 282–287

Keatinge WR 1986 Seasonal mortality among older people with unrestricted home heating. British Medical Journal 293: 732–733

Keatinge WR 1987 Hazards of cold weather. In: Maudgal DP (ed) Hypothermia: medical and social aspects. Pergamon, Oxford, pp 3–5

Keatinge W 2003 Death in heatwaves. British Medical Journal 327: 1228b

Keatinge WR, Coleshaw SRK, Cotter F, Mattock M, Chelliah R 1984 Increases in platelets and red cell counts, blood viscosity, and arterial pressure during mild surface cooling: factors in winter mortality from coronary and cerebral thrombosis in winter. British Medical Journal 289: 1405–1408

Keatinge WR, Donaldson GC, Butcher K et al. 1997 Cold exposure and winter mortality from ischaemic heart disease, cerebrovascular disease, respiratory disease, and all causes in warm and cold regions of Europe. Lancet 349: 1341–1346

Kenney RA 1989 Physiology of ageing: a synopsis, 2nd edn. Year Book, Chicago

Kenney L, Chiu P 2000 Influences of age on thirst and fluid intake. Medicine and Science in Sports and Exercise 33: 1524–1532

Kettner SC, Kozek SA, Groetzner JP et al. 1998 Effects of hypothermia on thermoelastography in patients undergoing cardiopulmonary bypass. British Journal of Anaesthesia 80: 313–317

Kunihiro A, Foster JDR 1998 Heat exhaustion and heat stroke. Available online at: www.emedicine.com/EMERG/topic236.htm

Kunihiro A, Foster J 2002 Heat exhaustion and heatstroke. Available online at: www.emedicine.com/EMERG/topic236.htm (accessed 20 February 2004)

Kunst AE, Looman CW, Mackenbach JP 1993 Outdoor air temperature and mortality in the Netherlands: a time series analysis. American Journal of Epidemiology 137: 331–341

Kurz A, Kurz M, Poeschl G 1993 Forced-air warming maintains intraoperative normothermia better than circulating water mattresses. Anesthesia and Analgesia 77: 89–95

Kurz A, Sessler DI, Lenhardt R 1996 Perioperative normothermia to reduce the incidence of surgical-wound infection and shorten hospitalization. New England Journal of Medicine 334: 1209–1215

Laszlo A, Sprung J, Polic S 1990 Effects of hypothermia and potassium variations on maximum diastolic potential. Anesthesiology 73: A263

Latman N 2003 Clinical thermometry: possible causes and potential solutions to electronic, digital thermometer inaccuracies. Biomedical Instrumentation and Technology 37: 190–196

Latman NS, Hans P, Nicholson L et al. 2001 Evaluation of clinical thermometers for accuracy and reliability. Biomedical Instrumentation and Technology 35: 259–265

Lawlor DA, Maxwell R, Wheeler BW 2002 Rurality deprivation, and excess winter mortality. Journal of Epidemiology and Community Health 56: 373–374

Lean M, James P 1986 Brown adipose tissue in man. In: Trayhun P, Nicholls D (eds) Brown adipose tissue. Edward Arnold, London, pp 339–365

Ledingham I, McA Mone JG 1980 Treatment of accidental hypothermia: a prospective clinical study. British Medical Journal 28: 1102–1105

Leinonen T, Leino-Kilpi H, Jouko K 1996 The quality of intraoperative nursing care: the patient's perspective. Journal of Advanced Nursing 24: 843–852

Lim WS, van der Eerden MM, Laing R et al. 2003 Defining community acquired pneumonia severity on presentation to hospital: an internal derivation and validation study. Thorax 58: 377–382

Lloyd EL 1986 Hypothermia and cold stress. Croom Helm, London

Mackowiak PA 2002 Diagnostic implications and clinical consequences of antipyretic therapy. Clinical Infectious Disease 31: 230–233

Maclean D 1987 Emergency management of hypothermia: a review. Journal of the Royal Society of Medicine 79: 528–531

Maclean D, Emslie-Smith D 1977 Accidental hypothermia. Blackwell Scientific, Oxford

MacMahon S, Peto R, Cutler J et al. 1990 Blood pressure, stroke, and coronary heart disease. Part 1: prolonged differences in blood pressure: prospective observational studies corrected for the regression dilution bias. Lancet 335: 765–774

Marrie TJ 1994 Community acquired pneumonia. Clinical Infectious Diseases 18: 501–515

Matsukawa T, Kurz A, Sessler DI et al. 1995 Propofol linearly reduces the vasoconstriction and shivering thresholds. Anesthesiology 82: 1169–1180

Matsuzaki Y, Matsuzaki T, Ohki K et al. 2003 Warming by resistive heating maintains perioperative normothermia as well as forced air heating. British Journal of Anaesthesia 90: 689–691

McAlpine C, Dall J 1987 Outcome after episodes of hypothermia. Age and Ageing 16: 115

McAlpine CH, Martin BJ, Lennox IM, Roberts MA 1986 Pyrexia in infection in the older. Age and Ageing 15: 230–234

McCarron K 1986 Fever – the cardinal vital sign. Critical Care Quarterly 9: 15–18

McCloskey B 2003 Ten tips for surviving summer sun. Available online at: www.dh.gov.uk/AboutUs/RelatedBodies/PublicHealthGroups/WestMidlands/W (accessed 12 November 2003)

McMichael AJ, Kovats RS 1998 Assessment of the impact on mortality in England and Wales of the heatwave and associated air pollution episode of 1976. Report to the Department of Health London. London School of Hygiene and Tropical Medicine, London

Miles JM, Thompson GR 1987 Treatment of severe accidental hypothermia using the Clinitron bed. Anaesthesia 42: 415–418

Miller D, Yoshikawa T, Castle SC 1991 The effects of age on fever responses to recombinant tumor necrosis factor alpha in a murine model. Journal of Gerontology 46: M176–M179

Monga M, Comeaux B, Roberts J 1996 Effects if irrigating fluid on perioperative temperature regulation during transurethral prostatectomy. European Urology 29: 26–28

Moore R, McIntyre T, Roper K et al. 2000 English house condition survey, 1996 energy report. Department of the Environment, Transport and Regions, London

Morgan LW 1997 Hypothermia. In: Ham JJ (ed) Primary care geriatrics: a case-based approach. Mosby, St Louis

Morris RH 1971 Operating room temperature and the anaesthetized paralysed patient. Archives of Surgery 103: 95–97

Morrison R 1988 Hypothermia in the elderly. International Anaesthiology Clinical 26: 124–130

Murdoch DR, Laing RTR, Mills GD et al. 2001 Evaluation of a rapid immunochromatographic test for detection of Streptococcus pneumoniae antigen in urine samples from adults with community-acquired pneumonia. Journal of Clinical Microbiology 39: 3495–3498

Murphy P 2003 Temperature homeostasis. In: Grimley Evans J, Franklin Williams T, Beattie B, Michel J, Wilcock G (eds) Oxford textbook of geriatric medicine, 2nd edn. Oxford University Press, Oxford, p 861

National Audit Office 2003 Warm front: helping combat fuel poverty. Report by the Comptroller and Auditor General, HC 769 session 2002–2003 June 25. National Audit Office, London

National Statistics 2003 Winter mortality. Available online at: www.statistics.gov.uk

Nayagam D, Shah S, Fairweather DS 1986 Which route for recording temperature in the old? Clinical Science 71 (suppl. 15): 16P

Negishi C, Hasegawa K, Mukai S et al. 2003 Resistive-heating and forced warming are comparably effective. Anesthesia and Analgesia 96: 1683–1687

Neild PJ, Syndercombe-Court D, Keatinge WR et al. 1994 Cold-induced increases in erythrocyte count plasma cholesterol and plasma fibrinogen of older people without a comparable rise in protein-C and factor-X. Clinical Science 86: 43–48

Neilsen H, Hasenkam JM, Pilegaard HK, Aalkjaer C, Mortensen FV 1992 Age-dependent changes in alpha-adrenoceptor mediated contractility of isolated human resistance arteries. American Journal of Physiology, Heart Circulation and Physiology 263: H1190–H1196

Norman DC 2000 Special section: aging and infectious. Disease Clinical Infectious Disease 31: 148–151

Norman DC, Yoshikawa TT 1996 Fever in the elderly. In: Cunha BA (ed) Fever. Infectious disease clinics of North America. WB Saunders, Philadelphia, PA, pp 93–101

Norman DC, Yamamura R, Yoshikawa TT 1988 Fever response in old and young mice after injection of interleukin-1. Journal of Gerontology 43: M80–M85

Oliver C 1983 Old and cold. Nursing Times 79: 8–9

Parker-Morris W 1961 Homes for today and tomorrow (Parker-Morris report). Ministry of Housing and Local Government, HMSO, London

Pattenden S, Nikiforov B, Armstrong BG 2003 Mortality and temperature in Sofia and London. Journal of Epidemiology and Community Health 57: 628–633

Pauleau A 2003 Death in heatwaves and injudiciously opening windows. British Medical Journal 327: 1228c

Pestana C 1989 Fluids and electrolytes in the surgical patient, 4th edn. Williams & Wilkins, Baltimore, MD

Rajagopalan S, Moran D 2000 Infectious disease emergencies. In: Yoshikawa TT, Norman DC (eds) Acute emergencies and critical care of the geriatric patient. Marcel Dekker, New York, pp 337–355

Ramsey J 1983 Heat and cold. In: Hockey R (ed) Stress and fatigue in human performance. Wiley, Chichester, pp 33–60

Roberts MJ 1975 Fever and survival. Science 188: 166–168

Roberts S, Bolton DM, Stoller ML 1994 Hypothermia associated with percutaneous nephrolithotomy. Urology 44: 832–835

Roghmann M, Warner MS, Mackowiak A 2001 The relationship between age and fever magnitude. American Journal of Medical Science 322: 68–70

Rooney C, McMichael AJ, Kovats RS, Coleman MP 1998 Excess mortality in Greater London, during 1995 heatwave. Journal of Epidemiology and Community Health 52: 482–486

Rosenthal TC, Silverstein CA 1988 Fever: what to do and what not to do. Post Graduate Medicine 83: 75

Royal College of Physicians 1966 Report of the committee on accidental hypothermia. Royal College of Physicians, London

Salive ME, Satterfield S, Ostfeld AM, Wallace RB, Havlik RJ 1993 Disability and cognitive impairment are risk factors for pneumonia-related mortality in older adults. Public Health Reports 108: 34–22

Salvage AV 1993 Cold comfort. A national survey of older people in cold weather. Age Concern Institute of Gerontology, research report no. 7. Age Concern England, London

Scannapieco F 1999 Role of oral bacteria in respiratory infections. Journal of Peridontology 70: 793–802

Schmied H, Kurz A, Sessler D, Kozek S, Reiter A 1996 Mild hypothermia increases blood loss and transfusion requirements during total hip arthroplasty. Lancet 347: 289–291

Schmitz T, Blair N, Falk M, Levine C 1995 A comparison of five methods of temperature measurement in febrile intensive care patients. American Journal of Critical Care 4: 286–292

Scott E, Buckland R 2004 The importance of temperature management in surgical patients. Nurse 2 Nurse Magazine 4: 59–62

Sessler DI 1994 Consequences and treatment of perioperative hypothermia. Anesthesia Clinics of North America 12: 425–456

Sessler DI 1997 Mild postoperative hypothermia. New England Journal of Medicine 336: 1730–1737

Sessler DI 2000 Perioperative heat balance. Anesthesiology 92: 578–596

Sessler DI 2001 Complications and treatment of mild hypothermia. Anesthesiology 95: 531–543

Sessler DI, Sessler AM 1998 Experimental determination of heat flow parameters during induction of general anesthesia. Anesthesiology 89: 657–665

Sessler DI, Sessler AM, Hudson S 1993 Heat loss during surgical skin preparation. Anesthesiology 78: 1055–1064

Shah S, Peacock J 1999 Deprivation and excess winter mortality. Journal of Epidemiology and Community Health 53: 499–502

Shelter 1997 Older people's housing. Cited in London research Centre Health Strategy for London rapid review on older people in London 1999. Shelter, London

Shiraki K, Konda N, Sagawa S 1988 Oesophageal and tympanic temperature responses to core blood temperature changes during hyperthermia. Journal of Applied Physiology 61: 98–102

Shua-Haim J, Ross J 2000 Pneumonia in the elderly. Clinical Geriatrics 8: 38–46

Sloan RE, Keatinge WR 1975 Depression of sublingual temperature by cold saliva. British Medical Journal 1: 718–720

Smitz S, Giagoultsis T, Dewe W, Albert A 2000 A comparison of rectal and infrared ear temperatures in older hospital inpatients. Journal of the American Geriatrics Society 48: 63–66

Stein D 1990 Managing pneumonia acquired in nursing homes: special concerns. Geriatrics 45: 39047

Stout RW, Crawford VLS, McDermott MJ, Rocks MJ, Morris TCM 1996 Seasonal changes in haemostatic factors in young and older subjects. Age and Ageing 25: 256–258

Styrt B, Sugarman B 1990 Antipyresis and fever. Archives of Internal Medicine 150: 158–159

Taylor G 1964 The problem of hypothermia in the older. Practitioner 193: 761–767

Todd MM, Warner DS 1992 A comfortable hypothesis reevaluated. Cerebral metabolic depression and brain protection during ischaemia. Anesthesiology 76: 161–164

Vankatesan P, Gladman J, Macfarlane JT 1990 A hospital study of community acquired pneumonia in the elderly. Thorax 45: 254–258

Vassallo M, Navarro G, Allen S 1995 Factors associated with high risk of marginal hyperthermia in older patients living in an institution. Postgraduate Medical Journal 71: 213–216

Vaughan MS, Vaughan RW, Cork RC 1981 Postoperative hypothermia in adult relationship of age anesthesia and shivering to rewarming. Anesthesia and Analgesia 60: 746–751

Watts AJ 1972 Hypothermia in the aged: a study of the role of cold sensitivity. Environmental Research 5: 119–126

Weiss M, Sitzer V, Clarke M et al. 1998 A comparison of temperature measurement using three ear thermometers. Applied Nursing Research 11: 158–166

Wicks M 1978 Old and cold. Hypothermia and social policy. Heinemann, London

Wilmshurst P 1994 Temperature and cardiovascular mortality. British Medical Journal 309: 1029–1030

Wolfe R 2003 Death in heatwaves: beware of fans. British Medical Journal 327: 1228b

Yoshikawa TT 1997 Perspective: aging and infectious disease: past, present, and future. Journal of Infectious Disease 176: 1053–1057

Chapter 19

Maintaining healthy skin

Gillian E. Pedley

INTRODUCTION

The skin is the part of ourselves which is visible to others and which can reflect our emotions, well-being and state of health. It performs a number of essential functions: protection, sensory, excretion, heat regulation and storage of fat and water. Normal ageing results in changes to these functions and the skin gives the most visible outward sign of this process. The effects of ageing on the skin are regarded, particularly in western societies, as negative, unwanted and to be avoided as long as possible.

The skin performs essential homeostatic, sensory and protective roles: impaired skin integrity will have an impact on these functions. Physiological, age-related changes and higher levels of morbidity in later life make the older person more vulnerable to skin damage, particularly from unrelieved pressure. Pressure damage occurs most commonly in those who are physically compromised and confined to bed or chair; it may delay a person's rehabilitation and if severe, have a devastating effect on recovery from illness.

Maintenance and restoration of healthy skin require a sophisticated knowledge base and the coordinated involvement of a range of health care professionals. This chapter provides an overview of general skin assessment in the older adult. Current knowledge on the causes of pressure damage, predisposing risk factors and risk assessment of the client is discussed. The principles of pressure ulcer prevention and related research evidence are considered, including the selection of support surfaces, seating and issues relating to education and practice development. An overview of wound healing and principles of wound management is given in the final section.

As well as performing sensory and homeostatic functions, the skin reflects systemic functioning. Assessment is therefore not just an appraisal of the functioning and integrity of the skin, but provides a visible summary of internal functioning. It can also indicate the ability to attend to personal care needs and indirectly reveal clues as to the client's level of functional ability. Skin assessment requires an understanding of normal changes in the skin and an ability to distinguish normal age-related changes from abnormal skin lesions and from signs of systemic disease in need of treatment. The assessment should include the past and present skin history, skin changes, medication and a visual assessment (Box 19.1).

Skin lesions are common in older people and observation should be made of their location, their structural characteristics, their size, colour and grouping. New lesions or lesions that have undergone changes and that are asymmetrical, have irregular borders, variable pigmentation or mottled appearance and if 6 mm or more in diameter will require further investigation. For a practical account of skin assessment of the older client, see McGovern & Kwaiser Kuhn (1992).

One of the greatest threats to skin integrity in the sick or frail older person is tissue necrosis and ulcera-

Box 19.1   Framework for the visual assessment of skin: key assessment areas, common findings and their possible significance

Colour and altered pigmentation
- Bruising/petechiae: vitamin deficiency; bleeding disorder; trauma
- Cyanosis: cardiovascular and/or pulmonary insufficiency
- Jaundice: gastrointestinal disease
- Pallor: anaemia; reduced vascularity; arterial insufficiency of limb
- Erythema: inflammation/infection; pressure-induced ischaemia
- Ankle flare, staining of lower limbs and varicosities: chronic venous hypertension/venous insufficiency

Texture
- Smooth, atrophic skin: arterial insufficiency
- Coarse skin: hypothyroidism
- Dry skin: reduced sebum and water content of skin

Turgor/oedema
- Reduced elasticity and resilience: reduced collagen; reduced hydration
- Taut, shiny and reduced skin mobility: oedema

Temperature
- Difference between trunk and extremities: maintenance of core and peripheral temperature
- Difference between lower limbs: vascular insufficiency
- Elevated temperature: inflammation; hyperthyroidism
- Low temperature: low core temperature; hypothyroidism

Lesions/rashes/scars/areas of discontinuity
- New growths: normal age-related changes; abnormal lesions
- Eczema: arthritis; chronic venous insufficiency
- Infection: bacterial; viral; fungal
- Cuts; abrasions
- Pressure ulcers and blisters
- Leg ulcers: venous/arterial insufficiency
- Rashes

Hygiene
- Odour: poor hygiene; self-care ability; loss of continence; infection
- Condition of skinfolds, feet, nails, genitalia and perianal area: self-care ability
- Infestation: head lice; body lice; scabies

tion due to sustained, unrelieved pressure. For this reason, skin assessment in this client group must include an inspection of the skin for early signs of pressure damage and pressure ulcers.

PRESSURE ULCERS

The Health of the Nation discussion document (Department of Health 1992) estimated a 6.7% pressure ulcer prevalence amongst UK hospital patients, with an estimated treatment cost of £60 million per year. Other sources have reported higher rates (O'Dea 1993). Hos-

pital treatment costs for pressure ulcers in England are between £180 million and £312 million (Department of Health 1993), with the treatment of a grade 4 pressure ulcer costing £40 000 (Collier 1999). Prevention can be equally expensive.

Pressure ulcers are localized soft-tissue injuries caused primarily by unrelieved pressure, shear or friction, or a combination of these. If sufficiently sustained, these mechanical stressors will impair the local microcirculation and will result in ischaemic changes or necrosis in the tissues served by the affected vessels. Visible skin changes occur, ranging from redness to localized tissue death and ulceration of the skin, sub-cutaneous fat and muscle.

Pressure ulcers can occur at all stages of the life cycle in both healthy individuals (for example, blisters from new shoes) and, most significantly, in those who are physically compromised and confined to bed or chair. The likelihood of disease and disability increases with advancing age; normal age-related changes also make soft tissues less resistant to pressure. For these reasons the occurrence of pressure-induced tissue damage is more common amongst the older population.

Aetiology: maintaining tissue perfusion

Tissue perfusion depends on an intact microcirculation; this is fundamental in maintaining tissue integrity and preventing pressure ulcers. The following section reviews the physiology of the microcirculation and its response to pressure, relevant soft-tissue anatomy and the impact of the ageing process on these.

Microcirculation

The microcirculation comprises arterioles, venules, thoroughfare vessels (metarterioles) and capillaries. The capillary walls are one cell thick and formed from endothelial cells. Their thin structure facilitates the diffusion of gases, nutrients and metabolites. This exchange of nutrients and waste products between the blood and tissues is achieved by an intermittent flow and stasis of blood through the capillaries and is controlled by the precapillary sphincters, their action mediated by the chemical composition of the capillary blood. When the sphincters are closed, blood flow ceases and an exchange of nutrients, oxygen, carbon dioxide and metabolites occurs. This accumulation of metabolites and carbon dioxide and a fall in oxygen triggers relaxation of the precapillary sphincters and oxygenated blood flows into the capillary, flushing out the deoxygenated blood and waste products.

Capillary blood pressure ranges from 32 mmHg at the arteriolar end of the capillary to 12 mmHg at the venous end. These values will vary according to systolic blood pressure and other factors influencing blood pressure. Compression of the microcirculation by external forces in excess of capillary pressure will, in theory, impede blood flow but the soft tissues and the microcirculation contained within are exposed to external pressures in excess of capillary pressure on a daily basis. A number of inbuilt anatomical and physiological mechanisms enable the soft tissues to resist the effects of pressure without incurring lasting ischaemic changes and cell damage: autoregulation, reactive hyperaemia, anatomical structures and pain.

Autoregulation

In response to external pressure, a process of autoregulation enables capillary pressure to rise and stabilize 10 mmHg above the external pressure, up to the pressure of the diastolic blood pressure. This protective response may be less dramatic in hypotensive clients and may be absent in those who develop ulcers (Schubert 1991).

Reactive hyperaemia

External pressure sufficient to occlude capillary blood flow will result in ischaemia and an accumulation of carbon dioxide, hydrogen ions and metabolites which produce local arteriolar dilatation. Removal of the external occluding pressure causes the dilated capillaries to experience a sudden increased blood flow which may be up to 30 times its resting value (Lamb et al. 1991). This increased blood flow, known as reactive hyperaemia, is visible on the skin as a clearly demarcated pink/red 'flush'. The reactive hyperaemic response lasts between half to three-quarters of the occlusion time; thus, clinical observation of the hyperaemic response gives an indication of the duration of ischaemia and the extent of the area affected. The patency of the capillaries in the affected area can be assessed by the application of light finger pressure to the hyperaemic area. Application of such pressure occludes the capillaries and this can be observed as a whitening of the area upon removal of the pressure – blanching hyperaemia. The white area rapidly turns deep pink as the capillaries refill with blood.

Anatomical structures

The structures of the dermis are supported in a matrix of collagen and elastin which protects blood and lymph vessels, nerves, glands and hair follicles against mechanical damage. Collagen has little extensibility but has high strength and resists deformation. Elastin has elastic properties and enables tissues to recover their shape after being stretched. Thus, collagen and elastin protect the tissues from the effects of pressure. The loose connective tissue underlying the dermis is composed primarily of fat cells. It is compressible, provides padding over bony prominences and permits the movement of the dermis over deeper structures. It contains little collagen and therefore lacks tensile strength and is vulnerable to mechanical stressors. Underlying the subcutaneous layer and surrounding the muscle is the fascia. Its high collagen content provides resistance to distortion and protects the soft muscle layer. The ageing process affects these protective mechanisms and makes the tissues less resistant to mechanical forces. For example, collagen synthesis gradually declines with age between the ages of 20 and 60 years, with a marked decline thereafter, and there is a steady fall in the total collagen from the age of 30 years (Hall et al. 1974, 1981). As collagen is removed from tissues more load is transmitted to the interstitial fluid and the cells. Elastin content of the tissues also declines (Krouskop 1983). Changes such as these may explain why epidemiological data reveal positive relationships between pressure ulcer development and increasing age.

Pain

Intact sensation and the ability to carry out spontaneous changes in position to alleviate pressure and redistribute weight are important protective mechanisms. A healthy person changes position approximately once every 15 min during sleep. These spontaneous body movements are triggered by the sensation of discomfort and pain from compressed ischaemic tissues. This continuous cycle of spontaneous movement relieves pressure deformation and permits reperfusion of the affected area, preventing permanent damage. Any neurological condition that impairs sensation or movement, including anaesthesia, sedation and mental ill health, will impair this protective mechanism. Neurological disorders are more common amongst older adults.

Aetiology: the role of sustained pressure, shear and friction

Excessive body loading, either as a perpendicular force or as shear, is widely acknowledged as the primary cause of pressure-induced necrosis. The role of pressure, shear and friction in the aetiology of pressure damage is outlined below.

Pressure

At levels exceeding capillary pressure, a load or force applied at right angles to the body acts to compress and occlude the blood supply, causing ischaemia. Accumulation of toxic metabolic by-products increases the rate of cell death; the surviving ageing cells are compromised and more susceptible to damage by mechanical forces such as pressure, hence persistent sustained pressure is more likely to result in tissue necrosis.

The hypoxia and accumulated metabolites act on the precapillary sphincters to trigger a marked hyperaemic response upon removal of the occluding pressure. This increases the amount of fluid which filters through the capillary wall into the interstitial space. Excess interstitial fluid is normally removed by lymph vessels, but under hypoxic conditions lymphatic

smooth muscle may be damaged, leading to loss of lymph motility and impaired lymph flow (Krouskop 1983). In addition to the effects of metabolic waste products on cells, the excess fluid separating capillaries from cells will make it more difficult for capillary oxygen to reach the tissues.

Application of pressure may cause interstitial fluid to be squeezed from between the cells, resulting in cell-to-cell contact pressure, known as the squeeze effect. This may be of sufficient magnitude to cause cell rupture. A sudden reduction in interstitial pressure associated with removal of the externally applied pressure, coupled with the rise in capillary pressure from the hyperaemic response, may result in capillary bursting. Damage to the lymph system will prevent removal of the products of capillary bursting from the interstitial space and this is thought to contribute to cell necrosis (Krouskop 1983). A reduction in the amount of collagen fibres in the tissues, as occurs with ageing, reduces the resistance to the squeeze effect.

Clinical signs of pressure-induced damage include a clearly defined, dull-red area of non-blanching hyperaemia overlying the pressure point, with associated oedema, induration or blister formation. Failure to relieve the pressure source will cause tissue necrosis to extend inwards through the dermis, into the subcutaneous layer, fascia and eventually the muscle.

Shear

Shear occurs when lateral forces are applied to the tissues, in conjunction with pressure, to create an opposite parallel sliding movement. As soft tissues are dragged over the rigid skeleton they are stretched and distorted. This commonly occurs when gravity causes a patient to slide down the bed or chair; the frictional forces of the skin against the chair surface cause the outer layers of tissues to remain static whilst the skeleton and deeper tissues slide forwards. The extent to which the tissues are subject to shearing depends on their consistency and structure. For example, the subcutaneous layer contains adipose tissue which provides padding and dissipates pressure but lacks tensile strength. Consequently, it provides little resistance to mechanical forces, and its mobility makes it particularly prone to shear. In contrast, the high collagen content of the underlying tough, firm fascia, and to a lesser extent the overlying dermis, enable these structures to resist mechanical deformation. It is at the interface of the subcutaneous layer and the fascia that the effects of shear are most pronounced, due to the angulation and distortion of the arterioles as they leave the mobile fat layer to penetrate the tough fascia. Disruption of the endothelial cells through angulation triggers the clotting process; platelets accumulate in the damaged vessels, causing occlusion and necrosis of the cells dependent on the vessel's blood supply. As this process usually occurs deep within the tissues, large areas of necrosis can occur with little initial outward sign other than discolouration of the overlying skin. Eventual skin breakdown reveals an often substantial area of necrotic tissue.

While pressure is the primary cause of occlusion, animal studies have shown that the presence of shear reduces by half the amount of pressure required to cause tissue damage (Bennett et al. 1979). Pressure combined with shear is therefore more damaging and this has important clinical implications for the moving, handling and positioning of patients, and in the choice of seating. Older people in particular tend to experience higher levels of shear whilst sitting (Bennett et al. 1981).

Friction

Friction may injure the epidermis and dermis, making these structures less resistant to pressure, or it may act in conjunction with shear and/or pressure as described above.

The preceding discussion illustrates how age-related changes reduce soft-tissue tolerance to pressure, making the older body more vulnerable to pressure damage. When disease states are superimposed on these changes, it becomes apparent how the sick older person may have a greater predisposition to pressure ulcers.

Diagnosis, classification and staging

Diagnosis

Diagnosis of pressure ulcers requires an unambiguous clinical consensus definition, which distinguishes pressure-induced soft-tissue damage from other forms of tissue destruction and from the body's normal hyperaemic response to pressure. Identification of early pressure ulceration from other forms of tissue damage can be particularly difficult and prone to controversy, yet prompt recognition and intervention are critical if its progression is to be prevented. Non-blanching hyperaemia is the definition of early pressure damage promoted by the UK consensus classification of pressure ulcers (Reid & Morrison 1994), the European Pressure Ulcer Advisory Panel (EPUAP [undated]) and the American National Pressure Ulcer Advisory Panel (1983). However, erythema and blanching hyperaemia have been used by earlier authors (Torrance 1983, Johnson 1985). Further controversy surrounds the length of time hyperaemia must persist before it can be classified as the first stage of pressure damage. Some authors apply the diagnosis if redness remains after 10 min of pressure relief (Sal-

vadala et al. 1992). As the duration of hyperaemia is proportional to the length of time the tissues have been subjected to pressure, this has resulted in over-diagnosis of pressure damage (Bergstrom 1993).

Lyder (1991) favours a 2-h time limit for resolution of erythema. She argues that longer periods of time are difficult to assess objectively as it is hard to know if the patient has been kept off the area. This should be possible if the time set is 2 h because this is the frequency with which most patients are turned. Bergstrom (1993) defines stage 1 ulcers as non-blanching erythema present on the same site on two consecutive observations made more than 24 h apart.

The use of blanching and non-blanching hyperaemia as diagnostic cues is further complicated for clients with dark skin. Heavily pigmented skin masks the pink/red hue of the hyperaemic response, making diagnosis of this stage of pressure damage more difficult. Alternative clinical signs indicative of early pressure damage include localized clinical purple/blue discolouration, induration, heat (due to the inflammatory process) or coolness (due to reduced perfusion in established tissue damage), oedema and/or pain (Bennett 1995).

The inconsistency in defining the early stages of pressure damage over the years has adversely affected the ability to compare findings of different studies, and accounts for the wide variations in the reporting of pressure ulcer incidence and prevalence. To eliminate error associated with misclassification some authors exclude not only blanching hyperaemia but also non-blanching hyperaemia (St Clair et al. 1995); however, it should be noted that superficial ulcers account for between 58% and 95% of all hospital-acquired sores (Allcock et al. 1994, Bridel 1995).

Ultimately, a consistent approach to the diagnosis and classification of pressure ulcers is required if nationally comparable pressure ulcer rates are to become a reality.

Classification

Numerous pressure ulcer classification or grading systems exist (Table 19.1), which are useful in the assessment of pressure ulcers, in the evaluation of treatment and for research and audit purposes.

Most current classification systems are derived from the work of Shea (1975) and describe the degree of tissue destruction (David et al. 1983, Torrance 1983, Lowthian 1987). Rather than measuring the depth of the ulcer in millimetres, classification requires the practitioner to identify the deepest layer of tissue damaged by pressure. This approach is used because individuals have differing amounts of muscle and fat, and different distributions of fat and muscle are found on different parts of the body. Thus a shallow ulcer of a heel may

Table 19.1   Pressure ulcer classification and grading systems

System and grade/stage	Definition
The Surrey system (David et al. 1983)	
Grade 1	Skin likely to break down (red, black and blistered areas)
	Healed areas still covered by a scab
Grade 2	Superficial break in the skin
Grade 3	Destruction of the skin without cavity
Grade 4	Destruction of the skin with cavity (involving underlying tissues)
The Torrance system (Torrance 1983)	
Stage 1	Blanching hyperaemia
Stage 2	Non-blanching hyperaemia
Stage 3	Ulceration progresses through the dermis
Stage 4	Lesion extends into subcutaneous fat
Stage 5	Infective necrosis penetrates down to the deep fascia
The Stirling system (UK consensus classification of pressure sore severity) (Reid & Morrison 1994)	
Stage 0	No clinical evidence of a pressure sore
0.1	Normal appearance, intact skin
0.2	Healed with scarring
0.3	Tissue damage, but not assessed as a pressure sore
Stage 1	Discolouration of intact skin – light finger pressure applied to the site does not alter the discolouration
1.1	Non-blanchable erythema with increased local heat
1.2	Blue/purple/black discolouration
Stage 2	Partial-thickness skin loss or damage involving the epidermis and/or dermis
2.1	Blister
2.2	Abrasion
2.3	Shallow ulcer without undermining of adjacent tissue
2.4	Any of the above with underlying blue/black purple discolouration or induration
Stage 3	Full-thickness skin loss involving damage or necrosis of subcutaneous tissue but not extending to underlying bone, tendon or joint capsule
3.1	Crater, without undermining of adjacent tissue
3.2	Crater, with undermining of adjacent tissue
3.3	Sinus, the full extent of which is not certain
3.4	Full-thickness skin loss, but wound bed covered with necrotic tissue which masks the true extent of tissue damage
Stage 4	Full-thickness skin loss with extensive destruction and tissue necrosis extending to underlying bone, tendon or joint capsule
4.1	Visible exposure of bone, tendon or joint capsule
4.2	Sinus assessed as extending to bone, tendon or capsule
The full classification system uses four digits	
The third digit describes the wound bed:	

Continued

Table 19.1 *Cont'd*   Pressure ulcer classification and grading systems

System and grade/stage	Definition
xx0	Not applicable, intact skin
xx1	Clean, with partial epithelialization
xx2	Clean, with or without granulation, but no obvious epithelialization
xx3	Soft slough, cream/yellow/green in colour
xx4	Hard or leathery black/brown necrotic tissue
The fourth digit classifies infective complications:	
xxx0	No inflammation surrounding the wound bed
xxx1	Inflammation surrounding the wound bed
xxx2	Cellulitis bacteriologically confirmed
The IAET system (International Association for Enterostomal Therapists 1988)	
Stage 1	Erythema not resolving within 30 min of pressure relief; epidermis remains intact; reversible with intervention
Stage 2	Partial-thickness loss of skin layers involving epidermis and possibly penetrating into but not through dermis. May present as blistering with erythema and/or induration; wound base moist and pink; painful; free of necrotic tissue
Stage 3	Full-thickness tissue loss extending through dermis to involve subcutaneous tissue. Presents as a shallow crater unless covered by eschar. May include necrotic tissue, undermining, sinus tract formation, exudate and/or infection. Wound base is usually not painful
Stage 4	Deep tissue destruction extending through subcutaneous tissue to fascia and may involve muscle layers, joint and/or bone. Presents as a deep crater. May include necrotic tissue, undermining, sinus tract formation; exudate and/or infection. Wound base is not usually painful
Shea classification (Shea 1975)	
Grade 1	Acute inflammatory reaction involving all soft-tissue layers with a moist irregular partial-thickness ulceration limited to the epidermis and exposing the underlying dermis
Grade 2	Full-thickness ulcer extending to the underlying subcutaneous fat
Grade 3	Necrotic, foul-smelling infected ulcer limited by the deep fascia but extensively involving the fat, with undermining of the skin
Grade 4	Lesion extends deep into the fascia, exposing bone and joint
Closed	Large bursa-like cavity extending to the deep pressure fascia or bone which drains through a small sore or sinus

reach the bone whilst an ulcer of similar depth located on the buttock may only reach the adipose layer. Classification requires not only visualization of the wound bed – often masked by slough and necrotic tissue – but also that the observer has sufficient knowledge to distinguish between the different tissues.

In reality, pressure ulcer gradings may not represent sequential stages in the severity of tissue damage; for example, discoloured, non-blanching unbroken skin may be the outward visible sign overlying and concealing serious pressure-induced necrosis of deep muscle, tendon and bone.

Most classifications have 4–6 stages, with a single descriptor per stage. Some systems start the scoring of grades at zero (Lowthian 1987), others at 1 (David et al. 1983, National Pressure Ulcer Advisory Panel 1983). Some include normal healthy skin as the first grade (David et al. 1983, Reid & Morrison 1994).

The need for a valid and reliable classification to enhance the quality of research and clinical practice has resulted in attempts, both in the UK and USA, to standardize the approaches used by developing a grading system by consensus agreement (National Pressure Ulcer Advisory Panel 1983). The UK consensus grading system, also termed the Stirling system (Reid & Morrison 1994), provides a four-stage system with 20 optional subcategories which add detail and function as descriptors. Although a positive step forward, there has not been widescale adoption of the scale within the UK. There is minimal literature addressing the reliability and validity of these classifications and, although the origin of these two scales suggests content and face validity, this does not guarantee their reliability, validity or ease of use.

Healey (1995) compared the interrater reliability of the Stirling, Torrance and Surrey pressure ulcer grading scales using 10 photographs of pressure ulcers. Overall, none of the three scales demonstrated great reliability. Healey's study is criticized on the grounds that it used photographs, some of which had been previously published, and that assessors need to see and touch real wounds if the assessment is to be valid and reliable. In all three scales the greatest interobserver reliability was obtained with the most severe ulcers. The lower grades, i.e. the 'superficial' ulcers, gave the least reliable levels of agreement, reaffirming that the differentiation of healthy tissue from pressure damage may be unreliable, leading to inaccurate diagnosis. Russell & Reynolds (2001) also used photographs to compare the consistency of ulcer gradings made by nurses and tissue viability specialists using the EPUAP and Stirling scales. They concluded that the EPUAP scale is simpler and more accurately used than the Stirling scale. These findings are not supported by a more recent clinically based evaluation of the EPUAP, one-digit and two-digit Stirling scales. This study used two experienced nurses to grade 35 pressure points on real patients (Pedley 2004). The study concluded that pressure ulcers were easier to grade using the two-digit Stirling scale. The subcategories in this version of the scale provided a more extensive choice of scale descriptors and this made it easier to identify a descriptor that matched the wound. Further studies are needed to clarify the accuracy of pressure ulcer grading scales. The ultimate solution to the issues of reliability and validity of these scales is to replace them with an objective physiological measure of tissue perfusion and pressure damage. Although physiological measures have been used experimentally, none is available for routine clinical use.

Incidence and prevalence

Two approaches are used to measure and monitor the occurrence of pressure ulcers: prevalence and inci-

dence. Incidence – the rate at which new ulcers develop – is defined as: 'the number of new cases of a disease that occur during a specified period of time in a population at risk for developing the disease' (Gordis 1996: p. 31) and prevalence – the proportion of people with ulcers at any one time – is defined as: 'the number of affected persons present in the population at a specific time divided by the number of persons in the population at that time' (Gordis 1996: p. 32).

The term *point prevalence* is often used to distinguish the number of people with pressure ulcers at a specified point in time from *period prevalence,* which describes the number of those with ulcers during a specified period of time.

Prevalence
Published pressure ulcer point prevalence rates across all specialty ranges show wide variations but, overall, rates appear to be falling. In 1993, O'Dea reported prevalence rates in acute-care hospitals within the UK to be between 14% and 22%. A repeat survey 6 years later showed that prevalence had declined to 10% (O'Dea 1999). Torrance (1999) also reports a similar downward trend in hospital prevalence from 14.7% to 8.5% over a 5 year period. Community prevalence rates of 3.0–6.1% are reported for the same period (Torrance 1999). Early prevalence studies indicate a positive relationship between increasing age and pressure ulcer prevalence (Barbenel et al. 1977). The highest hospital prevalence rates appear to be within the care of the older service (David et al. 1983, Allcock et al. 1994). Comparison of prevalence rates by specialty also reveals marked variation (David et al. 1983, Clark & Cullum 1992).

Prevalence is the most commonly reported measure but it is not always the most useful for evaluating care. When planning prevention policies, allocating resources and evaluating the effectiveness of prevention strategies, it is necessary to measure and distinguish between the number of existing ulcers and the number of new ulcers occurring since the introduction of the new policy or preventive measures.

Incidence
Incidence rates also vary by specialty and between care settings within specialties. A comparative study between orthopaedic, medical and surgical settings reports incidence rates of 10.9%, 3.8% and 1.8% respectively, with an overall rate of 4.03% (Clark & Watts 1994). St Clair et al. (1995) report a lower overall hospital incidence rate of 1.2%, while an incidence of 2.9% is reported within an elderly-care hospital setting (KS Gebhardt 1996, personal communication).

Incidence is influenced by the vulnerability of patients, the effectiveness of preventive care and by variations in the standard of care within specialties. Differences in dependency and frailty levels between similar groups of patients with apparently similar risk may be sufficient to affect rates and to cause variations across settings within the same specialty. Thus rates specific to each ward or team, rather than global specialty, hospital or community rates, will enable resources to be more accurately targeted to areas of need. Incidence calculations based on the population at risk also require a consistent, standardized definition of 'at risk' to be applied across all studies and audits. This is necessary to provide meaningful data with which to compare rates between settings and studies. Currently there is a lack of consistency in the denominator used to calculate incidence rates, and also inconsistency in the definitions of the denominators used.

In summary, the wide variations in reported incidence and prevalence rates are due to inconsistencies in the methodological approaches used to calculate incidence and prevalence, and to differences in defining and grading ulcers, particularly the grade 1 ulcer (Clark & Cullum 1992, Nuffield Institute for Health, NHS Centre for Reviews and Dissemination 1995). Most health care settings audit pressure ulcers as a means of monitoring the quality of care. However, until there is greater standardization in the approaches used to collect the data, the use of reported pressure ulcer rates for this purpose requires considerable caution. For further discussion, see Bridel (1995) and Allcock et al. (1994).

Location

Pressure ulcers occur most frequently on areas of the body where soft tissues are vulnerable to compression between two hard surfaces, usually the bony prominences or 'pressure points' where there is little opportunity for pressure to dissipate through fatty tissues, and another firm surface – usually a support surface – mattress, chair or floor. Prostheses and appliances may also exert pressure on soft tissue. Pressure ulcers can be caused by pressure from tubing, such as urinary catheters, nasotracheal and endotracheal tubes in and around body orifices.

The three most common sites for pressure ulcer development are, in descending order, the sacrum, the buttocks and the heels (David et al. 1983, Dealey 1991, St Clair et al. 1995). Dealey (1991) gives a 44.5% point prevalence rate for sacral ulcers and 13.1% for buttocks. An incidence rate of 76.3% and 18.2% for sacral ulcers and heels respectively is reported by Clark & Watts (1994). St Clair et al. (1995) report that 81% of hospital-acquired ulcers occur on the sacrum or buttocks, compared with 48.6% of community-acquired ulcers. This difference may reflect the extended periods of chair nursing commonly practised in many hospital settings.

Predisposing risk factors in pressure ulcer development

As previously noted, pressure and shear-induced soft-tissue damage can occur at all ages of the life cycle, in both healthy individuals as well as in those who are physically compromised. The reasons why some individuals have greater predisposition to pressure ulcers remain unclear. However, it is evident that pressure, shear and friction are mediated by a complex interrelationship of risk factors.

Risk factors are intrinsic or extrinsic characteristics that increase a person's susceptibility to the effects of pressure and/or decrease the tissue's ability to withstand pressure. Braden & Bergstrom (1987) present a schema for the aetiology of pressure ulcer formation (Fig. 19.1). They identify two critical causative factors of pressure ulcer formation: the intensity and duration of pressure and the ability of the skin and soft tissues to tolerate pressure; these, in turn, are influenced by risk factors. The model identifies three risk factors – reduced mobility, reduced activity and reduced sensory perception – as increasing the risk of prolonged, intense pressure. Tissue tolerance is influenced by intrinsic factors – nutrition, age, arteriolar pressure – and by extrinsic variables – moisture, friction, shear – which alter the structures of the skin and soft tissues and, in turn, their ability to withstand pressure. Braden & Bergstrom's conceptual framework on the aetiology of pressure ulcers has been developed further by Defloor (1999).

Risk factors have been the focus of much investigation, yet the exact role of many variables in pressure ulcer formation remains unclear. Further, the risk factors or combination of risk factors most significant in identifying patients at greatest risk remains uncertain. The Royal College of Nursing's *Clinical Practice Guidelines* (Royal College of Nursing 2000) lists 12 intrinsic risk factors as being influential in pressure ulcer development: (1) reduced mobility; (2) sensory impairment; (3) acute illness; (4) level of consciousness; (5) extremes of age; (6) previous history of pressure damage; (7) vascular disease; (8) malnutrition; (9) pressure; (10) shear; (11) friction; and (12) medication. In comparison, the National Pressure Ulcer Advisory Panel (1983) for the USA includes inactivity, faecal incontinence, reduced consciousness and, for some groups, fracture and systemic illness as important risk factors. An overview of some of the most frequently cited risk factors is given in the next section.

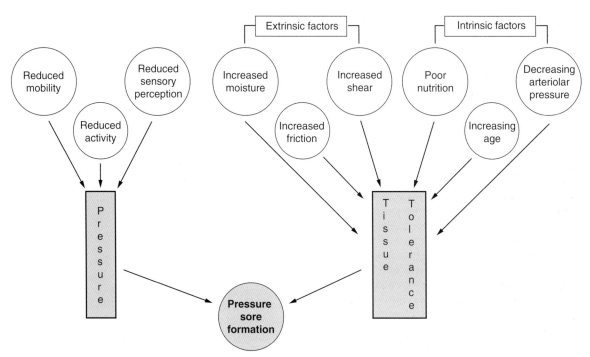

Fig. 19.1   Aetiology of pressure sore formation: Braden & Bergstrom's conceptual scheme. (After Braden & Bergstrom 1987.)

Intrinsic risk factors influencing tissue tolerance

Age   Serious illness of any kind, and associated medical interventions, may result in compromised physiological processes. The likelihood of disease and disability increases with advancing age and, coupled with the normal physiological processes of ageing, makes the occurrence of pressure ulcers more common amongst the older population. A statistically significant difference between the age of those who develop pressure damage and those who don't has been reported in the literature (Guralnik et al. 1988, Spector 1994, Bergstrom et al. 1996, Halfens et al. 2000).

Mobility   Any condition which reduces mobility or the sensation of pain, such as paralysis, anaesthesia, sedation, trauma or poor physical condition, can contribute to pressure ulcer development by interfering with the spontaneous movements normally made in response to ischaemic discomfort. A reduction in the number of spontaneous body movements made by older people during sleep has been shown to be directly related to an increase in the incidence of pressure ulcers (Exton-Smith & Sherwin 1961). More recently, Schubert & Heraud (1994) studied the effects of lying supine and semirecumbent for 30 min on the sacral microcirculation of older patients. Subjects tended to make more movements towards the end of the 30-min period, indicating the ability to sense discomfort from compressive forces. All patients made between one and seven spontaneous movements that restored blood flow to the pressure point, with the exception of three of the four patients with Parkinson's disease, who made no movements at all.

Continence   Incontinence is associated with an increased occurrence of pressure ulcers. Chemical irritation of the skin can result from prolonged contact with urine and faeces, while prolonged exposure to moisture may result in skin maceration; it is likely that chemical irritation and maceration will make the tissues less tolerant to mechanical stressors.

Norton et al. (1975) found that 38% of incontinent patients developed pressure ulcers compared with 7% who were continent. Subsequent investigation of Norton et al's work found incontinence to discriminate well between 'risk-free' and 'at-risk' patients (Goldstone & Goldstone 1982). Spector (1994) reports nursing-home older residents with faecal incontinence several times per week to be 2.5 times more likely to have pressure ulcers than those with few or no episodes of incontinence. Further, those with daily urinary incontinence are 80% more likely to have an ulcer. Other studies have found regular faecal incontinence to be strongly associated with pressure ulcers but have been unable to demonstrate a significant relationship with urinary incontinence (Brandeis et al. 1994, Allman et al. 1995). Allman et al. (1995) found a strong association between faecal incontinence and poor mobility, and it is possible that both these variables are indirect measures of a common underlying risk factor with major significance in the aetiology of pressure ulcer formation. Further research is needed to clarify the role of urinary and faecal incontinence as valid indicators of pressure ulcer risk.

Nutrition Nutrients are required to sustain and maintain body repair processes, such as the renewal of collagen. The literature makes frequent associations between pressure ulcers and poor nutritional status. Malnutrition may be more common in institutionalized older patients than is recognized, increasing susceptibility to pressure ulcers. A retrospective study by Cullum & Clark (1992) of older hospitalized patients aged between 69 and 97 years revealed serum protein concentrations to be lower in those with pressure ulcers on admission or in those who developed an ulcer while in hospital, in comparison with those who remained pressure-ulcer-free. Antony et al. (2000) also found serum albumin to be a significant predictor of pressure ulceration, although associations between serum albumin and pressure ulceration are not consistently supported by other studies (Guralnik et al. 1988, Allman et al. 1995). A nutritional intake less than the recommended daily allowance for protein, calories and zinc has been found to predict pressure ulcers (Bergstrom & Braden 1992), although this has not been shown in all studies (Halfens et al. 2000). There is some indication that the use of nutritional supplementation with protein, arginine, zinc and antioxidants may delay the onset of pressure ulceration and reduce the severity of tissue damage in patients with hip fractures (Houwing et al. 2002). Reduced incidence of pressure ulceration following nutritional supplementation in acutely ill older patients is also reported by Bourdel-Marchasson et al. (2000). For a review of the role of protein, vitamin C and zinc in the aetiology of pressure ulcers the reader is referred to the discussions by Lewis (1996a, 1996b).

Cullum & Clark (1992) also report weight to be lowest in patients admitted to hospital with ulcers or in those who developed ulcers, and highest in those remaining free of pressure ulcers; Allman et al. (1986) report similar findings. Decreasing body weight has been associated with increasing age; decreased body weight, depleted triceps skinfold and lymphopenia have been significantly associated with pressure ulcer formation in patients aged 55 years and over (Allman et al. 1995). Factors influencing feeding may also be

implicated: a nationally representative sample of 2803 American nursing-home residents found those needing help with feeding were 2.12 times more likely to have pressure ulcers. At greatest risk were those with cognitive impairment and who were unable to feed themselves. The findings showed that being underweight increased the likelihood of developing an ulcer by 50% (Spector 1994).

Blood pressure, vascular disease and anaemia Any condition that decreases the quality or quantity of blood reaching the tissues will increase the likelihood of pressure damage. Cardiac disorders, anaemia, peripheral vascular disease, arteriosclerotic disease and low blood pressure are thought to be predisposing factors in pressure ulcer development.

Schubert (1991) reports a significantly lower systolic blood pressure in older institutionalized patients with pressure ulcers compared with those without ulcers. Using a Doppler technique to obtain transcutaneous non-invasive continuous measurements of the microcirculation, the author reports that a low mean blood pressure and low systolic blood pressure were significantly correlated with an impaired hyperaemic reaction after ischaemia, and that a low systolic blood pressure was associated with pressure ulcers. The study concludes that blood pressure measurement is important in identifying patients at risk of developing pressure ulcers. The interpretation and classification of clinical blood pressure readings in order to identify those at risk require further development. A review of the role of blood pressure as a predictor of pressure ulcer development can be found in Pedley (2000).

Psychological factors The effects of the individual's emotional state on tissue breakdown is not fully understood. The emotional stress of illness and disability stimulates the adrenal glands to increase production of glucocorticoids. This leads to an inhibition of collagen formation and an increased risk of tissue breakdown (Maklebust 1987). Anderson & Andberg (1979) examined associations between psychosocial factors and the occurrence of pressure ulcers in a sample of quadriplegic and paraplegic patients aged 16–70 years. Contrary to the expectation that quadriplegics would have a greater incidence of pressure ulcers than paraplegics because of the greater degree of disability making pressure relief more difficult, the results of this study showed pressure ulcer incidence to be related to psychosocial variables, rather than the level of injury alone. Those patients who maintained an intact skin had higher levels of satisfaction with life and stronger feelings about taking responsibility for skin care, and this was unrelated to the level of injury. These findings reinforce the view that pressure, shear and friction alone do not fully explain the mechanism of pressure ulcer development.

Elevated temperature and infection   An increase in skin temperature of 1°C increases tissue metabolism by 10%. This, in turn, will increase the oxygen requirement of the tissues. It is hypothesized that local application of heat to 'at-risk' areas and pyrexial states which increase metabolic rate and oxygen demand will further endanger ischaemic tissues (Maklebust 1987).

Extrinsic factors

Skin hygiene   Dry skin is a problem commonly encountered with ageing due to reduced sebum production and reduced water content of the skin. Aggressive washing will further aggravate this problem and can act as a source of friction. Although frequent washing of the incontinent patient is necessary, overzealous use of soap and poor rinsing of the skin after washing can be harmful because protective oils are lost, the skin pH is altered and dehydration occurs, making the skin less resistant to friction (Lowthian 1982, Torrance 1983). Vigorous skin massage can be dangerous to vulnerable tissues. Dyson (1978) reported a reduction of 38% in the incidence of pressure ulcers in a group of older patients whose skin was not massaged, compared with those whose pressure areas were massaged. Postmortem examination of tissues from the massaged group showed extensive damage, compared with virtually none in the non-massaged group.

Patient handling and positioning   The positioning and moving and handling of patients can cause damage from pressure, friction and shear if undertaken incorrectly. The combination of these forces is particularly hazardous for patients positioned in a sitting or semi-sitting position in bed, and even more so for patients forced to endure long periods of sitting out in ill-fitting chairs, under the pretext of 'rehabilitation'. Bed-making can equally contribute to pressure damage: crumpled sheets can act as sources of friction and shear, while tight bedding can completely restrict the movement of a debilitated patient and can be sufficient to act as a source of pressure on vulnerable areas, such as the toes.

Drugs   Any drug which decreases sensation or mobility, for example sedatives, opiates and alcohol, can increase the likelihood of pressure ulcers. David et al. (1983) reported that 41% of patients with pressure ulcers were receiving sedatives or narcotics. Steroids have been shown to mimic and exacerbate the ageing process by reducing the collagen content of the dermis; for this reason the tissues of patients receiving steroids may be less tolerant of pressure. These effects are reversed when steroid therapy is withdrawn (Hall et al. 1974).

Identifying patients at risk

The nursing assessment of any older patient should include an assessment of the risk of pressure ulcers. This is necessary to target expensive resources appropriately at those who are most at risk and to avoid wastage associated with providing unnecessary prevention for those who do not need it. The assessment, and any required preventive actions, must be implemented at the earliest opportunity if they are to be effective. The aim is to achieve this within 6 h of the first point of contact with the health care services (National Institute for Clinical Excellence 2003). This timescale may not be achievable within community settings where pressure-relieving devices need to be ordered and delivered to the client's home. For professional and legal reasons the assessment must be documented and, because the client's condition may change, routine reassessment is necessary; the frequency of reassessment will reflect the patient's condition. The assessment strategies used for assessing pressure ulcer risk include clinical judgement and pressure ulcer risk assessment scales. Biomedical techniques have been devised for detecting early physiological indicators of pressure damage before visible signs are evident. These are currently only used in experimental studies but they may, in the future, offer a more objective clinical measure of pressure ulcer risk.

Risk assessment tools

The current trend is for standardized assessment and quantification of risk using a risk assessment scale. There are at least 17 published risk assessment scales (Clark & Farrar 1992). Risk factors form the basis of these risk assessment scales and a comparison of five commonly used published scales (Norton, Gosnell, Knoll, Waterlow and Braden scales) showed that mobility and incontinence occur in all five; activity, nutrition and mental state occur in four out of five of the scales; and general physical condition, skin appearance and medication occurred in three out of five. A number of the variables used to construct these scales are *assumed* risk factors, rather than *confirmed* risk factors identified by empirical investigation.

The Norton scale   The Norton scale, developed in the 1950s, was the first published pressure ulcer risk assessment tool, and the precursor to many subsequent scales (Table 19.2). It is intended for use with older people and was originally designed as a data

Table 19.2 Pressure ulcer risk assessment scales: the Norton scale

A		B		C		D		E	
Physical condition		Mental condition		Activity		Mobility		Incontinent	
Good	4	Alert	4	Ambulant	4	Full	4	Not	4
Fair	3	Apathetic	3	Walk with help	3	Slightly limited	3	Occasionally	3
Poor	2	Confused	2	Chair-bound	2	Very limited	2	Usually of urine	2
Very bad	1	Stuporous	1	Bedfast	1	Immobile	1	Doubly	1

Instructions for use:
1. Score the patient 1–4 under each heading (A–E), and total the scores.
2. A score of 14 or less was formerly taken to indicate the patient was at risk and in need of preventive care. A score of 16 or less is now used.
3. When sacral oedema is present, the patient might be at risk, even with a high score.
4. Assess the patient regularly.
Reproduced from Norton et al. (1975) with kind permission from Churchill Livingstone.

collection tool in an investigation into the role of skin products and skin care in preventing pressure ulcers in older people (Norton et al. 1975). It has five components: (1) physical condition; (2) mental state; (3) activity; (4) mobility; and (5) incontinence; the physical condition of the patient is assumed to reflect nutritional status (Norton 1989). Each category has four items, each weighted from 1 to 4, giving a minimum possible score of 5 and maximum score of 20. Originally a score of 14 or less indicated 'risk' but, owing to demographic changes, advances in medicine and drug therapy, Norton (1989) subsequently advises that patients with a score of 16 or less should be considered 'at risk'. However, this remains unsubstantiated by research.

Goldstone & Goldstone (1982) investigated the discriminant function of the five components of the Norton scale using a random sample of older orthopaedic trauma patients. Statistically significant correlations were found between physical, mental and mobility scores, indicating unnecessary duplication. The combined incontinence and physical scores discriminated 'at-risk' patients from 'risk-free' patients as effectively as the full scores.

Most of the more recently developed risk assessment scales are based on the Norton scale. Rather than attempt to identify those patient features most predictive of risk, their authors have included additional factors in an attempt to improve the applicability and predictive ability of the scale. This approach has increased their length and complexity without any real improvement in their predictive capacity. As illustrated by Goldstone & Goldstone (1982), the most valid approach to risk prediction is to identify the risk factor or combination of risk factors that best predicts risk, through the use of statistical techniques.

The Waterlow pressure sore prevention/treatment policy
The Waterlow assessment scale has evolved from a risk assessment card (Waterlow 1985) to a combined prevention and treatment policy (Waterlow 1991) and is one of the most common pressure ulcer risk assessment scales in use in the UK (Table 19.3). The scale contains many presumed risk factors grouped into seven categories, some of which reflect those devised by Norton et al. (1975); each category contains 4–7 weighted items. Scores of each category are summed and the total is used to identify whether the patient has a low, medium, high or very high risk: a high score indicates a high risk. It is intended for use on a wide range of patient groups, including older people, but it lacks discriminatory power when used to predict risk in this client group – most older inpatients are identified as high or very high risk. An appraisal of the scale's reliability when used in the care of older people has also shown interrater reliability to be poor (Cook et al. 1999). The variability in the risk scores allocated to each patient by different ward nurses was sufficient to place each patient in several risk categories – in some cases risk scores spanned three or four risk categories. The widest variations in subscores were obtained for the 'skin type', 'mobility', 'tissue malnutrition' and 'body build' risk factors. To date the published literature contains no satisfactory reports on the discriminatory ability of the risk factors, the testing and development of the risk factor weightings or the derivations of the thresholds classifying levels of risk.

The Braden scale The Braden scale (Table 19.4) is based on Braden & Bergstrom's conceptual schema (Fig. 19.1). It assesses mobility, activity, sensory perception, skin moisture, friction, shear and nutritional status (Bergstrom et al. 1987, Braden & Bergstrom 1987, 1989).

Table 19.3 Pressure ulcer risk assessment scales: the Waterlow pressure sore prevention/treatment policy; ring scores in table, add total. Several scores per category can be used

Build/weight for height		Skin type visual risk areas		Sex and age		Special risks	
Average	0	Healthy	0	Male	1	**Tissue malnutrition**	
Above average	1	Tissue paper	1	Female	2	e.g. terminal cachexia	8
Obese	2	Dry	1	14–49	1	Cardiac failure	5
Below average	3	Oedematous	1	50–64	2	Peripheral vascular disease	5
		Clammy	1	65–74	3	Anaemia	2
		(temperature ↑)		75–80	4	Smoking	
Continence		Discoloured	2	81+	5	**Neurological deficit**	1
		Broken/spot	3			e.g. diabetes, multiple	4–6
Complete/	0					sclerosis, cerebrovascular	
cateterized						accident, motor/sensory,	
Occasionally		**Mobility**		**Appetite**		paraplegia	
incontinent						**Major surgery/trauma**	
Catheter/incontinent	1	Fully	0	Average	0		
of faeces	2	Restless/fidgety	1	Poor	1	Orthopaedic-below waist,	
Doubly incontinent		Apathetic	2	Nasogastric	2	spinal	5
	3	Restricted	3	tube/fluids		On table > 2 h	5
		Inert/traction	4	only		**Medication**	
		Chair-bound	5	Nil-by-mouth/	3	Cytotoxics, high-dose	
				anorexic		steroids, anti-inflammatories	4

Score: 10+ at risk; 15+ high risk; 20+ very high risk.

Remember: tissue damage often starts before admission, in casualty. A seated patient is also at risk.

Assessment: if the patient falls into any of the risk categories, then preventive nursing is required. A combination of good nursing techniques and preventive aids will definitely be necessary.

Prevention

Preventive aids

Special mattress/bed	10+ overlays or specialist foam mattresses
	15+ alternating pressure overlays, mattresses and bed systems
	20+ bed systems: fluidized, bead, low air loss and alternating-pressure mattresses
	Note: preventive aids cover a wide spectrum of specialist features. Efficacy should be judged, if possible, on the basis of independent evidence
Cushions	No patient should sit in a wheelchair without some form of cushioning. If nothing else is available, use the patient's own pillow
	10+ 10-cm foam cushion
	15+ specialist gel and/or foam cushion
	20+ cushion capable of adjustment to suit individual patient
Bed clothing	Avoid plastic draw sheets, incontinence pads and tightly tucked-in sheets/sheet covers, especially when using specialist bed and mattress overlay systems
	Use duvet, plus vapour-permeable cover

Prevention

Nursing care

General	Frequent changes of position, lying/sitting. Use of pillows
Pain	Appropriate pain control
Nutrition	High protein, vitamins, minerals
Patient handling	Correct lifting technique – hoists – monkey pole – transfer devices
Patient comfort aids	Real sheepskins – bed cradle
Operating table	10-cm cover plus adequate protection

Continued

Table 19.3 *Cont'd*   Pressure ulcer risk assessment scales: the Waterlow pressure sore prevention/treatment policy; ring scores in table, add total. Several scores per category can be used

---

Prevention

Nursing care
Theatre/A&E trolley
Skin care   General hygiene. No rubbing, cover with an appropriate dressing
If treatment is required, first remove pressure

Wound classification
Stirling Pressure Sore Severity Scale (SPSSS)
Stage 0: No clinical evidence of a pressure sore
0.1 Healed with scarring
0.2 Tissue damage not assessed as a pressure sore. (a) see below
Stage 1: Discolouration of intact skin
1.1 Non-blanchable erythema with increased local heat
1.2 Blue/purple/black discolouration – the sore is at least stage 1 (a or b)
Stage 2: Partial-thickness skin loss or damage
2.1 Blister
2.2 Abrasion
2.3 Shallow ulcer, no undermining of adjacent tissue
2.4 Any of these with underlying blue/purple/black discolouration or induration. The sore is at least stage 2 (a, b or c + d for 2.3, + e for 2.4)
Stage 3: Full-thickness skin loss involving damage/necrosis of subcutaneous tissue, not extending to underlying bone, tendon or joint capsule
3.1 Crater, without undermining of adjacent tissue
3.2 Crater, with undermining of adjacent tissue
3.3 Sinus, the full extent of which is uncertain
3.4 Necrotic tissue masking full extent of damage
The sore is at least stage 3 (b ± e, f, g + h for 3.4)
Stage 4: Full-thickness loss with extensive destruction and tissue necrosis extending to underlying bone tendon or capsule
4.1 Visible exposure of bone, tendon or capsule
4.2 Sinus assessed as extending to same. (b ± e, f, g, h, i)

Guide to types of dressing treatment
a   Semipermeable membrane
b   Hydrocolloid
c   Foam dressing
d   Alginate
e   Hydrogel
f   Alginate rope/ribbon
g   Foam cavity filler
h   Enzymatic debridement
i   Surgical debridement

Reproduced with kind permission from Waterlow (1991; revised 1995).
A pressure ulcer prevention manual giving advice on the use of the scale is available from www.judywaterlow.fsnet.co.uk

Table 19.4   Pressure ulcer risk assessment scales: the Braden scale for predicting pressure sore risk

Patient's name			Evaluator's name	Date of assessment
Sensory perception Ability to respond meaningfully to pressure-related discomfort	1. Completely limited Unresponsive (does not moan, flinch or gasp) to painful stimuli, due to diminished level of consciousness or sedation or limited ability to feel pain over most of body surface	2. Very limited Responds only to painful stimuli. Cannot communicate discomfort except by moaning or restlessness or has a sensory impairment which limits the ability to feel pain or discomfort over half of the body	3. Slightly limited Responds to verbal commands, but cannot always communicate discomfort or need to be turned or has some sensory impairment which limits ability to feel pain or discomfort in one or two extremities	4. No impairment Responds to verbal commands. Has no sensory deficit that would limit ability to feel or voice pain or discomfort
Moisture Degree to which skin is exposed to moisture	1. Constantly moist Skin is kept moist almost constantly by perspiration and urine. Dampness is detected every time patient is moved or turned	2. Very moist Skin is often, but not always, moist. Linen must be changed at least once a shift	3. Occasionally moist Skin is occasionally moist, requiring an extra linen change approximately once a day	4. Rarely moist Skin is usually dry; linen only requires changing at routine intervals
Activity Degree of physical activity	1. Bedfast Confined to bed	2. Chairfast Ability to walk severely limited or non-existent. Cannot bear own weight and/or must be assisted into chair or wheelchair	3. Walks occasionally Walks occasionally during day, but for very short distances, with or without assistance. Spends majority of each shift in bed or chair	4. Walks frequently Walks outside the room at least twice a day and inside room at least once every 2 h during waking hours
Mobility Ability to change and control body position	1. Completely immobile Does not make even slight changes in body or extremity position without assistance	2. Very limited Makes occasional slight changes in body or extremity position but unable to make frequent or significant changes independently	3. Slightly limited Makes frequent though slight changes in body or extremity position independently	4. No limitations Makes major and frequent changes in position without assistance

Continued

Table 19.4 *Cont'd* Pressure ulcer risk assessment scales: the Braden scale for predicting pressure sore risk

Patient's name

Evaluator's name

Date of assessment

	1. Very poor	2. Probably inadequate	3. Adequate	4. Excellent
Nutrition *Usual* food intake pattern	Never eats a complete meal. Rarely eats more than one-third of any food offered. Eats two servings or fewer of protein (meat or dairy products) per day. Takes fluids poorly. Does not take a liquid supplement or is nil-by-mouth and/or maintained on clear liquids or intravenous fluids for more than 5 days	Rarely eats a complete meal and generally eats only about one-half of any food offered. Protein intake includes only three servings of meat or dairy products per day. Occasionally will take a dietary supplement or receives less than optimum amount of liquid diet or tube feeding	Eats over half of most meals. Eats a total of four servings of protein (meat, dairy products) each day. Occasionally will refuse a meal, but will usually take a supplement if offered or is on a tube-feeding or total parenteral nutrition regimen which probably meets most of nutritional needs	Eats most of every meal. Never refuses a meal. Usually eats a total of four or more servings of meat and dairy products. Occasionally eats between meals. Does not require supplementation
	1. Problem	**2. Potential problem**	**3. No apparent problem**	
Friction and shear	Requires moderate to maximum assistance in moving. Complete lifting without sliding against sheets is impossible. Frequently slides down in bed or chair, requiring frequent repositioning with maximum assistance. Spasticity, contractures or agitation lead to almost constant friction	Moves feebly or requires minimum assistance. During a move skin probably slides to some extent against sheets, chair, restraints or other devices. Maintains relatively good position in chair or bed most of the time but occasionally slides down	Moves in bed and in chair independently and has sufficient muscle strength to lift up completely during move. Maintains good position in bed or chair at all times	
				Total score

Unlike the previous scales, an operational definition of each subscale category is provided; this removes ambiguity and increases the likelihood of interrater agreement. Each dimension is rated from 1 (least favourable) to 3 or 4 (most favourable); the total score range is from 16 to 23. A score of 16 or less indicates pressure ulcer risk, although the authors recommend that each clinical area should determine its own cut-off point. The scale has been subjected to well-designed validation studies within acute and long-term older care settings, including nursing homes, as well as medical-surgical and intensive care settings. It is the most reliable of the four scales reviewed here and can be considered to be amongst the most reliable of the published scales. Halfens et al. (2000) identified only two variables from the scale – 'sensory perception' and 'friction and shear' – to be predictive of pressure ulcer development. In this study, these two variables, in conjunction with 'age' and a revised moisture variable (combining urinary, faecal incontinence and extreme sweating) predicted pressure ulcer development better than the original Braden scale. The 'moisture', 'mobility/activity' and 'nutrition' variables, as defined by Braden & Bergstrom, were not predictive of pressure ulceration.

The Walsall Community Pressure Sore Risk Calculator

The Walsall Community Pressure Sore Risk Calculator is derived from the Medley score and has been specifically designed for use in community settings. The original scale contained nine risk factors: (1) predisposing disease; (2) level of consciousness; (3) mobility; (4) skin condition; (5) nutritional status; (6) pain; (7) bladder incontinence; (8) bowel incontinence; and (9) the extent to which the patient has access to 24-h carer input. The validity of the scale has been assessed by Chaloner & Franks (1999). They investigated the relative importance of each risk factor in pressure ulcer development using multivariate analysis and found that some of the presumed risk factors in the original scale – pain, predisposing disease, broken skin and carer input – were not predictive of pressure ulcer development. The revised scale is shown in Figure 19.2. Although little association was found between carer input and pressure damage, this was considered an important risk factor and was retained in the revised scale.

All published scales identify a score which delineates the 'at-risk' from 'low-risk' groups. Clark & Farrar (1992) illustrate the need to determine threshold scores locally on the client group on which the scale is to be used, rather than using the published threshold score. They compared the accuracy of six risk assessment tools (Norton, Waterlow, Lowthian, Knoll; NPRU (Nursing Practice Research Unit), and Braden scales) on 257 patients admitted to a district general hospital. None of the published threshold scores achieved the best discrimination between 'at-risk' and 'risk-free' patients but all scales performed reasonably well when the threshold scores were set locally. The local setting of threshold scores is rarely done and this has implications for the accuracy of the risk scales.

A proper comparative assessment of the performance of each risk scale is hampered by the differences in the research design and poor quality of many of the validation studies undertaken to date; this includes inadequate operational definitions, particularly relating to the definition and diagnosis of the stage 1 pressure ulcer, and insufficient reporting of results. These scales may be useful as a teaching tool and aide-mémoire for students and inexperienced carers, but there is no conclusive evidence that they are more effective in identifying at-risk clients than the professional judgment of experienced nurses or that they improve outcomes (Nuffield Institute for Health, NHS Centre for Reviews and Dissemination 1995). While they have their place, they should not be used as a substitute for, or to override, clinical judgement (National Institute for Clinical Excellence 2003).

Many hospital and community trust pressure ulcer prevention policies identify the risk assessment score as a basis for planning care. In practice, however, the role of the pressure ulcer risk score in preventing pressure damage seems unclear. Research evidence suggests that preventive care – manual repositioning or the provision of pressure-relieving mattresses – may not depend on the risk score or the development of pressure ulcers (Abbruzzese 1985, Clark & Cullum 1992, Salvadala et al. 1992, Defloor & Grypdonck 2005). This raises some interesting questions as to how nurses determine the need for preventive care and the purpose of risk scores.

Prevention

Risk reduction strategies aim to reduce interface pressure and improve the soft tissues' ability to withstand compressive forces by removing external risk factors, such as friction and shear, and alleviating internal risk factors. A successful strategy requires collaborative, interprofessional working. The American guidelines, *Prediction and Prevention* (Panel for the Prediction and Prevention of Pressure Ulcers in Adults 1992), identify four overall goals for predicting and preventing ulcers: (Bergman-Evans et al. 1994: p. 20):

1. Identify at-risk individuals who need prevention and the specific factors that place them at risk
2. Maintain and improve tissue tolerance to pressure in order to prevent injury

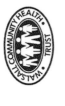

WALSALL COMMUNITY PRESSURE SORE RISK CALCULATOR

Name .... Date of Birth ....

RISK CATEGORIES		SCORE	ASSESSMENT DATES						
LEVEL OF CONSCIOUSNESS	ALERT	0							
	LETHARGIC/CONFUSED	3							
	SEMI-COMATOSE	3							
	COMATOSE	3							
MOBILITY AMBULATION	MOVES WITHOUT ASSISTANCE	0							
	MOVES WITH LIMITED ASSISTANCE	3							
	MOVES ONLY WITH ASSISTANCE	8							
	CHAIRFAST (8 HRS PLUS)	8							
	BEDFAST (12 HRS PLUS)	8							
SKIN CONDITION	HEALTHY	0							
	RASHES/DRYNESS	2							
	INCREASED TURGOR/FRAGILE	4							
	REDNESS	4							
NUTRITIONAL STATUS	WELL BALANCED DIET/STABLE WEIGHT	0							
	POOR APPETITE/WEIGHT LOSS	4							
	VERY POOR/FLUIDS ONLY/NIL BY MOUTH	4							
SUB-TOTAL RISK SCORE (A)									

RISK CATEGORIES		SCORE	ASSESSMENT DATES						
BLADDER INCONTINENCE	NONE	0							
	OCCASIONAL (<2/24 HRS) OR CATHETERISED	0							
	USUALLY (>2/24 HRS)	1							
	TOTAL (NO CONTROL)	4							
BOWEL INCONTINENCE	NONE	0							
	OCCASIONAL	4							
	TOTAL (NO CONTROL)	6							
CARER INPUT	NO CARER REQUIRED	0							
	ACTIVE CARERS (24HRS)	0							
	INTERMITTENT CARER (8HRS PLUS)	2							
	LIMITED CARER (3-8HRS)	2							
	OCCASIONAL CARER (0-3HRS)	2							
SUB-TOTAL RISK SCORE									
SUB TOTAL RISK SCORE (A)									
TOTAL RISK SCORE									
TICK IF PATIENT HAS PRESSURE SORE									
ASSESSOR'S SIGNATURE									

PEGASUS *Egerton*

WALSALL COMMUNITY PRESSURE SORE RISK CALCULATOR

The Walsall Community Pressure Sore Risk Calculator assists in the identification of the main contributing factors in the development of pressure sores. It is designed for use in the community.

This tool should be used only as a **guide**, following holistic patient assessment that includes:

- Professional Judgment
- Patient Choice

1. RISK ASSESSMENT

The columns allow for regular assessment, either at intervals indicated by the patient's level of risk, or should the patient's condition change.

2. RISK CATEGORIES

Score the patient in one area only in each risk category. Record the score in the appropriate column and total at the end. From the total risk score, determine the category as:

| < 4 not at risk | 4 – 9 low risk | 10 – 14 medium risk | 15 + high risk |

3. SHADED AREAS

A score in the shaded area denotes nursing intervention may be required. e.g. by improving nutritional intake, implementation of continence programme, etc.

4. EQUIPMENT GUIDE

Low risk	-	Fibre filled overlay Foam Overlay Foam mattress,	eg. SERENE™ eg. KEY 2 CARE SERENE™
Medium risk	-	Alternating pressure relieving overlay,	eg. VIACLIN™/OVERTURE™
High risk	-	Alternating pressure relieving mattress replacement,	eg. CAIRWAVE™ AIRWAVE™ TRINOVA™ BI=WAVE™ Carer/Plus

An appropriate seating system should also be provided for patients who are seated in a chair.

5. PRESSURE SORE GRADING SCALE [1]

STAGE 1 - Erythema not resolving within 30 minutes of pressure relief. Epidermis remains intact.

STAGE 2 - Partial thickness loss of skin layers involving epidermis and possibly penetrating into, but not through, dermis.

STAGE 3 - Full thickness tissue loss extending through the dermis to involve subcutaneous tissue. Presents as shallow crater unless covered by eschar.

STAGE 4 - Deep tissue destruction extending through subcutaneous tissue to fascia and may involve muscle layers, joint and/or bone. Presents as a deep crater.

[1] International Association for Enterostomal Therapy. Dermal Wounds: Pressure Sores. *Journal of Enterostomal Therapy.* 1988. 15: 4-17

© Walsall Community Health Trust.

The Walsall Risk Calculator is sponsored by Pegasus Egerton. For further information, or further copies of the scoring sheets, please contact:

Customer Services, Pegasus Egerton Ltd.
Pegasus House, Waterberry Drive,
Waterlooville, Hants., PO7 7XX
Tel: (023) 9278 4200 Fax: (023) 9278 4250
E mail: custserv@pegasus-uk.com
Website: www.pegasus-uk.com

PEGASUS EGERTON, PEGASUS, AIRWAVE, CAIRWAVE, BI=WAVE, OVERTURE, TRINOVA, VIACLIN, KEY 2 CARE SERENE, SERENE and the associated device marks are Trade Marks of Pegasus Egerton Limited.

Fig. 19.2 The Walsall Community Pressure Sore Risk Calculator. (Sponsored by Pegasus Egerton; Courtesy of the Walsall Community Health Trust.)

3. Protect against the adverse effects of external mechanical forces (pressure, friction, shear)
4. Reduce the incidence of pressure ulcers through educational programmes.

This offers a useful framework for developing a prevention plan. Strategies to improve tissue tolerance, reduce mechanical forces and improve education will be reviewed in the following sections.

Reducing mechanical forces

Relief of pressure is one of the fundamental aims of prevention and this applies as much to chair-bound patients as to those who are bed-bound. Two main principles underpin strategies used to alleviate pressure:

- reduction of the amount of pressure by redistribution over a wider surface area
- reduction of the duration of the pressure by regular repositioning and/or by alternating the amount of pressure exerted on the patient by the support surface.

Selection of an appropriate pressure-relieving support surface, of which the mode of operation is based on one or other of these principles, is the primary course of action in preventing pressure damage. There are an estimated 130 patient support surfaces (Clark 1994), making appropriate selection difficult. The ideal pressure-relieving support system should have the following characteristics and be comfortable and acceptable to the patient (Torrance 1983: pp. 29–30):

- distribute pressure evenly to avoid tissue distortion and disruption of the microcirculation, or
- provide frequent relief of pressure by varying the areas under pressure
- minimize friction and shear forces
- provide a comfortable ventilated interface environment
- be acceptable to the patient and not restrict movement
- not impede nursing procedures
- be easy to lift patients on and off
- be readily adaptable for external cardiac massage
- be easily maintained and cleaned
- be realistically priced.

The performance of equipment is most appropriately assessed using randomized controlled trials. The testing of pressure-relieving equipment is frequently undertaken using young volunteers, with an underlying assumption that pressure readings obtained on young individuals will be applicable to older people. The ageing process and the associated changes in fat-to-lean ratio, to collagen and water content and reduced muscle tone may alter the soft tissues' ability to withstand mechanical forces. Hence older individuals are likely to experience higher pressures (Maklebust 1987). Contact pressures at the patient–support surface interface are used as an indirect measure of the effectiveness of pressure relief but, because of the pressure gradient between the skin and deep tissues, this reading is likely to be less than the pressure immediately overlying the bony prominence. Inconsistency and measurement error in the methods used to determine contact pressures also limit the comparison of findings between studies.

Thirty randomized controlled trials evaluating the effectiveness of pressure-relieving support surfaces were conducted between 1966 and 1995, of which only one-third clearly reported a random allocation of patients. After evaluating these trials, the Nuffield Institute for Health and NHS Centre for Reviews and Dissemination (1995: p. 13) concluded that 'there is insufficient research evidence on clinical or cost effectiveness to guide equipment choice'. Nevertheless, research evidence to date indicates that pressure-relieving supports are generally more effective in relieving pressure than the National Health Service (NHS) standard foam mattress.

Torrance (1983) classified the numerous pressure-relieving support systems available into four types:

1. constant low-pressure devices
2. alternating-pressure devices
3. those which assist or simulate normal body movement
4. those which protect specific body areas.

Redistribution of pressure: constant low-pressure static support systems

Redistribution of pressure can be achieved using materials such as laminated foam or gel, or mechanically operated pressure-relieving support surfaces.

Foam mattresses The standard NHS foam mattress is made of single-density foam. The sides are reinforced with reconstituted foam. The depth of foam is frequently insufficient to prevent 'grounding' and the absence of a soft outer layer means there is no mechanism for limiting shear or for distribution of pressure over pressure points. The standard-issue mattress is covered by a tight-fitting, non-stretch waterproof cover. The tight-fitting cover prevents redistribution of body weight, creating a 'hammock effect' which increases tension and interface pressures, particularly over bony prominences. Reported interface pressures for patients lying supine on a standard hospital bed and mattress range from 50 to 150 mmHg (Redfern et al. 1973, Norman et al. 1995, Collier 1996). The standard NHS mattress and cover is therefore not a suitable support surface for patients at risk of pressure ulcers.

Pressure caused by the weight of the body on a surface is inversely proportional to the area of contact. It can be reduced by increasing the area of contact between the body and the support surface. In principle, this can be achieved by a laminated foam mattress combining layers of elastic foam of differing densities – a high-density, firm foam core for durability, covered by softer, low-density outer layers of foam which 'give' easily under areas of high pressure, such as the bony prominences, increasing the surface area of the support surface and redistributing the pressure to surrounding areas (Fig. 19.3; Rithalia 1996). Alternatively, cutting/scoring or profiling the surface of the mattress is used. Some foam mattresses also contain pockets of fluid or air in an attempt to enhance the moulding and pressure-redistributing performance. Viscoelastic foam is temperature-sensitive; when warmed by body heat it becomes softer, moulding around the patient. The performance between different mattresses remains unclear; in most instances clinical trials are small and reported differences are not always statistically significant. Gun-

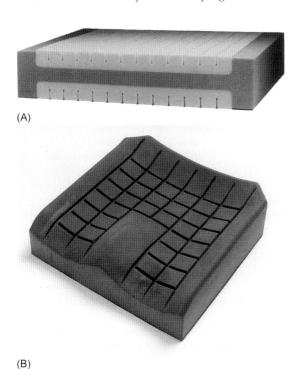

(A)

(B)

Fig. 19.3 (a) Cross-section of a contoured cut foam mattress. The inner core provides a firm base with two semirigid columns running the length of the mattress, giving support when the patient's weight is transferred to the edge. (b) Moulded foam cushion. (Courtesy of Medical Support Systems, Cardiff.)

ningberg et al. (2000) found no significant difference in the incidence of pressure ulcers between patients nursed on a viscoelastic mattress and those nursed on a standard foam mattress. However, the severity of pressure damage was greater for those nursed on the standard mattress. Six randomized controlled trials comparing the standard NHS mattress with non-standard pressure-reducing foam mattresses – Comfortex DeCube mattress, Beaufort bead bed, Softform, Clinifloat, Therarest, Transfoam and Vaperm – showed that the incidence and severity of pressure damage in high-risk patients may be less in patients nursed on non-standard foam mattresses (Nuffield Institute for Health, NHS Centre For Reviews and Dissemination 1995). These forms of pressure-reducing support surfaces tend to be used with clients at lesser risk.

The correct choice of mattress or cushion cover is of equal importance to the choice of support surface if interference with the performance of the support surface is to be avoided. A water-vapour-permeable, low-friction, two-way stretch cover should be used.

Foam holds moisture and humidity and should be used on an open-mesh bed base to promote air circulation and prevent mould formation. Some mattresses also require regular turning to prolong their life expectancy. Without proper care, both the mattress and cover can deteriorate; to prevent this, the manufacturers' instructions should be followed.

In general, foam mattresses have a life expectancy of approximately 3–5 years, depending on quality, after which a permanent compression-set occurs, with loss of the pressure-reducing support properties, often termed 'grounding' or 'bottoming out'. For this reason, a foam mattress replacement scheme is an essential part of any pressure ulcer prevention strategy.

Low–air–loss mattress This mattress is electrically operated and comprises a series of air sacs which lie edgeways across the width of the bed. Air within the sacs is constantly lost and replaced, and this process enables them to contour around the patient. The pressure within each sac can be set independently. Randomized controlled trials indicate that the low-air-loss bed may be more effective in preventing and treating pressure ulcers in the critically ill than the standard NHS foam mattress (Nuffield Institute for Health, NHS Centre for Reviews and Dissemination 1995).

Air–fluidized bed This is a motorized bed with a tank-like base containing ceramic or silicone beads. Pressure is reduced and redistributed by the circulation of the beads in warm air; this produces a fluidizing effect and an interface pressure of approximately 11 mmHg (Dealey 1995). The beads are retained within the base by a thin fabric cover upon which the patient 'floats'. When switched off, the beads settle to form a firm base, which is useful when administering nursing care or cardiopulmonary resuscitation. The circulation of air has a drying effect, advantageous for patients with burns or wet wounds, but for most other categories of patients an additional fluid intake is required to compensate for the extra fluid lost. Two hospital-based randomized controlled trials exploring treatment of existing pressure ulcers showed enhanced healing with the air-fluidized bed (Allman et al. 1987, Munro et al. 1989), in contrast to a community-based study which showed no statistical difference (Strauss et al. 1991). Patients require minimal repositioning on this type of bed but the design is not conducive to rehabilitating the patient. The bed is expensive and requires regular maintenance. For these reasons its use is usually restricted to high-risk patients in whom movement is best avoided, for example trauma or burns patients, the terminally ill and those in severe pain.

Alternating-pressure devices This category of support surface is made as an overlay, replacement mattress, bed or cushion. It consists of a series of air sacs or 'cells' which inflate and deflate in a series of two- or three-phase timed cycles, each of which includes a period of low or zero interface pressure. The size of the air cell, the weight of the patient and the robustness of the design influence the effectiveness of these devices. The amount of inflation is governed by the patient's weight: underinflation will cause grounding and over-inflation will produce high interface pressures. Designs vary in their degree of sophistication: some automatically adjust to the weight of the patient, others must be set manually. The air cells must also be large enough to lift the patient sufficiently clear of the bed. Whatever the range of options available, the manufacturer's instructions should always be consulted in order to select the most appropriate device and the correct settings.

Studies comparing the effectiveness of alternating pressure and constant low-pressure systems give conflicting results. A randomized controlled trial of constant low-pressure mattresses and alternating-pressure mattresses has been undertaken with intensive care patients with comparable physical characteristics, medical management and manual turning regimens. Of 23 patients nursed on the alternating-pressure mattresses, one developed persistent erythema and none developed a pressure ulcer. In comparison, pressure damage was noted in over half the patients nursed on constant low-pressure mattresses: three developed persistent erythema and eight developed grade 2 and 3 pressure ulcers. Of particular interest was the difference in cost between the two interventions; the cost of providing the more effective alternating-pressure intervention was

£44.50, half that of the constant low-pressure mattresses, costing £86.50 per patient (Gebhardt et al. 1996). Comparisons of 11 randomized controlled trials of alternating-pressure mattresses with constant low-pressure mattresses and the standard NHS foam mattress also indicate that the alternating-pressure mattresses are more effective in preventing ulcers (Nuffield Institute for Health, NHS Centre for Reviews and Dissemination, 1995). The Cochrane review of support surfaces for the prevention and treatment of pressure ulceration highlights the inadequate design of many studies investigating the performance of support surfaces (Cullum et al. 2004). The reviewers conclude that:

- The standard hospital mattress has been outperformed and should not be used for high-risk patients
- Low-air-loss mattresses are effective in preventing and treating pressure ulcers relative to foam mattresses
- The relative benefits of low-air-loss, air-fluidized and alternating-pressure air mattresses are unclear
- Cushions have not been adequately evaluated.

Other considerations
Degree of risk, treatment objectives, body weight and interface pressures are not the only considerations when selecting a support surface. Patient acceptance and ability to tolerate the proposed support are central to a successful preventive plan. Patients may reject pressure-relieving equipment because they find it uncomfortable, because the noise from the motor is disturbing or because the equipment hinders their ability to move independently. The movement of alternating-pressure mattresses can be sufficiently disconcerting to interfere with the patient's ability to rest. Thus, for some individuals the acceptance of a pressure-reducing or relieving support surface may depend on the selection of a less sophisticated option, which provides better comfort and rest but which affords lower levels of pressure relief. Additional considerations include ease of transportation, the size and weight of the equipment in relation to the room in which it is to be used and the ease of operation, maintenance and cost.

Replacement mattresses, overlays or cushions alter the overall dimensions of the support surface. The extent to which this affects the patient's ability to maintain good posture and independent mobility requires careful assessment. Most replacement mattresses are deeper than the standard mattress, increasing the overall height of the support surface. Similarly, the addition of a mattress overlay or cushion will also alter the total bed or seat height. Adjustable-height beds can minimize this, but where a fixed-height bed is being used, as in the patient's own home, or the range of chair sizes is limited, the effect of this increased height may impair the client's functional ability. As a general guide, the total height of the chair, inclusive of cushion, should not exceed the length of the patient's leg, from the popliteal fossa to the floor, and should enable the seated patient to maintain a 90° angle at the hips and knees.

Seating   As part of the rehabilitation plan, it is not uncommon for the rehabilitating patient to spend increasing periods out of bed. The totally chair-bound patient will be at greater risk of pressure ulcers because, when seated, the body weight is concentrated on a smaller surface area, whereas in the recumbent patient the weight is distributed over a much wider surface. Inadequate seating may not only increase the risk of pressure damage but may also give rise to poor posture, increased muscle tone and discomfort. For these reasons, careful attention should be given to the choice of seating.

Chairs should promote good posture, minimize pressure, friction and shear and facilitate independent access in and out of the chair. Ill-fitting chairs place excess stress on body structures, encourage poor posture, contribute to fatigue and ultimately may make it more difficult for those with limited movement to readjust their posture and body weight in response to pressure-induced discomfort. Seat depth should allow for a 2-cm gap behind the knee. Chairs which have seats that are too deep will place pressure on the popliteal fossa, impairing circulation to the extremities. To overcome the discomfort the patient slides forward, increasing the risk of shear and pressure on the sacral area. Chairs with deeply angled backs are still in use; they should be avoided as they also push the buttocks forward, encouraging the patient to slide forward, with the potential for shear. Seat width should allow for a 2-cm clearance on either side of the buttocks. Chairs that are too wide cause the patient to loll to one side, placing undue pressure on one side of the body. If the chair is too high, the patient's feet will not rest on the floor. Pressure which is normally taken through the feet will be transferred to the thighs and buttocks, increasing the risk of damage to these areas. Seating that is too low or too short in depth will prevent pressure being taken through the thighs and this will increase pressure and the risk of damage to the buttock area. The additional muscular effort required to rise from chairs which are too low can result in the less mobile and older person being stranded. Ill-fitting or poorly padded chairs may lead to pressure not only on

the sacrum and ischium but also on the spinous processes. Any form of seating which causes the person to slide forward or down the chair may result in excessive pressure on the heels and heel ulceration. For further background reading on seating principles and types of cushions, see Collins (2001a; 2001b; 2001c).

Cushions   Excessively high mean interface pressures of 226 mmHg have been reported in wheelchairs used without cushions (Rithalia 1989), highlighting the importance of cushions in pressure ulcer prevention. It is important that the cushion is appropriate to the patient and chair or wheelchair in which it will be used. The occupational therapist has particular expertise in this area and advice can be sought through the occupational therapy department. A wide range of foam, siliconized hollow-fibre, bead, gel, water and alternating-pressure cushions are now available, of varying degrees of sophistication. As with the pressure-relieving mattresses, the cushion cover can significantly impinge on the cushion's effectiveness and covers should be chosen with care. Despite significant improvements in design, most cushions cannot relieve pressure completely, thus additional pressure relief strategies will be required.

Protecting specific body areas: comfort aids
Heels   Heels are a frequent location for pressure damage. The small surface area of heels and their relative lack of subcutaneous tissue makes pressure redistribution difficult. Correct choice of seating may reduce the risk of heel damage in the seated patient and there is a range of commercially available heel protectors for use with patients nursed in bed. Ideally, these devices should lift the heels clear off the bed but, in doing so, should not put undue pressure on the surrounding area, for example, the Achilles tendon or calf. The effect of the device on limb position will need consideration in patients who have had orthopaedic surgery; patient comfort and the ability to decontaminate the equipment after use are other essential considerations. In the absence of commercially available heel protectors, pillows can be used but care in their positioning is essential to prevent pressure under the calf or knee. 'Doughnut' ring cushions or similar devices have been shown to impede blood and lymph flow in the surrounding area, thus contributing to tissue breakdown (Crewe 1987).

Comfort aids   There are a number of sacral and elbow protectors available made of foam, gel, siliconized hollow-fibres, bandages and artificial sheepskin. Many frail older people find them comfortable and of value in protecting friable skin from the friction of rough sheets or the sharp foot plates of wheelchairs. There is little evidence as to their pressure-relieving value; it is unlikely that they make a great contribution to the prevention of pressure ulcers and are best thought of as comfort aids. More significantly, some may be harmful by restricting the blood supply, such as the heel 'doughnut' made from bandages, or by creating very high friction values, such as fleeces.

Summary Very few of the aids available totally remove the need for continued preventive care by nurses and other members of the multidisciplinary team. At best, most reduce the frequency with which pressure relief is required, and if nurses do not appreciate the principles on which the device works and its limitations, the patient is at considerable risk.

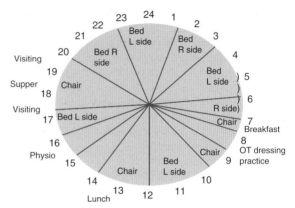

Fig. 19.4 A 24-h schedule of pressure relief. (After Lowthian 1979.)

Turning and positioning

Three principles can be used to minimize the effects of pressure, friction and shear in patients who are nursed in bed: (1) limiting the amount to which the head of the bed is elevated; (2) limiting the length of time the patient is nursed in a semirecumbent position; and (3) the use of positioning techniques, profiling beds and additional support with pillows to counter the effects of gravity and pressure. This includes careful positioning of the limbs to prevent contractures and pressure damage where bony prominences touch each other.

Risk reduction strategies for the vulnerable person should encompass a 24-h repositioning regimen. Despite being the traditional method of relieving pressure, there has been only a modest amount of research evaluating the effectiveness and required frequency of this approach (Clark 1998). The extent of manual repositioning needed for pressure-relieving purposes when using pressure-relieving support surfaces is unknown.

Traditionally, repositioning has been administered 2-hourly but the frequency should be based on individual assessment of need, and may be as much as half-hourly (Clark 1998). To be acceptable, the format of the regimen must be planned and agreed with the patient and carers, and should be constructed around the patient's daily routine and lifestyle. Lowthian's (1979) 24-hour turning clock is a simple aid used to record and communicate the repositioning regimen and can be individualized to suit the patient's needs and wishes (Fig. 19.4). A number of devices, such as electric profiling beds, turning and tilting beds, hoists and standing and raising aids, are available to assist with moving and repositioning.

To protect the vulnerable pressure points of the trochanter, a 30° tilt rather than a lateral 90° turn is advocated. High interface pressures and low transcutaneous oxygen tensions have been recorded when patients lie directly on the trochanter (Seiler et al. 1986). At an angle of 30°, direct pressure on the trochanter is avoided, being dissipated through the gluteal muscle, increasing the time the tissue can tolerate pressure (Fig. 19.5). In this position Seiler et al. found that neither the sacral nor the trochanteric skin became hypoxic. Similar results were reported by Colin et al. (1996). The extent to which the 30° tilt is effective in the older person with reduced muscle bulk and collagen content is not extensively discussed in the literature, but from a theoretical perspective it is conceivable that the age-related changes in the tissues would make them less able to dissipate pressure. Bliss (1996) has observed that the 30° tilt is less well tolerated than the lateral position by older people with poor balance or disorientation due to cerebrovascular disease. For an account of this technique, see Preston (1988).

Maintaining and improving tissue tolerance to pressure

Individual assessment will identify specific interventions required to enhance tissue tolerance to pressure. An interdisciplinary action plan should be established to alleviate the risk factors individually identified for each patient. The management of each risk factor demands expert knowledge and requires a range of interprofessional skills, highlighting the complexity of pressure ulcer prevention. Areas to consider are outlined below. An indepth review of prevention plans for all possible risk factors is beyond the scope of this text and the reader is directed to other specialist texts.

Multidisciplinary plan

A successful risk reduction plan will require dialogue between team members, the client and the family or carers, and will draw on the diverse skills and expertise of the multidisciplinary team. The assistance of additional specific specialist help beyond the expertise of the team may be required. These plans will include correction or restabilization of underlying disease processes, for example heart failure, diabetes and the management of associated symptoms which may make tissues more vulnerable to damage, such as oedema, and a review of the patient's drug regimen. The management of pain is equally important as this will influence the patient's psychological state and the desire to move.

Psychological care

The patient's psychological state should be considered and depression identified and treated. Adequate sleep and rest are important for psychological well-being and for tissue regeneration and repair.

Nutritional support

A formal assessment of nutritional status should feature as an integral component in the health assessment of the older individual, and this is now beginning to receive attention. Malnutrition and dehydration can result from many disease processes and older people are more at risk from malnutrition than many other client groups. Research on the role of nutrition in the aetiology of pressure ulcers is continuing and includes

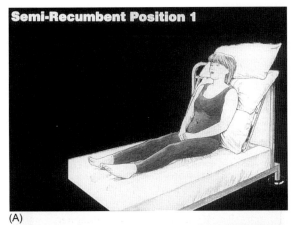
(A)

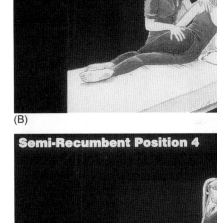
(B)

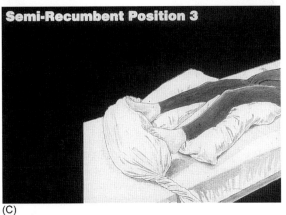
(C)

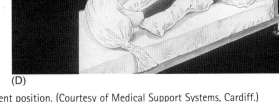
(D)

Fig. 19.5   (a)–(d) The semirecumbent position. (e)–(j) The recumbent position. (Courtesy of Medical Support Systems, Cardiff.)
Semirecumbent 30° tilt position
(a) The patient's lower back should be positioned as far into the pillow as possible to support the lumbar spine. Pump or fold the lower pillow if necessary.
(b) An additional pillow is placed underneath the other pillows. The corner is carefully positioned under the buttock to tilt the body and give clearance to the ischial tuberosities and sacrum.
(c) The legs are supported as in parts g and h showing the recumbent position. Ensure the heels are clear of the mattress and that the feet are correctly positioned. Note: the use of pillows against the soles of the feet is contraindicated in some clients, particularly stroke patients: seek advice from the physiotherapist.
(d) The full semirecumbent 30° tilt position.

Continued

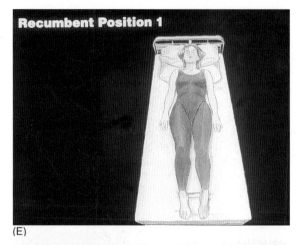

(E)

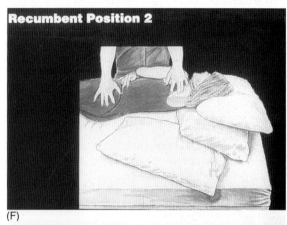

(F)

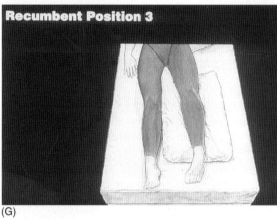

(G)

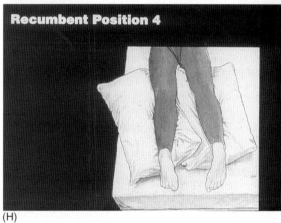

(H)

Fig. 19.5 Cont'd   *Recumbent 30° tilt position*
(e) Lie the patient in the centre of the bed. Use one or two pillows to support the head and neck.
(f) Use a further pillow to support the lumbar region and shoulder. This tilts the patient on to one buttock and lifts the sacrum clear of the mattress. Use your hand to check this clearance.
(g) Support the full leg by placing it centrally on another pillow. Ensure that the heel overhangs the edge of the pillow.
(h) An additional pillow gives further comfort to any unsupported areas of the other leg.

a Cochrane review (Langer et al. 2003); it appears likely that a nutritionally compromised patient is at greater risk of pressure ulcers. Those individuals not achieving a nutritional intake that meets the recommended daily requirements for their age and activity level, or who show evidence of being nutritionally compromised, will require a plan of nutritional support under the guidance of the dietician. For a discussion on nutritional assessment and nutritional problems in the older person, the reader is referred to Chapter 16.

Skin care

The principles of the skin care strategy are to minimize irritation and maceration of the epidermis by moisture and chemical irritants such as urine, and improve the quality and hydration of the skin. Dry skin and skin exposed to constant moisture is more susceptible to damage, particularly if the moisture contains chemical irritants, as found in body fluids. Dry skin also lacks suppleness and can fissure and crack, making the epidermis less resistant to injury. As dry skin is a common feature of ageing, due to a decrease in water content and sebum production, it would seem prudent to implement a skin care regimen aimed at maintaining natural skin oils and hydration. In addition to regular skin assessments, this should include the avoidance of repeated, prolonged exposure to moisture and prompt skin cleansing after soiling to reduce the potential of irritants to damage the epidermis. Warm rather than hot water and a mild cleanser rather than soap should

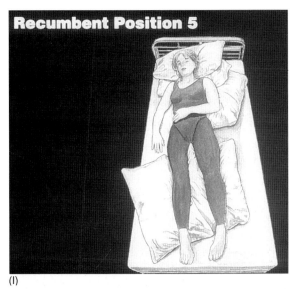

(I)

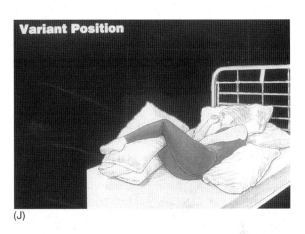

(J)

Fig. 19.5 Cont'd   (i) The full recumbent 30° tilt position.
(j) Variant position.

be used. pH-balanced skin cleansers may have a role in maintaining skin integrity in such patients. Applying a moisturizer after bathing will help retain the moisture absorbed by the skin during bathing and will improve its hydration. Dry skin which has lost its natural oils may also benefit from the application of oil-based creams. Barrier creams containing silicone or zinc can help prevent skin damage from repeated incontinence or diarrhoea but lanolin-based products should be avoided as some patients are sensitive to these. Cavilon® barrier film may also be used to protect intact or superficially damaged skin from irritation from urine or wound exudate. This is applied as a fluid, which rapidly dries to provide a colourless barrier lasting up to 72 h. Semipermeable film or hydrocolloid dressings can be useful in protecting vulnerable areas, such as heels, elbows and sacrum, from moisture or friction damage.

Promoting continence

Most forms of incontinence are amenable to correction or improvement and support from the continence adviser may be required when this is a problem. Plastic-backed incontinence pads encourage skin maceration through sweating, and if incorrectly applied can act as a source of pressure in the sedentary patient; ill-fitting incontinence pants can cut into and chafe the skin. Their indiscriminate use without an individualized assessment and continence plan is to be condemned. A review of the role of continence aids in maintaining skin integrity can be found in Hughes (2002).

Moving and handling

The principles of skilled handling techniques must include the avoidance of friction and shear on the sacrum and heels. The facilitation of normal movement should be the primary strategy for moving clients, supported, where necessary, by sliding sheets, hoists, standing aids, one-way glides and similar devices. This promotes self-care, minimizes trauma from careless handling and ensures adherence to the *Manual Handling Operations Regulations* (Health and Safety Executive 1992). Encouraging ambulation via physiotherapy and exercises designed to increase coordination, balance, flexibility and muscle strength will increase the patient's ability and confidence to readjust posture, move and mobilize independently. In addition to their lead role in re-educating the patient towards mobility, physiotherapists can advise on positioning, and back-care advisors on safe moving and handling techniques. A discussion of mobility can be found in Chapter 13.

Continuity of care

When patients are being transferred, liaison within and between community and hospital settings is essential if the prevention plan is to be maintained. To enable appropriate preparation of support surfaces, the prevention needs of individual patients require communicating to hospital departments, district nursing services and nursing homes in advance of the patient arriving. This is particularly important when the patient is being transferred into community settings, as sufficient time is needed for the ordering and delivery of equipment. Within the hospital setting, accident and emergency, operating theatre and radiology departments are areas where patients are often immobile for long periods and where pressure relief requires special consideration. Monitoring the length of time patients are required to wait for ambulance transfer or portering services may identify points in the patient trajectory which contribute significantly to pressure damage, and where greater continuity of care is needed.

Education and practice development

Patients are central to the prevention plan. Their involvement, together with that of their family or carers, in the planning process and in setting and agreeing objectives is essential for success. Motivation to accept and participate in the plan depends upon the patient's understanding of the cause and significance of pressure ulcers, the risk factors and means of prevention. For this reason, any prevention plan needs to incorporate a plan of education which takes account of the patient's and family's existing knowledge, cognitive abilities, specific needs and lifestyle, with the aim of motivating them to participate and ultimately take responsibility for preventive care in so far as condition and ability allow. This is particularly so if clients are living at home where they and/or their family may have primary responsibility for implementing the prevention plan.

The Royal College of Nursing *Clinical Practice Guidelines: Pressure Ulcer Risk Assessment and Prevention Recommendations* (2000) recommend interdisciplinary education and training in pressure ulcer risk assessment and prevention for all health care professionals in the following areas:

1. pathophysiology, risk factors and risk assessment, including the limitations and potential applications of risk assessment scales
2. skin assessment and care
3. selection, use and maintenance of pressure-redistributing equipment
4. patient positioning and manual handling
5. interprofessional roles and responsibilities
6. policies and procedures for the transfer of patients between care settings
7. documentation
8. patient education and information-giving.

Other initiatives for developing practice include the patient-focused benchmarking of eight fundamental areas of care (Department of Health 2001). The pressure ulcer benchmark covers nine factors:

1. the extent to which screening and detailed assessment take place
2. level/expertise of the practitioner undertaking the assessment
3. provision of information to clients and carers
4. the existence of individualized, documented, multidisciplinary plans for prevention, treatment and ongoing assessment
5. the assessment and documentation of the patient's need for repositioning
6. the assessment and documentation of the patient's need for pressure-redistributing support surfaces
7. availability of resources and equipment
8. the extent to which there is implementation of an individualized multidisciplinary plan
9. evaluation of interventions and patient participation by a registered practitioner.

The benchmarking process provides practitioners with a structured approach for comparing practice within and between settings. It aims to identify good practice and develop actions to improve poor care; comparison groups, networking and sharing best practice are used as a means of raising standards.

Summary
Physiological age-related changes may reduce the soft tissues' tolerance of external mechanical forces, placing the older compromised adult at greater risk of pressure ulcers. Despite the large volume of literature, current research knowledge on the causes and prevention of pressure ulcers is undermined by weaknesses in the research design of existing studies and there is a need for more methodologically sound empirical investigations, in particular randomized controlled trials, to confirm understanding and inform decision-making.

MANAGEMENT OF PRESSURE ULCERS

Meticulous attention to preventive care, both systemic and local, can avoid the development of pressure ulcers for most patients. Intensive preventive measures may not prevent the occurrence of pressure damage in significantly compromised patients, particularly those who are terminally ill. When severe, pressure ulcers can be life-threatening, and restoring skin integrity in patients with deep wounds presents particular challenges to the multidisciplinary team.

The general principles of pressure ulcer management are to relieve pressure, remove and avoid predisposing factors and to support and enhance the body's own wound-healing abilities. Selection of appropriate wound dressings is guided by a holistic patient assessment. To undertake this effectively, the practitioner requires a sound knowledge of the wound-healing process and factors influencing healing. The collection of wound assessment data is required in order to prescribe and deliver a holistic, individualized wound care plan.

The following section provides an overview of wound healing and the principles of wound assessment. A brief résumé of wound-dressing products is also included. For an indepth coverage and specialized literature on this complex subject the reader is directed to the list of recommended reading at the end of the chapter.

Wound healing

The healing of wounds involves a variety of complex mechanisms interlinked in a continuous process of repair. For convenience these can be grouped under three headings: inflammation, proliferation and maturation. There are two additional mechanisms that occur alongside these stages: contraction and epithelialization. A brief summary of the key features of each stage of normal adult wound healing is given below. Differences in these processes occur at both the early and later stages of the life cycle, and an account of these is given by Desai (1997a, 1997b).

Inflammation
Damaged tissues release histamine and other substances; the vasodilatation and increased permeability of capillaries resulting from this chemical response bring neutrophils and, later, macrophages, which have a major role in clearing bacteria and debris from the wound. Macrophages secrete a range of growth factors essential for wound repair, for example platelet-derived growth factor and transforming growth factor-beta which stimulate collagen deposition and which, in conjunction with other growth factors, initiate and control the repair process (Desai 1997a). These cells and substances are found in wound exudate, the fluid that collects in the wound bed. Any attempt to remove or dry this fluid, or chemically destroy its constituents, for example via inappropriate wound dressings or cleansing agents, will delay healing. Vasodilatation enhances the blood supply to the damaged area and, in so doing, provides the additional nutrients required in the rebuilding process. Patients who have a depressed inflammatory response as a result of disease or drug therapy may experience delay in this phase of healing.

The wound must be free of debris, clinical infection and devitalized tissue before tissue repair can begin. Under normal circumstances, neutrophils and macrophages achieve this, obviating the need for routine cleansing of all wounds. Only when the wound is visibly contaminated with dirt, or contains pus or large amounts of necrotic tissue, is cleansing necessary. This is often the case with deep pressure ulcers, which frequently contain necrotic tissue, slough or eschar.

Proliferation
New blood vessels and collagen strands develop to form granulation tissue. Under the influence of transforming growth factor-beta, fibroblasts are attracted into the wound where they proliferate to produce and deposit a matrix of collagen in the wound. Dietary amino acids, vitamins and trace elements are essential in this process, hence patients in a poor nutritional state are likely to experience delayed tissue repair.

Maturation
This is an ongoing process of collagen synthesis and degradation which continues for many months after the wound appears visibly healed. Cross-linking, remodelling and realignment of collagen occur to ensure maximum strength but the mature collagen scar never achieves the full tensile strength of the original tissue it replaces.

Contraction
Part of the healing process is achieved by contraction of the wound – an inward centripetal movement of the wound edges initiated by myofibroblasts. The effect of this process becomes evident if the dimensions of the mature scar tissue are compared with the initial size of the wound; the former is usually one-tenth of the original size of the wound (Thomas 1990). Contraction is an important healing mechanism for wounds with tissue loss, such as pressure ulcers, as this reduces the deficit to be repaired. It takes place most effectively in wounds which are free from debris, infection and eschar, and is delayed in the presence of adherent dressings and in wounds which have been permitted to dry out (Thomas 1990). Applications of chemicals such as cleansing agents can also impair this process. These are important considerations when managing pressure ulcers if healing by contraction is to be maximized.

Epithelialization
Hair follicles and the wound margins provide the main source of epidermal regeneration, and in shallow wounds which contain viable hair follicles, migration of epidermal cells across the wound surface can occur fairly rapidly. Winter (1976) demonstrated that it takes 7 days to bridge the gap between two hair follicles. For deeper wounds, healing is much slower because the sources of epidermal regeneration, other than at the wound margins, are lost.

The speed at which wounds progress through the above stages and events depends on the nature of the wound (incised surgical wounds versus cavity wounds), the amount of tissue loss and the condition of the patient. Sutured surgical wounds have little tissue loss and heal rapidly. In contrast, pressure ulcers have large areas of tissue damage with loss of the skin and subcutaneous layers. These wounds cannot be sutured and the body must replace the lost tissue by the process of granulation, which occurs from the base of the wound upwards. Once the deficit is repaired, epithelialization takes place. Healing in this type of wound is termed healing by secondary intention. Inevitably, wounds healing by secondary intention take longer to heal than sutured wounds.

The healing process is thought to slow with age, although the comparison of healing rates by age is made difficult due to a lack of standardization of research methods and definitions used, and difficulties in controlling for confounding variables such as nutritional status and disease states. As age advances, changes have been described at each stage of the healing process; some activities appear less intense, while others are enhanced, due in part to a reduction in the number of cells and an altered response to growth factors. For a review of age-related changes in the wound-healing process, see Desai (1997b).

From a clinical perspective, the most relevant considerations for wound repair are the influencing factors which affect healing, and which may be more pronounced in later life. Most individuals who develop pressure ulcers do so during times of ill health, and the effect of their compromised health status is likely to affect the body's healing ability: multipathology, polypharmacy and impaired nutritional state are more common amongst the older population, and influencing factors such as these may explain the slowed healing rate just as much as any age-related change in the healing mechanism.

Wound assessment

It is impossible to judge the rate of healing or deterioration of a wound or the effectiveness of local treatments without assessing the wound. While pressure ulcer grading systems provide some information on the degree of tissue loss, on their own they do not provide sufficient information on the size of the wound or factors influencing the healing process.

Holistic wound assessment and factors influencing healing

To be effective, wound assessment must encompass the whole patient and give consideration to the physi-

ological, psychological and social factors that might influence the wound-healing process. These include the underlying medical condition and related therapeutic interventions. Medical problems such as those which impair oxygen uptake, tissue perfusion, nutritional or fluid intake will compromise the body's ability to repair itself. Medical treatments may also impair the healing process, for example steroid therapy and cancer treatments. The location of the wound and activity level of the patient will influence the choice of wound dressing; location may also indicate the potential risk for infection, for example wounds on the buttocks and sacrum will be at greater risk of faecal and urinary contamination, particularly in the incontinent patient. Odour may be indicative of infection and can have a distressing psychological effect on the patient and the family. Pain assessment is an integral part of wound assessment. Pain may result from the underlying disease process, from the wound itself or the wound management regimen. Pain can limit the patient's ability to tolerate the plan of care and may interfere with sleep. As wound repair proceeds most rapidly during sleep, impaired sleep may, in turn, delay the healing process.

Wound measurement

In clinical practice it is customary to photograph and/or trace the circumference of the ulcer on to transparent film in order to monitor changes in the size of the wound and the condition of the wound bed. Tracing film forms an integral part of some wound dressing products (e.g. Opsite Flexigrid®). When tracing, the wound is covered with cling film to maintain hygiene, and the wound margins traced on to acetate or tracing paper using a permanent felt-tip pen. Areas of necrosis, slough, granulation and epithelial tissue can be marked. The photograph or tracing is dated and labelled with the patient's name and hospital number and filed in the patient's notes. Contraction will result in the wound changing shape as it heals; this process, in conjunction with debridement, can initially make the wound appear larger and this should be borne in mind when interpreting the wound assessment data.

Tracing or photography will not reveal the depth of the wound. The depth and amount of tissue loss are important in pressure ulcer wound assessment, as significant tissue destruction can occur without this being evident at the wound surface. It is therefore not uncommon for the diameter of the wound tracing to be significantly smaller than the underlying cavity. The presence and extent of any undermining must be gently and carefully assessed by an experienced practitioner using a sterile round-ended probe. Deep pressure ulcers which have penetrated the fascia and muscle can quickly extend along and around bones and joints and present a major risk of serious systemic infection. For this reason a skilled appraisal of deep cavity ulcers must be undertaken promptly and appropriate specialist help sought without delay.

Assessment of the wound bed

Inspection of the wound bed and wound margins is an essential part of wound assessment. This helps identify the stages of healing and the presence of factors which may delay the healing process and which need priority attention, for example, the presence of devitalized tissue and infection. By their very nature, pressure ulcers frequently contain dead tissue resulting from ischaemia and related responses. Skin affected in this way loses the ability to control evaporation of moisture and dehydration occurs, resulting in a dry, black, leathery area – an eschar. Continued evaporation will extend the dehydration process into the subcutaneous layers. Visualization of the wound bed will also identify specific features of the wound which will need to be considered when selecting an appropriate wound dressing. These include the shape and accessibility, condition of the surrounding skin, amount and type of exudate, the presence of slough, eschar, infection, and the presence of granulation tissue or epithelial tissue.

Structured wound assessment forms are increasing in popularity. These aim to encourage consistent and complete documentation of the wound assessment and, in some cases, measure healing rates; examples of such forms can be found in the literature (Morison 1992, Dealey 1994, Briggs & Banks 1996, Flanagan 1997, Stotts 2001). The benefits of providing specific forms for wound assessment and wound care planning, and the effects of their introduction on clinical practice, are described by Briggs & Banks (1996).

Principles of management

The general principles and priorities of wound care are to support the body's own mechanisms for wound cleansing and healing. Pressure ulcers are chronic wounds, and their management will also focus on correcting imbalances that occur within the microenvironment of the chronic wound (Romanelli & Mastronicola 2002). Due to factors such as the recurrence of necrotic tissue, repeated trauma (e.g. unrelieved pressure) and heavy bacterial loading, pressure ulcers exhibit prolonged and complex inflammatory processes, and produce high levels of exudate. These events cause biochemical and cellular changes within the wound, which have a negative effect on healing. In order to promote healing, preparation of the wound bed aims to debride necrotic tissue, control exudate and correct bacterial imbalance. This is achieved by the application of a primary wound dressing which creates an optimal healing environment, appropriate to the stage of healing, depth of tissue loss and condition of the wound bed. A thorough wound assessment will provide the information required to select an appropriate wound dressing and identify the specific factors affecting healing, enabling the relevant corrective interventions and referrals to be planned accordingly. In keeping with the natural sequence of healing, infection must be treated and necrotic, sloughy tissue removed before granulation can proceed effectively – initial care must focus on these priorities. The cause of the pressure ulcer must also be addressed as a matter of priority. Patients with pressure ulcers are at high risk of developing further pressure damage and, in addition to caring for the wound, management of patients with ulcers must also focus on pressure relief and the removal and avoidance of predisposing risk factors. Meeting psychosocial needs, maintaining quality of life and ensuring patient participation should be central features of the wound care plan.

The potential for healing may be limited in patients whose prognosis is poor. For these individuals improving the appearance of the wound, enhancing body image and the control of their symptoms (odour, exudate and wound pain) are essential to maintaining their quality of life; in such cases these become the goals of wound care. Particular care should be taken to discuss the goals of wound care with all members of the team, including the patient, in order to avoid subjecting patients to painful care regimens which have little chance of success, to the detriment of their comfort and quality of life.

Cleansing and debridement

Routine cleansing of wounds is unnecessary, and may delay the healing process due to mechanical or chemical trauma, or cooling the wound by the application of cold fluids. Where there is loose, superficial debris or remnants of dressing products to be removed from the wound, cleansing is best achieved by irrigating the wound with warm, potable tap water (Griffiths et al. 2001, Fernandez et al. 2002); sterile saline 0.9% should be used for very deep wounds with exposed tendon or bone, or if the patient is immunosuppressed. Irrigation can be achieved in a variety of ways: for a discussion of irrigation methods and fluids, and their effects on wound healing, see Lawrence (1997). On occasions mechanical swabbing with gauze may be justified in order to remove adherent tissue and debris from the wound bed; however, owing to the risk of mechanical trauma to granulating tissue and the potential for introducing gauze fibres into the wound, which in turn may act as foci for bacterial growth, this method should be avoided wherever possible. In wounds that show evidence of clinical infection, measures to reduce the bacterial load will be required: this will include systemic antibiotic therapy and the use of appropriate dressing products.

The term 'debridement' describes the removal of dead tissue from a wound. As already noted, debriding a pressure ulcer of all necrotic tissue is necessary before healing can begin. Some methods of debridement are summarized below; for more comprehensive reviews of wound debridement, see Bale (1997) and Vowden & Vowden (1999a, 1999b).

Surgical debridement Surgical excision of necrotic tissue and slough is the quickest and most effective method of debridement. The procedure is commonly performed under a general anaesthetic but in certain circumstances it may be possible to undertake small areas of surgical debridement at the bedside. Particular care is required with this procedure: anatomical structures within sloughy and necrotic wounds can be difficult for the inexperienced practitioner to identify and there is a real danger of accidentally severing nerves, blood vessels and tendons, particularly in areas such as the lower leg, where there is little soft tissue overlying the bone. For this reason surgical debridement should only be undertaken by surgeons or appropriately trained specialist practitioners.

Autolytic debridement The rehydration and softening of dry and devitalized tissue will enable the body's own enzymes to break down and liquefy dead tissue – termed autolysis. In time, the dead tissue will separate spontaneously from the healthy underlying tissue. Rehydration can be achieved by the application of a hydrogel water-containing dressing which will release its water content into the wound, or by the application of a dressing which prevents, or significantly reduces, water evaporation. There are a number of occlusive and semipermeable primary dressing products suitable for this purpose, for example, the hydrocolloids. Autolytic debridement is the safest and most comfortable means of debridement and for this reason may be considered the method of choice, particularly with frail older people. This approach does, however, take longer than other methods.

Enzymatic agents Proteolytic enzymes which liquefy necrotic tissue can be used as debriding agents. Varidase® contains the enzymes streptokinase and streptodornase which break down fibrin, collagen and elastin. It can be applied either directly on a soaked gauze swab or mixed with KY® jelly and applied after scoring the eschar with a scalpel until oozing occurs. It

can also be injected under the eschar. Other enzymatic treatments exist, for example, crab collagenase (Glyantsev & Adamyan 1997) and larval therapy.

Larval therapy There is renewed interest in larval therapy, using the larvae of the greenbottle fly *Lucilia sericata*. These larvae secrete proteolytic enzymes which dissolve dead tissue into a semiliquid which they then ingest. Applications not exceeding 10 larvae per 10 cm^2 are recommended (Bale 1997); excessive applications can result in an erythematous reaction caused by an excess of the proteolytic enzymes. For further discussion and case study review, see Thomas et al. (1996).

Chemical debridement Chemical debriding agents, such as the hypochlorites – for example, Edinburgh University solution of lime (eusol) and Milton – were once commonly used as antimicrobial and debriding agents. Hypochlorites are toxic to cells and delay wound healing by increasing the inflammatory response, interfering with collagen synthesis, and by damaging epithelial cells; their antimicrobial and debridement activity is now known to be weak (Brennan et al. 1986, Leaper 1986). For these reasons chemical debriding agents are rarely used today.

Wound dressings

The ideal dressing

Pressure ulcers at different stages of healing require different wound dressings. Modern wound products aim to create an 'ideal' environment which maximizes tissue repair. The properties of the 'ideal' dressing are described by many authors and include: maintenance of a moist wound–dressing interface; absorption of excess exudate; prevention of bacterial contamination; maintenance of an optimum temperature; promotion of patient comfort and prevention of trauma to the wound upon removal; free from toxins, residues and contaminants (Turner 1982, Johnson 1988, Thomas 1990).

Epithelialization occurs at a faster rate if dehydration and scab formation are prevented. Winter (1976) reported a two- to threefold increase in the rate of epithelial cell migration in moist wounds covered with an oxygen-permeable film dressing. Under a scab, this process is hindered by collagen fibres at the junction of the scab and the drying dermis (Thomas 1990). Maintenance of a moist wound can also prevent wound pain associated with dehydration of the sensory nerve endings. Preventing the dehydration of wound exudate also prevents adherence of the dressing, and associated pain and trauma to the wound upon removal. Furthermore, substances essential to wound repair are lost if dehydration of the wound and its exudate is permitted, and, as already noted, hydration of slough and necrotic tissue facilitates debridement by autolysis. Excess exudate can, however, cause maceration of the surrounding skin. The 'ideal' dressing therefore needs to absorb excess exudate away from the wound while maintaining a moist wound–dressing interface. A review of wound exudate, its role in wound healing and its implications for dressing selection is given by Thomas (1997).

Cell division and enzyme activity are influenced by the temperature of the wound. Exposed wounds are prone to heat loss and cooling, as are wounds exposed to frequent dressing changes and cold cleansing fluids. A fall of 2°C can be sufficient to arrest healing; wounds that have been cooled take approximately 40 min to regain their normal temperature, and up to 3 h for mitotic and leukocytic activity to recommence (Johnson 1988). Wound dressings which have good thermal properties to maintain the wound at body temperature and require infrequent dressing changes will help prevent delayed healing due to cooling.

Atmospheric oxygen was formerly believed to be essential for rapid wound healing. More recent studies indicate that the formation of granulation tissue and new blood vessels is enhanced by a slightly hypoxic environment (Johnson 1988), while epithelialization benefits from increased oxygen.

Occlusive and semipermeable dressings prevent the movement of bacteria into or away from the wound site and are advantageous in preventing delayed healing from wound contamination and cross-infection. Particulate matter from fibrous dressings can become embedded in the healing wound, delaying tissue repair. This is less common with modern wound products, but the potential for their contamination with residual chemicals from the manufacturing process is noted by Thomas (1990).

Choice of wound dressing

No product meets all the requirements of an 'ideal' dressing. A vast range of modern wound products are now available, each varying in its specific properties and ability to meet the 'ideal' criteria. In order to make an appropriate choice, the properties of the wound care product need to be matched to the type of wound, its specific needs, the extent of tissue loss and stage of healing. Products can be broadly classified into groups sharing some similarities in basic characteristics and constituents; some of these product groups are presented below. Increasingly, each product has individual and specific performance characteristics, therefore products within a particular category may not be interchangeable.

Ventilating, woven dressings   Ventilating, woven dressings such as gauze, expose the wound surface to dehy-

dration, so allowing scab formation. The dressing fibres often become entangled in the scab, resulting in pain and trauma to the granulating tissue when the dressing is removed. The fibres from these types of dressings have the potential to be shed into the wound, providing foci for bacterial growth. This is particularly relevant because they are not impermeable to bacteria. For these reasons ventilating dressings are no longer recommended as primary wound dressings for pressure ulcers.

Hydrogels   Hydrogels are hydrophilic, semipermeable water polymer gels which are conformable and non-adherent. In addition to being able to absorb small amounts of excess exudate from the wound, their high water content enables them to release water into the drier wound, making them particularly useful for rehydrating eschar and necrotic tissue. They exist as sheet dressings which have a stable cross-linked structure, enabling them to remain in this form as they absorb water, and as an amorphous hydrogel paste which, because it is not excessively cross-linked, loses its viscosity as it takes up water (Thomas & Jones 1996). The latter is more difficult to retain in situ on superficial areas such as heels. A secondary dressing is required to secure the hydrogel in place and prevent it from drying out.

Hydrocolloid dressings   Hydrocolloid dressings have an inner hydrocolloid layer that absorbs the wound exudate to form a gel which creates a moist environment. Most have a polyurethane film backing which renders them impermeable to liquids and bacteria. This characteristic can be used to prevent the spread of bacteria, such as methicillin-resistant *Staphylococcus aureus*, from infected wounds. Hydrocolloid paste is available for filling cavity wounds prior to the application of the adhesive wafer dressing. The dressings can be left in situ for 5–7 days. Aquacel® is a fibrous hydrocolloid dressing, similar to the alginates in appearance. It is highly absorbent and valuable for the heavily exuding wound.

Foam dressings   Foam dressings are highly absorbent while retaining a moist wound surface that enables rehydration and liquefaction of slough and necrotic tissue. They are soft and comfortable and are easy to shape to the contours of the wound. Some have an adhesive contact layer, while others need securing in place with a secondary dressing and/or tape. A small number of foam 'fillers' are specially designed for cavity wounds such as deep pressure ulcers. Cavi-Care® is made up from two pastes, which are mixed together and poured into the wound; the mixture expands into the wound and sets to a solid spongy foam which fits the contours of the wound exactly. This dressing can be removed, cleaned and replaced once or twice daily, as required. As the wound heals and becomes smaller, the foam will no longer fit the wound and a new dressing is required. Ready-made foam 'fillers' are available in a range of shapes and sizes.

Vapour-permeable films Vapour-permeable films are transparent, polyurethane dressings with an acrylic adhesive that are permeable to water vapour but impermeable to water and micro-organisms. Their transparency permits direct visualization of the wound bed, allowing healing to be monitored. Limited amounts of exudate can evaporate away from the wound through the film. This permeability (expressed as the moisture vapour transmission rate, g/m^2 per 24 h) varies between products. The dressings cannot accommodate medium or large amounts of exudate and have no ability to expand into cavities and are therefore inappropriate for these types of wounds. They are suitable for superficial grade 1 or 2 pressure ulcers, or for protecting healthy skin in high-risk areas, such as elbows and heels, from friction and as secondary dressings over alginates or gels. These dressings can remain in situ for approximately 7 days but their removal needs care to avoid damage to the new tissue. The technique for removal usually involves stretching the dressing to destroy the adhesive; the manufacturer's instructions should be followed carefully.

Alginates Alginates are soft, dry, fibrous dressings manufactured from brown seaweed. They exist in pad, ribbon and rope forms, the latter two being designed for filling cavity wounds such as pressure ulcers; some have an integral secondary dressing. Alginates are absorbent and react with wound exudate to form a hydrophilic gel at the wound surface, under which debridement and granulation can occur.

Heavily exuding wounds dressed with alginate will require a secondary dressing in the form of an absorbent dressing pad and may require daily dressing changes initially, but these can usually be quickly reduced in frequency as exudate production declines. A plastic secondary dressing, such as a film, will be required for wounds with only minimal exudate; this is to prevent dehydration of the wound and adherence of the dressing to the wound bed. If there is doubt as to whether there is sufficient exudate to enable a gel to form, either the dressing or the wound can be moistened with normal saline at the time of application. Since these dressings are dependent on exudate for creating a moist healing environment, they are contraindicated for application to dehydrated wounds or eschar.

The universal wound dressing does not exist and wound dressings should be thought of as 'wound-specific'. Rarely will a single product meet the needs of a wound throughout all the stages of healing; the wound dressing prescription will need to be changed as the wound progresses and its specific requirements change. This necessitates regular evaluation and reassessment of the wound.

Adjunct therapies

A range of treatments exists for use as adjunctive therapies, to initiate and accelerate healing in chronic wounds. Their effectiveness, however, remains unclear. These therapies include ultrasound, low-intensity laser therapy and electrical stimulation. For an account of these therapies, see Dyson & Lyder (2001). The Cochrane Library contains reviews of the effectiveness of electromagnetic therapy (Flemming & Cullum 2001) and hyperbaric oxygen (Kranke et al. 2004) as treatments for pressure ulcers.

Summary

Wound healing is a complex process and pressure ulcers are wounds which have a complex aetiology and pathology. Patients with pressure ulcers have particular needs, and the combined features of ageing and multipathology present particular challenges in the management of these wounds in the older adult. As with prevention, the assessment, care and evaluation of pressure ulcers require a holistic, multidisciplinary approach, in which the nurse plays a major role.

CONCLUSION

Skin care has traditionally been viewed as a basic, routine task that can be left to the least skilled staff, yet pressure necrosis is one of the greatest threats to skin integrity in the sick or frail older person. The maintenance and restoration of healthy skin require a sophisticated knowledge base and draw on a range of interprofessional skills. This aspect of care of the older adult presents specific and significant challenges to the multidisciplinary team.

Recommended reading

Bader DL (ed) 1990 Pressure sores: clinical practice and scientific approach. Macmillan, Basingstoke.
A classic multidisciplinary biomedical and nursing text on specific bioengineering, nursing and medical aspects of pressure ulcer prevention. For students seeking a broader perspective.

Bale S, Jones V 1997 Wound care nursing: a patient centred approach. Baillière Tindall, London.

An undergraduate nursing text giving broad coverage on a wide range of wound care issues across the lifespan, from wound assessment and wound healing to the management of specific wounds. Each chapter has an age-specific focus; the book includes a chapter on wound management in the older client.

Morison M J 2001 The prevention and treatment of pressure ulcers. Mosby, London.

Provides a focused review on the prevention and management of pressure ulcers. An accessible and well-referenced text, suitable for both undergraduate and postgraduate students.

Morison MJ, Moffatt C, Bridel-Nixon J, Bale S 1997 A colour guide to the nursing management of chronic wounds, 2nd edn. Mosby, London.

This book provides good coverage of wound healing, assessment and management of a range of wound types, including pressure ulcers. Although aimed at nurses, it is suitable for all senior students and qualified practitioners involved in the care of patients with wounds.

National Institute for Clinical Excellence 2003 Pressure ulcer prevention. Clinical guideline 7. NICE. Available online at: www.nice.org.uk.

All practitioners involved with patients who are vulnerable to, or at elevated risk of, pressure ulceration should ensure they are familiar with its content. It combines two earlier guidelines: pressure ulcer risk assessment and prevention, and clinical practice guideline for pressure-relieving devices: the use of pressure-relieving devices (beds, mattresses and overlays). The original guidelines can be obtained in full from the Royal College of Nursing website (www.rcn.org.uk) and NICE website (www.nice.org.uk) respectively.

The Cochrane wounds group. The Cochrane Library. Available online at: www.mrw.interscience.wiley.com/cochrane.

An excellent resource of systematic reviews and up-to-date information on evidence-based practice relating to tissue viability. The reviews are regularly updated and the library is published four times each year, in January, April, July and October.

Thomas S 1990 Wound management and dressings. Pharmaceutical Press, London.

Although in need of updating, this is a readable text and reference book giving historical, clinical and pharmaceutical detail on the major categories of wound dressing products which is not normally provided in nursing texts.

References

Abbruzzese RS 1985 Early assessment and prevention of pressure sores. In: Lee BY (ed) Chronic ulcers of the skin. McGraw-Hill, New York, pp 1–19

Allcock N, Wharrad H, Nicholson A 1994 Interpreting pressure sore prevalence. Journal of Advanced Nursing 20: 37–45

Allman RM, Laprade CA, Noel LB et al. 1986 Pressure sores amongst hospitalised patients. Annals of Internal Medicine 105: 337–342

Allman RM, Walker JM, Hart MK 1987 Air-fluidised beds or conventional therapy for pressure sores. Annals of Internal Medicine 107: 641–648

Allman RM, Goode PS, Patrick MM, Burst N, Bartolucci AA 1995 Pressure ulcer risk factors amongst hospitalised patients with activity limitation. Journal of the American Medical Association 273: 865–870

Anderson TP, Andberg MM 1979 Psychosocial factors associated with pressure sores. Archives of Physical Medicine and Rehabilitation 60: 314–346

Antony D, Reynolds T, Russell L 2000 An investigation into the use of serum albumen in pressure sore prediction. Journal of Advanced Nursing 32: 359–365

Bale S 1997 A guide to wound debridement. Journal of Wound Care 6: 179–182

Barbenel JC, Jordan MM, Nichol SM, Clark MD 1977 Incidence of pressure sores in the Greater Glasgow Health Board area. Lancet ii: 548–550

Bennett MA 1995 Report of the task force on the implications for darkly pigmented intact skin in the prediction and prevention of pressure ulcers. Advances in Wound Care 8: 34–35

Bennett L, Kavner D, Lee BY, Trainor FA 1979 Shear vs pressure as causative factors in skin blood flow. Archives of Physical Medicine and Rehabilitation 60: 309–314

Bennett L, Kavner D, Lee BY, Trainor FA, Lewis JM 1981 Skin blood flow in seated geriatric patients. Archives of Physical Medicine and Rehabilitation 62: 392–398

Bergman-Evans B, Cuddigan J, Bergstrom N 1994 Clinical practice guidelines: prediction and prevention of pressure ulcers. Journal of Gerontological Nursing 20: 19–26, 52

Bergstrom N 1993 Braden scale and clinical judgement (letter). Journal of Enterostomal Nursing 20: 133–134

Bergstrom N, Braden B 1992 A prospective study of pressure sore risk among institutionalised older. Journal of the American Geriatric Society 40: 747–758

Bergstrom N, Braden B, Laguzza A, Hollman V 1987 The Braden scale for predicting pressure sore risk. Nursing Research 36: 205–210

Bergstrom N, Braden B, Kemp M, Champagne M, Ruby E 1996 Multi-site study of incidence of pressure ulcers and the relationship between risk level, demographic characteristics, diagnoses and prescription of preventative interventions. Journal of the American Geriatric Society 44: 22–30

Bliss MR 1996 Letter. Journal of Tissue Viability 6: 127–128

Bourdel-Marchasson I, Barateau M, Rondeau V et al. 2000 A multi-center trial of the effects of oral nutritional supplementation in critically ill older inpatients. Applied Nutritional Investigations 16: 1–5

Braden B, Bergstrom N 1987 A conceptual schema for the study of the etiology of pressure sores. Rehabilitation Nursing 12: 8–12, 16

Braden BJ, Bergstrom N 1989 Clinical utility of the Braden scale for predicting pressure sore risk. Decubitus 2: 44–46, 50–51

Brandeis GH, Ooi WL, Hossain M, Morris JN, Lipsitz CA 1994 A longitudinal study of risk factors associated with the formation of pressure sores in nursing homes. Journal of the American Geriatric Society 42: 388–393

Brennan SS, Foster ME, Leaper DJ 1986 Antiseptic toxicity in wounds healing by secondary intention. Journal of Hospital Infection 8: 263–267

Bridel J 1995 Interpreting pressure sore data. Nursing Standard 1: 52–54

Briggs M, Banks S 1996 Documenting wound management. Journal of Wound Care 5: 229–231

Chaloner DM, Franks PJ 1999 Validity of the Walsall community pressure sore risk calculator. British Journal of Nursing 8: 1142, 1144, 1146, 1148, 1150, 1152, 1154, 1156

Clark M 1994 Problems associated with the measurement of interface (or contact) pressure. Journal of Tissue Viability 4: 37–42

Clark M 1998 Repositioning to prevent pressure sores – what is the evidence? Nursing Standard (Tissue Viability Supplement) 13: 58, 60, 62, 64

Clark M, Cullum N 1992 Matching patient need for pressure sore prevention with the supply of pressure redistributing mattresses. Journal of Advanced Nursing 17: 310–316

Clark M, Farrar S 1992 Comparison of pressure sore risk calculators. In: Harding KG, Leaper DL, Turner TD (eds) Proceedings of the 1st European conference on advances in wound management. Macmillan, London, pp 158–162

Clark M, Watts S 1994 The incidence of pressure sores within a national health service trust hospital during 1991. Journal of Advanced Nursing 20: 33–36

Colin D, Abraham P, Preault L, Bregeon C, Saumet JL 1996 Comparison of 90° and 30° laterally inclined positions in the prevention of pressure ulcers using transcutaneous oxygen and carbon dioxide pressures. Advances in Wound Care 9: 35–38

Collier ME 1996 Pressure reducing mattresses. Journal of Wound Care 5: 207–211

Collier ME 1999 Pressure ulcer development and principles for prevention. In: Miller M, Glover D (eds) Wound management theory and practice. NT Books, Emap, London, pp 84–95

Collins F 2001a An adequate service? Specialist seating provision in the UK. Journal of Wound Care 10: 333–337

Collins F 2001b How to assess a patient's seating needs: some basic principles. Journal of Wound Care 10: 383–386

Collins F 2001c Selecting cushions and armchairs: how to make an informed choice. Journal of Wound Care 10: 423–425, 427

Cook M, Hale C, Watson B 1999 Interrater reliability and the assessment of pressure sore risk using an adapted Waterlow scale. Clinical Effectiveness in Nursing 3: 66–74

Crewe RA 1987 Problems of rubber ring cushions and a clinical survey of alternative cushions for ill patients. Care Science and Practice 5: 9–11

Cullum N, Clark M 1992 Intrinsic factors associated with pressure sores in older people. Journal of Advanced Nursing 17: 427–431

Cullum N, McInnes E, Bell-Syer SEM, Legood R 2004 Support surfaces for pressure ulcer prevention. The Cochrane database of systematic reviews 2004, issue 3.

Article no. CD001735. DOI: 10.1002/14651858. CD001735. pub. 2. Available online at: www.mrw.interscience. wiley.com/cochrane (accessed 21 January 2005)

David JA, Chapman RG, Chapman EJ, Lockett B 1983 An investigation of the current methods used in nursing for the care of patients with established pressure sores. Report of the Nursing Practice Research Unit, University of Surrey, Guildford

Dealey C 1991 The size of the pressure sore problem in a teaching hospital. Journal of Advanced Nursing 16: 603–670

Dealey C 1994 The care of wounds. Blackwell Scientific, Oxford

Dealey C 1995 Mattresses and beds. A guide to systems available for relieving and reducing pressure. Journal of Wound Care 4: 409–412

Defloor T 1999 The risk of pressure sores: a conceptual scheme. Journal of Clinical Nursing 8: 206–216

Defloor T, Grypdonck MFH 2005 Pressure ulcers: validation of two risk assessment scales. Journal of Clinical Nursing 14: 373–382

Department of Health 1992 The health of the nation. A consultative document for health in England. HMSO, London

Department of Health 1993 Pressure sores. A key quality indicator. A guide for purchasers and providers. Department of Health, Lancashire

Department of Health 2001 The essence of care. Patient-focused benchmarking for healthcare practitioners. Department of Health, London

Desai H 1997a Ageing and wounds. Part 1: foetal and postnatal healing. Journal of Wound Care 6: 192–196

Desai H 1997b Ageing and wounds. Part 2: healing in old age. Journal of Wound Care 6: 237–239

Dyson R 1978 Bedsores – the injuries hospital staff inflict on patients. Nursing Mirror 146: 30–32

Dyson M, Lyder C 2001 Wound management: physical modalities. In: Morison MJ (ed) The prevention and treatment of pressure ulcers. Mosby, London, pp 177–193

European Pressure Ulcer Advisory Panel [undated] Pressure ulcer treatment guidelines. EPUAP, Oxford

Exton-Smith AN, Sherwin RW 1961 The prevention of pressure sores. The significance of spontaneous body movements. Lancet ii: 1123–1126

Fernandez R, Griffiths R, Ussia C 2002 Water for wound cleansing. The Cochrane database of systematic reviews 2002. Issue 1. Article no. CD003861. DOI: 10.1002/14651858. CD003861. Available online at: www.mrw.interscience.wiley.com/cochrane (accessed 21 January 2005)

Flanagan M 1997 Wound management. Churchill Livingstone, London

Flemming K, Cullum N 2001 Electromagnetic therapy for treating pressure sores. The Cochrane database of systematic reviews 2001. Issue 1. Article no. CD002930. DOI: 10.1002/14651858. CD002930. Available online at: www.mrw.interscience.wiley.com/cochrane (accessed 21 January 2005)

Gebhardt KS, Bliss MR, Winwright PL, Thomas JM 1996 Pressure-relieving supports in an ICU. Journal of Wound Care 5: 116–121

Glyantsev SP, Adamyan AA 1997 Crab collagenase in wound debridement. Journal of Wound Care 6: 13–16

Goldstone LA, Goldstone J 1982 The Norton score: an early warning of pressure sores? Journal of Advanced Nursing 7: 419–426

Gordis L 1996 Epidemiology. WB Saunders, London

Griffiths RD, Fernandez RS, Ussia CA 2001 Is tap water a safe alternative to normal saline for wound irrigation in the community setting? Journal of Wound Care 10:407–411

Gunningberg L, Lindholm C, Carlsson M, Sjoden PO 2000 Effect of visco-elastic foam mattresses on the development of pressure ulcers in patients with hip fractures. Journal of Wound Care 9: 455–460

Guralnik JM, Harris TB, White LR, Cornoni-Huntley JC 1988 Occurrence and predictors of pressure sores in the national health and nutrition examination survey follow-up. Journal of the American Geriatric Society 36: 807–812

Halfens RJG, Van Achterberg T, Bal RM 2000 Validity and reliability of the Braden scale and the influence of other risk factors: a multi-centre prospective study. International Journal of Nursing Studies 37: 313–319

Hall DA, Reed FB, Nuki G, Vince JD 1974 The relative effects of age and corticosteroid therapy on the collagen profiles of dermis from subjects with rheumatoid arthritis. Age and Ageing 3: 15–22

Hall DA, Blackett AD, Zajac AR, Switala S, Airey CM 1981 Changes in skinfold thickness with increasing age. Age and Ageing 3: 19–23

Healey F 1995 The reliability and utility of pressure sore grading scales. Journal of Tissue Viability 5: 111–114

Health and Safety Executive 1992 Manual handling guidance on regulations. Manual handling operations regulations. HMSO, London

Houwing RH, Rozendaal M, Wouters-Wesseling W et al. 2002 A randomised, double-blind assessment of the effect of nutritional supplementation on the prevention of pressure ulcers in hip-fracture patients. Clinical Nutrition 21(suppl. 1): 84(abstract)

Hughes S 2002 Do continence aids help to maintain skin integrity? Journal of Wound Care 11: 235–239

International Association for Enterostomal Therapists 1988 Dermal wounds: pressure sores. Philosophy of the IAET. Journal of Enterostomal Therapy 15: 4–17

Johnson A 1985 A blueprint for the prevention and management of pressure sores. Care Science and Practice 1: 8–13

Johnson A 1988 Criteria for ideal wound dressings. Professional Nurse 3: 191–193

Kranke P, Bennett M, Roeckl-Wiedmann I, Debus S 2004 Hyperbaric oxygen for chronic wounds. The Cochrane database of systematic reviews 2004. Issue 1. Article no. CD004123. DOI: 10.1002/14651858. CD004123.pub 2. Available online at:

www.mrw.interscience.wiley.com/ cochrane (accessed 21 January 2005)

Krouskop TA 1983 A synthesis of the factors that contribute to pressure sore formation. Medical Hypotheses 11: 255–267

Lamb JF, Ingram CG, Johnson TA, Pitman RM 1991 Essentials of physiology, 3rd edn. Blackwell Scientific, London

Langer G, Schloemer G, Lautenschlaeger C 2003 Nutrition for preventing and treating pressure ulcers (protocol for a Cochrane review). In: The Cochrane Library, issue 2, 2003. Oxford: Update Software. Available online at: www.update-software.com (amended August 2001)

Lawrence JC 1997 Wound irrigation. Journal of Wound Care 6: 23–26

Leaper DJ 1986 Antiseptics and their effect on healing tissue. Nursing Times 82: 45–47

Lewis B 1996a Protein levels and the aetiology of pressure sores. Journal of Wound Care 5: 479–482

Lewis B 1996b Zinc and vitamin C in the aetiology of pressure sores. Journal of Wound Care 5: 483–484

Lowthian P 1979 Turning clocks system to prevent pressure sores. Nursing Mirror 148: 30–31

Lowthian P 1982 A review of pressure sore pathogenesis. Nursing Times 78: 117–121

Lowthian P 1987 The classification and grading of pressure sores. Care Science and Practice 5: 5–9

Lyder CH 1991 Conceptualisation of the stage 1 pressure ulcer. Journal of Enterostomal Nursing 18: 162–165

McGovern M, Kwaiser Kuhn J 1992 Skin assessment of the older client. Journal of Gerontological Nursing 18: 39–43

Maklebust J 1987 Pressure ulcers: etiology and prevention. Nursing Clinics of North America 22: 359–390

Morison MJ 1992 A colour guide to the nursing management of wounds. Wolfe, London

Munro BH, Brown L, Heitman BB 1989 Pressure ulcers: one bed or another? Geriatric Nursing 10: 190–192

National Institute for Clinical Excellence 2003 Pressure ulcer prevention. Clinical guideline 7. NICE, London

National Pressure Ulcer Advisory Panel 1983 Pressure ulcers prevalence, cost and risk assessment: consensus development. Decubitus 2: 24–28

Norman D, Dunford C, Swain I 1995 Assessment of support surfaces: First Technicare Mistral mattress and Bodipillo foam chip overlay. Journal of Tissue Viability 5: 115–117

Norton D 1989 Calculating the risk. Reflections on the Norton scale. Decubitus 2: 24–31

Norton D, McLaren R, Exton-Smith AN 1975 An investigation of geriatric nursing problems in hospital, 2nd edn. Churchill Livingstone, Edinburgh

Nuffield Institute for Health, NHS Centre for Reviews and Dissemination 1995 The prevention and treatment of pressure sores. Effective Health Care 2: 1–16

O'Dea K 1993 Prevalence of pressure damage in hospital patients in the UK. Journal of Wound Care 2: 221–225

O'Dea K 1999 The prevalence of pressure damage in acute care hospital patients in the UK. Journal of Wound Care 8: 192–194

Panel for the Prediction and Prevention of Pressure Ulcers in Adults 1992 Prediction and prevention: clinical practice guidelines, no. 3. AHCPR publication no.92-0047. Agency for Health Care Policy and Research, Public Health Service, US Department of Health and Human Services, Rockville, MD

Pedley GE 2000 Is blood pressure a clinical predictor of pressure ulcer development? Journal of Wound Care 9: 408–412

Pedley GE 2004 Comparison of pressure ulcer grading scales: a study of clinical utility and interrater reliability. International Journal of Nursing Studies 41: 129–140

Preston KW 1988 Positioning for comfort and pressure relief: the 30 degree alternative. Care Science and Practice 6: 116–119

Redfern SJ, Jeneid PA, Gillingham ME, Lunn HF 1973 Local pressure with ten types of patient support systems. Lancet ii: 277–280

Reid J, Morrison M 1994 Classification of pressure sore severity. Nursing Times 90: 46–50

Rithalia SVS 1989 Comparison of pressure distribution in wheelchair seat cushions. Care Science and Practice 7: 87–92

Rithalia S 1996 Pressure sores: which mattress and why? Journal of Tissue Viability 6: 115–118

Romanelli M, Mastronicola D 2002 The role of wound-bed preparation in managing chronic pressure ulcers. Journal of Wound Care 11: 305–310

Royal College of Nursing 2000 Clinical practice guidelines: pressure ulcer risk assessment and prevention recommendations. Royal College of Nursing, London

Russell LJ, Reynolds TM 2001 How accurate are pressure ulcer grades? An image-based survey of nurse performance. Journal of Tissue Viability 11: 67, 70–75

St Clair M, Cooper S, Gebhardt K 1995 Measuring pressure sore incidence: a study. Nursing Standard 9: 50–51

Salvadala GD, Snyder ML, Brogdon KE 1992 Clinical trial of the Braden scale on an acute care medical unit. Journal of Enterostomal Nursing 19: 160–165

Schubert V 1991 Hypotension as a risk factor for the development of pressure sores in older subjects. Age and Ageing 20: 255–261

Schubert V, Heraud J 1994 The effects of pressure and shear on skin microcirculation in older stroke patients lying in supine or semi-recumbent positions. Age and Ageing 23: 405–410

Seiler WO, Allen S, Stahelin HB 1986 Influence of the 30 degree laterally inclined position and the 'super-soft' 3-piece mattress on skin oxygen tension on areas of maximum pressure: implications for pressure sore prevention. Gerontology 32: 158–166

Shea JD 1975 Pressure sores. Classification and management. Clinical Orthopaedics and Related Research 112: 89–100

Spector WD 1994 Correlates of pressure sores in nursing homes: evidence from the national expenditure survey. Journal of Investigative Dermatology 102 (suppl.): 42S–45S

Stotts NA 2001 Assessing a patient with a pressure ulcer. In: Morison M J (ed) The prevention and treatment of pressure ulcers. Mosby, London, pp 99–115

Strauss MJ, Gong J, Gary BD 1991 The cost of home air fluidised therapy for pressure sores. A random controlled trial. Journal of Family Practice 33: 52–59

Thomas S 1990 Wound management and dressings. Pharmaceutical Press, London

Thomas S 1997 Assessment and management of wound exudate. Journal of Wound Care 6: 327–330

Thomas S, Jones H 1996 Clinical experiences with a new hydrogel dressing. Journal of Wound Care 5: 132–133

Thomas S, Jones M, Shutler S, Jones S 1996 Using larvae in modern wound management. Journal of Wound Care 5: 60–69

Torrance C 1983 Pressure sores: aetiology, treatment and prevention. Croom Helm, London

Torrance C 1999 Pressure sore survey: part one. Journal of Wound Care 8: 27–30

Turner T 1982 Which dressing and why – 1. Wound care series no. 11. Nursing Times 78: 41–44

Vowden KR, Vowden P 1999a Wound debridement, part 1: non-sharp techniques. Journal of Wound Care 8: 237–240

Vowden KR, Vowden P 1999b Wound debridement, part 2: sharp techniques. Journal of Wound Care 8: 291–294

Waterlow J 1985 Pressure sores. A risk assessment card. Nursing Times 81: 49–55

Waterlow J 1991 A policy that protects. The Waterlow pressure sore prevention/treatment policy. Professional Nurse 6: 258–264

Winter G 1976 Some factors affecting skin and wound healing. In: Kenedi RM, Cowden JM, Scales JT (eds) Bedsore biomechanics. Macmillan, London, pp 47–54

Chapter 20

Sleep and rest

S. José Closs

'It's not enough to sleep – sleep must be organized!'
George Mikes

INTRODUCTION

Sleep is a highly complex and organized phenomenon, and its structure tends to change with advancing age. It is difficult to define and its function is poorly understood but it may be thought of as an altered state of consciousness in which the sleeper is in a state of reduced responsiveness to the outside world. Sleep is the natural state of unconsciousness (Horne 2001).

Although sleep is a normal state, it can be difficult to distinguish from abnormal states of stupor or coma, and sleep can be deliberately simulated. It is not uncommon for nurses who are caring for sick and older people to be faced with the problem of distinguishing between normal sleep, feigned sleep and incipient stupor. Indeed, if concern for the well-being of an older person is great, and doubt exists about the nature of his or her unresponsiveness, we almost automatically resort to vocal or tactile stimuli to test the state of affairs – much to the annoyance of the 'sleeper'.

In the course of everyday practice, nurses have informally gleaned a wealth of information about the sleeping patterns of older people. We have observed the sick and frail and, to a lesser extent, healthy older people in hospital and care homes. However, in recent years we have had more and more scientific knowledge about a wide range of aspects of sleep to inform our practice. Next to older people themselves and their families and friends, it is nurses who have the greatest vested interest in understanding sleep: first, to promote the optimal day-to-day functioning of older people in our care and, second, because their sleep–wake pattern could have important implications for the 24-h nursing workload and therefore for the way in which we choose to deploy the limited number of staff available in most care settings.

Individuals vary greatly in their apparent need for sleep, with the average duration being around $7\frac{1}{2}$ h. Some people take very little sleep, perhaps 2 h or less per night, while others sleep longer than the normal, needing 10 h or more if they are to feel refreshed. However, the majority become concerned if they fail to sleep as long as is normal for them. Efficient functioning of older people when they are awake is fundamentally dependent upon the quality and quantity of their sleep; and this in turn is related to the pattern of their sleep–wake circadian rhythm. It is necessary first to examine the state of knowledge about sleep generally in order to understand the particular problems of sleep in older people.

This chapter presents background information about normal sleep; how it changes with ageing; causes of sleep problems in older people; the assessment of sleep; and a brief mention of sleep therapies.

NORMAL ADULT SLEEP

Most research on sleep has used young healthy adults as subjects. The physiological functioning of the brain, muscles, heart, lungs and reproductive systems during sleep has been recorded, as well as the effects of total and partial sleep deprivation. Reviews of this research can be found in Colquhoun (1971, 1972), Minors & Waterhouse (1981), Morgan (1987) and Kryger et al. (1994). The monitoring of sleep classically uses scalp electrodes to measure electrical activity in the brain (the electroencephalograph, EEG) and the movement of the eyes (electro-oculograph, EOG), plus body electrodes to record muscle tone (electromyograph, EMG). Together these recordings are known as polysomnography. Hormone, electrolyte and other chemical levels in the blood can be monitored by the use of venous catheterization. Older equipment produces a paper printout of these recordings, but nowadays these extensive polygraphic records tend to be stored electronically.

Sleep stages

Findings from these complicated recordings during sleep have led to sleep being separated into two main types: non-rapid-eye-movement (non-REM or NREM) sleep (sometimes called orthodox) and rapid-eye-movement (REM) sleep (sometimes called paradoxical). These sleep states are distinguished by characteristic differences in the frequency and amplitude of the EEG and resting muscle tone as assessed by the EMG. Sleep begins from stage 0, corresponding with relaxed wakefulness with the eyes shut, with alpha rhythms (8–12 Hz) predominating on the EEG. This gradually changes into stage 1 (drowsiness) where EEG frequency is still quite high but muscle tone decreases. Further slowing of the EEG signals the entry into stage 2, the first stage of true sleep, where characteristic waveforms called sleep spindles and K-complexes are seen. This is the most common sleep stage throughout the night. Stages 3 and 4 together are known as slow-wave sleep (SWS), since they are characterized by large-amplitude slow electrical brain activity, 0.5–3 Hz, which is 5–10 times the amplitude of activity seen during wakefulness. Stages 2–4 comprise NREM sleep.

Once asleep, there is normally a repeated progression between the sleep stages from stage 2 to stages 3 and 4 and then into a period of REM, then back to stage 2 and through the sequence again. REM sleep is typically associated with rapid jerky eye movements, an almost complete absence of muscle tone and a return to low-amplitude fast EEG frequencies similar to those seen during wakefulness. People often report dreaming when woken up from REM sleep, and one theory about the concomitant loss of muscle tone is that it effectively prevents them from acting out their dreams and potentially harming themselves.

In a typical night it has been found that adults pass through a complete cycle from stage 2 through to REM approximately every 90 min, or 4–6 times per night. One complete cycle is illustrated in Figure 20.1. There is a gradual lengthening of the time spent in each episode of REM sleep which is usually greatest just before wakening.

Many other physiological changes occur within sleep and these are summarized in Table 20.1.

The purpose of sleep

There are a number of theories about the function of sleep. Some are philosophical and open to debate, some are formulated as scientific hypotheses which may be tested through research, while others are grounded in scientific evidence. Theories concerning why or whether sleep is needed by humans are regularly revisited or newly proposed. These include the suggestions that sleep is merely a hangover from evolutionary times when it was dangerous to move in the dark because of the risk from predators; it is an essential means of energy conservation, with metabolic rate falling during sleep; and that sleep is necessary for the restitution of brain and body functions. The only really convincing evidence for humans is that which indicates that the cerebral cortex undergoes recovery during sleep, and in particular during SWS (Horne 1988). The rest of the body appears to recover just as effectively during relaxed wakefulness as it does during sleep.

Most attention is focusing now on the role of sleep in replenishing brain stores of the carbohydrate energy reserve molecule glycogen. These levels are being related to the concentrations of the compound adenosine, the breakdown product of adenosine triphosphate (ATP), which provides the essential fuel for all cellular metabolism. As adenosine accumulates, the brain switches into deeper sleep, during which resynthesis of glycogen and ultimately increases in the level of ATP occur. Other chemicals appear to be important in this process and there is clear evidence that a chemical

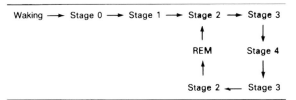

Fig. 20.1   Sleep cycle. REM, rapid eye movement. (Reproduced with permission from Sanford 1982.)

Table 20.1   Types of sleep

	Non–REM	REM
Electroencephalogram (EEG)	Sleep spindles and K-complexes appear in stage 2 and are considered diagnostic of sleep onset. Slow waves appear, their amplitude increases and frequency decreases from 8–15 Hz in stage 2 to 0.5–2 Hz in stage 4	Low-voltage, desynchronized waves, similar to wakefulness
Eye movement on electro-oculogram (EOG)	Absent, or slow rolling	Rapid jerky eye movements
Muscle tone	Reduced	Abolished
Heart and respiratory rate	Steady, regular, slow	Increased, irregular
Blood pressure	Lowered	Raised
Metabolic rate	Lowered	Raised relative to non-REM
Penile erection	Rarely	Yes
Vaginal blood flow	Lowered	Increased
Growth hormone	Secreted mainly in stage 4	No change
Dreaming	Infrequent	Frequent, vivid
Response to external stimuli	Diminishes as sleep progresses from stage 1 to stage 4	Less responsive than stage 4. Very difficult to awaken or awakens spontaneously

REM, rapid eye movement.
Adapted from Koreorgos (1980).

messenger, the cytokine tumour necrosis factor-alpha, promotes longer and deeper non-REM sleep in animals. This chemical is released in bacterial and viral infections and causes a febrile response to these illnesses. It should not be a surprise to find that feverish patients are usually sleepy.

The function of REM sleep and its relationship to dreaming have provoked endless, largely fruitless, speculation. REM sleep and dreaming may be independent of one another, even though they tend to occur at the same time. Dreaming seems to take place in the higher centres of the brain, the cortex, while REM is controlled in the brainstem and midbrain. Repeated selective REM sleep deprivation does not appear to harm those so deprived, and patients tolerate drugs like the tricyclic antidepressants, which specifically suppress REM, without producing any physical or mental ill health. REM is at its most plentiful in the fetus and the neonate, suggesting that it has an important role when rapid growth and development are taking place. It has been suggested that there is a lack of external stimulation within the uterus, and that REM provides substitute stimulation to aid brain development (Roffwarg et al. 1966).

At present, then, SWS seems to be important in restitution of the cerebral cortex, but the functions of other stages of sleep remain obscure.

SLEEP ARCHITECTURE OF OLDER PEOPLE

So far we have been discussing the sleep of adults in general. Does the sleep of the healthy older person differ? Is it normal for older people to sleep less well at night than younger adults? Research has shown age-related changes in depth, continuity and duration of sleep. The internal architecture of the sleep of older people is characterized by an increase in the number of shifts between different stages of sleep, a reduction in the amount of SWS, sometimes with the complete disappearance of stage 4, more episodes of intervening wakefulness during the night and more daytime napping.

These changes have been well documented by researchers. The prevalence of insomnia has been shown to increase with age, reported by as many as one-third of those aged over 65 (Morgan et al. 1988; Ford & Kamerow 1989; Brabbins et al. 1993; Newman et al. 1997). Questionnaire survey findings support the view that older people are generally dissatisfied with their sleep, and the use of sedative-hypnotic medication increases with age. McGhie & Russell (1962) surveyed 2466 subjects in the UK of all age groups and found that there was a significant increase in the pro-

portion of people over 65 years who claimed to sleep less than 5 h per night. Between 20% and 30% of these older people reported frequent night awakenings, 15% waking before 05.00 h; and 25% of men over 65 years and 40% of women over 45 years described themselves as light sleepers.

In this and similar studies, complaints of sleeping difficulties have tended to be higher for women than men. However, when objective measurements of sleep are taken, many research studies have found that older men have more disturbed sleep than older women (Dement et al. 1982a, Webb 1982; Rediehs et al. 1990). This may be due in part to the effects of nocturnal penile tumescence which occurs automatically during REM in healthy men (Gheorghiu et al. 1995).

Periods of wakefulness during the night are normal at all ages but become more common in older people. For example, Webb & Swinburne (1971) observed 19 people aged 66–96 years over 24 h and found that, although they spent 11–12 h in bed, they only averaged 8.5 h sleep, including daytime naps. It seems that the sleep of older people is not less than that of younger people but is more variable in distribution throughout the 24 h.

So although these early studies and also Feinberg (1968) suggested that the total sleep time declines with age, more recent studies report that the amount of sleep per day and the need for sleep do not decrease with age; rather it is redistributed over the 24 h. Only those studies which cover the whole 24 h can elucidate the relationship between night-time sleep and daytime naps. Many sleep researchers support the view that the daytime sleepiness of older people is the direct consequence of night-time sleep deprivation. Johns (1975) found that not only did the amount of time awake after initial sleep onset increase with age, but that night-time wakefulness was associated with increasing amounts of sleep during the day. His conclusion was that daytime naps were compensating for broken night-time sleep. Dement et al. (1982b: p. 31) stated categorically that 'fragmented sleep in persons of advanced years is not the result of decreased sleep need' since great individual variability in sleep has been found and significant ageing trends are rarely demonstrated. As with other age groups, older individuals cannot automatically be assumed to follow the general trend. On the whole, however, it seems that older people spend more time lying in bed at night without attempting to sleep, and more time unsuccessfully trying to sleep than younger people. They also spend more time in bed in the daytime resting or napping, but their total sleep time is not usually increased compared with the young, and it may be reduced. The explanation for this apparent discrepancy may lie in differences in natural body rhythms (see below).

The major changes in sleep stages with age are summarized in Table 20.2. There is an increase in stage 2 light sleep and a decrease in deep sleep stages 3 and 4. The relative amount of REM sleep is found to persist until extreme old age, although a decline in the proportion of REM sleep seems to correlate with reduced intellectual functioning and organic brain syndrome.

According to Dement et al. (1982b: p. 30), and in agreement with common belief, 'it is axiomatic that there is a relationship between sleep at night and the way we feel during the day'. Most of us have felt the general effects of lack of sleep, including tiredness, headache or sensation of a tight band around the head, 'prickling' or heavy eyelids, lack of muscle coordination, maybe even affecting speech (dysarthria), decreased facial expression and difficulty in maintaining attention. However, many of the symptoms attributed to lack of sleep in young people are labelled as part of the ageing process in older people. Amongst these, Dement et al. (1982b: p. 30) included:

> losses of abilities to perform highly skilled tasks in a rapid fashion, to resist fatigue, to maintain physical stamina, to unlearn or discard old techniques, and to apply the rapid judgement needed in changing and emergency situations.

Some studies have used a standard measure of sleepiness termed 'sleep latency'. This is how long it takes to fall asleep as measured by EEG recordings. This sleep latency can be measured at any time of the day or night and is a more valid and reliable measure of sleepiness than naturally occurring naps. Measurement is precise and objective, and the opportunity and environment for sleeping are controlled. In a study of healthy, older subjects who were in bed for 10 h per night, seriously fragmented and interrupted sleep was found (Carskadon et al. 1982). About 60% of the subjects had more than 100 brief or prolonged arousals during the night's sleep. The number of brief arousals per hour of nocturnal sleep was predictive of daytime sleepiness, as measured by sleep latencies. The sleep latency scores suggested that a substantial number of older people are pathologically sleepy in the daytime even when they do not complain of sleep problems.

CAUSES OF SLEEP PROBLEMS IN OLDER PEOPLE

If we aim to promote sleep in older people we need to examine all possible causes for sleep problems. We stand little chance of making logical decisions or taking helpful action unless we attempt to move beyond the signs and symptoms of poor sleep and to identify their cause.

Biological rhythms, ageing and sleep

One view of the ageing process is that it is characterized by the disorganization of biological rhythms. The sleep–wake activity pattern is a circadian rhythm (around a day) but most bodily functions display rhythmicity patterns with peaks and troughs occurring

Table 20.2   Sleep pattern and age

Age	REM (%)	Stage 1 (%)	Stage 2 (%)	Stages 3 and 4 (%)	Total (h)
Infant			50 (stages poorly differentiated)		14–18
Newborn	50		70–80		12–13
1 year	20–30				
Young, active, healthy adult	25	5–10	50	15–20	6–9
Older adults	20–25 (decline associated with impaired intellectual functioning)	Increased	Unchanged or increased	Decreased, stage 4 sometimes disappears altogether	Total variable – unchanged or reduced and fragmented

Adapted from Feinberg (1968).

at intervals of seconds, minutes, hours, days, months or years. Health and well-being are dependent, to a certain extent, upon these rhythms being synchronized with one another, and this synchronization is affected not only by internal events but also by external cyclic time cues (zeitgebers) such as light–dark, socially determined rest–activity cycles and eating times (Reinberg 1966). The regular alternation of sleep–wakefulness is regarded as a fundamental biological rhythm which in normal circumstances is able to entrain (synchronize) other circadian rhythms.

With ageing, there tends to be an uncoupling of the 24-h fluctuations in sleep and core body temperature from one another, such that the minimum temperature occurs earlier than normal during the night-time sleep period, at around 04.00 h (Czeisler et al. 1986). This desynchronization means that the core temperature is at its lowest about 90 min earlier than usual. Monk (1989) found that older healthy people have smaller responses to zeitgebers than do younger subjects. Since the response to usual time cues, e.g. sunrise and sunset, are much attenuated in older isolated individuals, they may explain some of the disordered pattern of daytime napping and consequent night-time wakefulness seen in older subjects. Consequently, one approach to the improvement of fragmented or irregular sleep in older people has focused on resynchronizing the different rhythms, in particular through the use of melatonin and bright light therapy. These are discussed later in the section concerned with sleep therapies.

The age-related changes associated with other circadian rhythms have not yet been fully explored. A reduction in the secretion of growth hormone has been found, as stages 3 and 4 sleep diminish, suggesting that night-time sleep may be less restorative in the aged than in the young. Wessler et al. (1976) found that institutionalized older patients had a high order of circadian regularity and synchronization, and they concluded that the strict institutional regimen was probably beneficial. There is some anecdotal evidence that a regular lifestyle plays a part in longevity and health. However, we should perhaps be wary of abruptly imposing a particular regimen of sleep–waking on older people, as their cycles are likely to be less adaptable and more easily disrupted than those of younger people and they need time to adapt to an unfamiliar routine. Regular daytime activities including both physical and mental stimulation undoubtedly help to maintain a healthy normal sleep–wake schedule for those whose rhythms are in synchrony, but abruptly enforced daytime activity is unlikely to help either the sleep-deprived or the desynchronized older person.

Sleep deprivation

Sleep deprivation has been studied in young rather than older adults, and to greater extremes in animals. Animals which are totally deprived of sleep eventually die after 14 days or so (Rechtschaffen 1998). However, the actual cause of death is not clear, and if those animals are allowed to sleep as they approach this point, they recover completely. When humans are sleep-deprived, particular types of activity are affected. Although traditionally it has been thought that it is mainly boring, repetitive tasks that suffer following sleep deprivation, more recently it has been shown that certain short and interesting types of task, such as of verbal fluency and non-verbal planning are also sensitive to sleep loss (Horne 1988). As mentioned earlier, a key function of sleep appears to be cerebral cortex recovery which is the area employed in stimulating tasks involving directing and sustaining attention, inhibiting distraction, aspects of working memory and flexible thinking. Short-term sleep deprivation has been shown to impair these abilities (Harrison & Horne 2000).

Recent developments in imaging confirm loss in function of the prefrontal cortex following sleep deprivation, while other areas of the cortex show greater activity, as if they are attempting to compensate (Drummond et al. 2000). When young adults are sleep-deprived for 36 h, the ability to perform neuropsychological tests becomes similar to that of a 60-year-old (Harrison & Horne 2000). Interestingly, healthy ageing also leads to impairment of the prefrontal cortex but, according to Horne (2001: p. 30), this 'does not imply that an aged brain is a sleep deprived brain, merely that regions of the waking cortex working the hardest are more vulnerable to both these factors'.

Total sleep deprivation can affect not only performance but also mood. Subjects tend to become irritable and disoriented, to slur speech, and even become deluded, paranoid and hallucinated. An apparently analogous phenomenon in sleep-deprived seriously ill patients has been described as the intensive care syndrome (Helton et al. 1980, Hewitt 2002).

Psychosocial and environmental context of sleep

There are a number of environmental factors that may increase sleep disturbance and deprivation in older people.

Hospital or institutional admission
Research on the effect of hospitalization on the sleep of older people has compared institutional and home sleeping patterns. Pacini & Fitzpatrick (1982) investi-

gated the sleep of 38 older people, half at home and half during the first 7 days of admission to medical/surgical wards. The hospitalized patients did not undergo surgery and were mainly cared for in private or semiprivate rooms. The findings from self-kept sleep charts and sleep pattern questionnaires were that nocturnal sleep time was reportedly shorter in hospital. This was attributed to being woken for recording of vital signs, medication or venesection. More daytime sleep occurred in the hospitalized and they both went to bed and were awakened earlier. However, the reported levels of anxiety, provoked by new medication and concern about impending investigations and discharge dates, were higher in hospital, and health and fatigue status was lower. So poor nocturnal sleep was not attributed solely or even primarily to the hospital environment, but to a significant extent to the health status and anxiety levels of the person admitted. This was corroborated by Closs (1990), who found that patients on surgical wards reported, on average, 1 h less sleep in hospital than at home. Noise, pain and anxiety were the main causes of sleep disturbance. People in long-term institutional care, on the other hand, may adapt to the pattern of life and sleep well, especially if they are neither acutely sick nor insecure. As mentioned earlier, Wessler et al. (1976) thought the strict institutional regimen beneficial.

Many environmental and psychosocial factors, including boredom, social isolation and physical confinement, are likely to result in excessive sleepiness, whereas heat, cold, light, movement and noise are liable to disturb sleep.

Noise effects on sleep

Auditory threshold awakening from stage 4 (deep) sleep has been found to be lower in old people, so they are more easily aroused from sleep than younger people (Roth et al. 1972; Zepelin et al. 1984). In a community setting noise may or may not constitute a disturbance to sleep, depending on adjustment. For example, one large study of the effects of noise around Heathrow airport suggested that sleep disturbances did not increase with age (Horne et al. 1994). The strangeness of noises in institutional settings, however, may be much more disturbing. Gress et al. (1981) observed the nocturnal behaviour of 11 persons (60–97 years) in an institution between 23.00 and 07.00 h on three nights. Their main findings were that sounds seemed to be amplified at night. Loud conversation, laughter and careless handling of supplies and equipment were observed to disturb some patients. Three subjects slept solidly each night, but the remainder were awake or up at least once. It seemed that 04.00 h was the only hour at which all patients were in bed

on all three nights, and 02.00 h was the most wakeful time.

Ogilvie (1980) compared the noise levels in a 'nightingale' ward and a cubicle 'race-track' ward. The nightingale ward was noisier than the cubicle but in both wards noise levels at night were comparable to 'a living room by day', and the average of noise levels on both wards consistently exceeded the recommended level of 35 dB (dB(A): a standard measure of intensity of sound) for a bedroom at night, often by as much as 15 dB. People – both staff and patients – were the most frequent source of noise, but the loudest noises came from equipment such as telephones, trolleys and doors. Noise has also been shown by Closs (1990) to be the greatest disrupter of sleep in hospitals.

In intensive care units patients are frequently sedated and paralysed, making it difficult to assess whether or not they are sleeping. However, the high level of noise and activity in these areas militates against the possibility of a good night's sleep. A small study of nine intensive care unit patients showed that patients enjoyed an average of only 1 h 51 min out of 24, and five of these patients did not sleep at all (Aurell & Elmqvist 1985). A more recent study indicated that environmental noise was responsible for a maximum of only 17% of awakenings from sleep, suggesting that, although noise is important, there are other factors responsible for the majority of disturbances (Freedman et al. 2001).

Confused patients and conversations with the hard of hearing can pose considerable problems when attempting to reduce noise at night. Indeed, increasingly high dosages of sedatives are sometimes requested for noisy patients in the hope that this will allow the other patients to sleep at night and reduce the night nurses' stress levels. While this may be an understandable reaction, other solutions should be explored:

- Can the physical condition of the patient be improved such that he or she is less liable to nocturnal confusion?
- Would a reduction in sedation be more efficacious than an increase?
- If the noisy patient's behaviour is intractable, what is the bed position in which he or she will cause least disruption?
- Should more staff be on night duty so that such individuals can be given continuous attention?

The mental health of older people in hospital settings is frequently neglected, with delirium, dementia and depression rarely identified and poorly treated (Holmes et al. 2002). A case could be made for specialized training of ward staff in order that patients exhibiting noisy and agitated night-time behaviours could be correctly diagnosed, referred (if necessary) and treated.

Night staff are not alone in shouldering the responsibility for reducing noise and other environmental irritants at night, although it is axiomatic that they should be vigilant about their own noise-making. Footsteps, talking and nursing procedures should be as quiet as possible and we should remember that being out of sight, in the kitchen, duty room or office, does not make us out of earshot. However, the day staff have many more resources available to them than the night staff. Oiling door hinges and trolley wheels, fixing windows, lights and heating can be accomplished by day. The services of administrators, carpenters and electricians may all need to be used to reduce the problem. It would not be beyond our wit to identify the major noise sources in our area and remove or reduce many of them.

Dietary effect on sleep

Dietary habits seem to have an important influence on sleep patterns. People who are gaining weight tend to sleep more and have a higher proportion of REM sleep, whereas those losing weight and anorexic persons sleep less and tend to have more disturbed sleep. The effect of diet on sleep is complex. Amino acids such as tryptophan and the brain transmitter 5-hydroxytryptamine (serotonin) are known to have effects upon mood regulation, pain sensitivity and sleep.

Certain foods are associated with sleep promotion, for example Horlicks. It may be that the continuation of a person's normal eating habits is more crucial than any particular food or drink. It is probable that the supper meal is too early for many people both in hospital and in institutional care. We may need to provide snacks later in the evening and ones that are similar to those which the person would take at home. Helping older people who are in an unfamiliar environment to follow familiar presleep routines, such as taking a drink or a snack, can aid relaxation and sleep onset.

Disturbed sleep may also be caused by intake of stimulants such as caffeine. Research on sleep following coffee intake found sleep to be disturbed within the first 3 h and the proportion of SWS reduced, although the total length of sleep was unchanged. More than 10 cups of caffeine drinks per day may result in dependence and tolerance. Early-morning drowsiness owing to caffeine withdrawal and the obligatory cup of coffee to wake up is a widespread phenomenon for all age groups. The elimination half-life of caffeine varies from around 3 h to 7 h and the sleep-disrupting effect of caffeine greatly increases with age (Karacan et al. 1976). It should be remembered that caffeine is also found in drinking chocolate and cola drinks, as well as being an ingredient of some mild analgesics.

Drugs associated with sleep disorders

Most central nervous system (CNS) stimulants and depressants affect functioning of older people and so are more likely to disturb sleep patterns (Coleman et al. 1981) and daytime efficiency (Morgan 1987). The effects of these drugs are well documented and are summarized below.

CNS depressants   These include sedatives, hypnotics, anticonvulsants, antihypertensives, antidepressants, antihistamines, beta-adrenergic blockers and alcohol.
Sustained use   Older people in particular are liable to develop excessive somnolence when these drugs are used therapeutically in moderate to high doses. In addition to sleepiness they feel groggy, depressed, unstable, shaky, agitated and may even have episodes of amnesia or paranoia. Regestein (1982: p. 167) stated that 'the chronic use of sedatives impairs the already diminished cortical functioning, rendering the older insomniac patient worse rather than better'. Use of large bedtime doses may result in alveolar hypoventilation.
Tolerance and withdrawal   With sustained use, CNS depressants become ineffective in inducing sleep, leading to physical and psychological dependence, increasing dosage, plus intermittent attempts to reduce or withdraw the drugs. The person who has become tolerant to sedatives – including barbiturates and non-barbiturates such as glutethimide, chloral hydrate, methaqualone, antihistamines, bromides, benzodiazepines and alcohol – develops long (more than 5 min) and frequent periods of wakening from sleep, especially during the second half of the night. The time to fall asleep also gets longer as the person becomes used to the drug. If the drug is omitted, sleep latency may be several hours. Residual (hangover) effects during the day include sluggishness, poor coordination, ataxia, slurred speech, visual problems, and in the late afternoon restlessness and nervousness. Gradual withdrawal from sedatives results in an improvement in sleep for many people, though after long habituation the individual may not return to an absolutely normal sleep pattern. Rapid reduction or abrupt withdrawal of CNS depressants almost completely disrupts sleep. REM sleep is suppressed by these drugs and REM rebound can precipitate terrifying nightmare attacks. Withdrawal symptoms of nausea, muscle tension, aches, restlessness and nervousness are likely to occur in the succeeding days and sleep-related myoclonus may appear.

There is general agreement that 'hypnotic medication should not be the mainstay of management for most causes of disturbed sleep' (National Institutes of Health 1991) because of these problems of tolerance and withdrawal. In older people the use of hypnotics should be avoided whenever possible, and low doses of drugs with short half-lives used if absolutely necessary. Usually drugs of this kind (such as benzodiazepines or pyrazolopyrimidines) are used for short-term problems only.

CNS stimulants These include thyroid hormone, amfetamines, methylphenidate, sympathomimetic drugs, analeptics, theophylline and caffeine. Apart from drug abusers, the majority of stimulants are prescribed to treat medical conditions, e.g. appetite-suppressant drugs for weight reduction, sympathomimetic drugs for asthma and chronic obstructive airway disease, analeptics for mood elevation of the depressed and stimulants for patients with somnolence, especially narcolepsy.

Use of these drugs leads to a delayed sleep onset and decline of total sleep time. To overcome the resultant daytime sleepiness more stimulants may then be taken. Sudden episodes of sleepiness by day – the 'crash' of the stimulant-dependent individual – occur from time to time. The person may also be anxious and irritable, have difficulty concentrating and even become severely depressed and suicidal.

Sustained use or withdrawal from other drugs Many drugs interfere with sleep. Two lists are particularly mentioned in the classification of sleep disorders, some of which are recognized for their psychotropic action, others not.

Group 1 includes antimetabolites and other cancer chemotherapeutic agents, thyroid preparation and anticonvulsants such as phenytoin, monoamine oxidase inhibitors (MAOI), adrenocorticotrophic hormone, alpha-methyldopa, propranolol and many others. Sleep onset is delayed by the drugs in group 1, and they also result in interrupted sleep and early awakening. The severity of the effect depends on the drug dosage.

Group 2 includes benzodiazepines, sedating tricyclic antidepressants and sometimes MAOIs, marijuana, cocaine, phencyclidine, opiates and even aspirin-containing drugs. Sleep is improved during the use of group 2 drugs, but sleep disturbance occurs during withdrawal in the same way as withdrawal from other CNS depressants.

Alcohol

The effectiveness of alcohol as an aid to sleep is less helpful than might be assumed by most older people. Just one glass of wine taken in the evening may produce drowsiness initially, but is likely to disturb sleep later in the night. Alcohol accelerates sleep onset but

allows wakefulness to return prematurely in the early hours of the morning with attendant disruption of the normal sleep–wake cycle. This may be due to partial tolerance to the effects of ethanol withdrawal during the night and/or the somatic effects of alcohol such as headache or gastric discomfort. Additionally, alcohol promotes excessive relaxation of the upper-airway muscles, which may convert simple snoring to frank sleep apnoea (see below). Arousal responses are generally blunted further, compounding the problems of a compromised upper airway during sleep. Some older people can be extremely secretive and defensive about the extent of their alcohol use, which in some cases increases insidiously for years before coming to medical or nursing attention. Enquiries about alcohol use should always be made in assessing any form of sleep disturbance in older people.

Illness and sleep disturbance

The majority of illnesses result in sleep disruption and further confound the sleep problems of older people. The sleep problem will only improve when the underlying medical condition is alleviated or cured.

Mental health

Mental health problems associated with sleep disorders include anxiety, depression, dementia and phobic, obsessive-compulsive and other neurotic disorders.

Anxiety Any acute emotional arousal or conflict caused by a loss or perceived threat can result in brief periods of sleep disturbance. Causes include bereavement of person or places, abrupt changes in lifestyle such as illness, hospital or institutional admission or discharge, and intense positive feeling, such as may result from the birth of a grandchild or the security of being cared for after a struggle to manage alone.

The majority of people respond with difficulty in falling asleep, intermittent awakening during the night and early-morning arousal. They may lose a substantial amount of sleep but are not truly sleepy by day, feeling fatigued, aching and 'washed out' but unable to nap. Some people respond with excessive difficulty in remaining awake, tending to stay in bed longer than usual and returning to bed frequently during the day to nap.

Both reactions to stress can be adaptive. The first maintains vigilance to cope with the new situation, the second conserves energy. They represent different coping styles which are likely to be typical of the individual. Usually after a few weeks the emotional reaction resolves and sleep returns to normal. As the lives of many older people are strewn with major and minor losses and threats, we should expect to see these sleep disruptions fairly frequently.

More persistent periods of sleep disturbance may arise from chronic tension–anxiety states. Sleep disturbance seems to be conditioned to chronic anxiety and the sleep problem and tension mutually reinforce one another. Such older people may stay in bed longer in an effort to resume sleep and try to nap with little success. High muscle tension may result in complaints of back and headache and pulse rates may be fast. They may complain of worried thoughts and anxious dreams, exhibit restless vigilant behaviour and regard tension as normal for themselves.

Depression Many studies have shown an association between poor-quality, unrefreshing sleep and depression (Habte-Gabr et al. 1991; Morgan 1996). Early-morning awakenings are the most common manifestation, but depression may also cause sleep-onset or sleep-maintenance difficulties. There is some evidence that the early treatment of sleep problems can prevent depression (Ford & Kamerow 1989).

The association between poor sleep and depression is frequently complicated, with high correlations not only between these two phenomena, but also with limitations of physical function, recent hospitalization, low self-perception of health, joint pain stiffness, emphysema, history of stroke or heart disease (Habte-Gabr et al. 1991). Clearly there are many physical factors that impact upon sleep and depressive symptoms, so any assessment and subsequent intervention need to be holistic in nature, considering all aspects of the problem and tackling it incrementally.

Dementia The kinds of sleep problems generally experienced as a consequence of ageing are frequently amplified in those who suffer from dementia (McCurry et al. 2000). These individuals take longer to fall asleep, wake more often and stay awake for longer than age-matched controls. They also tend to be more active when they are awake, but far more likely to fall asleep during the day. Their circadian rhythms may be severely disrupted, with individuals often sleeping more during the day and 'sundowning' (becoming agitated and wandering at night; Bliwise 1993). These behaviours create considerable difficulty for those looking after them, both informal carers in community settings, and formal carers in hospital and institutional settings. There has been some success in managing dementia-related sleep disruption by providing distractions during the day which prevent napping (Hinchcliffe et al. 1991).

Other mental health problems Patients with psychotic depression generally fall asleep readily, but have diffi-

culty in maintaining sleep and wake early in the morning feeling fatigued, achy and 'washed out'. Patients in the depressed phase of manic-depressive psychosis and those with mild depressive disorders tend to be excessively sleepy by day. Mania or hypomania results in difficulty in falling asleep and short sleep time. Such people may wake refreshed after as little as 2 or 4 h sleep. It should be noted that the older the patient with depression, the greater the sleep loss in the second half of the night. Schizophrenia and schizoaffective disorders can result in partial or complete inversion of the day–night sleep cycle, and extreme agitation in the first half of the night. The extent of sleep disruption will depend on the severity of the illness.

Physical pathologies
A daunting array of physical pathologies singly or in combination leads to disturbed and unrefreshing sleep in older patients (Calverley 1993). Damage to the CNS may result in pain, paraesthesiae and abnormal movements, or promote excessive drowsiness. Damage includes raised intracranial pressure from any cause, including tumours, subdural and subarachnoid haemorrhage and hydrocephalus (Roffwarg 1979). As already noted, many febrile illnesses, especially those involving the CNS, will promote excessive sleepiness and some, such as trypanosomiasis, are even known as sleeping sickness.

Endocrine disorders such as hypothyroidism, acromegaly and other problems associated with changes in body weight are often accompanied by excessive daytime drowsiness and loud snoring. These patients may have a significant degree of obstructive sleep apnoea (OSA). This is important to recognize, as appropriate treatment with replacement drugs, e.g. thyroxine, can produce dramatic improvements in daytime and social functioning.

Increasingly, respiratory and cardiac disorders are recognized as producing chronic sleep disruption. Younger patients with asthma have been shown to be more tired when they have performed mental arithmetic tests than educationally matched non-asthmatic subjects. Over 50% of patients with chronic congestive heart failure have evidence of alternating periods of hypo- and hyperventilation during sleep – so-called Cheyne–Stokes respiration. These episodes usually end in EEG arousal and it is not surprising to see an exhausted cardiac patient sitting dozing in a chair after such a disturbed night's sleep. Moreover, there is evidence that these events can contribute to the cardiac disease disorder itself, as treatment of nasal continuous positive airway pressure (CPAP) improves cardiac function (Naughton et al. 1994).

Sleep apnoea (sleep–related cessation of breathing)
This area of knowledge continues to expand rapidly but the significance of these periods of absent airflow (apnoea) or reduced airflow (hypopnoea) to the overall sleep pattern of the older patient is still debatable. An apnoea may be defined as a cessation of airflow for more than 10 s, while hypopnoea is defined as a 50% reduction in thoracoabdominal movement of at least 10 s (Gould et al. 1988).

Detailed population studies suggest that this problem is much more common than was previously thought. Thus the Wisconsin Sleep Cohort Study found prevalences of 4% of men and 2% of women with both symptoms of sleepiness and an abnormally high frequency of respiratory pauses during sleep (Young et al. 1993). In middle-aged patients treatment is now considered when there are 15 or more apnoeas or hypopneas per hour slept, accompanied either by loud snoring and/or significant daytime sleepiness. Studies in all the patients suggest that lesser numbers of apnoeas are very frequent and their impact on sleep architecture and relationship to daytime symptoms still need to be clarified.

Central apnoeas occur when airflow stops and the patient makes no effort to breathe. Apnoeic events, more common in older people, are OSA, when airflow stops while the patient continues to struggle to breathe. Signs and symptoms of OSA include snoring, and, less frequently, choking and excess body movements during sleep. During the day, there may be resulting headaches, excessive sleepiness, intellectual deterioration, fatigue and personality changes.

These events may be more common in older people but their clinical significance is still debated. The sudden onset of silence after hours of prolonged snoring is particularly alarming for the bed partner who often wakes the patient up to ensure he or she is still alive! The snoring itself can be extremely disruptive for everyone around the patient and may lead to much embarrassment and some reluctance to travel away from home. Patients with more than 30 events per hour are usually helped with nasal CPAP, which must be used for at least 3 h per night on a regular basis. This treatment is relatively cumbersome, requires both motivation and comprehension on the patient's part, but is extremely effective in improving wakefulness and general levels of energy (Engleman et al. 1994). How best to apply this to older patients who may have lower expectations of wakefulness and whose anxiety about treatment is higher than younger age groups is still to be properly addressed. As a result of these problems patients with milder disease (15–30 apnoeas per hour) are often not treated. Other available options include surgical therapy, but this tends to be reserved for people without much in the way of respiratory pauses where surgery to the soft palate is more likely to resolve the troublesome snoring. There may be some benefits from using modified dental plates which advance the lower jaw, but we are still not sure how comfortable older patients would find these when worn throughout the night.

The long-term consequences of sleep apnoea beyond increasing daytime drowsiness are still to be clarified (Wright et al. 1997). There are data that suggest that apnoea may be an independent risk factor for hypertension. Spriggs and colleagues (1992) found that loud snoring was an important predictor of the severity and indeed mortality of patients admitted to their general stroke unit, and larger prospective studies are now being conducted to confirm this potentially important observation.

Alveolar hypoventilation   In some circumstances the tidal volume during sleep fails to meet the level needed to maintain the normal elimination of carbon dioxide and replenishment with oxygen of the arterial blood. These problems differ from those associated with complete cessation of breathing as the patient usually does not snore. It is not clear whether they result from the interaction of normal sleep pathology and coexisting disease, e.g. in severe chronic obstructive airways disease, or whether there is a more specific defect in ventilatory control, e.g. in obesity–hyperventilation syndrome. Changes of this type occur especially in REM sleep and other causes include scoliosis, cordotomy, disease of the respiratory control centres, poliomyelitis and myotonic dystrophy.

Sleep-related leg movements   The causes of this relatively common problem during sleep remain largely unknown. The patients are usually middle-aged or older and they (and often their partners) complain of night-time wakenings, unrefreshing sleep and daytime sleepiness. Some notice leg cramps and in extreme cases they may even fall out of bed. These symptoms are the result of repetitive leg muscle jerking, occurring about every 20–40 s for a few minutes or even up to an hour at a time. The contraction comprises an extension of the big toe and a partial flexion of the ankle, knee and sometimes hip. They are accompanied by EEG features of arousal and the sleepiness is thought to be a consequence of the resulting sleep fragmentation. These movements are not usually accompanied by jerking of the rest of the body and so specific leg electrodes have to be used to pick up the EMG signal.

In some cases these problems extend into the day and such patients may be unable to sleep at night. Whilst neurological disorders such as motor neurone disease can present in this way, the worst-affected cases often have evidence of chronic renal failure. Dramatic improvements in well-being in all severities of disease can be produced by treatment with L-dopa, usually accompanied by a dopa-decarboxylase inhibitor, where low doses taken in the evening often produce satisfactory control.

Pain A range of painful physical pathologies disturb sleep, and older people tend to have more painful conditions than younger ones. For example, one-third of a group of nursing-home residents reported that pain was a major cause of sleep disruption (Gentili et al. 1997). Pain may disturb sleep directly, or in combination with mood changes such as depression (Cakirbay et al. 2004). Chronic conditions such as low-back pain, peripheral neuropathy, peripheral vascular disease, arthritis and fibromyalgia commonly disturb sleep, mainly by delaying sleep onset and increasing the frequency of awakening.

Some painful conditions, such as dyspepsia and ulcer pain, have a circadian rhythmicity whereby pain becomes worse during the night. Angina has been shown to produce worst chest pain between 23.30 h and 03.00 h and 06.30 h and 08.30 h (Thompson et al. 1991); sciatic pain is frequently at its worst during the night (Domzal et al. 1983); and cluster headaches often commence during REM sleep.

Exactly how different types of pain influence sleep quality and architecture is poorly understood. A study by Drewes et al. (1997) showed that muscle pain caused wakefulness and reduced REM; joint pain caused widespread changes throughout the whole EEG; and cutaneous pain produced poorly defined changes. It has been suggested that the duration of pain rather than pain intensity reduces sleep quality (Menefee et al. 2000). Some disease processes themselves cause sleep disruption; for example, rheumatoid arthritis produces cytokines which modulate sleep (Kreuger & Majde 1995).

Changes in sleep may also influence pain. A study of 12 healthy middle-aged women showed that SWS (orthodox) deprivation decreased the pain threshold (Lentz et al. 1999), and this was confirmed by Onen et al. (2001), who found that both REM and SWS deprivation decreased pain thresholds, but that this effect was most significant after total sleep deprivation.

In summary, the interplay between pain and sleep is complex, with pain disrupting sleep quality and architecture and sleep deprivation reducing pain thresholds.

Other disorders

A range of parasomnias (undesirable physical phenomena associated with sleep) may be exhibited by the old as well as the young. Sleep-walking in older people is more likely to be due to psychomotor epilepsy or fugue states than to true somnambulism. Nightmares are more prevalent at times of emotional stress and during REM rebound from drug withdrawal. Older individuals with sleep-related inadequacy in swallowing saliva are at risk of respiratory aspiration, and sleep-related gastrointestinal reflux may result in oesophageal stricture or aspiration pneumonia. The primary sleep disorders such as narcolepsy and idiopathic CNS hypersomnolence persist into old age, so may be occasionally seen. The habitual long and short sleepers will also continue this pattern into old age.

Conclusions

Sleep research has come a long way towards helping us understand the sleep problems of older people. We can use this knowledge to assess, care for, teach and sympathize with the people in our charge. It may help us and older people to overcome the prejudice that there is something lazy about sleeping during the day. There is now clear evidence that much of this daytime sleepiness is a result of physical problems disrupting normal sleep and these may be present whether or not the patient complains of insomnia. The subtle and complex interactions of normal ageing and increasing physical frailty explain much of the disruption to sleep rhythms seen in patients.

There is possibly greater variability in the sleep of older people than in that of the young adult, and sleep–wake cycles may be more easily disrupted in older people. Increased dissatisfaction with sleep is generally supported by objective (EEG) evidence of reduced duration, depth and continuity of sleep (Morgan 1987). Many current sleep researchers consider older people need to have the same amount of sleep as younger people and are at risk of becoming seriously sleep-deprived if they are not given lengthened opportunities to sleep compared with those of the young. All seem to agree that the potential causes of insomnia increase in old age, that the primary sleep abnormalities do not remit, that secondary sleep abnormalities increase and that hypnotic overuse is endemic in the older population with all its deleterious side-effects.

Gledhill (1985), in a questionnaire survey of 109 people living in the community either in sheltered accommodation or attending a day centre, found that 53% reported a moderate or severe sleep problem (insomnia) which they attributed primarily to worry, or pain and discomfort or lack of physical exercise. The most common causes of awakening reported by sleep observers are: sleep apnoea, nocturnal myoclonus, physical discomfort, especially distended bladder and urinary urgency, pain, 'restless legs' and dyspnoea.

The most common causes of sleep disturbance for adults include:

- chronic pain (especially due to rheumatism and arthritis)
- nocturnal dyspnoea
- nocturnal discomfort from pruritus
- peripheral neuritis
- enforced uncomfortable positions
- nocturia
- dyspepsia
- cerebral degeneration
- abnormal movements
- secondary disturbance of the circadian sleep–wake cycle
- environmental factors associated with hospitalization.

The most important and consistent finding regarding sleep problems for older people is the number and length of periods of awakening after sleep has started. However, as in all age groups, there are considerable individual differences. Research findings may reveal statistically significant differences between the sleep of the young and the old, but we can never assume that the individual person in our care conforms to a trend. Detailed assessment is essential before we plan our care.

ASSESSMENT OF SLEEP

The initial assessment of sleep or lack of it by either medical or nursing staff relies heavily on the subjective report of the sleeper. However, nurses have the inestimable advantage of being present night and day to assess the sleep and wake behaviour of individuals, whereas doctors and sleep researchers are able to undertake polygraphic recordings of internal events such as neurological and cardiovascular responses.

There are a number of potential problems which face us when assessing the quantity and quality of patients' sleep. To what extent do the person's subjective complaints about sleep correspond with objective measurable sleep problems? The correspondence is not absolute by any means. From some of the research discussed earlier it is obvious that some older people who have no sleep complaints in fact have multiple microarousals during their night's sleep and spend much time in light stages of sleep. Microapnoeic arousals and even nocturnal myoclonic attacks will not generally be visible, even to the most observant night nurse, but the aftermath of daytime sleepiness

and complaints of poor sleeping will be genuine. On the other hand, some older (and younger) people who complain of poor sleep do not exhibit EEG abnormalities when monitored in sleep laboratories.

An important distinction should be made between the person who is fatigued but tense and, although longing to sleep is rarely able to do so, and the person who is tired and suffering from sleep deprivation who, if given the opportunity, will be able to make up the sleep lack by spending a longer time in bed at night and taking daytime naps. Severely sleep-deprived persons will eventually fall asleep whatever the surrounding activities, whereas the fatigued tense person is likely to be vigilant of all that is happening.

What about individuals whose circadian rhythms are out of phase with surrounding society – wanting and able to sleep for long periods by day and having difficulty in sleeping by night? A detailed assessment of their sleep–wake patterns and social responses over the weeks before we meet them, plus a 24-h diary of sleeping should be kept day after day before we can be certain of this diagnosis. It is important not to dismiss complaints about poor night-time sleep and we should accept that we may not be able to improve the situation overnight. Apart from any other consideration, it is important that older people feel they have slept well and that we are willing to listen and do all in our power to provide an environment in which they have the opportunity to sleep.

Methods of assessment

There is a wide range of approaches to the assessment of sleep, some of which measure physiological concomitants of sleep (EEG, EOG, EMG, body movements); some which measure psychological aspects of daytime activity which are affected by the quality of sleep (reaction times, daytime sleepiness, and mood states); and, perhaps most importantly, subjective reports of sleep from the sleeper. In most clinical situations it is unlikely that nurses will use any physiological sleep indices, since they are not the most appropriate measures for the majority of people and the equipment required is cumbersome and expensive. It is likely that nurses will note daytime mood and sleepiness informally, not usually using a standardized measurement instrument such as the Stanford Sleepiness Scale (Hoddes et al. 1972). However, it is the sleep history recorded on admission (when the older person is in a hospital or nursing home) or on first assessing them in the community plus subjective assessments of sleep which provide the most important and useful information.

Sleep history

Taking a sleep history allows the nurse to elicit information about the usual sleep patterns of individuals, their usual timing and duration of sleep and daytime napping habits. A basic sleep history would be fairly simple, such as that shown in Box 20.1. Additional questions concerning individual preferences, such as presleep routines, bedding type and light levels, can help hospital nurses to create an environment as conducive to sleep as possible in hospital (Box 20.2). However, where there are obvious problems, greater detail can be sought. A far more detailed history, such as that indicated in Box 20.3 (Lacks 1987) may be used, but would not be appropriate for the majority. This approach includes 48 questions covering seven categories of information about sleep:

1. description of the symptoms, extent and duration of insomnia (questions 1–7)
2. psychological contributing factors (questions 8–16)
3. sleep hygiene (questions 17–27)
4. psychopathology (questions 28–32)
5. organic sleep pathology (questions 33–39)
6. serious medical problems (questions 40–45)
7. patient's self-help attitudes (questions 46–48).

Of these, the nurse may be able to give direct help in terms of sleep hygiene and psychological contributing factors, while referrals to other specialists may be required where psychopathology, organic sleep pathology or serious medical problems are identified. More detail on nursing interventions may be found in Morgan & Closs (1999: Chapters 6–9).

Box 20.1   Questions for a simple sleep history on admission

Usual sleep pattern at home
1. What time do you usually settle down for the night?
2. About what time do you usually fall asleep at night?
3. About how many minutes does it usually take you to fall asleep?
4. How many hours' sleep do you usually have at night?
5. How many times do you usually wake up during the night?
6. What wakes you during the night (if anything)?
7. What time do you usually wake up in the morning?
8. How well do you usually sleep throughout the night at home?
    Very well   Fairly well   Not very well   Not at all
9. Do you usually nap during the day at home?   Yes   No
    If yes, when?
    For how long?
10. Do you usually take any medicines to help you sleep at home?   Yes   No
    If yes, specify:

Box 20.2   Questions for a brief assessment of patient's sleep routine and preferences

Do you usually drink something before you go to sleep?   Yes   No
What?
Do you usually eat something before you go to sleep?   Yes   No
What?
What else do you like to do before retiring to bed (if anything)?
How many pillows do you like?
What bedding do you prefer (duvet, blankets, etc.)?
What position do you like to go to sleep in?
Do you like to sleep with the window open?
Do you prefer to sleep with a light on or off?
Do you need absolute quiet in order to sleep?
Do you prefer your bedroom to be warm or cold in order to sleep?

Box 20.3   Sleep history questionnaire

Name _____   Date _____

1. How many nights per week do you usually have difficulty falling asleep?

   _____

2. On nights when you *do* have difficulty falling asleep, how many *minutes* does it usually take you to fall asleep after going to bed?

   _____

3. On nights when you *do not* have difficulty getting to sleep, how many *minutes* does it usually take you to fall asleep after going to bed?

   _____

4. Do you ever wake up in the middle of the night and have difficulty falling back
   to sleep?   yes   no
   (a) If yes, about how many nights does this happen each week?

   _____

   (b) On average, how many times do you wake up each night?

   _____

   (c) How many minutes does it usually take you to get back to sleep each time you
       awaken?

   _____

5. How often do you wake up early in the morning, before your scheduled wake time,
   and are unable to return to sleep?

   _____

6. On nights when you have insomnia, approximately how long do you sleep each
   night?

   _____

7. How long have you had a sleep problem?   _____
8. How long would you like to be able to sleep each night?   _____
9. Is your sleep problem sometimes worse than other times?   yes   no
   If yes, explain: _____

   _____

   _____

10. Why do you think you have a sleep problem?

    _____

    _____

11. Was the onset of your problem related to any specific event?   yes   no
    If yes, describe: _____

12. Do you sleep better when you are away from home?   yes   no
13. What do you do when you can't sleep?

    _____

    _____

14. When you try to sleep, is it hard for you to turn off your mind?   yes   no
15. Have you been under stress more than usual recently?   yes   no
    If yes, explain: _____

    _____

16. Are you the kind of person who tends to worry a lot?   yes   no
17. How often is your sleep disturbed by environmental factors such as traffic,
    neighbours or family members?

    _____

Continued

Box 20.3   Sleep history questionnaire—*cont'd*

18. Is your bedroom adequately dark at night?   yes   no
19. On weekends or your days off, do you sleep more than an hour later than your usual
    wake-up time?   yes   no
20. How many times per week do you take naps?

    _____

21. Are you on a weight-loss programme?   yes   no
22. Do you engage in some kind of physical exercise?   yes   no
    If yes, describe the time, frequency and time of day:

    _____

23. How many cups or glasses of caffeinated beverages (e.g. coffee, tea or cola) do you
    drink in a day?
    coffee   tea   cola
24. How many days a week do you drink caffeinated beverages after 4 p.m.?

    _____

25. Do you take any medications that contain caffeine or stimulants (e.g. allergy medication
    or painkillers)?   yes   no
    (a) If yes, what medication and dose?

    _____

    (b) How often do you usually take it?

    _____

    (c) How soon before bed do you take it?

    _____

26. How often do you use alcohol to aid sleep?

    _____

27. How many cigarettes a day do you smoke?

    _____

28. Does difficulty sleeping ever affect your mood during the day?   yes   no
29. Would you describe yourself as an especially nervous person?   yes   no
30. Estimate how many nightmares you have had in the past year:

    _____

31. How often and what amounts of alcohol do you drink?

    _____

32. Have you ever been treated or hospitalized for mental, emotional, drug or alcohol
    problems?   yes   no
33. Does difficulty sleeping affect your functioning during the day?   yes   no
    If yes, describe how it affects your functioning:

    _____

34. Do you snore?   yes   no
35. Do you ever wake up in the night and feel unable to breathe?   yes   no
36. Do your legs ever jerk repeatedly or feel restless after you go to bed at night?   yes   no
37. Do you ever work the night shift? (11 p.m. to 7 a.m.)   yes   no
38. Do you work a rotating or split shift?   yes   no
    If yes, please describe:

    _____

39. Have you recently taken any prescription or over-the-counter medication for sleeping
    problems?   yes   no
    (a) If yes, what medication and amount are you taking?

    _____

Box 20.3   Sleep history questionnaire—*cont'd*

(b) How many nights a week do you usually take this medication?

_____

(c) How long have you been taking sleeping medication?

_____

40. Are you currently taking any other medication?   yes   no
    (a) If yes, what medication is it?

    _____

    (b) What illness was it prescribed for? _____
41. Do you have any other physical problems or illnesses?   yes   no
    If yes, describe: _____
42. Have you ever been hospitalized during the past 10 years?   yes   no
    If yes, please describe:

    _____

43. Have you ever had any convulsions or significant head injury?   yes   no
    If yes, please describe:

    _____

44. How many times per night do you wake up to use the bathroom?

    _____

45. How many nights per week do you have indigestion or heartburn?

    _____

46. Have you previously received treatment for sleeping problems?   yes   no
    If yes, describe

    _____

47. Have you tried any self-help remedies for your sleeping problems?   yes   no
    If yes, describe:

    _____

48. Would you be willing to devote 30 min per day to a programme of treatment to improve   yes   no
    your sleep?

    _____

Source: Lacks (1987)

Daily assessment

Where an older person has an ongoing sleep problem, daily monitoring of sleep may help in the assessment and management of insomnia. Sleep diaries are now widely used for this purpose, and vary according to the type of problem being investigated. They may focus on sleep quality and quantity, quantities and patterns of sleep and wakefulness, or perhaps sleep and its after-effects. Box 20.4 shows a basic sleep diary.

In many cases a lighter touch is needed, with one simple question to indicate satisfaction with the previous night's sleep. In the past visual analogue scales have been widely used for this, for example, a 10-cm horizontal line with the anchors 'best sleep ever' and 'no sleep at all' at each end. The sleep is scored by indicating the point on the horizontal line representing quality. This method has been shown to be conceptually difficult for some to use, particularly older people.

It is recommended that a simple format such as that in question 10 of Box 20.3 is used.

Patient objectives regarding sleep

Having made an assessment of sleep, it should be possible to use this as a basis from which to set objectives for sleep. These general objectives might be:

1. Older persons will sleep at their normal times and for their normal duration
2. The older person will have undisturbed sleep at night
3. The older person will have rest time during the day
4. The older person will feel and appear rested
5. The older person will understand the use of sedatives and analgesics
6. The older person will be able to plan a return to a healthy sleep–wake activity pattern.

Box 20.4   A simple daily sleep diary

Name   Date

1. At what time did you go to bed last night?
2. At what time did you settle down to sleep?
3. How long did it take you to fall asleep?
4. How many times did you wake up?
5. What woke you up?
6. For how long do you think you were awake on each of these occasions?
7. At what time did you finally wake up?
8. How did you feel when you woke up this morning (tick one)?
    Refreshed and alert
    Alert but not at peak
    Tired
    Absolutely shattered
9. At what time did you get up?
10. How would you rate last night's sleep (tick one)?
    Very good
    Good
    Average
    Poor
    Very poor
11. What medicines did you take yesterday?
12. How much alcohol did you drink yesterday?

Reproduced with permission from Morgan & Gledhill (1991)

Nursing intervention to promote sleep

With these general aims in mind, there is a range of interventions that nurses may use to improve the quality of sleep in institutional settings:

1. management of environment, e.g. position of beds, oiling door hinges and trolley wheels, ventilation, lighting and reduction of staff noise at night
2. planning 24-h sleep–activity patterns suitable for the individual
3. helping patients to achieve presleep rituals as near as possible to their normal pattern
4. provision of nutrition and fluids at times normal for that patient
5. organization of nursing, medical and other interventions to give patients undisturbed periods of time (at least 90 min for one complete sleep cycle)
6. relief of physical symptoms which interrupt sleep, e.g. pain, frequency, dyspnoea, cough
7. discussion and relief of psychological distress

8. review of the dosages and effects of sedatives and stimulants
9. patient teaching regarding sleep habits
10. treatment of any underlying medical/surgical condition.

The areas of intervention over which nurses have most control are the sleeping environment and nursing interruptions of sleep. However, the total management of factors likely to disrupt sleep patterns requires discussion, decisions and action to be undertaken jointly by nurses, medical, paramedical and administrative staff, as well as with help from engineers and porters.

Reassessment or continuing assessment of sleep

This requires the repeated assessment of all the factors that were originally assessed.

The primary question which is being asked in reassessment is: have the patient's goals been achieved or not? If not, why not? Have we or the patient failed to carry out the planned intervention?

We may also ask: were the goals unrealistic? For example, it may have to be accepted that disturbed nights are inevitable if the patient has irreversible CNS pathology, or were we trying to push the person into a pattern of sleep which suited our own needs? Key to this is the sleeper's own report. If he or she is refreshed and satisfied with sleep, then it can be considered normal for that individual.

SLEEP THERAPIES

Once nursing interventions such as optimizing the sleep environment, increasing older persons' understanding of their own sleep, managing expectations of sleep and the provision of sleep hygiene advice have been tried, there may still be difficulties that require further interventions. These may be considered in two main groups: pharmacological and non-pharmacological therapies.

Pharmacological therapies

The use of hypnotic drugs to treat chronic insomnia in older people is not recommended. UK clinical guidelines have stipulated that in primary care it is necessary to 'reduce the prescribing of long-term hypnotics for older people by asking older people if they would like to "come off" long-term benzodiazepines and providing support for them to do so' (Department of Health 2001). There are both pharmacological and psychological risks associated with hypnotic drug use, such that they are only considered to have an important role in the management of short-term insomnias which are 'severe, disabling, or subjecting the individual to extreme distress' (Committee on the Safety of Medicines 1988). Where these drugs are the only realistic option, it is preferable to provide those with the shortest half-lives (such as zolpidem), given at the lowest effective dose.

The use of herbal remedies is increasing in popularity in the UK, although it is not clear whether older people comprise a significant proportion of current users. Few herbal treatments have research evidence to support their efficacy and safety. However, valerian is one reportedly effective over-the-counter herbal medication which is commonly used in insomnia. A recent review found 18 studies of valerian's effectiveness, the majority of which had reported positive subjective effects from its use, although objective sleep indicators were less convincing (Pallesen et al. 2002). In spite of this, caution is needed when using these kinds of drug. Valerian can contain alkylating agents which may cause cell damage; and liver damage has been reported after using valerian in combination with other herbal sedatives (Ernst 1998). Given that older people often take several medications, the risk of interactions as well as other adverse effects means that more evidence concerning safety is needed before herbal remedies of this type can be recommended wholeheartedly.

Non–pharmacological therapies

For the most part, these comprise psychological management including stimulus control approaches, relaxation-based approaches and cognitive approaches. These are well established in clinical practice and have been used successfully in primary care (Espie et al. 2001).

Psychological interventions
Stimulus control aims to strengthen and maintain the association between bedroom and sleep onset. It involves only going to bed when tired, using the bedroom only for sleep (and sex), leaving the bedroom if sleep onset does not occur within 15–20 min and getting up at a predetermined time regardless of the amount of sleep gained.

Relaxation-based treatments include progressive relaxation, autogenic training and EMG feedback techniques for reducing physical tension. These have been successful in the general population but their effectiveness with older people is less clear. Painful conditions such as osteoarthritis would militate against the use of these, since relaxation techniques involve the use of muscle tension, which could cause unnecessary discomfort.

Cognitive treatments mainly aim to reduce cognitive arousal and focus presleep thoughts. They range from imagery training to paradoxical intention. The latter involves the insomniac attempting to stay awake so that anxiety about getting to sleep is reduced. These have been shown to be effective with older people (Morin & Azrin 1988), and may be successful both singly and in combination with relaxation therapies.

Approaches such as stimulus control and sleep restriction which target maladaptive sleep habits seem to be particularly beneficial for older people, while relaxation-focused approaches have more limited success (Morin et al. 1999). A systematic review of trials of cognitive-behavioural therapy for sleep problems in those aged over 60 years suggested that cognitive-behavioural therapy produces mild improvement in sleep, particularly in sleep maintenance insomnia (Montgomery & Dennis 2003b). A major proviso for the use of these kinds of approach is, of course, that the cognitive functioning of individuals is fairly intact, which will exclude those with degenerative brain conditions.

Strengthening of circadian rhythms
Sleep problems which are thought to be associated with circadian decay have been treated with therapies designed to strengthen and re-entrain circadian rhythms. Normally the hormone melatonin is secreted by the pineal gland, and acts as a chemical messenger of the primary circadian pacemaker, stimulating sleep. Trials have suggested that early-evening supplements improve general sleep quality and encourage sleep onset, but have produced conflicting reports on the effectiveness of melatonin on the maintenance of sleep (Haimov et al. 1995, Hughes et al. 1998, Pawlikowski et al. 2002).

There has been considerable investigation into the effects of bright light therapy, at various intensities, times, frequencies and duration. However, a Cochrane systematic review of relevant trials concluded that, up until 2003, there were no trials on which to base any firm conclusions, but that this was a promising area to pursue (Montgomery & Dennis 2003a). Whatever the outcome of future studies, we need not assume that sleep rhythm changes in older people are simply an inevitable consequence of the ageing process.

Exercise and body warming
Physical activity seems to have a role in improving sleep. A recent systematic review has supported claims for the efficacy of exercise as an intervention to treat sleep problems, and insomnia in particular (Montgomery

& Dennis 2003c). Regular physical exercise may promote relaxation and raise core body temperature, leading to the improved initiation and maintenance of sleep. Even low-intensity exercise has been shown to increase SWS and improve memory (Naylor et al. 2000). A little caution should be observed, however, since exercise is not appropriate for everyone. Physical health and well-being will influence what is desirable and possible.

Finally, there has been some interest in the effect of body warming alone as a method of improving sleep. Insomnia in older people is associated with changes in the circadian rhythm of body temperature. Characteristic of the insomnia of older people is a phase-advanced sleep pattern (falling asleep earlier) and a decreased amplitude of body temperature rhythms (Dijk et al. 2000; Weinert 2000). A warm bath in the early evening appears to improve sleep quality by decreasing sleep onset latency and enhancing restorative SWS (Liao 2002).

While these approaches provide a useful alternative to pharmacological interventions, care is needed in the matching of therapy with the individual. In particular, general health should be carefully assessed, including circulatory problems and skin condition, cognitive ability and painful conditions when selecting an intervention.

FINALLY, A WORD ON LONELINESS

There is an association between sleep and loneliness. Lonely individuals have reported poorer sleep than others, and this increases with age (Cacioppo et al. 2002). Many older people have to face bereavement of their nearest and dearest, perhaps living alone for the first time in their lives after the age of 60, 70 or later. Many older couples are separated when one needs institutional care and the other doesn't, or when they both find themselves in institutions of different kinds. Could we be more adventurous and enable institutional care to be more like home – where possible, allowing family members to settle their relatives for the night, and spouses (or partners) to sleep together if they wish?

Many older people have had the physical comfort and warmth of a spouse in their bed for decades and, either owing to bereavement or to hospital or institutional admission or both, have to face the night in solitude. Some have substituted their pets as bed companions while at home. Others may be in a state of mental regression in which they long once more to hold their children and babies in their arms or even to be held again in their own mother's arms. Night

nurses often have a closer relationship with wakeful patients than day nurses. The comfort of a person who will listen to the troubles and anxieties at the end of the day may be the best tranquilliser in the world.

CONCLUSION

In conclusion, sleep is an activity that needs to be considered on an individual basis. Many factors disturb sleep in later life; in particular, circadian decay, physical and mental health, and moving into unfamiliar institutions and other environments. The complex interactions between day and night-time behaviours all have a profound influence on the structure and efficacy of sleep. John Bailey's (1999) memoir of author Iris Murdoch describes movingly the importance of sleep in the case of someone with Alzheimer's disease: 'After an impossible night I turn on the light at five and start trying to write this. Iris is asleep. The sleeping draught did not work, but nature seems to have taken over at last. She lies peacefully, her face relaxed. But at half-past six she becomes restless again. The time just before was wonderful, like a pool of clear dark water, the sort of pool we used to dream of finding to swim in. She was asleep and I was tapping my typewriter. Total darkness in the sky outside, friendly darkness with no trace of dawn.'

In conclusion, it is crucial that any primary cause of sleep problems is identified, since symptomatic interventions can have only limited success. Careful assessment, realistic expectations and the provision of advice on both day and night-time activities, general comfort measures, therapeutic interventions and referrals to other specialists (where necessary) can all help. To revisit the quote from George Mikes at the beginning of this chapter, 'It's not enough to sleep – sleep must be organized!'

Recommended reading

Morgan K, Closs SJ 1999 Sleep management in nursing practice. An evidence-based guide. Churchill Livingstone, Edinburgh.
Probably the only book available specifically to guide nursing practice.

Kryger MH, Roth T, Dement WC 1994 Principles and practice of sleep medicine. WB Saunders, Philadelphia.
The major textbook of sleep medicine with authoritative accounts of the theoretical and practical management of sleep disorders in all ages.

Morgan K, Gledhill K 1991 Managing sleep and insomnia in the older person. Winslow Press, Oxon.
A simple guide which is useful for both nurses and informal carers of older people with sleep problems.

Reite M, Ruddy J, Nagel K 1997 Evaluation and management of sleep disorders, 2nd edn. American Psychiatric Press, Washington.
This is a very concise but comprehensive resource.
Horne J 1988 Why we sleep. Oxford University Press, Oxford.
Still the best general book on the reasons for sleep and their implications for sleep disorders.

References

Aurell J. Elmqvist D 1985 Sleep in the surgical intensive care unit: continuous polygraphic recording of sleep in nine patients receiving postoperative care. British Medical Journal 290: 1029–1032

Bailey J 1999 Iris and the friends: a year of memories. Abacus, London

Bliwise D 1993 Sleep in normal ageing and dementia. Sleep 16: 40–81

Brabbins CJ, Dewey ME, Copeland JRM et al. 1993 Insomnia in older people: prevalence, gender differences, and relationships with morbidity and mortality. International Journal of Geriatric Psychiatry 8: 473–480

Cacioppo JT, Hawkley LC, Crawford LE et al. 2002 Loneliness and health: potential mechanisms. Psychosomatic Medicine 64: 407–417

Cakirbay H, Bilici M, Kavakci O et al. 2004 Sleep quality and immune functions in rheumatoid arthritis patients with and without major depression. International Journal of Neuroscience 114: 245–256

Calverley PMA 1993 Medical problems during sleep. British Medical Journal 306: 1403–1405

Carskadon MA, Van den Hoed J, Dement WC 1982 Insomnia and sleep disturbances in the aged. Sleep and daytime sleepiness in older people. Journal of Geriatric Psychiatry 13: 135–151

Closs SJ 1990 Influences on patients' sleep on surgical wards. Surgical Nurse 3: 12–14

Coleman R, Miles SL, Guilleminault C 1981 Sleep–wake disorders in older people: a polysomnographic analysis. Journal of the American Geriatric Society 29: 289–296

Colquhoun WP (ed) 1971 Biological rhythms and human performance. Academic Press, New York

Colquhoun WP (ed) 1972 Aspects of human efficiency: diurnal rhythm and sleep loss. English University Press, London

Committee on the Safety of Medicines 1988 Benzodiazepine dependence and withdrawal. Current Problems 21: 1–2

Czeisler CA, Brown EN, Ronda JM et al. 1986 Phase advance and reduction in amplitude of the endogenous circadian oscillator correspond with systemic changes in sleep–wake habits and daytime functioning in older people. Sleep Research 15: 258

Dement WC, Miles LE, Carskadon MA 1982a Changes in the sleep and waking EEGs of non-demented and demented older subjects. Journal of the American Geriatric Society 30: 86–93

Dement WC, Miles LE, Carskadon MA 1982b 'White paper' on sleep and ageing. American Geriatric Society Journal 30: 25–50

Department of Health 2001 Medicines and older people: implementing the medicines-related aspects of the NSF (national service framework) for older people. HMSO, London

Dijk DJ, Duffy JF, Czeisler CA 2000 Contribution of circadian physiology and sleep homeostasis to age-related changes in human sleep. Chronobiological International 17: 285–311

Domzal T, Szczudlik A, Kwasucki J, Zaleska B, Lypka A 1983 Plasma cortisol concentration in patients with different circadian pain rhythm. Pain 17: 67–70

Drewes AM, Nielsen KD, Arendt-Nielsen L, Birket-Smith L, Hansen LM 1997 The effect of cutaneous and deep pain on the encephalogram during sleep – an experimental study. Sleep 20: 632–640

Drummond SPA, Brown GA, Gillin JC et al. 2000 Altered brain response to verbal learning following sleep deprivation. Nature 403: 655–657

Engleman HM, Martin SE, Deary IJ, Douglas NJ 1994 Effect of continuous positive airway pressure on daytime function in sleep apnoea/hypopnea syndrome. Lancet 343: 572–575

Ernst E 1998 Harmless herbs? A review of the recent literature. American Journal of Medicine 104: 170–178

Espie C, Inglis SJ, Tessier S, Harvey L 2001 The clinical effectiveness of cognitive behaviour therapy for chronic insomnia: implementation and evaluation of a sleep clinic in general medical practice. Behavioral Research Therapy 39: 45–60

Feinberg GI 1968 The ontogenesis of human sleep and the relationship of sleep variables to intellectual function in aged. Comprehensive Psychiatry 9: 138–147

Ford DE, Kamerow DB 1989 Epidemiologic study of sleep disturbances and psychiatric disturbances. Journal of the American Medical Association 262: 1479–1484

Freedman NS, Gazendam J, Levan L, Pack AI, Schwab RJ 2001 Abnormal sleep/wake cycles and the effect of environmental noise on sleep disruption in the intensive care unit. American Journal of Respiratory Critical Care Medicine 163: 451–457

Gentili A, Weiner DK, Kuchibhatil M, Edinger JD 1997 Factors that disturb sleep in nursing home residents. Aging Milano 9: 207–213

Gheorghiu S, Mulligan T, Veldhuis JD 1995 Lack of temporal association among REM sleep, LH secretion, testosterone secretion, and nocturnal penile tumescence (NPT) in healthy aged men. Journal of the American Geriatrics Society 43: SA81

Gledhill K 1985 Sleep and older people: some psychological dimensions and their implications for treatment. In: Butler A (ed) Ageing: recent advances and creative responses. Croom Helm, London, pp 263–277

Gould GA, Whyte KF, Rhind GB et al. 1988 The sleep hypopnea syndrome. American Review of Respiratory Disease 137: 895–898

Gress LD, Bahr RT, Hassanein RS 1981 Nocturnal behaviour of selected institutionalised adults. Journal of Gerontological Nursing 7: 86–92

Habte-Gabr E, Wallace RB, Colsher PL et al. 1991 Sleep patterns in rural elders: demographic, health and psychobehavioral correlates. Journal of Clinical Epidemiology 44: 5–13

Haimov I, Lavie P, Laudon M et al. 1995 Melatonin replacement therapy of older insomniacs. Sleep 18: 598–603

Harrison Y, Horne JA 2000 The impact of sleep loss on decision making: a review. Journal of Experimental Psychology: Applied 6: 236–249

Helton MC, Gordon SH, Nunnery SL 1980 The correlation between sleep deprivation and the intensive care syndrome. Heart and Lung 9: 465–468

Hewitt J 2002 Psycho-affective disorder in intensive care units: a review. Journal of Clinical Nursing 11: 575–584

Hinchcliffe AC, Hyman I, Blizard B, Livingston G 1991 The impact on carers of behavioural difficulties in dementia: a pilot study on management. International Journal of Geriatric Psychiatry 7: 579–583

Hoddes E, Dement WC, Zarcone V 1972 The history and use of the Stanford sleepiness scale. Psychophysiology 9: 150 (abstract)

Holmes JD, Bentley K, Cameron I 2002 Between two stools: psychiatric services for older people in general hospitals. Report of a UK survey, University of Leeds Academic Unit of Psychiatry and Behavioural Sciences, on behalf of Leeds Primary Care Trusts and the Royal College of Psychiatrists. University of Leeds, Leeds

Horne JA 1988 Why we sleep: the functions of sleep in humans and other mammals. Oxford University Press, Oxford

Horne J 2001 State of the art: sleep. Psychologist 14: 302–306

Horne JA, Pankhurst FL, Reyner LA, Hume K, Diamond ID 1994 A field study of sleep disturbance: effects of aircraft noise and other factors on 5742 nights of actimetrically monitored sleep in a large subject sample. Sleep 17: 146–159

Hughes RJ, Sack RL, Lewy AJ 1998 The role of melatonin and circadian phase in age-related sleep-maintenance insomnia: assessment in a clinical trial of melatonin replacement. Sleep 21: 52–68

Johns M 1975 Factor analysis of subjectively reported sleep habits and the nature of insomnia. Psychological Medicine 5: 83

Karacan I, Thornby JI, Anch AM et al. 1976 Dose response effects of coffee on the sleep of normal middle aged men. Sleep Research 5: 71

Koreorgos J 1980 Sleep and sleep disorders. Practitioner 224: 717–721

Kreuger JM, Majde JA 1995 Cytokines and sleep. International Archives of Allergy and Immunology 106: 97–100

Kryger MH, Roth T, Dement WC 1994 Principles and practice of sleep medicine. WB Saunders, Philadelphia

Lacks P 1987 Behavioural treatment for persistent insomnia. Pergamon, New York, pp 63–65

Lentz MJ, Landis CA, Rothermel J, Shaver JLF 1999 Effects of slow wave sleep disruption on musculoskeletal pain and fatigue in middle aged women. Journal of Rheumatology 26: 1586–1592

Liao W-C 2002 Effects of passive body heating on body temperature and sleep regulation in older people: a systematic review. International Journal of Nursing Studies 39: 803–810

McCurry SM, Reynolds CF, Ancoli-Israel S et al. 2000 Treatment of sleep disturbance in Alzheimer's disease. Sleep Medicine Review 4: 603–628

McGhie A, Russell S 1962 The subjective assessment of normal sleep patterns. Journal of Mental Science 108: 642

Menefee LA, Frank ED, Dogramji K et al. 2000 Self-reported sleep quality and quality of life for individuals with chronic pain conditions. Clinical Journal of Pain 16: 290–297

Minors DS, Waterhouse JM 1981 Circadian rhythms and the human. Wright, Bristol

Monk TH 1989 Circadian rhythm. Clinics in Geriatric Medicine 5: 331–346

Montgomery P, Dennis J 2003a Bright light therapy for sleep problems in adults aged 60+. Cochrane Database of Systematic Reviews, 1

Montgomery P, Dennis J 2003b Cognitive behavioural interventions for sleep problems in adults aged 60+. Cochrane Database of Systematic Reviews, 1

Montgomery P, Dennis J 2003c Physical exercise for sleep problems in adults aged 60+. Cochrane Database of Systematic Reviews, 1

Morgan K 1987 Sleep and ageing. Croom Helm, London

Morgan K 1996 Mental health factors in late-life insomnia. Reviews in Clinical Gerontology 6: 75–83

Morgan K, Closs SJ 1999 Sleep management in nursing practice. An evidence-based guide. Churchill Livingstone, Edinburgh

Morgan K, Gledhill K 1991 Managing sleep and insomnia in the older person. Winslow Press, Bicester

Morgan K, Dallosso H, Ebrahim S et al. 1988 Characteristics of subjective insomnia among older people living at home. Age and Ageing 17: 1–7

Morin CM, Azrin NH 1988 Behavioral and cognitive treatments of geriatric insomnia. Journal of Consulting and Clinical Psychology 56: 748–753

Morin CM, Mimeault V, Gagné A 1999 Review. Nonpharmacological treatment of late-life insomnia. Journal of Psychosomatic Research 46: 103–116

National Institutes of Health 1991 Consensus development conference statement: the treatment of sleep disorders of older people. Sleep 14: 169–177

Naughton MT, Bernard DC, Rutherford R, Bradley TD 1994 Effect of continuous positive airway pressure on central sleep apnoea and nocturnal PCO in heart failure. American Journal of Respiratory and Critical Care Medicine 150: 1598–1604

Naylor E, Penev PD, Orbeta L et al. 2000 Daily social and physical activity increases slow-wave sleep and daytime neuropsychological performance in older people. Sleep 23: 1–9

Newman AB, Enright PL, Manolio TA et al. 1997 Sleep disturbance, psychological correlates and cardiovascular disease in 5201 older adults: the cardiovascular health study. Journal of the American Geriatrics Society 45: 1–7

Ogilvie AJ 1980 Sources and levels of noises on the wards at night. Nursing Times 76: 1363–1366

Onen SH, Alloui A, Gross A, Eschallier A, Dubray C 2001 The effects of total sleep deprivation, sleep interruption and sleep recovery on pain tolerance thresholds in healthy subjects. Journal of Sleep Research 10: 35–42

Pacini CM, Fitzpatrick J 1982 Sleep patterns of hospitalised and non-hospitalised aged individuals. Journal of Gerontological Nursing 8: 327–332

Pallesen S, Bjorvatn B, Nordhus IH, Skjerve A 2002 Valerian as a sleeping aid? Tidsskrift for Den Norske Laegeforening 122: 2857–2859 (abstract)

Pawlikowski M, Kolomeda M, Wojtczack A, Karasek M 2002 Effects of six months melatonin treatment on sleep quality and serum concentrations of estradiol, cortisol, dehydroepiandrosterone and somatomedin C in older women. Neuroendocrinology Letters 23 (suppl. 1): 17–19

Rechtschaffen A 1998 Current perspectives on the function of sleep. Perspectives in Biology and Medicine 41: 359–390

Rediehs MH, Reis JS, Creason NS 1990 Sleep in old age: focus on gender differences. Sleep 13: 410–424

Regestein QR 1982 Insomnia and sleep disturbances in the aged: sleep and insomnia in older people. Journal of Geriatric Psychiatry 13: 153–171

Reinberg A 1966 Circadian rhythms (letter). Journal of the American Medical Association 196: 108

Roffwarg HP (ed) 1979 Diagnostic classification of sleep and arousal disorders. Sleep 2: 1–137

Roffwarg HP, Muzio JN, Dement WC 1966 Ontogenic development of the human sleep–dream cycle. Science 152: 604–619

Roth T, Kramer M, Trinder J 1972 The effects of noise during sleep on the sleep patterns of different age groups. Canadian Psychiatric Association 17: 197–201

Spriggs DA, French JM, Murdy JM et al. 1992 Snoring increases the risk of stroke and adversely affects prognosis. Quarterly Journal of Medicine 83: 555–562

Thompson DR, Sutton TW, Jowett NI, Pohl JEF 1991 Circadian variation in the frequency of onset of chest pain in acute myocardial infarction. British Heart Journal 65: 177–178

Webb WB 1982 Sleep in older persons: sleep structures in 50 to 60 years old men and women. Journal of Gerontology 37: 581–586

Webb WB, Swinburne H 1971 An observational study of the sleep of the aged. Perceptual and Motor Skills 32: 895–898

Weinert D 2000 Age-dependent changes of the circadian system. Chronobiological International 17: 261–283

Wessler R, Rubin M, Sollberger A 1976 Circadian rhythm of activity and sleep–wakefulness in older institutionalised patients. Journal of Interdisciplinary Cycle Research 7: 333

Wright J, Johns R, Watt I, Melville A, Sheldon T 1997 Health effects of obstructive sleep apnoea and the effectiveness of continuous positive airway pressure: a systematic review of the research evidence. British Medical Journal 314: 857–860

Young T, Palta M, Dempsey J et al. 1993 The occurrence of sleep-disordered breathing among middle aged adults. New England Journal of Medicine 328: 1230–1235

Zepelin H, McDonal CS, Zammit GK 1984 Effects of age on auditory awakening thresholds. Journal of Gerontology 39: 294–300

Chapter 21

Sexuality and relationships in later life

Denise Forte, Angela Cotter and Diane Wells

INTRODUCTION

The main focus of this chapter is on sexuality and its importance in later life. However, it also focuses on important aspects of sexuality within the broader context of relationships in later life, an area which appears to provide some difficulties, in practice, for health and social care workers. Setting the subject in context therefore is an important place to start. Throughout life much of our experience and knowledge is rooted in relationships. It is through relationships that we learn to be a member of a family, a group, or a community, and it is also in relating that we develop an identity. This identity or sense of self is sustained by relationships with friends and family members. With all the changes that are liable to take place in later life, relationships are particularly important. They can provide comfort and support and a sense of self or identity, especially during times of loss. This can be a loss of friends or family or loss of function and independence. It is through our relationships that we understand and come to value friendships and love. Within this, however, long-term one-to-one sexual relationships are usually a particularly valued part of the life experience. The question of the definition of sexuality is therefore important in the context of a relationship-centred approach.

WHAT IS SEXUALITY?

Sexuality is much more than the physical act of sex. It encompasses:

> the quality of being human, all that we are as men and women. . . encompassing the most intimate feelings and deepest longings of the heart to find meaningful relationships (Hogan 1980: p. 3).

Sexuality and sensuality go to make up our self-concept and how we see ourselves and are seen by others. Our sexual self-concept, like all other parts of our personality, is a social phenomenon, created through interaction with others.

In looking at the many definitions of sexuality there is no one definition that fully expresses its breadth and depth, but all definitions have as central some concept of sexuality being about the 'humanness of the individual', and suggest that human needs of close relationships, expressions of intimacy, identity and sexuality are important for good sexual health in all individuals, including older people. In practice this implies, firstly, that older people will experience sexuality in a way which is unique to them based on their own life experiences and, secondly, that there is continuity between the 'then and now' for individuals. The latter may not always be the case, for example in the situation where a person has dementia. Importantly, it means that 'there is no one way to love or to be loved, no one liaison which is superior to another, no one lifestyle in single-hood or marriage' (Garrett 1994: p. 25). However we learn, through living in a culture, what its expected and approved forms of behaviour are, and if we do not live up to these norms we may experience guilt and feelings of inadequacy.

WHAT DO WE MEAN BY RELATIONSHIPS AND RELATIONSHIP-CENTRED CARE?

Part of sexuality for the individual is the ability to form meaningful relationships. Person-centred care features highly in policy, practice and research into care of older people at present (Nolan et al. 2001). The idea of 'personhood', central to person-centred care for older people, is seen as a status implying respect, recognition and trust in the context of relationship and social being (Kitwood 1997).

The *National Service Framework (NSF) for Older People* (Department of Health 2001a) aims to provide guidance on the standards needed to ensure all older people have access to the same quality of care as everyone else and are enabled to lead a healthy and active life. Standard 2 in the NSF talks about person-centred care and standard 8 discusses active ageing and health promotion. Both standards, however, fail to focus on intimacy, sexuality or sexual health in older people. Person-centred care sets out to ensure that older people are treated as individuals and receive appropriate and timely packages of care which meet their needs regardless of health and social services boundaries. It includes important requirements for managers and professionals: to listen to older people; respect their dignity and privacy; recognize their indi-

vidual differences and specific needs, including cultural and religious; enable them to make informed choices; involve them in all decisions about their needs and care; and involve and support carers whenever necessary. However, it misses the opportunity to emphasize the importance of relationships and sexual health in older people. Similarly, the *National Minimum Standards* document (Department of Health 2001b) also discusses promoting privacy and dignity but fails to mention relationships and sexuality. Do these policies do enough to support an environment in which sexuality is acknowledged as part of the overall health care agenda or do they implicitly reinforce the myths about sexuality and older people? Arguably, this omission raises concerns that the very policies aimed at promoting equality in older people's services are in themselves inherently ageist and subscribe to the myth that older people are asexual beings. Health and social care managers and policy-makers will need to engage more fully in the debate about relationship-centred care and the ways in which sexuality, intimacy and relationship-centred care are effectively supported in practice.

SEXUALITY IN WESTERN SOCIETIES
Myths and stereotypes

Sexuality in western societies tends to focus on youth and physical attractiveness and is seen as belonging to our youth culture. Almost all professional articles about ageing and sexuality begin with the myth that older people 'are seen as asexual' before going on to debunk it (Drench & Losee 1996, Eliopoulos 1997, Grigg 1999). The question is: why does this myth persist, and why do people continue to see older people in this way? In part, it may be because the many myths surrounding ageing and sexuality are reinforced by media images of 'the sexual norm' as beautiful young women and handsome young men seen virtually 24 h a day in advertisements on television, in public transport, on billboards and in magazines. Delicate feminine features and slim bodies or rugged, sporty masculine leanness is what we are urged to strive for. Very few images of older people as sexually attractive appear in advertising (Fig. 21.1). Instead, mellowed, comfortable pictures of older people may sell thermal underwear or storage heaters, but there is nothing sexual or sensual about these. It is thought that libido and sexual needs decline along with loss of the culturally valued outer signs of beauty or handsomeness, and that at the same time sexual capacity fades (Kaye 1993, Hodson & Skeen 1994, Deacon et al. 1995, Hajjar & Hosam 2003). Hajjar & Hosam (2003) state that the

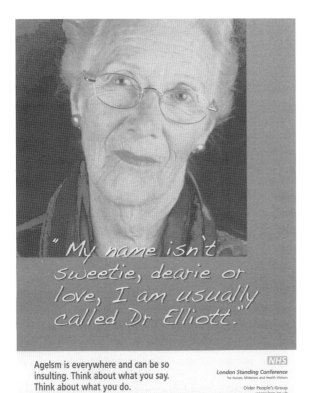

" My name isn't sweetie, dearie or love, I am usually called Dr Elliott."

Agelsm is everywhere and can be so insulting. Think about what you say. Think about what you do.

NHS
London Standing Conference
for Nurses, Midwives and Health Visitors
Older People's Group
www.lscn.co.uk

Fig. 21.1 "Don't call me dearie" – ageism. (Reproduced with permission: London Standing Conferences supports origins and roles of practitioner initiatives.)

people as sexual beings change our perception of older people or is the problem more deep-rooted?

It is notable that social usefulness is defined for men by productiveness at work, and retirement from work may be associated in people's minds with retirement from a sexual life as well (Kuhn 1976). Changes to the retirement age and a greater emphasis on more flexible working for older people will challenge the negative views of old age linked to productivity and may go some way towards combating the myths surrounding ageing and sexuality. For women the menopause is widely believed to herald this sexless, useless phase. In 1933 Havelock Ellis wrote that: 'There is a frequent well-marked tendency in women at the menopause to an eruption of sexual desire, the last flaring up of a dying fire, which may take a morbid form' (cited in Arber & Evandrou 1993: p. 105). This myth, as with many others about menopause, sees women as no longer interested in sexual activity (Gibson 1993, Kaye 1993, Drench & Losee 1996). In a survey of 441 postmenopausal women, only 19% felt that sex was worse than when they were younger, while over 40% felt it was better than in earlier years (Russell 1998), reinforcing the challenge to negative myths surrounding the menopause.

How do these myths affect health care in practice? Kaye (1993), drawing on a number of studies, including that of Butler & Lewis (1988), writes that it is often assumed that older people 'do not have any sexual desires; are unable to perform sexually even if they want to; are physically unattractive, therefore sexually unattractive; are fragile and therefore might harm themselves; or that any sexuality among the older is perverse' (Kaye 1993: p. 416). These are very negative sentiments and other studies, while not subscribing so overtly to such negative stereotypes, still find staff unconsciously adopting some of these beliefs. Nay (1992), when studying women and sexuality in nursing homes, found that staff saw older women as asexual, which suggests that infantalization may play some part in consciously or unconsciously influencing staff's attitudes to sexuality and autonomy in older adults, especially women. Indeed, some studies have found that staff often feel uncomfortable when confronted with older people's sexuality (Booth 1990, Gibson et al. 1999). Grigg (1999) suggests that one reason nurses feel embarrassed is the lack of training staff receive to address this important aspect of people's lives and that in some instances it is not even recognized as being relevant to older people's care. Other studies suggest that the comfort or discomfort felt by staff about their own sexuality is in some ways a predictor of their views on sexuality in older people and that staff attitudes need to be examined as a first step

myth about older people as asexual beings still persists and ignorance and prejudice still dominate western views of sexuality and old age.

However, the picture is changing. As the proportion of older people in the population increases, so does their value as consumers and the media are not slow to respond. Over the last decade we have seen an increase in the portrayal of older people in the media, including a more positive acknowledgement that sexuality is an important component of their lives. A recent movie *Something's Gotta Give* portrayed an older couple (Jack Nicholson and Diane Keaton) enjoying an active and varied sex life, a scenario normally reserved for younger people. Also a recent poster advertising Valentine's day consisted of an old couple holding hands and gazing intimately at each other. A review of the media and how older people are represented suggests that there is an increased willingness to see older people as ageing well, and hence sexually active (Walz 2002). Will this more realistic media portrayal of older to addressing questions of sexuality (Smook 1992, Doyle et al. 1999, Minichiello et al. 2000).

Double discrimination

Even within this discrimination against older people there is yet further discrimination in relation to gender. Men who still show signs of sexual activity are labelled 'dirty old men', but there is a 'good public relations' side to this (Sontag 1978). Men are supposed to maintain their 'manhood' for longer than women do their sexuality, and society lends approval and even celebrity to those who father children at an advanced age. Charlie Chaplin and Pablo Picasso were two of these famous fathers. But there are no lauded 'dirty old women'. Signs of wanting a sexual relationship, 'flirting' and dressing like 'lamb' when one is really 'mutton' are viewed as unseemly and distasteful or even disgusting in a woman. Older men may be described as handsome but older women are never beautiful (de Beauvoir 1973, Sontag 1978, Grigg 1999).

Balding in men is often said to be a sign of increasing virility, and greying hair denotes a distinguished man. Women's thinning hair is never seen as enviable, however, and certainly not as an indication of increased sexuality. Rather, women often colour-rinse their greying hair to make it more 'attractive'. It is noteworthy that the English language has no parallel term for virility to describe high levels of sexuality in women – the phenomenon is not supposed to exist and so a word is not needed (Webb 1983).

The bad faith involved in these two sets of standards for the old and young and for women and men is further evidenced in jokes. In a study of jokes related to ageing and sexuality, Palmore (1971) found that in general they reveal a hostile and negative view of ageing. However, jokes about women were negative in 77% of cases, while this was true of only 51% of jokes about men (Puner 1974). A quick review of birthday and other cards shows older people are still the butt of jokes, with an overemphasis on declining sexual powers. Other cultural myths about sexuality in old age promote the idea that it is acceptable for older men to marry younger women. Indeed, this is a cause for congratulation and envy of the man. Older women should not marry younger men, and such an act on the part of the woman would lead to accusations of 'cradle-snatching' as well as to doubts about the motives or psychosexual adjustment of the man (Kuhn 1976). Marriage or remarriage by old people is generally frowned upon, and studies suggest that this may be due to links between sexuality and procreation in our culture. Thus, once procreation is no longer feasible then, so the myth suggests, all sexual activity should cease. This myth has its origins in early religion, and more recently Victorian cultural taboos about sexuality and its role in the lives of older people, which can still influence behaviour today (Gibson 1993, Drench & Losee 1996).

Other studies have found that there is a gender bias when it comes to staff valuing older people's expressions of sexuality and that men's behaviour is often tolerated more than women's. They also suggest that sexual behaviour in men is more often recognized as sexual behaviour, whereas in women it may be missed. In 1998 Archibald carried out a study which aimed to explore a number of issues related to sexuality in people with dementia. She sent a postal questionnaire to managers of residential homes, in one area of Scotland, and found that gender permeated the responses. Despite most of the staff and residents being female, most of the incidents they chose to report were 'male residents directing their attention to female staff or other residents'. While there were some reported incidents of female residents expressing sexuality, staff responses tended to be protective, and these incidents were less likely to be reported (Archibald 1998, Gibson et al. 1999).

It is suggested that these myths and stereotypes may act as self-fulfilling prophecies for some older people. They are told that they are sexually unattractive, unwanted and useless and this information rebounds on their self-concept and adds to their negative self-view (Weg 1983, Drench & Losee 1996, Grigg 1999). As a result, when they experience sexual urges they think these are abnormal, and feelings of guilt, shame and embarrassment ensue. In 1989 Clark found that in some seminars he ran there was a reluctance by older people 'to acknowledge anything but an asexual role for themselves and their age peers' (cited in Arber & Evandrou 1993: p. 113). In contrast, research into attitudes of older women, when talking about sexuality and intimacy, found there was no such reluctance to acknowledge their sexuality and the importance it played in their lives (Jones 2002). A number of other studies have found older people freely expressing their views on their own experiences of sexuality when interviewed (Gibson 1993, Archibald 1998, Minichiello et al. 2000, Jones 2002). A study by Starr & Weiner (1981), looking at a sample of older people in the community, found that older women, even if they were less sexually active, expressed as much interest in sex as men. The researchers went on to suggest that, for the women who were less sexually active, it was more likely to be due to lack of opportunity rather than lack of desire (Archibald 1998).

In 1992 Gibson advertised for autobiographical accounts of older people undertaking new relationships in later life. The study suggests that the autobiographical accounts of new sexual relationships, for those volunteering to take part in the study, showed little difference to the pattern of those relationships experienced at any other stage of their life (Gibson 1993).

Although Itzen (1984) suggests that 'attitudes of sexism and ageism combine to make the lot of older women especially difficult' (cited in Arber & Evandrou 1993: p. 111), the reality of sexual experiences for older people suggests that attitudes are changing, albeit slowly. In a comparative study of literature available about 106 cultures, Winn & Newton (1982) found that in 70% of the cultures studied there were expectations of continued sexual activity by men as ageing advanced. The comparative figure for women was higher, at 84%. A majority of these references were to women's changed reproductive role after menopause and a consequent lessening of inhibitions in sexual behaviour, conversation, humour and gestures. Overall, however, many references were found to negative attitudes to the sexual desirability of older people.

The experts' prejudices

Even among the 'experts' there are prejudices to be found. Sexual relations may only be discussed in textbooks in terms of marital relations, implying that there is no place for sex unless people are married. Masturbation may be seen as acceptable in the absence of a marital partner but not as an activity which anyone might partake of by choice (Puner 1974, Costello 1975). In contrast, Neugebauer-Visano (1995) reports that two-fifths of women and half of men in their 60s masturbate, suggesting it is more acceptable to older people than previously thought.

Scully & Bart discovered in 1973 that few of the findings of Masters & Johnson's famous and extensive studies of sexual behaviour (1966b, 1981) had worked their way through into current textbooks in the 10 years following their publication. They found a widespread belief among medical writers in the 'normality' of vaginal orgasm and little reference to clitoral orgasm. Today, over 25 years later, the same observations can still be made of the literature on ageing and sexuality. The clitoris and its function are rarely mentioned, and marital sex is used as the standard for discussion of other forms, which are only of importance in the absence of a marital partner. This confirms a view of vaginal intercourse as the norm for women and the only way for men to achieve sexual satisfaction. Homosexuality and bisexuality are rarely discussed, making it hard for the voice of gay, lesbian and bisexual older people to be heard (Hayter 1996, Fullmer et al. 1999).

Sex can be good for you

After all this pessimism and simple inaccuracy, it is refreshing to learn that sex is good for older people. In a study of 70-year-old women and men in Sweden, Persson (1980) found that men who continued to have sexual intercourse slept better and had better mental activity and a more positive attitude towards sexual activity in old age. Similarly, women who continued to have sexual intercourse retained their former levels of emotional stability, had low levels of anxiety, had better mental health, felt generally more healthy and had a positive attitude towards sexual activity in old age.

Sexual activity has been said to help arthritis, reduce physical and psychological tensions and promote a good physical condition (Butler & Lewis 1973, Eliopoulos 1997, Bortz et al. 1999). Taking the wider concept of sexuality, the value of continuing to take account of this dimension of humanity into old age is sympathetically addressed by Eliopoulos (1997): '...love, warmth, caring and sharing between people, seeing beyond grey hair, wrinkles and other manifestations of ageing, and the exchange of words and touches by sexual human beings. Feeling important and wanted by another person promotes security, comfort, and emotional wellbeing' (Eliopoulos 1997: p. 209). This is a timely reminder of the importance of sexuality as more than penetrative sex.

In 1998 the US National Council on the Aging (www.sexualityandu.ca/eng/health/SOW/sexualactivity.cfm) conducted a survey of 1300 older Americans and asked about their sexual activities. They found that sexual activity is seen as an important component in the relationships of many older people. From the sample, 48% said they were sexually active and had sex at least once per month. Of this group, 74% of men and 70% of women said they were as satisfied or more satisfied with their sexual lives as they had been in their 40s. Over 70% of those who were sexually active felt that it was an important component of their relationship with their partner. In 2002 another study, the Pfizer Global Study, which looked at 26 000 people from around the world aged 40–80 years, found similar results, suggesting that if older people abstain from sex it is most likely to be because of a lack of a partner or illness rather than having reached a chronological age where they are no longer interested (www.sexualityandu.ca/eng/health/SOW/sexualactivity.cfm). It is important to remember that older people are no different from any other group and if they have been sexually active and had satisfying lives in their youth, then it is likely that they will continue to do so in old age. It will only be illness or a lack of a partner that forces an end to sexual engagement (Eliopoulos 1997, Minichiello et al. 2000, Heath 2002). Indeed, the study by Minichiello et al. (2000) found that those older people in a sexual relationship at the time of the study were more likely to feel that sexual activity had positive physiological and psychological benefits for older people.

On that positive note, myths and stereotypes will be left behind in order to consider the realities of sexuality and older people.

SEXUALITY AND OLDER PEOPLE

It is widely agreed that psychosocial factors have a much greater impact on sexuality in older people than physiological factors (Masters & Johnson 1981, Weg 1983, Sarrel 1990, Drench & Losee 1996, Jagus & Benbow 2002). However, there are some physiological changes that do occur with age, and it is important that older people are aware of the changes to prevent any negative impact these may have on relationships and sexual activity. In older women, vaginal lubrication is slower, vaginal expansion and contraction of the uterus are depressed, the labia are no longer elevated and the fat under the mons veneris is much reduced. The clitoris remains relatively unaltered but low levels of oestrogen may cause vaginal soreness, painful clitoral stimulation and uterine spasms during orgasm (Masters & Johnson 1981, Eliopoulos 1997, Heath 2002). Women remain capable of multiple orgasms and may experience an increase in sexual desire after the menopause, when androgens are minimally opposed by oestrogens (Weg 1983) and fear of unwanted pregnancy is gone (Eliopoulos 1997). Regular sexual activity by women will usually help to maintain sexual capacity, sexual orgasms can help maintain muscle tone and reduce urinary incontinence (Grigg 1999) but masturbation is less effective than coitus in counteracting vaginal dryness and irritation (Backman & Leiblum 1981).

Masters & Johnson (1981) report that men over the age of 60 years take longer to achieve full penile engorgement, and may have a decrease in expulsive pressure and a reduction in the volume of ejaculatory fluid expelled. Also, although levels of sexual interest may remain, the subjective desire for ejaculation may be reduced. Erection is more rapidly lost after ejaculation than in the earlier years. Men may be affected by 'performance anxiety' if they are unaware that these changes are normal and do not herald the termination of sexual activity. Women, too, may feel threatened if their partners do not ejaculate (Morgentaler 2003).

A lack of knowledge about sexuality may contribute to 'performance anxiety' and to giving up sexual activity altogether (Neugebauer-Visano 1995, Drench & Losee 1996, Minichiello et al. 2000). This suggests there is an urgent need for health professionals to recognize the importance of health education for older people on sexuality and the normal changes that occur with age. As Masters & Johnson (1966a) state, 'ignorance of the facts surrounding sex is the single greatest deterrent to the active enjoyment of sexuality' (Neugebauer-Visano 1995: p. 13).

Contrary to popular mythology, both older women and men report that factors in the man usually lead to the cessation of sexual activity, rather than lack of interest on the part of the woman (Hendricks & Hendricks 1978). The most common of these male factors are illness, lack of interest, premature ejaculation and inability to have an erection (impotence). In one study both men and their partners reported that premature ejaculation resulted in lower sexual satisfaction but had little impact on relationship satisfaction (Byers & Grenier 2003). Women's tendency to live longer than men and therefore to be left without a marital partner, the earlier decline in sexual function in men already noted, and the cultural prescription that men should take the initiative in sexual relations make women's position more unsatisfactory. Nevertheless, these studies report that, for those not in a current relationship with another person, masturbation may prove a satisfactory way of maintaining sexual identity. There is evidence that the frequency of masturbation declines less in women than men (Russell 1998). This increase in masturbation suggests that social mores are becoming more flexible. However, it has implications for older people in care homes where privacy may not be seen as an essential right of all older people and a lack of privacy may have a negative impact on an older person's ability to meet sexual needs. Thus the *National Service Framework*'s emphasis on privacy can be understood in a wider context.

Psychosocial factors, then, play a greater role in influencing sexuality and sexual function in older people – as indeed they do at other stages of adult life. Availability of a suitable partner, physical health, past sexual activity and living accommodation are among the strongest factors involved. Single older people face particular problems according to Corby & Zarit (1983) because they are not thought to have a legitimate right or need for sexual privacy, whether at home or in institutions.

Homosexuality

Gay, lesbian, bisexual and transgender older people may suffer from many of the same myths and stereotypes as their heterosexual counterparts. Added to this are the generalizations based on youth-oriented perspectives in the gay and lesbian communities which do not serve the older population well (Archibald & Baikie 1998). Lesbians who are old are hidden even from the lesbian community and it is difficult to identify them (Neugebauer-Visano 1995). Gay men in particular will suffer from a lack of potential partners as they grow old but for older lesbians life may be easier because the number of eligible partners will be larger and because of a commitment to longer-term relationships (Weg 1983). It is important to recognize that gay men, lesbians and bisexual and transgender groups are not socially cohesive. There is a tendency in society to see them as a homogeneous group with the same sexual and health needs, thus rendering them more invisible to policy and service providers (Age Concern 2003b).

Despite this timely reminder about the complexity of sexuality from Weg (1983) suggesting that 'there is no one way to love or to be loved; there is no one liaison that is superior to another. No one lifestyle in single-hood or marriage, heterosexual or homosexual, will suit all persons. Self-pleasuring, homosexuality, bisexuality, celibacy and heterosexuality are all in the human repertoire' (Weg 1983: p. 76). A study by Heapy et al. (2003) found, when exploring the experiences of lesbians, gay men and bisexuals aged between 50 and 80, that only a small proportion of the sample felt that health care workers were positive towards their sexuality and in general they were discriminated against on the basis of their sexuality. This view is echoed by Macdonald & Rich (1984) when they discuss the problems for older lesbian women and gay men and suggest the silence around sexuality holds powerful and repressive messages for these groups. It is still an unfortunate reality that the needs of older lesbians and gays are largely ignored by society at large, including by members of their own communities (Fullmer et al. 1999).

Many older lesbian, gay men, bisexuals and transgender individuals may feel their sexual orientation is a private issue and not one they feel comfortable talking about. For older men in this generation it was not until 1967 that homosexuality became legal in the UK so they may have become adept at keeping their sexuality secret (Jones 1994, MacGregor 1994). Many fear discrimination and prejudice if they 'come out'. Staff may hold quite negative attitudes to the sexual orientation of these groups but feel because they do not verbally express such views they are able to provide care without displaying prejudice. Research suggests that this is not the case and that the non-verbal language of staff, including facial expressions, tone of voice and touch, are significant in communicating to patients their judgemental attitude, leaving the patient feeling emotionally excluded (Hayter 1996). It is therefore essential that staff receive appropriate education and training to address such negative attitudes.

A problem for lesbians, gay men, bisexuals and transgender older people is that the lack of recognition of their sexual orientation may mean that when they become ill, need care or lose a partner from a long-term relationship, the depth of their loss is not recognized or supported. They may have weaker family or friendship networks to provide such support. Also there is evidence that if one partner is ill the other person, because he or she is not seen as family, may be excluded from visiting the partner if the partner is critically ill, and may not be given information or consulted about care options (Age Concern 1993b). This may be about to change with the passing in March 2004 of the Civil Partnership Bill which gives same-sex couples, who sign a register held at the registry office similar to marriages, the same rights as married couples, including the right to be nominated as next of kin (Ahmed & Hinsliff 2004).

The experience of lesbian, gay men, bisexual and transgender older people going into a care home is less than positive and many have called for the provision of services to meet the specific needs of these different groups (Archibald & Baikie 1998). In 1998 the Gay and Lesbian Humanist Association in its submission to the Royal Commission on the Funding of Long-Term Care pointed out that many older people have fought hard to have their sexuality validated and it would be unrealistic to find this denied on entering a care home. They made a number of recommendations to recognize the sexual needs of these communities, including having a gay awareness policy and antidiscriminatory training, and an environment in all care homes which supports gay people displaying affection without being considered offensive (www.galha.org/press/1998/04_02.htm). Counsel and Care have published a guide for staff in care homes on supporting older people's sexual and relationship needs. In it they identify the importance of treating 'gay relationships between residents . . . with the same respect as any other relationship' (Clarke et al. 2002).

Times are changing and older people from these groups are becoming heard more frequently in policy and health and social care agendas. The Department of Health's commitment to challenge age discrimination (Department of Health 2001a) and its attempts to involve service users of all sectors in policy and service delivery (Department of Health 2000, 2001c) have meant that there are increasing opportunities for the voice of older lesbian, gay men, bisexual and transgender groups to be heard and their views acted upon. The Age Concern Opening Doors campaign appears to be helping in the establishment of local groups to support, educate and ensure the needs of these groups are met (www.ageconcern.org.uk).

Research into the gay population has been limited and there is a need for more extensive research into this area. Age Concern found that research which has been done so far has tended to focus 'on the "young old" of 50–60 years, does not differentiate between men and women and tends to reflect the experiences of white, well educated, affluent individuals living in large urban communities' (Age Concern 1993b)

HIV, AIDS and older people

It seems worthwhile considering human immunodeficiency virus (HIV)-related problems affecting older people as a topic in itself in this chapter both because HIV/acquired immune deficiency syndrome (AIDS) is an increasing phenomenon in older people, and because much of what has been stated earlier in the chapter applies equally if not more to older people infected and/or affected by HIV (MacGregor 1994, Second World Assembly on Ageing 2002).

Stereotyping by doctors, nurses and other health professionals means that HIV is not usually considered in relation to older people (Whipple & Scura 1996). The reality is that it is an increasing problem for older people, with 18% of those with HIV aged over 50 years (Avert 1998) and a lack of understanding by health care professionals means that they are often misdiagnosed or not diagnosed until late in the virus trajectory (Wooten-Bielski 1999, Sellers & Angerame 2002). Over the last 5 years the incidence of new cases of HIV in older women has risen by 40% (Second World Assembly on Ageing 2002). The course of AIDS seems to be more rapid in older people (Ship et al. 1991), and this may be linked with later diagnosis, owing to health care professionals assuming that older people are not at risk of becoming HIV-positive because they are not sexually active and/or older people's reluctance to mention the possibility that they have been at risk.

Older people may have received their own socialization into sexual matters from those educated in Victorian times, and so are likely to be reluctant to take the initiative in mentioning any risk of HIV acquisition to health care staff. Older women left without a male partner due to men's earlier mortality rates may not realize that they are at risk of infection, and are unlikely to use a condom because pregnancy does not need to be avoided. They may also be at increased risk

because their diminished vaginal secretions and friable vaginal mucosa make infection more likely (Whipple & Scura 1996). Knowledge about HIV and AIDS in older people may still be limited by the fact that the majority of health education efforts and voluntary organizational activity focuses on much younger age groups (MacGregor 1994). A leaflet published by Age Concern (1993a) is a rare example of an attempt to reach out to this group. As a result, knowledge about HIV/AIDS and safer sex practices is likely to be lacking in older people.

Apart from questions of attitudes and prejudices, diagnosis of AIDS in older people may be difficult because it is the 'great imitator' (Sabin 1987). This can occur particularly with dementia, which might simply be thought to be Alzheimer's disease, for example. AIDS-related dementia is different, however, in that it is of sudden onset, may wax and wane, and may be accompanied by extrapyramidal symptoms mimicking parkinsonism without resting tremors (Whipple & Scura 1996).

The well-recognized opportunistic infections associated with HIV are more likely to occur in older people because their immune systems are less effective than those of younger people. Thus *Pneumocystis carinii* pneumonia (PCP), tuberculosis, oral and genital candidiasis and herpes zoster should give rise to a consideration of AIDS as a possible diagnosis, as should conditions such as non-Hodgkin's lymphoma and Kaposi's sarcoma. Indeed, the possibility should be considered in all cases of fatigue, weakness, anorexia and weight loss (Whipple & Scura 1996).

As far as the implications for nursing and other health care professionals are concerned, most important is the recognition of HIV/AIDS as a possible factor in older people's health, and sufficient and accurate knowledge that allows appropriate care to be delivered and health promotion to be carried out. The Royal College of Nursing (1994: p. 3) guidelines should always be followed with all patients: 'Since it is impossible to identify all those who are sero-positive to HIV or hepatitis B, it has been recommended that every patient be regarded as a potential biohazard'.

Universal precautions should be used in all cases, no matter what the age of the patient. However MacGregor (1994) found that nurses do not feel the need to use universal precautions with older people because they do not think of them as being at risk of acquiring the virus. In many ways, the care needs of AIDS patients do not differ from those of other patients with similar conditions (Turton 1995), but there are additional considerations related to age for older patients. For example, oral thrush always causes a sore mouth and difficulty in eating, but older people may be prevented from wearing their dentures and this will add to their problems. Malaise and general debility may make it more likely that they will become bed-ridden, and skin breakdown is a great risk. This will be exacerbated if the patient has AIDS-related diarrhoea. All the usual caring measures, such as good skin hygiene with soap and water washes followed by barrier-cream application, frequent changes of position and good nutrition (especially intake of protein, calories and potassium) and hydration, assume even greater importance. Risk of falling may be increased, and careful observation and supervision are needed because patients may be unable to call for assistance if they are confused (Schuerman 1994).

MacGregor (1994) points out that people with HIV/AIDS are living longer and AIDS is coming to be viewed as a chronic manageable condition. This makes it essential that health care workers in hospitals, care homes and in the community are aware that older people may be affected by HIV/AIDS and therefore have the necessary knowledge and skills to ensure that early diagnoses are made, appropriate support and treatment are given, and the necessary outreach work is done to inform and support patients and carers.

EFFECTS OF ILL HEALTH AND DISABILITY ON OLDER PEOPLE'S SEXUALITY

When it comes to ill health and sexuality a number of myths continue to influence older people's expectations of sexuality. These myths are often a result of a lack of information, knowledge and understanding of the normal ageing changes and the impact illness may have. A number of medical conditions will have an impact on sexuality in older people and, like any illness or disability, may disturb the person's self- or sexual concept (Fielo & Warren 1997, Russell 1998). General bodily disturbances, weakness, tiredness and malaise occur to varying degrees in all illnesses. The result is that there is less energy for investing in self-care, clothing, appearance and for home, leisure, social and sexual activities. This may lead to a rebound effect on self-esteem and falling energy levels.

The effects of illness on an individual's sexuality will be influenced by a number of factors outside the illness, including personality, coping mechanisms, previous experiences and attitudes to sex and the nature of ongoing relationships. In relation to sexuality, a further complication may arise because it is known that older people are less likely than younger people to restart sexual activity after a period of cessation, such as a break due to illness (Berman & Lief 1976, Grigg 1999, Schiavi 1999). Lack of information by

doctors and nurses about what to expect from an illness, and when it is safe to resume sexual activity, can lead to anxiety, confusion or ceasing sexual activity altogether (Yee & Sundquist 2003). It is essential that health care workers are alert and sensitive to the needs of older people and support them in maintaining sexual functioning and identity, thus promoting wellness and normality (Eliopoulos 1997, Russell 1998).

Cardiovascular conditions, especially myocardial infarctions, are a great source of anxiety in relation to sex, especially for men. If they are not given adequate information they may imagine that there is significant risk in resuming sexual activity whereas in reality it requires no more exertion than normal activities such as 'taking a brisk walk or climbing a flight of stairs', which are seen as criteria for resuming activity following myocardial infarction (Schiavi 1999). In fact, the benefits of intercourse, including a sense of well-being, less depression, gentle exercise and reduction of tension, outweigh the risks (Weg 1983).

Respiratory disorders may make it difficult for the person to participate comfortably in sexual activity and this in turn may lead to a sense of inadequacy and loss of self-esteem.

Nervous system changes in old age may affect perception and sensation, and thereby inhibit sexual response. Eyesight, hearing and touch all play a part in sensuality as well as in actual sex acts.

Musculoskeletal conditions and changes associated with ageing may cause weakness, limitation of movement, deformity and pain. Chronic pain such as that of arthritis can be extremely depressing and debilitating, and lead on to loss of interest in sex as well as decreased possibilities of performing satisfying sexual acts (Kraimaat et al. 1996). On the positive side, sexual activity increases adrenal corticoid production, which may relieve arthritic symptoms (Weg 1983).

Common endocrine disorders occurring in old age are hormonal disruption and diabetes mellitus. The most common hormonal problem in men is low levels of testosterone with subsequent loss of libido, reduced energy levels and mild depression, weak erection and reduced muscle mass. Also men with low testosterone may be at risk of osteoporosis. Low testosterone levels may occur in women leading to the same symptoms as men, including loss of sexual desire (Schiavi 1999, Morgentaler 2003). Treatment by increasing levels of testosterone with patches or injections will result in an increase in sexual interest and an increase in activity levels, leading the man to report he feels as good as he did when he was many years younger (Morgentaler 2003). Diabetes mellitus can cause specific complications for both women and men. For women, vaginal lubrication is delayed and scant, even when oestrogen levels are adequate. There is therefore an increased susceptibility to vaginal soreness and infection, which are disincentives to sexual activity. For men, retrograde and/or premature ejaculation may occur and as many as 50% of sufferers cannot have an erection which may be caused by changes in the arterial bed or neuropathy.

Genitourinary conditions in women and men have perhaps the most obvious link with sexual activity and sexuality. Men widely believe that prostatectomy means the end of sexual activity but this is not so in the majority of cases. Simple prostatectomy rarely affects potency (Schiavi 1999), although loss of potency increases the older the person is at the time of the prostatectomy. Incontinence, urinary infections and atrophic vaginitis involve local pain or discomfort which may inhibit feelings and responses as well as making the person feel unclean or unattractive (Getliffe & Dolman 1997).

Cessation of sexual activity has been attributed to ill health, particularly by men, but illness and disability do not necessarily mean that an active sex life is impossible or that sensuality and sexuality are compromised. Self-concept and confidence may be low and the sufferer may fear rejection, but desires and feelings continue (Hogan 1980, Weg 1983). It is imperative that health care workers are aware of the importance of taking a detailed sexual history of the older person which enables them to identify and deal with the effects of illness on sexual activity before they become intractable (Eliopoulos 1997, Andrews 2000, Gott & Hinchliff 2003, Swabo 2003, Yee & Sundquist 2003).

As Heath & White (2001) remind us: 'Acknowledging the impact of health care changes on sexual well-being is no longer a marginal activity for specialists in sexual health but integral to the practice of all registered nurses' (Heath & White 2001: p. 31). It is important, then, that health care workers support older people to enable them to be more creative sexually and to develop a more fulfilling relationship which if necessary replaces penetrative sex with intimacy, sensuality, companionship and friendship (Swabo 2003, Fielo & Warren 1997).

People sometimes joke about the treatment being worse than the disease, but with regard to sexuality this may be no joke. It can be devastating truth. Any surgical operation, for example, causes temporary disturbance of health which can also disrupt sexual activity. Particular operations, however, can have permanent effects on body image which in turn may have an impact on the person's self-concept as an intact and sexually desirable being (Russell 1998).

Many drugs, both social and medically prescribed, affect sexual function, either as part of their desired mode of action or by causing debilitating side-effects. An example of a social drug which compromises sexual activity is alcohol, which has a depressant effect on the central nervous system, with resulting impotence. In one study it was found that only about a third of the sample were aware of the effects medication and depression could have on sexuality (Minichiello et al. 2000). Narcotics, tranquillizers, sedatives and anxiolytic drugs depress the central nervous system and suppress libido. Numerous antihypertensive drugs such as chlorothiazide, hydralazine and methyldopa have the same effect, and tricyclic and monoamine oxidase inhibitor antidepressants can cause impotence. Other common drugs occasionally reported to have adverse effects on sexuality include cimetidine, which can cause impotence and gynaecomastia, and propranolol, which can lead to impotence (Hogan 1980, Weg 1983, Eliopoulos 1997, Russell 1998, Morgentaler 2003).

A relatively recent treatment for erectile dysfunction is the drug sildenafil, commonly known as Viagra. It was launched in 1998 and thought to be effective in treating older men with erectile difficulties. Results from a double-blind, multicentre trial using doses ranging from 25 to 100 mg have shown increased erectile function in men 65 years and over (Wagner et al. 1998). However, due to very clever marketing, and tapping into society's desire for 'certainty and a quick fix', it soon became seen as the wonder drug to cure all male sexual problems. It was thought Viagra was 'a fountain of youth, a sure cure, the real deal' (Morgentaler 2003: p. 2). The effectiveness of Viagra is in its effect on increasing the blood flow to the penis and hence a firm erection. It does not however have any effect in increasing libido unless loss of libido follows failure of erection (Morgentaler 2003). Viagra does not offer a solution to a couple who are experiencing relationship difficulties despite myths to the contrary. Potts et al. (2003) observe that there has been little research on the effect of Viagra on the sexual partners of men. The authors were particularly interested in the perspectives of women and how much they felt Viagra enhanced or detracted from the relationship. Morgentaler (2003) highlights the problems caused when the man does not tell his partner that he is taking Viagra and the negative effect this can have on the trust in a relationship when the partner finds out.

The situations described in the previous section on the effects of ill health, disability and sexuality assume even greater importance when it is remembered that older people may be experiencing multiple pathology and concomitant multiple medications and treatments. Health care workers can do much to help patients and clients in these circumstances to express their sexuality in the way they themselves choose as most appropriate. Studies suggest health care workers miss many opportunities to promote positive attitudes and experiences of sexuality in their older clients. This raises the need for a debate on normal sexuality and sexual health in older people and the best way to work with older people to meet sexual health needs (Evans 1999). The next section explores this in more detail.

PROMOTING RELATIONSHIPS AND SEXUALITY IN CARE HOMES

Care homes present many challenges and opportunities for older people to maintain intimate and sexual relationships. Much of the research suggests that there are a number of barriers to older people's sexual needs being recognized and met in care homes and a need for staff, residents and carers to engage in open debate about the culture of a home and ways in which it can meet the intimacy and sexuality needs of its residents (Archibald 1994, Garrett 1994, Bauer 1999, Doyle et al. 1999).

The rights to privacy and expressions of sexuality, discussed earlier, are extremely important in a care home where much of a resident's life is conducted in a space that is far more public than most of us are used to. Peace et al. (1997) discuss 'private lives in public places' (the title of an earlier publication in 1987), indicating that residents have to conduct much of their lives in public spaces accessible to other residents, staff and visitors, and where they are always on show. The public nature of everyday living in a care home has several facets. Living with 10, 20 or 40 other people makes eating a meal or even walking to the bathroom potentially an event to be shared with at least several others. In addition, disabilities and frailty may necessitate help with intimate care such as washing or toileting. These activities are usually part of our private selves but because of frailty or illness they may become someone else's task, albeit enacted with kindness and decorum. They are still an invasion of the older person's privacy and, if not handled sensitively, may be quite damaging to sense of self.

The intimate nature of personal care presents staff with a number of challenges if they are to foster the older person's sense of privacy, dignity and choice. Sometimes, especially when there is some cognitive impairment, a carer's provision of intimate care might be mistaken for sexual advances. Staff need to be sensitive to this possibility and ensure that the care they give is unambiguous. Staff work with touch and intimacy in this sense every day and the difficulty, and skill, needed to carry out this work with sensitivity seems to be another hidden aspect of care.

Older people moving into a care home may experience many disruptions to their former lifestyle and these may have a negative impact on their sense of self and their former relationships, including sexual relationships. Moving into a care home places the older person in the midst of others and yet the losses that have precipitated this move often lead to feelings of vulnerability and loneliness. Successful transition into the home will depend on many factors, but one of the most important is how all staff recognize the vulnerabilities new residents may be feeling and work alongside them to create a sense of welcome and community. This is an area of increasing concern to researchers and a number of studies have attempted to look at how sexuality, intimacy and relationships can be fostered in the care home environment (Smook 1992, Reed & Payton 1996, Steinke 1997, Walker et al. 1998, Nolan et al. 2001).

Case study 21.1 describes a resident's sense of isolation and loneliness from a group of short-term residents admitted to his care home for rehabilitation. He wants to make friends with them but feels that they are a separate group and inaccessible to the permanent residents.

Another case study (Case study 21.2) describes the importance of reminiscence with a resident about the loss of her partner.

First impressions are very important. One resident described how she felt comforted when she arrived at a care home because two nurses were standing just inside the front door, and as she came in, they said 'Welcome'. The warmth and friendship that she felt were being offered at the beginning seemed to form a basis for her future relations with these two members of staff. She went on to say how from that day she had always got on with Charles; they could always have a joke together. As for Rachel, the other staff member – she was lovely, so kind, she had a way of making you feel included. Listening to residents reminds us of the unique role of relationships in the care home and the importance of supporting staff. The research evidence suggests that this is not always easy and staff face many challenges and dilemmas in their day-to-day practice. Some of these come from their own feelings of discomfort when faced with the sexual needs of their older residents and others come from residents and family and friends (Fig. 21.2).

A survey looking at the attitudes of nursing-home staff illustrates some of the conflicts that arise in this area of care. When asked about acceptable forms of sexual behaviour they identified as acceptable only a limited number of sexual behaviours, which included hugging and kissing on the cheek. However, they also went on to say that residents probably needed 'more

---

Case study 21.1:   Relationships between short-term and long-term residents

Mr Rollo is sitting alone in the passageway of the nursing unit. He says he is lonely and you sit down and begin to talk to him. He is upset because he feels he and his fellow long-stay residents are ignored by the six older people who have come to the home as part of intermediate care services.

You are surprised by this as you felt they were enhancing the home's profile. Mr Rollo is very clear that there is little chance of developing any sort of relationship with this group of visitors to the home. He says 'because they are going out it bonds them and unites then in the common goal of going home whereas the other residents are unable to share the goal as the only way they leave is by a permanent move into hospital or death'. As a result he finds there is little communication between the two groups and that a 'them and us' mentality has developed which makes it unpleasant to live in the home.

Reflecting on this conversation with Mr Rollo you realize that the staff have probably contributed to this division by encouraging the rehabilitation group to sit together at meal times which in turn means they tend to remain together when they move to the sitting room. If you are honest you realize that it is easier to talk to this group about their rehabilitation and their plans to go back home and that you have paid little attention to the effect it is having on the permanent residents.

Relationships are essential to any care environment and Mr Rollo has reminded you that from his point of view this has been forgotten and has resulted in him feeling upset and excluded. This is a timely reminder of how fragile relationships are and how they need constant attention if they are to be positive. Staff will need to review the way they encourage more positive relationships between the residents whose home it is and the rehabilitation people who remain short-term guests in the home.

Case study 21.2:   Loss and reminiscence

Stella, a care assistant, helped Mrs Singh get into her favourite chair by the window. Mrs Anita Singh was pleased that her room was on the ground floor. She could look across the garden and car park, watching the flowers bloom and wither with the seasons and watching people come and go.

Stella finished tidying Mrs Singh's room and then turned to see if there was anything else she wanted. She saw tears rolling down Anita's face.

'What is it?' Stella asked. 'Has your pain come back?'

'Not *that* pain', replied Anita. 'It's just when I see that man, and he comes nearly every afternoon, I see him – taking his wife around in the wheelchair. He looks so nice, and they look so happy together. It's not that I begrudge them that, you know – I'm not that bad – it sounds silly, doesn't it? But it reminds me that my husband is not here to take me out like that'. Anita took a deep breath as the tears continued to trickle down her cheeks. 'But', she continued, 'I'm sorry, you must think me such a crybaby. Thanks, Stella, I know you have lots more to do – don't worry about me, you go.'

'No', said Stella, 'I don't have to go this minute. This is important. I don't like to think of you crying on your own like this.'

'Thanks', Anita said and held out her hand as if appreciating the comfort and asking for a little more. Stella took her hand and sat sideways on the window seat so that she could both look at Anita's face and also glance out to the garden to see what Anita was seeing.

'Oh, I know I'm lucky. I've got lots to be grateful for, but I can't help feeling sad sometimes. Of course we had our ups and downs but my husband was a very good man, you know, and we did enjoy being together.'

There was a pause. Stella asked, 'You lived around here, didn't you?'

Anita: 'Yes, for 40 years, we lived about 5 miles from here.'

Stella: 'If you went out together where did you used to go?'

Anita: 'It would depend on the time of year, but summertime we would often go to the sea.'

'I'd like to hear about that', said Stella, 'as well as what it's like for you to be here now, both the sad and the happy times. Would you like to tell me about those things?'

'Yes, sometime when you've got time, I would. It often helps to talk and to feel that someone wants to understand how my life has been as well as how it is now because it all kind of fits together I think.'

Stella and Anita arranged to continue the conversation the following day. Both seemed content with this arrangement. As Stella left, Anita thanked her.

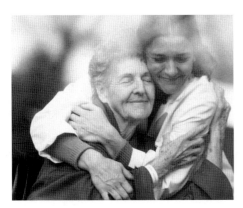

Fig. 21.2   Intimacy.

intimate touching and affection' (Szasz 1983). In other studies the most frequently reported forms of sexual expression are holding hands, kissing, touch and masturbation. According to Archibald (1998), holding hands is viewed as a 'safe' expression of sexuality to witness and to disclose. She goes on to state that Plummer (1995) 'discusses the culture around telling sexual stories, and indicates holding hands is an easy story to tell' (cited in Archibald 1998: p. 97). Public masturbation on the other hand is an area that causes both staff and other residents a good deal of discomfort. She goes on to suggest that, although expressions of sexuality are assumed to be a private affair, residential homes are arenas where the boundaries between private and public become blurred and this can have an impact on the way some older people meet their sexual needs. Perhaps many homes fail to provide the older person with the appropriate privacy needed for sexual expression, in part because of a lack of recognition of the needs, or as a way of minimizing the problems of sexual expression. These are seen as challenging issues for staff (Booth 1990, Kaye 1993, Steinke 1997, Archibald 1998).

It has been suggested that sexuality is often misunderstood by staff who see issues of sexual expression as 'behavioural problems' rather than a need for loving contact and that these attitudes create a barrier to the expression of sexuality and intimacy in institutions. In one study 60% of staff did not believe it was necessary for residents to maintain either a self-image or sexual activity. This response may be indicative of how ill-prepared staff are to deal with the issues (Steinke 1997).

Heath (1999) argues that sexuality 'can generate deep and powerful emotions of embarrassment and fear, longing and frustration' (Heath 1999: p. 1). Other studies which have looked at staff attitudes to intimacy and sexuality report staff feeling embarrassed, uncomfortable or not knowing what to say (Booth

1990, Gibson et al. 1999). In another study Smook (1992) found that the comfort/discomfort held by staff about their own sexuality was in some ways a predictor of their views on sexuality in older people. Some work has been critical of the idea that 'comfortableness' with sexuality is a state that is reached once and for all. Like anything else, our attitudes may change over the lifespan as we have to face different issues in our personal experience and as a result of society's perceptions (Savage 1987, 1989). However, if staff are going to help residents, they need to be able to talk about sexuality and relationships wherever they are on the spectrum of acceptance of their own sexuality. They need to be given opportunities to explore their own feelings before they will be in a position to influence changes in attitudes and practice towards creating a more open environment in which older people are free to express their need for intimacy and sexuality.

In the USA, federal nursing-home regulations make it obligatory for married residents to have privacy during their spouses' visits, and for married couples who are both residents to share a room (Branzelle 1987, Drench & Losee 1996). The same consideration of residents' rights should surely be afforded to unmarried couples and friends, whether their relationship is a heterosexual or homosexual one. In the UK, while this is seen as good practice, there is no legal requirement to do so. Therefore, support for people living together in a care home is variable and will rely on staff recognizing its importance and being prepared to do something about it. Case study 21.3 describes what happened when two people with dementia, who had met and formed a close relationship in hospital, were discharged by chance to the same care home.

As mentioned earlier, the literature indicates how ill-prepared care staff feel when dealing with issues related to sexuality. However there is considerable evidence suggesting that staff who have worked longer with older people, attended more educational programmes and had ongoing discussions about care issues are more sensitive to the sexual needs of residents (Steinke 1997, Mayers & McBride 1998, Walker et al. 1998). Indeed, many of the studies identify education as a predictor of how well older people's needs for intimacy, relationships and sexual expression are supported in the home; this is discussed more fully in the next section.

ROLES FOR HEALTH CARE WORKERS

Education

Education and training of workers are crucial for promoting satisfactory relationships amongst older

> **Case study 21.3:** Intimacy of two people with dementia
>
> Mr Jones, 89 years, and Miss Brown, 82 years, both suffer from dementia and first met while in hospital where they became close friends.
>
> They were subsequently discharged to the same care home, although this was not linked to the close relationship they had formed in hospital. Mr Jones was discharged first and it was some weeks before Miss Brown was ready for discharge. At the time of accepting Miss Brown the care home staff were unaware they had even known each other. The hospital staff had not really considered the relevance of this information despite the closeness of the couple.
>
> On Miss Brown's arrival at the care home it was obvious they recognized each other and were both really happy to be together again. Shortly after arriving at the home Miss Brown decided to share the same room with Mr Jones, who seemed delighted with the decision.
>
> The philosophy of the home was to respect the rights and choices of its residents. Miss Brown's decision posed a dilemma for staff as it was so obviously the wish of both Mr Jones and Miss Brown to share the same room.
>
> The staff talked through the issues and concerns it raised, recognizing that these were their concerns and not the residents'. Both families also agreed that the couple had the right to make their own decisions wherever possible.
>
> Mr Jones and Miss Brown were supported in maintaining the intimate relationship they first formed in the hospital many months before and continue to share a room. Neither has much speech these days but they continue to communicate and support each other.

people. Although the need for education is highlighted in much of the literature, the way it can be delivered is less well addressed (Garrett 1994, Waterhouse 1996, Steinke 1997). It is noteworthy that knowing the facts about the importance of relationships and sexuality in later life does not automatically lead to appropriate practice. Undoubtedly, the work is skilled, and may lead those without the requisite education and training to avoid it. It is indeed difficult to provide professional supportive relationship care; it requires a great deal of skill and support in the workplace. Staff need opportunities to talk about their interactions with older people and to feel listened to. This kind of approach is advocated by Selby (2000), who suggests the 'Balint approach could answer the requirements of educators ... It offers ways to help practitioners become alert and aware of the psychosocial needs of their patients. The insights gained in a Balint style seminar can encourage different ways of relating to patients' (Selby 2000: p. 224). She suggests that this approach challenges the medical model and prepares staff to work in a more person-centred way, encouraging them to support the older person in maintaining healthy relationships and sexuality. This approach has many similarities with reflective practice but the specific feature that is often absent in other forms of reflection is the study of emotion. Balint, in line with psychoanalytic thinking, points out that the feelings aroused within the practitioner when close to a resident often emanate from the resident's world (Balint et al. 1993). The study of stories told by practitioners, with particular reference to feelings, can alert the prac-

titioner to the resident's feelings. The benefits of this approach are that, by acknowledging feelings, the practitioner not only has the chance to become aware of the resident's emotional state, but also the chance to be aware of feelings within herself/himself and to develop this awareness as part of her/his own repertoire of skills. Another promising approach to education in this area is the use of narratives to enable staff to hear the voice of older individuals telling their story in a way that brings the issues to life. This is a powerful way to help staff to recognize the reality for the older person. As a methodology it has been used successfully in a number of educational packages aimed at helping staff to challenge their attitudes to working with older people (Cotter & Rowe 1999).

Further exploration of appropriate educational approaches to enabling nurses and health professionals to feel comfortable in discussing sexual issues with patients needs to be done and published to aid educators.

Sexual health

If older people are enjoying sexual activity, it is essential they are encouraged to practise safe sex and understand sexual health promotion. However, unless staff feel comfortable with the subject they will not be able to meet an important, and possibly the primary, need for older people themselves, which is for information regarding sexuality. Myths and stereotypes need to be stripped of their credibility and replaced with accurate information about sexual functioning and sexuality. Knowledge of how anatomy and physiology evolve with ageing would do much to dispel anxieties and shame in an age group which often feels that its sexual feelings are manifestations of oversexuality or sinfulness (Grigg 1999, Heath & White 2001).

The subject of sexuality and sensuality should be tactfully raised when taking a nursing history; it also provides the first opportunity for education about normal functioning and an excellent framework for launching any discussion on older people's concerns about sexual matters (Eliopoulos 1997, Fielo & Warren 1997, Peate 2004). A sexual history should be part of any health review but the evidence suggests that health care professionals are reluctant or uncomfortable to raise the issue of sexuality with older people, thus reinforcing the view that sexual matters are unimportant or insignificant (Russell 1998, Peate 1999, Andrews 2000). Subsequently, when carrying out care or working with clients, health care professionals need to be alert to cues pointing to covert requests for information or knowledge deficits, and to be able to discuss these in an open, accepting and informative style. In this way older people can come to accept and feel comfortable with their own thoughts, feelings, fantasies and urges. Whether they wish to be sexually active or not they may have insecurities which need to be brought out into the open. This may apply equally to their families, whose own anxieties may cause or add to those of older people themselves. A study by Gott & Hinchliff (2003) found that in their sample of older people, general practitioners (GPs) were seen as the main source of advice if the older person had a sexual problem. They also reported that there were a number of barriers in seeking help from GPs which included the attitudes of the GPs themselves, the older person's own feelings of shame/embarrassment and fear, beliefs held about the seriousness/lack of seriousness of sexuality and sexual problems and the degree of information held about appropriate support and services to help deal with such problems. Other studies have found that, while older people prefer any discussion about sexual issues to be initiated by nurses or other health care professionals, the reality is that this is rarely done (Waterhouse & Metcalfe 1991, Heath & White 2001). This suggests the need for a greater emphasis on the role of GPs and other health care professionals to see sexual health as part of any health promotion programme (Peate 2004). One group of health care professionals, in an ideal position to provide support and promotion of sexual health, is the practice nurse. However, as yet, such a role does not seem to be well established (Rathbone 1997).

Evans (1999) states: 'Just because they are older, people should not be denied the health advice on sexual issues that would routinely be given to younger people' (Evans 1999: p. 46).

Nurses and other health care workers as advocates

It is just as important to take account of sexuality with those who do not wish to be sexually active. While it would be undesirable to upset people by pressing them to behave in ways which others find liberating, sexuality is a much wider matter than sexual acts, as we have already discussed. People who are sexually inactive, whether by choice or circumstances, are still sexual beings in this broader sense and have needs of which nurses and other health care workers need to be aware (Weg 1983, Eliopoulos 1997, Doyle et al. 1999). The advocate role includes speaking for older people when they are not able to influence the situation themselves and working to provide services and facilities which they require. Nurses and other health care workers, whether working in clients' homes or in institutions, are in a potentially strong position to influence the care older people receive and to contribute to meeting their needs in relation to sexuality.

Older people, in health and illness, have the same needs in relation to sexuality and intimacy as every other adult. Acts of intimacy and warmth, companionship and love, self-respect and the respect of others help to maintain an intact self-concept at this stage of life as at any other. Indeed, close friendships may be more important because relationships with family and friends grow fewer as some of them die, and work and social roles are curtailed with retirement and decreased mobility (Weg 1983). Physical appearance and dress are fundamental and highly visible ways of expressing sexuality and individuality. Maintaining a dignified style of dress and presentation is essential to self-respect but this may not be easy for people who have a lower income than during their working lives and cannot so easily get about to make purchases and launder their clothes. Full, individually owned clothing, including underwear, with washing facilities, should be an obligatory provision in health care institutions. Impaired mobility and eyesight may make it difficult to keep hair clean and groomed. Attractive and comfortable dentures, spectacles and hearing aids are a necessity for older people, and functionality is not the only consideration. Help with keeping up appearances may be needed by older people, who will feel that this is not an added refinement or the 'icing on the cake', but is their basic right as human beings.

Privacy, too, is something we all need at times, as recognized in the NSF (Department of Health 2001a), whether to give an opportunity for quiet thinking, to attend to personal hygiene and grooming or to carry out sexual acts. When older people live with their younger families or in institutions this need is easily forgotten. Doors may be left open routinely and people may enter the room without knocking and waiting for permission to enter. Privacy is virtually absent when a room is shared with another resident or the old person sleeps in a downstairs room which the family uses as a living room during the daytime.

As well as assisting people to satisfy their needs in these respects, nurses may have opportunities to influence medical treatment in relation to sexuality. For example, an older woman suffering from atrophic vaginal changes will benefit from using oestrogen cream. Nurses may be the first to notice that a drug is adversely affecting a patient's sexuality or, through closer knowledge of individual patients or clients, may be able to draw a doctor's attention to the effect an illness or disability is having in this respect.

CONCLUSION

Clearly all nurses and health care workers cannot, and should not, be sex therapists. This is a role that requires extensive specialist training (Hogan 1980, Weinberg 1982). But all nurses and other health care workers need to be able to identify problems and intervene appropriately by teaching or counselling within the limits of their knowledge or by referring patients or clients to specialists for help. Our cultural norms and values in the realms of sexuality have changed enormously in the twentieth century, and continue to do so in the twenty-first century. Our future clients and patients are likely to be increasingly assertive about their needs and rights in relation to sexuality. It is our responsibility as professionals to ensure that we are educated and equipped with the knowledge and skills to fulfil our obligations to them. This chapter therefore concludes by reiterating a statement made in a recent article that:

> acknowledging the impact of health care changes on sexual wellbeing is no longer a marginal activity for specialists in sexual health but integral to the practice of all registered nurses and health care workers (Heath & White 2001: p. 31).

The work is challenging and we have a long way to go in providing holistic and comprehensive care in relation to sexual expression and practice for older people. This chapter has set out some of the issues and provided a number of pointers for educators of health care professionals.

Recommended reading

Clarke A, Bright L, Greenwood C 2002 Sex and relationships: a guide for care homes. Counsel & Care, London.
A valuable guide for care staff in developing a proactive approach to sex and relationships in care homes.
Gibson HB 1992 The emotional and sexual lives of older people. Chapman & Hall, London.
Indepth review of social research into a broad range of issues related to sexuality in older people.
Van Ooijen E, Charnock A 1994 Sexuality and patient care. A guide for nurses and teachers. Chapman & Hall, London.
A general textbook on sexuality as part of holistic care.
www.alznsw.asn.au/library/risex.htm Intimacy and sexuality issues in dementia: A guided and annotated resource list.
A valuable annotated resource list prepared by the Alzheimer's Association, New South Wales, Australia.
Wells D, Clifford D, Rutter M, Selby J (eds) (2000) Caring for sexuality in health and illness. Churchill Livingstone, Edinburgh.
A valuable resource for people who wish to develop their psychosexual skills, in particular using discussion and reflective seminars.
www.psychosexualnursing.org.uk.
This is the main website for the Association of Psychosexual Nursing. It includes information on study days and courses based on Balint seminars.

References

Age Concern 1993a HIV? AIDS? We're older gay men, it's not our problem. Lewisham Age Concern, London
Age Concern 1993b Issues facing older lesbians, gay men and bisexuals. Age Concern, London. Available online at: www.ageconcern.org.uk
Ahmed K, Hinsliff G 2004 Gay couple win full rights to 'marriage'. Sunday Observer, 28 March
Andrews W 2000 Approaches to taking a sexual history. Journal of Women's Health and Gender-Based Medicine 9: S-21–S-44
Arber S, Evandrou M (eds) 1993 Ageing, independence and the life course. Jessica Kingsley, London, pp 104–118
Archibald C 1994 Sex: is it a problem? Journal of Dementia Care 2(4): 16–17
Archibald C 1998 Sexuality, dementia and residential care: manager's report and response. Health and Social Care in the Community 6: 95–101
Archibald C, Baikie E 1998 In: Bernard M, Phillips J 1998 The sexual politics of old age (eds) The social policy of old age. Centre for Policy on Ageing, London, 222–236
Avert 1998 United Kingdom HIV/AIDS Statistics cited by Evans G (ed) 1999 Sexuality in old age: why it must not be ignored by nurses. Nursing Times 26: 46–47
Backman G, Leiblum S 1981 Sexual expression in menopausal women. Medical Aspects of Human Sexuality 15: 96B–96H

Balint E, Courtnay M, Elder A, Hull S, Julian P 1993 The doctor, the patient and the group. Routledge, London

Bauer M 1999 Their only privacy is between their sheets. Journal of Gerontological Nursing 25: 37–41

Berman EM, Lief HI 1976 Sex and the ageing process. In: Oaks WW, Melchiode GA, Ficher I (eds) Sex and the life cycle. Grune & Stratton, New York

Booth B 1990 Does it really matter at that age? Nursing Times 86: 50–52

Bortz W, Wallace W, Wiley D 1999 Sexual function in 1202 ageing males: differentiating aspects. In: Minichiello V, Plummer D, Loxton D (eds) 2000 Knowledge and beliefs of older Australians about sexuality and health. Australian Journal of Ageing 19: 190–194

Branzelle J 1987 Ensuring residents' rights to sexual desire and expression. Provider 13(10): 30: 33

Butler R, Lewis M 1973 Sex after sixty. Harper & Row, New York

Butler R, Lewis M 1988 Love and sex after sixty, 2nd edn. Harper & Row, London

Byers E, Grenier G 2003 Premature or rapid ejaculation: heterosexual couples' perceptions of men's ejaculatory behaviour. Archives of Sexual Behavior 32: 261–270

Clarke A, Bright L, Greenwood C 2002 Sex and relationships: a guide for care homes. Counsel & Care, London

Corby N, Zarit JM 1983 The unmarried in later life. In: Weg RB (ed) Sexuality in the later years: roles and behaviour. Academic Press, New York

Costello MK 1975 Sex, intimacy and ageing. American Journal of Nursing 75: 1330–1332

Cotter A, Rowe J 1999 The use of biographies in community nurse training. Paper presented to IPPR Seminar on the use of biographies from research. London

Deacon S, Minichiello V, Plummer D 1995 Sexuality and older people: revisiting the assumptions. Educational Gerontology 21(5): 497–513

de Beauvoir S 1973 The coming of age. Warner Paperback Library, New York

Department of Health 2000 National plan. HMSO, London

Department of Health 2001a National service framework for older people. Stationery Office, London

Department of Health 2001b Care homes for older people: national minimum standards. Care standards act 2000. Stationery Office, London

Department of Health 2001c The expert patient: a new approach to chronic disease management for the 21st century. Department of Health, London

Doyle D, Bisson D, Janes N, Lynch H, Martin C 1999 Human sexuality in long-term care. Canadian Nurse 95: 26–29

Drench M, Losee R 1996 Sexuality and sexual capacities of older people. Rehabilitation Nursing 21: 118–123

Eliopoulos C 1997 Gerontological nursing, 4th edn. Lippincott, Philadelphia, pp 207–217

Evans G 1999 Sexuality in old age: why it must not be ignored by nurses. Nursing Times 95: 49–50

Fielo S, Warren S 1997 Sexual expression in a very old man: a nursing approach to care. Geriatric Nursing 18: 61–64

Fullmer E, Shenk D, Eastland L 1999 Negating identity: a feminist analysis of the social invisibility of older lesbians. Journal of Women and Aging 11: 131–148

Garrett G 1994 Sexuality in later life. Older Care 6: 23–28

Getliffe K, Dolman M (eds) 1997 Promoting continence: a clinical and research resource. Baillière Tindall, London

Gibson HB 1993 Emotional and sexual adjustment in later life. In: Arber S, Evandrou M (eds) Ageing, independence and the life course. Jessica Kingsley, London, pp 104–118

Gibson M, Woodbury G, Beaton C, Janke C 1999 Expressing sexuality in an institutional setting. Journal of Gerontological Nursing 25: 30–39

Gott M, Hinchliff S 2003 Barriers to seeking treatment for sexual problems in primary care: a qualitative study with older people. Family Practice 20: 690–695

Grigg E 1999 Sexuality and older people. Older Care 11: 12–15

Hajjar R, Hosam K 2003 Sexuality in the nursing home. Part 1: attitudes and barriers to sexual expression. Journal of the American Medical Directors Association 4: 152–156

Hayter M 1996 Is non-judgemental care possible in the context of nurses' attitudes to patients' sexuality? Journal of Advanced Nursing 24: 662–666

Heapy B, Yip A, Thompson D 2003 The social and policy implications of non-heterosexuals ageing: selective findings. Quality in Ageing: Policy Practice and Research 4: 30–35

Heath H 1999 Sexuality in old age. Nursing Times monograph, vol 40. Emap Health Care, London, pp 1–14

Heath H 2002 Sexuality and later life: In: Heath H, White I (eds) The challenge of sexuality in health care. Blackwell Science, Oxford, pp 133–152

Heath H, White I 2001 Sexuality and older people: an introduction to nursing assessment. Nursing Older People 13: 29–31

Hendricks J, Hendricks CD 1978 Sexuality in later life. In: Carver V, Liddiard P (eds) An ageing population. Hodder & Stoughton/Open University, Sevenoaks

Hodson D, Skeen P 1994 Sexuality and aging: the hammerlock of myths. Journal of Applied Gerontology 13: 219–235

Hogan R 1980 Human sexuality: a nursing perspective. Appleton-Century-Crofts, New York

Itzen C 1984 In Arber S, Evandrou M (eds.) 1993 Ageing, independence and the life course, Jessica Kingsley, London, pp 104–118

Jagus C, Benbow S 2002 Sexuality in older men with mental health problems. Sexual and Relationship Therapy 17: 271–279

Jones H 1994 Mores and morals. Nursing Times 90: 55–58

Jones R 2002 'That's very rude, I shouldn't be telling you that': older women talking about sex. Narrative Inquiry 12: 121–143

Kaye R 1993 Sexuality in the later years. Ageing and Society 13: 415–426

Kitwood T 1997 Dementia reconsidered. Open University Press, Buckingham

Kraimaat F, Bakker A, Janssen E, Bijlsma J 1996 Intrusiveness of rheumatoid arthritis on sexuality in male and female patients living with a spouse. In: Schiavi R (ed) Ageing and male sexuality. Cambridge University Press, Cambridge

Kuhn ME 1976 Sexual myths surrounding ageing, In: Oaks WW, Melchoide GA, Ficher I (eds) Sex and the life cycle. Grune & Stratton, New York

MacDonald B, Rich C 1984 Look me in the eye. Women's Press, London

MacGregor H 1994 Risk exposure. Nursing Times 90: 58–59

Masters W, Johnson V 1966a Human Sexual Response. Little Brown Co., Boston

Masters WH, Johnson VE 1981 Sex and the ageing process. Journal of the American Geriatrics Society 29: 385–390

Mayers K, McBride D 1998 Sexuality training for caretakers of geriatric residents in long-term care facilities. Sexuality and Disability 3, 227–236

Minichiello V, Plummer D, Loxton D 2000 Knowledge and beliefs of older Australians about sexuality and health. Australian Journal of Ageing 19: 190–194

Morgentaler A 2003 The Viagra myth: the surprising impact on love and relationships. Jossey-Bass, San Francisco

National Council on Aging www.sexualityandu.ca/eng/health/SOW/sexualactivity.cfm (accessed February 2004)

Nay R 1992 Sexuality and aged women in nursing homes. Geriatric Nursing 13: 6312–6314

Neugebauer-Visano R (ed) 1995 Seniors and sexuality. Canadian Scholars' Press, Toronto

Nolan M, Davies S, Grant G 2001 Working with older people and their families. Open University Press, Buckingham, pp 75–98

Palmore E 1971 Attitudes to aging as shown by humor. Gerontologist 11(3): 181–6

Peace S, Kellaher L, Willcocks D 1997 Re-evaluating residential care. Open University Press, Buckingham

Peate I 1999 The need to address sexuality in older people. British Journal of Nursing 4: 174–180

Peate I 2004 Sexuality and sexual health promotion for the older person. British Journal of Nursing 13:188–193

Persson G 1980 Sexuality in a 70 year old urban population. Journal of Psychosomatic Research 24: 335–342

Potts A, Gavey N, Grace V, Vares T 2003 The downside of Viagra: women's experiences and concerns. Sociology of Health and Illness 25: 697–719

Puner M 1974 To the good long life. Macmillan/Open University, London

Rathbone S 1997 Do ya think I'm sexy? Nursing Times 93: 59

Reed J, Payton VR 1996 Constructing familiarity and managing the self: ways of adapting to life in nursing and residential homes. Ageing and Society 16: 561–578

Royal College of Nursing 1994 Guidance on infection control in hospitals. Royal College of Nursing, London

Russell P 1998 Sexuality in the lives of older people. Nursing Standard 11: 49–53

Sabin TD 1987 The new 'great imitator'. Journal of the American Geriatric Society 35: 467–468

Sarrel PM 1990 Ovarian hormones and the circulation. Maturitas 12: 287–98

Savage J 1987 Nurses, gender and sexuality. Heinemann Nursing, London

Savage J 1989 Sexuality: an uninvited guest. Nursing Times 85: 25–28

Schuerman D 1994 Clinical concerns: AIDS in the older. Journal of Gerontological Nursing 20: 11–17

Schiavi R 1999 Ageing and male sexuality. Cambridge University Press, Cambridge

Scully D, Bart P 1973 A funny thing happened on the way to the orifice. American Journal of Sociology 78: 1045–1049

Second World Assembly on Ageing 2002 Building a society for all ages. United Nations, Madrid, Spain www.un.org/ageing

Selby J 2000 Coaching for psychosexual awareness. In: Wells D, Clifford D, Rutter M, Selby J (eds) Caring for sexuality in health and illness. Churchill Livingstone, Edinburgh

Sellers C, Angerame 2002 HIV/AIDS in older adults: a case study and discussion. Advanced Practice in Acute and Critical Care 13: 5–21

Ship JA, Wolff A, Selik RM 1991 Epidemiology of acquired immune deficiency syndrome in persons aged 75 years or older. Acquired Immune Deficiency Syndrome 4: 84–88

Smook K 1992 Nurses' attitudes towards the sexuality of older people: an investigative study. Nursing Practice 6: 15–17

Sontag S 1978 The double standard of ageing. In: Carver V, Liddiard P (eds) An ageing population. Hodder & Stoughton/Open University, Sevenoaks, pp 72–80

Starr B, Weiner M 1981 The Starr–Weiner report on sex and sexuality in mature years. Stein and Day, New York

Steinke E 1997 Sexuality in ageing: implications for nursing facility staff. Journal of Continuing Education in Nursing 28: 59–63

Swabo P 2003 Counselling about sexuality in the older person. Clinics in Geriatric Medicine 19: 595–604

Szasz G 1983 Sexual incidents in an extended care unit for aged men. Journal of the American Geriatrics Society 31: 407–411

Turton AJP 1995 Developing a community nursing service for people with HIV disease: an action research project incorporating ethnographic methods. PhD thesis. University of Manchester, Manchester

Wagner G, Mayton M, Smith M et al. Analysis of the efficacy of sildenafil (Viagra) in the treatment of male erectile dysfunction in older patients. In: Schiavi R (ed) (1999) Ageing and Male Sexuality. Cambridge University Press, Cambridge

Walker B, Osgood N, Ephross P et al. 1998 Developing a training curriculum on older sexuality for long-term care facility staff. Gerontology and Geriatrics Education 19: 3–22

Walz T 2002 Crones, dirty old men, sexy seniors: representations of sexuality of older persons. Journal of Ageing and Identity 7: 99–112

Waterhouse J 1996 Nursing practice related to sexuality: a review and recommendations. NT Research 1: 412–418

Waterhouse J, Metcalfe M 1991 Attitudes towards nurses discussing sexual concerns with patients. Journal of Advanced Nursing 16: 1048–1054

Webb C 1983 Words fail me. Nursing Times 27: 62–66

Weg RB (ed) 1983 Sexuality in the later years: roles and behaviour. Academic Press, New York

Weinberg JS 1982 Sexuality: human needs and nursing practice. WB Saunders, Philadelphia

Whipple B, Scura K 1996 HIV in older adults. American Journal of Nursing 96: 23–28

Winn RL, Newton N 1982 Sexuality in ageing: a study of 106 cultures. Archives of Sexual Behaviour 11: 283–298

www.galha.org/press/1998/04_02.htm (accessed April 2004)

Wooten-Bielski K 1999 NGNA, HIV and AIDS in older adults. Geriatric Nursing 20: 268–272

Yee L, Sundquist K 2003 Older women's sexuality. Medical Journal of Australia 178: 640–643

Chapter 22

Pain and older people

Kate Seers

NATURE OF PAIN

Pain is a common experience and caring for patients in pain is often a central part of the nurse's role. Pain has been described, however, as 'one of the most challenging problems in medicine' (Melzack & Wall 1988: p. ix). This applies equally to nursing. Part of this challenge lies in the complexity of the pain experience. Pain is more complex and dynamic than purely a response to stimulation – it includes the interaction of physiological, psychological and social factors and thus each person's experience of pain is individual and unique. Since others cannot directly measure this experience, pain is also subjective.

The multifactorial nature of pain was highlighted by Melzack & Casey (1968), who described sensory, motivational and cognitive determinants of pain. Syrjala (1987) restated these and described the sensory dimension as including qualities such as burning, stabbing, pressure or tingling. Motivational or affective terms can describe how the pain affects the person; for example, it may be perceived as unpleasant and/or exhausting. Cognitive appraisal or evaluating the pain experience can include thinking about the meaning of pain. Although described separately, all these dimensions are interrelated and can all influence behaviour, including both verbal and non-verbal expressions of pain.

The description of pain as consisting of more than a purely sensory dimension (the sensation of pain) provides a framework that allows variables such as mood, culture, anxiety, the meaning of pain and past experiences of pain, amongst many other things, to influence the experience of pain.

The modulation of pain sensation by factors other than the actual potentially painful stimulus can be explained conceptually by the gate-control theory of pain, stated and updated by Melzack & Wall (1965, 1988). There are many discussions and disagreements about the exact neurophysiology involved, but the theory provides a way of understanding how pain can be influenced by factors other than the sensory stimulus.

Basically, Melzack & Wall propose that there is a gating mechanism in the substantia gelatinosa in the dorsal horn of the spinal cord. If the gate is shut, pain impulses can go no further. If it is partially or completely open, pain impulses can pass through the gate and ascend to the brain. The position of the gate can be influenced by activity in both the peripheral and central nervous systems. Thus potentially painful impulses can be modified by fibres descending from the brain. Ascending messages to the brain can also influence descending controls. For example, anxiety or fear could open the gate, thus increasing pain, whereas by reducing anxiety and closing the gate, pain may be relieved.

Many factors can act to open or close the gate, and this explains why the relationship between injury and pain is 'highly variable' (Melzack & Wall 1988: p. 165). Since there are so many potential influences on the experience of pain, it follows that the response of each individual will be unique. Dickenson (2002: p. 755) argues that the gate theory of pain has stood the test of time. He argues that: 'This plasticity, the capacity of the pain signalling and modulating systems to alter in different circumstances, has changed our ways of thinking about pain control.' His paper provides a very useful summary of recent developments in this area. The role of endorphins (the body's own morphine) and a variety of transmitters, receptors and channels in pain and pain relief is complex and an area in which much work is currently being undertaken.

It is difficult to define pain. If pain has several dimensions and can be influenced by many things, how can it be defined? This complexity of pain was summed up by the National Institutes of Health Consensus Development Conference (1987: p. 36):

> Pain is a subjective experience that can be perceived directly only by the sufferer . . . Pain does not occur in isolation but in a specific human being with psychosocial, economic, and cultural contexts that influence the meaning, experience, and verbal and non-verbal expression of pain.

This definition emphasizes the subjective and individual nature of pain.

ACUTE AND CHRONIC PAIN

A distinction is made between acute and chronic pain because what may normally work to control acute pain may not necessarily be so effective or appropriate for those with chronic pain (Fordyce 1978). Whereas anxiety is often associated with acute pain, depression is more commonly associated with chronic pain.

Acute pain

This refers to pain usually associated with trauma or disease and is of short duration or recent onset. Examples are stubbing your toe, or the pain of a myocardial infarct. Acute pain usually serves as a warning signal to stop further damage and/or make the person in pain seek help. Melzack & Wall (1988: p. 35) describe the characteristics of acute pain as 'the combination of tissue damage, pain and anxiety'. The anxiety could, for example, centre on worries about future consequences of the injury.

Chronic pain

This is usually defined as lasting for 6 months or more (McCaffery & Beebe 1989), although they point out that there is disagreement over how prolonged pain should be before it is called chronic. Chronic pain persists long after it can serve as a useful warning signal. Sternbach (1987) proposes that the difference between acute and chronic pain is much more than duration of pain. He argues that chronic pain is not a symptom or a warning signal or a need-state for rest, but a syndrome. By implication this syndrome could be treated in its own right.

IS PAIN ANY DIFFERENT IF YOU ARE OLD?

There are reviews in this area, to which the interested reader is referred for more detail (Ardery et al. 2003, focusing on acute pain; American Geriatrics Society 2002, focusing on persistent pain; Gibson et al. 1994, Gibson & Helme 1995, Melding 1995, Ferrell & Ferrell 1996). An overview of the area will be given here. The acceptance that pain and old age go together seems widespread. Closs (1994) found almost a third of the 208 nurses in her study felt pain and discomfort were unavoidable consequences of ageing. This perception also seems to be shared by some older people: a focus group study involving older people found age-related expectations included pain being a normal part of ageing (Davis et al. 2002). Certainly many disorders common in older people produce pain. Melding (1995) outlines certain types of pain common in older people, such as angina, arthritis, cervical spondylosis, collapsed vertebrae, fractures, intermittent claudication, osteoporosis, malignancy, neuropathies, Paget's disease, postamputation pain, postherpetic pain, sympathetic dystrophy, thalamic syndrome, trigeminal neuralgia and vasculitis. Other pains, such as those caused by rheumatic diseases, temporal arteritis, surgery and gout, are mentioned by McKenzie (1985), and Matteson & McConnell (1988) add coronary artery disease, osteomyelitis, osteoporosis, depression and constipation to this list.

It seems then that older people may have diseases that can cause pain. A systematic review by Fox et al. (1999) reported a prevalence of pain in older adults in nursing homes and long-term institutions of between 49% and 83%. However, they found there was a lack of studies evaluating interventions to manage this pain. There is some research that has looked at the incidence of pain in older people. For example, Sengstaken & King (1993) investigated the presence of pain in residents of nursing homes for old people. Although they found that 66% of the 76 communicative residents had chronic pain, the treating doctors did not detect pain (defined as any mention of pain in the problem list or progress notes, or if the patient had one or more analgesics) in 34% of those patients who had reported pain when interviewed. A higher incidence was found by Mobily et al. (1994); they studied over 3000 people aged 65 and over in the USA and found 86% reported having pain, and 59% had multiple pain complaints, during the previous year. Joint pain was the most prevalent, reported by 66% of people. In the same age group in France, Brochet et al. (1991) found a similar 68% reporting joint pain. A large survey of 662 people aged 85 and over in London found 70% reported aches, pains or stiffness in muscles or joints (Bowling & Browne 1991). Jakobsson et al. (2003) compared a large sample of older people with and without pain. They found pain was more common as people got older, and a lower quality of life was associated with being older and in pain.

Older people may have more than one pain from multiple pathology and their pain may be chronic, acute or both. Liebeskind & Melzack (1987: p. 1) note that: 'Pain in the elderly is often dismissed as something to be expected and hence tolerated'. There is, however, a growing body of opinion that pain is not an inevitable part of ageing, but demands diagnosis and treatment as it does at any age (Butler & Gastel 1980). Harkins et al. (1984: p. 112) state that: 'Pain, discomfort and suffering are not natural consequences of growing old'. Kwentus et al. (1985) highlight the need to understand age-related changes in how pain presents and how the older person perceives and tolerates pain. Pain in older people has been described by McCaffery & Beebe (1989) as a neglected area and they add that there are many gaps in our knowledge. Butler & Gastel (1980) remind the reader that the pain of older people is not others' pain but our own, as more of us survive into old age. Older people are not well represented at pain clinics according to Wells (1989), and he wonders if this is due to their complaining less, and to doctors assuming that their pain is acceptable in view of their age. From his experience he concludes that old people are more, not less, likely to experience chronic pain, especially neurological pain. Benbow et al. (1995) support the frequency of neurogenic diagnoses in older people; it was the most common pain condition in the elderly pain clinic population they studied.

Although sensory, motivational/affective and cognitive/evaluative dimensions of pain all overlap, these categories will now be used to examine whether pain for older people is any different from pain for other age groups.

Sensory dimensions

There is much debate over whether pain thresholds change in older people. Pain threshold is 'the least experience of pain which a subject can recognize', and pain tolerance is 'the greatest level of pain which a subject is prepared to tolerate' (International Association for the Study of Pain Subcommittee on Taxonomy 1986). Pain tolerance has also been defined as 'the duration or intensity of pain that a person is *willing* to endure' (McCaffery & Beebe 1989: p. 15).

A useful review of 280 papers in this area has been undertaken by Gibson & Helme (1995). They looked first at the effects of ageing on pain receptors and argued there was no conclusive evidence of changes in the density or structure of free nerve endings of myelinated fibres. However, there was evidence of age-related changes in the skin, which may reduce skin pain sensitivity and thus affect nociceptive input (information coming from receptors which respond preferentially to a noxious stimulus or a stimulus that could be noxious if it went on long enough). When considering the effects of ageing on peripheral nerves, they concluded there was age-related disturbance of primary afferent fibres. In the central nervous system, they describe slower central processing of incoming noxious input and a reduction in cortical activation. However, this is balanced by a reduction in function of endogenous pain-inhibitory systems. Gibson & Helme (1995) conclude there is a modest increase in pain threshold intensity with age, especially for thermal stimulation. However, in contrast, older people are more sensitive to strong levels of noxious stimulation and have a reduced ability to endure mechanical, electrical and cold pain sensation. They argue that, while an increased pain threshold may make it easier for older people to deal with an increase in minor pathology, the actual experience of any reported pain is not less. Thus when an older person does report pain, this needs to be considered exactly as for any other adult. Gibson & Helme (1995: p. 129) conclude that, 'to assume that altered threshold pain sensitivity means reduced suffering in the elderly is totally fallacious and will ultimately lead to inadequate management'.

Chakour et al. (1996), in a laboratory study of 15 young and 15 older subjects, found the older group relied on C-fibre input when reporting pain, while the younger group utilized additional information from A-delta fibres. When only C-fibre information was available, both groups responded similarly. This was interpreted as demonstrating an age-related change. Davitz & Davitz (1981) found that age of patients (65 years or more compared with younger adults) had little influence on nurses' inferences of physical pain or psychological distress. This view was supported by Harkins & Chapman (1976, 1977) who argued that perception was similar but that older people were less accurate in discrimination and less willing to label a sensation as painful. Harkins et al. (1994) argue that it is appropriate to conclude that age does not affect the discomfort and suffering associated with clinical, recurrent or chronic pains.

There is debate about the differences in pain experienced by older compared with younger patients in some specific conditions. A small selection of these conditions will now be discussed.

Myocardial infarction

In a study by Aronow (1987), which included 87 patients with acute myocardial infarction (MI) aged 62 years and over, 72% did not present with chest pain. The prevalence and symptoms of MI in older long-term care patients were studied by Wroblewski et al. (1986). They found that intense dyspnoea, syncope and weakness were more common than chest pain and that there was low diagnostic accuracy of acute MI in elderly people. Cocchi et al. (1988) concluded that the clinical diagnosis of acute MI was more commonly missed in older patients, with ageing, atypical presentation and the coexistence of several diseases accounting for most of the unrecognized acute MI.

This high incidence of painless MI in older people has not always been supported by other studies. Mac-Donald et al. (1983) studied 296 patients admitted to a coronary care unit who were aged less than 60 and 317 aged 70 or more. They found 77% of the younger group, as compared with 61% of the older group, had pain as the main presenting symptom. Thus in the majority of the 70+ age group, although chest pain was less common, it was still the most common presenting symptom. MacDonald et al. concluded that the incidence of painless MI had been overestimated in the past. This supported the work of Konu (1977), who found that chest pain was the most common symptom in over 65% of a sample of 226 MI patients aged 65+.

It has been found that atypical presentations of MI in older patients are associated with impaired mental scores on admission (Black 1987), and Kwentus et al. (1985) argue that an MI may present atypically if patients are confused or have communication difficulties.

Other studies have suggested that the presentation of MI may be different in very old people. Bayer et al. (1986) studied the symptoms associated with acute MI in 777 patients aged between 65 and 100 years. They reviewed discharge summaries and looked at original records, and found that the spectrum of presentation changed with increasing age. Chest pain was common and present in almost 70% of those aged 65–84. However, it tended to become less common with increasing age and the incidence of syncope, stroke and acute confusion increased. After age 84, shortness of breath was the most common symptom, present in 43%, and pain was the second most common symptom, present in 37.5%.

These findings were supported by Day et al. (1987), who found atypical presentation was common in 100 patients aged 85 years or more. They found 69% of those aged 65–84 had chest pain compared with 41% of those aged 85+. Those aged 85 years or more were significantly more likely to be acutely confused. Only 2% in the 65–84 and 4% in the 85% group had a silent or symptomless MI. However, while this study supports that of Bayer et al., it appears to be based on essentially the same sample of patients, extended by 2 years. Thus it can only be regarded as an extension, rather than a replication, of the study by Bayer et al. (1986). It is important to note that atypical presentation of acute MI can also occur in younger patients. MacDonald (1984) concluded that about 40% of older patients will present in a non-classical manner, as compared with about 25% of younger patients.

It seems that, while reports of the incidence of painless MI in older people may have been overestimated, the findings of Bayer et al. (1986), extended by Day et al. (1987), suggest that about 30% of those aged 65–84 and around 60% of those aged 85+ who have an acute MI may present without chest pain. Once an MI has been diagnosed, older patients may be treated differently: Tresch et al. (1996) found that older patients with MI were significantly less likely to have thrombolytic therapy and revascularization procedures than younger patients, even though both therapies are of benefit to older patients. Aronow (2003), in a review article, concluded that the prevalence of clinically unrecognized MI detected by routine electrocardiograms in older individuals varies from 21% to 68%. Atypical symptoms associated with acute MI in older persons include dyspnoea and neurological and gastrointestinal symptoms, as well as chest pain.

Appendicitis

McCallion et al. (1987) studied 30 older patients (average age 72) and 30 younger patients (average age 23) who presented with a confirmed diagnosis of appendicitis. They found that all the older patients had abdominal pain and the presentation was broadly similar between the two groups. The older patients had symptoms for significantly longer before they presented than the younger group, and there was a longer delay between admission and surgery. Although presentation was similar, only 54% of the older compared with 90% of the younger group were correctly diagnosed before surgery. This may partly explain the delay to surgery. Their finding of a similar presentation between the two age groups was not supported in a multicentre, international survey of acute abdominal pain by Telfer et al. (1988). They investigated patients with acute appendicitis and found 366 patients aged over 50 (who were termed 'elderly') presented differently from 1970 patients aged less than 50 years. Amongst other things they found that the 'elderly patients' were more likely to have general pain. The finding that pain was of a longer duration in the older group did support the results of McCallion et al. (1987).

It seems that appendicitis in older people is associated with pain. This conclusion differs somewhat from that of a study which investigated older patients with a peptic ulcer.

Peptic ulcer

Clinch et al. (1984) compared the presentation of peptic ulcer in 132 patients aged 60 or more with that of 67 younger patients aged 20–50. They found that abdominal pain was not present in a third of the older group. Thirty-five per cent of the older group, as compared with 8% of the younger group, had no abdominal pain at the time of referral or during the previous 6 months – a difference which was significant. Clinch et al. speculate that this may be due to decreased cutaneous pain sensitivity, decreased visceral sensitivity or an increase in the use of non-steroidal anti-inflammatory drugs (NSAIDs) by the older patients. The Bandolier (2004) website (www.jr2.ox.ac.uk/bandolier/booth/painpag/nsae/nsae.html) clearly highlights how a risk of an NSAID-related adverse event is age-related. For those over 75, an annual risk of a gastrointestinal bleed with an NSAID is 1 in 110 and the annual risk of death from a gastrointestinal bleed is 1 in 650.

Affective/evaluative dimensions

What pain means and the effect it has is a crucial part of the pain experience for all age groups. We should recognize the sort of questions pain may raise in the sufferer. Illich (1977: p. 149) outlines some of these questions: 'What is wrong? How much longer? Why must I/ought I/should I/can I suffer? Why does this kind of evil exist, and why does it strike just me?' Baken (1968) adds the question, 'Does this pain mean I will die?' Those questions may or may not be articulated. Some people may see some value in some pain some of the time, for religious or self-testing or self-growth reasons. Questions like this are very much part of the experience of pain.

Needless pain and suffering impoverish quality of life for patients and their families (Liebeskind & Melzack 1987). Ghose (1987) argues that socioeconomic factors, housing problems, social isolation and loneliness are all likely to influence pain sensitivity in older people. In an effort to minimize pain, activities of daily living can become time- and energy-consuming (Matteson & McConnell 1988). Pain may mean that the ability for self-care is reduced, and mobility is restricted; it may become difficult to go out independently and enjoyment of life can be limited. The ability to cope with pain is important. Harkins et al. (1984) suggest that the negative social or psychological aspects of ageing may reduce the older person's capacity to respond successfully to the negative consequences of chronic pain. The results of a study by Walker (1989) suggest the sort of factors that influence ability to cope. She studied 190 older patients in the community with painful conditions and found that factors such as 'having regrets', 'being occupied', 'pain under control', having 'personal problems' and 'feeling informed' were the best predictors of mood and coping. Walker suggested that all these predictors be included in pain assessment and intervention. The importance of ability to cope has also been emphasized by Wachter-Shikora & Perez (1988), who argued that older people reported pain less frequently or stated that they felt less pain since they knew what to expect and how to cope with their pain. Gibson & Helme (2000) investigated whether cognitive factors mediated pain and resultant suffering. They studied 169 older patients attending a pain management clinic. They concluded that cognitive beliefs were related to self-reported pain and psychological adjustment. Older people who believed that pain severity was controlled by chance reported greater depressive symptoms and more pain. Keefe & Williams (1990) found there were no significant age differences in use or perceived effectiveness of pain coping strategies. The role of expectations in coping may be important. For example, Williamson & Schultz (1995) found the restriction of routine activities due to pain and illness may be more distressing to younger than older patients, possibly suggesting a lower expectation of functional status and more experience with illness and disability amongst the older group. The likely importance of factors other than pain in influencing the impact of pain was suggested by Roy et al. (1996). They found that even sometimes severe pain seemed to interfere only marginally with the social life of 205 older people who belonged to a support group. Those choosing to belong to such a group could be different from other older people in the community.

A report of pain may have wider implications and involve more than may be immediately apparent. Increasing age may be associated with loss of physical health, loss of loved ones, decreased economic resources and lowered social status, and complaints of pain may be seen as an acceptable attempt to elicit some caretaking (Kwentus et al. 1985). Symptoms such as poor concentration, attention and memory dysfunctions can be ascribed to pain (Harkins et al. 1984), as can behavioural changes such as confusion or restlessness, or non-specific symptoms such as fatigue or anorexia (Butler & Gastel 1980). Moore & Whanger (1983) outlined how it is not uncommon for atypical pain to be the main, if not the sole, symptom of depression. Many studies have found an association between chronic pain and depression (Kramlinger et al. 1983, Doan & Wadden 1989), although the percentage reported to be depressed varies. Turk et al. (1995) studied 100 chronically ill patients divided into those aged 69 or less and those aged 70 or more. Younger patients showed a low and non-significant correlation between pain severity and depression. Conversely there was a strong association with older patients. It seems thus that the relationship between pain and depression may vary depending on age group. In contrast to younger patients, as pain intensity increased in older patients, they felt less in control of their lives and depressive symptoms increased. There were no differences in the level of disability or general activity levels or perceived life control between the two age groups.

There is also debate concerning the extent to which people are depressed because they are in chronic pain, or whether chronic pain is a manifestation of depression. Reid et al. (2003) found depressive symptoms were associated with the occurrence of disabling musculoskeletal pain in older people in the community. Lin et al. (2003), in a randomized controlled trial, concluded that when depression care for older people with arthritis was improved, depression and pain were reduced, and quality of life and functional status improved. Melzack & Wall (1988) argue that it is unreasonable to ascribe chronic pain to neurotic symptoms and, while psychological processes contribute to pain, they are only one factor influencing the complex experience of pain.

The effects that chronic pain can have on behaviour have been utilized by Fordyce (1978). He argued that people often receive positive reinforcement for having pain. For example, complaints of pain may elicit sympathy from family or friends and allow the avoidance of activities the person in pain would not normally want to do. Thus the individual receives rewards for having pain and this reinforces the pain behaviour. Fordyce argues that these people can be retrained by stopping rewards for pain behaviour and reinforcing only 'well' behaviours. This is known as operant conditioning. However, this technique has been the subject of much discussion. Melzack & Wall (1988) question whether it means that the patient feels less pain or simply complains less, for example. They also question whether this operant conditioning is any better than a placebo effect.

McCaffery (1983) highlights points to consider when using the operant conditioning technique, including that it only be used for *selected* patients in chronic pain, with their informed consent; that it has no place in the care of patients in acute pain; that learning to use pain for certain benefits does not occur on a conscious level; and that occasional use of pain to obtain certain benefits is not unusual and does not warrant any special treatment. Miller & Le Lieuvre (1982) used an operant conditioning approach in a small pilot study with four older residents in a nursing home. They found attention and praise reduced the required medication, pain behaviour and self-reports of pain, but they were unable to show an increase in the number of activities in which residents engaged.

So, knowing that pain is sometimes dismissed in older people as an inevitable consequence of ageing, that many disorders common in older people produce both acute and chronic pain, and that pain can reduce quality of life, it is how pain in old people is *managed*, as Eland (1988) argues, that influences the degree of activity, social isolation and the quality of life for the older person. Encouragingly, Closs (1996) found that awareness of the negative consequences of chronic pain was good in her study of 208 qualified nurses.

HOW CAN YOU MANAGE PAIN?

Your own feelings

Before you assess pain with any patient or intervene to help reduce pain, it is important that you examine your own feelings about pain and pain relief. Some factors to consider include whether you think patients/clients should put up with some pain, and if so, how much? What are your own feelings about taking or giving painkillers – both narcotic and non-narcotic? How do you decide whether a patient/client is in pain? Blomqvist (2003) collected 150 stories about older patients from health care staff. She found older people were seen as exaggerating pain, and those with care-related or self-caused pain frustrated the staff. Those seen as enduring their pain evoked satisfaction in the staff. Blomqvist concluded that it was important to base care on needs of older people rather than on staff attitudes and preferences. It is useful to bear in mind that Sloman et al. (2001) found nurses' knowledge about pain management in older people was not ideal and they recommended more education in this area. Turner & Weiner (2002) have developed expert-based guidelines for a medical student curriculum on chronic pain management in older people. This is a useful first step although, as the authors point out, the efficacy of these guidelines needs to be assessed.

The patient's perspective

The nurse and the patient may have different perspectives on pain and its management. For example, Walker (1994) found differences in the way nurses and older people saw the nurse's contribution to pain management. Patients emphasized qualities such as empathy, gentleness and quality of interpersonal care; nurses were more pessimistic and relied on medical referral. Older people placed a high value on caring aspects, whereas nurses emphasized curing and treating. The importance of the whole experience is further highlighted by Hall-Lord et al. (1994). They studied 18 older patients in an intensive care unit and found they needed help not only with the physical and emotional aspects of pain, but with spiritual (existential) aspects too. The views of older people with pain were also studied by Yates et al. (1995), who looked at the views of pain and pain management practices held by older people in long-term residential care settings. They conducted 10 focus group interviews, with an average of five people per group. They found that three themes emerged: (1) older people became resigned to their pain; (2) they felt ambivalent about any action for their pain; and (3) they were reluctant to express their pain. Zalon (1997), in a qualitative study of 16 postoperative older women, found the women tended to endure pain and trust the nurses to manage pain. However, others have found self-management and having a more active role in pain relief can be beneficial. For example, Ersek et al. (2003) found that self-management of chronic pain in older people in the community improved physical role function and pain intensity. McDonald et al. (2001) found that older people who had been taught pain management communication skills and had pain management information had less postoperative pain over the course of their hospital stay.

These studies, looking at the patient's perspective, can inform our discussions with patients as we then go on to assess and manage pain. Some general principles for managing pain and identifying possible barriers are outlined in Box 22.1. Pasero & McCaffery (1996) add some selected barriers to effective pain management in older people. These are divided into three categories (Box 22.2).

Titler et al. (2003) found that, for nurses caring for older patients with hip fractures, the greatest barriers to pain relief were difficulty contacting physicians and difficulty communicating with them about the type and/or dose of analgesic. Davis et al. (2002) looked at barriers to managing chronic pain from the perspective of the older person with arthritis, using focus groups. They identified nine themes: (1) personal decision-making about pain management; (2) pain and

---

Box 22.1   Ten principles of pain management for older people

1. Always ask older people about their pain
2. Acknowledge and accept what they say about their pain
3. Chronic pain can have a marked effect on quality of life and the ability to do everyday things
4. Always document pain assessment
5. Don't wait for a diagnosis to relieve suffering
6. Use drug and non-drug approaches as appropriate
7. Involve patients in their treatment
8. Use analgesic drugs correctly. Start with a low dose and increase slowly, titrating to effect. Anticipate side-effects
9. Anticipate and attend to anxiety and depression
10. Evaluate the effectiveness of any intervention to ensure you maximize quality of life

Adapted from Ferrell (1991).

Box 22.2 Barriers to effective pain management

Barriers relating to the older person
- Worried about interrupting or annoying caregivers
- Belief that health care team members know about the pain and will do something if they think it is needed
- Hesitation to use technical equipment, such as a patient-controlled analgesia (PCA) pump
- Cognitive impairment (Closs 1994)

Barriers relating to the health care team
- Belief that opioids should be avoided in older people
- Belief that older people will tell you if they have pain
- Belief that older people feel less pain than younger people

Barriers relating to patient, family and health care team
- Fear of addiction
- Lack of understanding and acceptance that the patient has a right to pain management
- Belief that pain is to be expected in older people
- Fears of side-effects of analgesic drugs

Adapted from Pasero & McCaffery (1996).

---

movement cycle; (3) diversional activities; (4) age-related expectations; (5) relationships with health care providers; (6) knowledge deficits; (7) lack of access to health care or treatment; (8) emotional distress; and (9) use of adaptive resources.

Assessing pain

The first step towards offering effective pain control is knowing about a patient's pain. To do this you need to assess the pain, but this is not always easy.

Misconceptions

McCaffery & Beebe (1989) outline 10 areas of pain assessment where misconceptions may exist that hamper assessment by causing us to doubt the patient's pain. An outline of these misconceptions follows. The interested reader is referred to the original reference, where each misconception is discussed in detail.

1. The first misconception concerns who is the authority about the patient's pain. McCaffery's (1972) definition, 'Pain is whatever the experiencing person says it is, existing whenever he says it does', emphasizes that the patient or client should be believed. McCaffery states that this belief covers both verbal and non-verbal pain behaviours. It is the patient, not the health professional, who knows how much pain he or she has, as well as the effectiveness of any pain relief measures. Although we all probably make some inferences about pain, McCaffery emphasizes that we do not necessarily see the situation as the patient does. In my own study (Seers 1987), I found that nurses consistently rated patients' pain as less severe than did the patient. We should be aware of the inferences we do make. Davitz & Davitz (1981) studied the effects of patient characteristics on nurses' inferences of physical pain and psychological distress. They concluded that stereotyped beliefs about the experiences of others in pain were bound to obscure individual differences. A recent correlational study by Tait & Chibnall (2002) looked at older adult and nurse ratings of pain. They found, over a 7-day period, that nurse and patient ratings were uncorrelated and nurse ratings tended to underestimate pain. They concluded that a more systematic assessment of pain was needed.

2. The second misconception that can hamper pain assessment is a reliance on personal values or intuition to judge whether a person is lying about the pain. McCaffery & Beebe (1989) point out that, while we may use this in our social life, it is not a professional approach.

3. That pain is largely an emotional/psychological problem is the third misconception. However, reacting to pain with emotion does not mean the pain was caused by an emotional problem.

4. Lying about pain or malingering is regarded as common, whereas McCaffery & Beebe argue that this rarely happens and is thus a misconception. They emphasize the importance of avoiding inaccurate labelling of patients as malingerers.

5. The fifth misconception is that patients who get benefits because of their pain are not in as much pain as they claim. However, using pain to one's advantage is not the same as malingering and it is not always easy to assess what does and what does not constitute using pain for advantage.

6. Another misconception is concerned with pain of unknown cause; if there is no obvious physical cause for pain, the existence of pain may be doubted. McCaffery & Beebe correct this by stating that all pain is the result of both physical and mental events. The point is that, whatever the cause of pain, the person still feels the pain.

7. The idea that pain is accompanied by reliable physiological and/or behavioural signs which can verify the existence and severity of pain is a misconception because physiological signs such as an increase in blood pressure and pulse can quickly adapt. Behavioural cues, such as cries, moans, wincing, guarding and so on can be unreliable and might not be present in cases of milder pain (Stewart 1977). Moreover, lack of pain expression does not necessarily mean a lack of pain. Patients/clients may take pride in self-control and may minimize their expression of pain in order to be a 'good' patient. Jacox & Stewart (1973) found that 41% of the 31 surgical patients they studied said they would remain outwardly calm when in pain. McCaffery & Beebe also point out that sheer fatigue can reduce expressions of pain.

8. The predictability of duration and severity of pain in different people is the eighth misconception. There is not an invariant relationship between stimulus and perception of pain. There can be large variations between individuals after, for example, identical operations (Seers 1987). So, severity and duration of pain cannot be predicted with certainty.

9. The ninth misconception is that patients/clients should have a high tolerance of pain. But how much pain 'should' a patient tolerate? Pain tolerance can differ between individuals and in the same individual at different times. Since pain is subjective and unique, tolerance to pain is likely to follow a similar pattern. Health professionals may tend to encourage a high tolerance. This in turn can encourage the patient to reduce the expression of pain in order to conform to these expectations.

10. The final misconception is that if a patient obtains pain relief from a placebo this must mean that the pain is not real. However, McCaffery & Beebe point out that there is no evidence for this and that using a placebo in this way raises legal and ethical questions and may destroy the patient's trust in health professionals.

Once you have considered the misconceptions and barriers that may hamper pain assessment and have thought about your own feelings concerning pain and pain relief, it is important to work out how you are going to assess pain.

Suggestions for assessing pain

Purely physiological or behavioural cues can be misleading. These signs may suggest the patient/client is in pain, but it is important to verify these impressions with the person in pain. However, Weiner et al. (1996) questioned the use of self-report if patients had impaired cognitive or communication skills. They suggested observation as an alternative and compared self-ratings of pain to observation in 39 older people living in the community. They concluded that pain behaviour observation, especially during activities of daily living, was a valid tool for use with older people. Simons & Malabar (1995) also observed pain behaviours in older patients who could not respond verbally. However, although they concluded that a pain intervention changed pain behaviours to non-pain behaviours, the assessment of this change could have been made by the same person making the original assessment, introducing the possibility of bias.

McCaffery (1972) argues that patients in pain should be believed, so it makes sense to ask them about their pain when this is possible. To obtain a comprehensive picture of any person in pain, you need to ask several questions in order to examine different aspects of the pain experience. These might include:

- How does the patient describe the pain? For example, is it burning, stabbing, throbbing, sharp, aching and so on?
- When did the pain start? Is it recent, or has it been there for months or years? What does the patient feel causes the pain?
- How long does it last – is it intermittent or constant?
- Where is the pain? There may well be more than one painful area, even if you think the site is obvious. The site of the pain may vary. A body outline could be a useful tool here
- How intense or severe is the pain? A pain scale (Figs 22.1–22.3) could be useful
- Does anything make the pain better or worse?

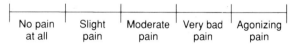

Fig. 22.1 Verbal rating scale.

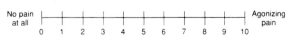

Fig. 22.2 Numerical rating scale.

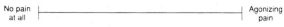

Fig. 22.3 Visual analogue scale.

- What impact does the pain have on the person's life? Does it affect activities of daily living such as mobility, concentration, sleeping, eating and socializing?
- How does the pain make the person feel? Anxious, depressed, angry?

Assessing pain is more than asking 'Any pain?' You need to sit down and discuss pain with the patient/client. You may not need to do a complete assessment of pain at every report of pain. McCaffery (1983) recommends that patients be asked to elaborate on any changes or difference in order to conserve time and energy, and to avoid an undue focus on pain.

Pain assessments should be documented, to provide a record which the patient and other health professionals can consult. How do you go about recording an assessment of pain? Pain history forms and pain charts can be useful tools. These scales or charts should be explained to patients to make sure they understand what you are asking them to do before they start to use them. Whenever possible, the patient rather than the nurse should complete the scale or chart, with help as necessary.

Allcock et al. (2002), in a questionnaire survey of 121 nursing homes with a 56% response rate, found that 37% of residents were identified as having chronic non-malignant pain. A pain assessment tool was not used in 75% of homes.

Pain scales

Verbal rating scale (Fig. 22.1) With this scale the patient is asked to make a cross on the line where the pain is now, and each category can be scored 0, 1, 2, 3 or 4 to give a pain score. The advantage of this scale is that it is easy to use and understand.

Numerical rating scale (Fig. 22.2) Again the patient marks on the line with a cross where the pain is, but other than the words at either end, there are numbers rather than words along the scale. This can be useful if patients feel they need a greater choice of categories than the verbal rating scale allows. The pain score can be taken either as the nearest number to the mark, or by measuring along the line from the left-hand side. Bourbonnais' (1981) pain scale incorporates elements of the verbal and numerical rating scales.

Visual analogue scale (Fig. 22.3) As with other scales, the patient marks on the line with a cross where the pain is now. The pain score is derived by measuring to the mark from the left-hand side. The drawback of this scale is that it can be difficult for patients to rate their pain on a line with no guideposts. Kremer et al.

(1981) found 11% of patients were unable to complete this scale, especially if they were old.

Some patients/clients have difficulty with these lines. Drawings of faces – usually eight faces from 'happy' to 'sad' – may be useful (Wong & Baker 1988: p. 11). With some patients it may only be possible to elicit whether pain is there or not there, or is bad or not too bad. It is important to be flexible and use a scale or chart that means something to the patient/client.

Herr & Mobily (1993) looked at the relationship between selected pain intensity measures, the ability to use the tools correctly and patient preferences in a group of 49 older people with leg pain who had responded to an advertisement. They found the highest failure rates with a visual analogue scale (8.2%) compared to 4.1% for a verbal descriptive scale. The older people preferred the verbal descriptive scale and found it easiest to complete. However, whether a group of people responding to an advertisement would respond similarly to those who did not is unknown. Gagliese & Katz (2003) argued that the reliability and validity of pain scales for the assessment of acute postoperative pain in older people remains to be demonstrated.

With all pain scales like these, the question of whether you can reduce the complex experience of pain to a single number on a scale is an issue for debate, but at least such scales are a start toward understanding the needs of the patient. Any of these scales could form the basis of a pain assessment chart.

Pain charts

There are several charts that can be used. A pain rating may be incorporated on to an observation chart as a numerical score. There may be a separate pain chart, which could include a rating scale, a body outline and space in which to note analgesics given, patient comments and nursing care given. This is especially useful if there is more than one pain.

- Sofaer's postoperative pain chart (adapted from the London Hospital chart; see Sofaer 1998: pp. 59, 60) is one example. A chart based on Sofaer's has also been used with orthopaedic patients by Davis (1988)
- A diary or home recording card can be used for patients/clients in the community (see McCaffery & Beebe 1989: p. 30).

In using these charts, it is important to return to the patient and evaluate the effect of any intervention.

An overview of some assessment tools has been presented. Matteson & McConnell (1988) point out that it is important to be familiar with a range of assessment methods, as choosing the right tool for the right person is the key to successful pain management. It is worth bearing in mind that a chart or scale is only a tool to help with assessment, planning and evaluating care. The information on it has to be used for it to make a contribution to the effective management of pain.

Special considerations with older people

Assessment tools and research examining special considerations for older people are lacking, as McCaffery & Beebe (1989) point out. So really we don't have much information at present which can help highlight specific tools or strategies that are appropriate specifically for older people. McCaffery & Beebe argue that active older people who have little or no memory or cognitive problems may be assessed in the same way as younger adults. If the patient/client has problems in communicating, or is confused or demented, then family and/or friends may be able to tell you the signs they use to tell them that their relative or friend is in pain. It is a particular challenge to assess pain with these patients/clients because we lack answers to many questions. McCaffery & Beebe argue that, based on your knowledge of physical pathology, on what other patients have experienced and on non-verbal cues, you can guess the patient's pain in these cases, but it is only a guess. They suggest that if self-reports of pain are unclear, a trial dose of analgesics, the effects of which are monitored, could be considered. Kaasalainen & Crook (2003) compared the faces pain scale, numerical pain scale and present pain intensity scale and a behavioural pain assessment scale in 130 older people in long-term care. They found reliability of the self-report tools decreased as cognitive impairment increased. Most of those with mild to moderate impairment could complete at least one of the scales. Closs et al. (2004) compared five pain assessment scales in 113 nursing-home residents with varying degrees of cognitive impairment. They found that the verbal rating scale was most successful, completed by 80.5% overall, and by 36% of those with severe cognitive impairment. Repeated explanation of the scales appeared to improve completion rates. It is more challenging to assess pain in people with severe dementia, but Manfredi et al. (2003) found clinical observations of facial expressions and vocalizations were an accurate means of assessing the presence of pain, but not its intensity. Other scales have been developed to assess pain in those with severe dementia, for example, that of Villanueva et al. (2003).

Weiner et al. (1999) developed a structured pain interview to complement a formal pain scale when assessing nursing-home residents, which included a pain map and also looked at aching and soreness as well as pain. They concluded there was considerable miscommunication about pain between residents and staff. Porter et al. (1996) looked at responses before, during and after venepuncture in 51 cognitively intact and 44 older people with dementia. They found that, independently of age, increasing severity of dementia was associated with blunting of physiological responses (it diminished the heart rate increase in the preparatory phase and heart rate increased with venepuncture, suggesting it had come as a surprise). It also interfered with the person's ability to respond to questions about anxiety and pain. Those who were able to respond gave relatively accurate self-assessments in that higher self-reported anxiety was associated with increases in heart rate. They concluded that dementia influenced both the experience and reporting of pain in older individuals. This conclusion has clinical implications as this group of people could be at risk of unidentified or inappropriately managed pain. Marzinski (1991) found that, of 60 patients with Alzheimer's disease, 26 had potentially painful conditions, yet only three received routinely ordered analgesics. However, she found it was difficult to identify pain behaviours in most of these 26 patients, so whether or not they were experiencing pain is unclear. Parmelee et al. (1993) found that pain complaints were reduced as cognitive impairment increased, suggesting cognitive status could interfere with pain reporting. Poor pain management may be a precursor of an acute decline in cognitive status; Duggleby & Lander (1994) found that mental status was reduced 1–2 days after total hip replacement in more than a third of patients, and the major predictor was pain, not analgesic intake.

Sight and hearing loss may cause problems. Ensure any eye glasses and hearing aids are to hand. The pain scales could be enlarged to enable them to be seen clearly. The verbal rating scale can be read out and a category chosen, or a number from 1 to 10 chosen if the patient/client has very poor or no sight. If hearing loss is a problem, as with all communication with that patient, sit so your face can be seen and don't rush. If the concentration span is short, try using a simple tool, like the faces scale or the verbal rating scale. For more information on communicating with older people with sight or hearing loss, see Chapters 12 and 11 respectively.

Planning/intervention

Is what you do about pain for older people any different from your approach with younger patients? For patients of all ages, basic considerations are very similar. When nursing care of a person in pain is planned, what is the aim of that care? Is complete relief or partial relief of pain the aim? Is the nurse's aim the same as the patient's? Davis, working to assess pain with patients in an orthopaedic ward, found the aim of using pain assessment charts was to control pain 'to a level acceptable to the patient' (Davis 1988: p. 326). The level acceptable to the patient should be reassessed regularly, as it can vary over time. What a person may be able to tolerate when there are the distractions of, for example, visitors, may be intolerable in the middle of the night when trying to sleep.

The plan should take into account usual methods of coping with pain. You may be able to help patients utilize and build on strategies that have worked in the past, as well as introducing them to new strategies.

Once pain has been assessed and the aim of pain relief decided, what are you going to do to achieve that aim? Pharmacological and/or non-pharmacological approaches may be used, and team work and good communication among all health professionals is important. The National Institutes of Health (1979) recommended a multidisciplinary approach to the treatment of pain in older people. Gibson et al. (1996) reviewed 14 studies of multidisciplinary management, 10 of which reported a benefit for older chronic pain patients. However, none of these studies used randomization or appropriate control groups in the evaluation of treatment efficacy, casting some doubt on the findings. Cutler et al. (1994) studied 153 patients aged 65+ and compared them with 317 who were less than 65 years old. They found as great an improvement in the older group as in other age groups in the majority of measures after treatment at a pain centre. They concluded that older people are good candidates for treatment in a pain centre setting. This supports Sorkin et al.'s (1990) conclusion that there are relatively few factors affecting pain based on age and that age should not be an important consideration when offering patients multidisciplinary treatment for chronic pain.

Pharmacological approaches

These can consist of analgesics and possibly antidepressants and anticonvulsants which are effective for some types of pain. A knowledge of onset and duration of drug action as well as of likely side-effects is important. This area has been reviewed by Popp & Portenoy (1996). When managing pain in older people, an awareness of their sensitivity to opiates and the margin between toxic and therapeutic doses of NSAIDs should be part of planning and evaluating care. Closs (1996) found that many nurses

had misconceptions about the pharmacological treatment of pain.

Kwentus et al. (1985) described older people as more sensitive to the pain relief effects of narcotics due to alterations in receptors, changes in plasma protein and prolonged renal clearance. They are thus more likely to develop narcotic side-effects such as a reduction in respiration rate, suppression of coughing, changes in level of consciousness and constipation. The studies in this area appear to corroborate this statement. Kaiko (1980), in a study involving 947 postoperative cancer patients, found that after intramuscular morphine, older patients (aged 70–89 years) obtained more pain relief for longer than did younger patients (aged 18–29 years). Whereas half the older group no longer obtained pain relief 5 h after the injection, half the younger group no longer obtained pain relief 3 h later. This supported the earlier work of Bellville et al. (1971), who found that older patients obtained more postoperative pain relief from intramuscular narcotics than did younger patients. They felt this was not purely the result of differences in absorption, distribution, metabolism and elimination of the drug, as the sedative side-effect did not correlate with age. In a study of 200 postoperative patients, Donovan (1983) found that dissatisfaction with pain relief was more common in younger than in older patients. Whether this was due to differences in pain threshold, pain tolerance or to the drugs being more effective or given more often to older patients is not known. Oberle et al. (1990) studied 41 patients aged 65+ and 249 aged less than 65 years. The older patients received fewer analgesics, but there were no significant differences in pain. They concluded that older people may require fewer analgesics for pain control.

Studies looking specifically at plasma level and excretion of narcotics in younger compared with older patients have tended to use small samples, and so results should be interpreted with caution.

Berkowitz et al. (1975) used intravenous morphine 10 mg/70 kg for 11 patients aged less than 50 years and for nine who were 50 years or older. In the older patients, serum morphine was increased compared with levels for the younger group at 2 and 5 min after administration, although it was only slightly elevated at 10 min. Berkowitz et al. suggested that the rapid entry of morphine to the brain after intravenous injection may explain why older people are sensitive to morphine, as initial serum levels are higher than in younger patients. Metabolism and excretion of pethidine were examined by Odar-Cederlof et al. (1985). They studied nine old (70–83 years) and seven young (18–29 years) patients. Pethidine 1 mg/kg was given intravenously. Excretion of the drug was similar in the two age groups, but its metabolism was slower in the older group because there was a slow disappearance of an active metabolite of pethidine from the plasma owing to slower renal clearance of this metabolite. The authors concluded that the presence of pharmacologically active metabolites will increase and prolong the response to medication and possibly increase the risk of side-effects. Portenoy & Farkash (1988) argue that, when using opioid analgesics for older people, there is a combination of a diminished volume of distribution, a longer half-life and reduced clearance – leading to a high peak or a more prolonged plasma level after a dose. They report few data for NSAIDs, but suggest a similar phenomenon for at least some of these drugs. Kwentus et al. (1985) also state that the margin between toxic and therapeutic doses of NSAIDs in older people is reduced. However, Rochon et al. (1993) point out that older people are often omitted from randomized controlled trials of NSAIDs. From 1987 to 1990 10 000 patients were involved in 83 such trials, yet only 203 were over 65 and none was over 85 years of age. Bandolier (2004) reviews age-related changes in risk with NSAIDs.

It is thus necessary to be vigilant for side-effects from any of these drugs, and the differences in metabolism and clearance in older patients should be borne in mind when assessing appropriate dosages. McCaffery & Beebe (1989) argue that this does not mean that the potential side-effects of narcotics make them too dangerous to use to relieve pain in older patients: these drugs may be used safely if response to medication is carefully monitored and the pharmacokinetics are recognized. For further information on medication and older people, see Chapter 27.

Non-pharmacological approaches

Other techniques are available to complement pharmacological treatments for pain. Health professionals such as nurses, physiotherapists, occupational therapists, clinical psychologists and doctors, amongst others, may be able to provide advice with these techniques. Techniques include positioning, exercise, deep breathing, relaxation, distraction, imagery, heat/cold, massage, and transcutaneous electrical nerve stimulation (TENS). These techniques have been reviewed in detail by McCaffery (1983) and Ferrell (1996). They all involve helping the patient to cope with pain. Patients or clients may already use some of these techniques and the nurse can help the patient build on past successful coping strategies. These techniques can help patients to have some control over their pain. The importance of this control had been emphasized by Walker et al. (1989: p. 242), who argue that to cope with pain the patient has to 'gain or maintain control over it even though the pain itself may persist'.

The key to successful management of pain is to use a variety of techniques and to persist with them, as a technique may require practice and may not work to its full potential on the first attempt.

There is much to learn about whether and how people who have dementia can use some or all of these non-pharmacological approaches.

Evaluation

The effectiveness of any pain relief intervention should be evaluated with the patient whenever possible. If communication is problematic, changes in behaviour may suggest that pain has been reduced. Lekan-Rutledge (1988) emphasizes that you should ask yourself what advantage, if any, the patient has gained from the intervention to relieve discomfort. Good pain control can improve comfort, mobility and independence. This is important for all patients. Portenoy & Farkash (1988) emphasize that the goals of pain therapy to be evaluated include improved mood, normal sleep, reduction in isolation and better nutrition.

CONCLUSION

Pain relief is affected by the complexity of nurse–patient and nurse–nurse relationships as well as by workload and organizational setting (Fagerhaugh & Strauss 1977). Understanding the individual nature of pain and pain relief, making and recording thorough assessments and giving pain relief a high priority in care will go some way towards providing adequate pain relief.

Principles of care for patients in pain are similar for most adult age groups, but we lack a great deal of information about assessing and reducing the pain of older people. If nursing care is delivered that takes account of the patient as a person, the specific problems and pains that an older person may have will be included in this assessment, as they would for any patient/client. A thorough and systematic assessment and documentation of pain and its treatment can lead not only to the reduction of pain but also to an improved quality of life. This will go some way to building up our knowledge of older people in pain. As Liebeskind & Melzack (1987: p. 1) state: 'By any reasonable code, freedom from pain should be a basic human right, limited only by our knowledge to achieve it'.

Recommended reading

Ferrell BR, Ferrell BA (eds) 1996 Pain in the elderly. International Association for the Study of Pain Press, Seattle, pp 35–44.

This publication, produced by an International Association for the Study of Pain taskforce, is a useful collection of research and expert opinion synthesized by those with considerable expertise in the area. It covers a range of types of pain and ways of managing pain.

Gagliese L, Melzack R 1997 Chronic pain in elderly people. Pain 70: 3–14.

This useful review identifies commonly used assessment instruments and examines the efficacy of psychological pain management strategies.

Gibson SJ, Helme RD 1995 Age difference in pain perception and report: a review of physiological, psychological, laboratory and clinical studies. Pain Reviews 2: 111–137.

A wide-ranging and comprehensive review, with useful coverage of physiological changes associated with ageing and age-related changes in the reporting of pain.

Keefe FJ, Williams DA 1990 A comparison of coping strategies in chronic pain patients in different age groups. Journal of Gerontology 45: 161–165.

A study which examined coping strategies across age groups and concluded that there were few age-related differences in coping.

Lang Porter F, Malhortra KM, Wolf CM et al. 1996 Dementia and response to pain in the elderly. Pain 68: 413–421.

A study which concluded that dementia influenced both the experience and the reporting of pain in older individuals.

Walker JM 1994 Caring for elderly people with persistent pain in the community: a qualitative perspective on the attitudes of patients and nurses. Health and Social Care 2: 221–228.

A helpful insight into what it means to older people to have chronic pain and what they expect from nurses. The contrast between older people's perspective and that of the nurses is interesting.

References

Allcock N, McGarry J, Elkan R 2002 Management of pain in older people within the nursing home: a preliminary study. Health Social Care Community 10: 464–471

American Geriatrics Society 2002 The management of persistent pain in older persons. AGS panel of persistent pain in older persons. Journal of the American Geriatrics Society 50 (suppl. S): 205–224

Ardery G, Herr KA, Titler MG, Sorofman BA, Schmitt MB 2003 Assessing and managing acute pain in older adults: a research base to guide practice. MedSurg Nursing: the journal of adult health 12: 7–19

Aronow WS 1987 Prevalence of presenting symptoms of recognised acute myocardial infarction and unrecognised healed myocardial infarction in elderly patients. American Journal of Cardiology 60: 1182

Aronow WS 2003 Silent MI. Prevalence and prognosis in older patients diagnosed by routine electrocardiograms. Geriatrics 58:24–26, 36–38, 40

Baken D 1968 Disease, pain, sacrifice: toward a psychology of suffering. University of Chicago Press, Chicago

Bandolier 2004 NSAIDs and adverse events. Available online at: http://www.jr2.ox.ac.uk/bandolier/booth/painpag/nsae/nsae.html (accessed 12 March 2004)

Bayer AJ, Chadha JS, Farag RR, Pathy MSJ 1986 Changing presentation of myocardial infarction with increasing old age. Journal of the American Geriatrics Society 34: 263–266

Bellville JW, Forrest WH, Miller E, Brown BW 1971 Influences of age on pain relief from analgesics. Journal of the American Medical Association 217: 1835–1841

Benbow SJ, Cossins L, Bowsher D 1995 A comparison of young and elderly patients attending a regional pain centre. Pain Clinic 8: 323–332

Berkowitz BA, Ngai SH, Yang MD, Hempstead BS, Spector S 1975 The disposition of morphine in surgical patients. Clinical Pharmacology and Therapeutics 17: 629–635

Black DA 1987 Mental state and presentation of myocardial infarction in the elderly. Age and Ageing 16: 125–127

Blomqvist K 2003 Older people in persistent pain: nursing and paramedical staff perceptions and pain management. Journal of Advanced Nursing 41:575–584

Bourbonnais F 1981 Pain assessment: development of a tool for the nurse and patient. Journal of Advanced Nursing 6: 277–282

Bowling A, Browne PD 1991 Social networks, health, and emotional wellbeing among the oldest old in London. Journal of Gerontology 46: S20–S32

Brochet B, Michel P, Barberger-Gateau P, Dartigues JF, Henry P 1991 Pain in the elderly: an epidemiological study in south-western France. Pain Clinic 5: 73–79

Butler RN, Gastel B 1980 Care of the aged: perspectives on pain and discomfort. In: Ng LKY, Bonica JJ (eds) Pain, discomfort and humanitarian care. Elsevier, New York

Chakour MC, Gibson SJ, Bradbeer M, Helme RD 1996 The effect of age on A delta and C fibre thermal pain perception. Pain 64: 143–152

Clinch D, Banerjee AK, Ostick G 1984 Absence of abdominal pain in elderly patients with peptic ulcer. Age and Ageing 13: 120–123

Closs SJ 1994 Pain in elderly patients: a neglected phenomenon? Journal of Advanced Nursing 19: 1072–1081

Closs SJ 1996 Pain and elderly patients: a survey of nurses' knowledge and experiences. Journal of Advanced Nursing 23: 237–242

Closs SJ, Barr B, Briggs M, Cash K, Seers K 2004 A comparison of five pain assessment scales for nursing home residents with varying degrees of cognitive impairment. Journal of Pain and Symptom Management 27: 196–205

Cocchi A, Franceschini G, Inclazi RA et al. 1988 Clinicopathological correlations in the diagnosis of acute myocardial infarction in the elderly. Age and Ageing 17: 87–93

Cutler RB, Fishbain DA, Rosomoff RS, Rosomoff HL 1994 Outcomes in treatment of pain in geriatric and younger age groups. Archives of Physical Medicine and Rehabilitation 75: 457–464

Davis PS 1988 Changing nursing practice for more effective control of post operative pain through a staff initiated educational programme. Nurse Education Today 8: 325–331

Davis GC Hiemenz ML, White TL 2002 Barriers to managing chronic pain of older adults with arthritis. Journal of Nursing Scholarship 34:121–126

Davitz JR, Davitz LL 1981 Inferences of patients' pain and psychological distress. Studies of nursing behaviors. Springer, New York

Day JJ, Bayer AJ, Pathy MSJ, Chadha JS 1987 Acute myocardial infarction: diagnostic difficulties and outcome in advanced old age. Age and Ageing 16: 239–243

Dickenson AH 2002 Editorial I. Gate control theory of pain stands the test of time. British Journal of Anaesthesia 88: 755–757

Doan BD, Wadden NP 1989 Relationships between depressive symptoms and descriptors of chronic pain. Pain 36: 75–84

Donovan BD 1983 Patient attitudes to postoperative pain relief. Anaesthesia and Intensive Care 11: 125–129

Duggleby W, Lander J 1994 Cognitive status and postoperative pain: older adults. Journal of Pain and Symptom Management 9: 19–27

Eland JM 1988 Pain management and comfort. Journal of Gerontological Nursing 14: 10–15

Ersek M, Turner JA, McCurry SM, Gibbons L, Kraybill BM 2003 Efficacy of a self management group intervention for elderly persons with chronic pain. Clinical Journal of Pain 19:156–167

Fagerhaugh SY, Strauss A 1977 Politics of pain management: staff patient interaction. Addison-Wesley, California

Ferrell BA 1991 Pain management in elderly people. Journal of the American Geriatric Society 39: 64–73

Ferrell BR 1996 Patient education and nondrug interventions. In: Ferrell BR, Ferrell BA (eds) Pain in the elderly. International Association for the Study of Pain Press, Seattle, pp 35–44

Ferrell BR, Ferrell BA (eds) 1996 Pain in the elderly. Taskforce on pain in the elderly. International Association for the Study of Pain Press, Seattle

Fordyce WE 1978 Learning processes in pain. In: Sternbach RA (ed) The psychology of pain. Raven Press, New York

Fox PL, Raina P, Jadad AR 1999 Prevalence and treatment of pain on older adults in nursing homes and other long-term care institutions: a systematic review. Canadian Medical Association Journal 160(3):329–333

Gagliese L, Katz J 2003 Age differences in postoperative pain are scale dependent: a comparison of measures of pain intensity and quality in younger and older surgical patients. Pain 103: 11–20

Ghose K (ed) 1987 Pain and the elderly. In: Ghose K (ed) Drug management of pain in the elderly. MTP Press, Lancaster

Gibson SJ, Helme RD 1995 Age differences in pain perception and report: a review of physiological, psychological, laboratory and clinical studies. Pain Reviews 2: 111–137

Gibson SJ, Helme RD 2000 Cognitive factors and the experience of pain and suffering in older persons. Pain 85: 375–383

Gibson SJ, Katz B, Corran TM, Farrell MJ, Helme RD 1994 Pain in older persons. Disability and Rehabilitation 16: 127–139

Gibson SJ, Farrell MJ, Katz B, Helme RD 1996 Multidisciplinary management of chronic non-malignant pain in older adults. In: Ferrell BR, Ferrell BA (eds) Pain in the elderly. International Association for the Study of Pain Press, Seattle, pp 91–99

Hall-Lord ML, Larsson G, Bostrom I 1994 Elderly patients' experiences of pain and distress in intensive care: a grounded theory study. Intensive and Critical Care Nursing 10: 133–141

Harkins SW, Chapman CR 1976 Detection and decision factors in pain perception in young and elderly men. Pain 2: 253–264

Harkins SW, Chapman CR 1977 The perception of induced dental pain in young and elderly women. Journal of Gerontology 32: 428–435

Harkins SW, Kwentus J, Price DD 1984 Pain and the elderly. In: Benedetti C, Chapman CR, Moricca G (eds) Advances in pain research and therapy, vol 7. Recent advances in the management of pain. Raven Press, New York

Harkins SW, Price DD, Bush FM, Small RE 1994 Geriatric pain. In: Wall PD, Melzack R (eds) Textbook of pain, 3rd edn. Churchill Livingstone, Edinburgh, pp 769–784

Herr KA, Mobily PR 1993 Comparison of selected pain assessment tools for use with the elderly. Applied Nursing Research 6: 39–46

Illich I 1977 Limits to medicine. Medical nemesis: the expropriation of health. Pelican, London

International Association for the Study of Pain Subcommittee on Taxonomy 1986 Pain terms: a current list with definitions and notes on usage. Pain 27: S220–S221

Jacox A, Stewart M 1973 Psychosocial contingencies of the pain experience. University of Iowa, Iowa

Jakobsson U, Klevsgard R, Westergren A, Hallberg IR 2003 Older people in pain: a comparative study. Journal of Pain and Symptom Management 26: 625–636

Kaasalainen S, Crook J 2003 A comparison of pain-assessment tools for use with elderly long-term-care residents. Canadian Journal of Nursing Research 35(4): 59–71

Kaiko RF 1980 Age and morphine analgesia in cancer patients with postoperative pain. Clinical Pharmacology and Therapeutics 28: 823–826

Keefe FJ, Williams DA 1990 A comparison of coping strategies in chronic pain patients in different age groups. Journal of Gerontology 45: P161–P165

Konu V 1977 Myocardial infarction in the elderly: a clinical and epidemiological study with one year follow-up. Acta Medica Scandinavica Supplement 604: 7–68

Kramlinger KG, Swanson DW, Maruta T 1983 Are patients with chronic pain depressed? American Journal of Psychiatry 140: 747–749

Kremer E, Atkinson JH, Ignelzi RJ 1981 Measurement of pain: patient preference does not confound pain measurement. Pain 10: 241–248

Kwentus JA, Harkins SW, Lignon N, Silverman JJ 1985 Concepts of geriatric pain and its treatment. Geriatrics 40: 48–57

Lekan-Rutledge D 1988 Gerontological nursing in long term care facilities. In: Matteson MA, McConnell ES (eds) Gerontological nursing: concepts and practice. WB Saunders, Philadelphia

Liebeskind JC, Melzack R 1987 The International Pain Foundation: meeting a need for education in pain management (editorial). Pain 30: 1–2

Lin EH, Katon W, vonKorff M et al. 2003 Effect of improving depression care on pain and functional outcomes among older adults with arthritis: a randomised controlled trial. Journal of the American Medical Association 290: 2428–2429

MacDonald JB 1984 Presentation of acute myocardial infarction in the elderly – a review. Age and Ageing 13: 196–200

MacDonald JB, Baille J, Williams BO, Ballantyne D 1983 Coronary care in the elderly. Age and Ageing 12: 17–20

Manfredi PL, Breuer B, Meier DE, Libow L 2003 Pain assessment in elderly patients with severe dementia. Journal of Pain and Symptom Management 25: 48–52

Marzinski LR 1991 The tragedy of dementia: clinically assessing pain in the confused, nonverbal elderly. Journal of Gerontological Nursing 17: 25–28

Matteson MA, McConnell ES 1988 Geronotological nursing: concepts and practice. WB Saunders, Philadelphia

McCaffery M 1972 Nursing management of the patient with pain. Lippincott, Philadelphia

McCaffery M 1983 Nursing the patient in pain. Lippincott nursing series. Adapted for the UK by B Sofaer. Harper & Row, London

McCaffery M, Beebe A 1989 Pain. Clinical manual for nursing practice. Mosby, St Louis

McCallion J, Canning GP, Knight PV, McCallion JS 1987 Acute appendicitis in the elderly: a 5 year retrospective study. Age and Ageing 16: 256–260

McDonald DD, Freeland M, Thomas G, Moore J 2001 Testing a preoperative pain management intervention for elders. Research in Nursing and Health 24: 402–409

McKenzie GJ 1985 Pain. In: Cormack DF (ed) Geriatric nursing: a conceptual approach. Blackwell Scientific, Oxford

Melding PS 1995 How do older people respond to chronic pain? A review of coping with pain and illness in elders. Pain Reviews 2: 65–75

Melzack R, Casey KL 1968 Sensory, motivational, and central control determinants of pain: a new conceptual model. In: Kenshalo DR (ed) The skin senses. Thomas, Springfield

Melzack R, Wall PD 1965 Pain mechanisms: a new theory. Science 150: 971–979

Melzack R, Wall PD 1988 The challenge of pain, 2nd edn. Penguin, London

Miller C, Le Lieuvre RB 1982 A method to reduce chronic pain in elderly nursing home residents. Gerontologist 22: 314–317

Mobily PR, Herr KA, Clark MK, Wallace RB 1994 An epidemiologic analysis of pain in the elderly. Journal of Aging and Health 6: 139–154

Moore JT, Whanger AD 1983 Functional psychiatric disorders. In: Cape RDT, Coe RM, Rossman I (eds) Fundamentals of geriatric medicine. Raven Press, New York

National Institutes of Health 1979 Pain in the elderly: patterns change with age. Journal of the American Medical Association 241: 2491–2492

National Institutes of Health Consensus Development Conference 1987 The integrated approach to the management of pain. Journal of Pain and Symptom Management 2: 35–44

Oberle K, Paul P, Wry J, Grace M 1990 Pain, anxiety and analgesics: a comparative study of elderly and younger surgical patients. Canadian Journal of Aging 9: 13–22

Odar-Cederlof I, Boreus LO, Bondesson U, Holmberg L, Heyner L 1985 Comparison of renal excretion of pethidine (meperidine) and its metabolities in old and young patients. European Journal of Clinical Pharmacology 28: 171–175

Parmelee PA, Smith B, Katz IR 1993 Pain complaints and cognitive status among elderly institution residents. Journal of the American Geriatric Society 41: 517–522

Pasero C, McCaffery M 1996 Postoperative pain management in the elderly. In: Ferrell BR, Ferrell BA (eds) Pain in the elderly. International Association for the Study of Pain Press, Seattle, pp 45–68

Popp B, Portenoy RK 1996 Management of chronic pain in the elderly: pharmacology of opioids and other analgesic drugs. In: Ferrell BR, Ferrell BA (eds) Pain in the elderly. International Association for the Study of Pain Press, Seattle, pp 21–34

Portenoy RK, Farkash A 1988 Practical management of nonmalignant pain in the elderly. Geriatrics 43: 29–47

Porter FL, Malhorta KM, Woilf CM et al. 1996 Dementia and response to pain in the elderly. Pain 68: 413–421

Reid MC, Williams CS, Gill TM 2003 The relationship between psychological factors and disabling musculoskeletal pain in community dwelling older persons. Journal of the American Geriatric Society 51: 1092–1098

Rochon PA, Fortin PR, Dear KBG, Minaker KL, Chalmers TC 1993 Reporting of age data in clinical trials of arthritis. Archives of Internal Medicine 153: 243–248

Roy R, Thomas M, Cook A 1996 Social context of elderly chronic pain patients. In: Ferrell BR, Ferrell BA (eds) Pain in the elderly. International Association for the Study of Pain Press, Seattle, pp 111–117

Seers CJ 1987 Pain, anxiety and recovery in patients undergoing surgery. PhD thesis. University of London, London

Sengstaken EA, King SA 1993 The problems of pain and its detection among geriatric nursing home residents. Journal of the American Geriatrics Society 41: 541–544

Simons W, Malabar R 1995 Assessing pain in elderly patients who cannot respond verbally. Journal of Advanced Nursing 22: 663–669

Sloman R, Ahern M, Wright A, Brown L 2001 Nurses' knowledge of pain in the elderly. Journal of Pain and Symptom Management 21: 317–322

Sofaer B 1998 Pain: principles, practice and patients, 3rd edn. Stanley Thornes, Cheltenham

Sorkin BA, Rudy TE, Hanlon RB, Turk DC, Stieg RL 1990 Chronic pain in old and young patients: differences appear less important than similarities. Journal of Gerontology 45: P64–P68

Sternbach R 1987 Mastering pain: a twelve step regimen for mastering chronic pain. Arlington, London

Stewart ML 1977 Measurement of clinical pain. In: Jacox AK (ed) Pain: a source book for nurses and other health professionals. Little, Brown, Boston

Syrjala KL 1987 The measurement of pain. In: McGuire DB, Yarbro CH (eds) Cancer pain management. Grune & Stratton, Orlando

Tait RC, Chibnall JT 2002 Pain in older subacute care patients: associations with clinical status and treatment. Pain Medicine 3: 231–239

Telfer S, Fenyo G, Holt PR, De Dombal FT 1988 Acute abdominal pain in patients over 50 years of age. Scandinavian Journal of Gastroenterology 23: 47–50

Titler MG, Herr K, Schilling ML et al. 2003 Acute pain treatment for older adults hospitalised with hip fracture: current nursing practices and perceived barriers. Applied Nursing Research 16: 211–227

Tresch DD, Brady WJ, Aufderheide TP, Lawrence SW, Williams KJ 1996 Comparison of elderly and younger patients with out of hospital chest pain. Archives of Internal Medicine 156: 1089–1093

Turk DC, Okifuji A, Scharff L 1995 Chronic pain and depression: role of perceived impact and perceived control in different age cohorts. Pain 61: 93–101

Turner GH, Weiner DK 2002 Essential components of a medical student curriculum on chronic pain management in older adults: results of a modified Delphi process. Pain Medicine 3: 240–252

Villanueva MR, Smith TL, Erickson JS, Lee AC, Singer CM 2003 Pain assessment for the dementing elderly (PADE): reliability and validity of a new measure. Journal of the American Medical Directors Association 4: 1–8

Wachter-Shikora N, Perez S 1988 Unmasking pain. Geriatric Nursing 3: 392–393

Walker J 1989 The management of elderly patients with painful conditions. Nursing Times 85: 53

Walker J 1994 Caring for elderly people with persistent pain in the community: a qualitative perspective on the attitudes of patients and nurses. Health and Social Care 2: 221–228

Walker JM, Akinsanya JA, Davis BD, Marcer D 1989 The nursing management of pain in the community: a theoretical framework. Journal of Advanced Nursing 14: 240–247

Weiner D, Pieper C, McConnell E, Martinez S, Keefe F 1996 Pain measurement in elders with chronic low back pain: traditional and alternative approaches. Pain 67: 461–467

Weiner D, Peterson B, Ladd K, McConnell E, Keefe F 1999 Pain in nursing home residents: an exploration of prevalence, staff perspectives, and practical aspects of measurement. Clinical Journal of Pain 15: 92–101

Wells JCD 1989 If you prick them, do they not bleed? Geriatric Medicine 19: 65–70

Williamson GM, Schultz R 1995 Activity restriction mediates the association between pain and depressed affect: a study of younger and older adult cancer patients. Psychology and Aging 10: 369–378

Wong DL, Baker CM 1988 Pain in children: comparison of assessment scales. Pediatric Nursing 14: 9–17

Wroblewski M, Mikulowski P, Steen B 1986 Symptoms of myocardial infarction in old age: clinical case, retrospective and prospective studies. Age and Ageing 15: 99–104

Yates P, Dewar A, Fentiman B 1995 Pain: the views of elderly people living in long-term residential care settings. Journal of Advanced Nursing 21: 667–674

Zalon ML 1997 Pain in frail, elderly women after surgery. Image, Journal of Nursing Scholarship 29: 21–26

Chapter 23

Delirium (acute confusional states) in later life

Hamish Thomson and Ian J. Norman

INTRODUCTION

The word 'confusion' has been used in at least three ways in the medical and nursing literature: as a diagnosis, a syndrome and a description. As a diagnosis the term 'confusion' should be avoided (Lipowski 1992, Byrne 1994, 1997) because it is ambiguous (means different things to different people: Simpson 1984), and distinguishing between well-validated syndromes of global cognitive impairment, such as delirium and dementia, is both possible and important.

More commonly confusion has been used, as by Roberts & Caird (1990), to refer to a syndrome characterized by: degrees of disorientation in time, place and person; difficulty in concentrating; short-term memory loss; and decline in cognitive abilities. Inouye & Charpentier (1996: p. 853) defined an acute confusional state (ACS) as 'a transient state of cognitive impairment'. It is a syndrome manifested by simultaneous disturbances of consciousness, attention, perception, memory, thinking, orientation and psychomotor behaviour that develop abruptly and fluctuate diurnally. The primary deficit is one of attention.'

This use of confusion and ACS may be helpful during initial assessment of patients, for describing in simple terms a dominant problem but one for which a more detailed formulation may be difficult or premature and so potentially prejudicial – for instance, applying the label of dementia (implying irreversibility) or delirium (implying reversibility).

The third use of confusion is as a descriptive term, for example by Lishman (1987: p. 4) who defines it as 'thinking with less than accustomed clarity'. Confusion, in this sense, may be a feature of many syndromes affecting not just older people, the cause of which may be either organic or functional. Thus, 'confusional state' may refer simply to those syndromes in which 'confusion' (thinking with less than accustomed clarity) is a feature. When prefaced by the word 'acute', this implies that the confusional state has a sudden onset, and because of this the term 'acute confusional state' has become synonymous with 'delirium'. We note, though, that other syndromes, such as depression in old age (discussed in Chapter 25), might also be consistent with this description of an ACS, but we find that 'delirium' is the most consistent term used in current literature.

In the sections which follow, we consider: disease classification, the presentation and prevention of delirium, the prevalence and causes of delirium in late life, aspects of assessment, and principles of management of the older patient experiencing delirium in hospital.

DISEASE CLASSIFICATION

One of the problems in this area is the plethora of terms which are used interchangeably with ACS, including acute brain failure, acute organic brain syndrome, acute organic psychosis and postoperative psychosis (Meagher 2001a). To avoid terminological confusion, Byrne (1997) advises reference to current nosological (disease classification) systems, which provide precise descriptions of changes in mental state consistent with different syndromes. Following Byrne, this chapter discusses delirium as defined in DSM-IV (American Psychiatric Association 1997) and ICD-10 (World Health Organization 1992); at the time of writing the World Health Organization has yet to publish the revised ICD-11. Chapter 24 discusses confusional states with gradual onset and prolonged course, which is almost always due to the dementia syndrome of various aetiologies.

Cole et al. (2003) compared the sensitivity and specificity of DSM-IV criteria for delirium with the sensitivity and specificity of DSM-III and ICD-10 criteria among older medical inpatients with or without dementia in Canada. They also examined the effect of changing the definition of criterion A, on sensitivity and specificity and compared the sensitivity and specificity of different numbers of symptoms of delirium. A total of 322 older patients who had been admitted as emergencies to medical areas were classified into one of four groups using DSM-III-R criteria: delirium and dementia ($n = 128$), delirium only ($n = 40$), dementia only ($n = 94$) and neither ($n = 60$). The sensitivity and specificity of DSM-IV, DSM-III, and ICD-10 criteria were compared against DSM-III-R criteria using three

definitions of criterion A (clouding of consciousness only, clouding of consciousness and inattention, clouding of consciousness or inattention). When criterion A was defined as clouding of consciousness or inattention, the sensitivity and specificity of DSM-IV, DSM-III and ICD-10 criteria were 100% and 71%, 96% and 91%, and 61% and 91%, respectively. The results were similar among patients with or without dementia. The lower specificity of DSM-IV was accounted for by its inclusion of patients who did not show disorganized thinking. They concluded that DSM-IV criteria for delirium are the most inclusive criteria to date for older medical patients with or without dementia.

PRESENTATION OF DELIRIUM IN LATE LIFE

The key features of delirium are captured in the following definition from Lipowski (1990: p. 490): 'a transient organic mental syndrome of acute onset and featuring concurrent disturbance of consciousness, a global cognitive and attention disorder, reduced or increased psychomotor activity and a disrupted sleep–wake cycle'. This definition reflects the diagnostic criteria for delirium listed in DSM-IV (American Psychiatric Association 1997) and ICD-10 (World Health Organization 1992). The clinical features of delirium derived from DSM-IV and ICD-10 criteria are summarized below. Presenting features of delirium may include the following (Byrne 1997):

- acute onset over several hours or a few days
- fluctuating course: symptoms vary within the day, from day to day and are often worse at night
- reduced attention, showing an inability to concentrate or to switch attention appropriately, or being easily distracted
- perceptual abnormalities, typically manifesting as misinterpretations, illusions or hallucinations
- impaired memory, particularly reduced recall of recent events, lesser impairment of remote memory and a reduced capacity for new learning
- disorientation, often of time and place, but rarely for person
- disorganized thinking, displayed as reduced comprehension, rambling or irrelevant speech, often appearing to be perplexed
- altered sleep–wake cycle, sleep reversal, daytime drowsiness, insomnia and vivid dreams/nightmares, often very disturbing for relatives
- altered mood, fluctuating between anxiety, depression, euphoria, apathy, irritability and fearfulness

- altered psychomotor activity, can be hypoactive or hyperactive, or swinging between the two, with noticeably increased reaction time.

Acute onset and course

In older people the onset of delirium may often be missed and so information on its time course may be limited (Byrne 1994). Many patients, possibly as high as 81%, however, do exhibit a prodromal phase (an early symptom indicating the onset of a disease or illness) lasting a few hours or up to 2–3 days, during which they experience a change in their cognitive functioning and usual behaviour (Morse & Litin 1969). Prodromal symptoms derived from Lipowski (1990) include: difficulty in concentrating, difficulty in thinking, disturbed sleep with vivid dreams or nightmares, drowsiness, insomnia, increased sensitivity to light and noise, restlessness, irritability and anxiety, tiredness and fatigue, and perceptual abnormalities including hallucinations and illusions (Lipowski 1990).

Research studies have indicated the mean duration of delirium in patients over 65 years to range between 19 and 21 days (Thomas et al. 1988, Koponen & Riekkinen 1993). Byrne's (1994) clinical experience leads her to suggest that patients with previously intact cognitive function and good health are likely to experience delirium of shorter duration than those with pre-existing cognitive impairment and poor health; but this impression requires confirmation. There is evidence, though, that patients with pre-existing poor health are more likely to suffer further cognitive decline on recovery from the initial episode (Koponen & Riekkinen 1993).

A careful history, usually obtained from relatives or friends, should elicit information about features of the prodromal syndrome, which are often more marked at night. Relatives may also describe fluctuations in the symptoms over time and periods of relative lucidity. Some patients do not progress beyond the prodromal stage; others may develop more severe symptoms, which are described below. Change is a key feature of delirium and so these features are not always present in one patient at any one time.

Disorder of attention

Patients may seem awake but find concentration difficult and are easily distracted. In part this is a consequence of drowsiness, but even when alert the patient's mind tends to lack focus. They may drift in and out of awareness of their surroundings, and communication may be fragmented and disrupted. Byrne (1994) points out that it is as if the patient's cognitive filtering mechanism, which we all use to prevent ourselves from being bombarded with extraneous stimuli, has broken down. When concentrating on work, for instance, we are able to ignore the sounds of the workplace until someone calls our name; then we are immediately alert and we are able to make a considered response. Patients experiencing delirium have lost the capacity to do this. They suffer from deficit selective attention; that is, they cannot separate out incoming stimuli that are relevant from those that are not, nor can they respond to relevant stimuli in a considered way, either automatically or through voluntary effort. Nursing interventions, which clearly seek to limit incoming extraneous stimuli and orient patients to those that are relevant to them, may be seen as one way of seeking to compensate for patients' faulty filtering processes.

The phrase 'clouding of consciousness' can be used to describe the patient experiencing delirium who slips back and forth from sleep to alertness and exhibits altered mental activity. However, disturbance or clouding of consciousness has become less prominent as a diagnostic feature of delirium over the years. This may be because of the difficulties of definition and objective measurement; it is relatively easy to define and assess disordered consciousness in patients experiencing delirium who are active but not in those who sit or lie quietly and are out of touch with their surroundings (Byrne 1997). More important diagnostically than clouding of consciousness is disordered attention, which is now required for a diagnosis of delirium under DSM-IV. Patients with disordered attention have difficulty attending to a conversation or questions, or shifting the focus of their attention appropriately. Perseveration may occur, where the patient repeats or prolongs an action, thought or utterance after the stimulus that prompted it has ceased.

Global cognitive impairment

Patients experiencing delirium may find it difficult to process information due to problems of perception, memory, orientation and thinking.

Perceptual abnormalities

These range from illusions, which cannot be corrected (as when a patient mistakes a dressing gown hanging behind the door for an intruder and is unable to reinterpret what is seen) to full-blown hallucinations, which are most commonly visual or auditory. As the day draws on and night-time falls, perceptual difficulties may be exacerbated by fatigue and reduced light levels.

Byrne (1994) reports that visual hallucinations occur in between 15% and 70% of cases of delirium and so are very common. She points out that visual hallucinations are unreliable diagnostically on their own and it is their presence together with other features of delirium that makes them significant.

Memory impairment

Recent memory is often impaired, as is remote memory, although to a lesser extent. Even when, in moments of lucidity, life events are recalled, they are often placed in the wrong time sequence. The capacity for new learning may also be reduced.

Disorientation

Patients may become disoriented sequentially in time, place, and, rarely, in person.

Disturbed thinking

Reduced comprehension may mean that information and ordinary events are misunderstood and patients may seem perplexed. Disturbed thought may lead to rambling, irrelevant or incoherent speech. Thoughts may have a dream-like quality, or may be impoverished or dominated by perceptual abnormalities (illusions and hallucinations) or delusional paranoid ideas.

Altered mood

This may be part of the prodrome or of the full-blown syndrome of delirium. Patients may be fearful or even terrified and show symptoms of physiological stress associated with increased sympathetic drive and catecholamine production, for example, increased heart rate, sweating palms, dry mouth and restlessness. Fear may be focused on real or psychotic events. Danger may be seen to lurk everywhere and patients may react with suspicion and aggressive outbursts.

Depression may occur and, if intense, may lead to suicide attempts. Unlike idiopathic depressive illness though, the depressed mood in delirium is rarely sustained over time. Bitter weeping on one occasion may be followed by apathy and lack of concern the next.

Altered activity

Increase or decrease in the speed of thought and movement is common in delirium. Some patients may exhibit episodes of both; others may be consistently under- or overactive. Byrne (1994) states that activity levels often mirror the other features of delirium. Thus patients who are experiencing florid hallucinations and delusions, often associated with fearful affect, are behaviourally overactive. While patients who are out of touch with their surroundings are often behaviourally underactive, overactive patients, particularly those in acute general hospital wards, demand attention and may be described by nurses rather vaguely as 'demanding', 'disturbed' or 'uncooperative'. In contrast, those who are underactive, sitting quietly and not drawing attention to themselves, may not be noticed and their delirium may remain undiagnosed.

Altered sleep–wake cycle

Daytime drowsiness and insomnia at night are common features of delirium and, in severe cases; there is a complete reversal of the normal pattern of daytime alertness and night-time sleep. Dreams are often vivid and may be followed by wakefulness with a dream-like quality.

PATHOPHYSIOLOGY OF DELIRIUM

The pathophysiology of delirium is still not fully understood. The main theory has been that the clinical syndrome of delirium arises from diffuse, reversible impairment of cerebral oxidative metabolism and neurotransmission (Lindesay et al. 1990, Lipowski 1990). Thus, delirium can result from interference by any drug or disease with neurotransmitter function or the supply or use of substrates for metabolism. This would explain the generalized slowing of the electroencephalogram (EEG) trace in most patients experiencing delirium and the stereotyped clinical picture in response to a range of underlying causes.

The characteristic symptoms of delirium that occur as a result of a wide diversity of causes could now be considered to support the concept of a 'final common pathway' (FCP). This may involve particular brain regions or circuits and certain neurotransmitters. Neuroanatomical data derived from neuroimaging and lesion reports suggest the importance of pathways in the prefrontal cortex, thalamus, fusiform cortex, posterior parietal cortex and basal ganglia (Trzepacz 2000). The neurotransmitters that are most implicated in delirium could mediate the characteristic symptoms of delirium, as well as producing the characteristic EEG changes; these are most likely to be acetylcholine and dopamine. Acetylcholine deficiency and dopamine excess, absolute and/or relative to each other, appear to be critical in the FCP. These neurotransmitters may affect each other, depending on the receptor subtype, and their receptor distribution among layers of cortex in areas such as the prefrontal cortex and temporal lobe, suggesting that cholinergic and dopaminergic neurons could interact with each other during delirium.

Van der Mast et al. (2000) examined the interrelationships between plasma levels of amino acids, physical condition as indicated by plasma cortisol, albumin and thyroid hormone concentrations, and postoperative delirium in 296 patients undergoing elective cardiac surgery. Both plasma tryptophan and the ratio of tryptophan to the other large neutral amino acids were reduced in patients experiencing delirium. The lower availability of tryptophan in the brains of patients experiencing delirium may lead to decreased serotonergic function. The ratio of phenylalanine to the other large neutral amino acids was increased, which may result in a higher synthesis of cerebral dopamine and noradrenaline (norepinephrine). These patients were also in poor physical condition, having decreased albumin levels and increased ratio of inactive reverse triiodothyronine (T_3) to active T_3. This suggests that decreased tryptophan and increased phenylalanine availability may give rise to the imbalance in cerebral neurotransmitters that is believed to contribute to delirium. Van der Mast (2000) also found large neutral amino acid changes associated with delirium in febrile older medical patients.

Zakriya et al. (2002) studied postoperative delirium following hip surgery in patients with no preoperative history. Their results suggest that preoperative medical conditions and an inability to mount a stress response (normal rather than raised white blood cell count) may influence the patient's postoperative mental status. In particular, two of the risk factors they identified that may be amenable to therapy were abnormal serum sodium and lack of an increase in white blood cell count during the stress of trauma and surgery.

Neurotransmitters

Acetylcholine was the first neurotransmitter to be identified (Marieb 2004). Deficiency of acetylcholine in the cerebral cortex may contribute to some of the behavioural, cognitive and memory changes seen in older people with Alzheimer's disease.

The biogenic amines include the catecholamines such as dopamine and the indolamines, which include serotonin. Dopamine (as well as adrenaline (epinephrine) and noradrenaline) are synthesized from the amino acid tyrosine. Serotonin is synthesized from the amino acid tryptophan. Increased levels of dopamine may be associated with hallucinations and psychotic episodes. Decreased levels of serotonin may affect sleep, appetite, nausea, headaches and regulation of mood; however, drugs which block its uptake such as Prozac are associated with the relief of anxiety and depression.

SUBTYPES

Two distinct subtypes of delirium can be recognized on the basis of the behaviour and alertness of the patient (Liptzin & Levkoff 1992). The agitated (hyperalert-hyperactive) variant of delirium (Lipowski 1990) is characterized by increased alertness to stimuli, psy-

chomotor hyperactivity and signs of overactivity of the sympathetic nervous system. Overactivity may be purposeless and repetitive. These patients may be observed picking constantly at their sheets or rolling their bedclothes into a ball. When approached or touched they may become startled, or be verbally or physically aggressive. They may wander, sleep very little and have insufficient rest, and this can lead to exhaustion.

Patients in quiet (or hypoalert-hypoactive) delirium are withdrawn and exhibit decreased responsiveness to stimuli. There is evidence that these patients are more severely cognitively impaired and remain longer in hospital than agitated patients experiencing delirium (Ross et al. 1991, Liptzin & Levkoff 1992). Some patients have a mixed psychomotor pattern, which changes unpredictably from lethargy to agitation.

Subacute confusional state is usually of the hypoalert-hypoactive type with a less acute onset and a less florid clinical picture.

Meagher et al. (2000) examined 46 patients with delirium who were consecutive referrals to a consultation-liaison psychiatry service. They examined the relationships between symptoms, as rated on the Delirium Rating Scale, and delirium motoric subtypes, as defined by Liptzin & Levkoff (1992). Most cases were of the mixed subtype (46%); 24% were hypoactive and 30% were hyperactive. Overall scores differed significantly among motoric subtype groups, being highest in the hyperactive, lowest in the hypoactive and intermediate in the mixed. On item scores, the hypoactive group scored lower than the hyperactive group for delusions, mood lability, sleep–wake cycle disturbances and variability of symptoms, but lower than the mixed group only for mood lability. Their results suggest that delirium presents as motoric subtypes that differ according to symptom profile and severity of delirium.

DIFFERENTIAL DIAGNOSIS

Identifying the underlying cause(s) of delirium is crucial because many cases are treated easily and failure to treat can significantly increase morbidity. Dementia is the main differential diagnosis. As discussed in Chapter 24, some dementias may have a rapid or relatively rapid onset (days to weeks, or weeks to a few months) and be of short duration (months to a year or two). But most dementias have a gradual onset over months or years. Marked impairment of consciousness or attention does not feature in most dementias, unlike delirium. However, delirium may often be superimposed on dementia, and dementia is a predisposing factor for delirium.

Mood disorders may also be mistaken for delirium, particularly hypomania and, rarely, severe depression which is, though, more likely to resemble dementia.

PREVALENCE IN OLDER PEOPLE

Prevalence, expressed as a percentage, refers to the number of people with a particular disorder within a given population. Most evidence for the prevalence of delirium in old age comes from hospital studies, which indicate that delirium occurs in about 15–30% of all general admissions to hospital (Trzepacz 1996); it occurs with higher frequency in older people and in those with pre-existing cognitive impairment (American Psychiatric Association 1999); 10–15% have delirium on admission and a further 10–40% develop delirium during the course of their hospital stay (Bucht et al. 1999, Fann 2000). Rates vary according to the population assessed, study setting and identification methods used, but overall, delirium is always more frequent in older populations (Meagher 2001b).

Delirium is especially common in older patients: this can be seen in high prevalence rates ranging from 14% to 56% of older hospitalized medical patients with an associated increase in morbidity and length of stay (Inouye & Charpentier 1996) and even higher prevalence rates if older surgical patients are included, particularly those with hip fractures, when rates of up to 61% have been found (Byrne 1994). However, more recently, Franco et al. (2001), in an investigation of postoperative delirium, found that, of 500 patients assessed, 57 (11.4%) developed delirium during the study.

Prevalence rates in older people living in residential care have received less attention from researchers, but Byrne (1994) quotes two North American studies (Rovner et al. 1986, Bienenfield & Wheeler 1989) which suggest a prevalence of about 6% in residential homes. Studies of older people living in their own homes are rare and show low prevalence; for example, Folstein et al. (1991) found only six cases of delirium in a sample of 810 individuals from Boston aged over 55 years, who were intensively screened. In all six cases delirium was associated with taking multiple medications.

We can draw three main conclusions from these surveys of delirium. Firstly, the resource implication: in the USA alone, the financial cost of delirium to health care has been estimated to be more than $4 billion (in 1994 dollars) per year (Inouye et al. 1999). Costs are also carried over into the community after discharge from hospital with the need for increased care of the confused patient in institutions, rehabilitation programmes or social care.

Secondly, patients experiencing delirium suffer significant morbidity and prolonged hospital stays and have a higher mortality rate than non-patients experiencing delirium. High mortality is probably due to the seriousness of associated illness(es) in most cases. Byrne (1994) reports that death follows delirium within 1 month for between 15% and 40% of cases and Inouye (1994) cites studies which indicate an even higher associated mortality rate, ranging between 10% and 65%.

Finally, delirium is underdiagnosed. Past studies suggested that between 32% and 67% of older patients experiencing delirium go unrecognized by doctors (Inouye 1994). There are several reasons for underdiagnosis, including: (1) ageism in health professionals (and society), which means that delirium is misattributed to the normal ageing process; (2) the often altered presentation of delirium in older people which goes against expectations (specifically, nurses and doctors expect delirium to present with agitation, hallucinations and agitated behaviour, whereas in older patients the hypoactive form of delirium may often present with lethargy and decreased activity and be frequently overlooked); (3) the fluctuating nature of delirium, which may lead clinicians to fail to appreciate lucid intervals as characteristic of the syndrome; and (4) overreliance on cross-sectional assessments of cognitive status, which do not highlight one of the most important features of delirium: changeability of the symptoms over time. Related to this we know from North American studies that cognitive function is often not formally assessed in routine medical examinations (McCarthy & Palmateer 1985) and, particularly in hospital, clinical staff have minimal knowledge about the previous cognitive status or the course of any cognitive changes (Inouye 1994).

CAUSES IN LATE LIFE

The pathway into delirium for many older people is likely to be complex and multifactorial, involving the interaction of precipitating factors superimposed on a vulnerable patient with predisposing conditions. This is perhaps especially true of hospitalized older patients, many of whom suffer from more than one medical condition. One study of delirium in this group of patients found more than one cause of delirium in 44% of the sample (Francis et al. 1990).

Inouye (1994) reviewed seven prospective studies that systematically examined predisposing or risk factors present at baseline for delirium in hospitalized older patients. There are disparities between the studies, but four common risk factors were identified:

1. advanced age
2. pre-existing underlying cognitive impairment
3. severe chronic illness
4. functional impairment.

Predisposing factors, in addition to those above, identified in relation to postoperative delirium in older people include (Whittaker 1989, O'Keefe & Ni Chonchubhair 1994):

- vitamin (especially thiamine) deficiency
- psychological factors (particularly depression, possibly due to treatment with drugs with anticholinergic activity and structural subcortical lesions)
- alcohol and benzodiazepine dependence
- prolonged surgical operations
- anticholinergic medications
- trauma (e.g. fat embolism caused by fractures of long bones, traumatic asphyxia, cerebral concussion and contusions, subdural haematoma).

Lipowski (1990) suggests four factors, which are likely to increase the severity or prolong the course of delirium in older people:

1. psychosocial stress
2. sleep deprivation
3. sensory underload or overload
4. immobilization.

Precipitating factors include many different diseases and metabolic imbalances. Common causes of delirium in older people are (Byrne 1994):

- cardiovascular disease (especially heart failure, i.e. left ventricular failure and congestive cardiac failure)
- infection (particularly urinary tract and respiratory infection)
- carcinomatosis
- transient ischaemia and the drugs of treatment
- almost any drug (particularly anticholinergic medications such as tricyclic antidepressants and benhexol, drug interactions, drug withdrawal)
- metabolic disorders (including hypoglycaemia, disorders of fluid and electrolyte imbalance and renal or hepatic failure)
- anoxia from whatever cause (including respiratory problems, anaemia, reduced cerebral perfusion).

Evidence for the role of some important factors is discussed below. For a more detailed review, refer to Liston (1982), Beresin (1988), MacDonald et al. (1989), Byrne (1994, 1997) and Meagher (2001a).

Advanced age is one of the most important predisposing factors for the development of delirium. Seymour & Pringle's (1983) study of postoperative confusion, for example, found that it was three times more common in patients aged 75 years and older than patients aged 65–75 years. The underlying mechanisms are unknown, but may include reduced cholinergic transmitters in normal ageing, impaired peripheral senses and a reduced capacity for homeostatic regulation in response to stresses such as surgery and anaesthesia. Age is also associated with increased prevalence of other risk factors, such as multiple disease states and degeneration of the central nervous system.

It has been estimated that up to two-thirds of cases of delirium are superimposed on dementia (Francis & Kapoor 1990). Some studies suggest that delirium in many hospitalized older patients may, in fact, be previously unrecognized dementia revealed by close observation in hospital or by an acute illness, but some researchers suggest that delirium itself may lead to chronic cognitive impairment (Francis & Kapoor 1990). Inouye (1994) highlights the complex relationship between dementia and delirium as a priority for research.

Medication is the most common reversible cause of delirium in older hospitalized patients (Moses & van Kaden 1986). Delirium can arise as a side-effect or a withdrawal effect and even quite small doses of some drugs may induce toxicity. Drugs with psychoactive side-effects, such as sedative-hypnotics, narcotics and drugs with anticholinergic side-effects, are most commonly associated with delirium. Other common drugs, which deserve special mention, include digitalis and its derivatives, which may be toxic in older people; also beta-blockers, non-steroidal anti-inflammatory drugs, some antibiotics (Inouye 1994), theophylline and warfarin (Tune et al. 1992).

A prospective study of a small sample of 78 older surgical patients by Platzer (1988) found that patients receiving glycopyrronium bromide, an anticholinergic drug that does not cross the blood–brain barrier, were less likely to become confused postoperatively than those receiving similar drugs which cross the blood–brain barrier, such as atropine and hyoscine. Platzer also found that most medical and nursing staff she spoke to were unaware that atropine could cause delirium in older patients and that glycopyrronium bromide was less likely to do so. Research to see how extensively atropine is still used for older surgical inpatients may highlight an area in which prevention of confusion is possible.

Iatrogenic causes of delirium associated with hospitalization suggested by research studies include sleep deprivation, unfamiliar environment, frequent room changes, lack of windows, pain, decreased mobility, and use of intravenous infusions or indwelling catheters (Inouye 1994). The role of these factors in delirium is uncertain, though, because most studies do not control for confounding factors, such as age and underlying illness. Overall, there has been only limited systematic study of psychosocial and environmental factors contributing to delirium in hospitalized older people, and inconsistent findings and small sample sizes do not allow definite conclusions to be drawn (Inouye 1994).

Studies of older patients with hip fracture (Gustafson et al. 1988) have found pre-existing cognitive impairment to be the most important predictor of delirium following surgery, and several studies have confirmed that cerebrovascular disease greatly increases the risk of developing delirium. This finding emphasizes that older people who have pre-existing cognitive impairment are particularly sensitive to changes in the homeostatic milieu of the brain caused by changes such as sensory impairment or deprivation, environmental changes, thermoregulation difficulties and metabolic abnormalities. These people are particularly prone to delirium when they develop a urinary tract or chest infection, for instance. They are also prone to aggravation of their cognitive impairment, so increasing their confusion, but without developing delirium.

Byrne (1997) points to the importance of distinguishing between delirium and an increase in pre-existing confusion so that management is appropriate. Factors identified by Byrne & Arie (1990), which may aggravate pre-existing cognitive impairment in older people, include:

- discomfort (e.g. pain, wetness, corns, constipation)
- environmental change (e.g. a move or holiday) or stress (e.g. excessive noise, extremes of temperature)
- sensory impairment (particularly impaired sight or hearing)
- alcohol, even in small amounts
- drug treatment (especially cholinergic agents)
- almost any physical illness
- psychological factors (e.g. anxiety, depression, anger, frustration, psychotic experiences, bereavement, insight into declining mental faculties).

ASSESSMENT

Assessment of older people is discussed in detail in Chapter 28. Here we highlight those aspects of assessment relevant to the diagnosis of delirium and the formulation of a comprehensive plan of care. Whether the assessment is carried out in hospital, at home or in a residential or nursing home, it is likely to involve more than one profession. Effective multidisciplinary working is therefore essential.

The diagnosis of delirium relies mainly on: knowledge of its key features; a careful history, especially of the onset and progression of the condition; examination of mental state through conversation with the patient and standard tests of cognition; a physical examination; and investigations. Byrne (1994) discusses history-taking and examination of older confused patients. Here we draw from her work in considering patient assessment.

History

Many people experiencing delirium are gravely ill and so diagnostic assessment will often take place in hospital. Wherever possible, though, there are great advantages to assessing patients in their own homes. Confusion and disorientation can be engendered through older people attending the hospital or health centre, so giving a falsely pessimistic picture of patients' mental functioning. In most cases a clear history cannot be obtained from the patient because of memory deficits, attention deficits or clouding of consciousness, and neighbours, friends or relatives are often the best informants.

Byrne (1994) suggests asking and pursuing three questions (Fig. 23.1):

1. How and when did the problem start? Was it related to a life event?
2. How did the problem progress?
   (a) Did it become gradually worse?
   (b) Did it fluctuate markedly? (within a day – worse in the morning/evening, from day to day or week to week) or
   (c) Did it worsen in a stepwise course?
3. How has the patient's physical health been?
   (a) previously well or ill?
   (b) past illnesses?
   (c) extent of alcohol and drug use (including smoking and prescribed and over-the-counter medication)?
   (d) experience of a recent trauma, or falls?

The answers to these questions will enable the assessor to make a likely syndrome diagnosis of delirium, depression or dementia. For example, if progress fluctuates markedly, and if the patient has previously been in good health, delirium is more likely than depression and either is more likely than dementia. Delirium and depression may overlay dementia. Further depression may occur with delirium because depression is often associated with physical illness. Byrne (1994) points out that her third question about the patient's previous health may clarify the coexistence of both syndromes.

Family history should establish the age and cause of death of family members and also family history of

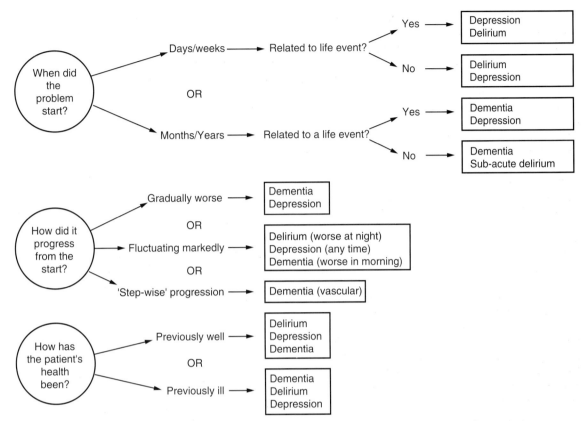

Fig. 23.1 Likely syndrome diagnosis indicated by three cognitive impairment questions. (After Byrne 1994.)

hypertension, stroke, dementia, depression and movement disorder.

Examination of mental status

Mental (and physical) status can be assessed through informal conversation with the patient and observation of gait, movement and physical signs. Anything the patient does or says may be a clinical sign of diagnostic significance; for Byrne (1994), this is an important principle of assessment.

Byrne (1994) highlights assessment of patients' abilities as being as important as their cognitive deficits. She gives the case of two older men, both of whom scored poorly on formal tests of mental status, but one of whom was able to live independently, whereas the other required round-the-clock care. The former was managing day-to-day living despite giving responses that were not quite right. The latter thought 'my mother will look after me' and his responses to questions on the test were wildly inaccurate.

Assessment of mental status involves examination of cognition, including:

- orientation (time, place, person). It is advisable to write down the patient's exact responses to all questions. This provides a baseline for future tests and assesses ability (i.e. orientation is higher for an individual whose response is out by 1 month in the year than someone whose response is out by 6 months). Also establish if the patient can use cues (e.g. by providing a list of years to choose from)
- memory (recent and remote)
- attention and concentration. These are best assessed through the process of taking a history
- grasp and judgement. The focus here is on patients' grasp of the reality of their situation inferred through their history, their attempts to manage their situation (e.g. being aware of cognitive failure and attempting to compensate for this by writing reminder notes) and information from key informants (neighbours, relatives)
- calculation. The 'serial-sevens test (counting backwards in sevens from 100, allowing 2 min and three errors) is useful as a test of perseveration and of the degree of cognitive slowing which may be

marked in severe depression, for example. Simplifying to 'serial-threes' (counting back in threes from 100) can be substituted in case of difficulty

- visual–spatial function. Byrne (1994, 1997) recommends the clock-drawing test of Schulman et al. (1986) as a simple bedside test of changing cognitive function. This test has been validated by its authors against standard instruments of cognitive function, and also evaluated on medical wards (Huntzinger et al. 1992). It involves asking patients to draw a clock within a predrawn circle and then to put in the hands (if they have not done so) to show a standard time. Simple scoring schemes have been devised and the test can be administered repeatedly to monitor cognitive change over time. Qualitative aspects of the test (e.g. how the patient approaches the task, carries it out and responds to it once completed) may also indicate the nature of the confusional state.

Screening instruments

Formal assessment of mental status is valuable but only within the context of the examination as a whole. Older people have a low tolerance for batteries of formal tests and such tests may produce similarly low scores for delirium, depression and dementia. Hence, they are best regarded as screening rather than diagnostic instruments (although some diagnostic tests of delirium have been developed). Repetition of the test is recommended if there is any doubt and, even when there is no doubt, repeated testing may illuminate fluctuation, which characterizes many confusional states.

Many brief cognitive tests are available to establish the patient's baseline status, for example: the Mini-Mental States Examination (MMSE) (Folstein et al. 1975), the Mental States Questionnaire (MSQ) (Kahn et al. 1960) and the Clifton Assessment Procedures for the Elderly (CAPE) (Pattie & Gilleard 1975).

Inouye (1994) cited 18 published instruments specifically designed or used for the diagnosis of delirium, but states that only two – the Confusion Assessment Method (CAM) (Inouye et al. 1990) and the Delirium Rating Scale (DRS) (Trzepacz et al. 1988) – fulfil four essential criteria for usefulness: (1) validated specifically for use in delirium; (2) capable of distinguishing delirium from dementia; (3) able to assess multiple features of delirium; and (4) feasible for use with patients experiencing delirium. In further work, Trzepacz et al. (2001) compared the DRS-R-98, (the 1998 revision, including a 16-item clinician-rated scale with 13 severity items and three diagnostic items), with the Cognitive Test for Delirium (CTD), Clinical Global Impression (CGI) scale, and DRS using five diagnostic groups ($n = 68$): (1) delirium; (2) dementia;

(3) depression; (4) schizophrenia; and (5) other. DRS-R-98 scores successfully distinguished delirium from each of the other diagnostic groups. DRS-R-98 total scores correlated highly with DRS, CTD and CGI scores. Interrater reliability and internal consistency were very high. The researchers concluded that the DRS-R-98 is a valid measure of delirium severity over a broad range of symptoms and is a useful diagnostic and assessment tool.

Such instruments are valuable as a means of standardizing and recording observations, but they require further testing on larger samples and are no substitute for clinical acumen. One of the most important features of delirium is the changeability of the symptoms, and because of this, both rating scales require observations over time.

Examination of physical status

Physical status examination focusing on any conditions which may be aetiologically significant is important for all patients with a suspected confusional state. Neurological examination is particularly important; readers are referred to Godwin-Austen & Bendall (1990) for details.

Investigations

Routine investigations for identifying people experiencing delirium include:

- full blood count
- erythrocyte sedimentation rate
- electroencephalography
- blood chemistry – calcium, electrolytes
- thyroid function tests
- urea and creatinine
- serology for syphilis.

Other investigations may be indicated by the previous medical history and the results of these initial tests. Which patients should undergo cerebrospinal fluid examination or brain imaging are areas for debate. Inouye (1994) concludes that cerebrospinal fluid examination should be prescribed for febrile patients experiencing delirium in whom meningitis is suspected but its benefits are less certain with afebrile patients, even when no other organic cause of delirium can be found. The value of brain imaging (such as computed tomography or magnetic resonance imaging) remains uncertain, and may be most useful for patients with new focal neurological signs, history or signs of head trauma or those in whom another cause cannot be identified.

PRINCIPLES OF CARE AND TREATMENT

Successful management of the delirious older patient requires prompt investigation and diagnosis, treatment of the underlying cause and supportive measures. In this section we focus on supportive measures, which are, in the main, the province of skilled nursing care.

Physiological care

Many patients experiencing delirium will be gravely ill. They may be unable to attend to their own physiological needs because of disorientation and agitation, and the highest priority should be given to supportive measures designed to maintain life. In the UK, patients with delirium may give informed consent during lucid periods, but for patients deemed incompetent, urgent interventions are governed by common-law doctrine, that is, interventions may be made without informed consent if medical colleagues would generally consider it appropriate and a reasonable person would want it. The competitive benzodiazepine antagonist flumazenil has been used to restore mental capacity temporarily in patients with delirium and hepatic failure to allow them to participate in decisions about treatment or personal affairs (Bostwick & Masterson 1998).

Inadequate sleep and rest may exacerbate delirium. Sedation is a double-edged sword. In cases in which the diagnosis has not been established, sedatives may mask the symptoms and so ideally should not be prescribed. Also, it is easy to oversedate and sedatives may prolong delirium, particularly for patients who fluctuate between agitation and lethargy (Lichtigfeld & Gillman 1990). For agitated and hallucinating patients for whom sedation is necessary, haloperidol has been the drug of choice (Lipowski 1990, Taylor & Lewis 1993). Low doses (0.5 mg twice or three times in 24 h) will produce a good effect in some patients; others may require more. Hypnotics are best avoided. Clomethiazole can be helpful if sleep is disrupted (Byrne 1997).

Olanzapine may also be useful in the treatment of delirium in younger adults. Breitbart et al. (2002b) looked at a sample of 79 hospitalized cancer patients. These patients all met DSM-IV criteria for a diagnosis of delirium. Fifty-seven patients (76%) had complete resolution of their delirium on olanzapine therapy. No patients developed extrapyramidal side-effects, though 30% experienced sedation (usually not severe enough to interrupt treatment). Several factors were found to be significantly associated with poorer response to olanzapine treatment for delirium, including age over 70 years, history of dementia, central nervous system spread of cancer and hypoxia. The authors concluded that age over 70 years is the most powerful predictor of poor response to olanzapine treatment for delirium. Olanzapine appears to be a clinically safe drug for the treatment of the symptoms of delirium in the hospitalized medically ill up to the age of 70 years.

Patients' sleep patterns during the day should be recorded and also the quality of their sleep and effectiveness of medications. Sleep, especially at night, should be interrupted as little as possible by timing clinical observations, medication and other nursing interventions at the beginning and end of the nighttime shift.

Patients with anorexia require help and encouragement to take a light nutritious diet; liquid nutritional supplements can be useful in such situations. To avoid dehydration – particularly a problem for hyperalert-hyperactive patients – they should be offered small drinks frequently; these patients may not easily tolerate intravenous infusions. Although there is no evidence that B-complex vitamins shorten the duration or severity of delirium, multivitamin supplements should probably be added to the nutritional and fluid regimen of all patients experiencing delirium (Delaney & Goldfrank 1987).

Disturbances of cholinergic metabolism are implicated in cases in which delirium is caused by hypoxia, traumatic brain injury or hypoglycaemia or is drug-related. Anticholinergic delirium is generally treated conservatively by withdrawing the offending agent and occasionally by administering physostigmine (American Psychiatric Association 1999). Other procholinergic agents used to counter cholinergic deficits in dementia have theoretical potential but are not recommended owing to the risk of causing adverse effects. Current smoking has been identified as a possible protective factor against delirium (Culp et al. 1997) but the usefulness of nicotine replacement treatment in protecting against delirium has not been tested (Meagher 2001a). Trazodone and mianserin are antidepressant compounds that share antagonistic actions at 5-hydroxytryptamine (serotonin) receptor sites. Studies of low-dose treatment of delirium with these compounds have found a rapid reduction of non-cognitive symptoms in particular. This effect is independent of the mood-altering actions of the drugs (Okamoto et al. 1999). Other reports have advocated the use of light therapy, but the usefulness of this treatment needs to be more fully evaluated before it is used routinely (Meagher 2001a).

Environmental measures

The physical and social environment for patients experiencing delirium has been little researched, although there is some evidence of benefits (Tesar & Stern 1986, Richeimer 1987). Thus most of the nursing interventions described below are based on clinical experience. If they are to be beneficial, environmental measures should relate to the core features of the delirium syndrome. Thus, for example, hyperalert-hyperactive patients may require a quieter environment than patients who are less aroused and may be able to tolerate more stimulation. The factors specified earlier in this chapter, which may aggravate pre-existing cognitive impairment, also demand attention.

Physical environment

Most hospitalized patients suffering from acute delirium are probably best nursed in single rooms where possible, which are kept reasonably quiet and in which the environment can be kept constant to ensure familiarity. Since darkness is likely to increase confusion it is often recommended that patients experiencing delirium are nursed in a well-lit room (Lipowski 1990), but there is no evidence to support this and it may be better to retain the semblance of the day–night cycle by dimming lights at night. Windows in a room will also help to maintain the day–night cycle. Some clinicians suggest that lighting be concealed to promote rest. Rooms should also contain orientation cues such as clocks, calendars, familiar objects and personal photographs.

Patients should be encouraged to wear their customary spectacles and hearing aids to support sensory perception and reduce the possibility of paranoid ideas. Background noise from the radio, television and conversations are best kept to a minimum, as this constitutes random stimuli, which present a challenge to patients' faulty cognitive filtering processes and so may exacerbate their confusion.

Restlessness and wandering require investigation and may sometimes be reduced by measures to relieve pain or constipation, for example. Ensuring safety is an important goal of care. Patients who do wander require close observation within a safe and reasonably enclosed environment. However, restrictions should be kept to a minimum since they are likely to result in patients becoming frustrated and angry. Particularly if hallucinating, patients experiencing delirium can be unpredictable and may need to be protected from hurting themselves or others. Sensible safety precautions, such as securing the windows and removing unnecessary furniture, may be necessary, and occasionally one-to-one observation is required. Physical restraints are inhumane: they increase agitation and may increase mortality (Evans & Strumpf 1989). They should not be used.

Social environment

Effective communication is essential if nurses are to reduce patients' emotional distress. Patients experiencing delirium share the fears and anxieties common to many older patients in hospital: concern about the past (regret about missed opportunities, memories of traumatic events, perceived wrong-doing) and worries about their illness and its outcome, about dependency, and their family and pets. In addition, patients experiencing delirium have difficulty processing information; they need statements and instructions delivered in a clear, calm, kindly and concerned manner, and plenty of information about what is going on around them. Byrne (1997) suggests that a good model is the way in which skilled handlers work with frightened animals; offering and repeating reassurance and information in a firm and clear voice may substantially reduce arousal and anxiety. Hallucinations present a particular challenge. Nurses can best respond by remaining with patients, reassuring them of their safety, explaining the hallucination as part of their illness which will subside as they get better, and acknowledging the emotional impact of such experiences.

Occasional lucid moments used to establish rapport and careful listening may reveal important information to guide future nursing management. Choice should be restricted, as patients experiencing delirium will be unable to determine priorities and think of alternatives and this may generate anxiety. However, relevant and timely closed questions requiring yes/no answers may help nurses to understand patients' needs and may give patients some sense of control over their chaotic perceptual world.

The same nurse(s) should care for individual patients whenever possible, because familiar faces are likely to be more reassuring. Reorientation may be helpful but requires repetition and is best carried out personally by nurses introducing themselves and orienting the patient to the care setting (home, hospital or residential home). Case study 23.1, based on nursing studies in Sweden (Andersson et al. 2002, 2003), illustrates a skilled nurse's handling of a patient with confusion.

Role of the family/supporters

Patients experiencing delirium are often gravely ill and family members and supporters may feel powerless to help them. Explaining the reasons for patients' confusion should help to increase families' ability to cope and, by role-modelling how to interact with individual patients, the nurse can try to promote the family's ability to participate in the plan of care. Friends and family members need to know that simply being with the patient introduces another familiar element into the patient's perceptual world and promotes reassurance. Also they are best placed to capitalize on lucid moments to provide the patient with orienting information and reassurance. The wider role of informal carers with older people and the burden of care are

Case study 23.1

Mrs T, a community psychiatric nurse working in south-east London, recalls her experience of caring for 84-year-old Mrs Dora Brown who had problems with recurrent episodes of depression. Despite a long-standing relationship with Mrs Brown, Mrs T remembers how challenging it was to communicate with her during a period of delirium that coincided with development of a chest infection.

Mrs T characterized her encounters with the client as if a wall had been built between herself and Mrs Brown, and that it had become more difficult to understand the changed situation. Sometimes Mrs Brown listened to the information and explanations that Mrs T gave, while at other times she did not. Mrs T could see Mrs Brown moving between lucidity and confusion and was conscious of using her own verbal and non-verbal skills in an attempt to understand Mrs Brown's experiences and feelings. Mrs T was aware that her client had all her senses functioning and responded to many stimuli in her surroundings but she thought that she could discern in Mrs Brown's eyes feelings of being scared, lost, worried and sad.

Mrs T says she responded to this situation in two main ways: by being a companion or acting as a surrogate. Being a companion meant that she tried to understand Mrs Brown's perception of reality by listening and just being there in her attempt to find meaning in Mrs Brown's thoughts. When acting as a surrogate, Mrs T took over some of Mrs Brown's responsibilities in order to protect her. In this approach she used a form of reality orientation with information and explanations to bring Mrs Brown back to the nurse's sense of reality. Mrs T was aware of the need for getting the balance right between protecting Mrs Brown and not insulting her integrity and the possible future loss of independence.

Once the chest infection had been successfully treated, Mrs Brown's delirium resolved. She remembered and could report in great detail about her delirium. She recalled that impressions of all kinds invaded her mind and were experienced as reality, making her feel like a victim of these impressions rather than the one who controls what comes into her mind. While in the middle of these experiences she simultaneously sensed that the impressions were unreal, thus indicating that she was in some sort of borderland between understanding and not understanding. The things that came into her mind were mainly frightening but some were neutral or enjoyable scenarios that seemed to be familiar but also unknown, rather like a dream. These scenarios seemed to be a mixture of past and present, of events and people, which seemed to float from location to location.

This account suggests that what takes place during delirium is not nonsense but probably a mix of the client's life history, her present situation and a form of communication concerning her emotional state and inner experiences in this new situation. It also indicates the need for understanding and support on the part of the nurse caring for a client who is experiencing delirium, whatever the care setting. This involves accurate assessment, good communication skills and not a small measure of experience and intuition.

discussed in Chapter 33. It is not surprising that delirium is a highly distressing experience for spouses/caregivers and nurses who are caring for these patients. Breitbart et al. (2002a) examined the experience of delirium in a sample of 154 hospitalized patients with cancer. These patients all met DSM-IV criteria for delirium. Of the 154 patients assessed, 101 had complete resolution of their delirium. Fifty-four (53.5%) patients recalled their delirium experience. Short-term memory impairment, delirium severity and the presence of perceptual disturbances were significant predictors of delirium recall. The presence of delusions was the most significant predictor of patient distress. Patients with hypoactive delirium were just as distressed as patients with hyperactive delirium. Delirium severity and the presence of perceptual disturbances were the most significant predictors of nurse distress. The authors concluded that the majority of patients with delirium recall their delirium as highly distressing.

PREVENTION

Understanding the predisposing factors, combined with careful observation, may identify individuals at greatest risk so that supportive and orienting environments can be emphasized as part of their care. For example, a dry bed at night for an older patient who is usually incontinent may indicate dehydration, which may not be noted until delirium is evident.

Few research studies have focused specifically on preventing confusion, but two are noted here. Both compared the incidence of postoperative confusion before and after medical and nursing interventions to reduce risk factors for older patients with hip fracture. In one study (Gustafson et al. 1991) interventions included a pre- and postoperative specialist geriatric assessment, oxygen therapy during surgery and the first postoperative day, prevention and early treatment of perioperative hypotension and prompt detection and treatment of postoperative complications. In this study, the incidence of delirium was reduced from 61% to 48%, the mean length of stay was reduced from 17 to 12 days, and episodes of delirium in the intervention group were milder and shorter than those of the controls. Williams et al. (1985) report the benefits of postoperative nursing interventions, such as repeated orientation and explanation, ensuring spectacles and hearing aids are worn, and improved continuity of care, in preventing delirium. This research team reports a reduced incidence of acute confusion from 52% in a previous study to 44% in the intervention group. Further research is needed to confirm these findings.

CONCLUSION

Delirium is an important condition affecting substantial numbers of older people, which remains relatively poorly detected (Meagher 2001b). It is associated with increased mortality and prolonged hospital stays, which are at least partly attributable to the delirium itself rather than to the seriousness of the associated physical illness(es). Delirium has, though, been relatively neglected by research and the inadequate knowledge base has hindered the development of robust evidence-based guidelines for the diagnosis and assessment of patients experiencing delirium and their nursing care and treatment (Inouye 1994). Recent developments in neuroscience, specifically in relation to delirium classification and assessment, have now reduced the methodological limitations that previously hindered delirium research and herald an exciting period of further study (Meagher 2001b). There is now some evidence that vigorous treatment of reversible causes of delirium and supportive nursing measures can ameliorate its effects, and that nursing interventions to promote orientation can reduce the incidence of delirium in older people.

Recommended reading

Byrne EJ 1994 Confusional states in older people. Edward Arnold, London.
An excellent concise text for the general reader, covering the major forms of confusion in old age from a medical viewpoint. Covers dementia as well as delirium and includes a helpful account of patient assessment.
Inouye SK 1994 The dilemma of delirium: clinical and research controversies regarding diagnosis and evaluation of delirium in hospitalized older medical patients. American Journal of Medicine 97: 278–288.
A relatively comprehensive review of the debates surrounding the problem of delirium in hospitalized older patients.
Lipowski ZJ 1990 Delirium: acute confusional states. Oxford University Press, New York.

The most authoritative text yet on delirium. Covers pathophysiology, causation, treatment and care management.
MacDonald AJD, Simpson A, Jenkins D 1989 Delirium in the older: a review and suggestion for a research programme. International Journal of Psychiatry 4: 311–319.
A critical account of management strategies for patients experiencing delirium, which sets out some suggestions for future research.
Meagher DJ 2001 Delirium: optimising management. British Medical Journal 322: 144–149.
A timely review of the day-to-day management of patients with delirium.
Meagher DJ 2001 Delirium: the role of psychiatry. Advances in Psychiatric Treatment 7: 433–443.
Discusses the role of the psychiatrist in the diagnosis and management of delirium.
O'Keefe ST, Ni Chonchubhair A 1994 Post-operative delirium in the older. British Journal of Anaesthesia 73: 673–687.
A valuable review of postoperative delirium in old age.

References

American Psychiatric Association 1997 Psychiatric diagnosis and the diagnostic and statistical manual of mental disorders (fourth edition), DSM-IV. American Psychiatric Association, Washington, DC

American Psychiatric Association 1999 Practice guidelines for the treatment of patients with delirium. American Psychiatric Association, Washington, DC

Andersson EM, Hallbert IR, Norberg A, Edberg AK 2002 The meaning of acute confusional state from the perspective of elderly patients. International Journal of Geriatric Psychiatry 17: 652–663

Andersson EM, Hallbert IR, Edberg AK 2003 Nurses' experiences of the encounter with elderly patients in acute confusional state in orthopaedic care. International Journal of Nursing Studies 40: 437–448

Beresin EV 1988 Delirium in the older. Journal of Geriatric Psychiatry and Neurology 1: 127–143

Bienenfield D, Wheeler BG 1989 Psychiatric services to nursing homes: a liaison model. Hospital and Community Psychiatry 40: 793–794

Bostwick JM, Masterson BJ 1998 Psychopharmacological treatment of delirium to restore mental capacity. Psychosomatics 39: 112–117

Breitbart W, Gibson C, Tremblay A 2002a The delirium experience: delirium recall and delirium-related distress in hospitalized patients with cancer, their spouses/caregivers, and their nurses. Psychosomatics 43: 183–194

Breitbart W, Tremblay A, Gibson C 2002b An open trial of olanzapine for the treatment of delirium in hospitalized cancer patients. Psychosomatics 43: 175–182

Bucht G, Gustafson Y, Sandberg O 1999 Epidemiology of delirium. Dementia and Geriatric Cognitive Disorders 10: 315–318

Byrne EJ 1994 Confusional states in older people. Edward Arnold, London

Byrne EJ 1997 Acute and sub-acute confusional states (delirium) in later life. In: Norman IJ, Redfern SJ (eds) Mental health care for older people. Churchill Livingstone, Edinburgh, pp 175–181

Byrne EJ, Arie T 1990 Coping with dementia in the older. In: Lawson DH (ed) Current medicine 1. Churchill Livingstone, Edinburgh

Cole M, Dendukuri N, McCusker J, Han L 2003 An empirical study of different diagnostic criteria for delirium among older medical inpatients. Neuropsychiatry and Clinical Neurosciences 15: 200–207

Culp K, Tripp-Reimer T, Wadle K et al. 1997 Screening for acute confusion in older long-term care residents. Journal of Neuroscience Nursing 29: 86–100

Delaney KA, Goldfrank L 1987 Delirium: assessment and management in the critical care environment. Problems in Critical Care 1: 78–94

Evans LK, Strumpf N 1989 Tying down the older: a review of the literature on physical restraints. Journal of the American Geriatrics Society 37: 65–74

Fann JR 2000 The epidemiology of delirium: a review of studies and methodological issues. Seminars in Clinical Neuropsychiatry 5: 64–76

Folstein MF, Folstein JE, McHugh PR 1975 Mini-mental state: a practical method for grading the cognitive state of patients for the clinician. Journal of Psychiatric Research 12: 189–198

Folstein MF, Bassett SS, Romanoski AJ, Nestadt G 1991 The epidemiology of delirium in the community: the Eastern Baltimore mental health survey. International Psychogeriatrics 3: 169–176

Francis J, Kapoor WN 1990 Delirium in hospitalized older. Journal of General Internal Medicine 5: 65–79

Francis J, Martin D, Kapoor WN 1990 A prospective study of delirium in hospitalized older. Journal of the American Medical Association 263: 1097–1101

Franco K, Litaker D, Locala J, Bronson D 2001 The cost of delirium in the surgical patient. Psychosomatics 42: 68–73

Godwin-Austen R, Bendall J (eds) 1990 The neurological examination of the older patient. In: The neurology of the older. Springer, London, pp 1–11

Gustafson Y, Berggren D, Brannstrom B et al. 1988 Acute confusional states in older patients treated for femoral neck fractures. Journal of the American Geriatrics Society 36: 525–530

Gustafson Y, Brannstrom B, Berggren D 1991 A geriatric-anesthesiologic program to reduce acute confusional states in older patients treated for femoral neck fractures. Journal of the American Geriatrics Society 39: 655–662

Huntzinger JA, Rosse RB, Schwartz BL, Ross LA, Deutsch SI 1992 Clock drawing in the screening assessment of cognitive impairment in an ambulatory care setting: a preliminary report. General Hospital Psychiatry 14: 142–144

Inouye SK 1994 The dilemma of delirium: clinical and research controversies regarding diagnosis and evaluation of delirium in hospitalized older medical patients. American Journal of Medicine 97: 278–288

Inouye SK, Charpentier PA 1996 Precipitating factors for delirium in hospitalized older persons. Predictive model and interrelationship with baseline vulnerability. Journal of the American Medical Association 275: 852–857

Inouye SK, van Dyck CH, Alessi CA et al. 1990 Clarifying confusion: the confusion assessment method; a new method for detection of delirium. Annals of Internal Medicine 113: 941–948

Inouye SK, Bogardus ST Jr, Charpentier PA et al. 1999 A multicomponent intervention to prevent delirium in hospitalized older patients. New England Journal of Medicine 340: 669–676

Kahn RL, Goldberg AI, Pollock M, Peak A 1960 Brief objective measures for the determination of mental states in the older. American Journal of Psychiatry 107: 326–328

Koponen HJ, Riekkinen PJ 1993 A prospective study of delirium in older patients admitted to a psychiatric hospital. Journal of Neurology, Neurosurgery and Psychiatry 52: 980–985

Lichtigfeld FJ, Gillman MA 1990 Dangerous synergism between sedatives and a hyponatremic state. Journal of the Royal Society of Medicine 83: 185–186

Lindesay J, Macdonald A, Starke I 1990 Delirium in the older. Oxford University Press, Oxford

Lipowski ZJ 1990 Delirium: acute confusional states. Oxford University Press, New York

Lipowski ZJ 1992 Delirium and impaired consciousness. In: Evans JG, Williams TF (eds) Oxford textbook of geriatric medicine. Oxford University Press, Oxford

Liptzin B, Levkoff SE 1992 An empirical study of delirium subtypes. British Journal of Psychiatry 161: 843–845

Lishman WA 1987 Organic psychiatry. Blackwell, Oxford

Liston EH 1982 Delirium in the aged. Psychiatric Clinics of North America 5: 49–66

MacDonald AJD, Simpson A, Jenkins D 1989 Delirium in the older: a review and suggestion for a research programme. International Journal of Psychiatry 4: 311–319

Marieb EN 2004 Human anatomy and physiology, 6th edn. San Francisco. Pearson Education

McCarthy JR, Palmateer LM 1985 Assessment of cognitive deficit in geriatric patients. Journal of the American Geriatrics Society 33: 467–471

Meagher DJ 2001a Delirium: optimising management, British Medical Journal 322: 144–149

Meagher DJ 2001b Delirium: the role of psychiatry. Advances in Psychiatric Treatment 7: 433–443

Meagher DJ, O'Hanlon D, O'Mahony E, Casey PR, Trzepacz PT 2000 Relationship between symptoms and motoric subtype of delirium. Journal of Neuropsychiatry and Clinical Neurosciences 12: 51–56

Morse RM, Litin EM 1969 Post-operative delirium: a study of aetiological factors. American Journal of Psychiatry 126: 388–395

Moses H, van Kaden BA 1986 Neurologic consultations in a general hospital: spectrum of iatrogenic disease. American Journal of Medicine 81: 955–958

Okamoto Y, Matsuoka Y, Sasaki T et al. 1999 Trazadone in the treatment of delirium. Journal of Clinical Psychopharmacology 19: 280–282

O'Keefe ST, Ni Chonchubhair A 1994 Postoperative delirium in the older. British Journal of Anaesthesia 73: 673–687

Pattie AH, Gilleard CJ 1975 A brief psychogeriatric assessment schedule: validation against psychiatric diagnosis and discharge from hospital. British Journal of Psychiatry 127: 489–493

Platzer H 1988 A study into the causes of post-operative confusion in the older. MSc dissertation. King's College, University of London, London

Richeimer SH 1987 Psychological interventions in delirium. Postgraduate Medicine 81: 173–180

Roberts MA, Caird FI 1990 The contribution of computerised tomography to the differential diagnosis of confusion in older people. Age and Ageing 19: 50–56

Ross CA, Peyser CE, Shapiro I, Folstein MF 1991 Delirium: phenomenologic and etiologic subtypes. International Psychogeriatrics 3: 353–371

Rovner BW, Kafonek S, Filipp L, Lucas MJ, Folstein MF 1986 Prevalence of mental illness in a community nursing home. American Journal of Psychiatry 143: 1446–1449

Schulman KI, Shedletsky R, Silver IL 1986 The challenge of time: clock drawing and cognitive function in the older. International Journal of Geriatric Psychiatry 1: 135–140

Seymour DG, Pringle R 1983 Post-operative complications in the older surgical patient. Gerontology 29: 262–270

Simpson CT 1984 Doctors' and nurses' use of the word confused. British Journal of Psychiatry 145: 441–443

Taylor D, Lewis S 1993 Delirium. Journal of Neurology, Neurosurgery and Psychiatry 56: 742–751

Tesar GE, Stern TA 1986 Evaluation and treatment of agitation in the intensive care unit. Journal of Intensive Care 1: 137–148

Thomas RI, Cameron DJ, Fahs MC 1988 A prospective study of delirium and prolonged hospital stay. Archives of General Psychiatry 45: 937–940

Trzepacz PT 1996 Delirium: advances in diagnosis, pathophysiology, and treatment. Psychiatric Clinics of North America 19: 429-448

Trzepacz PT, 2000 Is there a final common neural pathway in delirium? Focus on acetylcholine and dopamine. Seminars in Clinical Neuropsychiatry 5: 132–148

Trzepacz PT, Baker RW, Greenhouse J 1988 A simple rating scale for delirium. Psychiatry Research 23: 89–97

Trzepacz PT, Mittal D, Torres R et al. 2001 Validation of the delirium rating scale–revised-98: comparison with the delirium rating scale and the cognitive test for delirium. Journal of Neuropsychiatry and Clinical Neurosciences 13: 229–242

Tune L, Carr S, Hoag E, Cooper T 1992 Anticholinergic effects of drugs commonly prescribed for the older: potential means for assessing risk of delirium. American Journal of Psychiatry 149: 1393–1394

van der Mast RC 2000 Commentary on 'Large neutral amino acid changes and delirium in febrile older medical patients': do amino acids play a role in the pathophysiology of delirium? Journals of Gerontology Series A: Biological Sciences and Medical Sciences 55: 253–254

van der Mast R, van den Broek WW, Fekkes D, Pepplinkhuizen L, Habbema J 2000 Is delirium after cardiac surgery related to plasma amino acids and physical condition? Journal of Neuropsychiatry and Clinical Neurosciences 12: 57–63

Whittaker JJ 1989 Postoperative confusion in the older. International Journal of Geriatric Psychiatry 4: 321–326

Williams MA, Campbell EB, Raynor WJ, Mlynarczyk SM, Ward SE 1985 Reducing acute confusional states in older patients with hip fractures. Research in Nursing and Health 8: 35–40

World Health Organization 1992 ICD-10 Classification of mental and behavioural disorders. WHO, Geneva

Zakriya KJ, Christmas C, Wenz JF et al. 2002 Preoperative factors associated with postoperative change in confusion assessment method score in hip fracture patients. Anesthesia and Analgesia 94: 1628–1632

Chapter 24

Person–centred dementia care

Sue Davies, Barry Aveyard and Ian J. Norman

CHAPTER CONTENTS

INTRODUCTION

'Dementia' is a term used to describe a range of brain disorders that have in common a loss of brain function that is usually progressive, irreversible and eventually fatal. Collectively, these conditions represent the most common serious mental illnesses affecting older people. The experience of dementia can be devastating for older people and their carers; however, there is increasing evidence to suggest that, with appropriate support, older people with dementia can be helped to achieve a good quality of life. Our main aim within this chapter is to present a summary of information that will help nurses and other caregivers to provide appropriate and effective support to older people with dementia and their families.

There are different ideas about the nature and causes of dementia. Although it results from a number of medical conditions, the experience of dementia cannot be fully explained by physical changes. According to some authorities, dementia is socially constructed. In other words, it is not simply a relentless disease process of the central nervous system in which personality and identity are progressively destroyed. Rather, dementia results from the ways in which some older people are treated by those who care for them and by society at large, and also from the unique ways that people with dementia deal with their altered world. These ideas draw upon well-established theoretical traditions in the social sciences; in particular, on the work of social psychologists and interpretive sociologists who emphasize the importance of understanding people's intentions and interpretations of the actions of others when seeking to explain human action. But the development, application and popularization of the notion of social construction in relation to dementia are comparatively recent. In the UK the social construction of dementia thesis owes much to the work of the late Tom Kitwood and his colleagues in the Bradford Dementia Group. Kitwood described what he called 'the new culture of dementia care', a term that captures changes in beliefs and attitudes towards dementia and in the organization of care for people with dementia.

Kitwood's approach to dementia care has been well established within the field since the early 1990s and it is perhaps time to move on from referring to it as a 'new' culture. A key element within this approach is the notion of person-centred dementia care. Person-centredness was first articulated by Carl Rogers, the US therapist and psychologist (Rogers 1959), and has now permeated many aspects of health and social care practice (Department of Health 2001). Morton (1997) suggests that person-centredness in the context of dementia care has the following key features:

- a shift in traditional power relations towards the client (the person with dementia or members of his or her family) and away from the health care professional
- increased attention to clients' feelings, emotions, experiences and perception of their own reality
- emphasis on the act of successful communication as central to high-quality care.

Accordingly, the responsibility is on the caregiver to recognize and encourage attempts by the person with dementia to communicate, resulting in increased self-esteem and enhanced quality of life.

The 'new' culture of dementia care arose, to some extent, as a reaction to the traditional medical viewpoint that the condition was associated with inevitable decline with no treatments or cure, and therefore often little interest was expressed in developing ways of caring for the person with dementia. Arguably, however, a biomedical perspective is not incompatible with the new culture of dementia care: as new pharmocological interventions promote enhanced cognition, albeit for a limited time, the importance of person-centred care is increasingly apparent. Accordingly, this chapter begins with an outline of the condition of dementia and its underlying disease processes from a biomedical perspective. We consider the signs and symptoms of dementia, including cognitive and non-cognitive features. Discussion of the causes of dementia focuses upon the three most common types: (1) Alzheimer's disease (AD); (2) vascular dementia (VAD); and (3) diffuse Lewy body disease (DLBD). We explore the recognition and assessment of dementia and outline the main pharmacological treatments.

Attention is then shifted to psychosocial perspectives of dementia, focusing on Kitwood's theory of dementia in particular. Emergent ideas about the importance of relationship-centred care to the well-being of older people with dementia and their carers are also discussed. The experience of dementia is considered from the perspective of people with the condition, their families and paid staff working with them. Finally we suggest four important foci that should help care providers to move in the direction of enabling older people with dementia and their carers to enjoy the best possible quality of life.

WHAT IS DEMENTIA?

There are many definitions of dementia but the following is often regarded as definitive:

> Dementia is the global impairment of higher cortical functions, including memory, the capacity to solve problems of day-to-day living, the performance of learned perceptual-motor skills, the correct use of social skills and control of emotional reactions in the absence of gross 'clouding of consciousness'. The condition is often irreversible and progressive (World Health Organization 1986, cited in Jones & Miesen 1992: p. 9).

Definitions of dementia tend to emphasize the cognitive aspects of the condition, although from the point of view of people with dementia and their carers, it is often the non-cognitive aspects that present the biggest challenges.

Although the features of dementia have been precisely identified, it is important not to treat the term 'dementia' as a diagnosis. There are many individual diseases which create the experience of dementia, while fitting into the broad definition above. These diseases have differing pathology and specific symptoms, and will respond to medication in different ways. It is important that people with dementia receive a definitive diagnosis of the condition causing their dementia so that care and treatment can be developed appropriately.

Prevalence and incidence of dementia

The prevalence of dementia is the frequency with which it occurs in a population. Mild dementia is difficult to diagnose and therefore it is difficult to be accurate about prevalence (North of England Evidence Based Guideline Development Project 1998). The Alzheimer's Society suggests that around 775 000 people in the UK are living with dementia, with AD being the most common diagnosis. Table 24.1, reproduced from McKeith & Fairbairn (2001), shows the distribution of the main causes of dementia.

The prevalence of dementia is very similar in studies carried out in the UK, USA and continental Europe, at about 5% of those over 65 years. However, Kendrick & Warnes (1997) point out that this figure is likely to be an underestimate because studies usually fail to include older people living in some form of residential care. When these people are included, prevalence rises to around 7–8% of the population over 65. The point prevalence of dementia (proportion of all people of that age who are affected) increases sharply with age from about 2.5% at age 65 to 10% at age 75 and 40% at age 85 (McKeith & Fairbairn 2001).

The prevalence of dementia among hospitalized patients is difficult to determine because most patients are admitted for reasons other than the dementia itself.

Table 24.1 Distribution of the main causes of dementia

Cause	%
Alzheimer's disease	50
Dementia with Lewy bodies	20
Vascular dementia	10
Mixed Alzheimer's/vascular dementia	10
Other dementias	10

Park et al. (2004) found that 8.5% of patients admitted to a community hospital also had a diagnosis of dementia. Tolson et al. (1999) found that 66% of patients over 65 consecutively admitted to general medical wards were found to have cognitive impairment, with 40% experiencing severe problems. Prevalence figures for dementia amongst residential care populations are fairly similar: Borman et al. (2004) found that 31% of residential home residents and 38% of nusing home residents were admitted with dementia. In addition to these cases, prevalence studies have consistently found numbers of people with dementia symptoms which cause problems for them and their families.

The incidence of dementia is the number of new cases within a given time period:

- It is estimated that by 2010 there will be about 840 000 people with dementia in the UK
- This is expected to rise to over 1.5 million people with dementia by 2050 (Alzheimer's Society 2003d)

Byrne (1994) estimates that, for an average health district (population of 250 000 with 15% aged over 65 years), there will be around 700 new cases of dementia annually.

Features of dementia

The clinical features of dementia vary according to the physiological basis of the condition, characteristics of individuals and their care environment. The features of dementia which may be apparent are listed in Box 24.1 and discussed below.

Impaired memory

Many of us have experienced walking upstairs and being unable to remember what we went upstairs for. We will probably remember if we stop to think but we may need to retrace our steps to jog our memory. The experience of early dementia may be like this, but the ability to respond to cues is lost. Short-term memory impairment is a marked problem for many people with dementia but will vary in severity. Memory problems are often exacerbated by loss of familiar cues, as occurs when moving from home into residential care. Eventually long-term memory may also be affected. Individuals forget the temporal order of events in their lives and then the events themselves. People with dementia may have difficulty naming objects (dysphasia) but experience problems defining words and concepts which go well beyond this. They may be prone to 'concrete thinking', that is the literal interpretation of abstract concepts. Byrne (1994) suggests that this

---

Box 24.1   Common features of dementia

Cognitive features
- Impaired memory
- Impaired abstract thinking
- Impaired judgement and insight
- Impaired higher cortical functions (e.g. aphasia, apraxia, agnosia)

Non-cognitive features
- Disorders of mood
- Hallucinations
- Delusional ideas
- Personality change
- Behavioural features (e.g. frustration, activity disturbances, changes in eating behaviour, disturbances in diurnal rhythm and changes in sexual behaviour)
- Decline in social competence
- Impaired abstract thinking

---

may help to explain everyday errors such as putting salt in tea rather than sugar; the person with dementia may be unable to realize that all white granular substances are not sugar.

Altered judgement and insight

People with dementia may be progressively unable to organize their lives or deduce the consequences of their actions. As a result they may neglect themselves and be unaware of the effects of this on those around them, or they may enter dangerous situations, wandering into a busy main road for example, and appear oblivious to the risks involved. This kind of behaviour can be especially difficult and challenging for carers to come to terms with and manage. Judgement is related to insight into the illness, which is very variable. Some people with dementia may seem unaware and be unconcerned about their increased difficulties, whereas others may have transient periods of awareness and become distressed. Anxiety and sometimes panic are not uncommon if things go wrong and individuals will often seek reassurance. In some instances catastrophic reactions may occur, as when the person with dementia encounters a problem that he or she cannot overcome and reacts with extreme distress and agitation. Cheston & Bender (1999) clearly articulate the emotional hardship these experiences place, both on the person with dementia and those around him or her.

Changes in the ability to communicate

People with dementia sometimes have difficulty in finding the right words in conversation. An early com-

munication problem is the inability to identify objects by their proper name, although the person may still be aware of the object's purpose. For instance, when asked to name a coat the person may say it is for putting on to go out. Later individuals with dementia may develop non-fluent aphasia, when speech becomes less spontaneous and contains fewer words. Alternatively, they may develop fluent aphasia. Here individuals with dementia do not have difficulty in finding words, but the words that they use are not clearly associated, making speech difficult to understand.

Changes in ability to make purposeful movement (apraxia and dyspraxia)

The person with dementia may experience difficulty in making purposeful movements or sequences of movements (including speech) voluntarily, but without associated muscle weakness. So, for example, individuals may be unable to pick up an object from the table on request, although they may be observed picking it up later. Another example is the difficulty experienced by some people with dementia when dressing; for example, putting clothes on inside out, or back to front, or in an unusual sequence. Inability to assemble objects in their correct spatial relationship to each other becomes apparent in difficulties in carrying out simple tasks such as laying the table or copying a simple drawing. Communication may also be affected since the person with dementia may experience restricted oral movement and be unable to gesture purposefully.

Other features

Difficulties in recognizing familiar things   Agnosia is the failure to recognize, and therefore to understand and name, familiar objects. Some people with dementia may also be unable to differentiate the right and left sides of their body and this may contribute to the dressing difficulty described above. Eventually the individual may be unable to recognize relatives and friends. This can be an extremely painful and frustrating experience.

Other psychological symptoms   Symptoms of depression such as loss of interest, decreased energy and agitation can be associated with dementia. However, given the frustrations of the symptoms of early dementia it is perhaps inevitable that people sometimes experience profound symptoms of depression.

Psychotic features (hallucinations and delusions) are more common in the middle stages of dementia (20–40% of cases; McKeith & Fairbairn 2001), with auditory hallucinations more common than visual hallucinations (Allen & Burns 1995). Research suggests that, as with delirium, hallucinations are more frequent during the evening and night than the daytime (Allen & Burns 1995). There is also evidence to suggest that hallucinations and delusions are particularly experienced by people with Lewy body dementia (Holden & Stokes 2002).

Personality changes   The characteristic way in which a person with dementia responds to events may alter to the extent that relatives may say that the person is different from the one they had known. Personality change may be of two types: (1) an exaggeration of previous character traits, so that the previously quiet person hardly utters a word; or (2) a dramatic reversal of previous characteristics, so that a previously quiet and reserved person becomes highly talkative and garrulous.

Changes in behaviour   From the perspective of carers, alterations in the behaviour of a person with dementia are often the most difficult aspects to cope with. Certainly, there is evidence that behavioural disturbances in the person with dementia often contribute to the decision to seek specialist help or even some form of residential care (Davies & Nolan 2003). It is sometimes helpful to classify such behaviour changes in order to identify the most appropriate way to support individuals with dementia and their carers. A useful categorization is provided by Hope & Patel (1993), who have identified six important aspects of behaviour:

1. 'Aggressive' behaviour. This is a difficult term and needs careful consideration before it is used. Other terms that are commonly used in this context include 'problem behaviour' and 'challenging behaviour'. However both these terms might imply that the problem is for the person with dementia rather than those who have to cope with the behaviour. The most common types of aggressive behaviour demonstrated by people with dementia are being uncooperative or resisting help, irritability and forms of verbal aggression. Biting, scratching, kicking and hitting are the most common forms of physical aggression, although serious injury to others is rare. It is thought that the form of aggression, whether it is physical or verbal, for instance, is of less significance in terms of providing support than understanding the context in which the aggression occurs: for example, whether the person becomes aggressive during intimate care or at mealtimes, or in response to poor care practices. Behavioural approaches to managing challenging behaviours are discussed later.

2. Changes in activity. People with dementia may engage in an altered pattern of activity, including repetitive actions and wandering, particularly at night. Some individuals demonstrate reduced activity and experience apathy. McShane et al. (1998) question whether behaviour often labelled as 'wandering' is, in the perception of the person with dementia, purposeful 'walking', a natural and healthy thing to do which would be encouraged in the lives of many older people.

3. Changes in eating behaviour. Decreased food intake is the most common alteration in eating behaviour in dementia. People with dementia may have difficulty in concentrating sufficiently to eat and in recognizing food and its significance (Parsons 2001). This often leads to weight loss and nutritional deficiency (Alzheimer's Society 2000). Other alterations in eating behaviour include changes in food preference (particularly for sweet foods), disturbances of chewing and swallowing, and eating inedible food (including faeces). Between 10% and 20% of people with dementia experience increased appetite (Allen & Burns 1995); Hope et al. (1989) suggest that damage to food intake control mechanisms in the brain may be an important factor in explaining this. Marshall (2003) suggests that there are many reasons why nutrition may be problematic for the person with dementia. She suggests that issues include: distraction from food by noisy dining environments, not recognizing the usual clues associated with food such as the smell of food and not recognizing feelings of hunger and fullness. Manthorpe & Watson (2003) suggest that providing nutrition is an essential element of dementia care-giving, the importance of which is sometimes unrecognized. They argue that it is an area of care where nurses need much more support to be able to care for nutritional needs effectively.

4. Changes in sleeping and waking. Problems commonly reported by family carers of people with dementia are often related to changes in the sleep–wake cycle (Rabins et al. 1982). Most older people sleep less than younger people and experience more daytime fatigue. In dementia these patterns are exacerbated and there may also be an increased frequency of night-time wakening. These changes may appear even in early mild dementia. Rapid eye movement sleep decreases and daytime sleep increases as dementia progresses (for more information on sleep in older people, see Chapter 20). Other

behaviours related to disturbances of diurnal rhythm include 'sundowning' (the worsening of activity disturbances in the latter part of the day), nocturnal activity disturbances (e.g. frequent night-time waking) and inappropriate dressing and undressing.

5. Changes in sexual behaviour. Under-reporting by female carers may explain in part the relatively low incidence of changes in sexual behaviour. These changes are reported in about 5% of men and are less frequently reported in women (Allen & Burns 1995). Reduced sexual drive with impotence may occur in men, but of more concern to carers is inappropriate sexual behaviour, such as masturbation in public, inappropriate sexual speech, kissing, hugging, and self-exposure and attempted fondling (Hope & Patel 1993) (see Chapter 21 for further details of sexuality in older people).

6. Other miscellaneous behavioural disturbances. Examples of these behaviours include screaming, picking at clothes or furniture and moving objects from place to place while walking around the house. These behaviours do not fit easily into the above categories and their significance is unclear.

Impact of changes in behaviour for the person with dementia and carers

Cognitive impairment will interfere with work, social activities and relationships. Typically, social abilities decline when dementia is more than mild. People with dementia are likely to experience difficulties with usual daily activities (such as shopping, cooking, dressing and personal hygiene) and, if insight is lost, they may be unable to appreciate what is happening to them, and attempts by well-meaning carers to help them may be resented.

Coping with environmental demands becomes increasingly difficult and the tendency is for people with dementia to try to restrict these to maintain control. Interests may be given up and people with dementia may be increasingly reluctant to meet people or even to leave the house for fear of getting lost. Eventually the individual's range of thought may diminish until it becomes restricted to a total concern with immediate considerations – eating a piece of cake, smoking a cigarette. Performing activities of daily living – dressing, washing, going to bed – may become haphazard or be forgotten completely. Without appropriate support the person with dementia may withdraw and become socially isolated.

Physical causes of dementia

Table 24.2, reproduced from Byrne (1994), lists physical causes of dementia categorized according to the speed of onset and possible progression of the condition. Most of the conditions listed here are irreversible, but some are examples of so-called 'reversible' (or treatable) dementias, i.e. those conditions that follow the course of dementia as long as their cause is present. For example, people with neurosyphilis will continue to decline mentally until treated with antibiotics. Likewise, surgery for hydrocephalus or a brain tumour can halt the progress of dementia. However, most older people presenting with dementia will experience a gradual onset (over months) and prolonged course (over years). The most common cause of dementia is AD.

Alzheimer's disease

AD generally has a gradual onset with a smooth downhill progression. The mean survival of people with AD is 5–6 years from initial onset, although most studies show a wide range from 1 year to 20 years or more. Death is usually attributed to accompanying conditions and events, such as pneumonia, vascular disease or accidental trauma, rather than the disease itself.

Stages of AD are described by some authors such as Blondin (1988) (Box 24.2) but these are controversial since the stages appear to reflect experience poorly. Furthermore, there is insufficient information at present to predict reliably the rate of deterioration and length of survival in individual cases (Tobiansky 1994). Other objections to stage theories of AD include their neglect of the social psychology of dementia care (Kitwood 1997b) (discussed later). Also, stage theories can create a self-fulfilling prophecy, and feelings of hopelessness and helplessness for people with dementia and their carers (Bell & McGregor 1995), so reinforcing historical stereotypes.

Traditionally a definitive diagnosis of AD has only been made on autopsy, when the distinctive neurological changes in the brain can be observed directly. However, advances in brain-scanning techniques and interpretation of these has led to increased confidence of being able to diagnose AD by scanning (Smith & Jobst 1996). The full causes of AD are not known, in spite of the considerable resources devoted to this field of research, and it may be that AD constitutes a group of related disorders, each with a different cause. The most important risk factors for AD revealed by epidemiological studies are old age, family history of dementia, Down's syndrome and Parkinson's disease (van Duijn et al. 1991).

A familial risk of AD has been recognized for many years, but estimates of risk have differed. Studies have

Table 24.2   Some physical causes of dementia

Onset and course	Type of damage	Disease
Rapid or relatively rapid onset (days to weeks).	Degenerative	Diffuse Lewy body disease
Duration and progression depend on underlying cause		Alzheimer's disease (rarely)
	Vascular	Cerebral infarction/embolus
		Cerebral aneurysm
		Cerebral vasculitis
	Transmissible dementias	Creutzfeldt–Jakob disease
		Gerstmann–Straussler syndrome
	Infection	Encephalitis (particularly herpes simplex)
		Whipple's disease
	Other	Severe cerebral trauma (course may be prolonged)
		Neuropsychiatric systemic lupus
		Rheumatoid, sarcoid, temporal arteritis
Gradual onset (months) and prolonged course (years)	Degenerative	Alzheimer's disease
		Pick's disease
		Wilson's disease
		Huntington's chorea
		Progressive supranuclear palsy
		Diffuse Lewy body disease
		Dementia of the frontal lobe type
		Corticobasal degeneration
		Multisystem atrophies
		Multiple sclerosis
		Motor neurone disease
		Thalamic dementia
	Vascular	Binswanger's disease
		Multiple lacunar infarction
		Cerebral infarction/embolus
	Infections	Neurosyphilis
	Space-occupying lesions	Primary intracranial tumours
		Meningioma
		Chronic subdural haematoma
	Metabolic and endocrine disorders	Uraemia
		Chronic hepatic encephalopathy
		Carcinomatosis
		Hypothyroidism
		Hypopituitarism
		Addison's disease
	Other	Communicating hydrocephalus
	Alcoholic dementia	

shown that between 50% and 80% of people diagnosed with AD have at least one affected first-degree relative (parent, sibling, offspring) with the disease, but controlled studies show that 50–60% of patients with AD have no family history (Fitch et al. 1988). Some studies (Katzman et al. 1989) show that the risk of first-degree relatives developing the disease is minimal if the individual's onset of the disease occurs after the age of 75.

The current state of knowledge about genetic causes of AD can be summarized as follows:

- There is no single gene responsible for all cases of AD

Box 24.2 Stages of Alzheimer's disease and typical family responses

Stage 1 Early confusion
- Forgetfulness interferes with routine
- Difficulty concentrating and learning new things
- 'Bad days' outnumber good ones
- Those around lose patience
- Family members irritated by forgetfulness
- Prompts are received about chores and routine

Stage 2 Late confusion
- Familiar places are no longer familiar – person gets lost in them
- Deterioration in recent memory: forgets appointments, forgets to pay bills, leading to frustration and embarrassment
- Loss of interest in social affairs
- Chores (shopping, cooking) become difficult
- May deny problems
- Disagreements with others over current and recent events – debates on who is right

Stage 3 Early dementia
- 'Good days' become less frequent
- Dietary imbalance as mealtimes become chaotic
- Names of significant others are forgotten (e.g. grandchildren and friends)
- Word-finding difficulty

- Sequential tasks (e.g. meal preparation) difficult to manage
- May wander

Stage 4 Middle dementia
- Disrupted sleep–wake pattern
- Needs supervision of basic life tasks
- Outbursts of fear and anger
- Increasing feelings of restriction and disappointment with loss of equal partnership with spouse

Stage 5 Middle-middle dementia
- Needs help with all daily living activities
- Meaning of speech is no longer intelligible: garbled
- Mobility difficulties
- Urinary (sometimes faecal) incontinence
- Carer exhausted, exasperated and may feel trapped: seriously considers admission of dementia sufferer to institutional care

Stage 6 Late-stage dementia
- Needs total care (incontinence, feeding)
- Communicates non-verbally or not at all
- Complications arise from immobility
- Carer grieves at loss of spouse; relief at prospect of release through admission to institutional care/death; guilt associations

---

- Genetic factors cause the disease in only a small number of cases
- Inherited factors alone do not explain why some people develop AD and others do not (Alzheimer's Society 2003b).

The neurotransmitter acetylcholine, associated with the processing of memories, can be reduced by 50% in the brain of a person with AD. Increasing the availability of acetylcholine within the brain of AD is the focus of the currently available cognitive-enhancing drugs.

Diffuse Lewy body disease

DLBD is now recognized as a relatively common cause of progressive cognitive decline in older people, accounting for up to 15% of people who have dementia (Alzheimer's Society 2003a). The clinical features of the illness are not those typically found in people with AD or VAD. They include: a fluctuating cognitive state, episodes of acute confusion with no clear physical cause, visual hallucinations and disorder of movement characteristic of Parkinson's disease (including

slowness to initiate movement, muscle rigidity and, less frequently, resting tremor; McKeith & Fairbairn 2001, Alzheimer's Society 2003a). Consequently, people with DLBD are prone to falls.

These features are associated with the presence of tiny spherical protein deposits known as Lewy bodies in both cortical and subcortical areas of the brain. Some individuals show histological changes similar to those seen in AD and so raise the possibility that DLBD is a subtype of AD. But the fact that DLBD shares clinical and neuropathological features of both AD and Parkinson's disease suggests that it is a spectrum disorder, with typical AD at one end of the spectrum and typical Parkinson's disease at the other (Harrison & McKeith 1996).

Vascular dementia

The term 'vascular dementia' incorporates several important causes of dementia. Multi-infarct dementia (cortical VAD) is the best known. Other types are VAD of acute onset, subcortical VAD (Binswanger's disease) and mixed cortical and subcortical dementia (ICD-10, World Health Organization 1992). In VAD the underlying pathology is infarction of the brain due to vascular disease. The cause of the dementia is presumed to be the result of small infarcts arising from occlusion of blood vessels supplying the neurones due to thromboembolism or haemorrhage, or disease of cerebral blood vessels. Areas of infarction can be detected on computed tomography (CT) examination, and magnetic resonance imaging (MRI) is particularly sensitive in detecting vascular brain lesions.

The risk factors for VAD are those also associated with strokes, with hypertension the most significant risk factor. Others include cigarette smoking, cardiac arrhythmias, coronary heart disease and vasculitic disorders. As with AD, VAD becomes more common with increasing age. Hachinski (1992) has described VAD as 'preventable senility' and advocates control of cerebrovascular risk factors (e.g. treatment of arrhythmias, anticoagulation therapy, appropriate diet, smoking cessation, treatment of hypertension) for risk groups and for those with VAD to limit further damage.

Recognizing dementia

Ideally, dementia should be identified at an early stage so that support can be mobilized. In reality, though, support services are more frequently oriented towards intervention in the later stages of the illness and during crisis periods (Alzheimer's Disease Society 1995, Keady & Nolan 1995a). Early detection relies upon the person and members of the family recognizing signs and symptoms for what they are and not discounting them as features of normal ageing (Pollitt et al. 1989). This is complicated by the fact that people living through the early stages of dementia will often adopt strategies to deny the difficulties they are experiencing and maintain a veneer of normality (Nolan et al. 1996). However, there comes a stage when signs and symptoms can no longer be ignored. Formal confirmation is normally provided by the individual's general practitioner, who faces the challenge of distinguishing mild dementia from the effects of normal ageing, or cognitive impairment associated with other conditions. It has been suggested that general practitioners can be reluctant to diagnose dementia and that many do not recognize the importance of early diagnosis (Audit Commission 2002). As it is clear that the cognitive-enhancing drugs work best the earlier they are prescribed, the need for early identification is an important issue.

The diagnosis of dementia relies mainly on: (1) a careful history, especially of the onset and progression of the condition; (2) examination of mental state through conversation and standard tests of cognition;

(3) a physical examination; and (4) investigations. These same factors are also relevant to the assessment of delirium, and most of them have been covered in Chapter 23. Here, we discuss specific aspects of assessment relevant to the diagnosis of dementia. Ways in which assessment contributes to individualized plans of care and approaches to assessing quality of care for people with dementia are discussed later in the chapter. Assessment of older people in general is discussed in Chapter 28.

Tests of cognitive function

There are no formal tests for dementia and tests of cognitive function should be considered in the context of overall assessment of the individual. Accordingly, tests of cognitive function should be seen as screening rather than diagnostic instruments. Four of the most popular and widely used are:

1. Clifton Assessment Procedures for the Elderly (CAPE) (Pattie & Gilleard 1975). This provides a practical cognitive rating scale designed mainly for brevity but is rather clumsy and insensitive in identifying symptom severity. As a measure of functioning it is somewhat limited, as well as requiring good motor coordination by the person being assessed
2. Mini-Mental State Examination (MMSE) (Folstein et al. 1975). This is a widely used screening test for dementia. It has particular significance, as scoring of the MMSE has a clear impact under the National Institute for Clinical Excellence (NICE) guidelines as to whether cognitive-enhancing drugs can be prescribed or not. However, the MMSE has been criticized for its lack of sensitivity to mild cognitive impairment (Miller 2003)
3. Comprehensive Assessment and Referral examination (CARE) (Gurland et al. 1979). This instrument was originally designed for use with people with dementia living in the community but it has also been validated for residential populations. It has been used extensively in research studies of older people and incorporates subscales, including the 10-item Organic Brain Score, which is used to detect levels of dementia
4. GMS/AGECAT (Dewey & Copeland 1986). This is one of the most recent and most promising assessment scales. It is a totally computerized package providing a wide range of indices, including a separate diagnostic subscale. It has been used in studies of prevalence and incidence of dementia and has been shown to be a sensitive and reliable instrument.

One difficulty in identifying dementia is to know whether cognitive skills have declined from their pre-morbid level (i.e. before the onset of the disease). Self-ratings of decline may be used (Rabbitt 1982): however, the validity of such methods has been questioned (Sunderland et al. 1986). In practice, assessment tends to rely on reports of decline by family members and a number of measurement scales are available. For a more detailed discussion, see Burns et al. (1999).

Assessment of the extent to which the older person with dementia is independent in areas such as personal hygiene, safety, mobility, cooking and eating is best carried out in the person's usual environment. This aspect of assessment indicates the level of support needed and identifies the value of aids and environmental adaptations. A number of structured assessment tools are available. These include:

- Everyday Living Skills Inventory (ELSI) (Barker 1985): designed by nurses for use across a range of patient groups and a variety of care settings, this inventory emphasizes individual strengths as well as deficits
- CAPE (Pattie & Gilleard 1975): this widely used instrument (mentioned previously as a screening measure) covers most potential problem areas of everyday living and provides a guide to change in overall levels of disability over time. However, it is of limited value in evaluating change in specific aspects of behaviour.

A problem with these assessment tools is that they tend to focus on the difficulties that a person has without considering the strengths and attributes that remain (Miller 2003). Unless used sensitively, this can have a negative impact on the person's self-esteem.

Research efforts have also been directed at ways of involving informal carers in the preliminary assessment of their older relative's social, behavioural and cognitive levels of functioning. Jorm et al. (1989), for instance, produced a questionnaire for completion by family carers, the IQCODE, to assess cognitive decline in older people over a 10-year period. Responses on this measure were found to correlate closely with the MMSE (Folstein et al. 1975) and, importantly, with the level of support required by the carer.

A further example of research in this area has been the development of the Dementia Stress Management Model (DSMM) (Zarit et al. 1985) which involves carers in assessment in an attempt to identify and prioritize problems for the family and plan relevant support for family carers. The DSMM has two components:

1. information-giving, in which the practitioner provides carers with information about the type, nature and cause of their relative's dementia, research information relevant to the problems faced by carers and local resources and financial support
2. problem identification and solution-finding within the family unit.

The DSMM has been developed for use in the UK by Keady & Nolan (1994a) in their Carer Led Assessment Process (CLASP).

Physical investigations

Routine investigations include a range of blood tests to screen for anaemia, thyroid disorders, inflammatory disorders and metabolic, renal and liver dysfunction. Chest and skull X-rays, electrocardiography and CT examination may also be carried out. CT is most helpful in patients with a reasonably high probability of VAD (to help confirm the diagnosis) or in those with a low probability (to exclude the diagnosis). Enlargement of the ventricles is the usual finding of CT in people with AD; this is reasonably sensitive but not specific to the disease. The use of neuroimaging with CT and increasingly MRI scanning is becoming more widespread and is seen as a useful aid to providing a diagnosis of dementia (Smith et al. 1996). However this can be problematic because of regional variations in availability of equipment.

Pharmacological treatments

Pharmacological intervention in dementia care falls into two main approaches: drugs used to relieve behavioural symptoms (e.g. agitation, aggression, psychosis, depression, apathy); and antidementia/cognitive-enhancing drugs. Until cognitive-enhancing drugs became widely available in the late 1990s, the main use of drugs was to relieve behavioural symptoms.

There has been increasing awareness that drugs used to control behaviour in dementia care can be open to abuse, resulting in the notion of 'the chemical cosh' (Burstow 2003). It is suggested that in order to prevent 'behavioural problems' people with dementia have been heavily sedated with little regard for the impact that this might have on their well-being (Burstow 2003). Many drugs that have an impact on behavioural symptoms also have side-effects which may make experiences of the condition worse. The drugs traditionally used are antipsychotic drugs and neuroleptics. These drugs were originally developed for the management of the hallucinatory and delusional symptoms associated with schizophrenia. Commonly used drugs include risperidone and olanzapine. However, recent evidence suggests that these drugs, previously considered relatively safe, can in fact induce strokes in people with dementia (Duff 2004). The use of antipsychotic medication in dementia care is therefore increasingly controversial and a guiding principle should be that these drugs should be avoided if at all possible, used only to treat hallucinations and delusions, and then for short periods of time (Alzheimer's Society 2004). It goes without saying that any decision to prescribe should be based upon a person-centred assessment.

Arguably, many of the so-called problem behaviours in dementia are a result of feelings of distress and anxiety. Consequently, it is considered that anxiety-relieving drugs may be more effective in relieving behavioural symptoms than antipsychotic drugs. However, associated side-effects, including unsteadiness and sedation, can contribute to an increased likelihood of falling (Hopker 1999).

While it is important to be clear that there are currently no treatments to cure dementia, cognitive-enhancing drugs developed for use in AD are playing an increasingly important role. In the brain of a person with AD there is not enough of the neurotransmitter acetylcholine, which is associated with the processing and storing of memory. In order to promote effective memory processing, acetylcholine is broken down in the brain by the enzyme acetylcholinesterase. The drugs Aricept and Exelon, which are acetylcholinesterase inhibitors, reduce the amount of acetylcholinesterase in the brain and therefore increase the concentration of acetylcholine. This is effective in temporarily improving cognitive ability in the early stages of AD.

The drug Reminyl works in the same way as the other acetylcholinesterase inhibitors but also has the effect of stimulating the nicotinic neuronal receptors in the brain, making them produce more acetylcholine. The latest of the cognitive-enhancing drugs, Ebixa, works in a different way and is more complex in its action. It blocks the neurotransmitter glutamate. Glutamate is released in excessive amounts in the brain of a person with AD, causing further damage to brain cells. Ebixa appears to be of use even in the middle stages of AD (Alzheimer's Society 2003c).

Within England and Wales the prescription of cognitive-enhancing drugs is covered by guidelines from NICE. These guidelines try to ensure equity of availability of the drugs to all who meet the criteria set by NICE. Within the guidelines the drugs are only used in AD, although there is evidence that they may also have a role in Lewy body dementia and VAD.

THE ROLE OF MEMORY CLINICS

Memory clinics were first established in the USA in the 1970s and were developed specifically to provide diagnostic, treatment and advisory services to people with early dementia. Since their introduction within the UK in the early 1980s their numbers have increased steadily (Thompson et al. 1997). The purpose of memory clinics is to provide a multidisciplinary outpatient service to diagnose and provide early detection of neurodegeneration. They may also provide assessment and follow-up (Lamers 2002).

Assessment in a memory clinic usually considers an individual's medical history, personal biography and insights into his or her relationships, beliefs and attitudes (Page 2003). Screening tools for cognitive function are also used. Memory clinics provide opportunities for comprehensive assessment and may contribute to an early diagnosis of dementia as well as identifying the underlying cause. Early diagnosis is particularly important since anti-dementia drugs are only effective in the early stages of the illness. A key role of memory clinics is to ensure that people with memory impairment are provided with information in a sensitive way that recognizes the potential impact of a diagnosis of dementia for the individual and the family. As well as comprehensive assessment, memory clinics may facilitate early intervention to limit the impact of dementia, particularly in the early stages. In addition to drug treatments, a number of behavioural interventions are available. For example, Wood (2001) highlights the growing interest in applying cognitive rehabilitation techniques with people with dementia, in order that they may 'hold on' to important information. Techniques include the use of internalized mnemonics to aid retrieval of information, reducing cognitive load, for example through environmental adaptations and memory aids, and enhancing learning. There is some evidence, particularly from single case studies, that these techniques can be helpful (Zanetti et al. 1997, Clare et al. 1999).

So far in this chapter, we have focused on the physical causes and features of dementia as a backdrop for considering some of the strategies and interventions that may be useful in helping people with dementia and their carers to cope with the condition. We now turn to some alternative ideas about ways in which dementia is experienced in order to extend the consideration of helping strategies further.

PSYCHOSOCIAL PERSPECTIVES OF DEMENTIA

The 'new' culture of dementia care reflects the view that there is much that can be done to improve the quality of life for people with dementia and their supporters while waiting for the 'magic bullets' of bio-medical science to effect a cure (Bond 1999). Without a doubt the most influential advances in thinking about ways to support people with dementia have arisen from the Bradford Dementia Research Group and the work of the late Tom Kitwood.

Kitwood's theory of dementia

The quality of support and care provided for people with cognitive impairment has been the focus of a body of work undertaken by Kitwood and the Brad-ford Dementia Research Group who highlight the role of social attitudes and care practices in the social con-struction of dementia. This work has been supported and extended by other researchers and theorists, such as Sabat & Harré (1992), working independently and reaching similar conclusions.

Earlier in this chapter some of the disease processes that are thought to contribute to the development of dementia were described. The implication of many bio-medical texts is that there is a direct causal relationship between these disease processes and dementia; that is, the disease process inflicts neurological damage on the brain, which results in dementia in its various forms. Kitwood and colleagues argue convincingly that this model is oversimplified. They suggest that, in reality, the presentation and experience of dementia in an individual arise from a complex interaction between five main factors (Bradford Dementia Group 1997):

1. neurological impairment (changes in the struc-ture and function of the neuron systems)
2. personality (including temperament, psycho-logical defences, coping style)
3. biography and recent life events
4. physical health and sensory awareness
5. an individual's social psychology, that is the set of relationships with individuals and groups with which we are all involved and which sur-round each of us in our day-to-day life.

Of these factors, it is the individual's social psychol-ogy that is most prominent in Kitwood's writings. He suggests an interplay between neurological impairment and 'the social psychology' that surrounds people with dementia and becomes increasingly 'malignant' as the disease progresses.

Malignant social psychology

In the course of his work Kitwood identified 17 aspects of malignant social psychology (MSP) (Kit-wood 1997b) that describe how carers, professionals and others unwittingly act towards people with dementia in ways that rob them of their confidence, self-esteem, sense of agency and eventually their per-sonhood. These aspects are summarized in Box 24.3.

Box 24.3   Aspects of the malignant social psychology of dementia

1. Treachery: using a form of deception to distract or manipulate people with dementia or force them to comply
2. Disempowerment: the person is not allowed to use retained abilities; failing to help in completing activities he/she has initiated
3. Infantilization: being patronizing (or matronizing)
4. Intimidation: threats or physical force being used to induce fear
5. Labelling: using a category, such as 'dementia', as the main basis upon which to interact with a per-son or explain his/her actions
6. Stigmatization: treating a person with dementia as if a diseased object
7. Outpacing: putting people with dementia under pressure to do things (e.g. make choices, perform activities) more rapidly than is possible for them; providing information at too fast a pace for them to understand
8. Invalidation: not acknowledging people's feelings or, more generally, their subjective reality

9. Banishment: physical or psychological exclusion of a person
10. Objectification: treating people as an object with-out regard to their status as sentient beings
11. Ignoring: carrying on (a conversation or action) in the presence of individuals as if they are not there
12. Imposition: forcing individuals to do something: overriding their desire, or denying them the possi-bility to make choices
13. Withholding: not meeting an evident need; refus-ing to give attention when asked
14. Accusation: blaming people for their actions or lack of action, which arise from lack of ability or misunderstanding of a situation
15. Disruption: breaking in on a person's action or reflection
16. Mockery: teasing or humiliating; making jokes at a person's expense
17. Disparagement: giving messages (e.g. implying worthlessness, incompetence) that are damaging to self-esteem

Many of the processes that comprise the MSP as described by Kitwood have also been identified in other research studies examining interactions between staff and older people in a range of care settings (Lanceley 1985, Armstrong-Esther et al. 1994, Davies et al. 2000).

Why should neurological impairment attract to itself an MSP? Kitwood (1990) identifies four reasons. Firstly, he argues that caregivers and service providers lack insight into their own actions, seeing care-giving as just common sense, as 'doing unto others as you would be done by'. Kitwood argues that this is an inadequate basis for the provision of high-quality care for people with dementia who are often less able to express their views and communicate their needs. As a consequence, carers of people with dementia need to go beyond common sense, and to empathize and seek to gain insight into the conceptual world of the person with dementia, then to draw upon their imagination and creativity to meet the needs of that person. Kitwood and others (Nolan et al. 2001) point out that the complex skills that these processes require are rarely acknowledged.

Secondly, Kitwood proposes that caring effectively for the person with dementia requires caregivers to cultivate an 'inner quietness' so that they are able to give their undivided attention to the messages given by the person with dementia. Unfortunately, exhaustion and depression among informal carers, and staff shortages and pressure of work in the health and social care services, mean that carers of people with dementia are not always able to cultivate such self-awareness. Thirdly, and more speculatively, Kitwood points to the MSP as a possible psychological defence against the anxiety of cognitive impairment that we all have to some extent. This defence lessens our ability and desire to form close relationships with those we care for. Fourthly, there is a tendency for carers to accept dominant stereotypes of people with dementia as 'non-persons', and thus to fail to treat them with the respect accorded to sentient beings, with social value and holding a distinct place in a social group.

These reasons suggest that MSP does not arise from any malicious intent on the part of carers, but rather from the routine, thoughtless activity of everyday caring in which people with dementia are dealt with in an overprofessional, overhelpful, patronizing manner, leading eventually to loss of 'personhood'. Kitwood suggests that the key to improving the care of people with dementia lies in improving the MSP. Strategies for improving the care experience of people with dementia based upon Kitwood's work are considered later in this chapter.

While undoubtedly influential, Kitwood's theory of dementia has been criticized for relying on limited empirical research which does not meet standard criteria of rigour (Adams 1996). More fundamental, though, is criticism directed at the concept of the MSP itself. Morton (1997) points out that Kitwood's description of the MSP could be applied in varying degrees to the social psychology of a range of people who are subject to social discrimination, and is not specific to people with dementia. In other words, aspects of the MSP are simply vivid descriptions of social relationships in which there is an imbalance of power. As such, Morton argues that the MSP provides an inadequate explanation of how the *specific* social psychology surrounding people with dementia develops.

Morton also argues that Kitwood's account of the social construction of dementia is insufficiently grounded in the structure of society and fails to take sufficient account of power relations. For Morton the MSP is, in fact, a general term which refers to the ways in which people relate to those with dementia. Consequently he argues that a proper focus of dementia care should be to improve these relations.

Relationship–centred care

Recognition of the complexity of relationships in health and social care has led to concerns about the adequacy of 'person-centred care' as the main outcome for health and social care services (Packer 2000, McCormack & McKenna 2001, Kizer 2002). Such concerns arise from the recognition that the notion of person-centredness fails to embrace explicitly the interdisciplinary and sociocultural nature of health care (Kizer 2002). Caring for older people with dementia is complex and requires a team approach to both identification of needs and therapeutic intervention. It also requires service providers to work in partnership with older people and their carers, drawing on each other's knowledge and experience (Brown et al. 2001, Nolan et al. 2002b). Focusing exclusively on the needs of the person with dementia runs the risk of overlooking the role of 'communitarian values' (Evans 1999) and the delicate interdependencies that characterize the best caring relationships (Nolan et al. 2002b, Brechin 1998). In a residential context, for example, the best care homes are 'communities' in a true sense, with high levels of interdependence between service users and service providers. This suggests a need to consider the experiences of all major stakeholders – residents, paid carers and family caregivers – in planning care for people with dementia (Gjerberg 1995, Stanley & Reed 1999).

More recently, commentators have highlighted the relevance of relationship-centred care as a concept to guide care practice with older people (Nolan et al. 2001). It has been argued for some time that caregiving can only be fully understood within the context of a relationship (Nolan et al. 1994, Brechin 1998) and yet the important dimensions of caring relationships have yet to be fully understood. Brechin argues that care is *primarily* about relationships, and any account which fails to consider these relationships will 'only reveal part of the story':

> If we want to understand 'good care' in the sense of care which brings positive consequences for those who are involved, then we must take account of the person and the relationship itself and not just see care as an instrumental means to an end (Brechin 1998: p. 177).

Brechin believes that care can only be seen as 'good' if it is good from the perspectives of all parties involved. This requires a construction of care which recognizes and acknowledges different perspectives, but which is underpinned by relationships based on mutual respect and a sense of equality.

These ideas are particularly relevant in the context of care provision for people with dementia and their families. Historically, dementia has been seen as having a destructive effect on relationships and the subject has received little attention. In particular, the potential therapeutic value of relationships between people with dementia and their caregivers has been neglected by researchers. A number of authors are now popularizing an approach to dementia care that explicitly recognizes the needs and contribution of three parties: (1) the person with dementia; (2) family carer(s); and (3) health and social care providers (Nolan et al. 2001, Adams et al. 2003). The remainder of this chapter is structured in order to reflect these diverse needs and contributions

In summary, theorizing and research which support dementia as a social construction challenge the view that dementia is the end-point of a relentless disease process over which individuals and their carers have little control, and propose a radical rethink about how dementia is managed at all stages. High-quality care for people with dementia requires carers to develop empathic understanding into the experience of dementia and to work imaginatively and creatively with people with dementia and their families. Interpersonal skills which help people with dementia to communicate with their carers are particularly important. Furthermore, Morton's critique of Kitwood's concept of MSP implies that nurses and other care workers should work not only with individuals and families, but also at a societal level to seek to reduce social discrimination generally and to improve the resources allocated to the care of people with dementia and their informal carers. Further research is also needed to test social constructionist theory for dementia care practice. A first step is to explore experiences of dementia from the perspective of people with the condition and their carers.

Experiences of dementia

The most important development in dementia care over the last decade has been a new awareness of the significance of the experience of the person with dementia (Wood 2001), and it is now recognized that understanding the nature of the subjective world of people with dementia is a prerequisite to humane, sensitive and individualized care. The dilemma for researchers and carers is how to gain access to the subjective experiences of people with dementia, when their capacity to communicate them is often disrupted. To date, our knowledge of the experience of dementia relies mainly on graphic accounts of the emotional, physical and social disruption associated with early dementia as described by individuals with the condition (see, for example, McGowin 1993, Hall 1994, DeBaggio 2002) and research involving interviews with people with dementia who are able to participate (Goldsmith 1996, Nygard & Borrell 1998, Keady & Gilliard 1999, Aggarwal et al. 2003). The most powerful accounts of dementia are undoubtedly those in the words of people experiencing the condition themselves:

> To me it's like knitting with a knotted ball of wool. Every now and then I come to a knot. I try to unravel it but can't so I knit the knot in. As time goes by there are more knots (Alzheimer's Society 2003f).
>
> I don't know where my head is, it's driving me mad. I can't remember anything (Aggarwal et al. 2003).
>
> I decided to cook a meal, which doesn't happen very often. I put the chops in the oven but couldn't remember how long to cook them. I looked in my cookery books but they didn't tell me. We have been married for 39 years and I had to ring my daughter to ask how long to cook chops. That made me feel very useless (Alzheimer's Society 2003).

What is clear from these accounts is that experiences of dementia are diverse and the meaning of these experiences uniquely individual (Russell 1996). However, there are some recurring themes. For example, several studies suggest that the experience of dementia changes over time. On the basis of interviews with 38 people with dementia Keady & Nolan (1994b, 1995a, 1995b, 1995c) identify the following stages: slipping, suspecting, covering up, revealing, confirming, surviving/maximizing, disorganization, decline and death. The notion of 'maximizing' reflects continual adaptation by individuals to their situation and environment, together with continual appraisal of personal coping strategies. A second theme within personal accounts of dementia is that of loss. In interviews with 27 people at various stages of dementia, Aggarwal et al. (2003) found numerous descriptions of loss, including loss of independence, dignity, and friends and relatives, as well as the more obvious loss of memory.

More recently there have been attempts to access the world and experiences of people with moderate to severe dementia directly, using a range of approaches. Hubbard et al. (2003) describe an ethnographic approach using extended periods of observation and repeated informal interviews with older people with dementia in residential settings. They identified exercising control and rights, maintaining and developing relationships and having meaningful activity and interaction within the context of the care home as particularly important to their quality of life. Similarly, Killick describes powerfully how he developed insights into the life-world of older people with dementia by living alongside them in a residential home and engaging them in indepth conversations that were tape-recorded and then analysed for meaning (Killick & Allen 2001). Killick also uses a degree of 'poetic licence' to develop poems based on the words of people with dementia. These convey a 'feeling' of what the person might be trying to communicate rather than focusing on the precise meaning of the words used (Innes & Capstick 2001). However, Innes & Capstick (2001) caution that interpretation of such constructions may be complex:

> The words of a person with dementia may be concrete statements of fact, but they may also be allusive, referring only briefly or indirectly to the person's true cause for concern. Communication may also have metaphorical significance, linking events, people or places somehow connected in the person's mind (Innes & Capstick 2001: p. 141).

Other approaches to understanding the lived experience of people with dementia include the use of video (Cook 2002), which allows access to the non-verbal strategies used by people with dementia in their attempts to communicate. Murphy et al. (2005) describes the use of 'talking mats', a low-technology communication resource to help frail older people, including those with dementia, to express their views and feelings. This technology has proved particularly useful in identifying factors that promote and inhibit quality of life for frail older people living in care homes (Tester et al. 2003).

Communicating with people with dementia about their experiences is further complicated if the ethnic and cultural background of the person is not fully understood (Innes & Capstick 2001). Little is known about cultural and ethnic differences in the experience of dementia. However, it would appear that dementia is often construed as 'normal ageing' (Patel et al. 1998). In a qualitative study of awareness and understanding of dementia symptoms in families of South Asian and African/Caribbean descent in the UK, Adamson (2001) found that knowledge of dementia was limited, both in terms of awareness of the condition and understanding of the causes. Difficulties in caring relationships could be attributed to a lack of understanding of the condition, particularly when family members blamed the person with dementia for his or her symptoms. The provision of accurate information about dementia in an accessible format is an important task for health and social care practitioners, particularly when caring for people from different cultures. Bowes & Wilkinson (2003) explored the experiences of South Asian people with a diagnosis of dementia through interviews with professionals working with them and four case studies. The case studies demonstrated overwhelmingly negative experiences of dementia, with poor quality of life, desperate needs for support, lack of access to appropriate services, little knowledge of dementia and isolation from community and family life. The Audit Commission report on mental health services (Audit Commission 2002) also reinforced the need for urgent attention to the mental health needs of older people from ethnic-minority groups.

In summary, creative methodologies are enabling us to develop new insights into the lived experience of dementia that will help to shape service provision in the future. What is currently clear is that experiences of dementia are diverse and individual. However, it is vital that service developments also take into account the views and experiences of family caregivers and it is to these that we now turn.

Family caregiver perspectives

Whereas the number of personal accounts of dementia are limited, there has been a wealth of research exploring the experiences of family members caring for a person with dementia. The difficulties family caregivers experience at each stage of the caregiving 'career' have been well documented (Dellasega & Mastrian 1995, Kellett 1999, Butcher et al. 2001, Davies 2001, Aggarwal et al. 2003):

> It's awful. A terrible situation. Each phase is a terrible phase. You sort of have a plateau going along and then something else stops and it's a big hurdle you have to get over and then you go along on another plateau (Aggarwal et al. 2003).

> When the diagnosis was confirmed at the hospital, we had little support compared to the support a person with cancer receives at the point of diagnosis. There was no specialist nurse, no referral to the help-group, not even a telephone number. Like hundreds of others, we were simply dropped into thin air (Alzheimer's Society 2003e).

Family caregivers report their most frequent unmet needs as:

- to know that someone will provide care when they are unable to do so
- a telephone hotline
- time away from caring duties
- ways to deal with stress
- time for physical rest
- ways to deal with feelings of being trapped (Leong et al. 2001).

However, even when services to meet these needs are provided, family caregivers do not always make use of them (Nolan et al. 2002a). This can be due to a lack of flexibility in service provision, or to the carer's judgement about the relative 'costs and benefits' of accepting help (Davies & Nolan 2003). For example, carers may find that the person with dementia is so disoriented and distressed by a period of respite care that they decide that any benefits to themselves are outweighed by the cost to the person they are caring for. The inability of formal service providers to respond to the needs of people with dementia and their carers in ways they will find helpful is succinctly captured by the husband of an older lady with dementia, interviewed as part of a study of relatives' experiences of nursing-home entry (Davies 2001: p. 113):

> SD: Did you get any help from the social services?
> No, no, they offered. But I didn't know what they could do and I said 'What can you do?' She said: 'Well, we can get her dressed in the morning', because that's where I was having a problem. I says: 'Fair enough, but what time are you going to come and get her up?' She says: 'Well what time do you want me?' I says: 'I don't know, she gets up any time; pick a time from two o'clock in the morning onwards'. I says: 'I know you can't come' (Reg, husband).

Despite the extensive literature in the field of family care, there is remarkably little evidence for the effectiveness of interventions to support family caregivers (Pusey & Richards 2001, Zarit & Leitsch 2001). This is attributed to the dominance of the stress-coping model in the majority of studies, which emphasizes the burden and difficulties faced by family carers whilst failing to acknowledge and build upon the satisfactions and rewards of caregiving. An increasing body of research is suggesting that family caregivers particularly appreciate attempts by formal caregivers to create partnerships with them and recognize their knowledge and experience (Lundh et al. 2003). However, evidence suggests that such positive experiences are not yet the norm and that care staff frequently fail to acknowledge and draw upon the expertise of family caregivers in planning and implementing care for the person with dementia (Naleppa 1996, Hertzberg & Ekman 2000). This is in spite of evidence demonstrating the benefits for all concerned of involving family members (McDerment et al. 1997, Specht et al. 2000, Pillemer et al. 2003). In Box 24.4, Una Martin describes her experiences of caring for her husband Ernest after he developed AD. Una's story illustrates the best and worst in relationships with service providers.

Paid carer perspectives

Nurses will encounter people with dementia in a wide range of care settings. For example, the development of community-based services for people with dementia is resulting in new challenges for health and social care providers. Caring for people with dementia in any care setting, and ensuring that this care is of a high quality, requires a sophisticated level of skill and knowledge and staff need support if disaffection and burnout are to be avoided (Marshall 2001). Graham (1999) described how a process of clinical supervision enabled a team of six community psychiatric nurses to improve patient-centred care and relieve feelings of burnout, stress and tedium when caring for people with dementia. Findings of this study suggest that the education of community psychiatric nurses needs to enable them to develop 'emotional competence' and to adopt a reflexive and self-questioning approach within their work. Certainly, the contribution of 'emotion work' to the care of people with dementia is emerging as an important area for further research. Berg et al. (1998), for example, discuss how nurses described a 'mutual interdependency' with patients with dementia during the caring process, resulting in

Box 24.4 Una's story

Ernest and I had been married for 35 years when I began to notice subtle changes in his personality. He was 59 years old. We had a very happy marriage and Ernest was the funniest, kindest, loveliest man you could ever wish to meet, extrovert, outgoing with a wicked sense of humour and very popular with everyone. A truly good man and my best friend. We had raised two lovely daughters and we were looking forward to a long and happy retirement together. We were financially secure and had everything we could possibly need. Ernest worked for British Steel as a departmental foreman having responsibility for some 30 men. He had started work there 35 years earlier as a general labourer and had worked his way up.

The first sign I had that something was wrong was when Ernest didn't want to go to work. He had always been a conscientious worker, never taking time off, but the time came when he never got a full week in, taking odd days off for no apparent reason. I suspected that there might be problems at work but when I tried to discuss this with him he just became abusive and refused to talk about it, saying that the problem was in *my* head and there was nothing wrong with *him*.

He began to have frequent unexplained illnesses, none of them conclusive, culminating in a stay in hospital under investigation for abdominal pain. During his time in hospital he became very confused and aggressive, but despite voicing my concerns to the staff, I was assured that this was quite common in 'elderly' patients in hospital. Ernest was 60 years of age. Elderly? I don't think so. They never did find the cause of his illness and he was subsequently discharged.

Things carried on very much the same, but Ernest was becoming more and more reliant on me. Although he had always been very self-sufficient, gradually he could no longer care for himself – he couldn't even make himself a cup of tea. At one time he could have prepared and cooked a three-course meal without batting an eyelid!

I was so worried that eventually I consulted our GP and explained the situation to him. He didn't want to know! So back to square one. If only he had known how much courage it had taken for me to admit to another person that there was something wrong with my beloved husband. I hadn't even confided in my family. I felt so alone. I felt as though I had betrayed Ernest's trust, although he was rapidly becoming a stranger to me.

After 2 years of pestering the doctor and more or less pleading with him, he eventually agreed to see Ernest on the pretext of carrying out routine blood tests. He diagnosed that Ernest was suffering from 'a bit of depression' and he prescribed an antidepressant.

From that point onwards, over a period of a few weeks, things went from bad to worse, to the point when I was afraid to leave Ernest alone because I feared for his safety. By this time I was desperate and eventually the doctor agreed to refer Ernest to a geriatric consultant.

In 1999 Ernest was diagnosed with Alzheimer's disease. The consultant arranged for him to attend a day hospital two mornings a week, and then the dementia support service at the hospital provided a sitter for one full day a week. In addition Ernest went into respite care for 2 weeks in every 8.

It was at this time that I became a member of the local branch of the Alzheimer's Society. I attended a caring and coping course and they also guided me through the financial minefield. They helped me to obtain attendance allowance, a council tax reduction and a power of attorney. They also kept in regular contact with me to see if I needed any help or advice, and without them I don't think I would have got through.

I was advised by the consultant and the social worker to start looking at care homes, and this I did over the next 12 months. I was appalled by some of the homes I saw and would not have entertained them as I wanted the best for Ernest. I only found one that I was truly happy with, but they were unable to take him because he was too active and challenging. However, at that stage I was in no hurry because I wanted to keep Ernest for as long as possible and I knew that I would know when it was time to let go.

As time went by Ernest became more and more demanding and unpredictable.

I vividly remember one occasion when he took the car keys from my handbag and drove the car away. I had already surrendered his driving licence when it became clear that it was unsafe for him to drive. I immediately rang the police, but it was 2 hours before they found him – the longest 2 hours of my life. He had no idea where he had been, although the police found him in Derbyshire. I now realized that I would have to be two steps ahead of him all the time and doubly vigilant. The strain was taking its toll.

Eventually things became so bad that I knew the time had come when I had to do something. I was having very little sleep because Ernest was getting up several times during the night and trying to get out of the house. At other times he would want to go to bed at 6 in the evening, or else he would refuse to go to bed at all, so we both had to spend the night downstairs because I was afraid to leave him on his own. He was also becoming violent. I was at rock bottom, and but for the help of

Continued

Box 24.4   Una's story (*Continued*)

Alzheimer's Society and Cedars (a day hospital within an NHS mental health trust), I think I would have gone under. What would have happened to Ernest then?

It was then that the consultant stepped in and admitted Ernest for assessment. He strongly advised me to consider full-time care, and to let him know when I had found a suitable care home.

And so my search began again, without success. Then, quite by chance, I heard about Birch Avenue. I went along without an appointment and was very impressed by what I saw. The staff were very open and answered any questions which I had. I was taken on a detailed tour of the home, including a couple of the residents' rooms, the kitchen and bathrooms. I saw food being prepared and was able to inspect menus. I was most impressed by the variety and quality of food provided. I came away knowing that Birch Avenue was the right home for Ernest, and I felt as though a load had been lifted from my shoulders. Ann Powell, the manager, went across to Pinecroft (an assessment unit within an NHS mental health trust) to assess Ernest, and I am happy to say that he was accepted.

A few days before he moved into Birch Avenue, I was invited to go along and personalize his room. I was made very welcome by everyone I met and I knew that Ernest would be made to feel at home when he moved in.

Ernest has been at Birch Avenue now since October 2001 and after the initial period he settled in well. I can visit whenever I want to and there are facilities for me to make a cup of tea for us to enjoy together. I can also have a meal with him at any time and I feel this adds a touch of normality to his life.

The decision to put Ernest into care is the hardest decision I have ever had to make and I spent many sleepless nights and shed bitter tears at a very frightening and traumatic time of my life. However, in retrospect, I can honestly say that I have never for one moment regretted my decision and I know now that it was the right one. I don't think the guilt will ever go away, but I am learning to live with it and each day it gets easier.

Unless you have lived with the hell that is dementia you cannot imagine how destructive it can be, and my heart goes out to anyone who is caring for their loved one alone.

Seek all the help you can and don't be too proud to ask. Be open about your loved one's illness because people do understand. The guilt never goes away but don't let it destroy your life. Your loved one would not want you to be tearing yourself apart and you owe it to them to live your life to the full.

---

an 'intertwined life'. Similarly, Rundqvist & Severinsson (1999) report that nurses caring for older people with dementia described the most important aspects of their relationships with their patients as touching (including caressing and hugging), confirmation (involving mutuality and sensitivity) and promoting positive values within the caring culture such as consideration, patience and compassion. Such 'emotional labour' can be very demanding and is inevitably linked to the well-being of the nurse carer (Gattuso & Bevan 2000). These arguments resonate with Brechin's assertion (Brechin 1998), mentioned earlier, that any analysis of care must address the experiences of all those involved so as to tease out the tensions and pressures which militate against good care in order to help identify and build appropriate support.

Nurses have highlighted the particular challenges of caring for people with dementia in acute care environments (Davies et al. 1999, Tolson et al. 1999). A number of strategies have been found to be useful, including:

- avoiding long waits in casualty by admitting straight to a ward if possible

- finding out from family members what normally helps to calm the person
- involving family members in direct caregiving when appropriate
- liaising with specialist staff for advice and support (Davies et al. 1999).

While recognizing the demands of caring for people with dementia, it is important to consider the sources of satisfaction and reward in caregiving for paid staff if person-centred and relationship-centred dementia care are to be achieved. Ryan et al. (2004) identified high levels of job satisfaction among community-based dementia care workers, enhanced by the ability to maintain relationships with people with dementia and their families, and feelings of contributing to and improving the status and quality of life of people with dementia. Innovative approaches to service provision are enabling practitioners to use their skills and creativity to ensure that older people with dementia receive the care and services they need. In Box 24.5, Ann Powell, leader of a community-based assessment team, describes the satisfaction of enabling an older person with dementia to return home following admission to hospital.

Box 24.5   A nurse's story

Ann Powell is nurse leader of the Accelerated Discharge Dementia (ADD) team, part of Sheffield Care Trust. She describes how the team worked to enable a 75-year-old man, Mr James, to return home.

I first met Mr James [when he] had been admitted to hospital during a visit to the falls clinic. He had fallen at home 2 weeks previously and the clinic staff suspected a subdural haematoma. Mr James had been admitted to the admissions ward and was awaiting a computed tomography (CT) scan. The ward staff felt he was confused. Mr James was not happy to be kept in hospital and could not understand what all the fuss was about. He kept requesting to go home.

I introduced myself to Mr James and explained my role and how I work with people who have memory problems and help them to return to their own home as soon as possible. I explained that before I could become involved with his care we would have to know the results of his CT scan, but I would be contacting his family if that was all right with him; he said it was. He did acknowledge that his memory was not as good as it used to be.

Later that day I met Mr James and his daughter. I took a full history and identified that Mr James's memory had been deteriorating for a number of years. The memory problems had only come to his daughter's attention following her mother's death 3 years ago, but Mr James had managed very well with her help. He had routines and was fiercely independent.

Mr James had had several falls over the last year and that is how he had come to be referred to the falls clinic. He was also being treated for hypertension. I discussed with Mr James and his daughter that he would be transferred to a specialist medical ward for people who had memory problems and this was arranged for the following day.

Mr James's CT scan results showed no subdural haematoma and I discussed with him and his family that the team would now be working with them to enable Mr James to return home as soon as possible. I introduced two support workers to Mr James and his family and they spent time getting to know each other. I performed the standardized Mini-Mental State Examination and Mr James scored 18/30, indicating moderate cognitive impairment. He told me that his memory problems were better some days than others. Mr James and his family were given his diagnosis of vascular dementia, but he didn't seem to take much notice of this. He said he was never happy to be in hospital. I contacted the falls clinic and informed them of Mr James's admission and proposed discharge date. They had already referred him to a community occupational therapist and they said they would send him his next appointment to clinic 2 weeks after discharge from hospital. I made them aware I would do a home visit risk assessment and let them know what I had found.

I met with the support workers, Mr James and his daughter to discuss the home visit. We agreed that Mr James would not go on the home visit as he was adamant he would not return to the ward afterwards, even though he said he liked all the staff; so one of the support workers came with me. During the home visit, we identified that an extra banister was required on the stairs and a nursing night light was needed to light the way to the bathroom for Mr James at night. His family felt that they did not require any other aids or help at this time, apart from an alarm on the front door so that Mr James's daughter could be alerted if he left the house without her knowing. All these modifications were arranged.

During the twice-weekly home visits following his discharge, the support workers were able to arrange a number of additional services, including a referral to the Alzheimer's Society for carer support and a referral to a sitting service to provide sensory stimulation and respite care. They also arranged for attendance allowance forms to be sent. Mr James was quite happy for someone to visit him and take him out to the places he wanted to go to and do the things he wanted to do. Following discharge from the team, a letter about our involvement was sent to his GP.

Working with Mr James was a very positive experience for the team. At first we were not sure how long it would take to get him home but we were pleased that we were able to achieve this within 7 days. The two team members allocated to work closely with him worked very hard to build up a relationship with Mr James, so that he could trust them. We were all apprehensive about Mr James's discharge and tried not to think too much about the risks, but we were able to discuss this as a team. It was frustrating at times because other services took longer to get involved or provide aids and adaptations than we would have liked. However, once he had been discharged from the team we were able to look back and think that we had done a good job.

Within continuing care settings there is evidence that relationships with residents are key factors in determining job satisfaction for staff (Moyle et al. 2003). Nursing assistants have identified their relationships with residents as the most important work issue and their major reason for staying in the job (Parsons et al. 2003). However, staff within care homes also need a clear therapeutic direction for their work if they are to experience job satisfaction. Hansebo & Kihlgren (2002) suggest that one of the main challenges for carers of people with cognitive frailty is to feel that their communication with residents is worthwhile, which is a prerequisite if they are to experience their caring as meaningful. Furthermore, staff need to feel that they are appreciated by residents and their families (Campbell 2003).

Collectively, these findings suggest that preparation for emotion work and working in partnership are essential prerequisites for working effectively with people with dementia and their carers.

CREATING POSITIVE ENVIRONMENTS FOR CARE

There is now considerable agreement about the principles upon which high-quality care for people with dementia and their families is based. For example:

- People with dementia have the same human value as anyone else, irrespective of their degree of disability or independence
- People with dementia have the same varied human needs as anyone else
- People with dementia have the same rights as other citizens
- Every person with dementia is an individual
- People with dementia have the right to forms of support that do not exploit family and friends (King's Fund 1986).

In a positive care environment where care is underpinned by such principles, there is evidence that people with dementia can maintain high levels of well-being (Bruce et al. 2002, Weaks & Boardman 2003). Care practices can positively influence the course and experience of dementia in two main ways: (1) by enabling each resident to remain in the best possible physical health, including full use of the senses of sight and hearing; and (2) by providing a physical and social environment which meets their needs and so empowers and sustains them.

The needs of people with dementia

Kitwood (1997a) identifies five core needs that must be met if any human being is to function as a person.

These needs are present in all human beings, but are likely to be more obvious in people with dementia, who are more vulnerable than the rest of us and usually less able to take the initiative to ensure their needs are met. These needs are for:

1. Comfort. This entails providing a feeling of security, warmth and strength which comes from feeling close to another person. For people with dementia this need is likely to be associated most acutely with loss, which may arise from a number of factors, such as bereavement, failing abilities or finishing a long-established pattern of life. Kitwood suggests that the heightened sexual desire of some people with dementia may be, at least in part, an expression of this need

2. Attachment. Forming bonds or attachments with others is evidence that we are a social species. In the early years of life attachments form a safety net in a perceptual world characterized by uncertainty. In dementia life is overshadowed by many uncertainties and anxieties, and memories of past secure attachments may be lost. Miesen (1992) suggests that the strangeness of the world as experienced by people with dementia is likely to invoke the attachment need

3. Inclusion. The need for inclusion is shown by the fact that human beings have always lived as members of social groups, but social isolation is all too frequently integral to the experience of dementia. For many people, social activity and interaction diminish as the dialectic interplay between the malignant social psychology and neurological impairment takes its course. The need for inclusion may be expressed in dementia in the form of so-called 'attention-seeking' or 'disruptive' behaviours, forms of protest and clinging or hovering behaviours. In traditional care environments the need for inclusion is often overlooked; residents may be cared for together, but no effort is made to foster a sense of group cohesion. Individual packages of care, although a great step forward, may also overlook the need for inclusion

4. Occupation. People may be occupied in the company of others or alone. Occupation might involve working on a project, playing, reflecting or relaxing. Whatever form it takes, occupation is a sense of feeling involved with life that draws on abilities and interests in a way that is personally satisfying. The opposite is a

sense of boredom and apathy. The need for occupation is overlooked in many care settings

5. Identity. Having a sense of identity entails having a sense of continuity with one's past and across the different roles and contexts of life in the present, and having a story to tell about one's life. In dementia a person's sense of identity is under threat from failing memory and mental agility. It is also threatened by institutional care regimens when familiar objects, people and routines are removed. Kitwood suggests that two things are essential if carers are to help the person with dementia to maintain his or her identity: (1) detailed knowledge of the person's past history; and (2) empathic understanding, that is, the ability to respond to the uniqueness of each individual.

An alternative framework for thinking about the needs of older people, including older people with dementia, is being developed by Mike Nolan and colleagues at the University of Sheffield. The Senses Framework (Nolan et al. 2002b, 2003) overlaps in many areas with the needs identified by Kitwood, but differs in that it also provides a way of thinking about the needs of families and staff working with older people. In this way, it provides a framework for considering how 'relationship-centred care' might be achieved. Nolan first developed the framework as a response to the lack of a therapeutic rationale for work with older people in long-term care settings (Nolan 1997). He identified six 'senses' which he believed might provide direction for staff and improve the care older people received. The term 'sense' was deliberately chosen to reflect the subjective and perceptual nature of the important determinants of care for both older people and staff. These 'fundamentals' were termed: a sense of security, belonging, continuity, purpose, achievement and significance. The Senses Framework has now been refined and developed within a series of research projects exploring the needs of older people and family caregivers within a range of contexts (Davies et al. 1999, Nolan et al. 2001, 2002b) and the main elements of each 'sense' are shown in Box 24.6. One advantage of the Senses Framework is that it prompts consideration of the important components of care from the perspective of older people, family members and staff working with them. Furthermore, by linking the experiences of older people, their families and staff, the Senses Framework has the potential to promote understanding of the experiences of others, thus enhancing communication and the ability to work in partnership.

Box 24.6   Six senses to guide practice with older people and their families

1. A sense of security – feeling safe
2. A sense of continuity – experiencing links between the past, the present and the future
3. A sense of belonging – having a 'place'
4. A sense of purpose – having direction
5. A sense of fulfilment –feeling you're getting somewhere
6. A sense of significance – feeling you matter

While Box 24.6 includes a broad definition of the senses for older people and for family caregivers, the way in which each sense can be achieved will vary according to the context and caregiving situation. Table 24.3 provides some suggestions for achieving the senses for older people living in care homes and their family caregivers. These are based on group discussions with nurses, care assistants, older people and family caregivers undertaken within the context of a series of research projects (Davies 2001, Nolan et al. 2001, Davies et al. 2002).

The focus of care

The needs of people with dementia identified within the previous section suggest four important foci if positive environments for dementia care are to be created and sustained:

1. Shaping the values of carers. It is crucial that carers perceive people with dementia as valuable and complete human beings deserving of respect, and not simply 'objects of care'. The importance of careful recruitment of care staff, training, supervision and support is paramount

2. Promoting individualized care. This is care which is relevant to each person who is a product of a unique set of life experiences, preferences, values, abilities and needs. This requires individual assessment and time spent getting to know people with dementia as individuals. It also involves working closely with family caregivers

3. Creating a supportive physical and social environment. People with cognitive disability are more dependent upon supports within their physical and social environment than most people and, paradoxically, are less able than the rest of us to take steps unaided to adapt to and control their environment

Table 24.3   Examples of factors within continuing care environments that create the 'senses' for older people, their family carers and staff

Sense	Older people	Family carers	Staff
Security	Staff introduce visitors to the home to residents Staff respond promptly to requests for help Staff make sure that a resident's call bell is within reach	Relatives are kept informed about a resident's condition and well-being Staff are approachable There is a clear procedure for complaints	Staff have access to training New staff have an induction period Staff feel able to raise concerns in an open and honest manner
Significance	Staff show interest in residents' former lives Staff ask permission before touching residents' personal belongings Staff always knock and wait to be invited in before entering residents' rooms	Staff value relatives' contribution to care planning Staff are interested in the needs and well-being of relatives	Staff members have a say in the way the home is run Staff members have a regular appraisal
Belonging	Residents can have their own place in the dining room if they wish Staff help residents to build relationships with other residents Residents are consulted about the running of the home	Relatives are welcomed on arrival at the home Relatives are offered refreshments during their visit Relatives are invited to social events within the home	Staff work as a team There is a regular newsletter There are regular staff meetings
Purpose	Residents are encouraged and supported to enjoy their interests and hobbies Staff help residents to plan for the future Residents have the opportunity to carry out tasks around the home	Relatives are encouraged to contribute to the care of their resident Relatives have an opportunity to influence what goes on in the home, for example through a relatives' committee or action group	Therapeutic goals of care for individual residents are explicit within care plans Staff members have individual specialist roles within the home There are opportunities to pursue personal career goals and aspirations
Continuity	The same staff members work with each resident Staff involve family members in a resident's care Residents can choose their daily activities	A primary nurse and/or keyworker are identified for each resident Staff assist relatives to continue to enjoy valued activities with residents	Expected standards of care are made explicit There is a stated philosophy of care Staff members are enabled to work with the same residents and their families
Achievement	Staff encourage residents to feel proud of their achievements during their lives Staff provide feedback on progress towards goals	Relatives receive feedback from staff on their contribution to care within the home	Staff receive regular feedback on their performance from managers and peers Staff have opportunities to receive feedback from residents and relatives

4. Enabling effective communication. Effective communication is a prerequisite for good relationships and the quality of the relationships between people with dementia and those around them is an important influence on how they cope with their illness.

While there is overlap between these areas, each will now be considered in more detail in order to highlight recent research contributing to our understanding of ways in which a positive culture of care for people with dementia and their families can be created and sustained.

Shaping the values of carers and making shared values explicit

It could be argued that attempts to create and strengthen awareness among care staff of the potential to enhance the life quality of people with dementia currently holds the greatest prospect for improving the day-to-day experiences of people with dementia and their carers. Furthermore, the interrelationship between the experiences of residents, their families and staff indicated by notions of relationship-centred care suggests that approaches that seek to create a shared set of values within care environments are likely to have the most impact on care experiences. On the basis of an indepth ethnographic study of a single nursing home in the USA, Powers (2001) highlights four domains in which shared values can enhance quality of life for residents with dementia and those who care for them. These domains are:

1. preserving the integrity of the individual
2. defining community norms and values
3. learning the limits of intervention
4. tempering the culture of surveillance and restraint.

Although in need of further development and testing, Powers suggests that this typology provides an ethical framework that can be used to support decision-making in relation to everyday issues concerning people with dementia in residential settings. Stanley & Reed (1999) also highlight the importance of shared values in moving care forward within residential settings. They propose a system of 'ethical audit' involving a range of stakeholders, an investigation of the values within a care home and an exploration of how those values are manifested in practice. This, they suggest, should then lead into an explicit agenda for change. Davies et al. (2002) describe how a similar approach was adopted with staff and relatives of residents at a nursing home for people with dementia in Sheffield, England. The importance of ensuring that services are developed and evaluated on the basis of shared values that are made explicit also emerges on the basis of a review of the literature on research with family carers and people with dementia (Nolan et al. 2002a). It is argued that the reason why many services for older people with dementia have not been as successful as might have been anticipated lies in the failure to recognize 'the intersubjectivity of dementia' and lack of attention to the relational aspects of care.

In Chapter 9, Claire Goodman and Sally Redfern highlighted the limited opportunities for education and training for staff working in long-term care settings. Training in the care of people with dementia has been found to improve staff attitudes and caring behaviours, but this may be insufficient to produce good outcomes for the recipients of care where there are organizational obstacles holding back positive change (Lintern et al. 2000). On the basis of group interviews with community practitioners, Iliffe & Manthorpe (2004) suggest that education for dementia care needs to encourage practitioners to reflect on their own emotional responses to dementia and the value of learning from the person with dementia in order to create the right approach.

Promoting individualized care

One of the best indicators of high-quality care for older people with dementia, whether they live in a care home or in their own home, is the extent to which the individuality of the person with dementia is respected and care strategies enable them to maintain their dignity, personality and personal relationships, and promote their self-esteem. In addition to the shared values already discussed, factors relating to these issues include careful assessment (discussed earlier and in Chapter 28), the development of individualized care plans based on personal biography, creating positive relationships and successful communication.

The importance of personal biography   Individual care plans rely upon paid carers having a sound knowledge of the person's unique and personal biography. Understanding a person's past and knowing what causes aggravation, what brings happiness and what makes a day meaningful all help to preserve the individual's identity (Powers 2001). For people with severe dementia this usually relies on close consultation with relatives and friends, who may be asked to develop a written (possibly illustrated) history of the person with dementia. Clarke et al. (2003), for example, describe a developmental project to investigate the introduction of a biographical approach to care on a unit within a National Health Service hospital. Findings revealed that life stories helped practitioners to see patients as people, to understand individuals more fully and to form closer relationships with their families. Reichman et al. (2004) have developed a guide to compiling life-history resources for older people living in care homes.

Maintaining personal contacts Continuing contact with family and friends is important for older people with dementia and these people should be encouraged to be involved in the life and activities of the hospital ward, care home or residential unit. In addition to providing affection and continuity for the person with dementia (Fleming 1998), relatives have the potential to provide a source of support for care staff, as well as contributing to the sense of community within a care home (Hertzberg & Ekman 2000, Davies 2001). Relatives may wish to continue to be involved in the day-to-day care of the person with dementia; for example, by assisting them at mealtimes. Some may wish to continue to be involved in more intimate care tasks and this should be encouraged and supported if this is in accord with the wishes of the person with dementia.

At times, visiting may be difficult for relatives, particularly if the person with dementia no longer recognizes them or becomes distressed when they are about to leave. Paid carers have an important role in supporting relatives and helping them to enjoy their visits. A relatives' support group is a feature of some

residential units and may provide valuable peer support. The best care homes go further and involve family members and volunteers in the life of the home in a range of creative ways (Burton-Jones 2001). Box 24.7 describes the work of the Support 67 Action Group, a group of staff and relatives of residents at a nursing home for older people with dementia in Sheffield, who meet regularly to plan ways to enhance the care home as an environment for living, working and learning (see also Davies et al. 2002).

Promoting choice and opportunity The continuing importance of maintaining personal control in day-to-day activities as far as possible is apparent within several studies of the views of older people with dementia about their care (Bamford & Bruce 2000, Tester et al. 2003). On the basis of focus groups involving people with dementia, Bamford & Bruce identified a series of desired outcomes at which care services should be aiming (Box 24.8). Their findings confirm the importance of 'having a say' in the development of services and maintaining their personal autonomy as far as possible.

To some extent, routine and order are important to people with dementia because these increase the predictability of events and so allow them more control over their lives. However, because people with dementia may find it difficult to express their wishes, they are particularly at risk if care routines become

---

Box 24.7   The Support 67 Action Group

67 Birch Avenue in Sheffield is a nursing home providing care for up to 40 older people with dementia. Since 2001, researchers at a nearby university have been working in partnership with staff, residents and relatives at the home with the aim of developing care practice and creating a positive environment for living, working and learning. The main principle guiding this work is the need to ensure that all participants – residents, relatives and staff – feel that they are valued members of the nursing-home community.

The project is using an action research approach to plan and evaluate developments. Initially, questionnaires were completed by staff and relatives and these provided the basis for discussion at a series of staff away-days. A feedback report highlighted areas that would most improve the experiences of residents, relatives, staff and students and this was circulated to everyone involved. Following the identification of needs and priorities, an action group was established to take ideas forward. The Support 67 Action Group meets monthly and includes

relatives of residents and representatives of all staff groups within the home, including domestic and catering staff. Senior managers of the care trust and housing association jointly responsible for managing the home also attend, ensuring that decisions can be acted upon quickly.

Achievements to date include:

- establishing an activities programme for residents, including assessment of each individual's abilities and interests
- production of a booklet for relatives aimed at easing the transition to life within the home
- setting up an information and support group for relatives
- developing resources to support student nurses on placement at the home.

Early evaluation suggests that the partnership project has enhanced communication and provided a renewed sense of purpose and achievement for relatives and staff alike.

Box 24.8   Desirable outcomes for community services identified by older people with dementia

Service-process outcomes
- Having a say in services
- Feeling valued and respected
- Being treated as an individual
- Being able to relate to other service users

Quality-of-life outcomes
- Access to social contact and company
- Having a sense of social integration
- Access to meaningful activity and stimulation
- Maximizing a sense of autonomy
- Maintaining a sense of personal identity
- Feeling safe and secure
- Feeling financially secure
- Being personally clean and comfortable

---

inflexible and fail to respond to individual needs and preferences. Graneheim et al.'s (2001) account of interactions between care staff and an older woman with dementia residing in a nursing home provides a powerful example of ways in which staff can unknowingly restrict or limit a resident's choices. Within residential settings, it is desirable to allow people with dementia to establish their own routine as far as possible, and then to support this through a structured and dependable programme of care to which changes are introduced slowly and only after careful preparation.

Individualized care at the end of life   The experiences and needs of people with dementia who are dying are beginning to be explored and the important contribution of specialist palliative care at this time is now recognized (Seymour & Hanson 2001). People with dementia may die at any stage during their illness and, like other older people, would prefer a homely and peaceful death. Wherever possible, moving individuals with dementia from their familiar environment when they are dying should be avoided and this may involve providing additional support to the carers who know them best. For people with dementia, the issues of pain and communication are likely to be central (Cox & Cook 2002). People with advanced dementia are often unable to report their level of pain and carers should be alert for other signs of pain, such as restlessness and agitation. Palliative care should be interdisciplinary, involving pain and symptom management, emotional and spiritual care and bereave-

ment support for families and care staff (Zerzan et al. 2000). Family carers are also likely to find decision-making about treatment options at the end of life difficult and emotionally stressful, and will need careful support (Hurley & Volicer 2002).

Creating an appropriate physical and social environment

Marshall (2001) suggests that the built environment is less important than care in achieving person-centredness for people with dementia. Nonetheless, the physical layout and fabric of a care environment can have significant consequences for the way in which relationships develop (Davies 2003, McKee et al. 2004). Marshall (2001) suggests consensus in relation to a number of design features for appropriate environments for people with dementia. These are shown in Box 24.9.

Issues of safety and security   There is a growing awareness that older people, including those with dementia, have the right to take risks as a part of everyday normal living. In the case of people with dementia this principle raises particular problems, as many may be unaware of the risks that they are taking and may have lost the ability to make rational choices. As a consequence, family carers and care staff are forced to make choices between personal autonomy and safety for the person with dementia on a daily basis.

One behaviour that particularly highlights this issue is 'wandering'. Care staff and family carers are

---

Box 24.9   Consensus on appropriate design features for environments for people with dementia

- Small size
- Familiar, domestic, homely
- Scope for ordinary activities (for example, kitchens in care units, washing lines, garden sheds)
- Unobtrusive concern for safety
- Different rooms for different functions
- Age-appropriate furniture and fittings
- Safe outside space
- Single rooms big enough for lots of personal belongings
- Good signage and multiple clues where possible
- Use of objects for orientation
- Enhancement of visual access
- Controlled stimuli, especially noise

---

often concerned that people with dementia who 'wander' will come to harm and some carers find the apparent searching activity of some wanderers upsetting. However, in designing interventions to reduce wandering, the emphasis has been on safety and little consideration has been given to the meaning of this behaviour for the person with dementia. Algase et al. (2003) suggest that the expression of wandering is unique to a given person in a particular context or situation and that interventions need to be individually planned, rather than introducing measures that affect everyone, such as 'baffle locks' and door alarms. Holmberg (1997) describes an innovative programme involving volunteers who 'walked with' wanderers under the supervision of clinical staff, thus increasing opportunities for physical and social stimulation.

In spite of such innovations, most care environments will have insufficient human resources to ensure that people who wander can be accompanied and sufficiently supervised to ensure their safety at all times and consequently, there is a need to identify alternative strategies. Some formal care settings have introduced tagging systems in which people with dementia who 'wander' have tags attached to their clothes which activate a buzzer should they attempt to leave the environment. Tagging may enhance safety and reduce anxiety for carers in some situations but still raises questions about liberty and personal autonomy (Hughes & Louw 2002). Furthermore, tagging does not offer a solution when the person with dementia insists on leaving, or having left, refuses to return. If coaxing fails, care staff may be tempted to lie to residents to persuade them to return. However, this runs the risk of destroying the older person's confidence and trust in the care providers and could be seen as an example of the 'treachery' described in Kitwood's theory of MSP.

Few people with dementia living in formal care environments are subject to compulsory care or treatment provisions under the law. An honest, gentle explanation pitched at the person's level of understanding may reduce distress. A subsequent offer of a realistic alternative may be acceptable as many people with dementia have a limited attention span and can often be distracted. Failing this, the carer may accompany the person on a walk which finally leads 'back home'. If all else fails carers may exercise their duty of care under common law to prevent the resident from coming to harm. In all cases carers should be able to give good reasons for their actions.

In spite of general acknowledgement that the use of physical restraints for people with dementia should be kept to a minimum, these continue to be used to varying degrees. A recent study of restraint use in the Netherlands, for example, found that 48% of residents of three care homes were regularly restrained: lap belts, seat trays and cot sides were the most frequently used forms of restraint (Hamers et al. 2004). Molasiotis (1995) argues that the need for restraint can be reduced by careful attention to environmental stressors that are prompting agitated or restless behaviour. Environmental modifications such as placing a resident's mattress on the floor, if acceptable to the resident, can be an alternative to 'cot sides'. Purposeful occupation and exercise can also reduce boredom and hence agitation. Visual barriers, such as mirrors, camouflage of exits and stripes of tape have been evaluated in a number of quasiexperimental studies; however, a Cochrane review concluded that there is insufficient evidence that such interventions prevent or reduce wandering behaviour (Price et al. 2001). Lai & Arthur (2003) have produced a useful review of wandering behaviour in people with dementia, including discussion of causes and interventions.

Managing the balance of rights and risks for people with dementia living alone at home can be particularly challenging. Wandering into the street in nightclothes, leaving the gas on and opening the door to strangers are examples of potential risks that give families and caregivers cause for concern. Readers are referred to Fennell's (1997) discussion of practical issues which arise in the care of older people with dementia and their legal and ethical implications.

Supporting relationships   Contrary to many people's expectations, older people with dementia are capable of developing a range of social bonds (Moore 1999). For example in a study of residential care homes for people with dementia, 36% of residents in seven care homes were reported by staff to associate regularly with another resident (Netten 1993). However, some older people may resist close friendships to protect themselves from the grief associated with another loss. In a recent study of quality of life for older people living in care homes, including people with dementia, Tester et al. (2003) found that being able to maintain a sense of one's self is important in sustaining relationships with other residents and with their families. Factors that contribute to a sense of self include being able to pay attention to personal appearance and taking pride in possessions.

Opportunities to develop new relationships may be restricted by limited interaction within care settings. Certainly observational studies conducted in a range of settings suggest low levels of contact between staff and people with dementia (Armstrong-Esther & Browne 1986, Nolan et al. 1995). Armstrong-Esther & Browne (1986) found that nurses on specialist hospital wards for older people spent only 10.7% of their time interacting with patients. Moreover, they spent a significantly greater amount of time interacting with lucid as opposed to confused patients (15% compared with 5.6%).

Relationships between people with dementia within care settings can extend to intimacy. However, there are a number of barriers to sexual expression, particularly for residents of long-term care facilities. These include lack of privacy, effects of chronic illness, lack of a willing partner, loss of interest, attitudes of staff and feelings of unattractiveness (Richardson & Lazur 1995). Staff can help remove barriers to sexual expression for older people with dementia by improving privacy, educating staff and facilitating conjugal or home visits if appropriate. However, it is important that decision-making capacity is assessed to ensure that older people with dementia are not exploited or abused. More commonly, staff may complain that older people with dementia express their sexuality in ways that are inappropriate within a communal living environment.

The use of structured therapies with people with dementia
A number of psychological therapies for people with dementia have been developed which are often conducted in small groups, although they may also be provided on an individual basis. Three of the most widely used are reality orientation, validation therapy and reminiscence therapy. While these approaches have been embraced enthusiastically by many practitioners, evidence of their effectiveness is limited, although anecdotal accounts suggest some benefits.

As its name suggests, *reality orientation* involves attempts to re-provide information that people with dementia have lost through neurological impairment, primarily in order to orient them to place, time and person. The technique involves correcting disoriented statements at each interaction and this is reinforced by memory aids such as clocks, signposts and calendars. Many studies have attempted to identify the impact of reality orientation and a Cochrane review (Spector et al. 1999a) concluded that it may improve behaviour and cognition for people with dementia. In recent years, the popularity of this technique has waned alongside concerns that the approach had become prescriptive and was often practised without respect for the individual. However, Brooker (2001: p. 148) suggests that there is still much to recommend the sensitive use of reality orientation, particularly during the early stages of dementia when people are 'struggling to keep a grip on present reality'.

Validation therapy aims to reduce distress and maximize self-esteem by communicating with disoriented

older people in whatever reality they are in, rather than attempting to orient them to a more generally perceived reality. The use of touch, eye contact, body movement, mirroring the voice rhythms and empathic understanding of feelings are among the techniques employed. A Cochrane review of the effects of validation therapy (Spector et al. 1999b) identified three studies that met experimental criteria and concluded that they provide insufficient evidence to make any conclusion about the efficacy of validation therapy for people with dementia or cognitive impairment. The review does however indicate that observational studies suggest there may be some positive effects.

Reminiscence therapy consists of employing a range of audiovisual aids, such as old photographs, music and mementos from the past, to encourage older people to recall the past and to reminisce. The assumption is that this has positive benefits in itself or that the stimulation of long-term memory will in turn stimulate short-term memory. In a recent study of 142 older people living in nursing and residential homes, McKee et al. (2002b) found that older people who took part in activities involving reminiscence (talking or writing about the past) or disclosure (talking or writing about meaningful events in the present) had a better psychological morale and less psychological ill health. They showed more positive and less negative emotion than people who had not taken part in these activities. The psychological benefits were the same regardless of whether people were engaged with the past or the present. The findings suggest that the benefits to older people relate more to the process of engagement in meaningful activity than to specific aspects of the activities.

In summary, attempts to evaluate the psychological therapies for dementia outlined here have shown at best that some change is possible, but the significance of such change, in terms of improved quality of life, has yet to be established. It may be that the main value of such therapies lies in the extent to which they increase opportunities for meaningful interaction. Alternative approaches to providing meaningful activity for people with dementia are now considered.

Providing meaningful activity
In spite of evidence to suggest the protective effects of purposeful and meaningful activity for people with dementia (Ballard et al. 2001), observational studies suggest that older people with dementia, both in residential settings and in their own homes, spend much of the time in passive inactivity. According to Ballard et al. (2001), for example, almost 50% of residents' time is spent asleep, socially withdrawn or inactive, with only 14% spent in some form of communication with others. Only 3% involves

constructive activity. Similarly, Lawton et al. (1995) found that older people with dementia living at home spent very little time in interaction with others.

Marshall & Hutchinson (2001) reviewed 33 studies evaluating the use of activities with people with AD, including music, art, reminiscence, physical activity, life review, reading and games. Although the overall impact of such activities was difficult to assess because of methodological weaknesses within the studies considered, the review provides some evidence that purposeful organized activity can make an important contribution to the quality and quantity of activity and can promote social interaction in formal care environments. Brooker & Duce (2000) used a within-subjects design to explore levels of well-being for individuals with mild to moderate dementia during three types of activity. They found higher levels of well-being for residents engaged in reminiscence therapy and group activities than unstructured time. However, many carers, both paid and unpaid, lack awareness of the kinds of activities that people with dementia will find enjoyable and meaningful and there is an expectation that, in order to be useful, activities must be highly structured. On the contrary, one-to-one activities for a short period of time may be more appropriate and beneficial. These might include looking at a newspaper or magazine together, hand or foot massage or listening to music together. The Pool Activity Level Instrument (Pool 1999) is one approach to assessing an individual's ability to take part in different activities. Completion of a structured checklist indicates whether the person with dementia is operating at one of four activity levels: planned, exploratory, sensory and reflex. Appropriate activities can then be arranged accordingly. Hutchinson & Marshall (2000) highlight the importance of ensuring that activities are tailored to the individual needs and likes of the individual with dementia and there are obvious links to the use of biography and life-story work.

There has been a great deal of interest in recent years in the potential for multisensory environments such as Snoezelen rooms to enhance well-being for older people with dementia (Baker et al. 2003, Cox et al. 2004). However, a review of the literature concluded that, overall, multisensory stimulation is no more effective than any other form of activity. Two exceptions are aromatherapy and bright light treatment, which appear to be effective in alleviating agitation and sleep disturbance for people with severe dementia (Burns et al. 2002).

Volicer (1997) has suggested that the crucial factor for persons with dementia is involvement in *meaningful* activity and Acton et al. (1999) found that 60% of people diagnosed with AD or probable AD expressed the need to be useful. Few studies have addressed the impact of providing meaningful *productive* activities, even though many persons with dementia have difficulty coping with traditional programmes of leisure-type activities. To feel useful, individuals need to engage in meaningful activities, not just during the few hours of special programmes, but all the time by doing housekeeping and general chores such as folding laundry (Brooker 2001). Being creative in relation to day-to-day events is likely to increase opportunities for meaningful engagement beyond those available in organized activities. For example, in an observational study of 27 residents, Mallott et al. 2001 (cited in Beck 2001) showed that making a meal in the dining room where residents could observe the food preparation, smell the food cooking and choose their favourite food resulted in residents with dementia eating significantly more and staying in the dining room longer.

Enabling effective communication

People with dementia need their carers to acknowledge and encourage their attempts to seek meaning and to continue to try to make sense of their experiences (Bruce et al. 2002). Hansebo & Kihlgren (2002), for example, describe how carers' attempts to understand and interpret the often incoherent utterances of patients with severe dementia were one way of protecting their self-respect. Kitwood's model of interpersonal communication (Kitwood 1993) emphasizes the importance of caregivers seeking to understand people's intentions and their interpretations of the actions of others if the act of communication is to be successful. The model is valuable to carers because it highlights dementia as a communication difficulty, helps to explain why communication between people may break down and alerts carers to the importance of recognizing gestures and utterances as attempts by the person with dementia to communicate and so deserving of a response. Hansebo & Kihlgren (2002) describe carers' interactions with people with severe dementia as 'a balancing act', constantly considering the progression of the dementia and the consequences for the person with dementia in managing daily life. Their paper is a good illustration of the sometimes intuitive skills that carers bring to bear in their interactions with people with dementia.

People with dementia may engage in a variety of what have been termed 'challenging behaviours', for example, wandering, screaming and shouting. Kitwood (1997b) suggests that these behaviours are best seen primarily as attempts at communication related to need, with the most appropriate response being to attempt to understand the message, and engage with the unmet need. Crisp (1999) identifies some useful strategies for communicating in such circumstances. These include:

- listening for the feeling behind the words – the person's tone of voice, posture and body language may give clues to his or her general mood
- looking for clues in the immediate context – for example, something in the immediate surroundings may be causing the person with dementia to become agitated
- looking for clues from the person's past – to indicate a frame of reference
- interpreting what is said – for example, looking for links of likeness, links in common usage (hot may become cold) and links to broader categories ('dog' might be used to describe any four-legged animal)

Normann et al. (2002) found that effective communication and periods of lucidity for people with dementia could be promoted through a number of strategies, including sharing the person's view, repeating and reformulating the person's utterance, reinforcing the person by using positive utterances, not emphasizing errors and avoiding making demands. Kitwood has attempted a more detailed description of successful strategies for communication based upon observations made during Dementia Care Mapping (DCM: see below). Twelve different types of positive interaction are identified by Kitwood (1997b) and these are summarized in Box 24.10. Kitwood refers to these strategies as 'positive person work' and suggests that they are important in preserving personhood.

In summary, there is a growing body of evidence identifying a number of strategies for enhancing our ability to interpret and understand meaning and intention for people with dementia, and these strategies should be used as a matter of course to inform our attempts to communicate. While this body of research highlights the potential for carers to improve and promote communication with people with dementia, it also demonstrates what a highly skilled and demanding activity this can be.

Approaches for ensuring person–centred dementia care

As the potential for enabling older people with dementia to maintain an acceptable quality of life begins to be realized, methods for assessing the quality of care for people with dementia are emerging.

Box 24.10   Strategies for effective communication with people with dementia

1. Recognition. This involves the use of verbal and non-verbal behaviour which acknowledges the person with dementia as a unique individual. It may involve an act of greeting by name, eye contact or listening to the person's story over the longer term

2. Negotiation. This involves consulting people with dementia about their preferences, desires and needs. Typically negotiation is over everyday activities (e.g. getting up in the morning, going out) and skilled negotiation takes account of the slower speed with which people with dementia handle information, and their sense of insecurity. Negotiation can empower the person with dementia and increase the sense of control

3. Collaboration. This involves two or more people sharing a task towards a definite end. It may involve literally working together (as in performing household chores) or one person helping another to compensate for disabilities (e.g. giving help to another to dress or take a bath). The hallmark of collaboration is the provision of care that harnesses the initiative and abilities of the person with dementia, and does not treat him or her as an object of care

4. Play. In contrast to work, which is goal-directed, play, in its pure form, is inherently valuable and has no goal beyond the activity itself. A high-quality care environment provides opportunities for such spontaneous self-expression

5. Timalation. Kitwood uses this term to refer to activities such as massage or aromatherapy which are sensuous or sensual. Such activities are undemanding for the recipient but can provide contact, reassurance and pleasure. Thus they are of particular value for people with severe cognitive impairment

6. Celebration. This refers to moments of life (special occasions and other moments) which are intrinsically joyful, moments at which the division between carer and cared-for comes nearest to vanishing as both are caught up in a similar mood

7. Relaxation. This refers to low-intensity interaction at a slow pace. Kitwood notes that, whereas some people relax best when alone, most people with dementia have strong social needs and so find

Continued

Box 24.10   Strategies for effective communication with people with dementia (*Continued*)

relaxation easier when they are near others or in physical contact with them

8. Validation. This involves accepting and acknowledging the reality and power of another's experience, emotions and feelings. Popularized in dementia care by Feil (1992), who developed validation therapy (outlined in the text, earlier), it involves the exercise of empathic understanding in an attempt to understand the resident's frame of reference, even when it is chaotic and deluded. The effect is to make the person with dementia feel more alive and connected with the world

9. Holding. As used here, holding means providing a safe psychological space within which hidden trauma, conflict and vulnerability are exposed and contained. When holding is secure the person with dementia will know that devastating emotions (e.g. terror, fear, anger) will pass. Psychological holding, as with children, may involve physical holding too

10. Facilitation. Facilitation is similar to collaboration in that it may involve helping people with dementia to perform actions that they are unable to carry out unaided. But in a more psychotherapeutic sense, facilitation occurs when the person's sense of agency is depleted, so that all that is left is a gesture or a hesitant move towards action. Facilitation in this context involves helping people with dementia get started, sustain their action and fill it with meaning

11. Creation. As when a person with dementia spontaneously begins to sing or dance, creation involves the resident offering something to others in their environment which draws upon his or her reservoir of abilities and social skills

12. Giving. As well as presenting a gift, giving may involve the person with dementia showing affection, concern or gratitude in a way that demonstrates sensitivity, sincerity and warmth

---

Most of these approaches involve direct observation and recording of activity and interactions (Brooker 1995). For example the Quality of Interaction Schedule (QUIS) scale (Dean et al. 1993) is designed for use with residents of care homes and classifies interactions with staff members into six categories (Box 24.11). However, currently, the most widely used tool for assessing the quality of dementia care is DCM, which is based on Kitwood's theory of dementia. DCM is increasingly used in formal care settings to assess the quality of care for people with dementia and identify areas for improvement. DCM does not purport to provide a comprehensive evaluation of care, but to provide the service user's point of view through detailed, skilled and empathic observation of the person with dementia's activities and interactions with staff. Thus it complements assessment of structural factors of the care environment.

DCM has been revised several times since it was developed (Bradford Dementia Group 1997). The method as currently described involves structured observation of between four and eight people with dementia over a 4–6-h period in the communal areas of a formal care environment. Observational data are recorded within three 'coding frames':

1. Behaviour category coding (BCC): this provides a summary of the behaviour of the person during each successive 5-min time period

and rates his or her state of relative well-being or ill-being (WIB) on a six-point scale. In assigning this score, the 'mapper' takes account of the 12 indicators of well-being and seven indicators of ill-being identified by the Bradford Dementia Group (1997) and listed in Box 24.12. These indicators have been developed by Kitwood and his team through extensive observation of people with dementia. A WIB value can be calculated for individuals or groups

2. Personal detraction coding (PDC): drawing upon the 17 aspects of MSP listed in Box 24.3, this records episodes in which the person is demeaned or discounted in his or her interactions.

3. Positive event coding: a recent development of DCM introduced in the seventh edition (Bradford Dementia Group 1997), this coding frame introduces a record of episodes of good care practice to balance the coding of personal detractions. These data may be used in feedback to care workers and for developing their skills.

A dementia care index (DCI) is calculated from the WIB values and behaviour categories taken together to provide an overall quality of care score. The DCI can be weighted to take into account factors related to staffing levels and patient mix.

Box 24.11   Coding categories for the Quality of Interaction Scale (QUIS)

1. No staff interaction
2. Positive: social interaction principally involving 'good, constructive, beneficial conversation and companionship'. For example, greetings directed towards individuals, general chat and conversation and offering choices
3. Positive care: interactions during the appropriate delivery of physical care such as verbal explanations and encouragement during toileting, bathing and feeding
4. Neutral: brief, indifferent interactions not meeting the definitions of the other categories, such as putting plates down without verbal or non-verbal contact and undirected greetings
5. Negative restrictive: interactions that oppose or resist the resident's freedom of action without good reason or which ignore the resident as a person; for example, being moved without warning or explanation or being told that the resident cannot have something without good reason or explanation
6. Negative protective: providing care, keeping safe or removing from danger, but in a restrictive manner, without explanation or reassurance; for example, being told to wait for medication or being fed too quickly

In addition, the behaviour of residents will be recorded in terms of representing the following four behaviours:

1. Disengaged: resident is inactive, sitting passively or sleeping, or involved in unpurposeful activity such as fiddling with clothes or aimless walking
2. Non-social engagement: resident is engaged in purposeful activities which do not involve social interaction with others; for example, combing hair, reading, watching television, actively listening to music, knitting
3. Social engagement: resident is engaged in some form of communication with others where there is a state of reciprocity with at least one other person or the resident is initiating contact with another person. This includes recognizable speech, attempts to speak, vocalizations, signs or gestures, physical prompting in a manner which gains, attempts to gain or maintains the attention of another person. It also includes clearly giving attention (as evidenced by eye contact or orientation of the head) to another person who has begun to interact with the subject
4. Challenging behaviour: resident is engaged in solitary repetitive, non-functional motor activity (e.g. body-rocking, pacing), verbal activity (e.g. crying out, grunting, continuous swearing), self-injury, aggression to others, damage to property or other inappropriate behaviour such as spitting, pestering others or stripping

---

Box 24.12   Indicators of well-being and ill-being for people with dementia suggested by the Dementia Care Mapping Approach

Indicators of well-being
1. Able to express wishes in an acceptable way; being assertive
2. Bodily relaxation
3. Sensitive to the emotional needs of others
4. Humour
5. Dancing or singing, or other forms of creative self-expression
6. Being helpful
7. Initiating social contact
8. Being affectionate
9. Finding pleasure in some aspects of daily life
10. Concern about hygiene, tidiness or appearance, or other indicators of self-respect
11. Expressing a full range of positive and negative emotions
12. Accepting others who also have dementia

Indicators of ill-being
1. Anxiety
2. Boredom
3. Withdrawal and apathy
4. Despair
5. Physical pain/discomfort
6. Anger that is sustained
7. Unattended sadness or grief

Most accounts of the use of DCM have been enthusiastic about its potential to raise awareness of poor practice (Brooker et al. 1998, Martin & Younger 2000), although there have been some suggestions that it can have a negative impact on staff morale, unless feedback is sensitively handled. A recent review of the efficacy of DCM, both as a tool to improve practice and as an outcome measure in research, concluded that the method has high face validity and reliability (Beavis et al. 2002). However, these authors also conclude that other aspects of the validity of DCM remain unexplored. Given the time-consuming nature of the method, they argue that further evaluative research is urgently required.

An obvious limitation of all approaches to quality assurance that make use of observation is that the observational procedures could cause staff to behave differently from their normal practice. Nonetheless, in combination with methods that seek to access individual views and experiences of care, observational methods have the potential to raise awareness of ways in which care practices can be improved. For people with severe dementia, who are no longer able to communicate, observational methods may provide the only way of gaining access to their experiences of care. Useful reviews of these approaches are provided by Brooker (1995) and McKee et al. (2002a).

CONCLUSION

Within this chapter we have attempted to provide an overview of current issues in caring for older people with dementia and their families. We have tried to demonstrate that blending knowledge from different disciplines and perspectives is likely to result in the most positive experiences of care. Advances in biomedical research are raising the possibility of understanding the complex risk factors for dementia and suggesting appropriate therapeutic interventions. At the same time, techniques for exploring and understanding the experience of dementia are being developed and are allowing an appreciation of ways in which care providers can enhance quality of life for people with the condition. However, our understanding of the techniques and strategies that are most effective in this respect suggests that these require a high level of skill and are demanding in terms of resources, both economic and personal. These factors are incompatible with the often low level of resources that are afforded to dementia care, particularly within residential settings. Until those who work closely with older people with dementia are valued and rewarded in a way that recognizes the complexity and skill involved, it is unlikely that the potential for ensuring optimal quality of life in dementia will be achieved.

Acknowledgement

We thank Una and Ernest Martin and Ann Powell for providing the personal accounts in this chapter.

Recommended reading

Cantley C (ed) 2001 A handbook of dementia care. Open University Press, Buckingham.
This readable text provides a wide-ranging overview of the current state of knowledge in the field of dementia care. It demonstrates the value of a range of perspectives, is multidisciplinary and critically reviews approaches to practice and development of services.
Journal of Dementia Care. Published by Hawker Publications, 13 Park House, 140 Battersea Park Road, London SW11 4NB; tel: 020 7720 2108.
An accessible publication written for a wide readership which keeps abreast of developments in person-centred dementia care.
Keady J, Clarke C, Adams T 2003 Community mental health nursing and dementia care. Open University Press, Maidenhead.
Although designed specifically for community mental health nurses, this edited volume includes a wealth of information and insight that will be of value to anyone working with older people with dementia and their families. As well as presenting an overview of the evidence underpinning community practice with people with dementia, the text argues for a new approach based on partnership with service users and their families.
Killick J, Allen K 2001 Communication and the care of people with dementia. Open University Press, Buckingham.
This book presents a creative approach to establishing and developing communication with people with dementia. Drawing extensively on conversations with people at all stages of dementia, it suggests ways of interpreting their words and actions and facilitating effective communication. This is essential reading for anyone working in this field.
Kitwood T 1997 Dementia reconsidered: the person comes first. Open University Press, London.
This text provides a clear account of Kitwood's theory of dementia and person-centred care. Essential reading for all involved in the dementia care field.

References

Acton GJ, Mayhew PA, Hopkins BA et al. 1999 Communicating with individuals with dementia. The impaired person's perspective. Journal of Gerontological Nursing 25: 6–13

Adams T 1996 Kitwood's approach to dementia and dementia care: a critical but appreciative review. Journal of Advanced Nursing 23: 948–953

Adams T, Keady J, Clarke C 2003 Introduction. In Keady J, Clarke C, Adams T (eds) Community mental health nursing and dementia care. Open University Press, Maidenhead, pp xvii–xxvii

Adamson J 2001 Awareness and understanding of dementia in African/Caribbean and South Asian families. Health and Social Care in the Community 9: 391–396

Aggarwal N, Vass AA, Minardi HA et al. 2003 People with dementia and their relatives: personal experiences of Alzheimer's and of the provision of care. Journal of Psychiatric and Mental Health Nursing 10: 187–197

Algase DL, Beel-Bates C, Beattie ERA 2003 Wandering in long-term care. Annals of Long Term Care 11: 33–9

Allen NHP, Burns A 1995 The noncognitive features of dementia. Reviews in Clinical Gerontology 5: 57–75

Alzheimer's Disease Society 1995 Right from the start: primary health care and dementia. Alzheimer's Disease Society, London

Alzheimer's Society 2000 Food for thought: eating and nutrition. Alzheimer's Society, London

Alzheimer's Society 2003a What is dementia with Lewy bodies (DLB)? Information Street. Alzheimer's Society, London

Alzheimer's Society 2003b Genetics and dementia. Information sheet. Alzheimer's Society, London

Alzheimer's Society 2003c Drug treatments for Alzheimer's disease – Aricept, Exalom, Reminyl and Ebixa information street. Alzheimer's Society, London

Alzheimer's Society 2003d Position Paper – Demography. Available online at: http://www.alzheimers.org.uk/News_and_Campaigns/Policy_Watch/demography.htm (accessed 23 December 2003)

Alzheimer's Society 2003e Quote from Alzheimer's web address. Available online at: www.alzheimers.org.uk/Real_lives/Carers_lives/diagnosis/index.htm (accessed 23 December 2003)

Alzheimer's Society 2003f Quote from Alzheimer's web address. Available online at: www.alzheimers.org.uk/Real_lives/People_with_dementia/index.htm (accessed 23 December 2003)

Alzheimer's Society 2004 Risperidone and olanzapine: restrictions on use for people with dementia. Information Sheet, Alzheimer's Society, London

Armstrong-Esther CA, Browne KD 1986 The influence of elderly patients' mental impairment on nurse–patient interaction. Journal of Advanced Nursing 11: 379–387

Armstrong-Esther CA, Browne KD, McAfee JG 1994 Elderly patients: still clean and sitting quietly. Journal of Advanced Nursing 19: 264–271

Audit Commission 2002 Forget me not. Audit Commission Publications, Wetherby

Baker R, Holloway J, Holtkamp C et al. 2003 Effects of multi-sensory stimulation for people with dementia. Journal of Advanced Nursing 43: 465–477

Ballard C, O'Brien J, James I et al. 2001 Quality of life for people with dementia living in residential and nursing home care: the impact of performance on activities of daily living, behavioral and psychological symptoms, language skills, and psychotropic drugs. International Psychogeriatrics 13: 93–106

Bamford L, Bruce E 2000 Defining the outcomes of community care: the perspectives of older people with dementia and their carers. Ageing and Society 20: 543–570

Barker P 1985 Patient assessment in psychiatric nursing. Croom Helm, Beckenham

Beavis D, Simpson S, Graham I 2002 A literature review of dementia care mapping: methodological considerations and efficacy. Journal of Psychiatric and Mental Health Nursing 9: 725–736

Beck C 2001 Identification and assessment of effective services and interventions: the nursing home perspective. Aging and Mental Health 5 (suppl. 1): S99–S111

Bell J, McGregor I 1995 A challenge to stage theories of dementia. In: Kitwood T, Benson S (eds) The new culture of dementia care. Hawker, London, pp 12–14

Berg A, Hallberg IR, Norberg A 1998 Nurses' reflections about dementia care, the patients, the care and themselves in their daily caregiving. International Journal of Nursing Studies 35: 271–282

Blondin M 1988 Alzheimer disease stages. Alzheimer Information and Support Service, 517N Segoe Road, Madison, WI

Bond J 1999 Quality of life for people with dementia: approaches to the challenge of measurement. Aging and Society 19: 561–579

Bowes A, Wilkinson H 2003 'We didn't know it would get that bad': South Asian experiences of dementia and the service response. Health and Social Care in the Community 11: 387–396

Bowman C, Whistler J, Ellerby M 2004 A national census of care home residents. Age and Ageing 33: 561–566

Bradford Dementia Group 1997 Dementia care mapping manual, 7th edn. University of Bradford, Bradford

Brechin A 1998 What makes for good care? In: Brechin A, Walmsley J, Katz J, Peace S (eds) Care matters: concepts, practice and research in health and social care. Sage, London, pp 170–187

Brooker D 1995 Looking at them, looking at me. A review of observational studies into the quality of institutional care for elderly people with dementia. Journal of Mental Health 4: 145–156

Brooker D 2001 Therapeutic activity. In: Cantley C (ed) A handbook of dementia care. Open University Press, Buckingham, pp 146–159

Brooker D, Duce L 2000 Well-being and activity in dementia: a comparison of group reminiscence therapy, structured goal-directed group activity and unstructured time. Aging and Mental Health 4: 356–360

Brooker D, Foster N, Banner A et al. 1998 The efficacy of dementia care mapping as an audit tool: report of a 3-year British NHS evaluation. Aging and Mental Health 2: 60–70

Brown J, Nolan M, Davies S 2001 Who's the expert? Redefining lay and professional relationships. In: Nolan M, Davies S, Grant G (eds) Working with older people and their families. Open University Press, Buckingham, pp 19–32

Bruce E, Surr C, Tibbs MA, Downs M 2002 Moving towards a special kind of care for people with dementia living in care homes. NT Research 7: 335–344

Burns A, Lawlor B, Craig S 1999 Assessment scales in old age psychiatry. Martin Dunitz, London

Burns A, Byrne J, Ballard C et al. 2002 Sensory stimulation in dementia: an effective option for managing behavioural problems. British Medical Journal 325: 1312–1313

Burstow P 2003 Keep taking the medicine 2. Liberal Democrats, London

Burton-Jones J 2001 Involving relatives and friends: a good practice guide for homes for older people. Relatives and Residents Association, London

Butcher HK, Holkup PA, Park M et al. 2001 Thematic analysis of the experience of making a decision to place a family member with Alzheimer's disease in a special care unit. Research for Nursing and Health 24: 470–480

Byrne EJ 1994 Confusional states in older people. Edward Arnold, London

Campbell S 2003 Empowering nursing staff and residents in long-term care. Geriatric Nursing 24: 170–175

Cheston R, Bender M 1999 Understanding dementia: the man with worried eyes. Jessica Kingsley, London

Clare L, Wilson B, Breen K et al. 1999 Errorless learning of face–name associations in early Alzheimer's disease. Neurocase 5: 37–46

Clarke A, Hanson E, Ross H 2003 Seeing the person behind the patient: enhancing the care of older people using a biographical approach. Journal of Clinical Nursing 12: 697–706

Cook A 2002 Using video observation to include the experiences of people with dementia in research. In: Williamson H (ed) The perspectives of people with dementia: research methods and motivations. Jessica Kingsley, London

Cox S, Cook A 2002 Caring for people with dementia at the end of life. In: Hickley J, Clark D (eds) Palliative care for older people in care homes. Open University Press, Buckingham, pp 86–103

Cox H, Burns I, Savage S 2004 Multisensory environments for leisure: promoting well-being in nursing-home residents with dementia. Journal of Gerontological Nursing 30: 37–45

Crisp J 1999 Towards a partnership in maintaining personhood. In: Adams T, Clarke C (eds) Dementia care: developing partnerships in practice. Baillière Tindall, London

Davies S 2001 Relatives' experiences of nursing home entry: a constructivist inquiry. Unpublished PhD thesis. University of Sheffield, Sheffield

Davies S 2003 Creating community: the basis of caring partnerships in nursing homes. In: Nolan M, Lundh U, Grant G, Keady J (eds) Partnerships in family care: understanding the caregiving career. Open University Press, Maidenhead, pp 218–237

Davies S, Nolan M 2003 'Making the best of things': relatives' experiences of decisions about care home entry. Ageing and Society 23: 429–450

Davies S, Nolan M, Brown J, Wilson F 1999 Dignity on the ward: promoting excellence in care. Help the Aged, London

Davies S, Ellis L, Laker S 2000 Promoting autonomy and independence for older people within nursing practice: an observational study. Journal of Clinical Nursing 9: 127–136

Davies S, Powell A, Aveyard B 2002 Developing partnerships in care: towards a teaching nursing home. British Journal of Nursing 11: 1320–1328

Dean R, Proudfoot R, Lindesay J 1993 The quality of interaction schedule (QUIS): development, reliability and use in the evaluation of two domus units. International Journal of Geriatric Psychiatry 8: 819–826

DeBaggio T 2002 Losing my mind: an intimate look at life with Alzheimer's. Free Press, New York

Dellasega C, Mastrian K 1995 The processes and consequences of institutionalising an elder. Western Journal of Nursing Research 17: 123–136

Department of Health 2001 The national service framework for older people. Department of Health, London

Dewey ME, Copeland JRM 1986 Computerized psychiatric diagnosis in the elderly: AGECAT. Journal of Microcomputing Applications 9: 135–140

Duff G 2004 Atypical antipsychotic drugs and stroke. Committee for Safety of Medicines. Medicines and Healthcare products regulatory agency (MHRA). Available online at: http://www.mhra.gov.uk

Evans M 1999 Ethics: reconciling conflicting values in health policy, Policy futures for UK health no. 9. Nuffield Trust, London

Feil N 1992 V/F validation: the Feil method. Feil Productions, Cleveland

Fennell P 1997 Legal and ethical issues in mental health care of elderly patients. In: Norman IJ, Redfern SJ (eds) Mental health care for elderly people. Churchill Livingstone, Edinburgh, pp 527–545

Fitch N, Becker R, Heller A 1988 The inheritance of Alzheimer's disease: a new interpretation. Annals of Neurology 23: 14–19

Fleming AA 1998 Family caregiving of older people with dementing illnesses in nursing homes: a lifeline of special care. Australasian Journal on Ageing 17: 140–145

Folstein MF, Folstein JE, McHugh PR 1975 Mini-mental state: a practical method for grading the cognitive state of patients for the clinician. Journal of Psychiatric Research 12: 189–198

Gattuso S, Bevan C 2000 'Mother, daughter, patient, nurse': women's emotion work in aged care. Journal of Advanced Nursing 31: 892–899

Gjerberg E 1995 Nursing home quality: different perspectives among residents, relatives and staff, a qualitative study. Vard i Norden. Nursing Science and Research in the Nordic Countries 15: 4–9

Goldsmith M 1996 Hearing the voice of people with dementia: opportunities and obstacles. Jessica Kingsley, London

Graham IW 1999 Reflective narrative and dementia care. Journal of Clinical Nursing 8: 675–683

Graneheim UH, Norberg A, Jansson L 2001 Interaction relating to privacy, identity, autonomy and security. An observational study focusing on a woman with dementia and 'behavioural disturbances', and on her care providers. Journal of Advanced Nursing 36: 256–265

Gurland B, Cross P, Defiguerido J et al. 1979 A cross-national comparison of the institutionalised elderly in the cities of New York and London. Psychological Medicine 9: 781–788

Hachinski VC 1992 Preventable senility: a call for action against the vascular dementias. Lancet 340: 645–647

Hall EB 1994 What is it like to have Alzheimer's disease? Alzheimer's Disease Society Newsletter September 3

Hamers J, Gulpers M, Strik W 2004 Use of physical restraints with cognitively impaired nursing home residents. Journal of Advanced Nursing 45: 246–251

Hansebo G, Kihlgren M 2002 Carers' interactions with patients suffering from severe dementia: a difficult balance to facilitate mutual togetherness. Journal of Clinical Nursing 11: 225–236

Harrison RWS, McKeith IG 1996 Senile dementia of Lewy body type – a review of clinical and pathological features implications for treatment. International Journal of Geriatric Psychiatry 10: 919–926

Henderson AS 1992 The epidemiology of mental illness. In: Evans JG, Williams TF (eds) Oxford textbook of geriatric medicine. Oxford University Press, Oxford, pp 617–620

Hertzberg A, Ekman S 2000 'We, not them and us?' Views on the relationships and interactions between staff and relatives of older people permanently living in nursing homes. Journal of Advanced Nursing 31: 614–622

Holden U, Stokes G 2002 The dementias. In: Stokes G, Goudie F (eds) The essential dementia care handbook. Speechmark, Bicester, pp 11–21

Holmberg SK 1997 A walking program for wanderers: volunteer training and development of an evening walker's group. Geriatric Nursing 18: 160–165

Hope RA, Patel V 1993 Assessment of behavioural phenomena in dementia. In: Burns A (ed) Ageing and dementia: a methodological approach. Edward Arnold, London

Hope RA, Fairburn CG, Goodwin GM 1989 Increased eating in dementia. International Journal of Eating Disorders 8: 111–115

Hopker S 1999 Drug treatments and dementia. Jessica Kingsley, London

Hubbard G, Downs MG, Tester S 2003 Including older people with dementia in research: challenges and strategies. Aging and Mental Health 7: 351–362

Hughes J, Louw S 2002 Electronic tagging for people who wander. British Medical Journal 325: 847–848

Hurley A, Volicer L 2002 Alzheimer's disease: 'Its okay mama, if you want to go, its okay.' Journal of the American Medical Association 288: 2324–2331

Hutchinson SA, Marshall M 2000 Responses of family caregivers and family members with Alzheimer's disease to an activity kit: an ethnographic study. Journal of Advanced Nursing 31: 44–50

Iliffe S, Manthorpe J 2004 The recognition of and response to dementia in the community: lessons for professional development. Learning in Health and Social Care 3: 5–16

Innes A, Capstick A 2001 Communication and personhood. In: Cantley C (ed) A handbook of dementia care. Open University Press, Buckingham, pp 135–145

Jones G, Miesen BML 1992 Care giving in dementia: research and applications. Routledge, London

Jorm AF, Scott R, Jacoby A 1989 Assessment of cognitive decline in dementia by informant questionnaire. International Journal of Geriatric Psychiatry 4: 35–39

Katzman R, Aronson M, Fuld PA et al. 1989 Development of dementia in an 80-year-old volunteer cohort. Annals of Neurology 25: 317–324

Keady J, Gilliard J 1999 The early experience of Alzheimer's disease: implications for partnership and practice. In: Adams T, Clarke C (eds) Dementia care: developing partnerships in practice. Baillière Tindall, London

Keady J, Nolan M 1994a The carer-led assessment process (CLASP): a framework for the assessment of need in dementia caregivers. Journal of Clinical Nursing 3: 103–108

Keady J, Nolan M 1994b Younger-onset dementia: developing a longitudinal model as the basis for a research agenda and as a guide to interventions with sufferers and carers. Journal of Advanced Nursing 19: 659–669

Keady J, Nolan M 1995a A stitch in time: facilitating proactive interventions with dementia caregivers – the role of community practitioners. Journal of Psychiatric and Mental Health Nursing 2: 33–40

Keady J, Nolan M 1995b IMMEL: assessing coping responses in the early stages of dementia. British Journal of Nursing 4: 309–314

Keady J, Nolan M 1995c IMMEL 2: working to augment coping responses in early dementia. British Journal of Nursing 4: 377–380

Kellett UM 1999 Transition in care: family carers' experience of nursing home placement. Journal of Advanced Nursing 29: 1474–1481

Kendrick T, Warnes T 1997 The demography and mental health of elderly people. In: Norman IJ, Redfern SJ (eds) Mental health care for elderly people. Churchill Livingstone, Edinburgh, pp 3–20

Killick J, Allen K 2001 Communication and the care of people with dementia. Open University Press, Buckingham

King's Fund 1986 Living well in old age. King's Fund, London

Kitwood T 1990 The dialectics of dementia: with particular reference to Alzheimer's disease. Ageing and Society 10: 177–196

Kitwood T 1993 Towards a theory of dementia care: the interpersonal process. Ageing and Society 13: 51–67

Kitwood T 1997a The experience of dementia. Ageing and Mental Health 1: 13–22

Kitwood T 1997b Dementia reconsidered: the person comes first. Open University Press, Buckingham

Kizer KW 2002 Patient centred care: essential but probably not sufficient. Quality in Health Care 11: 117–118

Lai C, Arthur D 2003 Wandering behaviour in people with dementia. Journal of Advanced Nursing 44: 173–178

Lamers C 2002 Memory clinics. In Stokes G, Goudie F (eds) The essential dementia care handbook. Speechmark, Bicester, pp 46–56

Lanceley A 1985 Use of controlling language in the rehabilitation of the elderly. Journal of Advanced Nursing 10: 125–135

Lawton M, Moss M, Dunamel L 1995 The quality of life among elderly care receivers. Journal of Applied Gerontology 14: 150–171

Leong J, Madjar I, Fiveash B 2001 Needs of family carers of elderly people living in the community. Australasian Journal on Ageing 20: 133–138

Lintern T, Woods B, Phair L 2000 Before and after training: a case study of interventions. Journal of Dementia Care 8: 15–17

Lundh U, Nolan M, Hellstrom I et al. 2003 Quality care for people with dementia: the views of family and professional carers. In: Nolan M, Lundh U, Grant G, Keady J (eds) Partnerships in family care: understanding the caregiving career. Open University Press, Maidenhead, pp 72–89

Mallott OW, Whifield K, Oliver T 2001 Enhancement of the breakfast eating experience in a dementia care unit. University of Waterloo, Ontario

Mann AH, Graham N, Ashby D 1984 Psychiatric illness in residential homes for the elderly: a survey in one London borough. Age and Ageing 13: 257–265

Manthorpe J, Watson R 2003 Poorly served? Eating and dementia. Journal of Advanced Nursing 41: 162–169

Marshall M 2001 Care settings and the care environment. In: Cantley C (ed) A handbook of dementia care. Open University Press, Buckingham, pp 173–185

Marshall M 2003 Nutrition. In: Hudson R (ed) Dementia nursing: a guide to practice. Radcliffe Medical Press, Abingdon, pp 60–69

Marshall MJ, Hutchinson SA 2001 A critique of research on the use of activities with persons with Alzheimer's disease: a systematic literature review. Journal of Advanced Nursing 35: 488–496

Martin GW, Younger D 2000 Anti-oppressive practice: a route to the empowerment of people with dementia through communication and choice. Journal of Psychiatric and Mental Health Nursing 7: 59–67

McCormack B, McKenna H 2001 Challenges to quality monitoring systems in care homes. Quality in Health Care 10: 200–201

McDerment L, Ackroyd J, Tealer R et al. 1997 As others see us: a study of relationships in homes for older people. Relatives Association, London

McGowin DF 1993 Living in the labyrinth: a personal journey through the maze of Alzheimer's disease. Mainsail Press, Cambridge

McKee K, Houston DM, Barnes S 2002a Methods for assessing quality of life and well-being in frail older people. Psychology and Health 17: 737–751

McKee K, Wilson F, Elford H et al. 2002b Evaluating the Impact of Reminiscence on the Quality of Life of Older People, Economic and Social Research Council, Growing Older Programme: Research Findings No. 8, University of Sheffield, Sheffield

Mckee K, Parker C, Barnes S, Morgan K, Tregenza P, Torrington J (2004) Supporting successful ageing in residential homes – the role of the physical environment. Psychology and Health 19(suppl): 111–112

McKeith I, Fairbairn A 2001 Biomedical and clinical perspectives. In: Cantley C (ed) A handbook of dementia care. Open University Press, Buckingham, pp 7–25

McShane R, Gedling K, Keene J et al. 1998 Getting lost in dementia: a longitudinal study of behavioural symptoms. International Psychogeriatrics 10: 253–260

Miesen B 1992 Attachment theory and dementia. In: Jones G, Miesen B (eds) Caregiving in dementia: research and applications. Routledge, London

Miller L 2003 Assessment and therapeutic approaches for community mental health nursing dementia care practice. In: Keady J, Clarke C, Adams T (eds) Community mental health nursing and dementia care. Open University Press, Maidenhead, pp 77–87

Molasiotis A 1995 Use of physical restraints 2: alternatives. British Journal of Nursing 4: 201–202

Moore KD 1999 Dissonance in the dining room: a study of social interaction in a special care unit. Qualitative Health Research 9: 133–155

Morton I 1997 Beyond validation. In: Norman IJ, Redfern SJ (eds) Mental health care for elderly people. Churchill Livingstone, Edinburgh, pp 371–391

Moyle W, Skinner J, Rowe G et al. 2003 Views of job satisfaction and dissatisfaction in Australian long-term care. Journal of Clinical Nursing 12: 168–176

Murphy J, Tester S, Hubbard G et al (2005) Enabling frail older people with a communication difficulty to express their views: the use of Talking Mats™ as an interview tool. Health and Social Care in the Community 13: 95–107

Naleppa MJ 1996 Families and the institutionalised elderly: a review. Journal of Gerontological Social Work 27: 87–111

Netten A 1993 A positive environment? Physical and social influences on people with senile dementia in residential care. Ashgate, Aldershot

Nolan MR 1997 Health and social care: what the future holds for nursing. Keynote address at the Third Royal College of Nursing Older People European Conference and Exhibition, Harrogate, 5th November. Royal College of Nursing, London

Nolan M, Grant G, Keady J (1996) Understanding family caregiving. Open University Press, Buckingham

Nolan MR, Grant G, Caldock K, Keady J 1994 A framework for assessing the needs of family carers: a multi-disciplinary guide. BASE Publications, Stoke-on-Trent

Nolan M, Grant G, Nolan J 1995 Busy doing nothing: activity and interaction levels amongst differing populations of elderly patients. Journal of Advanced Nursing 22: 528–538

Nolan M, Davies S, Grant G 2001 Quality of life, quality of care. In: Nolan M, Davies S, Grant G (eds) Working with older people and their families: key issues in policy and practice. Open University Press, Buckingham, pp 4–18

Nolan M, Ryan T, Enderby P, Reid D 2002a Towards a more inclusive vision of dementia care practice and research.

Dementia: International Journal of Social Research and Practice 1: 193–211

Nolan M, Brown J, Davies S et al. 2002b Advancing gerontological education in nursing: final report of the AGEIN project. Report to the English National Board for Nursing, Midwifery and Health Visiting, University of Sheffield, Sheffield

Nolan M, Grant G, Keady J, Lundh U 2003 New directions for partnerships: relationship-centred care. In: Nolan M, Lundh U, Grant G, Keady J (eds) Partnerships in family care: understanding the caregiving career. Open University Press, Maidenhead, pp 259–291

Normann H, Ketil N, Asplund K 2002 Confirmation and lucidity during conversations with a woman with severe dementia. Journal of Advanced Nursing 39: 370–376

North of England Evidence Based Guideline Development Project 1998 Evidence based guideline for the primary care management of dementia. Centre for Health Services Research, Newcastle upon Tyne

Nygard L, Borell L 1998 A life-world of altering meaning: expressions of the illness experience of dementia in everyday life over 3 years. Occupational Therapy Journal of Research 18: 109–136

Packer T 2000 Does person-centred care exist? Journal of Dementia Care 8: 19–21

Page S 2003 From screening to intervention: the community mental health nurse in a memory clinic setting. In: Keady J, Clarke CL, Adams T (eds) Community mental health care nursing and dementia care. Open University Press, Buckingham, pp 120–133

Park M, Delaney C, Maas M et al. 2004 Using a Nursing Minimum Data Set with older patients with dementia in an acute care setting. Journal of Advanced Nursing 47: 329–339

Parsons M 2001 Living at home. In: Cantley C (ed) A handbook of dementia care. Open University Press, Buckingham, pp 123–134

Parsons S, Simmons W, Penn K et al. 2003 Determinants of satisfaction and turnover among nursing assistants: the results of a statewide survey. Journal of Gerontological Nursing 29: 51–58

Patel N, Mirza NR, Lindblad P et al. 1998 Dementia and minority ethnic older people. Managing care in the UK, Denmark and France. Russell House Publishing, Lyme Regis

Pattie AH, Gilleard CJ 1975 A brief psychogeriatric assessment schedule: validation against psychiatric diagnosis and discharge from hospital. British Journal of Psychiatry 127: 489–493

Pillemer K, Suitor J, Henderson C et al. 2003 A cooperative communication intervention for nursing home staff and family members of residents. Gerontologist 43 (special issue II): 96–106

Pollitt PA, O'Connor DW, Anderson I 1989 Mild dementia: perceptions and problems. Ageing and Society 9: 261–275

Pool J 1999 The pool activity level (PAL) instrument: a practical resource for carers of people with dementia. Jessica Kingsley, London

Powers BA 2001 Ethnographic analysis of everyday ethics in the care of nursing home residents with dementia: a taxonomy. Nursing Research 50: 332–339

Price JO, Hermans DG, Grimley Evans J 2001 Subjective barriers to prevent wandering of cognitively impaired people. The Cochrane Database of Systematic Reviews, Issue 1, Art. No. CD 001932, DOI: 10.1002/14651858. CD 001932

Pusey H, Richards D 2001 A systematic review of the effectiveness of psychosocial interventions for carers of people with dementia. Aging and Mental Health 5: 107–119

Rabbitt P 1982 Development of methods to measure changes in activities of daily living in the elderly. In: Corkin S et al. (eds) Alzheimer's disease: a report of progress (aging), vol 19. Raven Press, New York

Rabins PV, Mace NL, Lucas MJ 1982 The impact of dementia on the family. Journal of the American Medical Association 248: 333–335

Reichman S, Leonard C, Mintz T et al. 2004 Compiling life history resources for older adults in institutions: development of a guide. Journal of Gerontological Nursing 30: 20–28

Richardson JP, Lazur A 1995 Sexuality in the nursing home patient. American Family Physician 51: 121–124

Rogers C 1959 A theory of therapy, personality and interpersonal relationships as developed in the client-centred framework. In: Koch S (ed) Psychology: a study of science. McGraw-Hill, New York

Rundqvist EM, Severinsson EI 1999 Caring relationships with patients suffering from dementia an interview study. Journal of Advanced Nursing 29: 800–807

Russell C 1996 Passion and heretics: meaning in life and quality of life of persons with dementia. Journal of the American Geriatrics Society 44: 1400–1402

Ryan T, Nolan M, Enderby P, Reid D 2004 'Part of the family': sources of job satisfaction amongst a group of community-based dementia care workers. Health and Social Care in the Community 12: 111–118

Sabat SR, Harré R 1992 The construction and deconstruction of self in Alzheimer's disease. Ageing and Society 12: 443–461

Seymour J, Hanson E 2001 Palliative care and older people. In: Nolan M, Davies S, Grant G (eds) Working with older people and their families: key issues in policy and practice. Open University Press, Buckingham, pp 99–119

Smith AD, Jobst KA 1996 Use of structural imaging to study the progression of Alzheimer's disease. British Medical Bulletin 52: 575–586

Smith AD, Jobst KA, Edmonds Z et al. 1996 Neuroimaging and early Alzheimer's disease Lancet 348: 829–830

Specht JP, Kelley LS, Manion P et al. 2000 Who's the boss? Family/staff partnership in care of persons with dementia. Nursing Administration Quarterly 24: 64–77

Spector A, Orrell M, Davies S, Woods RT 1999a Reality orientation for dementia (Cochrane review). Cochrane Library issue 3. Update Software, Oxford

Spector A, Orrell M, Davies S, Woods RT 1999b Validation therapy for dementia (Cochrane review). Cochrane Library issue 5. Update Software, Oxford

Stanley D, Reed J 1999 Opening up care: achieving principled practice in health and social care institutions. Arnold, London

Sunderland A, Watts K, Baddeley AD et al. 1986 Subjective memory assessment and test performance in elderly adults. Journal of Gerontology 41: 376–384

Tester S, Hubbard G, Downs M et al. 2003 Perceptions of quality of life of frail older people in care homes. Unsettling the ordinary: changing ideas about ageing. 32nd Annual Conference of the British Society of Gerontology, Newcastle upon Tyne, 4–6 September 2003. British Society of Gerontology, Newcastle upon Tyne

Thompson P, Ingilis F, Findlay D et al. 1997 Memory clinic attenders: a review of 150 consecutive patients. Aging and Mental Health 1: 181–183

Tobiansky R 1994 Understanding dementia: the clinical course of dementia. Journal of Dementia Care 2: 26–28

Tolson D, Smith M, Knight P 1999 An investigation of the components of best nursing practice in the care of acutely ill hospitalised older patients with coincidental dementia: a multi-method design. Journal of Advanced Nursing 30: 1127–1136

van Duijn CM, Stijnen T, Hofman A 1991 Risk factors for Alzheimer's disease: overview of the EURODEM collaborative re-analysis of case control studies. International Journal of Epidemiology 20 (suppl. 2): S4–12

Volicer L 1997 Goals of care in advanced dementia: comfort, dignity and psychological well-being. American Journal of Alzheimer's Disease 12: 196–197

Weaks D, Boardman G 2003 Normalisation as a philosophy of dementia care. In: Keady J, Clarke C, Adams T (eds) Community mental health nursing and dementia care. Open University Press, Maidenhead, pp 186–198

Wood RT 2001 Discovering the person with Alzheimer's disease: cognitive, emotional and behavioural aspects. Aging and Mental Health 5 (suppl. 1): S7–S16

World Health Organization 1992 The ICD-10 classification of mental and behavioural disorders: clinical descriptions and diagnostic guidelines. WHO, Geneva

Zanetti O, Binetti G, Magni E et al. 1997 Procedural memory stimulation in Alzheimer's disease: impact of a training programme. Acta Neurologica Scandinavica 95: 152–157

Zarit SH, Leitsch SA 2001 Developing and evaluating community based intervention programmes for Alzheimer's patients and their caregivers. Aging and Mental Health 5: S84–S98

Zarit S, Orr N, Zarit M 1985 The hidden victims of Alzheimer's disease. New York University Press, New York

Zerzan J, Stearns S, Hanson L 2000 Access to palliative care and hospice in nursing homes. Journal of the American Medical Association 284: 2489–2494

Chapter 25

Depression in older people

Colin Hughes

INTRODUCTION

In this chapter the role of nurses in the care and treatment of older people with depression is described. Reference is made where possible to the growing evidence base on which nurses can base their contemporary practice. Case histories illustrate the common presentations of depression and the settings in which it is especially common are highlighted. Some recent evidence on causative factors is presented. The role of nurses in prevention and detection is emphasized.

Ways to improve management are discussed, including public and professional education and screening. For effective management of depression in older people nurses will work as a member of a multidisciplinary team and are well placed to coordinate the multidimensional approach to assessment and care that is needed. The role that nurses have in the medical, psychological and social aspects of this approach is described. A generic nursing approach is discussed which will be of particular relevance to general nurses. Psychiatric nurses will have roles in more specialist interventions, which are also described. The prognosis for older people with depression depends greatly on the service provided: nurses have important roles in initial care and treatment and in follow-up to maintain improvement and prevent relapse.

Depressive disorder in older people is a major public health problem. It is very common but often goes undetected in primary care, general medical units and in care homes. When it is detected, it is not always treated adequately. When this happens the prognosis is poor with increased mortality rates. Depressive disorder is a cause of disability in its own right and also adds to the disability of physical disorder. It accounts for increased use of health and social services of all kinds and reduces quality of life. However, there is now a substantial evidence base showing how depressive disorder in older people should be treated. This chapter is concerned with depression in older people and the role that nurses have in the process leading to effective care and treatment.

PRESENTATION OF DEPRESSION IN OLDER PEOPLE

The following case histories illustrate how depression in older people may present.

Major depression

Mary Smith (Case study 25.1) has major depression. She is experiencing a number of key depressive symptoms of depression and as a consequence her usual daily life is adversely affected. In isolation some of the symptoms she is experiencing could be part of a reaction to the difficulties often associated with older age. An older person might feel some sadness or demoralization as health deteriorates and some interests have to be given up. Normal biological ageing might result in reduced vitality. Physical illness might affect sleep and appetite. However. a person will only be considered to be suffering from a depressive disorder when a significant number of key depressive symptoms are experienced, that is, when the depressive syndrome is present. In consequence, the person will usually have difficulty continuing with usual activities, and relationships are likely to be affected.

The key symptoms of depression in a person of any age are described in the World Health Organization *International Classification of Diseases*, tenth edition, known as ICD-10 (World Health Organization 1992). Box 25.1 shows the ICD-10 guidelines on how a depressive episode can be classified as mild, moderate or severe. The alternative classification system is

---

Case study 25.1

Mary Smith is 85 years old and lives in her own house, a quarter of a mile from the village shops. Her husband died 3 years ago. He had strokes and suffered from dementia. She has two daughters who live in nearby villages. She has become increasingly depressed over the past 2 months. She experiences considerable pain from her left hip and has been more and more disabled by this for the past 6 months. She is on the waiting list for a hip replacement. She feels miserable and no longer enjoys reading or gardening. She feels irritated and restless when in the company of her family. She has no energy, finds everything an effort and has no interest in household chores. She rarely walks into the village for shopping, relying on family to do this for her. She spends most of the day just sitting on the settee, glancing at the newspaper, but not being able to concentrate on it for long. She has little appetite for food and feels nauseous much of the time. The general practitioner can find no physical cause for this. She sleeps fitfully at night and takes a sleeping tablet occasionally to get a better night's sleep. She cannot see anything to look forward to in the future and cannot see himself getting better. She feels guilt-ridden about the occasions she became irritated with her husband's difficult behaviour when she was tired and stressed in looking after him at home. She thinks that life is not worth living but denies any suicidal intent. Mrs Smith had been to see her general practitioner with complaints of poor sleep and nausea but depression was then recognized and she was prescribed an antidepressant and referred to the community mental health team for psychological therapy.

Box 25.1   ICD-10 guidelines for depressive episode

1. Depressed mood
2. Loss of interest and enjoyment
3. Reduced energy leading to increased fatigability and diminished activity
4. Reduced concentration and attention
5. Reduced self-esteem and self-confidence
6. Ideas of guilt and unworthiness
7. Bleak and pessimistic views of the future
8. Ideas or acts of self-harm or suicide
9. Disturbed sleep
10. Diminished appetite

Mild depressive episode: at least two of 1, 2 or 3, plus at least two of the others (i.e.: at least four out of 10 symptoms)

Moderate depressive episode: at least two of 1, 2 or 3, plus at least three (preferably four) of the others (i.e. at least five out of 10 symptoms)

Severe depressive episode: all of 1, 2 and 3 plus at least four others (i.e. at least seven out of 10 symptoms)

Symptoms should usually have been present for about 2 weeks

published in the *Diagnostic and Statistical Manual of Mental Disorders*, 4th edition, known as DSM-IV (American Psychiatric Association 1994). In this system major depressive episode is defined by the presence of five or more of the following symptoms: depressed mood, markedly diminished interest or pleasure, decrease or increase in appetite with significant weight loss or weight gain, insomnia or hypersomnia, psychomotor agitation or retardation, fatigue or loss of energy, feelings of worthlessness or excessive or inappropriate guilt, diminished ability to think or concentrate and recurrent thoughts of death or suicidal ideation. At least one of either depressed mood or loss of interest or pleasure should be present. Severe depressive episode, and possibly moderate depressive episode, are equivalent to major depressive disorder under the DSM system. A severe depression meeting these criteria is commonly referred to as major depression.

In major depression, mood is depressed to a degree that is abnormal for the person and is mainly uninfluenced by circumstances. The depressed mood is present for most of the day, nearly every day. The depressed mood can vary somewhat during the day (diurnal variation) and is characteristically worse in the morning in more severe depression. The person describes not being as interested in usual activities as previously or not being able to experience pleasure (anhedonia). Reduced energy is experienced as sustained fatigue even in the absence of physical exertion. Psychomotor retardation may result, with slowed monotonous speech, increased pauses before answering, slow body movements and decreased amount of speech (poverty of speech) or even muteness. In the most severe cases depressive stupor may develop. The person may complain of memory problems and indecision and may appear distracted.

People have negative thoughts about themselves, saying, for example, 'I am not as good as other people' or 'I am not a very interesting person anymore'. They have distorted beliefs about current or passed failings or blame themselves for some untoward event or for their illness. They may believe that they do not deserve the attention of their family or the concern of the doctor or nurse. Ideas of guilt and unworthiness can be delusional in intensity. They believe that the future will be unpleasant, that something bad will happen or that there is not a future for them. They may believe that the treatment will not help and that they will not recover. They feel hopeless and helpless. Often, they think that they would be better off dead. They may have thoughts of self-harm, with or without a specific plan, or may have attempted suicide.

There may be problems in getting to sleep, waking in the middle of sleep or waking early in the morning. Waking early, 2 h or more before the usual time, is also especially characteristic of severe depression. People no longer enjoy food so eat less and often lose weight. Psychomotor agitation may be prominent instead of diminished activity. They cannot sit still and will pace about, wringing their hands or pulling at their hair or clothes.

The clinical presentation of depression in older people is much the same as in younger adults. In general, similarities in presentation are more important than any differences. However some differences might distract the unwary from the correct identification of depression. Older people may complain less of depressed mood or sadness even when appearing depressed (Baldwin 2002). Note that the presence of depressed mood per se is not needed for a diagnosis of a depressive episode by ICD-10 and DSM-IV criteria; loss of interest and enjoyment have equivalent diagnostic significance. Anxiety may be a dominant feature or the person may have some obsessional symptoms. Hypochondriasis is more common. If depressed older people also have a physical problem, they may complain more about that, especially if their pain threshold has been lowered by the depression.

Complaints of asthenia, headache, palpitations, pain (especially abdominal pain), dizziness and shortness of breath are not uncommon (Rasmussen et al. 1999).

Depression presents in a range of severity. The consensus is that most depressive disorders lie on a continuum rather that being discrete categories (Lebowitz et al. 1997). Nonetheless, it is important for nurses to be aware of the terminology currently applicable to different levels of severity.

Psychotic depression

A major depression can present with psychotic symptoms, that is, with delusions or hallucinations. Reginald Evans (Case study 25.2) suffered with psychotic depression. Delusions may be paranoid, with individuals believing that they are being poisoned, for example. Others may involve ideas of guilt, sin, poverty or impending disaster. They may believe that their body is rotting away or that they are dead (a nihilistic delusion) or that they have a serious illness such as cancer (a hypochondriacal delusion). They may experience hallucinations such as hearing voices saying derogatory things about them or accusing them of doing evil things (auditory hallucinations). They may perceive an unpleasant smell (an olfactory hallucination), especially if they believe that they are also physically ill.

Milder depressions

These are far more common than major depression and will usually be seen in primary care. When a person does not quite fulfil criteria for major depression but has some symptoms and significant functional impairment, the term 'minor depression' is being increasingly used. It is suggested that the criteria for minor depression are the presence of at least two (but fewer than five) of the symptoms for a major depressive episode (American Psychiatric Association 1994). It is commonly associated with physical illness.

Betty Watson (Case study 25.3) has a more chronic milder depression. In this disorder the mood disturbance is chronic and variable. Mrs Watson feels well for periods but most of the time she feels depressed and everything is an effort. She tends to brood and complain. She does not fulfil the criteria for a major depression and would be diagnosed as suffering from dysthymia, a chronic mild depression. However, episodes of major depression may develop. The diagnostic criteria for dysthymia are shown in Box 25.2.

Case study 25.2

Reginald Evans, aged 82, lives with his wife and had become increasingly depressed in the past month. He has become convinced that they have no money. He also believes that there is a fault with the power supply to the house and that they should not be using electricity, so will switch off domestic appliances if not supervised by his wife. He believes that something terrible is going to happen to them both so will not let his wife leave the house. He feels upset that he has somehow let his wife down. His condition worsened so that he was neglecting his self-care, was eating little and drinking only with much persuasion. He did not want people visiting him as he thought that he had something wrong with his bowels and that he had a contagious disease and did not want to infect anyone. He was seen by a psychiatrist at home who prescribed an antidepressant and an antipsychotic drug. However, he accepted admission to hospital a week later and consented to having electroconvulsive therapy.

Case study 25.3

Betty Watson is 80 years old. Her husband died 10 years ago. She has arthritis in her knees and hips and has angina. Her mood has been somewhat depressed since her husband died. She gets tearful sometimes, although her mood is brighter for a few days at a time, especially when in company. She no longer enjoys the garden and greenhouse, partly through loss of interest and partly through the pain she gets from her arthritis. She has become particularly anxious about her angina and grumbles that the doctor does not visit often enough. Two months ago she stopped going to the local day centre which she would usually attend one day a week and enjoy. She still walks to the local shops several times a week. Her appetite has remained good and her sleep pattern has not changed. Because of the persistence of her relatively mild depressive symptoms, the general practitioner prescribed an antidepressant and also referred her to the community mental health team for further advice and support.

Box 25.2   DSM–IV criteria for dysthymia

A. Depressed mood for most of the day, for more days than not, for at least 2 years
B. The presence while depressed of two or more of the following:
   1. poor appetite or overeating
   2. insomnia or hypersomnia
   3. low energy or fatigue
   4. low self-esteem
   5. poor concentration or difficulty making decisions
   6. feelings of hopelessness
C. During the 2-year period the person has never been without the symptoms for more than 2 months at a time

---

When depressed mood occurs as part of a period of adjustment to some significant life change, such as moving into a residential home for example, but few other symptoms occur, it would be described as an adjustment disorder with depressed mood. We shall see that depression can sometimes be due to systemic disease or drugs used to treat physical problems; the term 'organic mood (depressive) disorder' is then used.

A new category of vascular depression has been proposed (Baldwin & O'Brien 2002). It is suggested that damage to end-arteries supplying subcortical structures may disrupt neurotransmitter circuitry involved in mood regulation, thus causing or predisposing a person to depression. The presumed basis is of vascular disease, though this is not yet proven. Its features are shown in Box 25.3.

Depressive episodes usually occur as either a single first episode or in the context of previous depressive episodes (recurrent depressive disorder). Experience of a manic episode in the past would be said to be bipolar disorder. Another distinction which is often made is that of late-onset depression, the first episode being in older age, and early-onset, when recurrent depression started in earlier life. Box 25.4 summarizes the types of depressive disorder in later life.

PREVALENCE AND INCIDENCE

Prevalence

An average prevalence in community samples across many European countries has been found to be 12.3%: 14.1% for women and 8.6% for men (Copeland et al. 1999). In an analysis of studies worldwide the average prevalence was 13.3% for all depressive syndromes (major and milder depressions), with rates of major depression averaging 1.8% (Beekman et al. 1999). Although the prevalence of major depression either remains static or perhaps decreases with age, when the whole range of depression is considered, it is likely that overall prevalence rises with age (Baldwin et al. 2002). It appears that ageing per se is not a risk factor for developing major depression (Roberts et al. 1997). Any associations are accounted for by increased health difficulties which, as we shall see, are an important risk factor.

When samples other than community samples have been studied, especially high prevalence rates have been found, as Table 25.1 illustrates.

Also, depression occurs at especially high rates in some physical disorders. Table 25.2 shows the prevalence of depression in older people in the context of a range of physical illnesses or degenerative conditions. The rate of major depression is usually much lower than the overall prevalence. The key message is that nurses working in these settings or with these populations should have a particularly high index of suspicion for depression.

Box 25.3   The vascular depression hypothesis: proposed features

- Late-onset depression (but not always)
- Increase in vascular risk factors
- Reduced depressive ideation
- Reduced insight
- Increased apathy and psychomotor retardation
- Cognitive impairment (particularly executive function)
- Neuroimaging abnormalities, notably affecting white matter and subcortical areas.

Box 25.4   Types of depressive disorder in later life

- Major depression
- Minor depression
- Dysthymia
- Adjustment disorder with depressed mood
- Mixed anxiety and depressive disorder
- Organic mood (depressive) disorder
- Bipolar disorder
- Vascular depression

Table 25.1 Studies of prevalence of depression in older people in different settings

Study	Setting	Prevalence of depression (%)
Banerjee & Macdonald 1996	Clients receiving home care from social services	26
Coope et al. 1995	Carers of dementia sufferers	28
Burn et al. 1993	Acute medical inpatients	23
Evans & Katona 1993	General practice attenders	37
Neville et al. 1995	Residential-home residents	17
Godlove Mozeley et al. 2000	New admissions to residential and nursing homes	45

Table 25.2 Studies of prevalence of significant depressive symptoms in older people with physical illness or degenerative condition

Study	Physical illness/degenerative condition	Prevalence of depression (%)
Cummings & Masterman 1999	Parkinson's disease	40
Allen & Burns 1995	Alzheimer's disease	20
Burvill et al. 1996	Poststroke	23
Massie & Holland 1990	Cancer	25
Holmes & House 2000	Hip fracture	9–47
Frasure-Smith et al. 2000	After myocardial infarction	31
Koenig 1998	Congestive heart failure	59
Yohannes et al. 1998	Chronic obstructive pulmonary disease	40

Incidence

Incidence refers to the number of new cases that arise within a given population in a given time period. Community studies have found rates of incidence between around 3% and 12% per year (Blanchard et al. 1994, Prince et al. 1998). The lower figure is found in studies of longer follow-up periods and may reflect the finding that those who develop depression are more likely to be lost to follow-up (due to increased physical and other mental health problems and mortality) before the onset can be detected. The study of different populations may also account for some of the differences in rates.

CAUSES OF DEPRESSION IN OLDER PEOPLE

No single theory adequately explains the development of depression. A dynamic stress-vulnerability model is particularly useful for understanding depression in older people (Ormel et al. 2001). This is an integrated model that incorporates evidence from the biological, psychological and social domains. In any individual depression will usually,

but not always, result from an interaction of a number of risk factors in one or more of these domains. According to the model, vulnerability factors may influence the risks of onset of depression by the amplification of the effects of acute life events (known as modification). Studies of causation of depression in older people are finding increasing evidence in support of such a model (Schoevers et al. 2000, Ormel et al. 2001). Importantly, these and other recent studies have a prospective design. Much current knowledge has been derived from cross-sectional design studies. These have a number of limitations, most notably concerning temporal relations, so that a characteristic found to be associated with depression may have caused the disorder or it may be a consequence of the depression.

The more important risk factors are briefly described here. For further discussion, readers are referred to Baldwin (2002).

Predisposing factors

Box 25.5 shows risk factors which can be regarded as predisposing or vulnerability factors.

Box 25.5   Predisposing factors to depression

- Female gender
- Past history of depression
- Family history of depression
- Widow(er)hood; being divorced
- Poverty
- Living in a residential or nursing home
- Physical health problems
- Lack of social support
- Personality
- Medication and alcohol
- Brain changes

Depression in older people is consistently found to be more common in women than in men. A number of possible reasons for this have been suggested (Evans 1996):

- loss of the traditional homemaker's role due to physical disability
- retirement of husband and his 'intrusion' into the home
- grief and loneliness following death of husband
- lack of family support, e.g. for spinsters or when children have moved away
- financial constraints or difficulty travelling causing social isolation
- loss of motherhood and role as domestic head of family when the family home is lost in a move to alternative accommodation.

It is generally regarded that genetic factors are less important as age of onset increases (Baldwin 2002). However, older individuals with a previous history of depression are more vulnerable to relapse (Schoevers et al. 2000).

Given that depression has been found to occur at high rates in residential and nursing homes (Neville et al. 1995), living in an institution must be regarded as a risk factor. Although this is likely to be linked to high levels of disability in some homes, the psychosocial environment will have an important impact if choice and control are restricted and there is limited opportunity for meaningful interaction and activity. As can be seen from Table 25.1, people who have recently entered a care home have especially high rates of depressive symptoms (Godlove Mozeley et al. 2000).

Personality and lifestyle can affect the likelihood of developing depression. For example, Ormel et al. (2001) found an association between neuroticism and depression. Also, previous heavy alcohol consump-

tion has been found to be a risk factor for depression in men (Saunders et al. 1991).

Depressive symptoms or a depressive disorder have been reported to be associated with many different drugs (Dhondt et al. l999). Such organic mood disorders due to drugs are usually caused by antihypertensives, steroids or analgesics.

There is increasing evidence that structural change in the brain increases some older people's vulnerability to depression. Evidence is often complex and the significance of some changes remains controversial (Baldwin 2002). Brain changes of interest include mild cerebral atrophy, white-matter lesions, reduced regional cerebral blood flow, alteration in brain neuroamines and receptors and neuroendocrine disturbance. Interestingly, then, Ormel et al. (2001) in their study of risk factors found that 7.2% of new depressive episodes were not preceded by any of the psychosocial risk factors they were studying. They suggested therefore that vascular and other organic changes might account for such episodes.

Precipitating factors

Risk factors which are best regarded as precipitating factors include a range of acute life events and chronic stressors and are shown in Box 25.6.

Box 25.6   Precipitating factors for depression

Acute life events
- Bereavement and separation
- Medical illness or threat to life of someone close
- Negative interaction with family member or friend
- Financial crisis or theft
- Sudden homelessness or having to move into an institution
- Acute physical illness

Chronic stressors
- Declining physical health, disability and handicap
- Sensory loss and cognitive decline
- Problems at work; retirement
- Housing problems
- Being a carer
- Major problems affecting family member
- Marital difficulties
- Social isolation and experience of loneliness

The experience of life stress is associated with the onset of depression in older people. Again, in a prospective study, Brilman & Ormel (2001) found that health-related events and difficulties were the most common life stresses, followed by deaths of loved ones and problems in non-partner relationships. Women reported more difficulties, especially health-related, than men. More severe events were strongly associated with onset of a first episode of depression, but milder events only triggered a recurrent episode. Ormel et al. (2001) found that a high level of neuroticism (a vulnerable personality trait) and long-term difficulties (chronic stressors) increased the risk of depression in the presence of an acute life event.

In their prospective study Schoevers et al. (2000) found that spousal bereavement was the strongest predictor of incident depression. Turvey et al. (1999) found the rate of significant depressive symptoms was nearly nine times higher in recently bereaved over-70s than in those still married (15.3% versus 1.9% in men and 13.2% versus 3.4% in women). Such depressive symptoms shortly after a bereavement would usually be seen as part of a normal grieving process. However 12% were still experiencing such symptoms 2 years after bereavement: many of these older people would have developed a depressive disorder.

We have seen that depression is associated with many physical conditions such as chronic obstructive pulmonary disease, heart disease, stroke and cancer. For some conditions, such as myocardial infarction, for example, the depression may be an important cause whereas in others the physical illness causes the depression by changes in body chemistry or by brain damage (Mulley 2001). However, psychological factors such as increased social isolation or embarrassment may also contribute to depression. For example, the depletion of the neurotransmitter serotonin in Parkinson's disease may be linked to the development of depression (Cummings & Masterman 1999) but psychological factors are also likely to be important. Endocrine and metabolic disturbances such as pernicious anaemia and disorders of thyroid function can also cause organic mood (depressive) disorder.

In another prospective study Prince et al. (1998) found that the strongest predictor for the onset of depression was disablement, especially handicap. Disablement is the long-term consequence of chronic limiting disease resulting in the restriction or lack of ability to perform a particular task. Handicap is the disadvantage for an individual in the performance of a normal role. As we have seen above, certain chronic diseases are associated with depression. Prince et al. (1998) suggest that the aspect of the poor physical health that confers risk of depression is not the type of disease or impairment but the manner in which it disadvantages the performance of normal roles, i.e. handicap. That is, how it disadvantages the individual in mobility, orientation, occupation, social integration, physical independence and economic self-sufficiency. Lack of contact with local friends was the only social support measure that was a risk factor for onset of depression. Conversely, higher levels of social support of this kind acted as a buffer, reducing the risk for depression in the presence of handicap. Also, the subjective experience of loneliness (which is different to living alone) was a strong risk factor. Marriage protected against depression for men but increased the risk for women compared to never-married women. It was low levels of social support and participation, not disablement, that predicted the maintenance of depression. This study therefore points to disablement being an important chronic stressor.

Sensory problems such as visual or hearing impairment often contribute to depression (Evans et al. 1991).

There are also factors which may protect or buffer against depression. These include good medical care, positive coping styles and social support (Baldwin et al. 2002). Again, in keeping with the dynamic stress-vulnerability model, Schoevers et al. (2000) found that being married had a protective modifying effect on functional disability as a risk factor for developing depression in the future. Social support had a similar effect in those not married.

MENTAL HEALTH PROMOTION AND THE PREVENTION OF DEPRESSION

Mental health promotion is any action to enhance the mental well-being of individuals, families, organizations and communities. It is also a set of principles which recognize that how people feel has a significant influence on health (Department of Health 2001a). Mental health promotion clearly has a role in preventing mental health problems. However, by improving mental well-being generally, it has a wider range of health, social and economic benefits.

It is clear from the summary of causative factors above that a wide range of physical, psychological and social factors can be implicated. It can be argued therefore that much physical health promotion activity is likely to impact on the risk of developing depression. Likewise, it can be argued that much health promotion activity that improves the social welfare of older people will impact similarly. The same applies to activities which enhance psychological well-being, for instance in providing bereavement support and encouraging active coping styles.

The UK *National Service Framework for Older People* (Department of Health 2001b) stresses the importance that maintaining physical health has on general well-being of older people. Older people should have access to mainstream health promotion and disease prevention programmes such as those described in the *National Service Framework for Coronary Heart Disease* (Department of Health 2000a) and *The NHS Cancer Plan* (Department of Health 2000b). Older people will benefit from health promotion activities such as increased physical activity (exercise), improved diet and nutrition, immunization and management programmes for influenza and strategies for preventing falls and their consequences and for preventing stroke (Department of Health 2001b).

Nurses have an important role in teaching older people about these interventions and encouraging their participation in them. Older people should be encouraged to consult their general practitioner (GP or family doctor) about physical problems at an early stage. The provision of aids and adaptations in the home to minimize the impact of disabilities will be important. Patients and carers need clear information about physical illnesses such as heart disease or stroke to encourage necessary adaptation and minimize disability and handicap. Carers also need to be helped to access the full range of support services available to maximize their morale.

The financial status of older people should be optimized. In 2000–2001 27% of older people of pensionable age lived on incomes below the poverty line (Help the Aged 2002). Nurses should always think to check a patient's entitlement to welfare benefits if circumstances suggest a need. Referral to the social services department might be appropriate. Help with form filling will often be needed.

In their public health role nurses can influence developments in the local environment and its amenities. This will involve improvements in housing and transport, access to leisure facilities, libraries and adult education, for example.

It is clear from the evidence above on causes of depression that social support can have an important role in acting as a buffer to the development of depression and might aid recovery in those who are already depressed. Nurses can be involved in the development of local support services for older people, such as befriending services, luncheon clubs or day centres. The social support derived from having a network of friends and other relationships should help to protect an older person from some of the stresses of old age. More specifically there is good evidence of the value of social support in aiding adjustment to bereavement over the long term (Long et al.

2002). This literature review also points to the beneficial effects, certainly in the short term, of individual psychologically based interventions such as bereavement counselling. It is important therefore that the usefulness of such an intervention is explained to an older person and encouragement and help offered to access such services.

BARRIERS TO EFFECTIVE MANAGEMENT OF DEPRESSION IN OLDER PEOPLE

Community surveys have consistently found that only small proportions of depressed older people are receiving treatment for their depression. For example, Prince et al. (1998) found that only 12% of their depressed community sample were prescribed antidepressants. Wilson et al. (1999) report a figure of 11%, but do note that this had risen from 4% over the 8 years of their follow-up study. Further surveys will inform us if such a trend has continued. Antidepressants are not the only treatment for depression. However, Blanchard et al. (1994) found that only 5% of their London sample were receiving counselling or supportive therapy over and above the 14% prescribed antidepressants.

A crucial barrier to treatment is that depression in older people is often not recognized in the first instance. Primary care services have a central role here. GPs and community nurses will see many older people in the GP practice and at home and have the opportunity to detect the presence of mental health problems. Also workers of the social services departments will have many contacts with older people. A study of GPs' awareness of depressed older people living at home in one electoral ward found that they were aware of 32 out of 62 (51%) older people found to be depressed by a psychiatric screening interview (Crawford et al. 1998). Those not recognized were more likely to be male, married, have high levels of physical handicap, have visual impairment and be less well educated. Banerjee & Macdonald (1996) found low recognition of depression by social services care workers. Also, Mullan et al. (1994) found that only 20% of surgery attenders judged to be depressed by the researcher had a diagnosis of depression recorded currently in their case notes. Junior doctors and general nurses have also been found to have problems detecting depression in older medical patients (Jackson & Baldwin 1993).

Depression in older people may go unrecognized for a number of reasons:

1. Older people may be less likely to present with overt feelings of depression and may present

more often with insomnia or somatic complaints such as pain

2. Depression may be expressed in an unusual way, as hypochondriasis, complaints of loneliness, or as a behaviour problem such as persistent requests to be helped to the toilet or food refusal

3. Older people and their relatives may not go to see their doctor or nurse because they do not recognize the problem as depression or know that it is treatable. Only 38% of depressed older people in one community survey said that they had discussed their psychiatric symptoms with their GPs (Blanchard et al. 1994)

4. Many professionals may lack knowledge and confidence in recognizing depression

5. Some depressive symptoms may be regarded as part of the normal ageing process

6. Depression may be overlooked when physical illness is also present: depressive symptoms may be considered 'understandable' in terms of the person's physical state

7. Similarly, depressive symptoms may be considered 'understandable' in terms of the person's psychosocial background

8. It is possible that some professionals collude with patients in not mentioning depression to avoid the stigma of mental illness

9. Screening tests are not used routinely. The Audit Commission reports of services nationally for older people with mental health problems found that the majority of GPs do not use screening tests or protocols (Audit Commission 2002).

Nurses need to take note of the above factors so as to ensure that possible depression in older people is detected.

Another key issue militating against effective management is undertreatment of depression. In the Crawford et al. (1998) study, of the 32 known to be depressed, only 12 had active treatment (38%). Why do some older people who are found to be depressed appear not to be receiving treatment? It is possible that a GP has instituted an initial trial of treatment but that inadequate follow-up arrangements were in place to monitor continued compliance and response. Antidepressants may have been stopped too soon after recovery, resulting in relapse which is not reassessed for treatment. Denihan et al. (2000), in a study of prognosis in the community, found older people with more severe depressions to be twice as likely as those with milder depressions to be treated with antidepressants. Perhaps milder depressions were seen not to warrant

antidepressant treatment. Recent research is indicating that this widely accepted stance may need reviewing in certain instances (Oxman & Sengupta 2002). Perhaps for an older person seeing the GP for a number of physical and possible mental health problems, the management of serious physical illness is prioritized over possible depression.

Certainly, many GPs report that they need more information and training on how to treat depression in older people (Rothera et al. 2002). Orrell et al. (1995), in a national questionnaire study, found that many GPs would often choose subtherapeutic doses of antidepressants, particularly of the older tricyclics. Also, antidepressants would be stopped too soon after recovery, thereby increasing the risk of relapse, and many would not refer to a psychiatrist or other mental health professional. Many GPs feel they do not have ready access to specialist advice so treatment may be delivered with little confidence (Audit Commission 2002).

TOWARDS MORE EFFECTIVE MANAGEMENT OF DEPRESSION

There is a need for more awareness of the nature of depression in older people amongst the public and professionals. Nurses have an important part to play in this mental health education role. Older people need to be made aware that depression is not a normal part of ageing, that there is no stigma attached to developing depression, and that it is an illness that is very treatable. Older people may then be more ready to go to their doctor or nurse to discuss their psychological symptoms. All professionals who come into contact with older people regularly in their work need more education about depression. Clearly, level of knowledge needed will vary depending on professional responsibilities. Nurses in all specialisms and in all settings should have the opportunity to become familiar with the key symptoms of a depressive disorder and with a screening instrument such as the Geriatric Depression Scale (GDS), discussed in the next section. They should also have some understanding of the range of treatment options and an awareness of the role of different professionals in providing comprehensive care.

Screening and education need to influence management and outcome. Routine screening alone, with increased detection, in primary care or on a general medical unit for example, does not necessarily lead to treatment and improved outcome (Iliffe et al. 1994, Weatherall 2000). Education on management generally may improve skills depending on how it is offered. For example, an educational package delivered to GPs by old-age psychiatrists has shown improvements in clinical knowledge and attitudes (Butler et al. 1997). However, one delivered by a nurse to GPs failed to generate results due to poor attendance and low return of evaluation questionnaires (Livingstone et al. 2000).

The adoption of a care pathway approach by the whole team, primary care or hospital ward, can be a way forward. The results of initial screening proceed to the next stage of physical screening and mental state examination and diagnosis and then, importantly, to treatment and follow-up. Other factors that should improve overall management are the integration of primary care with the specialist mental health services, the use of care coordinators and the use of liaison psychiatric services in hospital. A number of studies have shown how nurses in the role of care coordinators can positively influence the outcome of depression in older people (Waterreus et al. 1994, McCurren et al. 1999). The linking of a community psychiatric nurse (CPN) to a general practice should provide opportunities for education of primary care staff, ongoing advice and support, and a care coordinator role for certain patients. The importance of such a role for members of the specialist mental health services is emphasized in the *National Service Framework for Older People* (Department of Health 2001b).

Screening is most efficient when targeted at high-risk populations. Baldwin et al. (2002) recommend screening in primary care in the following instances:

- recent major physical illness
- chronic handicapping illness
- receiving high level of personal care at home
- recent bereavement
- socially isolated
- those who persistently complain of loneliness or sleep difficulties.

Also, patients in acute general hospital wards, people in residential and nursing homes and carers of people with stroke, dementia or depression would be useful targets (Wattis 2001).

As emphasized above, screening is only effective when it leads to appropriate care and treatment by being part of a care pathway approach, for example.

ASSESSMENT OF DEPRESSION IN OLDER PEOPLE

The Geriatric Depression Scale

Nurses in different settings will be helped in detecting depression by the routine use of the GDS, developed specifically for detecting probable depression in older people.

The GDS consists of 30 questions which concentrate on the thoughts and feelings of depression as they have been experienced over the past week (Stiles & McGarrahan 1998). The GDS avoids asking about physical symptoms as these could readily be of physical illness rather than depression. Its simple yes/no answer format is easy to complete and can also be administered by interview for further ease if eyesight or manual dexterity is poor. A cut-off score of 11 or more indicates probable depression. The original validation study was with psychiatric outpatients and inpatients (Yesavage et al. 1983). The GDS adequately detects depression in medical patients (Jackson & Baldwin 1993) and it has been found to be effective in primary care (Evans & Katona 1993).

A short form of the GDS has been developed with just 15 questions (Sheikh & Yesavage 1986) (Box 25.7). This is especially useful when fatigue and poor concentration are problems, with physically ill patients for example. Scores of six or more indicate probable depression. A number of studies now point to its usefulness as a screening instrument for older people living at home (Arthur et al. 1999), for primary care attenders (D'Ath et al. 1994), for psychiatric outpatients (Almeida & Almeida 1999) and for medical patients (Pomeroy et al. 2001). It also remains effective for those over 85 years of age (De Craen et al. 2003). The total score on the 15-item version appears to correlate with severity of depression (Almeida & Almeida 1999).

A 12-item version (GDS-12R) has been developed for use in residential and nursing homes (Sutcliffe et al. 2000). Items 9, 10 and 15 were omitted as they were frequently misunderstood by residents of care homes. The scale's performance was not affected by moderate to high levels of cognitive impairment. A four-item version (comprising questions 1, 3, 6 and 7) will identify most primary care patients with significant depression (D'Ath et al. 1994). However this is recommended for rapid screening only (Baldwin et al. 2002). There is a website dedicated to the GDS with details of current versions and translations (www.stanford.edu/~yesavage/GDS.html).

Assessment of depression by nurses

Nurses will assess older people with depression in a variety of settings. Whether the assessment is taking place in hospital, at home or in a residential or nursing home, the assessment will usually need to involve more than one profession. Effective multidisciplinary working is therefore essential to the process. For

---

Box 25.7   The Geriatric Depression Scale (short form)

Choose the best answer for how you have felt over the past week

1. Are you basically satisfied with your life? yes/no
2. Have you dropped many of your activities and interests?   yes/no
3. Do you feel that your life is empty? yes/no
4. Do you often get bored?   yes/no
5. Are you in good spirits most of the time? yes/no
6. Are you afraid that something bad is going to happen to you?   yes/no
7. Do you feel happy most of the time? yes/no
8. Do you often feel helpless?   yes/no
9. Do you prefer to stay at home, rather than going out and doing new things? yes/no
10. Do you feel you have more problems with memory than most?   yes/no
11. Do you think it is wonderful to be alive? yes/no
12. Do you feel pretty worthless the way you are now?   yes/no
13. Do you feel full of energy?   yes/no
14. Do you feel that your situation is hopeless? yes/no
15. Do you think that most people are better off than you are?   yes/no

The following answers score one point:
  No to 1, 5, 7, 11, 13
  Yes to 2, 3, 4, 6, 8, 9, 10, 12, 14, 15
A score of six or more indicates probable depression (this cut-off can be changed depending on aims of use)

(Reproduced with permission from Sheikh & Yesavage 1986.)

- risk assessment
- main problem areas as seen by the client
- social network
- current and past physical problems
- current medication and compliance

Severity can be judged on ICD-10 diagnostic guidelines (Box 25.1). Possible causative factors in the development of the depression should be noted as these may require specific intervention, in the case of deteriorating physical health or bereavement, for example. The same applies to maintaining factors such as avoidance of going out or abuse of alcohol. Family dynamics should be assessed as inappropriate interactions may have developed during the development of the depression which will now work against the treatment plan. For instance, a carer might have become frustrated and irritated by the lack of interest and motivation of the sufferer. As a result the carer may have withdrawn somewhat, thereby unwittingly intensifying the lack of motivation and withdrawal of the sufferer. Enquiries should be made of any previous depressive or manic episodes and the response to any treatment. Any family history of such problems should be sought as should a description of usual personality.

As we have seen, an older person may not complain of depressed mood as such so it is particularly important to assess for anhedonia (the inability to experience pleasure) and psychological symptoms. This is especially so for patients with physical illness when symptoms of sleep disturbance, appetite change, fatigue and psychomotor retardation may equally be due to a depression or the physical illness. In assessing for the presence of anhedonia it is important to ask about activities the person usually engages in and enjoys, and whether such activities have been dropped, and why. Psychological symptoms include self-perception, how the patient sees the world and how he or she sees the future. Marked negative thinking in any of these areas is indicative of a depressive disorder.

Often we need to assess the significance of depressive symptoms in someone who has been bereaved in recent months. Depressed mood, loss of interest, poor concentration, poor sleep, poor appetite, weight loss and agitation are all common features of normal grieving in older people. However, grief can be complicated by the development of a depressive disorder (Worden 1991). How can we tell when this might be the case? Specifying no particular age group, DSM-IV suggests that even though such symptoms might meet criteria for major depression, they should be considered as bereavement unless they persist for more than

further discussion of nursing assessment readers are referred to Neal et al. (2001).

In addition to using an appropriate screening tool, an assessment should cover the following main areas:

- severity of current episode
- duration, development and maintaining factors
- past history of mood disorder and response to treatment
- previous personality and family history of mood disorder
- current symptom profile

2 months or include marked functional impairment, morbid preoccupation with worthlessness, suicidal ideas, psychotic symptoms or psychomotor retardation (American Psychiatric Association 1994). Turvey et al. (1999) suggest that, given that widows and widowers in later life have lost a – possibly lifetime – companion, a period longer than 2 months may be expected. The most severe symptoms should normally have improved after 6 months or so.

Some older people who present with depression also have some cognitive impairment. This then should also be assessed, including use of the Mini-Mental State Examination (Folstein et al. 1975). It is possible that some have a dementia and have become depressed. Interestingly, however, it has been suggested that in some patients depression (in association with some cognitive impairment) may be a prodrome to dementia (Schweitzer et al. 2002). In other words, the depressive syndrome is seen as an early manifestation of a developing dementia. In their review Schweitzer et al. (2002) conclude that it is patients with late-onset depression who are more likely to have cognitive impairment and are more likely to progress to dementia. The implication for nurses is that such patients should have close follow-up. Importantly, though, not all patients with late-onset depression will inevitably go on to develop dementia. The link between the depression and the dementia may be due to the sharing of a common aetiological pathway (e.g. via vascular pathology). Alternatively, it has been hypothesized that persistently raised levels of cortisol damage the hippocampus, the brain structure which is central to memory function (Steffens et al. 2000). Raised cortisol levels result from hyperactivity of the hypothalamic–pituitary–adrenal axis which is associated with depression.

A detailed risk assessment must be undertaken. Areas of risk are clearly important to assess as they have implications as to whether the person may need to be treated urgently in hospital, or whether an intensive supportive package needs to be arranged urgently to maintain the person safely in the community. It is essential to assess for thoughts of suicide. Asking about suicidal thoughts does not encourage suicidal acts. 'Do you ever think that life is not worth living?' is a useful initial question. Increasing levels of severity of suicidal ideas are indicated by the following thoughts:

'Life is not worth living' – without any thoughts of self-harm.

'I think I would be better off dead', and the most serious: 'I can't go on, I'm going to end it all' – the means of self-harm is likely to have been considered.

The following factors would indicate higher risk (Baldwin et al. 2002):

- older age (especially over 80), male gender, isolation, recent bereavement
- history of previous suicide attempt(s)
- chronic and painful physical disorder, abuse of alcohol or sedatives
- clinical picture of severe depression with agitation, guilt, hopelessness, insomnia and hypochondriasis

Possible self-neglect is the other main risk area. Neglect of food, and particularly fluids, can soon put an older person in danger. Neglect of self-care and heating of accommodation also need assessment. Risk assessment should be ongoing so that risk is monitored by regular reviews of the patient.

Assessing people's view of the situation and the main problem areas as seen by them are important in planning care. Their social network should be carefully assessed. Particularly supportive relationships should be noted as these can be used to help in treatment. It is not always the tangible support that is most important; a particular source of support may have more meaning to a person's situation and problems and be perceived as more supportive. A change in overall pattern of social network may be needed in acute treatment and for relapse prevention. The effect of the current problems on family and other carers should be assessed as they may require support themselves. Carers can also become depressed.

Many physical illnesses can present with symptoms of depression such as fatigue, loss of appetite, psychomotor retardation or depressed mood. Examples are disorders of thyroid function, electrolyte disturbances, anaemia, vitamin deficiencies and malignancy (Wattis & Curran 2001). It is important therefore that medical examination and indicated investigations are carried out in all persons being assessed for depression. Also, the disabling effects of conditions such as arthritis or stroke should be assessed as supportive measures to maximize understanding and independence and counter handicap will contribute to treatment of the depression.

Note should be made of any medication being taken. The person may be taking medication that can contribute to depressive symptoms such as antihypertensives, steroids or analgesics. An antidepressant may have been prescribed but at a subtherapeutic dose. Level of adherence to current medication should be assessed as this will help guide any further prescribing and monitoring.

CARE AND TREATMENT OF DEPRESSION AND THE ROLE OF THE NURSE

Nurses from different specialisms will see depressed older people in a variety of settings. District nurses and health visitors are likely to have some depressed older people on their caseloads whom they see at home. Practice nurses will see depressed older people in their work in the GP surgery or at home. As hospital inpatients or day patients, depressed older people will be seen by other general nurses. In my own practice as a CPN for older adults, depression accounts for around a third of my caseload at any one time. Older people with the most severe problems will be nursed by mental health nurses in psychiatric units.

Although different nurses will have somewhat different roles and levels of involvement with their depressed older patients, there are a number of important principles to care and treatment which will apply in all settings. There are also some fundamental elements to the nursing approach which can be applied in varying degrees by different nurses in different settings. I will call this the generic nursing approach. It is recognized that in most situations the priorities of the general nurse will be in the more physical aspects of nursing care. However, most general nurses will have sufficient knowledge and skills to implement this generic approach with depressed, physically ill patients. As discussed in the next section, this approach involves relationship building, giving support and information and enabling change in thinking patterns, activity and skills.

Specialist mental health nurses will use the generic approach but will also develop it in terms of:

- more specialist assessment, including risk assessments
- more indepth and intensive interventions, including psychological therapy and medication management
- care coordination functions
- advice to, and supervision of, other professionals.

Specialist mental health nurses are likely to be involved therefore when reassessment is needed, when depression is more severe with significant risk or psychosis present, or when initial treatment has failed so that more specialist intervention is required.

Principles of care and treatment of an older person with depression

The following important principles apply when nursing any depressed older person:

1. It is a problem-solving exercise based on a thorough assessment
2. It is usually a multidimensional approach with some combination of physical, psychological and social interventions
3. A multidisciplinary approach is therefore usually needed
4. Care needs to be coordinated
5. The timing of interventions is important
6. Physical condition should always be monitored and problems treated
7. Family members and other carers should be involved where appropriate.

Fundamental elements of the nursing approach

The therapeutic relationship

Nurses often form close relationships with their patients. Also, they are usually well aware that the quality of the relationship is an important element in their patient's recovery. Such a close relationship is fundamentally important in nursing people with mental health problems. A key ingredient of the therapeutic relationship is the personal qualities of the nurse. These personal qualities are those described by Carl Rogers in his work on client-centred counselling as the key personal qualities of the 'effective helper' (Rogers 1967). These personal qualities are not simply counselling techniques that can be learnt. They are said to be more of the order of personal convictions and these need to be communicated to the patient at least to some degree.

Key personal qualities

Warmth   Nurses should have a warm, positive and accepting attitude to patients. They should realize that patients have an inherent worth and dignity deserving of respect. This warmth will be conveyed to the patient in general manner, tone of voice and way of phrasing words.

Empathy   Empathy is the ability to see and understand the world as the patient sees it. Nurses need, to some degree, to be able to understand how the patient is feeling and communicate this understanding to the patient.

Genuineness   This refers to the quality of the nurse in having genuine professional interest in patients and their problems. Nurses need at times to be able to share their own feelings with the patient in an open honest manner and not hide behind the professional facade.

The establishment of a therapeutic relationship encompassing the above qualities is the foundation for nursing older people with depression.

The generic nursing approach

Nurses can help depressed older people by being with them and listening to them. Rapport and understanding will only be established by spending time with the person. The overall approach should generally be gentle and accepting. A light-hearted approach aimed at trying to 'cheer the person up' is not helpful. It will merely communicate a lack of understanding and lack of respect for the person's feelings. It may often be necessary to speak more slowly and allow more time for the person to respond. If individuals are severely depressed and say very little then just being with them can be of comfort and communicate a genuine concern for their well-being.

A depressed person should be encouraged to express thoughts and feelings. Clearly, counselling skills are important here. The person is likely to feel some relief from expressing any concerns about the past or present. Also, such expression will allow the nurse to monitor the person's current mental state. The individual may feel in a hopeless situation with no future. Information-giving is important. The nurse can gently reassure the person that, although recovery from the depression may be slow and possibly take many weeks, improvement will occur. Again such reassurance needs a gentle considered approach so as not to communicate a lack of understanding of the person's situation. All the above aspects of care detail the supportive role that nurses have.

The generic nursing approach involves care which enables changes in thinking patterns, activity and skills. When depressed, a person often neglects usual interests and activities, including those that were previously enjoyable. People also commonly think that they cannot resume such activities until their depression has lifted. However, it is clear that engaging in enjoyable activity which also gives a sense of achievement is a powerful antidepressant. It is important, therefore, for the nurse gradually to engage the person in potentially enjoyable activity. It will be important to negotiate realistic goals at each stage of treatment. The depressed person should also gradually be encouraged to resume previous social contacts. Family involvement in care is important here.

Nurses should also be aware that there is increasing evidence for the positive effects of exercise on depressive symptoms in older people (Mather et al. 2002, Penninx et al. 2002). Older people can be encouraged to attend established groups as part of their treatment plan or nurses can develop new exercise programmes in hospital and community settings.

Negative thinking very often dominates a depressed person's perception of reality. Negative evaluations of events and situations may occur automatically so that the person is quite unaware of the process. Negative thinking will perpetuate the depressed mood. The nurse can gently help the person to identify such thoughts and help to examine them so as to see them in a more rational light. Distraction from preoccupation with negative thinking is also important at times so the person can be encouraged to socialize or take part in activities.

Depending on individual circumstances, including the severity of the depression, the following physical aspects of care will need consideration:

- monitoring of fluid and food intake
- offering preferred foods with regular small meals
- monitoring weight
- bowel care
- enhancing sleep by avoiding frequent daytime naps and planning activities according to energy levels
- assisting with personal care and promoting independence by positive reinforcement.

For further discussion of the above aspects of care readers are referred to Stuart (1998).

Physical treatments and the role of the nurse

Antidepressant drugs

The pharmacological treatment of depression is usefully conceptualized as having an acute phase followed by a continuation and a maintenance phase, as illustrated in Figure 25.1. Successful acute treatment should be followed by 12 months of continuation treatment in order to prevent relapse (Anderson et al. 2000). Longer-term maintenance treatment, possibly indefinitely, is recommended for individuals with a history of several depressive episodes, chronic depression or bipolar disorder in order to prevent recurrence.

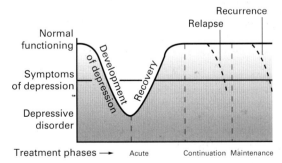

Fig. 25.1 Phases in the pharmacological treatment of depression.

In summarizing the evidence base for the treatment of depression, Baldwin et al. (2002) offer the following guidance:

- for psychotic depression – antidepressant and antipsychotic drug
- for severe depression – antidepressant plus psychological therapy if possible
- for moderate depression – antidepressant or psychological therapy
- for dysthymia – antidepressant (Williams et al. 2000)
- for recent-onset minor depression – education, support and re-evaluation
- for minor depression when functional impairment is severe or if symptoms persist or worsen after a 4–6-week period of support – antidepressant (Williams et al. 2000)
- for grief or bereavement – as for moderate depression if indicated.

A recent review of the treatment of minor depression showed that the response to active control conditions across all age groups ranges from 35% to 68% (Oxman & Sengupta 2002). These authors suggest therefore that amplification of non-specific treatment factors may be an important strategy for management: these include therapeutic empathy, contact and social support, providing a treatment rationale, talking about one's problems to an attentive professional and behavioural activation. Interestingly, the generic nursing approach described earlier encompasses all of these factors and so may arguably be very helpful in treating many older people with milder depressions. Many such people will be seen by primary care nurses, and by general nurses in medical and surgical settings where, as we have seen, non-major depression can be very common. Psychological therapy is discussed further in the next section.

Table 25.3 shows some of the antidepressants prescribed for older people. Side-effects and dosages are shown. It is not a comprehensive list but it illustrates the classes of antidepressants that may be prescribed.

In moderate to severe depression up to around 60% of patients significantly improve with antidepressants (Mittman et al. 1997). The response to placebo is often up to 30%. There is no difference in efficacy between different classes of antidepressant. Older people usually take longer to recover. There appear to be no differences between antidepressant drugs in terms of speed of onset. A therapeutic trial may last up to 12 weeks. Older drugs such as the tricyclic antidepressants have more dangerous side-

Table 25.3 Some antidepressants for older people

	Type of action	Antimuscarinic effect	Antiadrenergic effect	Antihistamic effect	Starting dosage (mg)	Average daily dose (mg)
Lofepramine	Newer TCA	1	1	1	70–140	70–210
Fluoxetine	SSRI	0–1	0	0	10	20
Paroxetine	SSRI	0–1	0	0	10–20	20–30
Sertraline	SSRI	0–1	0	0	25–50	50–100
Citalopram	SSRI	0–1	0	0	10–20	20–30
Venlafaxine	SNRI	0–1	0–1	0	25–75	75–200
Trazodone	SSRI/blocks 5HT	0	1	3	100	300
Nefazodone	SSRI/blocks 5HT	0	1	1	50–100	150–300
Moclobemide	RIMA	0–1	0	0	300	300–450
Mirtazepine	NaSSA	0	0	2	7.5–15	15–30

TCA, tricyclic antidepressant; SSRI, selective serotonin reuptake inhibitor; SNRI, selective serotonin and noradrenaline (norepinephrine) reuptake inhibitor; 5HT, 5-hydroxytryptamine (serotonin); RIMA, reversible inhibitor of monoamine oxidase; NaSSA, noradrenergic and specific serotonergic antidepressant.
Notes: Effect size on an arbitrary scale from 0 (least effect) to 5 (most effect).
Antimuscarinic effect: dry mouth, blurred vision, constipation, urinary retention, sweating, confusion, worsening of glaucoma.
Antiadrenergic effect: postural hypotension, dizziness, falls.
Antihistamic effect: oversedation, weight gain.
SSRIs: more common side-effects include: nausea (15%), diarrhoea (10%), insomnia (5–15%), restlessness or anxiety (2–15%), headache, weight gain and hyponatraemia.
Starting and average daily dosages are only a guide; they may vary depending on individual circumstances

effects. Newer drugs, as listed in Table 25.3, are safer in overdose (Wilson & Curran 2001). For medically ill patients newer drugs have much fewer contraindications. It is therefore not surprising that in primary care selective serotonin reuptake inhibitors (SSRIs) are now favoured as the first line of treatment in many countries (e.g. Rothera et al. 2002).

There are a number of potential strategies for the patient who does not respond to first-line treatment:

- increasing dose if not optimal
- extending the length of treatment
- switching class of antidepressant
- prescribing lithium salts alongside the antidepressant (lithium augmentation)
- using electroconvulsive therapy (ECT) (Baldwin et al. 2002).

Nurses have an important role in caring for someone prescribed an antidepressant. The nurse needs to teach the patient and family about important aspects of antidepressant therapy including the rationale for taking the medication alongside other interventions. Antidepressants can take up to 4–6 weeks to produce any benefit. It is especially important therefore to support patients through these early weeks. They might experience side-effects, making them feel worse, but with little change in depressive symptoms. They then might be tempted to stop taking the medication because 'it was not working'. Adherence can always be a problem. Packaging in drug drawers or Dossett boxes or in blister packs can help adherence, especially if the patient has memory problems. Carers may need to prompt the patient to take medication. The patient should be informed of possible side-effects. These need to be closely monitored by the nurse and reported to the doctor. Patients taking lithium should be warned about the risk of toxicity and told to stop taking the lithium if they become unwell, particularly with diarrhoea, nausea or vomiting, and inform their doctor. Clearly, overall response, or non-response, to medication should be monitored as dosage may need to be gradually increased. The nurse also needs to ensure that the patient does not stop taking the drug when feeling better. As we have seen, the drug should be continued into the continuation phase and possibly a maintenance phase. It is particularly important to monitor a patient with suicidal ideas closely. An antidepressant that is considered to be safer in overdose may be prescribed and it should be prescribed in smaller quantities.

Electroconvulsive therapy

The main indication for ECT is severe depression, particularly when antidepressants have failed (Benbow

2001). It may be the treatment of choice for patients who have a history of not responding to antidepressants but responding to ECT. It may also be the first-line treatment for patients whose lives are threatened by high suicide risk or if refusing to eat or drink. It is often considered as the treatment of choice in psychotic depression. The response rate in patients for whom it is indicated is 70–80%. It has been used for people with a range of concurrent physical illnesses and for the very old. Although there are no absolute contraindications, older people with cardiovascular and neurological conditions need particular attention given to management of the physical condition and treatment technique.

The procedure involves passing a small current through the brain, either longitudinally through the non-dominant hemisphere (unilateral ECT) or across the brain through both hemispheres (bilateral ECT). The patient is given a short-acting general anaesthetic and a muscle relaxant. The grand mal-type fit that is induced by the passage of current is then hardly noticeable. It is suggested that bilateral ECT is usually the method of choice, often being more rapidly effective, but that unilateral ECT is preferred in the presence of pre-existing cognitive impairment. ECT is usually administered twice weekly with a course length of between 6 and 12 treatments.

Side-effects of ECT which occur occasionally and are usually only mild include headaches, muscular aches, drowsiness, weakness, nausea and anorexia (Benbow 2001). Cognitive side-effects may occur. ECT can affect memory for events prior to treatment (anterograde amnesia) and which take place after treatment (retrograde amnesia). Acute confusional states may develop between treatments.

The role of the nurse in ECT involves the physical and psychological preparation of the patient, preparation of equipment, safe handling of the patient during administration of treatment and recovery of the unconscious patient afterwards. ECT arouses much anxiety. Nurses particularly have an important role in teaching patients and their relatives about the nature and procedures of ECT.

Psychosocial interventions

In the multidimensional approach to treatment a range of psychosocial interventions have an important role either on their own or alongside physical treatments. When social isolation, poor housing or bereavement, for example, have contributed to the development of the depression, a complete and lasting recovery is unlikely unless these psychosocial factors are dealt with in their own right. A person may be able to receive psychological therapy for depression if indicated or preferred. Nurses have an important role in delivering psychosocial interventions.

Psychological therapy

A number of research reviews (Pinquart & Sorensen 2001) have now provided evidence for the efficacy of the following interventions for depression in older people:

- cognitive-behavioural therapy (CBT)
- interpersonal therapy (IPT)
- brief psychodynamic therapy
- problem-solving therapy
- life review

Of these, the strongest evidence of efficacy exists for CBT and IPT (Hepple et al. 2002). These are therefore described in more detail below. There is some evidence that problem-solving therapy may be effective for minor depression (Williams et al. 2000).

Cognitive-behavioural therapy and interpersonal therapy

Both are structured forms of psychological therapy aimed at alleviating symptoms and helping the patient to deal more effectively with the problems associated with the depression. They are time-limited problem-solving and focus on the 'here and now'.

In CBT the emphasis is on the negative thinking that is characteristic of depression. The contemporary theoretical view is that negative thinking is part and parcel of the depressive syndrome but is a particularly important symptom. Negative thinking does not cause the depression but it may be important in shaping and maintaining it. Thinking is often distorted in a negative way so that the person has a negative view of self (I'm useless), the world (the world is a terrible place to live in) and the future (I'll never get better). Underlying such negative automatic thoughts are beliefs, attitudes and assumptions about the self and the world which are, in the case of depressive thinking, 'dysfunctional' or unhelpful in that they are fixed, excessive and difficult to change. An example of a dysfunctional belief might be 'unless I can always be physically well, I cannot be happy'. The cognitive model explains depression at one level without negating biological and sociological elements and cognitive distortions are important entry points into the depressive system for therapy. CBT aims to alleviate depressed mood and other symptoms of depression by changing this pattern of negative thinking and so allow other problems to be tackled. Therapy usually involves a range of behavioural as well as cognitive techniques to achieve this end. Behavioural techniques are often used early in therapy to counteract inactivity

and loss of motivation. For example, activity scheduling is a technique which involves the patient and therapist agreeing on tasks to be done (scheduled) on an hour-to-hour basis throughout the day so as to increase general activity levels. The patient is then encouraged to monitor and rate the activities on giving a sense of mastery and pleasure. As well as increasing activity levels the patient is providing evidence that can be used to challenge negative thinking such as 'I never get anything done' or 'I can't enjoy myself any more'. In graded task assignment, challenging tasks (e.g. walking into town for shopping) are initially broken down into small achievable parts which are practised as homework (e.g. walking to the end of the street) and then the task is gradually built up.

Cognitive techniques involve identifying negative automatic thoughts and the related emotion and recording the situations in which they arose. The aim then is to modify negative thinking by active challenge by, for example, examining the evidence for and against the thought or collecting alternative information through behavioural experiments. It is also important that any unhelpful underlying rigid beliefs are identified and also challenged, not to change them but to add some flexibility to them.

In IPT the emphasis is on the connection between the onset of depressive symptoms and current interpersonal problems. It is based on the research evidence that close interpersonal relationships play a role in preventing depression and that disruption of those relationships can have a causal role in depression. Attention is on current interpersonal relationships as a focus for treatment. Indepth exploring of early life events is avoided. The therapist formulates a proposed focus for treatment in one of four broad areas: (1) grief; (2) role transitions; (3) interpersonal role disputes; and (4) interpersonal deficits. Techniques involve exploration and direct elicitation of the problem area, encouragement and acceptance of painful affect related to this, examining problems in communication in the area and behaviour change techniques. Education is an essential function of IPT in that ultimately all interventions are aimed at teaching patients about their interactions with others. Patients are taught to analyse situations, solve problems for themselves and make their own choices.

Other psychological approaches

Grief work Grief work is mentioned here separately because in working with depressed older people it is a very common part of therapy. It involves expressing emotions (catharsis) and letting go of lost loved ones. It can be a focus of IPT, as above, and cognitive-behavioural interventions may be appropriate (Ricketts 1995). Also, a person may grieve for lost physical functioning due to stroke, for example. However, as Knight (1996: p. 126) succinctly points out, the processes and goals are quite different: 'In brief, lost functioning is often recovered or compensated, but deceased people stay deceased'.

Non-directive client-centred counselling Counselling is an important intervention when a patient needs help in resolving specific problems, making decisions, coping with crises, working through conflict or improving relationships with others (Department of Health 2001c). This will often be needed as part of the multidimensional approach to the treatment of depression. However, research evidence for the effectiveness of non-directive counselling in treating depression in older people is still lacking. Nonetheless, nurses usually spend a lot more time with patients than other professionals and so have opportunities to use their counselling role to help patients in many ways. In relation to depression a counselling approach will probably be most appropriate alongside social and practical interventions in the milder depressive disorders.

Family work Family issues commonly arise in treatment and, although some can be resolved fairly easily, others may require formal family therapy, especially when family discord, for example, is maintaining depression and preventing recovery. Readers are referred to Pearce (2002) for an account of the development of family (or systemic) therapy with older people. However, this approach to depression still requires further evaluation in older people.

Social and practical interventions

In the multidimensional approach to depression described here nurses have a role in implementing other psychosocial interventions. These might include: arranging transport to the optician or chiropodist, for example; referral to check on welfare benefit entitlement; referral to a day centre, luncheon club or support group; referral for domiciliary services such as home care and delivery of meals; and help with rehousing. The timing of social interventions such as referral to a day centre needs careful consideration. Severely depressed people will probably need antidepressant or psychological therapy to begin to lift mood and energy levels; only then might they be able to consider changes in their social network.

In the light of the above it is useful to reflect on the case studies presented earlier. Mary Smith (Case study 25.1) had major depression. As there were no significant risks she was treated successfully at home with antidepressant medication and CBT by a CPN. Reginald Evans (Case study 25.2) had major depression with psychotic symptoms and needed hospital treatment. He was supported through ECT by the ward nurses and he was discharged home on continuation antidepressant medication and CPN follow-up. Betty Watson (Case study 25.3) had dysthymia, chronic mild depression. Again, antidepressant medication was indicated alongside CPN support. In each case nurses made a significant contribution to effective care and treatment.

Research into the effectiveness of nursing interventions

A small number of research studies have examined nursing interventions for depression in older people. These studies contribute to the evidence base of nursing but they do vary in the rigour of experimental design. Studies of the effectiveness of community mental health teams are also relevant as mental health nurses usually constitute the majority of the workforce in such teams.

In Waterreus et al.'s (1994) study, older depressed patients found in a community survey in London were allocated to either CPN intervention directed by a multidisciplinary team or a control condition of routine GP management. At 3 months there was significant improvement in depression scores in the intervention group versus the control group. The greatest improvement was seen in the more chronic depressions. Overall benefit seemed to be associated with the nursing activities of counselling and behavioural work.

McCurren et al. (1999) examined the intervention of a psychiatric nurse on depressive symptoms in residents of three UK nursing homes. The nurse made comprehensive assessments, developed treatment plans and provided therapeutic interventions augmented by older adult volunteers in the role of mental health paraprofessionals. She trained and supervised the volunteers. Individual strategies included provision of emotional and social support, identification and capitalization of strengths, development of diversional activities and enhancement of the social network. After 24 weeks of treatment depressive symptoms were significantly reduced in the treatment but not in the control group.

In Proctor et al.'s (1999) study, staff of residential and nursing homes in the UK selected residents who were difficult to manage. Intervention consisted of training staff in seven 1-h seminars by a hospital outreach team and weekly psychiatric nurse visits to the home to give advice and support in the development of care planning skills. At the 6-month follow up, the mean decrease in depression scores was significantly larger for residents in the intervention homes than for those in the control homes.

Rabins et al. (2000) studied psychiatric nurses in a mobile outreach programme for residents of three public apartment buildings in the USA: three other buildings formed the control group. In the intervention group, building staff were trained to be case-finders; nurses carried out assessments in residents' apartments and provided care as indicated. Most frequent interventions were counselling, patient education about their illness and positive health behaviours, and ensuring medication compliance. The mood disorder group showed significant improvement in depressive symptom score compared to the control group.

Kurlowicz (2001) reports on the work of a psychiatric consultation liaison nurse (PCLN) in a US teaching hospital. The nurse was consulted by staff in medical and surgical wards and assessed and developed a joint care plan with ward staff. Interventions by the PCLN were ongoing assessment, supportive and IPT, advice to ward staff, daily review of medications, recommendations for referral to a psychiatrist, family support and nursing care plan modifications. At follow-up before discharge, patients referred with depression showed a significant decrease in mean depression scores, but there was no control group.

Finally, a randomized controlled trial has demonstrated the effectiveness of a multidisciplinary team approach in the UK. Banerjee et al. (1996) examined the approach to depressed older people receiving home care from a local authority in inner London. A management plan was implemented by an assigned team member (including nurses) with a range of interventions being implemented. At 6 months 58% had recovered versus 25% in the control group of usual GP care.

THE PROGNOSIS OF DEPRESSION IN OLDER PEOPLE

What is the outcome for depression in older people in the community if it is not treated? A 5-year follow-up study in Liverpool, UK is worrying (Sharma et al. 1998). Over that period 41 (34%) out of an original 120 cases had died, 33 (28%) dropped out of the study and 46 (38%) had complete follow-up. Of these 46 cases, only 22% had recovered, 24% had been continuously depressed and the remaining 54% had fluctuating levels of symptoms. Importantly, the majority of people with depression were not receiving treatment.

A 3-year follow-up study in Dublin showed the outcome of depressed older people detected in the community when GPs were informed of depressed cases and treatment recommended (Denihan et al. 2000) (Table 25.4). Only just over 10% had fully recovered. Of those still alive at 3 years, 50% were still depressed. Undertreatment appears to be a significant factor in the poor prognosis. Of those who had recovered at 3-year follow-up (i.e. well or subclinical cases), 63% were or had been prescribed antidepressants. Of those still depressed, the figure was only 38%, and 29% of these had received subtherapeutic doses.

The prognosis for older people whose depression has required hospital treatment as an outpatient or inpatient is shown in Table 25.5. These are the results of a meta-analysis of a number of hospital-based studies of major depression (Cole & Bellavance 1997). In the long term it is clear that less than half of those treated will remain well, with relapse and chronic symptoms being common.

Another significant finding of outcome studies is that the death rate in older people who have become depressed is often higher than normally expected at that age (Saz & Dewey 2001). Suicides only account for a small number of deaths at follow-up. Poorer physical health contributes to increased mortality but is not the sole explanation. The main causes of death reported are vascular disease (cardiovascular or cere-

Table 25.4 Three-year outcome of depression in older people in a Dublin community sample (expressed as %)

	Fully recovered	Depressed	Died	Other case	Subclinical case of depression	Other subclinical case
All cases (n = 106)	10.4	34.9	30.2	4.7	8.5	11.3

Subclinical case, some symptoms present but below case-level threshold.
Adapted from Denihan et al. (2000) with permission.

Table 25.5 The prognosis of major depression in older people following hospital-based treatment

Length of follow–up	Well (%)	Recovered after relapse (%)	Continuously depressed (%)	Other (e.g. death, dementia) (%)
< 2 years	44	16	22	23
> 2 years	27	33	14	31

Data from Cole & Bellavance (1997).

brovascular), carcinoma and respiratory disease. It is not clear why this should be, although it is possible that stressful life events contribute to heart disease and depression and that depression has an adverse effect on the immune system.

A number of factors are associated with a poorer prognosis. These include slower initial recovery, severity and chronicity of the depression, psychotic symptoms, dementia, chronic stress, a new physical illness and poor perceived social support (Baldwin 2002).

Improving prognosis and the role of the nurse

The studies reviewed here again emphasize the importance of detecting and comprehensively treating depressions in older people. Otherwise a chronic course will follow or relapses will be common. Nurses have an important role in improving prognosis:

1. The initial episode of depression should be adequately treated whatever the setting. Nurses will have a role in delivering psychological and social interventions as an adjunct or alternative to physical treatments
2. When antidepressants are used adherence should be carefully monitored in the acute, continuation and maintenance phases of treatment
3. New physical illness should be promptly treated
4. Patients with dementia who become depressed should be recognized and treated appropriately
5. Nurses can be involved in support groups which will be important in preventing relapse.

Nurses can coordinate the plan of care and treatment. A coordinated care plan should ensure that everyone involved in the person's care knows to report changes in mood and behaviour to the care coordinator so as to detect early signs of possible relapse. Antidepressant medication may need reviewing, the person may need to attend the day hospital again or a new concern over finances or family, for example, may need a psychological or social intervention.

SUICIDE IN OLDER PEOPLE

It is beyond the scope of this chapter to give a detailed account of suicide in older people. Readers are referred to Harwood (2002) for a good introduction.

As discussed earlier, it is crucial that suicide risk is assessed in a depressed older person since the majority (up to 87%) of older people who commit suicide will have been suffering from a depressive disorder prior to death (Harwood et al. 2000). Similar rates are found in older people who have attempted suicide. Physical illness and complaint of pain are also strongly related to suicide in older people.

The rate of suicide in older people in England and Wales has been declining in both sexes, with the exception of the 85-year-plus age bands (Shah et al. 2001). In 1998 the annual rate in males aged 65–69 years was 14 per 100 000 population and in females 7 per 100 000. This compares with rates of 21.3 and 6.8 in the 85–89 age groups. Harwood et al. (2000) found the commonest methods of suicide were hanging in men and drug overdose in women. A total of 49.8% had seen their GP in the month before death and 15.4% were under psychiatric care.

In working with depressed older people nurses always need to assess for suicidal thoughts and the risk of a suicide attempt. This is especially so in those depressed patients who are in the higher-risk group: that is, older males, the recently bereaved, the socially isolated, those suffering from a painful physical illness and those who have a history of previous attempts. With high suicide risk a person may be admitted to hospital and be closely supervised. Nurses need to be aware that some changes in behaviour may indicate the possibility of suicidal thoughts: these include altering wills, giving away possessions, changes in religious interest or the hoarding of medications. Depression should be treated. Any physical problems should be reassessed and appropriate care given, with special attention to any painful conditions. If the person is living at home the GP and family need to be educated about risk factors present. The CPN will have a key role here. Any medications should be carefully monitored. Prescriptions covering short periods of time, the use of blister packs of medication and avoiding the prescription of particularly toxic drugs will be part of the management plan.

CONCLUSION

This chapter has shown how nurses can make significant contributions to the process leading to the effective care and treatment of depression in older people. Nurses can have a key role in preventing much depression. Nurses see many older people in a variety of settings and are therefore in a unique position to ensure that depression is detected and treated adequately. This chapter has also referred to some of the substantial evidence base that now exists in this field on which nurses can base their contemporary practice.

Recommended reading

Anderson IM, Nutt DJ, Deakin JFW et al. 2000 Evidence-based guidelines for treating depressive disorders with antidepressants: a revision of the 1993 British Association of Psychopharmacology guidelines. Journal of Psychopharmacology 14: 3–20.
This substantial paper reviews the evidence on which to base treatment of mild to moderate depression in adults with antidepressants. The guidelines contain special reference to older people as is needed.
Baldwin RC, Chiu E, Katona C, Graham N 2002 Guidelines on depression in older people: practising the evidence. Martin Dunitz, London.
This excellent text provides an overview of current evidence and best practice on the classification, prevalence, causation and management of depressive disorder in older people. Recommendations for practice are made on the basis of the strength of evidence in each of these areas.
Curran S, Wattis JP, Lynch S (eds) 2001 Practical management of depression in older people. Arnold, London.
This multidisciplinary text is an excellent contemporary overview of practice. The chapter by Graham Mulley on depression in physically ill older patients will be of particular interest to registered nurses in primary care and general hospital settings.
Hepple J, Pearce J, Wilkinson P (eds) 2002 Psychological therapies with older people: developing treatments for effective practice. Brunner-Routledge, Hove.
Psychological therapies should be as available to older people as to any other age group. The authors describe the therapies most likely to be useful in a mental health service for older people. It is an important source for all disciplines offering psychological therapy.
Jacoby R, Oppenheimer C (eds) 2002 Psychiatry in the elderly, 3rd edn. Oxford University Press, Oxford.
This major text includes substantial chapters on topics relevant to depressive disorder. In particular: liaison old age psychiatry in

the general hospital by Michael Philpot, Declan Lyons and Tom Reynolds, depressive disorders by R C Baldwin and suicide in older persons by Daniel Harwood.

References

Allen NHP, Burns A 1995 The non-cognitive features of dementia. Reviews in Clinical Gerontology 5: 57–75
Almeida OP, Almeida SA 1999 Short versions of the geriatric depression scale: a study of their validity for the diagnosis of a major depressive episode according to ICD-10 and DSM-IV. International Journal of Geriatric Psychiatry 14: 858–865
American Psychiatric Association 1994 Diagnostic and statistical manual of mental disorders (DSM-IV), 4th edn. American Psychiatric Association, Washington
Anderson IA, Nutt DJ, Deakin JFW 2000 Evidence-based guidelines for treating depressive disorders with antidepressants: a revision of the 1993 British Association of Psychopharmacology guidelines. Journal of Psychopharmacology 14: 3–20
Arthur A, Jagger C, Lindesay J et al. 1999 Using an annual over-75 health check to screen for depression: validation of the short geriatric depression scale (GDS15) within general practice. International Journal of Geriatric Psychiatry 14: 431–439
Audit Commission 2002 Forget me not 2002: developing mental health services for older people in England. Audit Commission, London
Baldwin RC 2002 Depressive disorders. In: Jacoby R, Oppenheimer C (eds) Psychiatry in the elderly, 3rd edn. Oxford University Press, Oxford, pp 627–676
Baldwin RC, O'Brien J 2002 Vascular onset of late-onset depressive disorder. British Journal of Psychiatry 18: 157–160
Baldwin RC, Chiu E, Katona C et al. 2002 Guidelines on depression in older people: practising the evidence. Martin Dunitz, London
Banerjee S, Macdonald A 1996 Mental disorder in an elderly home care population: associations with health and social service use. British Journal of Psychiatry 168: 750–756
Banerjee S, Shamash K, MacDonald AJD et al. 1996 Randomised controlled trial of effect of intervention by psychogeriatric team on depression in frail elderly people at home. British Medical Journal 313: 1058–1106
Beekman ATF, Copeland JRM, Prince MJ 1999 Review of community prevalence of depression in later life. British Journal of Psychiatry 174: 307–311
Benbow S 2001 ECT in the treatment of depression in older people. In: Curran S, Wattis JP, Lynch S (eds) Practical management of depression in older people. Arnold, London, pp 61–75
Blanchard MR, Waterreus A, Mann AH 1994 The nature of depression among older people in inner London, and the contact with primary care. British Journal of Psychiatry 164: 396–402
Brilman EI, Ormel J 2001 Life events, difficulties and onset of depressive episodes in later life. Psychological Medicine 31: 859–869

Burn WK, Davies KN, McKenzie FR et al. 1993 The prevalence of psychiatric illness in acute geriatric admissions. International Journal of Geriatric Psychiatry 8: 171–174

Burvill PW, Johnson GA, Jamrozik KD et al. 1996 Prevalence of depression after stroke: the Perth community stroke project. British Journal of Psychiatry 166: 320–327

Butler R, Collins E, Katona C et al. 1997 Does a teaching programme improve general practitioners' management of depression in the elderly? Journal of Affective Disorders 46: 303–308

Cole MG, Bellavance F 1997 The prognosis of depression in old age. American Journal of Geriatric Psychiatry 5: 4–14

Coope B, Ballard C, Saad K et al. 1995 The prevalence of depression in the carers of dementia sufferers. International Journal of Geriatric Psychiatry 10: 237–242

Copeland JRM, Beekman ATF, Dewey ME et al. 1999 Depression in Europe: geographical distribution in older people. British Journal of Psychiatry 174: 312–321

Crawford MJ, Prince M, Menezes P et al. 1998 The recognition and treatment of depression in older people in primary care. International Journal of Geriatric Psychiatry 13: 172–176

Cummings JL, Masterman DL 1999 Depression in patients with Parkinson's disease. International Journal of Geriatric Psychiatry 14: 711–718

D'Ath P, Katona K, Mullan E et al. 1994 Screening, detection and management of depression in elderly primary care attenders. I: The acceptability and performance of the 15 item geriatric depression scale (GDS 15) and the development of short versions. Family Practice 11: 260–266

De Craen AJM, Heeren TJ, Gussekloo J 2003 Accuracy of the 15-item geriatric depression scale (GDS-15) in a community sample of the oldest old. International Journal of Geriatric Psychiatry 18: 63–66

Denihan A, Kirby M, Bruce I et al. 2000 Three year prognosis of depression in the community-dwelling elderly. British Journal of Psychiatry 176: 453–457

Department of Health 2000a National service framework for coronary heart disease. Department of Health, London

Department of Health 2000b The NHS cancer plan: a plan for investment, a plan for reform. Department of Health, London

Department of Health 2001a Making it happen: a guide to delivering mental health promotion. Department of Health, London

Department of Health 2001b National service framework for older people. Department of Health, London

Department of Health 2001c Treatment choice in psychological therapy and counselling. Department of Health, London

Dhondt T, Derksen P, Hooijer C et al. 1999 Depressogenic medication as an aetiological factor in major depression: an analysis in a clinical population of depressed elderly people. International Journal of Geriatric Psychiatry 14: 875–881

Evans M 1996 Depression in older women. In: Defeat depression: articles reprinted from Geriatric Medicine 1991–1996. Medpress, Sevenoaks, pp 84–91

Evans S, Katona C 1993 Epidemiology of depressive symptoms in elderly primary care attenders. Dementia 4: 327–333

Evans ME, Copeland JRM, Dewey ME 1991 Depression in the elderly in the community: effect of physical illness and selected social factors. International Journal of Geriatric Psychiatry 6: 787–795

Folstein MF, Folstein SE, McHugh PR 1975 Mini-mental state: a practical method for grading the cognitive state of patients for the clinician. Journal of Psychiatric Research 12: 189–198

Frasure-Smith N, Lesperance F, Gravel G et al. 2000 Depression and health care costs during the first year following myocardial infarction. Journal of Psychosomatic Research 48: 471–478

Godlove Mozeley C, Challis D, Sutcliffe C et al. 2000 Psychiatric symptomatology in elderly people admitted to nursing and residential homes. Aging and Mental Health 4: 136–141

Harwood D 2002 Suicide in older persons. In: Jacoby R, Oppenheimer C (eds) Psychiatry in the elderly, 3rd edn. Oxford University Press, Oxford, pp 677–682

Harwood DMJ, Hawton K, Hope T et al. 2000 Suicide in older people: mode of death, demographic factors, and medical contact before death in one hundred and ninety-five cases. International Journal of Geriatric Psychiatry 15: 736–743

Help the Aged 2002 Tackling pensioners' poverty today: Help the Aged policy statement 2002. Help the Aged, London

Hepple J, Pearce J, Wilkinson P (eds) 2002 Psychological therapies with older people: developing treatments for effective practice. Brunner-Routledge, Hove

Holmes JD, House AO 2000 Psychiatric illness after hip fracture. Age and Ageing 29: 537–546

Iliffe S, Mitchley S, Gould M et al. 1994 Evaluation of the use of brief screening instruments for dementia, depression and problem drinking among elderly people in general practice. British Journal of General Practice 44: 503–507

Jackson R, Baldwin B 1993 Detecting depression in elderly medically ill patients: the use of the geriatric depression scale compared with medical and nursing observations. Age and Ageing 22: 349–353

Knight BG 1996 Psychotherapy with older adults, 2nd edn. Sage Publications, London

Koenig HG 1998 Depression in hospitalised older patients with congestive heart failure. General Hospital Psychiatry 20: 29–43

Kurlowicz LH 2001 Benefits of psychiatric consultation–liaison nurse interventions for older hospitalised patients and their nurses. Archives of Psychiatric Nursing 15: 53–61

Lebowitz BD, Pearson JL, Schneider LS et al. 1997 Diagnosis and treatment of depression in late life: consensus statement update. Journal of the American Medical Association 278: 1186–1190

Livingstone G, Yard P, Beard A et al. 2000 A nurse coordinated educational initiative addressing primary care professionals' attitudes to and problem-solving in depression in older people – a pilot study. International Journal of Geriatric Psychiatry 15: 401–405

Long AF, Godfrey M, Randall T et al. 2002 Developing evidence based social care policy and practice. Part 2: effectiveness and outcomes of preventive services for older people: risk factors, coping strategies and outcomes of interventions in bereavement. Nuffield Institute for Health, Leeds

Massie J, Holland J 1990 Depression and the cancer patient. Journal of Clinical Psychiatry 51 (suppl. 7): 12–17

Mather AS, Rodriguez C, Guthrie MF et al. 2002 Effects of exercise on depressive symptoms in older adults with poorly responsive depressive disorder. British Journal of Psychiatry 180: 411–415

McCurren C, Dowe D, Rattle D et al. 1999 Depression among nursing home elders: testing an intervention strategy. Applied Nursing Research 12: 185–195

Mittman N, Herrman N, Einarson TR et al. 1997 The efficacy, safety and tolerability of antidepressants in late life depression: a meta-analysis. Journal of Affective Disorders 46: 191–217

Mullan E, Katona P, D'Ath P 1994 Screening, detection and management of depression in elderly primary care attenders. II: Detection and fitness for treatment: a case record study. Family Practice 11: 267–270

Mulley G 2001 Depression in physically ill older patients. In: Curran S, Wattis JP, Lynch S (eds) Practical management of depression in older people, Arnold, London, pp 89–103

Neal M, Hughes P, Bell M 2001 The role of the nurse in the assessment, diagnosis and management of depression in older people. In: Curran S, Wattis JP, Lynch S (eds) Practical management of depression in older people. Arnold, London, pp 123–145

Neville PG, Boyle A, Brooke S et al. 1995 Time for change – psychiatric morbidity in residential homes for the elderly. International Journal of Geriatric Psychiatry 10: 561–567

Ormel J, Oldehinkel AJ, Brilman EI 2001 The interplay and etiological continuity of neuroticism, difficulties, and life events in the etiology of major and subsyndromal, first and recurrent depressive episodes in later life. American Journal of Psychiatry 158: 885–891

Orrell M, Collins E, Shergill S et al. 1995 Management of depression in the elderly by general practitioners: I. Use of antidepressants. Family Practice 12: 5–11

Oxman TE, Sengupta A 2002 Treatment of minor depression. American Journal of Geriatric Psychiatry 10: 256–264

Pearce J 2002 Systemic therapy. In: Hepple J, Pearce J, Wilkinson P (eds) Psychological therapies with older people: developing treatments for effective practice. Brunner-Routledge, Hove, pp 76–102

Penninx BW, Rejeski WJ, Pandya J et al. 2002 Exercise and depressive symptoms: a comparison of aerobic and resistance exercise effects on emotional and physical function in older persons with high and low depressive symptomatology. Journal of Gerontology: Psychological Sciences and Social Sciences 57: 124–232

Pinquart M, Sorensen S 2001 How effective are psychotherapeutic and other psychosocial interventions with older adults? A meta-analysis. Journal of Mental Health and Ageing 7: 207–243

Pomeroy IM, Clark CR, Philp I 2001 The effectiveness of very short scales for depression screening in elderly medical patients. International Journal of Geriatric Psychiatry 16: 321–326

Prince MJ, Harwood RH, Thomas A et al. 1998 A prospective population-based cohort study of the effects of disablement and social milieu on the onset and maintenance of late-life depression. The Gospel Oak Project VII. Psychological Medicine 28: 337–350

Proctor R, Burns A, Stratton Powell H et al. 1999 Behavioural management in nursing and residential homes: a randomised controlled trial. Lancet 354: 26–29

Rabins PV, Black BS, Roca R et al. 2000 Effectiveness of a nurse-based outreach program for identifying and treating psychiatric illness in the elderly. Journal of the American Medical Association 283: 2802–2809

Rasmussen J, Findlay D, Hindmarch I et al. 1999 Health and ageing: guidelines for depression. Wyeth Laboratories, Maidenhead

Ricketts T 1995 Grief: a cognitive-behavioural perspective. British Journal of Nursing 4: 992–998

Roberts RE, Kaplan GA, Shema SA et al. 1997 Does growing old increase the risk for depression? American Journal of Psychiatry 154: 1384–1390

Rogers C 1967 A therapist's view of psychotherapy: on becoming a person. Constable, London

Rothera I, Jones R, Gordon C 2002 An examination of the attitudes and practice of general practitioners in the diagnosis and treatment of depression on older people. International Journal of Geriatric Psychiatry 17: 354–358

Saunders PA, Copeland JRM, Dewey ME 1991 Heavy drinking as a risk factor for depression and dementia in elderly men: findings from the Liverpool longitudinal community study. British Journal of Psychiatry 159: 213–216

Saz P, Dewey ME 2001 Depression, depressive symptoms and mortality in persons aged sixty-five and over living in the community: a systematic review of the literature. International Journal of Geriatric Psychiatry 16: 622–630

Schoevers RA, Beekman ATF, Deeg DJH et al. 2000 Risk factors for depression in later life; results of a prospective community based study (AMSTEL). Journal of Affective Disorders 59: 127–137

Schweitzer I, Tuckwell V, O'Brien J et al. 2002 Is late onset depression a prodrome to dementia? International Journal of Geriatric Psychiatry 17: 997–1005

Shah A, Elanchenny N, Collinge T 2001 Trends in age band specific suicide rates among elderly people in England and Wales. Medicine, Science and Law 41: 102–106

Sharma VK, Copeland JRM, Dewey ME et al. 1998 Outcome of the depressed elderly living in the community in Liverpool: a five year follow-up. Psychological Medicine 28: 1329–1337

Sheikh JI, Yesavage JA 1986 Geriatric depression scale (GDS): recent evidence and development of a shorter version. Clinical Gerontologist 5: 165–173

Steffens DC, Byrum CE, McQuoid DR et al. 2000 Hippocampal volume in geriatric depression. Biological Psychiatry 48: 301–309

Stiles PG, McGarrahan JF 1998 The geriatric depression scale: a comprehensive review. Journal of Clinical Geropsychology 4: 89–110

Stuart GW 1998 Emotional responses and mood disorders. In: Stuart PW, Laria MT (eds) Stuart and Sundeens's principles and practice of psychiatric nursing, 6th edn. Mosby, St Louis, pp 348–379

Sutcliffe C, Cordingley L, Burns A et al. 2000 A new version of the geriatric depression scale for nursing and residential home populations: the geriatric depression scale (residential) (GDS–12R). International Psychogeriatrics 12: 173–181

Turvey CL, Carney C, Arndt S et al. 1999 Conjugal loss and syndromal depression in a sample of elders aged 70 years and older. American Journal of Psychiatry 156: 1596–1601

Waterreus A, Blanchard M, Mann A 1994 Community psychiatric nurses for the elderly: well tolerated, few side-effects and effective in the treatment of depression. Journal of Clinical Nursing 3: 299–306

Wattis JP 2001 Getting the measure of depression in old age. In: Curran S, Wattis JP, Lynch S (eds) Practical management of depression in older people. Arnold, London, pp 1–14

Wattis J, Curran S 2001 Practical psychiatry of old age. Radcliffe Medical Press. Oxford

Weatherall M 2000 A randomised controlled trial of the geriatric depression scale in an inpatient ward for older adults. Clinical Rehabilitation 14: 186–191

Williams JW, Barrett J, Oxman T et al. 2000 Treatment of dysthymia and minor depression in primary care: a randomised controlled trial. Journal of the American Medical Association 284: 1519–1526

Wilson S, Curran S 2001 The pharmacological treatment of depression in older people. In: Curran S, Wattis J P, Lynch S (eds) Practical management of depression in older people. Arnold, London, pp 44–60

Wilson KCM, Copeland JRM, Taylor S et al. 1999 Natural history of pharmacotherapy of older depressed community residents: the MRC-ALPHA study. British Journal of Psychiatry 175: 439–443

Worden JW 1991 Grief counselling and grief therapy: a handbook for the mental health practitioner, 2nd edn. Routledge, London

World Health Organization 1992 The ICD-10 classification of mental and behavioural disorders: clinical descriptions and diagnostic guidelines. World Health Organization, Geneva

Yesavage JA, Brink TL, Rose TL et al. 1983 Development and validation of a geriatric depression screening scale: a preliminary report. Journal of Psychiatric Research 17: 37–49

Yohannes AM, Roomi J, Baldwin RC et al. 1998 Depression in elderly outpatients with disabling chronic obstructive pulmonary disease. Age and Ageing 27: 155–160

Chapter **26**

Dying, bereavement and loss

Margaret Johnson

We are such stuff as dreams are made on; and our little life is rounded with a sleep.

(William Shakespeare: *The Tempest*)

CHAPTER CONTENTS

INTRODUCTION

For many of us, death seems incomprehensible and our mortality will perhaps only be challenged by serious accident, life-threatening disease, the death of a close partner, relative or friend. And yet it is argued that doctors and nurses who find themselves caring for dying people will experience difficulty unless they explore their attitudes to death and come to terms with their own mortality (Twycross 1982). Evidence suggests that for most people the real concern about mortality lies in the manner in which we might die rather than death itself (Garrett 1983, Mak 1992). Older people are no exception. Studies have indicated that they rarely concern themselves with death, although there is a need, as there is in all of us, to make sense of living in the face of dying. Only the integrity of old age, however it is achieved, will help those who are old and dying to accept their mortality. Irrespective of age and social circumstance, dying is a unique experience. Complex and changing needs have therefore to be embodied in a dynamic care plan which, when implemented, will convey the message, 'You matter because you are you; you matter to the last moment of your life and we will do all we can to help you not only to die peacefully but also to live until you die' (Saunders 1976).

Contemporary attitudes towards death and dying in western societies are marked by apprehension, fear and avoidance (Field 1989). Changes in patterns of mortality have made deaths outside the older age range a relatively rare event, with the majority of us reaching our middle years with little or no personal experience of bereavement (Littlewood 1992). It is perhaps this lack of experience, coupled with the medicalization of dying and death, that accounts for the problems we in western societies seem to have in coping with the end of life. It is perhaps an anomaly that the one thing certain to happen to us, death, remains mainly a taboo aspect of life.

In spite of the difficulties we have in coping with death, there seems to be a general assumption that, with respect to older people, death is 'natural' and marks the end of what may have been a full and productive life. Older people are often thought to be used to losses and therefore do not feel a loss as intensely as a younger person (Scrutton 1995, Siddel et al. 2001, S Thompson 2002a). S Thompson (2002) sees this as reflecting an expression of ageism that Doka (2001) termed 'disenfranchised grief': the discrimination by society of older people's needs at times of loss. S Thompson (2002) identifies this discrimination as existing in personal dealings with older people that can be seen in nurses' attitudes (Armstrong-Esther et al. 1989). It is also seen in areas such as on films, TV and advertising and in using first names when this may not be comfortable for older people who would not have expected this when they were young. This ageism is also evident in the structural way society fails to take notice of older people's views. This may change as the number of older people increases and the 'grey' vote starts to make a difference. Any system or care setting that denies older people their own personal history, losses that they have experienced and coping strategies they have developed fails to see older people as individuals in their own right.

Field (1989) believes that there is a direct relationship between caregivers' attitudes towards death and dying and the well-being of those who are dying in their care. Some of the difficulties patients and their families experience during the terminal phase of life may be exacerbated by professional health carers being unable to deal effectively with their own feelings and beliefs about death and dying (Neuberger 2003). There is much evidence that professional carers use blocking tactics when dealing with patients who have life-threatening disease (Webster 1981, Wilkinson 1995). This can result in patients being ill-informed about their diagnosis and prognosis, which in turn can lead them to becoming socially isolated (McIntosh 1978, Bond 1983, Field 1989, Bliss & Johnson 1996). However, there is evidence of a shift in medicine and nursing towards being more honest and open with dying patients, the perceived benefits of which include reducing suspicion, anxiety and loneliness in patients and their carers (Seale 1995).

CAUSES OF DEATH IN OLDER PEOPLE

In the UK, in 1900 about 25% of deaths were of those dying over the age of 65 years but today this figure is 83% (Seale et al. 1997). It has been predicted that this upward trend is likely to continue, which has serious implications not only for social policy-makers but also for those responsible for the provision of health and social care. Understanding and meeting the needs of these older dying individuals becomes a necessity.

When considering mortality in people aged 65–84 years, the most common cause of death continues to be circulatory disease (40%: this includes cardiac and cerebrovascular diseases), followed by cancer (23%) and respiratory disease (13%). However, comparing causes of death between the age groups 65–84 years and 85 and over indicates there are some differences. In those over 85 years, whilst circulatory disease remains the most common cause of death, the overall composition changes within this category, with cardiac disease decreasing and cerebrovascular disease increasing. Respiratory diseases (19%) overtake cancers (16%) as the second most common cause of death (National Statistics Online).

At a United Nations Symposium on Health and Mortality (United Nations 1997), it was reported that health had improved significantly in the preceding two decades for those over 65 years. The statistics concurred with those above, stating that those aged between 60 and 80 years died mainly of cardiovascular disease and cancers and that these tend to incur higher and more prolonged medical costs at the end of life than those dying later whose terminal illnesses tended to be of shorter duration. Those over 85 years tended to die of senescence (the deterioration of normal bodily functions) and succumbing to influenza, pneumonia, acute bronchitis, congestive heart failure and acute digestive disorders.

Thus, bearing in mind the nature of the diseases most commonly associated with mortality amongst older people, there can be a protracted journey often accompanied by increasing physical and psychosocial distress such as chronic pain, frailty, immobility, loss of continence, loss of independence and perhaps mental changes prior to the final, possibly short, terminal phase in their life. Planning good care and support for older people includes planning for a 'good' death.

DYING A GOOD DEATH

Aries (1974, 1983) argues that the history of dying from the Middle Ages to the present time has been marked by two changes: control of the dying process and the place of death.

A 'good death' is often seen to be culturally determined or varying from individual to individual (Bloch & Parry 1982, Badbury 2000, Neuberger 2003, Saunders et al. 2003). From a non-industrial or non-western society's point of view a 'good death' arises when there is some kind of control over events; death occurs with dignity, is prepared for and occurs in accordance with social and spiritual rituals and rites. A 'bad death' is one which was not prepared for and happens at the wrong place or time. In many cultures suicide is considered to be the worst form of death.

From a current British society point of view, Badbury (2000) identified three ideal types of 'good death'. The first is a traditional 'sacred good death' with similar features of a good death described above. The second is a 'medicalized good death' where medical techniques and technologies allow some control over death, for instance by controlling pain, prolonging and increasing quality of life. The third is a 'natural good death'. Here the dying person actively takes control over the events, negotiating with the medical team what treatments to use, where death is to take place and even extending into the funeral arrangements as well. This last view has arisen with the changes in emphasis in health and social care over the last decade or so from a medical paternal approach to an empowered, autonomous and person-centred approach (Randall & Downie 2000). This latter view may not be a widely held view in the oldest section of our society but is likely to become more evident as time goes by. A natural good death may also be perceived as one in which a person dies suddenly without distressing symptoms or in a manner that the deceased would have appreciated, such as participating in a much-loved activity.

Although there is a definite cultural aspect to what is considered a good death, there appear to be some similarities across cultures. Most views of a good death seem to include a notion of control, dying peacefully without pain or other distressing symptoms and with family or significant others nearby (Badbury 2000, Kikule 2003, Saunders et al. 2003). However, professional people caring for dying people should be aware that individual and cultural differences do exist. For instance, Kikule (2003) describes a study in Uganda where dying at home is seen as a part of a good death not only because of the familiar surroundings with family members present, but also because it is less expensive than a hospital death which many find difficult to afford. Walter (2003) describes how dying on the floor is part of a good death for a Hindu. Dealing with what are seen as bad deaths can be difficult for professionals and may lead to some reticence in being completely open with relatives (Badbury 2000). Neuberger (2003) identifies the deficiencies in some institutions caring for people with Alzheimer's disease where palliative care is frequently missing and spiritual care left unaddressed.

WHERE DO OLDER PEOPLE DIE?

When considering the place of death of older people, perhaps the first question to ask is: where do older people live and with whom? The answer to this question varies between men and women according to age. For women between 65 and 84 years, 45% are married and nearly half are widowed. For women over 85 years only 10% are married, with 80% being widowed. Of women over 85 years old, about 70% live on their own, 10% live with others (spouses, siblings, children, friends) and 18% live in residential or nursing homes. The picture for men is very different, with 70% of men between 65 and 84 years remaining married. For men over 85 years, 45% remain married and living with their spouses, 42% live alone, 7% live with others and only 11% live in communal homes (National Statistics Online).

People die in a variety of settings, especially when they become older. The main settings include hospital, private and residential homes, nursing homes and hospices. Few now die at home. From the 2001 Registrar General statistics for the place of death, about half die in hospitals. This continues the trend for place of death that is in direct contrast to the situation before the end of the Second World War when the majority of people were still dying in their own homes (Victor 1995).

However, while more than half the deaths actually occur in hospital, prior to the actual moment of death much of the care given to the person who is dying occurs in the home or in some other 'social setting', such as a residential or nursing home (Cartwright & Seale 1990). As shown above, many of these older people live alone, with more men than women dying at home (13% of men versus 9.5% of women in the over-85s). Meanwhile, increasingly, those living in residential or nursing homes die in communal homes – 15% of men and 20% of women over 85 years die in nursing homes and 20% of women and 10% of men die in residential homes.

Whilst hospices are considered as a place of dying, as people become older fewer die in hospices. For those aged 65–74 years, about 7% die in hospices but for those over 85 years this drops to only about 1%. This is despite cancer remaining a major cause of death even in this older age group, although this diagnosis may be compounded by other chronic diseases (Office of National Statistics 2001). Thus the variety of agencies involved in the care of the dying can be highly diverse and may include both public and voluntary agencies (Victor 1995).

There has been considerable debate about where the best place for a person to die might be but this debate has mainly been between deaths in hospital versus those at home. Concerns about the hospitalization of death and people dying alone have been voiced by several authors. Hospitals can be stressful environments where staff distance themselves from dying patients, thus leaving them to die in isolation (Glaser & Strauss 1965, Illich 1977, McIntosh 1978, Bond 1983). Those who die at home will perhaps feel more wanted because they may be less likely to be rejected by their family or the community in which they live (Bowling 1983). However, Seale (1995) contends that this kind of argument locates institutional care as being outside the caring community and points out that people are in fact less likely to die alone in an institution (Seale & Cartwright 1994) than people who live alone and die at home.

The nature of health and social care, however, has moved on since the debate outlined above. The statistics given earlier show that care homes are becoming increasingly the last 'home' of many frail, older people, especially for women. These institutions, therefore, are likely to be increasingly the place where older people will also die, alongside hospitals. However, Siddel et al.'s (2001) study into palliative care in care homes identifies some problems. These include identifying when a person is dying; meeting the needs of the living and the dying at the same time; and issues of education and training and support for bereaved residents and carers. Hospices still offer a place to die for some individuals but this becomes less likely for the oldest dying person. However, more nursing homes are offering terminal care beds for people who need them.

Hospitals are now places for acute care and interventions, with little resources for rehabilitation or care for those dying of chronic conditions or because of their age. They are appropriate places for interventions for older people with acute crises when their medical condition requires stabilizing. Some may still die in such acute settings when interventions are unsuccessful and death is rapid or when the person is so weak that relocation would be inappropriate and cruel. The introduction of intermediate care beds (see Chapter 9) following publication of *The NHS Plan* (Department of Health 2000) and National Health Service core principles (www.nhs.uk/aboutTheNHS/coreprinciples.cmsx#d) has opened up a more appropriate place for older people who need assessment or reassessment of their care as chronic conditions deteriorate, home circumstances change or the person is no longer able to cope. Terminal care beds may be available if necessary or an alternative care package can be organized at home, or in a community home or hospice. It appears likely that more care will continue to

be given within the community, either in care homes or the individual's own home. Appropriate resources and support will be required to enable this transfer of care for dying people away from the acute hospital.

The household circumstances of those who are dying will affect their need for care and, given that the majority of people who die are older, their household circumstances will reflect those of older people. The 2001 census shows that, of men and women over 75 years living alone, 5000 have neither central heating nor sole use of a bathroom. There is a trend for both younger adults and those who have retired to establish and maintain independent households. Similarly, these households of retired people may have adequate resources initially but it may become increasingly difficult for ageing householders to update and modernize their properties because of financial difficulty, a lack of energy required to organize major work, feelings of security in a familiar environment and a dislike, even fear, of having strangers in their homes. The implication of this trend is that an increasing number of older people will find themselves alone, or at best with an ageing partner, during the final stages of their lives in living conditions which may be amongst the poorest in the population.

Not only does the home environment need to be considered when planning care for older dying people but also the availability of carers, both professional and lay. With demographic changes in the population (discussed in Chapter 3), a falling birth rate and an ageing population result in a reduction of people working in any capacity and especially in health and social care. The rising numbers of older, but more especially, frail people will increase the need for greater numbers of health and social professionals to meet the increasing need. Also a greater financial budget will be required. In Scotland, it is estimated that the long-term cost for statutory care for older people will increase from £11.1 billion in 1995 to £14.7 billion in 2051 (Levy 2003). Both the World Health Organization (2002, www.who.int/chronic_conditions/en/icccexecsummary.pdf, Whelan 2002) and the UK government in its *NHS Plan* (Department of Health 2000) identify the need for a change in emphasis from acute care to chronic care. The World Health Organization framework emphasizes the need for involvement of the patient and family; building integrated rather than fragmented health services; encouraging evidence-based and team approaches; providing services and support in the community; and putting an emphasis on active lifestyle and preventive medicine. *The NHS Plan* provides for a *National Service Framework (NSF) for Older People* (Department of Health 2001) that aims to address these issues. The NSF aims to provide an integrated, coordinated service that is person-centred but also addresses the problem of age discrimination so that older people are treated with dignity and respect.

Much of the care of both dying and older people who remain in their own homes is carried out by lay carers, that is, spouses, other family members or friends and members of voluntary groups. The 2001 census shows that more than an eighth of over-90-year-olds give over 50 h of informal care a week and more than half of these carers are men, despite making up only a quarter of this population. Such support, however, especially in a protracted final illness, often with increasing immobility, incontinence and perhaps confusion, places a great strain on the informal carer or carers whatever their age. These carers may be less than healthy themselves, or have other demanding responsibilities, for example young children and/or employment. The informal carers' physical, emotional and social needs must also be assessed, in that they may require considerable support from the primary care team, social services and/or voluntary agencies. Admission to hospital in the early stages of the final illness may be necessary to confirm a diagnosis and treat distressing symptoms or to plan a package of care to facilitate home care. Later, short-term hospital admissions may be necessary, ranging from a few days to a week to prevent longer-term admission precipitated by exhaustion in the carers (Garrett 1983).

It is important that the carer's wishes, as well as those of the dying person, should be given full consideration when trying to reach a decision concerning the best place to die. Equally the carer should not be left with the burden of responsibility for the ultimate decision as to where a person might die. The health care professional should be prepared to support both the patient and the relatives in their wishes in a way that does not leave the carers or the patient feeling responsible and therefore guilty if subsequently any of them feel a wrong decision was made (Chalmers 1980).

The development of 'community care' policies, which include the negotiation of lay involvement (Finch & Mason 1992), has laid emphasis on providing a moral structure which channels love and obligation. Thus caring teams are needed which include a range of expertise in palliative medicine and nursing, bereavement counselling and complementary therapies in an attempt to confront death and manage it as an active part of life. The 'best place to die' is likely to be different for different individuals, thus each individual's needs, circumstances and desires should be carefully considered before a decision is reached. This implies that much more careful and proactive care is needed for older people, in both their care and support as their health deteriorates but also in recognizing end-of-life issues in good time so that a planned, appropriate and controlled transfer to care for the individual dying person is achieved. Those offering support and giving professional care must be well educated about people's reactions to facing imminent death, in basic palliative care skills and understanding bereavement and supporting those who are bereaved.

REACTIONS TO IMMINENT DEATH

From the 1960s, an upsurge in interest in death and dying seemed to occur. There have been various theories about how people generally react to the realization that they are dying and how they cope in facing their own imminent mortality.

Glaser & Strauss (1967) are remembered most famously for their work on grounded theory but not everyone is aware of the work that introduced their methods when they studied dying patients, their relatives and professional carers (Glaser & Strauss 1965). They described four contexts of awareness of the closeness of death in these patients. There were those who were aware of the proximity of death and discussed this openly with their relatives and professional carers. This was termed the 'context of open awareness' when awareness and open and free communication occur between individuals because everyone is as aware of the situation as everyone else.

When there is not open awareness, often the patient is the one who has not been told that death is approaching. However, patients often figure this out for themselves from their state of health and the communications and actions of those around them who are trying to conceal the prognosis. This is termed the 'context of suspicious awareness'. Patients in this situation will often try to confirm their suspicions and trap those around them into revealing the true state of affairs. Case study 26.1 illustrates an example of suspicious awareness which a nursing student was able to turn into one of open awareness after being approached by the patient.

Another situation described by Glaser & Strauss arises when everyone knows the prognosis and everyone suspects that the others all know but all pretend that nothing is wrong or needs to be discussed. This is the 'context of mutual pretence'. Again this situation can lead to a strain on relationships and communications between those involved.

Finally there is the 'context of closed awareness'. In this instance, the dying person is not told of the poor prognosis and is unaware of the seriousness of the condition. This situation rarely remains for very long. At

Case study 26.1   Mr Andrews: suspicious awareness

Mr Andrews, aged 75, was admitted to hospital for investigations into symptoms of loss of appetite, weight loss and persistent, epigastric discomfort. To those around him, it was known that it was probably a gastric malignancy that was unlikely to be treatable. However this was not revealed to him (a context of closed awareness for Mr Andrews).

He had built up a good relationship with a mature nursing student allocated to assist in caring for him. He respected her because she had an open and honest approach and seemed to understand him.

One morning when this student was on duty, Mr Andrews asked her to help him in taking a bath despite the fact that usually he was self-caring. The student found the time to assist him during the course of her morning's work.

Once in the bathroom it became apparent that having a bath was not the main reason for Mr Andrew's request. He revealed to the student that no one had been forthcoming with the test results and their implications, despite having had tests both during the previous week and before he was admitted to hospital. Everyone seemed to be avoiding him. He was sure that this was because the news was not good. He had had a work colleague who had similar symptoms and tests. This colleague was found to have cancer and died not long afterwards. Mr Andrews asked the student if this was what was wrong with him (a context of suspicious awareness for him).

Mr Andrews had approached the student because she was usually open and frank and less likely, he thought, to be 'in league' with the more senior nurses and doctors.

The student explained that this was not really an appropriate issue for her to deal with directly but she discussed the situation with the staff nurse on duty and by the end of the afternoon Mr Andrews had been approached by his doctor and the situation regarding his test results and their implications discussed with him.

The context had become one of open awareness. The situation had become easier for all concerned. Trying to hide information from another individual puts a strain on those concerned as they avoid discussing the topic and are always on their guard in their mannerisms and facial expressions so as not to let the secret out.

---

some point the person realizes that the disease is progressing and treatments are failing and either becomes suspicious or maintains a mutual pretence, even if not open awareness. In a retrospective survey of people who had died in the previous year, Seale et al. (1997) found that the number of people dying in a state of closed awareness had decreased when compared with a similar study in 1969, suggesting that communication with those who are dying has improved over time.

Another approach to understanding how individuals cope with their imminent mortality is through a proposal of stages or phases that people move through in order to come to turns with their dying. The most famous of these theories is put forward by Kubler-Ross (1969), but Wiseman (1979) also proposed such a theory. The Kubler-Ross theory is well known and is sometimes used to account for people coming to terms with bereavement but, in fact, her theory was developed to understand people's reactions to knowing they are dying. Her theory involves five stages of reaction, although some people may not progress through them all.

The first stage on learning that they are dying is denial. People are shocked and unbelieving, as they often are when hearing bad news for the first time. This can turn, in the second stage, to other emotions as the realization that the news is true occurs. Kubler-Ross suggests that anger is the main emotion in this second stage. The anger may be directed at themselves, their family, the health care professionals, God or anyone or anything else they may think is responsible for such a turn of events.

Once their anger has subsided, the next stage of bargaining may commence. Bargaining may be with doctors to try one last treatment or with God to allow them to live for some future event. In return the person may promise to do something in return. However, the finality of the situation eventually sinks in and depression occurs. This is the fourth stage. From this position the person finally moves into accepting the situation, the fifth stage.

There have been various criticisms levelled against this theory. Although Kubler-Ross did not anticipate that it was necessary for all individuals to pass through each stage in turn, the theory has been interpreted in this way and observation has found this not to be the case. Dying people can be seen to vacillate between stages or miss a stage out and may never achieve a state of acceptance. Others have questioned the validity and adequacy of the evidence that underlies the theory and still more see the theory as one-dimensional (Copp 1999).

Another approach suggests that how individuals cope with other critical events in their lives determines how they cope when faced with their own mortality (Schneidman 1980). Buckman (1992) suggests a combination of approaches and agrees with Schneidman that people will cope with impending death in their own way. This depends on their personalities and previous coping strategies. Buckman goes on to suggest three stages that people will go through to accept their own death. The initial stage is 'facing the threat', when they become aware of their prognosis and approaching death. A mixture of characteristic emotional reactions that the individual experiences to critical events will be in evidence. These may include denial, anger and bargaining, identified by Kubler-Ross, but also fear, anxiety, shock, disbelief, guilt, humour, hope or despair.

After this initial stage the person reaches the chronic stage of 'being ill'. There is resolution of those emotions that are resolvable that were experienced in the initial stage and a reduction in intensity of any other emotions. The final 'acceptance' stage occurs when the person accepts that he or she is dying or at least is not distressed and can communicate normally with significant others. Buckman suggests that help is offered to those who are unable to resolve or accept their emotions within the chronic stage and so help them to move on. Whilst this model incorporates elements from different perspectives, it remains one-dimensional (Copp 1999).

Finally Copp's (1999) study of cancer patients looked at the personal perspective of individuals facing death and their understanding of the meanings involved and their redefinition of themselves. She also considered how nurses support and facilitate this process, remarking on how labour-intensive emotionally and physically this work is for nurses. Despite every person being individual and having their individual reactions, Copp was able to identify some common themes from respondents' reactions of a psychological, emotional and social nature. People internalize the time-scale that doctors give them for their approaching death and compare themselves to where they should be on this trajectory. From nurses' descriptions of the state of dying hospice patients, Copp could identify four categories of situations patients found themselves in. In the first situation the patient's body is ready to die and the person is mentally ready to die, having come to terms with life and death. These patients tend to die peacefully.

The next situation occurs when the person has come to terms with death but the body continues to live on. This is often seen as a lingering death. These people see themselves living beyond their time, 'beyond their sell-by date'. Older people can sometimes be heard saying similar things, that they have

outlived their time, beyond their three score years and ten. When physical deterioration takes place these people also tend to die without a struggle. In a study into carers of older people over 85 years who have a 'lingering' death, Seale & Addington-Hall (1995) found that younger, informal carers thought that it would have been better for the person to have died earlier. However, spouses who were carers did not agree and thought their spouse had died at an appropriate time. This was especially true when the bereaved person was lonely.

When individuals have not accepted imminent death but their body deteriorates anyway, they often show anguish as they approach death. These are the people who are seen as fighting against their death and are often said to have a difficult death. Finally, on occasions a person is still unprepared for death and the body also rallies and maintains a steady state. Often these people become more confident and start planning for future life again.

Hospice nurses aim to help people die a peaceful death and often they succeed. This may be an unrealistic and unattainable goal, however, as it can depend as much on the patient's reaction to impending death as the support and care the nurse can give.

People do not know how to die because no one can come back to say what it was like; those who observe people dying, often carers, both professional and lay, do not talk about it because it is seen as morbid. However, Copp reports some of these observations and notes that some people seem to withdraw physically and psychologically and become emotionally 'disorganized' as they approach death. Others hold on to life for as long as possible despite their physical deterioration, doing as much as they can until the last possible moment. A minority vary between holding on to life and appearing to let go of it with fluctuations between denial and acceptance. Some people withdraw altogether from others, imposing on themselves a kind of 'social dying'.

How do these theories apply to older people? None was based on studies specifically of older people so it is difficult to say how representative these theories are for older people in particular. Copp does note that older people appear no more accepting of death despite the common belief to the contrary, so such work may apply equally to older people. No doubt most nurses involved in looking after dying people will be familiar with the reactions to imminent death that Copp describes.

Glaser & Strauss (1965) emphasize the importance of good communication skills required by those caring for dying people. This is also a particular necessity for older people who often have sensory deficits or are slower at collecting their thoughts, especially if anxious. Time invested in communicating adequately repays itself as their condition deteriorates. Nurses will then have some idea of the wishes of their patients directly from the patients themselves rather than through the go-between of their relatives or friends. Many older people want to know what is going on even if they wish to let others make decisions on their behalf. For information on communication challenges and skills in general, see Chapter 10.

Kubler-Ross can help us to understand some of the emotions that people who are dying may pass through at one time or another, although it is probably the case that people vacillate between these emotions at different times rather than progress systematically through them. This view can be compared with a recent dual-process theory of bereavement in which Stroebe & Schut (1999) identify two orientations between which bereaved people oscillate. 'Loss orientation' is the grief that is seen in bereaved people and is discussed in traditional bereavement theories, whereas 'restorative orientation' occurs when the bereaved person is able to manage the everyday aspects of living and can deal with the affairs of the deceased person.

Buckman (1992) suggests ways to communicate with people when bad news has to be given to them. His six-step protocol can be adapted to finding out another's understanding of a situation and helping those people to explore the issues involved. The six steps commence by giving advice on how a carer can 'get started' by getting the context and environment appropriate for such a sensitive exchange. The second step is to find out what the person knows or understands about the circumstances, in this case the prognosis. This can be achieved by the use of appropriate open questions. The third step is to find out what the person wants to know. If the wish is to know very little then the person should be left in the knowledge that more information is available and will be given in a sensitive manner. If the wish is to have information then the carer needs to have prepared how to give this information and could share the plan with the recipient (the fourth step). Buckman advises carers to 'align' themselves with the person by reinforcing the information the person has already understood and using that person's language. Further information should be given in a similar style of language, in small, easily assimilated steps starting with a 'warning shot' that indicates the kind of news to be given. Clarifying the person's understanding should be monitored regularly and use of diagrams or other techniques can be used. As people respond with various emotions when hearing bad news, the fifth step is to acknowledge and respond to those feelings. The final step involves agreeing what plans are to be made, the timescale and when reassessment of issues will be undertaken.

'Anticipatory grief' is a term introduced by Lindemann (1944, cited by Littlewood 1992), who observed that people who showed no overt manifestations of grief at the time of death had in fact experienced a period of 'normal' grief prior to the death occurring. While there has been some controversy over whether or not anticipatory grieving is helpful to people during their post-death bereavement, there is some evidence that when people have some warning of pending death they are less likely to present with psychological difficulties. This is probably because during a gradual 'leave-taking' there is an opportunity for grief to be shared with the dying person, as well as an opportunity to address deficiencies in the relationship and feelings of guilt to be eased (Stroebe & Stroebe 1987).

Copp agrees with Rando (1988) that the term 'anticipatory grief' is a more complex concept than the oversimplified view that losses are to come in the future. The anticipation of future losses is certainly a central part of anticipatory grief but it is difficult to separate this from the grief of connecting past with present losses. Copp identifies three foci as central to anticipatory grief, that is past, present and future losses, and three variables that influence this grief, namely the physical, the psychological and the social.

Caring for people with chronic conditions who are entering the final stages of life comes into the category of palliative care, discussed next.

PALLIATIVE CARE

Over the years there have been a variety of definitions of palliative care. The World Health Organization's definition of 1990 states that 'Palliative care is the active and total care of patients whose disease is not responsive to curative treatment. Control of pain, of other symptoms and of psychological, social and spiritual problems is paramount. The goal of palliative care is achievement of the best possible quality of life for patients and their families' (cited by National Council for Hospice and Specialist Palliative Care Services 2001: p. 3; a definition can also be found at www.who.int/cancer/palliative/definition/en/html accessed 24 August 2004).

The National Council for Hospice and Specialist Palliative Care Services identifies the aims that palliative care sets out to achieve. Palliative care perceives dying and death as normal processes that affirm life and living. Palliative care does not seek to prolong or hasten death but it does aim to help patients to live as actively as possible when near to death. Whilst providing adequate symptom control, palliative care integrates psychological, social and spiritual aspects of patient care. This includes supporting families and other carers to cope during the patient's illness and in their own bereavement (National Council for Hospice and Specialist Palliative Care Services 2001).

Palliative care can include a range of interventions and advanced diagnostic techniques. These interventions may involve chemotherapy, antibiotic therapy, radiotherapy and surgery, including percutaneous and endoscopic intervention techniques (Salamange 2001). Many new and more effective treatments are being introduced and researched each year. Better scanning and improved blood tests can diagnose and monitor changes in the patient's condition more closely than in the past. When these interventions are less invasive or have fewer side-effects than the more conventional treatments, they may provide more acceptable interventions for older patients whose declining health may preclude invasive monitoring or treatment. This assumes that access and funding are provided to all and that people are not discriminated against because of their age.

Palliative care has grown out of the modern hospice movement that developed in the UK following the foundation of St Christopher's Hospice in south London by Dame Cicely Saunders in 1967. The specialty of palliative medicine was recognized by the Royal College of Physicians (London) in 1987 (Hockley 1997). This development of care in hospices, and thus palliative care, was originally only provided to adult persons who were dying of cancer. Moreover, these people were usually at the end of their cancer trajectory and were admitted to receive good care and aid in achieving a 'good death'. Care of the dying at this time was not really thought about as a separate kind of care but was assumed to be given as any other care was. However, the care received was often poor, as Dame Cecily Saunders and others have described (Glaser & Strauss 1965, Kubler-Ross 1969, Saunders 1976). Indeed, Illich (1977) compared a historical, past acceptance of mortality with the then contemporary view of denial of death. He described attitudes to death as at best 'primitive', arguing that rather than seeing death as a natural end to life, we seek to blame someone or something when it occurs. Death was something ultimately to be avoided. Such attitudes were undoubtedly reinforced by a lack of sensitization to dying and death until later in our lives. This kind of attitude was seen to increase the institutionalization of the care of dying people, when a terminal prognosis was rarely disclosed (Field 1989). Seale (1995) criticizes the argument that modern society denies death and points out that calls to 'cease denying death' have

been heeded and are reflected in the philosophy of the hospice movement, where death is anticipated, prepared for and perhaps, more importantly, accompanied by life and living.

The limiting of palliative care solely to the person with cancer close to death has been discussed and debated in recent years. Within cancer care, palliative care teams developed in hospices and hospitals now intervene in care at a much earlier stage of the cancer trajectory (Field & Addington-Hall 1999). Palliative care can be instigated when unwanted symptoms from the disease or medical interventions occur and participation in care prior to the final stage of life is seen as important. Indeed, many patients may return for short stays in a hospice or receive interventions from an inpatient palliative care unit or a home care team on various occasions prior to death. Up to 45% of patients admitted to hospices or inpatient palliative care units are discharged (Eve & Smith 1996). This earlier intervention in care is not only so the expertise of these teams in symptom control can help deliver appropriate interventions at any appropriate stage of cancer trajectory but also so that a relationship can be developed at an early stage between the individual and the team who may take over more and more of the care.

Over the past few years it has seemed inequitable that the specialist palliative care offered to people dying of cancer care is denied to those dying of other diseases. Questions have been asked such as 'who should be entitled to palliative care?' and 'in what form and by whom should this care be delivered?' These issues have been debated by government, professionals and specialists in palliative care (NHS Executive 1996, Standing Medical Advisory Committee and Standing Nursing and Midwifery Advisory Committee 1992, National Council for Hospice and Specialist Palliative Care Services 2001) and in specialist journals (*Social Science and Medicine, European Journal of Palliative Care*). Reviews have taken place to identify other chronic and incurable disease processes where unwanted symptoms occur towards the end of life and thus identify those patients who would benefit from palliative care expertise (Chavannes 2001, Gibbs et al. 2002).

The National Council for Hospice and Specialist Palliative Care Services (2001) proposed different categories of care dying people may require in the form of palliative care prior to death and argued that these services should be extended to 'ensure all patients with palliative care needs, together with their carers, have equitable access to a range of specialist palliative care services appropriate to those needs' (p. 2).

For people with low to moderate complexity of palliative care need, in whatever setting, general palliative care can be provided by the usual professionals who would be caring for them in that setting. Knowledge and practice of palliative care principles should be an integral part of these professionals' routine clinical practice. This care focuses on quality of life and encompasses good symptom control, a holistic and sensitive approach to care that takes account of the person's history and current situation and offers respect and autonomy for that person and the family and other carers. Open and sensitive communication is required by all professionals whatever their field of expertise. Skills that these professionals require to fulfil this role include assessment in palliative care needs. This may appear to be obvious and nurses may assume that they are good at assessing their patients' needs. However, Siddel et al. (2001) found that those nursing older patients in nursing homes were poor at identifying residents who had pain and required analgesia. Meeting palliative care needs of low to moderate complexity should be within nurses' competence, including basic symptom control and open communication skills. Skill is required in recognizing when more expert palliative care skills are necessary and knowing where these skills can be sought. More education and training may be required in these areas to support those who at present do not have the more basic skills.

Specialist palliative multidisciplinary care teams will be required to advise non-specialist carers and to be more involved in the care of those who have highly complex palliative care needs. These teams should have a full range of trained and specialized palliative care professionals (doctors, nurses, physiotherapists, occupational therapists, social workers, chaplains or other religious or spiritual supporters and bereavement counsellors) who can offer a full range of services from inpatient hospital and hospice services, day care or home care and who can also take on an educational role in supporting non-specialists.

Nearly 20% of cancer patients now die in a hospice or specialist palliative care unit and a further 40% die under the care of specialist home care teams. However, only 3.3% of referrals to inpatient hospice or specialist palliative care services and 3.9% of referrals to home care teams do not have a diagnosis of cancer (Eve et al. 1997). As discussed earlier, older people, especially the very old, fail to receive hospice care for cancers they may have, let alone for conditions other than cancer, such as heart failure or respiratory problems and, as death is most likely when we are old, many more would benefit from this care.

Field & Addington-Hall (1999) appraised the possibility of extending specialist palliative care services to all who might require them. They identified five barriers. The first concerns the availability of caregivers with skills required for managing the palliative care needs of those with non-malignant conditions. All care settings should be able to offer holistic care to patients and manage common areas of symptom control.

The second barrier concerns the identification and then referral of patients to specialist palliative care services. The difficulty for general practitioners (GPs) and other doctors in predicting survival times of patients with non-malignant diseases is much greater than for cancers and makes judging the time of referral difficult. There is also evidence that, even with cancer patients, doctors are overoptimistic about survival times (Glare et al. 2003). Severs & Wilkins' (1991) study showed that when a palliative care unit for older people accepted admissions to patients with a predicted 2–4 weeks of survival time, the actual survival times varied. Out of 128 patients admitted under this procedure approximately one-third did not meet the prediction. Others confirm similar difficulties in predicting the end-of-life phase for people dying of diseases other than cancer (O'Brien et al. 1998, Gibbs et al. 2002).

The third barrier identified was the lack of information on the acceptability of these services to non-cancer conditions. Cancer has long been a taboo condition and hospices have been associated with the care of cancer patients. People with other conditions may be prejudiced against admission to hospice services. This fear may be gradually decreasing as more people have been exposed to the good care received by family members or friends in hospices.

The fourth barrier concerns the resources required to implement a policy of extending palliative care services to all who might benefit from them. Although, officially, there has been a move for better access to palliative care, this does not mean that it will or can be rapidly turned into reality. The idea must not only become recognized and accepted by all health professionals but also the facilities have to be available. Initially there may need to be some form of rationing of the services until facilities increase. George & Sykes (1997) suggest that older people in need of palliative care provision have different needs than those of the, often, younger cancer patient receiving palliative care. Older people have multiple diagnoses and multisystem pathologies; identifying the terminal stage of an older person's life generally only comes when all treatments fail, which is often at a point much closer to death than for younger patients; communication becomes more difficult when older people reach this stage of their lives; and older people often have reduced social and support networks. Therefore, setting up palliative care services to meet older people's needs may take more time and may cost more than is the case for younger people. Field & Addington-Hall (1999) estimated that there would be an increase of 79% in specialist palliative services to meet all the needs of those dying of non-malignant diseases.

The final barrier concerns those who have a vested interest in services remaining as they are. Some professionals may not wish to allow their patients to be transferred to another team as the patient approaches death, as this is the final care the non-specialist team can offer the patient. These professionals may feel that they will be deskilled in this area of practice. Specialist palliative care teams may also resent the extra workload that suddenly becomes their responsibility. A more coordinated and consultative approach to the care of the dying might be more appropriate.

Field & Addington-Hall (1999) searched for evidence of patients with non-malignant conditions with unmet needs that would benefit from palliative care services. The current remit for palliative care teams needs to be identified and compared with those dying from other causes. The needs the authors identified include alleviating physical, psychological and spiritual distress associated with the process of dying; managing and controlling distressing symptoms; and supporting family, friends and other carers.

Field & Addington-Hall (1991) suggest that the original remit for admittance to a hospice concentrated on relieving physical, psychological and spiritual distress associated with dying from cancer and allowing people to live as full a life as possible for as long as possible. The remit has since included symptom control and a greater emphasis in earlier involvement in the disease trajectory. In reviewing studies of people dying from other diagnoses than cancer they state that the studies 'demonstrate considerable symptom burden, psychological distress and family anxiety' (p. 1273) and conclude that the unmet needs of these patients fall within the remit of specialist palliative care. Those dying of progressive chronic diseases need more psychological support, increased communication with health care professionals and more support for informal carers than they currently receive.

Other reviewers consider specific patient groups such as patients with heart failure (Gibbs et al. 2002) and with heart failure and chronic obstructive pulmonary disease (COPD) (Chavannes 2001). These conditions, as discussed earlier, are those from which older people often die. Gibbs' group reviewed studies that identified people who had died of heart failure and demonstrated that they had the following symptoms in the last year of life: pain (50%), dyspnoea (43%), low mood (59%) and anxiety (45%). It was observed that pain and urinary incontinence were the most distressing symptoms.

Another study showed that, in the last 3 days of life, patients with heart failure suffered severe pain (41%) and dyspnoea (63%). Koenig's (1998) study confirmed that 60% of those dying of heart failure had suffered from depression (major 35.5%, minor 25.5%) and that those who had suffered from depression were more likely to be readmitted to hospital and had an increased chance of dying. Other problems reported were cognitive, such as short-term memory problems, confusion, and mobility difficulties. The issue of approaching death was not often discussed, although many patients had worked this out for themselves. However, patients found this subject difficult to raise themselves but often would have appreciated the chance to do so. Chavannes (2001) reports similar findings and also quotes from a study of patients with heart failure in GP practices in west London over a 16-month period. Within the first month, 19% had died and only 57% were alive 18 months later.

When it comes to COPD, Chavannes found little literature to review. However, the frequency of exacerbation and quality of life could be predicted by daily cough, wheeze, sputum and frequency of exacerbations the previous year. When compared with patients with lung cancer, those with COPD had more difficulty with activities of daily living and physical, emotional and social functioning. Furthermore, 90% had anxiety or depression compared with 52% with lung cancer. This identifies the need for increased psychological support for these patients. Another study showed that COPD patients suffered from severe breathlessness (61%), fatigue (32%) and severe pain (25%) which seriously affected physical and social functioning. There are differences between the end-of-life trajectories and characteristics of cancer patients and those dying of heart failure or COPD. Cancer patients are younger and the trajectory of their illness tends to be a little more predictable and generally of shorter duration. Older people, although they also die of cancer, are more likely to die of heart failure or COPD or of multiple, interacting causes.

MANAGING THE PROBLEMS OF DYING OLDER PEOPLE

When considering the older person with palliation needs some other factors must be taken into account. The detailed management of symptoms is not discussed here but management for particular aspects that may be of particular relevance for the older person is.

As they move to the end of life, older people may begin to present with a range of symptoms that need to be carefully identified and assessed. Thus, they can be treated effectively in order to achieve a good quality of life. Continuous monitoring of the effects of treatment, with appropriate modifications, is essential to ensure continuous symptom control and to reduce treatment toxicity. Pain, insomnia, loss of appetite and dyspnoea are symptoms which both patients and their carers have reported to be distressing for the patient during the final stage of life (Cartwright et al. 1973, Field & Addington-Hall 1999, Gibbs et al. 2002). Evaluation of long-standing medications and consideration of other beneficial interventions in reducing new symptoms may be necessary in order to ensure the most appropriate and effective regime is reached. The unwanted effects of medications should be acknowledged and any side-effect produced by medication should not outweigh the beneficial effect of that medication. When side-effects of a medication are well-known (for instance, constipation caused by opiates) then preventive interventions should be commenced at the same time. Older people's capacity to break down and excrete medication is generally slower than in a younger person and therefore smaller doses should be started and gradually titrated to maximum effect. Increasing the frequency of a smaller dose of medication may enhance efficacy with a reduction in troublesome side-effects (O'Brien et al. 1998, Colleau 2004). Interaction between medications in the older person is more likely simply because they tend to be prescribed more medications at one time and are less able to remove them from their system as efficiently (see Chapter 27 for more information on drugs and older people). Careful monitoring is needed, particularly with older people with renal and liver disease (Colleau 2004). Quality of life is the most important consideration at the end of life.

Pain

Historically, pain has been seen to be a difficult and sometimes impossible symptom to manage effectively. It is perhaps the reason why pain is something people fear above all else, and many people who are ill have an expectation that they will die in pain. This can lead to a situation where people who are dying 'don't know how much pain they are supposed to have' (Saunders 1976). However, during the past 30 years the hospice movement has been largely responsible for the development of strategies to deal with pain effectively and thus it is now argued that people should not expect to die in pain; dying can be painless if approached in the appropriate manner (McKenzie 1985).

Numerous definitions of pain have been offered in the literature, ranging from the purely physical to a more holistic interpretation of its meaning. For example, McCaffery (1972) perceives pain to be whatever people experiencing it say it is and exists whenever they say it does (see Chapter 22 for comprehensive information on pain in older people). 'Total pain', a concept introduced by Saunders (1978), is an attempt to encourage those assessing pain to give careful thought and consideration not only to the physical, but also to the emotional, social and spiritual dimensions of pain. More recently, Atkinson & Davies (1993) built on this concept by arguing that pain is more than a feeling of discomfort but rather it envelops emotional, social, psychological and behavioural factors, which may mean that the severity of the disease causing the pain is not directly linked to the intensity of the pain as described. However, no one has really been able to define succinctly exactly what pain is and the effects that it has but everyone has experienced pain, though can never experience other people's pain.

Older people appear to be reluctant to tell health professionals they have pain or will make light of their pain. However if asked about discomfort, soreness or aching they may be more forthcoming (Colleau 2004). Colleau also suggests that older people underreport their pain, often assuming that pain is a natural part of ageing and something that must be endured. They may also fear that complaining of pain may divert the attention of the doctor or nurse from treating their underlying condition or that the admission of pain will signify progression of their disease. The limited reserves older people have means that long-standing pain can have severe consequences to their functioning and possibly survival by reducing mobility, inducing depression and decreasing appetite. Also, older people were not brought up in a culture of over-the-counter medications for pain relief so may not understand the concept of pain control as much as younger people do. Teaching older people about the principles of good pain management and emphasizing that they do not need to suffer pain and that effective pain management will not cause addiction to the medications is important (Ferrell et al. 1994, Clotfelter 1999).

Older people are often undertreated for pain by professional carers. Bernabei et al. (1998) report a study which showed that people over 85 years are 50% less likely to receive weak opiates or morphine than those in the 65–74-year age group. The over-85s were also more likely to receive no analgesia at all. Cleeland et al. (1994) showed that 42% of older patients were not given adequate analgesia therapy, with physicians underestimating patients' pain when compared with patients' reports of the severity of their pain. The older the patient, the more likely this was to be the case.

In developing an effective strategy to manage pain in older people it is therefore important to consider both the subjective assessment of pain, that is, the patient's description of the pain with no observer bias, and objective assessment by the nurse or doctor based on the patient's appearance and comments. It is important to consider a whole-body perspective to managing pain. The older person with multipathology may have pain resulting from many physiological, and indeed psychological and emotional, causes (Colleau 2004). Someone dying of heart disease may have pain from arthritis and oedema in the lungs but the pain may also be affected by insomnia, breathlessness, anxiety and fears for the future. Reassessment of each different pain and contributing symptoms and their effects on functioning will be necessary in order to monitor and manage the pain effectively.

Assessment strategies used for older people should be gauged by their physical condition and energy level, their current cognitive abilities and their ability to communicate. Factors such as pain, distress and anxieties about their condition, effects from insomnia, breathlessness or other symptoms, and maybe anxieties for a spouse who is worried for them, will reduce older people's capabilities to a greater extent than for younger people. Detailed information on perception, assessment and management of pain can be found in Chapter 22.

Management of pain should consider both pharmacological and non-pharmacological approaches. In terms of pharmacological interventions the approach could follow the three-step analgesic ladder (World Health Organization 1990). When pain begins to be bothersome, the first type of analgesia would be non-opioid analgesia: paracetamol, aspirin if tolerated or non-steroidal anti-inflammatory drugs (NSAIDs) such as ibuprofen. However, NSAIDs should only be used with caution in older people as they can have more serious, sometimes fatal, reactions to them (Heath 1997, Colleau 2000).

If pain persists or increases, analgesia on the next step of the ladder, weak opioids, such as codeine or dextropropoxyphene, could be substituted or used in addition to the non-opioid analgesia. Should the pain continue to persist or increase further despite increased doses of weak opiates and/or non-opiate analgesia, the next step is to take strong opioids such as morphine, fentanyl or diamorphine. Because of their effect on older people strong opiates should be commenced at one-third to one-half normal adult doses and titrated until pain relief is obtained (Jacox et al. 1994). Titration of all medication should be carried out slowly because opiates are eliminated from the body more slowly in older people and monitoring of renal and hepatic functioning should be maintained. Analgesia should be given at regular intervals to maintain adequate blood levels of the drug rather than on an as-required basis. If side-effects interfere with the beneficial effects of an opiate, then it is worth reducing the dose of opiate given but increasing the frequency of doses so that the same total dose of drug is maintained in 24 h. Once a regime that controls the pain adequately is reached, sustained-release medications can be introduced related to the dosage being given. Provision should be made for additional analgesia to be available for any 'breakthrough' pain should this occur.

The rule should be to give as few medications in the lowest dose to achieve satisfactory pain control whilst also taking into account appropriate treatment of unwanted effects. In the older person this can become a complex issue. However there are useful adjuncts that may be used depending on the type of pain; for instance, for neuropathic pain, small doses of one of the following may be effective: tricyclic antidepressant (e.g. amitriptyline) or an anticonvulsant (e.g. carbamazepine).

Generally, analgesia should be given orally as sustained-release tablets if at all possible. Sublingual preparations or liquids may also be possible routes of administration but will need to be given regularly and may cause some peaks and troughs in blood levels. These modes of administration are more suitable for breakthrough pain. When oral medication becomes impossible transdermal patches or a self-administered subcutaneous syringe driver may be used to give continuous levels of analgesia.

Side-effects of opiate administration are well known and should be anticipated and, when occurring, treated. The most commonly known one is constipation. Constipation can cause not only much misery for dying patients but also make them feel most undignified. The combining effects of opiates, weakness, poor mobility and lack of fluid intake make it necessary to manage constipation successfully (see Chapter 17). Drinking more fluids and eating more fibre helps. Prunes and figs are beneficial if liked and the modern trend for fruit 'smoothies' can give fruit fibre as well as fluids.

Sedation is another common side-effect encountered in an older person who is taking strong opiates. Tolerance often develops to this and no other action is needed. Reducing the dose of opiate but increasing the frequency will help to reduce the peak blood levels and not the total dose of analgesia. If sedation remains a problem a small dose of stimulant may be tried (Colleau 2000). Respiratory depression is often feared when opiates are given to older people. It is better to avoid this by starting opiates at low doses and gradually increasing doses. Extra care is required for those with significant pulmonary disease and decreasing the dose may be required (O'Brien et al. 1998). Nausea and vomiting may also be a side-effect of opiate medication and can be treated with metoclopramide for the first few days, but tolerance should occur.

Much emphasis is placed on pharmacological control of pain but non-pharmacological methods can contribute to the comfort of the person who is dying and enhance the action of the medications taken. Simple physical measures such as helping the person change position are helpful. The application of warmth, and occasionally cold, can have a soothing effect on pain and is easily applied. Extreme heat and cold should, of course be avoided. Vibration has also been shown to be of use for older people (Rhiner et al. 1993). Information on the role of complementary therapies, such as massage, in managing pain is given in Chapter 31.

The emotional aspects of pain, for example, anxiety, anger and fear, can lower pain thresholds, while diversion, sympathy and understanding can raise them (Twycross 1978). Alleviating fear and anxiety with simple communication skills can help; time spent finding out these things repays itself in the improved quality of life. In the management of pain, communication is also of paramount importance.

Breathlessness and cough

Alongside pain, breathlessness and cough can be the most distressing symptoms suffered at the end of life (see Chapter 15). Breathlessness in people who are dying can provoke a vicious cycle of anxiety, fear, stress and increased breathlessness. All known causes of breathlessness should be considered and treated accordingly, but if these measures fail, then small doses of oral morphine or diamorphine with or without an antiemetic given 4-hourly (or just at night for some people) can reduce anxiety without depressing respiration. Alternatively, a small dose of the short-acting benzodiazepine, lorazepam, may help (Hockley 1991) and oxygen may also help.

A persistent cough can be tiresome and exhausting for the person who is dying. Again small doses of morphine can be useful, as may a linctus. Linctus codeine is usually effective but, if the sputum is thick and tenacious, bromhexine tablets or elixir will be more effective (Hockley 1991). Linctus methadone is not suitable as it has a long duration of action and tends to accumulate, neither of which is advised for older people (British National Formulary Joint Formulary Committee 2004).

Excessive respiratory secretions (death rattle) may accompany the breathing of one close to death.

Although the individual may not be aware of this, it is very distressing for relatives, friends and carers. The symptom can be controlled with the judicious use of a subcutaneous injection of hyoscine bromide but this will have the adverse effect of inducing a dry mouth (O'Brien et al. 1998).

Insomnia

Insomnia in those who are dying is more common than is generally realized and is often accepted by both patients and nurses as a normal reaction to being ill and in hospital. In the dying patient insomnia is commonly seen amongst those who are suffering from respiratory or malignant disease (Cartwright et al. 1973). Pain, breathlessness, anxiety, depression, urinary frequency and being confined to bed all day can militate against natural sleep at night. It is therefore important to identify and treat the causes of insomnia, but in those cases where intervention fails to reduce sleeplessness then medication such as temazepam can be offered. Often the mistake is made of omitting night sedation for patients receiving opiates (Hockley 1991) but opiate medication is not a sedative and will not therefore deal with insomnia. It is also worth emphasizing the benefits of human contact, in that a wakeful patient will often benefit from being able to talk with someone and perhaps having a warm drink. For more information on insomnia, see Chapter 20.

Pressure sores

Nurses need to be alert to the high risk of pressure sores developing in dying older people and pressure area management should be reviewed regularly throughout the 24-h period. It is salutary that, while the prevention of pressure damage is fundamental to nursing care, and despite the amount of literature available, the prevalence and the incidence of pressure sores do not appear to be diminishing (Land 1995). Pressure area breakdown can be a source of great distress to both the person who is dying and to carers.

Immobility, paralysis, malnutrition and incontinence are some of the factors predisposing to pressure sores. Furthermore, the healing process slows down towards the end of life and this can be further compounded by interventions such as steroids, chemotherapy and radiotherapy. An additional problem is that a dying person who is experiencing pain will be afraid to move or be moved by carers and it may be that a particular position is the only one that affords relief from pain. Explaining to the patient and carers the importance of repositioning in reducing the risk of a pressure sore developing may help relieve some of the distress for those experiencing pain. However, in the final stage of life such repositioning may be intolerable to the patient and therefore the benefits may need to be weighed against the distress it can induce. Special mattresses and the use of soft sheepskins will help to reduce the risk of further breakdown of pressure areas and reduce discomfort. Chapter 19 provides more information on maintaining healthy skin.

Incontinence

When the dying older person has a history of good bladder control, incontinence often becomes a problem only in the last few hours of life (Hockley 1991). There are many incontinence-alleviating products available, with usually something suitable for most people and, with specialist continence nurses employed by hospital and primary care trusts, guidance can easily be sought. See Chapter 17 for detailed information on the assessment and management of incontinence.

Confusion and terminal restlessness

It is not uncommon for older people to become confused during the final stages of life. Because of the complexity of definition and cause, confusion can be a difficult problem to deal with, especially if the patient is restless at the same time. Confusional states can be acute (delirium) and chronic (dementia) and readers are referred to Chapters 23 and 24, respectively, for detailed information.

While it is difficult to determine the cause of confusion in dying patients, management must be specific and the blanket use of sedatives and tranquillizers avoided. Support, including explanations of the causes of confusion, offered to both the patient and relatives, can lessen anxiety and concern. Efforts should be made to orient patients in both time and place by talking with them, encouraging relatives actively to engage with them and ensuring that they are not left in isolation for any length of time. Meanwhile the physical needs of the patient, such as adequate hydration and elimination, must not be overlooked.

Restless and agitated patients may become a danger to themselves and to others and sometimes the symptoms of confusion can only be controlled by sedation. Drugs which may be helpful, but which should only be used if the symptoms are causing distress to patients and their relatives, include diazepam, haloperidol, chlorpromazine or trifluoperazine. If muscle-twitching occurs during the final day or so,

lorazepam can be effective. Should a crisis occur, for example, acute breathlessness, haematemesis or haemoptysis, an injection of diamorphine 2.5 mg and hyoscine 0.4 mg with or without chlorpromazine can be effective (Hockley 1991). Staying with and comforting the patient will greatly add to the effectiveness of the drug intervention.

Confusion and restlessness in people who are dying can be extremely distressing, not only for the patient but also for family, friends and health care professionals. Good communication, including explanations about the cause of the symptoms and reassurances that they can be managed effectively, will help provide mutual support not only for patients and relatives but for staff as well (for more information on communication with older people, see Chapter 10).

The final phase of life

Perhaps one of the greatest fears the dying person has is of dying alone (Seale 1995). As previously mentioned, it is not so much death itself but the process of dying that most people fear. But with effective management the reality when it comes is almost always painless and peaceful. Mental and physical pain usually recede during the last few hours of life and in many cases during the previous few days (Saunders 1976). Patients and relatives may need to be told this and to be reassured that every effort will be made to ensure that the patient does not die alone.

When patients are confined to bed, usually they do not like to lie flat on their backs but prefer to be propped up or lying on one side with plenty of support using pillows. Because they are often unable to move by themselves, they will need to be turned and moved gently at fairly regular intervals. It is better for the patient if the range of nursing care (including medical interventions) can be carried out at the same time so that the patient can have reasonable periods of undisturbed rest. Dying patients are often afraid of the dark and may need soft light and fresh air. Gentle sponging and massage may help to ease both physical and mental discomfort and some carers have reported that the burning of essential oils has brought relief and comfort to the dying patient. Although thirst is the least of their concerns they appreciate sips of iced water and regular mouth care. Most patients drift in and out of consciousness some time before the moment of death. Even if patients linger in this stage and appear not to recognize anyone, it is believed that they are aware of those who are with them. Hearing is the last sense to go and therefore relatives and health professionals should be aware of this and not assume patients cannot hear because they are drifting in and out of consciousness.

BEREAVEMENT AND LOSS

Loss, grief, bereavement and mourning are often considered together and their meanings may not always be distinguished from each other. Loss can be defined as 'the fact of losing someone or something, deprivation of or failure to keep a possession, attribute or faculty etc.' (*New Shorter Oxford English Dictionary* 1993). Bereavement is the very specific loss of a person through death. Grief, according to Worden (1983), 'encompasses a broad range of feelings and behaviours that are common after a loss' (p. 19) and Feifel (1998) shows how broad and diverse these responses may be, by stating that grief is 'multifaceted and manifests numerous faces' (p. 3). Payne et al. (1999: p. 7) suggest the terms 'mental pain, distress and deep or violent sorrow' to describe the effects of grief. People may have a grief reaction to losses other than bereavement and these emotions may be reactions to other severe stresses. 'Mourning' is a term usually used for the time following bereavement. Mourning is defined by the social structures of the culture in which the

bereavement takes place and the mourning process is usually guided by social expectations and rites. Mourning is culturally dependent and people caring for the bereaved must have an understanding of mourning practices of those cultures with which they are likely to come into contact but, above all, they need awareness of and sensitivity to the wishes of the bereaved, whatever their background. Two examples of bereavement are given in Case studies 26.2 and 26.3, both illustrating complicated grief reactions and including a comment on why the bereavement may have taken this form in each case.

To return to the concept of loss, this concept is important for the understanding of older people who will have suffered many losses during their lives and possibly more in their older years than at any other time. Bailey & Clarke (1989) suggest that loss is a concept that 'underlies all change throughout an individual's life' (p. 290) and that each progression during maturational development involves loss. Paradoxically, each loss is often followed by change. For each substantial loss or change in life, there is a process or period of adaptation. This can be seen from the moment of birth when we are ejected from the safe and comforting security of the womb into a world to

---

Case study 26.2   Mr Roberts: severe grief reaction

Mr Roberts, 80 years old, was admitted to an elderly care assessment unit in a confused and dishevelled state. He was dehydrated, had a urinary tract infection and appeared very weak. His mood seemed very low.

As his physical state stabilized the story behind his admission emerged. Four weeks previously he had gone downstairs to make his wife her usual morning cup of tea. On returning upstairs he found her collapsed on the floor, unable to move and having difficulties in speaking. She was admitted to hospital but her condition deteriorated and she died of a cerebrovascular accident.

They had been married for nearly 60 years and had been very close, particularly since he had retired 15 years ago. They had done everything together. They shopped, cooked and looked after the house and garden together. They would even walk to the post box together. They had no children or close relatives still alive. Many of the older neighbours had died or moved away or into care homes. Their next-door neighbours at present were, on one side, a young couple who had not long moved in, who worked full-time and were out most of the time and, on the other side, a couple with a small child. Mr Roberts found it difficult to relate to children as he had never had any of his own. He and his wife had had two or three couples

that they socialized and played bridge with. It was one of these friends who had helped him to make the funeral arrangements when his wife died and who had visited him and called the doctor prior to his admission.

Mr Roberts had found it very difficult since his wife died. He had appreciated the help of his friend as for the first week or so he had felt very numb and had acted 'on autopilot'. He had tried to continue as before but found that everything he did reminded him of his wife. He had become tearful and embarrassed by this. For instance, when shopping, the check-out girl had asked him how his wife was, he had broken down in tears, rushed from the shop and was too embarrassed to return. Similarly with his friends, it did not seem right without his wife; being with them made him tearful and he had made excuses not to see them. In fact he had withdrawn into himself. He was unaware that he had neglected himself so much.

Comment
What had caused Mr Roberts to have such a severe grief reaction? First, he had an obvious, close attachment to his wife with very few outside social ties or support. Those he did have were all shared with her. It is not surprising that he should have had such a deep grief when she died.

Case study 26.2   Mr Roberts: severe grief reaction (*Continued*)

Second, Parkes (1997) points out that earlier in life a stable attachment is prognostic of a favourable outcome to bereavement when compared with ambiguous or fraught relationships. However, for older people, a happy, stable marriage can cause very severe reactions.

Other predictors associated with a poor outcome of bereavement that could apply to Mr Roberts are the sudden and unexpected nature of his wife's death, the trauma of finding her on the floor and his lack of social support. It is unclear how Mr Roberts had reacted to previous bereavements, although it appeared he had been an only child and his parents had been dead for over 40 years. It is also unclear how much he contributed to the running of the house or how dependent he had been on his wife, that is, how able he was in looking after himself without her support.

Mr Roberts was referred to the occupational therapy department for an assessment of daily living skills and to the psychiatric service for assessment of his grief reaction and some residual confusion he showed.

Case study 26.3   Mrs Williams: complicated grief reaction

Mrs Williams was referred to the local bereavement service after the death of her husband and was visited over a period of time by bereavement support worker, Sue. The initial information that Sue gained about Mrs Williams was that she was 79 years old, living on her own in the large house she and her husband had lived in for the last 45 years. She had a son and a daughter who gave her some support.

Mrs Williams was very distraught at the death of her husband who had died of lung cancer but she said she had not realized that he was dying of cancer until it was suggested that the local hospice be contacted to help care for him. She did know that he had been having chemotherapy but did not think his situation was so serious. She continually returned to this theme through the contact with Sue. It became evident that she was very angry with her husband for dying and leaving her on her own. She had arthritis, recurrent urinary tract infections and epigastric problems and had relied on her husband to support her. There were no photos of her husband on display in the house in the early visits and she volunteered very little spontaneously about her husband.

Sue gathered some more information when Mrs Williams' son visited his mother on a couple of occasions to mow the lawns or deliver shopping he had done for her. One day Sue was able to have a long conversation with the son when they both left the house at the same time. It appeared Mr Williams had been unwell for much of the last year of his life, suffering from chest pains and weight loss that increased as time went by. Mrs Williams' children had continually tried to persuade Mr Williams to seek medical advice and return to the general practitioner when the antibiotics given for chest infections were of little help and the weight loss was more apparent. Both Mr and Mrs Williams seemed unconcerned about Mr Williams' problems. Eventually, 2 months before his death, he had been seen by a chest consultant and admitted for some more tests, had the diagnosis confirmed, had a chest aspiration and was offered chemotherapy as a palliative measure. After coping well with two courses of chemotherapy, Mr Williams' condition suddenly deteriorated over the course of a week and he died at home with his children and grandchildren around him.

The son confirmed that his mother had been very angry that his father had died and would continually ask the children how long they had known their father had had cancer. His mother had put everything that had belonged to his father in rubbish bags and put them out for the rubbish collection. Fortunately for the son, he had visited before the bags were collected and offered to take them away. Inside were all the photographs and memorabilia of his father, much to the distress of the son. The son returned the photos gradually and, although they did not return to the rubbish bins, they were put into drawers rather than displayed. It was obvious that Mrs Williams' children offered her more support than she would admit to.

Over a period of months Mrs Williams became less angry, some photographs began to be displayed and she began coping better with life on her own.

Comments
What can the theories of bereavement tell us about this case?

First, anger is a common emotion exhibited at a time of loss (Buckman 1992, Parkes 1993, Payne et al.

Continued

Case study 26.3   Mrs Williams: complicated grief reaction (*Continued*)

1999) and during stressful periods (Lazarus 1966). Anger is often directed at the perceived source of the distress.

Second, Worden suggests that the disposal of all possessions is a sign that the bereaved person is finding it difficult to accept the reality of the loss of the deceased – if reminders of the deceased person are not visible then there will be less hurt, they think. This may also be a way of trying to deny the death. However, according to Parkes (1993) and Worden (1991), these strategies do not work

because working through the pain of grief is a necessary part of the grief process.

There may have been a process of denial in both Mr and Mrs Williams' ignoring of Mr Williams' health problems and so avoiding seeking help earlier. Mrs Williams may also have denied the seriousness of her husband's illness. Alternatively, she may never have had this explained to her in terms she could understand at the time. In either case, to her the death had been as if it was a relatively sudden death.

---

which we must constantly adapt and learn to survive. From the dictionary definition, it can be seen that older people are not immune from losses. Indeed they occur all too frequently. Older people suffer losses not just from bereavement of spouses, siblings, children, even grandchildren and friends, but if any of these people acted as a support for that older person the loss will be compounded (Parkes 1997).

The degree of loss of faculties increases with age just because of the ageing process, let alone the effects of any pathological change or disease process. Payne et al. (1999) quote from the work of Le Poidevin who suggests that loss has a variety of dimensions. These include physical, social, emotional, lifestyle, spiritual and identity dimensions. Loss of mobility, sensory deficits and cognitive deterioration can lead to major changes in life. Social roles may be more difficult to fulfil as older individuals may no longer be able to manage their own shopping let alone that of a friend or sibling; looking after grandchildren or greatgrandchildren may no longer be possible and even their visits can become tiring and may be confusing. Much-loved social activities may become impossible, for instance, difficulties in hearing and sight make it more difficult to interact and to recognize those being interacted with, thus making attendance at social functions an ordeal rather than a pleasure. Being unable to manage one's own household and being moved to either a smaller accommodation or a communal home can be an almost unbearable loss. Not only does it advertise a loss of independence and competence in daily living but also a loss of familiar daily routines and surroundings. Furthermore, there is a loss of all the memories and possessions that have contributed to a lifetime's identity.

S Thompson (2002) builds on this theme and identifies some of the losses experienced when an individual moves into a community care home. The first of these is identity, as described above. Aspects of identity that were assumed now become lost and the few

possessions taken into the care home now define the person's identity as the majority of the past life, other than memories, is left behind. Control over when to get up, the daily routine, diet and so on is taken away and previously enjoyed activities may no longer be available. When staff are busy, the spontaneity of having drinks or snacks outside set times or going into the garden or to a shop is usually precluded. Because of the responsibility of care that staff have over the residents, the right to make one's own decisions and take risks, such as making a cup of tea for oneself, is often not allowed. For more information on living in a care home, see Chapter 9.

The losses described above often go unnoticed and unaddressed. N Thompson (2002) points out that these losses do not have the same rites attached to them that would alert others to the effects of these losses and guide our social and cultural practices in these situations. Frequently, people supporting these older people may also have losses. Children and grandchildren, siblings and friends may all be mourning too. A house that an adult child may have known all his or her life, with its associated attachments and memories, may need to be sold at the same time as settling a parent into new surroundings or having a care package organized. Children may feel guilty that they can no longer support their parent in the family home. Understanding loss is a fundamental task if one is to understand bereavement. Even people who have not had a personal bereavement have had losses throughout their lives and so can understand bereavement to some extent. My nursing students, whether pre- or post-registered, identified similar reactions to loss although to a less severe extent than older people did when asked to think of a recent loss unconnected with the death of a person and then write down their reactions to that loss.

Theories, models and literature about bereavement have been evolving over most of the last century.

Much has been written on this subject, which is beyond the scope of this chapter. An overview of the major theories that have influenced work in the UK is provided, however. Rarely does one theory fit all situations but aspects of different theories or models may help explain what is happening to a patient or client. Later a discussion will take place that uses aspects of these theories to help older people in their bereavement.

Freud (1917, cited in Saunders 1989) was probably the first to put forward a theory of bereavement and this was based on his psychodynamic (also called psychoanalytic) theory of psychology. The main tenet of Freud's theory was that the energy that was invested in the person who died needs to be gradually retrieved during a period of grief and then new energy could be invested in a new relationship. This notion of having to give up the love for the deceased person before another relationship could be successfully embarked on seems to be the basis of many later theories. Many of the theories put forward before the 1990s encourage the practice of 'letting go' and 'getting over' the relationship with the deceased person. Although Walter (1999) noted that Freud in his own experience of bereavement did not find this to be the case, Freud did not update his theory, although Saunders (1989) argues that he did in private letters. Freud was important because his work laid the basis of much of the work that followed, even though there is much criticism of his work.

John Bowlby (1980, cited in Saunders 1989, Payne et al. 1999) initially studied attachment and separation of young children from their parents and proposed a theory of attachment. Bowlby suggested that attachment of infants to their mother acts as a prototype for the child's relationships in the future. Unsatisfactory attachment or separation at an early age can lead to difficulties with later relationships and with separations due to bereavement. When separated from their parents Bowlby (1980) noted the pattern of distress that he termed separation anxiety, involving the infant protesting loudly, despairing and becoming apathetic and finally detached. This seems similar to the distress of the bereaved. Bowlby's emphasis on the importance of our early attachments and the attachment to the deceased will influence the nature of our bereavement. Understanding the nature of the relationship or attachment the bereaved person had with the deceased may give us an insight into how bereaved people may grieve. A secure and stable attachment may lead to uncomplicated bereavement whereas an insecure relationship may alert us to a more difficult bereavement. It should also be borne in mind that the death of a spouse after many years of close attachment leads to separation and bereavement that may cause much distress. Indeed, Parkes (1997) cites studies where younger people who have an ambiguous relationship with the deceased are likely to find bereavement difficult. For older people it may be those who were securely attached who have more severe difficulties, including severe depression, tearfulness, loneliness and hallucinations.

An alternative approach, that of phases, has been offered by Bowlby (1980), Parkes (1993) and others. Parkes describes the first phase as a period of 'numbness' which in some ways draws parallels with 'denial' as described by Kubler-Ross (1969). During this phase, bereaved people are able to disregard their loss for hours or days. For Parkes this can be seen as adaptive as it acts as a barrier to the immediate pain and allows the individual to deal with any immediate duties of mourning. The numbness gives way to the second phase, that of 'searching and pining'. Searching behaviour is a restless hyperactivity, with inability to concentrate on anything and going over the context of the death of the bereaved person. At the same time the person pines for the lost one, yearns for him or her with 'pangs' of grief and may display other emotions, such as anger. Feelings of despair and an inability to function normally in their environment describes the third phase of the grieving process. Finally, in the fourth phase, behaviour is reorganized and life is 'pulled back together'. While Bowlby and Parkes argue that the bereaved person must pass through a series of phases before grief is finally resolved, there are clearly overlaps between the various phases, as there are with Kubler-Ross's stages of grief. Parkes identifies the strong emotional effect that bereavement, especially in the early days, has on an individual.

Worden (1983, 1991) takes a more developmental approach to bereavement and believes that people 'must' work through four tasks of mourning to achieve satisfactory resolution of grief. During the first task, 'accepting the reality of the death', Worden believes that the person must cognitively acknowledge the death and that the deceased person has died and is not coming back. Worden suggests that some people may react by minimizing the loss, for instance by saying 'he was not a good husband' or 'I don't miss him'; still others may remove everything about the deceased person from the home so they will not have to face the reality of the individual's death (see Case study 26.3).

Worden describes the next task as 'experiencing the pain of grief' and suggests that one cannot grieve properly without any pain being involved. The level of pain may be different for different individuals and circumstances. People may try to avoid facing the painful side of grief but Worden believes that at some point they will need to give in to this.

The third task that people need to address is 'adjusting to the environment in which the deceased is missing'. It takes time to realize all that has changed with a death. It may take a while for a widow to come to grips with all the tasks her husband did; what bills are due to be paid and when; where to get an electrical appliance mended, and so on. Often bereaved people recognize the new skills they have developed.

The final task is 'withdrawing emotional energy and reinvesting in another relationship'. This echoes Freud's belief that bereaved people must 'let go' of the relationship and move on and be able to start new relationships. This may be an unreal task for someone over 80 years as the energy involved may seem to them to be unwarranted for the short time the new relationship may last, and the bereaved person may want to avoid a new loss if the new friend dies first.

Besides providing us with a theory of bereavement, Worden also recognizes cognitive, physical and behavioural aspects of a normal bereavement, listed in Table 26.1. These aspects can help us to understand the wide range of reactions a bereaved person may have.

Table 26.1   Manifestations of normal grief

Physical sensations	Feelings
• Hollowness in the stomach	• Sadness
• Tightness in the chest	• Guilt and self-reproach
• Oversensitivity to noise	• Anxiety
• Sense of depersonalization	• Loneliness
• Breathlessness	• Numbness
• Weakness of the muscles	• Shock
• Lack of energy	• Anger
• Dry mouth	• Yearning
	• Emancipation
	• Relief

Cognitions	Behaviours
• Disbelief	• Sleep disturbance
• Confusion	• Appetite disturbance
• Preoccupation	• Absent-minded
• Sense of presence	behaviour
• Hallucinations	• Restless overactivity
	• Crying
	• Sighing
	• Social withdrawal
	• Dreams of the deceased
	• Searching, calling out
	• Reminders of the deceased: visiting places, carrying objects, treasuring objects

In the last decade these theories and models have been re-evaluated in terms of the criticisms levied at previous theories and models and their limitations in practice in social and health care services. Criticisms of the use of phases and tasks are similar to those directed toward Kubler-Ross' theory discussed earlier. N Thompson (2002) criticizes these theories for being too narrow in their approach to loss and concentrating mainly on psychological and emotional aspects. Important social and cultural dimensions are ignored. More recent theories have tried to address this imbalance.

Stroebe & Schut (1999) evaluated research into grief and bereavement and came to the conclusion that grief was both helpful and a problem. Although they do not reject earlier models and theories, they add a new concept to the debate. They suggest that there are two processes that occur alongside each other. The first is the 'loss orientation' which includes all the grief reactions described by the traditional theories of grief. However this 'grief work' consumes much energy and prevents the bereaved person from working towards adapting to the changed world that now exists. The other orientation is the 'restorative orientation'. Restorative orientation allows the bereaved person to take time off from grieving and to deal with the practicalities of the world without the deceased person, to master new skills, develop new roles and adapt to the changed world. Both these processes are important and the bereaved person will oscillate between the two orientations. Initially the balance will be towards loss orientation and gradually it will shift to a more restorative orientation. There will also be individual differences to the balance between each orientation. This theory explains how bereaved people have good and bad days, days when they can cope and days when they find life very difficult. It also explains why particular times (anniversaries), places or situations can precipitate the loss orientation even years after the death. Visiting or assessing bereaved people on one occasion only is unlikely to give the full picture of how they are coping.

Walter (1999) looks at bereavement from a more sociological than psychological perspective, and queries the belief that bereaved people must 'let go' of their relationship with the deceased, maintaining that the practice of insisting on this in bereavement counselling is unhelpful. He suggests that what is more important is that the individual must reconstruct or rebuild the relationship, or private bond, with the dead person so that life can continue without him or her. These bonds can be maintained by sensing the presence of the deceased through religious beliefs or spiritualist medium, by talking to the dead person and through symbolic places such as visiting the grave or reminiscing with family photos and possessions. Walter implies that the dead person should not be forgotten but kept alive for the bereaved person.

Walter's approach can be viewed in conjunction with the 'meaning reconstruction' theory of Neimeyer & Anderson (2002). The death of a significant person disrupts the normal equilibrium of our lives and understanding of the world. After the death bereaved people have to make sense not only of their loss or losses, but of their changed situation, routine and lifestyle and their changed relationship with the dead person. They need to seek a new meaning for their future and their self-identity. This will take time as the sense of meaning evolves over time.

Finally, N Thompson (2002) suggests using PCS (personal, cultural, structural) analysis as a framework for appreciating the complexities of loss and bereavement. This approach analyses events at these three different levels and also the interactions between these levels. The 'personal level' relates to the aspect of the bereaved individual, including personality, psychological reactions, attitudes, emotions and feelings. The 'cultural level' relates to the shared assumptions or the social group and culture in which the individual lives. The 'structural level' relates to the structure society puts on loss and bereavement and includes the interactions of law, bureaucracy, class, gender and race. It can be seen that the more recent theories, models and frameworks, like Thompson's, help to put bereavement and loss into the context of the social and cultural world of the bereaved person.

The main issue in the context of this chapter is to consider if and how bereavement is different for older people and how we might assess those who need help and how those who are at risk might be helped. Few studies exist of older people, let alone of the very old. Parkes (1997) reviewed the literature in terms of the mental health of the bereaved older person. For the majority of older people, bereavement is 'less devastating than expected' (p. 47). However, a minority may suffer from various mental health problems. For the 10–17% of older bereaved people who suffer from depression, this can be as severe as for someone who attends a psychiatric clinic. Of those between 65 and 74 years who become depressed, they tend to remain depressed, but for those over 75 years with depression they seldom remain depressed for more than a year. For those with vulnerability to psychiatric illness then bereavement may precipitate other psychiatric problems. Increasing intake of alcoholic can lead to alcohol dependency; anxiety can progress into panic attacks or anxiety states; and a perfectionist may become obsessional. In addition, Parkes notes that some people may develop pathological grief reactions. There are several of these grief reactions that Parkes identifies particularly. First of all, there is 'chronic grief', when the grief exists for a longer duration than usual. Some people may have 'delayed grief', when there is an initial absence of overt grieving that is followed by distorted or inappropriate responses. Still others may have 'conflicted grief': because of the ambivalent nature of the past relationship, abnormal anger or guilt may follow which complicates recovery.

Various studies show that, after bereavement, people increase their number of visits to the GP in the following 18 months but, unlike younger people who tend to complain of psychological problems, those over 65 years report more physical symptoms (e.g. arthritic pain). Mortality may increase in bereaved people but this is mainly restricted to the first 6 months of bereavement in over-75-year-olds.

Before one can assess the needs and consider a plan for intervention, it is necessary to be aware of the factors or determinants that could affect bereavement, both positive factors that may predict a likely favourable outcome and the factors that may predict a negative outcome. Using the terms 'could' and 'may' is quite deliberate here as an individual's reactions will not always occur as predicted. However, if we could identify those we think are most at risk from complicated grief or those who would most benefit from our interventions, then the provision of appropriate services can be planned.

Parkes' (1997) review identifies some determinants of the mental health outcomes of bereavement. The first risk factor Parkes identifies is the extent of anticipated adaptation needed to cope in the new world without the deceased person and the magnitude of change needed. Next, the presence of a support system is needed to help bereaved people through their grief and to rebuild, or reconstruct, their world. Parkes suggests that older people may need a period of dependency whilst they adapt and learn the new skills they need in their changed circumstances. This needs to be taken into account by those supporting the bereaved older person. Limited views of the capabilities of, or negative attitudes to, older bereaved people can hinder the progress of adaptation.

Worden (1983) also sets out factors or determinants that will influence the course of the bereavement. The first of these is who the bereaved person is and the nature of the attachment to the deceased person. Obviously the death of a spouse is a severe blow but there is agreement that the death of an adult child or of a grandchild or greatgrandchild can be equally devastating as it can be considered a death out of the normal order of things. Parents and grandparents are supposed to die first (Worden 1983, Koop & Strang 1997, Parkes 1997). Next, Worden suggests that the mode of death is important, especially a sudden and unexpected death, and particularly if some form of violence was involved or the death was suicide. The awareness of the impending death and avoidance of thinking of the possibility were reported as factors by Koop & Strang (1997). Parkes (1997) also highlights length of final illness: if the last illness lasted for more than 6 months, then this can cause difficulties for the older person. Other determinants include historical antecedents and personal variables such as the way the person has coped with previous bereavements and stressful events and if depression occurred in the period prior to the death (Koop & Strang 1997). Social, religious and cultural variables will interact with these determinants and need equal consideration. Additional factors described by Koop & Strang (1997) include financial difficulties, low educational level, the main language not being English and the nature of support given by professional carers.

There are some assessment tools that can be used and these have been reviewed by Walshe (1997). She identifies from these studies that personality and relationship factors as well as the circumstances of the death are all predictors of bereavement outcome whereas demographic factors (age, gender, social class) are not. There are tools that assess the risk of poor bereavement outcome and others that measure grief.

In reviewing the risk assessment tools available, no one tool stands out from the rest as the best tool to use. Both the tools devised by Ley (1992) and Parkes & Weiss (1983) (Bereavement Risk Index: BRI) found that skilled nurses' judgement has good predictive value, though this fails to offer an objective test or auditable outcome.

Also there are no grief measurement tools, according to Walshe, that appear suitable for all situations, but Walshe suggests that users take into account the population the tool was tested on and the ease of use of the different tools. Walshe makes three recommendations. First, that those who assess the risk or want to measure and monitor grief should have good education and training in the determinants of bereavement outcome, bereavement assessment and an exploration of appropriate tools. Second, that the use of tools should not replace clinical assessment and finally, that there should be an awareness of timing of assessment as this would also have a bearing on the most appropriate tool to use.

SPIRITUALITY AND CARING FOR DYING AND BEREAVED PEOPLE

During the latter part of the twentieth century society developed both a heightened awareness of its own mortality and an interest in the meaning and purpose of life (Garcia & Maitland 1983, King 1989, Moss 2002). Coupled with the changing pattern of health needs (Cox 1982), the increase in the number of older people and the recognized importance of spiritual well-being for this group (Forbis 1988), attention has focused on the role of the nurse in identifying and meeting the spiritual needs of patients (Granstrom 1985, Soeken & Carson 1987). As people age, their need for 'inner serenity' becomes increasingly important (Forbis 1988) and spirituality can offer not only a means of reconciliation but also meaning and purpose to life. It is often the spiritual dimension that helps older people cope with problems associated with illness and ageing (Harrison & Burnard 1993).

Holistic care means the provision of care in respect of physical, psychological, social and spiritual well-being, but perhaps the most challenging aspect of care is the spiritual dimension. All those working in caring services will have encountered the questions 'why?' and 'why me?'. Searching for meaning is aroused when critical events occur, such as when facing our own mortality or faced with the death of a close relative or friend, or on joyous occasions, such as the birth of a child. Thus, questions involving 'why?' are always difficult to deal with as there is no one answer and one person's answer to the meaning of life will be different from another's. Those of us who watch these events may be asking the same questions of ourselves. For those who manage to find an answer, these will always be individual responses. Even those who see spirituality in religious terms interpret their religion in their own way, hence the numerous sects that are found in all the major religions.

For these reasons care professionals often avoid addressing these questions or supporting people in seeking an answer for themselves, especially if they have not found their own answers. Professionals leave it to someone else. Those who have an answer need to be careful about evangelizing their own point of view as it may not be aligned with the bereaved individual's philosophy to life.

What then is spirituality? Moss (2002) suggests that the meaning of spirituality depends on the point of view of the person defining it – a little like *Alice in Wonderland*, where words mean what Alice wants them to mean. These range from those with strong, unerring convictions of what spirituality is to those who are much less convinced and dismiss it as 'gobbledegook and psychological flawed metaphysics' (Moss 2002: p. 34) that has little to do with the modern world. In between these two extremes lie numerous other definitions and understandings of the word. At a basic level, Moss (2002) reduces definitions to a search for meaning, in particular, the profound meanings about life and purpose in life. However, Moss then identifies different sets of definitions for different people. First, for those with religious beliefs, they will have their own specific principles that can help them make sense of life and death. If they have faith in a deity then often people will trust in their god. Their god will take care of them. They also have an identified person who care professionals call upon to support the individual, that is, the religious leader. This may be the individual's religious representative or one attached to the care setting. These may be seen as the easiest people to help address their spirituality; however when deep-seated beliefs are challenged, it may be a very distressing time for some individuals. Religious representatives may be the last people that the distressed individual wants to see.

Moss (2002) quotes from Lloyd (1997: 185) who gives a definition of spirituality as a person's values, beliefs and attitudes but recognizes that spirituality 'reaches beyond the wholly rational and material'. Another approach comes from Canda & Furman (1999) who suggest that spirituality underpins the acts of helping, empathy, compassion and caring and that the drive behind those who care is part of their spirituality, although often unacknowledged. Yet another dimension of spirituality can be seen in seeking some sense of justice and truth.

Highfield & Cason (1983) identified spiritual need as falling into one of four categories: (1) the need for meaning and purpose in life; (2) the need to receive love; (3) the need to give love; and (4) the need for hope and creativity.

Spiritual assessment requires the effective use of verbal and observational skills and should be a continuous process. Harrison & Burnard (1993) draw our attention to the importance of listening for cues and suggest that open questions be used to respond to non-verbal and verbal cues, particularly when they indicate spiritual need. Spiritual need or distress may be expressed in behavioural ways, for example, extremes of behaviour, mood changes and anger (which can be directed at staff). The authors point out the importance of a trusting, empathic relationship with the patient built on acceptance, sensitivity and a respect for the patient's values and beliefs. Saunders (2002) stresses the skills of reflective attention to give space for such a search. A safe and secure relationship and environment can also encourage such exploration.

This can be achieved through active listening as well as the offer of love, kindness, mercy, understanding and any quality which will add meaning to life and bring solace and comfort to those who are spiritually distressed (O'Brien 1982). The use of therapeutic touch may also offer some support and comfort during spiritual distress (Shaffer 1991), although nurses need to be aware of its appropriateness and be sensitive to the way in which patients may react to its use.

For spiritual issues in clinical practice to be addressed more effectively, nurses need to develop not only their theoretical knowledge but also their own self-awareness regarding spirituality, spiritual care and support (Granstrom 1985, McSherry 1996). By being clear about their own position in relation to their feelings and beliefs, nurses will then be helped to differentiate the patient's problems from their own (Labun 1988).

Irrespective of the nurse's spiritual affiliation, it is argued that being helped to worship according to their faith is a basic right of all patients (Henderson 1969). Increasingly, however, patients fail to fit neatly into a 'religious pigeon-hole' (Myco 1985) and at many levels doubts may occur, which can be expressed in many different ways. Moreover, 'non-believers' also like to discuss religion and philosophy and may wish to clarify their beliefs no less than those who believe in religion. Nurses need to be aware that human life is open to a wide range of possibilities right until the moment of death. Each human life must complete itself, as judged from within, not from without (Myco 1985). Thus the nurse has a responsibility to help patients, however disabled or distressed they may be, to identify the possibilities open to them. If the patient has a declared religion then this can be used as a source of support rather than simply an end in itself. Through the development of 'self' patients can be helped to achieve what they are capable of achieving, whether in their last years or the final stages of life.

While the emphasis has been on nurses fulfilling their role in holistic care, it is of equal importance that nurses acknowledge their limitations in helping patients with their spirituality. It may become necessary to involve someone else such as a counsellor, chaplain or religious adviser. Indeed, it is believed (Carson 1989) that when nurses can approach a patient knowing that they do not have all the answers this is a mark of humility, which in turn allows nurses to accept both patients and themselves as they are. In offering this kind of support to patients, nurses themselves may be in need of support and it is therefore important they develop networks to help them to form personal coping strategies. Unless they do, they may become unable to give spiritual support to others (Harrison & Burnard 1993).

EMOTIONAL SUPPORT FOR PEOPLE WHO ARE DYING AND THEIR CARERS

Caring for dying patients requires commitment and often considerable involvement, but without the loss of objectivity. As mentioned earlier, nurses who feel unable to confront the situation are known to use a variety of blocking tactics and in consequence communication remains at a very superficial level (Webster 1981, Wilkinson 1995). There are also a number of other barriers to effective communication and these include isolation of the patient, dishonesty amongst health professionals and relatives, age and gender of doctors and nurses, class, health of carers, education and 'being too busy' (Chalmers 1980). Moreover, to label patients who withdraw and who do not apparently want to talk about their prognosis as being 'in denial' is dangerous and could miss vital cues. For some patients, and their relatives, the acceptance of impending death is a gradual process (Saunders 1976) during which strategies for coping are developed and sustained. The nurse is well placed to develop a trusting empathic relationship within which a patient may feel encouraged and safe to talk of innermost feelings about dying and death. However, we also need to recognize and respect that patients will choose the time and place to share their feelings (Egan 1986). Death is something about which many older people will have given considerable thought and therefore some of the emotional reactions to dying and death may be less acute than for younger people (Carr 1982).

It is a commonly held yet mistaken belief that nurses require specialized skills in counselling to be able to support people who are dying and their carers. There may be special cases but, on the whole, if nurses demonstrate a willingness to stay near, listen and try to understand, this will be adequate. Wilkinson (1995) suggests the following steps to help patients express their feelings (for example, in dealing with feelings of anxiety):

- *Recognition.* The nurse recognizes either from verbal or non-verbal cues that the patient is anxious
- *Acknowledgement.* Use of reflection: 'I can see you are anxious'
- *Permission.* The nurse gives permission for feelings of anxiety: 'It is all right/OK to feel anxious'
- *Understanding.* The nurse provides the opportunity for the patient to discuss why he or she is feeling anxious: 'I would like to try and find out what is making you feel anxious'
- *Empathic acceptance.* The nurse reflects from the patient's viewpoint why he or she is feeling anxious: 'From what you've said it seems you're anxious because . . .'
- *Assessment.* The nurse tries to establish the extent to which the anxiety is affecting the patient's normal activities
- *Alteration* (or intervention). It may not be possible to alter the patient's anxiety state but when possible the cause of the anxiety should be removed.

Caring for a dying older person is both complex and challenging. In planning care, nurses need to consider not only the physical needs of patients and their relatives but also their less obvious emotional, social and spiritual needs. It is important that nurses are aware of both patients' and carers' reactions to dying and provide an opportunity for them to express their hopes and fears, which are then accepted and respected rather than ignored or, at worst, suppressed. To do this effectively we may need seriously to address our own attitudes towards dying and death and be prepared to engage in issues such as euthanasia and spirituality. We cannot choose to focus only on those aspects of care we feel comfortable with if they do not square with the needs of our patients and their families. Our aim must be to relieve suffering in all its dimensions, ranging from effective clinical intervention to 'just being there'.

Recommended reading

Death and dying

Buckman R 1992 How to break bad news: a guide for health-care professionals. Papermac, London.
This book not only gives an account of his theory about those facing death but also gives very useful practical advice for communicating about sensitive issues such as occur when people are faced with dying.
Copp G 1999 Facing impending death: experiences of patients and their nurses. Nursing Times Books, London.
The whole of Copp's work on cancer patients facing impending death can be found in this book. It also gives a chapter on theories about those facing death.
Dickensen D, Johnson M, Katz JS 2001 Death, dying and bereavement. Sage Publications, London.
A useful book that covers many aspects of death, dying and bereavement, including psychological, sociological, cultural, personal and ethical aspects.

Palliative care

Fallon M 1998 ABC of palliative care. British Medical Journal, London.
Publication of a series of articles in the British Medical Journal *on palliative care issues that covers 17 different relevant topics.*

Loss and bereavement

Thompson N (ed) 2000 Loss and grief; a guide for human services practitioners. Palgrave, Basingstoke.

Although written mainly with social workers in mind, this book has much to offer any health care professional who cares for patients who have suffered a loss. It takes a wider perspective on loss than just bereavement but does address more recent perspectives. It has a section on education and training needed to help those who have suffered a loss and a chapter that gives advice on how to put theory into practice.

Walshe C 1997 Whom to help? An exploration of the assessment of grief. International Journal of Palliative Nursing 3: 132–137.

This article has useful details of available tools that are used to identify those who may need professional help in coming to terms with their grief. It also gives a good critique of these tools.

Walter T 1999 On bereavement: the culture of grief. Open University Press, Buckingham.

In this book Walter critiques the literature and theories of bereavement and then gives his perspective on bereavement, including the findings from his research. This is a sociological approach to bereavement.

Worden JW 1991 Grief counselling and grief therapy, 2nd edn. Routledge, London.

Worden writes an easily understood text about his theory of bereavement and how to help those who are having problems during bereavement.

Useful websites

www.statistics.gov.uk/census2001/default.asp
The website for the Census 2001 results, presented in an easily assimilated format.
www.statistics.gov.uk/STATBASE
From this website the more detailed tables of information can be retrieved for national and local information.
www.whocancerpain.wisc.edu
A website for the World Health Organization journal Cancer Pain Release *that has useful articles on different matters related to cancer pain from around the world.*

References

Aries P 1974 Western attitudes towards death. John Hopkins University Press, Baltimore

Aries P 1983 The hour of our death. Peregrine, Aylesbury

Armstrong-Esther CA, Sandilands ML, Miller D 1989 Attitudes and behaviour of nurses towards the elderly in adult acute settings . Journal of Advanced Nursing 14: 34–41

Atkinson R, Davies G 1993 Issues in pain management. In: Clarke D (ed) The future for palliative care. Open University Press, Milton Keynes, pp 148–166

Badbury M 2000 The good death? In: Dickensen D, Johnson M, Katz JS (eds) Death, dying and bereavement, 2nd edn. Sage Publications, London

Bailey R, Clarke M 1989 Stress and coping in nursing. Chapman and Hall, London

Bernabei R, Gambassi G, Lapane K et al. 1998 Management of pain in elderly patients with cancer. Journal of the American Medical Association 279: 1877–1882

Bliss J, Johnson BM 1996 CRMF study. International Journal of Palliative Nursing 3: 126–133

Bloch M, Parry J (eds) 1982 Death and the regeneration of life. Cambridge University Press, Cambridge

Bond S 1983 Nurses' communication with cancer patients. In: Wilson-Barnett J (ed) Nursing research – ten studies in patient care. Wiley, Chichester, pp 57–80

Bowlby J 1980 Loss, sadness and depression, vol 3. Hogarth Press, London

Bowling A 1983 The hospitalisation of death: should more people die at home? Journal of Medical Ethics 9: 158–161

British National Formulary Joint Formulary Committee 2004 British national formulary, 47th edn. British Medical Association and Royal Pharmaceutical Society of Great Britain, London. Available online at: www.bnf.org

Buckman R 1992 How to break bad news: a guide for health-care professionals. Papermac, London

Canda E, Furman L 1999 Spiritual diversity in social work practice. Free Press, New York

Carr AT 1982 Dying and bereavement. In: Hall J (ed) Psychology for nurses and health visitors. Macmillan, London, pp 217–236

Carson VB 1989 Spirituality and the nursing process. In: Carson VB (ed) Spiritual dimensions of nursing practice. WB Saunders, Philadelphia

Cartwright A, Seale CF 1990 The natural history of a survey: an account of the methodological issues encountered in a study of life before death. Kings Fund, London

Cartwright A, Hockey L, Anderson JL 1973 Life before death. Routledge & Kegan Paul, London

Chalmers GL 1980 Caring for the elderly sick. Pitman Medical, Tunbridge Wells

Chavannes N 2001 A palliative approach for COPD and heart failure? European Journal of Palliative Care 8: 225–227

Cleeland CS, Gonin R, Hatfield AK et al. 1994 Pain and its treatment in outpatients with metastatic cancer. New England Journal of Medicine 330: 592–596

Clotfelter CE 1999 The effect of an educational intervention on decreasing pain intensity in elderly people with cancer. Oncology Nurses Forum 26: 27–33

Colleau SM 2000 Pain in the elderly with cancer. Cancer Pain Release 13 (2). Available online at: www.whocancerpain.wisc.edu

Colleau S M (ed) 2004 Ageing, pain and cancer: the role of geriatrics, oncology and palliative care. An interview with Dr Janet Abraham and Dr Ludovico Balducci. Cancer Pain Release Vol. 17(1–2)

Copp G 1999 Facing impending death: experiences of patients and their nurses. Nursing Times Books, London

Cox C 1982 Frontiers of nursing in the 21st century. Lessons from the past and present for future directions in nursing education. International Journal of Nursing Studies 19: 1–9

Department of Health 2000 The NHS plan: a plan for reform. Department of Health, London

Department of Health 2001 National service framework for older people. Department of Health, London

Doka K J (ed) 2001 Disenfranchised grief, 3rd edn. Lexington, New York

Egan G 1986 The skilled helper: a systematic approach to effective helping, 3rd edn. Brooks Cole, Monterey, California

Eve A, Smith AE 1996 Survey of hospice and palliative care inpatient units in the UK and Ireland. Palliative Medicine 10: 13–21

Eve et al. 1997 Hospice and palliative care 1994–1995, including a summary of trends 1990–1995. Palliative Medicine 11: 31–34

Feifel H 1998 Grief and bereavement. Bereavement Care 7: 2–4

Ferrell BR, Ferrel BA, Ahn C, Tran K 1994 Pain management for elderly patients with cancer at home. Cancer 74: 2139–2146

Field D 1989 Nursing the dying. Tavistock/Routledge, London

Field D, Addington-Hall J 1999 Extending palliative care to all? Social Science and Medicine 48: 1271–1280

Finch J, Mason J 1992 Negotiating family responsibilities. Routledge, London

Forbis PA 1988 Meeting patients' spiritual needs. Geriatric Nursing 9: 158–159

Freud S 1957 Mourning and melancholia. In: Strachey J (ed) Standard edition of the complete works of Sigmund Freud, vol 14. Norton, New York

Garcia J, Maitland S 1983 Walking on water. Virago, London

Garrett G 1983 Health needs of the elderly. Macmillan, London

George R, Sykes J 1997 Beyond cancer. In: Clark D, Ahmedzai S, Hockley JM (eds) New themes in palliative care. Open University Press, Buckingham, pp 239–294

Gibbs JRS, McCoy ASM, Gibbs LME, Rogers AE, Addington-Hall J 2002 Living with and dying from heart failure: the role of palliative care. Heart 88 (suppl.): ii36–ii39. Available online at: www.heartjnl.com

Glare P, Virik K, Jones M et al. 2003 A systematic review of physicians, survival predictions in terminally ill cancer patients. British Medical Journal 327: 195. Available online at: bmj.com

Glaser BG, Strauss AL 1965 Awareness of dying. Aldine, Chicago

Glaser BG, Straus AL 1967 The discovery of grounded theory. Adeline, New York

Granstrom S 1985 Spiritual care for oncology patients. Topics in Clinical Nursing 7: 35–45

Harrison J, Burnard P 1993 Spirituality and nursing practice. Avebury, Aldershot

Heath ML 1997 The use of pharmacology in pain management. In: Thomas VN (ed) Pain: its nature and management. Baillière Tindall, London, pp 95–103

Henderson V 1969 Basic principles of nursing care, revised. ICN, Geneva

Highfield M, Cason C 1983 Spiritual needs of patients. Are they recognised? Cancer Nursing 6: 187–192

Hockley J 1991 Death and dying. In: Redfern SJ (ed) Nursing elderly people, 2nd edn. Churchill Livingstone, Edinburgh, pp 391–401

Hockley J 1997 The evolution of the hospice approach. In: Clark D, Hockley J, Ahmedzai S (eds) New themes in palliative care. Open University Press, Buckingham

Illich I 1977 Limits to medicine: medical nemesis and the expropriation of health. Penguin, Harmondsworth

Jacox A, Carr DB, Payne R 1994 Management of cancer pain. Clinical practice guideline no 9. AHCPR (Agency for Health Care Policy and Research, now Agency for Healthcare Research and Quality) Supported Clinical Practice Guidelines publication No 84–0592 National Center for Biotechnology Information, US National Library of Medicine, Bethesda, MD

Kikule E 2003 A good death in Uganda: survey of needs for palliative care for terminally ill people in urban areas. British Medical Journal 327: 192–193

King V 1989 Women and spirituality. MacMillan, Basingstoke

Koenig HG 1998 Depression in hospitalised older patients with congestive cardiac failure. General Hospital Psychiatry 20: 29–43

Koop PM, Strang V 1997 Predictors of bereavement outcomes in families of patients with cancer: a literature review. Canadian Journal of Nursing Research 29: 33–50

Kubler-Ross E 1969 On death and dying. Macmillan, New York

Labun E 1988 Spiritual care, an element in nursing care planning. Journal of Advanced Nursing 13: 314–320

Land L 1995 A review of pressure damage prevention strategies. Journal of Advanced Nursing 22: 329–337

Lazarus R 1966 Psychological stress and the coping process. McGraw-Hill, New York

Levy S 2003 Using technology to support older people. Royal College of Nursing, London

Ley D 1992 Spiritual care in hospice. In: Cox GR, Fundis RJ (eds) Spiritual, ethical and pastoral aspects of death and bereavement. Baywood, Amityville, NY, pp 207–215

Lindemann E 1944 Symptomatology and management of acute grief. American Journal of Psychiatry 101: 141–148

Littlewood J 1992 Aspects of grief: bereavement in adult life. Routledge, London

Lloyd M 1997 Dying and bereavement, spirituality and social work in a market economy of welfare. British Journal of Social Work 22: 175–190

Mak MHJ 1992 Psychological responses to death and dying. Senior Nurse 12: 48–51

McCaffery M 1972 Nursing management of the patient with pain. Lippincott, Philadelphia

McIntosh J 1978 Communication and awareness on a cancer ward. Croom Helm. London

McKenzie GJ 1985 Death and dying. In: Cormack D (ed) Geriatric nursing: a conceptual approach. Blackwell Scientific, Oxford, pp 182–194

McSherry W 1996 Raising the spirits. Nursing Times 92: 48–49

Moss B 2002 Spirituality: a personal view. In: Thompson N (ed) (2000) Loss and grief; a guide for human services practitioners. Palgrave, Basingstoke, pp 34–44

Myco F 1985 The non believer in the health care situation. In: McGilloway O, Myco F (eds) Nursing and spiritual care. Harper & Row, London, pp 36–52

National Council for Hospice and Specialist Palliative Care Services 2001 What do we mean by palliative care: a discussion paper. Briefing no 9 May 2001

National Statistics Online: Older people – living arrangements, population, life expectancy. Available online at: www.statistics.gov.uk/census2001/default.asp (accessed May 2004). www.statistics.gov.uk/STATBASE (accessed May 2004)

Neimeyer RA, Anderson A 2002 Meaning reconstruction theory. In: Thompson N (ed) Loss and grief; a guide for human services practitioners. Palgrave, Basingstoke, pp 45–64

Neuberger J 2003 A healthy view of dying. British Medical Journal 327: 207–208

New Shorter Oxford English Dictionary 1993 Oxford Univerity Press, Oxford

NHS Executive 1996 A policy paper for commissioning cancer services. EL(96)85. Palliative Care Services, Department of Health, London

O'Brien ME 1982 The need for spiritual integrity. In: Yura H, Walsh WB (eds) Human needs and the nursing process. Appleton Century Crofts, Norwalk, CT, pp 286–289

O'Brien T, Welsh J, Dunn FG 1998 ABC of palliative care: non-malignant conditions. British Journal of Medicine 316: 286–289

Office of National Statistics 2001 Mortality statistics: review of the Registrar General on death in England and Wales. Office of National Statistics, London

Parkes CM 1993 Bereavement as a psychosocial transition: processes of adaptation to change. In: Dickenson D, Johnson M (eds) Death, dying and bereavement. Open University/Sage, London, pp 241–247

Parkes CM 1997 Bereavement and mental health in the elderly. Review of Clinical Gerontology 7: 47–53

Parkes CM, Weiss RS 1983 Recovery from bereavement. Basic, New York

Payne S, Horn S, Relf M 1999 Loss and bereavement. Open University Press, Buckingham

Randall F, Downie RS 2000 The main tradition. In: Dickensen D, Johnson M, Katz JS (eds) Death, dying and bereavement. Sage Publications, London, pp 263–269

Rando TA 1988 Anticipatory grief: this term is a misnomer but the phenomenon exists. Journal of Palliative Care 4: 70–73

Rhiner M, Ferrell BR, Ferrell BA et al. 1993 A structured non-drug intervention program for cancer pain. Cancer Practitioner 1: 137–143

Salamange M 2001 Palliative medicine for all. European Journal of Palliative Care 8: 234–236

Saunders C 1976 Care of the dying, 2nd edn. Nursing Times 72: 3–4

Saunders C 1978 The management of terminal disease. Edward Arnold, London

Saunders CM 1989 Grief: the mourning after – dealing with adult bereavement. John Wiley, London

Saunders C 2002 The philosophy of hospice. In Thompson N (ed) Loss and grief: a guide for human services practitioners. Pargrave, Basingstoke, pp 23–33

Saunders Y, Ross JR, Riley J 2003 Planning for a good death: responding to unexpected events. British Medical Journal 327: 204–207

Schneidman ES 1980 Voices of death. Harper & Row, New York

Scrutton S 1995 Bereavement and grief: supporting older people through loss. Edward Arnold, London

Seale C 1995 Dying alone. Sociology of Health and Illness 17: 374–392

Seale C, Addington-Hall J 1995 Dying at the best time. Social Science and Medicine 40: 589–595

Seale C, Cartwright A 1994 The year before death. Avebury, Aldershot

Seale C, Addington-Hall J, McCarthy M 1997 Awareness of dying: prevalence, causes and consequences. Social Science and Medicine 45: 477–484

Severs BM, Wilkins PSW 1991 A hospital palliative care ward for elderly people. Age and Ageing 20: 361–364

Shaffer J 1991 Spiritual distress and critical illness. Critical Care Nurse 11: 42–45

Siddel M, Katz JS, Komaromy C 2001 The case for palliative care in residential and nursing homes In: Dickenson D, Johnston M, Katz JS (eds) Death, dying and bereavement. Sage Publications, London also in Ageing and Society

Soeken K, Carson V 1987 Responding to the spiritual needs of the chronically ill. Nursing Clinics of North America 22: 603–611

Standing Medical Advisory Committee and Standing Nursing and Midwifery Advisory Committee 1992 The principles and practice of palliative care. Standing Medical Advisory Committee and Standing Nursing and Midwifery Advisory Committee, London

Stroebe W, Schut H 1999 The dual process model of coping with loss: rationale and description. Death Studies 23 (3): 197–226

Stroebe W, Stroebe MS 1987 Bereavement and health. Cambridge University Press, Cambridge

Thompson N (ed) 2002 Loss and grief: a guide for human services practitioners. Pargrave, Basingstoke

Thompson S 2002 Older people. In: Thompson N (ed) Loss and grief: a guide for human services practitioners. Pargrave, Basingstoke, pp 162–173

Twycross RG 1978 Relief of pain. In: Saunders CM (ed) The management of terminal illness. Arnold, London, pp 65–92

Twycross RG 1982 Euthanasia – a physician's viewpoint. Journal of Medical Ethics 8: 86–95

Victor CR 1995 Health policy and services for dying people and their carers. In: Dickenson D, Johnson M (eds) Death, dying and bereavement. Sage/Open University Press, Milton Keynes, pp 56–63

Walshe C 1997 Whom to help? An exploration of the assessment of grief. International Journal of Palliative Nursing 3: 132–137

Walter T 1999 On bereavement: The culture of grief. Open University Press, Buckingham

Walter T 2003 Historical and cultural variants of the good death. British Medical Journal 327(7408): 218–220

Webster ME 1981 Communicating with dying patients. Nursing Times 77: 23

Whelan J 2002 WHO calls for countries to shift from acute to chronic care. British Medical Journal 32; 1237

Wilkinson S 1995 Communication. In: David J (ed) Cancer care: prevention, treatment and palliation. Chapman & Hall, London, pp 204–223

Wiseman AD 1979 Coping with cancer. McGraw-Hill, New York

Worden JW 1983 Grief counselling and grief therapy. Routledge, London

Worden JW 1991 Grief counselling and grief therapy, 2nd edn. Routledge, London

World Health Organization 1990 Cancer pain relief and palliative care: a report of WHO expert committee, technical report series no 804. WHO, Geneva

World Health Organization 2002 Innovative care for chronic conditions: building blocks for action. WHO, Geneva

Chapter 27

Drugs and older people

Dinah Gould

INTRODUCTION

With advancing age the likelihood of developing a chronic illness will increase or an existing complaint may be exacerbated. An individual in the prime of life is able to respond to environmental fluctuations through homeostatic control but with advancing years this ability declines. Thus the older adult is able to adjust to changes of temperature and posture less effectively. Accidents are more common, the risk of infection is greater and the tissues heal more slowly than in the younger person. Many of these conditions can be treated with drugs, allowing the older person years of comfortable, independent living. In other cases medication is unnecessary providing changes are made to lifestyle. For example, including fibre in the diet on a regular basis may reduce the need for aperients as gut motility decreases. Similarly, alterations to the carbohydrate and fat content of the diet may obviate the need for drugs for the patient who has developed non-insulin-dependent diabetes mellitus.

At one time the symptoms of age-related disorders were regarded by patients and health professionals as an inevitable part of life. Today they are treated routinely. In consequence older people and their families have higher expectations from doctors, nurses and the National Health Service (NHS), a situation which, while it is desirable, also proves expensive. At the present time older people (those over the age of 65 years) make up a high and growing proportion of the population and consume the highest proportion of the NHS drugs budget. The number of older people within the UK population is increasing, so nurses can expect to care for increasing numbers in the future and more of them will be taking medication. In the past most of this care took place in hospital, but with the trend towards care in the community now firmly established, nurses will be required to look after increasing numbers of acutely as well as chronically ill older people in community settings. It is also likely that in future a smaller, but more intensively qualified nursing workforce will be involved in assessing and monitoring the care of these patients, while much of the 'hands-on' day-to-day care will be devolved to health care assistants and to lay carers whose activities will be supervised by the nurse. As part of their extended role many nurses are now responsible for prescribing a range of pharmaceutical products and it is accepted that in future the scope of nurse-prescribing will expand. Every nurse thus needs to develop a sound knowledge of pharmacology and to be particularly aware of age-related changes that alter the body's response to drugs (Otway 2002).

PROBLEMS ASSOCIATED WITH DRUG USE BY OLDER PEOPLE

The first problem related to the use of medication by older people is selecting the appropriate drug because symptoms of disease often differ from those presenting in younger age groups. For example, urinary tract infection in a young woman will typically manifest itself as urinary frequency, with pyrexia and dysuria. Older people are less likely to respond with pyrexia. Instead the nurse may become aware that something is wrong when a previously cooperative, lucid patient shows signs of disorientation. Further indicators may include loss of continence. Clearly this type of assessment is only possible when the nurse already knows

the patient. However, infection should always be suspected if the urine appears cloudy and has an offensive odour. This example illustrates how the signs and symptoms of illness frequently become vague and non-specific with age, a problem that may be compounded by communication difficulties and the coexistence of more than one medical condition. Some people develop side-effects to medication which they may fail to recognize and report. In other cases the cause of side-effects is difficult to pin down because people take over-the-counter (OTC) medication which they have forgotten about or do not mention in the mistaken belief that anything which can be purchased without prescription cannot have any untoward effects and will not interact with drugs that have been prescribed.

Dangers of polypharmacy

Some older people have multiple health problems. For example, the prevalence of hypertension in people over 60 years is 50% (Ramsey 1999) and it has been suggested that the number of people with diabetes, another condition affecting older people, will double by 2010 (Department of Health 2002). Hypertension, diabetes, obesity and smoking are all risk factors for cardiovascular disease, ischaemic heart disease and stroke. Risk increases with age and when the same individual has a range of medical conditions, each will need specific treatment. The amount of medication taken by the individual will therefore also increase. It has been established that older people receive more prescriptions per head than any other group (Department of Health 2001).

Polypharmacy is defined as the practice of prescribing four or more medications for the same person (Department of Health 2001; Fig. 27.1). The *National Service Framework for Older People* (Department of Health 2001) showed that 5–17% of hospital admissions are caused by adverse reactions to medicines and that 6–17% of older people in hospital experience adverse drug reactions. This is because several drugs taken simultaneously give greater scope for mistakes and misunderstandings and because drug interactions are more likely to occur. Sometimes a patient who has received medication for a long-established condition will develop a new, unrelated health problem for which additional drugs are prescribed or purchased. This can lead to drug interactions or even to a situation in which one drug is used to treat the side-effects caused by another. The addition of more drugs to the patient's existing regimen leads to confusion, mistakes and muddled reports from the patient or family and may culminate in hospital admission (Case study 27.1).

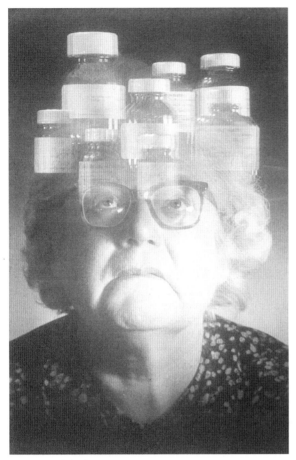

Fig. 27.1   Polypharmacy.

Changes in drug response with age

The body's response to drugs changes with age. The amount recommended and expected response of a given dose of drug are both calculated from data obtained concerning the dose–response of healthy young adults. There have been few studies comparing the responses of typical young volunteers and older subjects, hence decisions concerning the most appropriate dosage for older people have been determined largely on a trial-and-error basis, according to the general physiological changes known to accompany ageing (Ramsey 1988). Clearly this situation is far from ideal and it is important to observe the older patient for signs of toxicity. It is known that young individuals of the same age handle drugs differently depending on their genetic make-up and other complex metabolic factors. The same variations in response are exhibited by older people but in addition the rate of ageing will also vary between individuals.

Case study 27.1

Mr M, aged 81 years, was admitted to hospital following a 'funny turn' which included the inability to walk. A civil servant who had retired from work at the age of 61 years with hypertension, he was prescribed at that time Decaserpyl plus a reserpine alkaloid by his general practitioner, who also suggested a change of lifestyle (early retirement). Over the following years the patient moved house and transferred to a new general practitioner, who continued his drug by repeat prescription, in spite of the advent of beta-blocking drugs, and without regular check-up. When he was 75 years old Mr M's wife complained of his unsteadiness, fidgety movements and withdrawal. During a hospital consultation parkinsonism was diagnosed and Sinemet (levodopa with carbidopa) was prescribed. Both drugs were then supplied on repeat prescription and no further consultation made until the present admission.

On Mr M's admission to hospital a cardiac monitor was set up and all drugs stopped. Blood pressure was only slightly raised and subsequently fell to within a normal range. No abnormality was detected and after 10 days the patient was discharged on a small dose of Sinemet to reduce slight rigidity. At an outpatient follow-up the drug was withdrawn and the patient remains well and drug-free.

This problem was due to both side-effects and interactions; firstly, reserpine alkaloids (Decaserpylplus) deplete dopamine; secondly, the addition of the drug levodopa (Sinemet) rectified the condition – one drug nullified the effect of the other. The patient's 'turn' was most probably due to postural hypotension, a known side-effect of levodopa, and an increasing sensitivity to the drug.

Changes in the ability to absorb drugs

Most drugs are administered orally because it is the most straightforward route. Before they can exert their required pharmacological effect they must be absorbed effectively by the body, enter the circulation and be transported to the site of action. Changes in the gastrointestinal tract which occur with ageing probably contribute to the differences in the amount and timing of drug absorption.

Reduced gastric acid secretion is indicated by a reduction in the basal rate of gastric acid and histamine-stimulated secretion. These factors may reduce the solubility of acidic drugs (e.g. aspirin). Conversely other drugs normally destroyed by gastric acid may be protected (e.g. penicillins).

Gut motility and the rate of gastric emptying are reduced. This increases the overall transit time of drugs to the site of absorption. A slower peak and prolonged absorption of medication may result. This is not usually a problem when drugs are given on a long-term basis but when a high concentration is needed rapidly the desired effect may not be achieved. Examples would be the administration of analgesia for sudden acute pain and antimicrobial therapy. Gastric irritants such as the non-steroidal anti-inflammatory drugs (NSAIDs) and levodopa may cause excessive discomfort if gastric emptying is marked. In consequence the patient may become reluctant to take them. Reduced gut transit time can result in an overall increase in drug absorption. This may be overcome by prescribing smaller doses. In other cases the drugs themselves alter gastric emptying. An example is atropine, sometimes used to treat diverticular disease, a commonly occurring condition in older people. Metoclopramide, often given to help reduce nausea, also speeds gastric emptying.

Reduction in the number of actively absorbing cells in the gastrointestinal mucosa may occur with age as general cellular turnover and replacement slow down. This may reduce the efficiency with which actively absorbed drugs such as the amines, methyldopa and levodopa enter the circulation. However, most drugs are absorbed passively so their uptake will not be affected.

The physical properties of the drug affect absorption; these include modifications in the formulation deliberately introduced by the manufacturer (such as slow-release tablets) and whether such medication is taken as advised.

It is apparent that the effects of ageing on drug action and absorption may be subtle and unpredictable. When individual problems arise, assays of the drug concentrations in the plasma during absorption can be undertaken. Even then, more than one change may occur and the effects of one age-related change may counter those of another. For example, a reduced ability to absorb may remain undetected because decreased transit time allows a prolonged period for slower absorption to take place.

Absorption of drugs from other sites

Changes in drug absorption from other sites may also be affected with age.

Drugs administered by injection depend on the subcutaneous or muscular circulation to carry them into the systemic circulation. Reduction in muscle tone through inactivity may cause the fluid to pool at the site of entry, delaying its action. Older people have delicate skin, especially if taking steroids, and bruise easily; it is vital to rotate the site when injections are administered frequently.

Locally administered drugs Drugs instilled into the eye, nose or ear and those applied to the surface of the skin, mouth or vagina produce their effects locally. They are not generally absorbed into the systemic circulation to any great extent. With age, the elasticity, moisture and turnover of epithelial cells are reduced and repeated application may result in irritation, soreness or breakdown of the epithelial layer. The area should be carefully inspected before each application and patients' reports of discomfort should be taken seriously. When individuals are responsible for administering their own medication they should be warned about possible side-effects and know where to seek help.

Changes in drug distribution

The value of any drug lies both in its specific action against the condition for which it has been prescribed and its ability to concentrate in the part of the body that is affected. Alterations in the composition of the tissues and in physical activity which result during ageing can affect the distribution of drugs and consequently their effectiveness.

The relative proportions of muscle and fat in the body change with age. The proportion of fat increases, producing a larger depot for lipid-soluble drugs such as the benzodiazepines and barbiturates to accumulate. These are taken up readily by adipose tissue and released slowly for metabolism and excretion. As a result older people recover from the effects of treatment slowly. Problems are exacerbated if they have to undergo general anaesthesia because the agents normally used are also fat-soluble. The patient becomes confused and may remain disoriented for several days (Platzer 1989). This is distressing for friends and relatives and a major difficulty for staff working in acute hospital settings. If an old person is admitted in an emergency, typically after falling, staff will have no yardstick against which to measure usual behaviour.

The amount of body water declines by up to 15% between the ages of 20 and 80 years. This reduction in fluid, with a parallel reduction in size, leads to higher concentrations of some drugs recorded for older patients following the administration of a standard dose. This can result in unexpected signs of overdose after what would be considered a normal dose. This effect is particularly likely to occur during long-term therapy when the concentration of drug has accumulated.

Changes in plasma proteins occur in older people. This has consequences for the distribution of drugs because they are poorly soluble in plasma and are transported attached to plasma proteins, chiefly albumin, which is the most abundant plasma protein in the body. In older people the amount of circulating albumin is reduced, so more of the drug is carried freely in the plasma (Montamat et al. 1989). Figure 27.2 shows that it is the amount of free drug in the circulation that determines rate of diffusion into the tissue fluid and ultimately its pharmacological action, which thus tends to be greater in older people.

Changes in vascularization caused by reduced cardiac output have been reported in older people: approximately 30% between the ages of 30 and 65 years. The consequent reduction in blood flow to different parts of the body is not uniform. It appears that there is little change in supply to the cardiac and skeletal muscles but marked reduction in supply to the liver and kidneys. It is probable that these changes reduce the speed at which drugs are detoxified and excreted from the body.

Changes in metabolism in the liver

Drugs are treated by the body as foreign substances. They are actively destroyed and rendered harmless before being excreted. Those absorbed from the gastrointestinal tract are carried via the portal vein to the liver before gaining access to the systemic circulation (Fig. 27.3). This is of clinical significance as most drugs are metabolized in the liver, explaining why only a proportion of the amount absorbed enters the systemic circulation. Destruction of a drug by the liver before it gains access to the general circulation (and target tissues) is known as the 'first-pass effect'. The first-pass effect tends to be increased in older people for two reasons: (1) the reduction in hepatic blood supply, discussed above; and (2) reduced activity of hepatic enzymes. The net result is a lower rate of metabolism, accumulation of the drug and the possibility of overdose if the signs and symptoms are not recognized and reported. This often falls to a relative

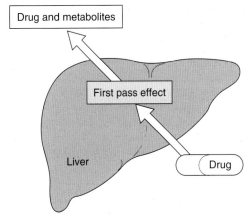

Fig. 27.3 First-pass effect in drug metabolism.

who must be taught what to look out for, or should be done by a health professional.

Changes in excretion

Renal excretion is the main route for the removal of toxins and waste products from the body. Drugs and their breakdown products are mainly excreted via the kidney. The speed of elimination is clinically important as it is the chief factor determining the duration of action of the drug. The length of time that active drug remains in the circulation is known as its plasma half-life. Chronic conditions affecting the renal system are more common in older people, but even in the physically well older person there is marked decline in renal function. Glomerular filtration rate and tubular absorption fall, so that by 80 years of age renal function is only half that at 40 (Montamat et al. 1989). For drugs such as digoxin, which have only small differences between concentrations that are therapeutic and toxic and are excreted unchanged in the urine, accumulation could be dangerous.

The older patient is thus vulnerable to the risk of unintentional overdose effects. Patients on long-term therapy will, as they grow older, become more at risk so that dose adjustment becomes necessary. Many older people regulate their drug intake themselves according to side-effects or by forgetting to take the occasional dose. When admitted to hospital the full prescribed dose will be administered, leading to the possibility of toxic response.

Other routes of excretion than via the kidneys are possible. As with any other products of metabolism, excretion via the bile, skin, lung or body fluids may occur with drugs. These routes are only of major significance when renal function becomes impaired. For older

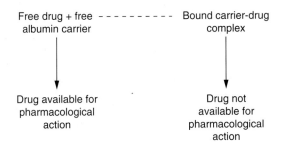

Fig. 27.2 Plasma carriage of pharmacologically active substances.

people, a general decline in the efficiency of these other routes makes the consequences of renal failure even more disastrous.

Changes in receptor sensitivity

The changes in physiology of the gut, skin, circulation and liver account for the variations in drug concentration seen in older people and hence the unexpected symptoms of overdosage or underdosage to what is considered a standard dose. For older people, a number of responses have been recorded which do not fit into the accepted categories of toxicity and which are probably explained by differences in sensitivity. For example, a single dose of a barbiturate can produce a wide range of responses, from restlessness to frank psychosis. Sensitivity may also be altered with diseases of the cardiovascular system, when increased sensitivity to warfarin can be expected. On the whole, the unexpected symptoms of drug sensitivity are vague: rashes, dizziness, confusion and agitation are common manifestations which unfortunately may be simply dismissed as signs of 'getting old' and not investigated.

Transdermal medication

In recent years pharmaceutical manufacturers have increased the range of medications which can be delivered via this route into the systemic circulation. Many people now receive their daily doses of analgesics, hormone replacement therapy, antianginals and nicotine replacement therapy through stick-on patches that deliver a constant amount of the drug over 12 or 24 h.

Adverse reactions

Older people experience a much higher rate of adverse reactions to drugs than people in other age groups. This is explained because the older person is more likely to be prescribed a cocktail of drugs so that the regimen is more complicated, with more scope for errors, and because they are less likely to be informed about the increased number of possible side-effects. A number of drugs commonly prescribed for older people are well-known for causing side-effects (e.g. NSAIDs), while others have a narrow therapeutic range and readily produce toxicity in overdose (e.g. digoxin). Although there is no evidence that older people intentionally fail to comply with the instructions to take their medication more often than younger patients, their drug-taking habits may increase their vulnerability to adverse reactions (Cargill 1992). When knowledge and understanding of the treatment are lacking and memory is needed to take medication, mistakes are liable to occur.

Adverse reactions fall into three broad classes: (1) dose-related; (2) hypersensitivity; and (3) idiosyncratic.

Dose-related reactions become apparent as symptoms of overdose. These are due either to exceeding the dose or to changes in the individual's handling or sensitivity to the drug.

Hypersensitivity reactions are due to genetic or immunological abnormalities. Even though present from birth, the existence of a genetic defect may not become apparent until old age because the individual has not taken the drug before.

Idiosyncratic responses may also result from a combination of genetic, disease and age-related causes. These may be the result of lifestyle, especially diet, or response to the drug itself. This is an area which has so far attracted little research. However, genetic differences in the hepatic enzymes responsible for metabolizing drugs are known to exist, resulting in individual variations in plasma concentration. If the individual has never taken the drug before, the reaction will not be known.

Tolerance

With repeated use some drugs are metabolized more effectively by the liver – the phenomenon of tolerance. Increasingly larger doses become necessary to produce a therapeutic effect. This may occur with narcotic analgesia such as morphine.

Organ sensitivity

There is evidence that some systems become increasingly sensitive to certain drugs as the individual ages. In particular, functions of the brain tend to become disturbed in older people, with the result that hypnotic drugs readily produce confusion during the night and excessive drowsiness or hangover effects the next day.

Effects of drugs on general health

The effect of drugs on the general health of the individual should not be overlooked. Taking large numbers of tablets may reduce the appetite, especially in hospital where they are usually presented immediately before a meal, or if taking them makes the mouth sore. Nutritional deficiency can result from prolonged use of drugs that suppress appetite or reduce absorption. Amfetamines and anticonvulsants may behave in this way. It is not unknown for the responsibility of managing a complex regimen of drugs to generate marked anxiety, either in the individual taking them or in a lay carer supervising medication at home. In other cases side-effects from the drugs themselves may lead to problems. Sometimes apparent mental illness may prove to be the result of physiological disturbance arising through the action or interaction of drugs.

Pathophysiological reactions may result from either dose-related or hypersensitivity reactions. In addition there are individual variations in the presentation of disease from the same drug. Drug-induced disease usually develops with prolonged use of the same medication. The risk of developing a gastric ulcer from repeated use of NSAIDs increases with age (Griffiths & Jordan 2002). Nutritional defects are also more likely when prolonged use of the same drugs is necessary. Some drugs cause problems because they dull appetite or reduce absorption (e.g. digoxin, anticonvulsants, amfetamines). Others interfere with absorption (e.g. mineral oil, phenolphthalein, phenytoin) or increase the loss of ions in the urine (diuretics, cortisone, alcohol). Some medication required long-term by older people antagonizes the effects of vitamins: warfarin (vitamin K), levodopa (vitamin B_6) or trimethoprim (folate).

Most deaths resulting from adverse drug reactions are due to commonly used medications such as digoxin, antimicrobials, insulin or diuretics. They occur through overdosage or from predictable side-effects. The most common adverse reactions reported for older people are shown in Table 27.1.

Drug interactions

Drug interactions are particularly common among older people for the following reasons:

- They are more likely to be prescribed several drugs, often to treat a number of different complaints. There is an established relationship between the number of different drugs taken and the number of adverse reactions reported (Montamat et al. 1989). Many people take OTC medicines which may interact with those that have been prescribed (Conn 1991). For example, many proprietary cough mixtures contain mild sedatives. This effect is then added to that of hypnotics they are already taking
- Deterioration in renal function alters the plasma half-life of drugs. Elimination is impaired,

Table 27.1 Problem drugs for older people

Drug group	Problems/symptoms
Cardiac glycosides	Overdosage easy – little difference between toxic and therapeutic dose
	Overdose effects more common when combined with potassium-depleting diuretics, hypercalcaemia and hypothyroidism
	Adverse symptoms – nausea, vomiting, confusion, depression, gynaecomastia and acute abdominal syndrome
	Any sort of arrhythmia may occur
Diuretics	Thiazides – potassium deficiency, digoxin toxicity
	Furosemide and etacrynic acid – homeostatic upsets, transitory or permanent deafness, impaired glucose tolerance
Benzodiazepines	Reduced reaction time. Build-up of sedation with repeated dosage
Antidepressants	Tricyclics – accentuated side-effects, dry mouth, hypertension, drowsiness
	Many interactions possible
	Monoamine oxidase inhibitors – potential hazard due to interactions with food and self-administered drugs
Anti-inflammatories	Age-related increase in incidence of gastric ulcer, bleeding and dyspepsia with both steroid and non-steroid drugs
	Interactions with anticoagulants
Phenothiazines	Induce parkinsonism, lethargy and hypotension. May cause cholestatic jaundice or reduce liver and thyroid function. Contribute to accidental hypothermia
	Interact with alcohol – effects enhanced
Oral anticoagulants	Increased anticoagulant response (warfarin), possibly due to reduced clotting factor production
	Unpredicted haemorrhagic complications
	Possible interactions, non-steroidal anti-inflammatories, steroids, barbiturates, quinidine, thyroxine

exposing older people to higher concentrations for reaction if dosages are not adjusted

- Concurrent illness may interfere with drug metabolism. For example, many old people suffer some degree of congestive cardiac failure. This reduces hepatic blood supply, so metabolism in the liver is reduced over and above any normal age-related effects, contributing to build-up and overdose
- Problems taking medication as instructed.

ADHERENCE TO TREATMENT REGIMENS

Clearly no drug can be effective unless it is taken; thus non-compliance is recognized as a major cause of treatment failure. Compliance is regarded as the extent to which an individual's behaviour coincides with instructions from health professionals (Haynes et al. 1987). Use of the term 'compliance' has fallen from favour because it represents the perspective of the health professional without taking account of the patient's view (Oseasohn et al. 1989), generating the impression of coercion, with the distribution of power lying firmly in the hands of the professional (Kolton & Piccolo 1988). For this reason the term 'adherence' is frequently used to promote the beneficial partnership between the provider of medication and its recipient (Carey 1984).

Non-adherence with medicine-taking by patients is described as either unintentional, when patients want to follow the prescribed regime but, for some reason do not do so, or intentional, when they choose not to follow the regime (Lowe & Raynor 2000). Only about 50% of medicines are taken as prescribed (Haynes et al. 1996, Knapp 2002). Non-adherence is a complex issue, as demonstrated by a study that found it to be related to 14 categories of misunderstanding between patient and doctor (Britten et al. 2000). Misunderstandings identified relate to patient information unknown to the doctor, doctor information unknown to the patient, conflicting information, disagreement about cause of side-effects, failure of communication about the doctor's decision and what Britten's group called 'relationship factors'. The authors emphasize that all the misunderstandings were associated with lack of participation by patients in the prescribing decision.

Recent literature shows that more than 70% of non-adherence is intentional in that patients choose to ignore advice or alter doses because of their concerns about side-effects or becoming dependent on the drug (Westbury 2002), or because they alter their drug-taking to fit in with their own priorities, such as fulfilling family and social obligations (Townsend et al. 2003). The language is changing from the emphasis on compliance, when health professionals expect and strive to keep patients on the professionally determined medication regime, to the notion of 'concordance' and involvement of the patient in treatment decisions (Pollock et al. 2002). Concordance acknowledges the position of patients as partners in prescribing decisions. As Britten (2003: p. 840) puts it: 'The integration, within the consultation, of best evidence and the patients' priorities is at the heart of concordance.' Doctors and other prescribers who take a concordance approach recognize that patients are competent to judge the appropriateness of medications in their individual circumstances even when their view is at variance with professional judgement. Recent Department of Health policy supports the idea of concordance. In 2002 the Department of Health announced a 2-year initiative called Medicines Partnership to put the principles of patient partnership and concordance into practice with different patient groups, including older people and residents of sheltered housing (*Pharmaceutical Journal* 2002). Further information on this initiative is on the Medicines Partnership website: www.medicines-partnership.org.

In hospital it is the nurse's responsibility to ensure that drugs are administered as prescribed and that the patient actually receives the drug. Omissions are possible and, in the author's experience, audit has revealed that the majority of cases where this happens occur either because the drug was not available when required or because the patient was not present at a time when it was offered. In other cases administration may be difficult because the patient has difficulty swallowing tablets. The patient should be offered a glass of water, adding more liquid if several are to be taken at once. Rushing does not help. If the patient fails to swallow, the tablet should be removed with a spoon and the patient offered a drink before starting again. A drink of water should be offered after liquid drugs have been taken as these are often sticky and leave an unpleasant feeling, as well as an unpleasant taste, in the mouth. Injections may be difficult, oozing out of flabby skin. Bruising frequently occurs with older patients. Such difficulties should be discussed with the pharmacist so that, where possible, other routes of administration can be used on a temporary or permanent basis. It is not advisable to crush tablets without first checking with the pharmacist as this may interfere with the action of the drug. For example, the delayed action of slow-release preparations will be lost if they are crushed.

For many patients in the community, the nurse does not need to be responsible for ensuring that each dose of medication is taken. For others, however, aids such as the Dossett box (a box with time-labelled compartments which contain all tablets for the day) are used in an attempt to increase the likelihood that medication is taken according to prescription. Non-adherence has been declared a significant problem in primary care, though there is no evidence that it is greater in older than younger people (McGraw & Drennan 2000). McGraw & Drennan point to a lack of knowledge about the effectiveness of medication adherence devices such as the Dossett box, stating that frequency and type of medication error are unknown, particularly when these devices are used by older people who are receiving complex care packages from multiple service providers.

The nurse in the community setting plays an important role in teaching patients about their medication and in promoting correct use. Drugs which have been hoarded instead of taken are a potential hazard (Watson 1989). Every year, cases of accidental poisoning are reported in children who have mistaken tablets for sweets, and there is the additional risk that hoarded supplies may be taken inappropriately by other frail family members. If a supply of medication is not used the nurse should ensure that it is disposed of safely by flushing it down the lavatory or returning it to the pharmacist.

Refusal of treatment

Occasionally patients will openly refuse treatment. Where this situation is known it can be more easily dealt with. In most cases explanation of the reason for treatment and its benefits, with persuasion to try the drug for a few days, will win confidence sufficiently to initiate treatment. If the patient dislikes the drug because of its taste or form, a change may be possible. For example, an antibiotic may be administered as a suspension rather than in tablet form. Often the reason for refusal is simple and addressing the problem from the patient's perspective will make all the difference. In some cases refusal may be legitimate. The patient may judge the side-effects to outweigh the advantages of medication. Codeine prescribed to control mild to moderate pain may have such an unpleasant constipating effect that the patient may prefer the pain. Clearly the success or otherwise of medication should be discussed with the patient soon after treatment begins and at regular intervals afterwards because it is often possible to find a solution. Another analgesic can be used or the addition of bran or extra fruit to the diet may help prevent constipation. Non-adherence is much more difficult when it is concealed. As discussed above, tablets that have been spat out or hidden can be a potential danger to others.

Covert medication

The practice of concealing medication in food or drink has been described as 'covert medication'.

It represents a legal and ethical minefield and has been harshly criticized by groups concerned with the welfare of older people such as Help the Aged and the Alzheimer's Society. Some authorities believe that under common law as laid down by the Law Commission, nurses and doctors have a duty of care to treat people who are incapacitated in their best interests and the least restrictive fashion (Treloar 2001). Thus, in extreme circumstances (for example, when a patient has become very aggressive), it may be admissible to deliver covert medication (in this example tranquillizers) because the only alternative would be to restrain the patient and administer an injection, a practice which could be construed as cruelty. However, the charity Help the Aged believes that reliance on common law does not adequately protect patients from potential abuse. Instead they would prefer legislation to allow older people to give power of attorney that would cover health care. This would enable them to nominate someone else to take decisions when they are no longer able to do so themselves. Although sound in principle, this practice would not afford protection to the many older people who have no one to take power of attorney for them. From a pharmaceutical perspective, covert medication is definitely to be avoided. Crushing tablets and mixing them with food or liquid may alter the rate of release of the active ingredient or prevent it being absorbed, thus defeating the purpose of medication.

Medication errors

Five categories of non-adherence have been identified (Wade & Bowling 1986):

1. errors of omission
2. errors of dosage
3. taking medication for the wrong reason
4. mistakes in timing
5. taking additional OTC medication.

It is not always easy to determine precisely which problems have arisen. However, the research evidence indicates that omission and mistiming are the most common (Parkin et al. 1976), probably because most individuals feel that they have to take too many medicines (Morrow et al. 1988). Problems may arise if drugs are ordered by repeat prescription over long periods without the patient seeing the doctor, as there is no opportunity for the regimen to be reviewed (Case study 27.2). Nurses in the community who visit

Case study 27.2

Mrs N was originally prescribed nembutal as a sedative during a US Air Force (USAF) alert in Norfolk, England – the noise of the planes kept her awake. The drug was added to those on her repeat prescription card by the general practitioner's secretary and on all subsequent occasions she was issued with a repeat prescription which included nembutal with her other drugs. When the USAF alert was over she only took the drug on 'bad nights' and accumulated quite a backlog of capsules. One day a friend complained of not sleeping well, so Mrs N kindly gave her a few capsules and then a bottle. Other customers followed and the prescription was subsequently accepted, so that she could supply her friends' needs. All these barbiturate-takers were older people and fortunately well, and not taking much alcohol or many drugs which might interact. Mrs N was amazed when she was told of the problems which could have developed.

Case study 27.3

Mr W, aged 70 years, came to the outpatients department with his wife, who complained that he kept her awake all night and then went to sleep in the morning when she 'had all her work to do'. Mr W was being treated for cardiac failure and had been discharged from hospital 3 weeks before on a drug regimen of digoxin, thiazide diuretic with potassium supplement and nitrazepam. He had kept very well but admitted that he did have to get up several times at night to urinate. The pharmacist checked his tablets with him, except for the sleeping tablets which he kept by his bed. He explained that he had 'little white ones' (heart tablets) twice a day and the 'white ones' (water tablets) in the morning, together with the 'oblong ones' which 'were to put back what went out with the water'.

Unfortunately all the containers were the same and the print rather small, otherwise he might have noticed that he was in fact taking his sleeping tablets, white round tablets, in the morning instead of his 'water tablets', also white and round, which he had by his bed and took at night. The problem was solved by putting a different-coloured label on the sleeping tablets and making sure that they, and not the diuretic tablets, were by his bed.

on a regular basis play an important role in monitoring the number and range of medications the individual is expected to take. Muddling tablets is another common problem (Case study 27.3). Many patients keep all the day's drugs in one bottle then take them randomly, or identify different bottles with a system that is inefficient and dangerous; for example, marking one of two bottles with an elastic band which may easily slip off and become lost. It should also be made clear that swapping drugs with other people or 'trying out' someone else's medication is extremely dangerous.

Measures to promote adherence

There is no doubt that people who receive information about their drugs comply better with their regimens of medication when they go home (Bird & Hassall 1993). Box 27.1 indicates the type of information required.

In addition to the practical information suggested in Box 27.1, patients should be able to discuss problems of medication with their nurse, pharmacist or general practitioner and may require help obtaining medication. There is also scope for improving professional practice in relation to medication.

Acceptance

Making treatment acceptable to the patient is the first step in ensuring cooperation. Occasionally patients harbour odd ideas about taking medication or have

---

Box 27.1   Information essential for patients receiving prescribed medication

- Name of the drug
- Strength
- Appearance (pink pills, red capsules, etc.)
- Purpose
- Dose
- Frequency with which it must be taken
- Storage (safety, how to dispose of unused medication if discontinued)
- The importance of expiry dates
- Common side-effects
- Common adverse reactions and early signs that they are occurring
- Common interactions and the need to mention existing medication when seeing a doctor
- Avoidance of over-the-counter prescriptions when this is relevant
- Special instructions – maybe related to the route of administration or foods to avoid

been influenced by 'old wives' tales'. Although these notions may seem quaint and ludicrously unfounded to health professionals, they must nevertheless be dealt with honestly, with opportunities for individuals to express their beliefs without having them dismissed out of hand.

Helping patients to obtain their medication

Patients leaving hospital are supplied with drugs to take with them but subsequent prescriptions must be obtained through the general practitioner. This should be made clear to the patient and reassurance should be given that the doctor will have been informed about the drugs which they have to take. The patient also needs to be made aware that tablets supplied by the hospital pharmacy may look different from those later received with a general practitioner's prescription and that, in many health centres, a new prescription must be requested at least a week before it can be collected. Frequently it is necessary for a relative or home help to collect prescriptions. Directly questioning patients about their intended method of obtaining supplies before discharge is a useful method of drawing attention to this need (Coombes & Horne 1994). For people in the UK over the age of 60 years prescriptions are free of charge. To qualify the individual must fill in and sign the reverse of the prescription form. Those eligible should be reminded if necessary.

Improving professional practice

Today it is considered essential that health professionals discuss medication with their patients and include them as partners in care. It is also desirable for nurses, doctors, pharmacists and other health professionals to liaise in the management of the patients who make up their caseloads so that all are informed about the medication regimen prescribed in terms of its aims, any possible disadvantages and individual problems. This is particularly important in the community where team work between health professionals is considered to be of key importance in securing patients' understanding and adherence with their medication (Ross 1991). The nurse may well be aware that the patient is taking a large number of different medications, some of which may not be strictly necessary, but this information will be of no value unless feedback is supplied to the person responsible for prescription. Likewise liaison between hospital and community staff is essential. In some cases general practitioners may discontinue medication initiated while the patient was in hospital (Coombes & Horne 1994).

Accurate administration

Labelling

Since 1984 it has been a requirement of the British Pharmaceutical Society that all containers for medication are marked with large, typed labels so that all members of the public, including older people, can read them. Instructions must be explicit. The label should contain clear details for administration and the purpose of the medication. 'Two tablets to be taken four times a day if necessary for pain' is acceptable. Vague general instructions such as 'Take as directed' are not acceptable.

Memory aids

Routines for drug administration vary between hospitals. However, apart from wards and units which are operating patient self-medication schemes (see below), when a new drug is started the patient will become familiar with the general routine. On discharge from hospital, this routine may need to be adapted to fit in with home circumstances. Remembering when to take drugs can be difficult for everyone, old and young. The problem is increased in proportion to the number of drugs to be taken and the different regimens of administration. Wherever possible patients should be taught to administer their drugs before discharge (Bird & Hassall 1993). Simple measures such as linking drug-taking to events in the daily routine (e.g. getting up, mealtimes) may be effective. Other devices include marking a diary when the drug is taken or using a calendar with tear-off strips (Entwhistle 1989). Another memory aid is to give the patient a treatment card with a sample tablet stuck down with transparent tape against an easily comprehended description of what it is intended for (e.g. 'water' tablet, pain tablet, breathing tablet). For patients with greater difficulties it may be necessary to make use of dose boxes such as the Dossett box. These are compartmentalized boxes or collections of tablet containers which are filled with a supply of drugs, usually weekly (Watson 1989). Each dose is placed in an individual compartment and the patient can check that the drug has been taken by seeing that the compartment is empty. This method requires the help of a relative, neighbour, friend or health professional to prime the box if the older person is unable to do so. The value of this type of system has been evaluated in numerous studies. Kennedy (1991) recommended the Dossett box as a safe and effective method of administration, allowing the patient to remain independent. Others have found that some older people dislike memory aids (Coombes & Horne 1994). The use of such aids needs to be monitored for individual patients.

The final resource for a patient who cannot remember to take drugs is to employ someone else to administer them. This could be difficult, however, because friends and relatives may themselves have memory problems. Relatives often begin to help when they observe signs of cognitive and physical impairment in the patient. Because they may spend more time with their older relative than a health professional, they can offer valuable insight into potential problems and the degree of coping that can be expected (Conn 1995).

Aids for people with physical disabilities

Many adults have difficulty opening 'child-proof' drug containers and this problem increases with age. The greatest difficulties are experienced by patients with physical disabilities, such as arthritis, resulting in stiff, swollen finger joints and loss of manual dexterity. Tablets can be dispensed in conventional containers or with winged caps; these are very helpful for stiff hands. Standard instructions may be given to pharmacists to provide a specific type of medication container for a patient (Entwhistle 1989). Small tablets may be difficult to handle and wide-necked bottles or tablet dispensers can help with this problem. Calendar packs can be snipped with scissors if the patient cannot tear foil.

Poor sight can be compensated for with large print or identifiable symbols to help the patient recognize the container. Different-coloured lids are available for easy identification. They are preferable to elastic bands and other 'home-made' remedies which may become detached, leading to confusion and errors (Watson 1989). Braille labels are also available, although not all blind people read braille. Dose boxes can be helpful in this situation as the patient can feel which compartments are empty. For liquid medication a measure marked clearly to the level of the exact dose or a fixed-volume syringe may be useful. These can be bought inexpensively from pharmacy stores. Special eyedrop dispensers and inhalers are also obtainable (Connolly 1995). Nurses are often surprised at the range of aids available and the amount of practical help that can be provided by the pharmacist (Bird & Hassall 1993). This is an indication of the need for multidisciplinary collaboration between different health professionals, noted earlier.

Whatever the method selected, it should be tried out with the patient, checking that it is appropriate. Once patients have been launched on a scheme of medication, their ability to cope should be monitored; as patients get older they may begin to need more help. For example, a nurse who can give an injection in a now inaccessible site would be welcomed by an older person with diabetes. Assessment at repeated intervals is important.

Absolute adherence is only possible with patients who are obsessive about their medication. For most drugs the occasional omission has only a minor effect and may at times be useful in avoiding side-effects (e.g. digoxin). Additional doses can, however, be dangerous, especially for older people (e.g. digoxin, levodopa, sedatives). Patients should be advised *not* to take an additional tablet to make up for one which they think they may have forgotten (Case study 27.4).

Self-administration of medication for inpatients

Patients in hospital can be encouraged to take responsibility for looking after their tablets and taking them at the appropriate times. They are then less likely to make mistakes when they go home because they have been involved in their own care and are not suddenly overwhelmed with too much information shortly before discharge (Bird & Hassall 1993). The benefits of such schemes are widely acclaimed. They include improved adherence to treatment, greater knowledge, better patient satisfaction and enhanced opportunities for individualized care (Graveley & Oseasohn 1991, Proos et al. 1992). Thus self-administration of medication has been promoted as a method of improving quality of care (United Kingdom Central Council for Nursing, Midwifery and Health Visiting

---

Case study 27.4

Mr J is a very fit, independent 78-year-old, successfully treated with Sinemet (levodopa and carbidopa) for parkinsonism. One morning he had an important meeting to attend at his local club and in his anxiety not to be late he suddenly wondered, 'Have I taken my morning dose of Sinemet?' Being very conscious of the benefits of the drug, he took another dose to be sure before he went out and drove to the club in his car. On arrival he felt dizzy and had to sit in the car again (postural hypotension), and on entering the club he rushed to the toilet and was sick (gastric irritation). The dizziness remained and a friend telephoned his wife. She suggested phoning the doctor, to which her husband responded by angrily knocking the telephone on the floor (aggression). All these manifestations, postural hypotension, gastric irritation and aggression, are symptoms of levodopa overdose. Mr J had, of course, taken his drug as normal with his breakfast.

1992). However, the proponents of these schemes may have been more enthusiastic than discerning in their interpretation of findings possible from the very small-scale research studies which have so far taken place. Furlong (1996) has suggested that, although self-administration may increase knowledge, the opportunities to acquire it may not be unique to such programmes, concluding that more work in this area is required.

OVER-THE-COUNTER MEDICATION AND THE OLDER PERSON

Selecting and purchasing drugs for one's own use has an important role in self-care and maintaining independence. Traditionally the treatment of common ailments such as colds, coughs, headaches, constipation and mild aches and pains, together with first aid in the home, have rested with the individual or the family caregiver (usually the mother). The purchase of OTC medicines also rests with the individual or the one in charge of shopping. Choice of drugs may be traditional, influenced by advertising or by advice from neighbours and friends. The range of products available is enormous. OTC medication can be obtained from pharmacies where the advice of a pharmacist is readily available, and from supermarkets where no information will be forthcoming apart from the instructions included with the packaging. Controls placed by the Medicines Act 1968 are related to the number and strength of tablets on sale through different outlets. The sale of large quantities of most OTC drugs is only permitted when a pharmacist is present. This is important, as many OTC drugs, including the large number of 'cold cures' sold every day, contain aspirin, paracetamol, antihistamines and alcohol; all these may interact with prescribed drugs.

Problems associated with over-the-counter medication

The potential for problems is enormous. It appears that members of the public do not consider patent medicines to be drugs or realize that they may cause problems with medication that has been prescribed. The results of an interview study with 186 people aged 65+ revealed that the majority were using almost twice as many OTC as prescribed drugs (Conn 1992). Those most commonly taken were aspirin, aperients, antacids and vitamins. These were often used over long periods and were taken inappropriately, especially aperients. Few of those interviewed were aware that the OTC medication could interact with drugs that had been prescribed and did not know of any contraindications

to taking them. The chief dangers to accrue from frequent and careless use of OTC drugs include overdose, drug interactions, masking symptoms and abuse.

Overdose may result from patients 'doubling up' on drugs already issued on prescription. For example, a patient might take a cold cure containing aspirin in addition to soluble aspirin which has been prescribed for rheumatic pain. This could result in frank overdose symptoms such as tinnitus or accentuated side-effects such as gastrointestinal bleeding.

Interactions with prescribed medication may result if the patient is not advised of the possibility that they may occur. Cold cures may interact with drugs belonging to the monoamine oxidase inhibitor group (MAOIs). Aspirin and anticoagulants may interact.

Masking symptoms can be a problem; the symptoms of illness in older people often present in a vague, atypical manner. Pain which might be diagnostic of myocardial infarction in younger people is often mild or absent in the old. Thus the taking (or giving) of analgesia for mild pain or discomfort could rob the clinician of a useful diagnostic indicator.

Abuse of OTC drugs is common, as explained above. This is primarily because OTC drugs can only relieve symptoms; their value in prophylaxis has not been confirmed by conventional randomized controlled trials. For example, the habitual taking of aperients by older people who believe that a daily bowel motion is normal can lead to dependence verging on addiction. The patient is only happy if he or she has taken an aperient and the bowel becomes incapable of evacuation without it. In time this may lead to fluid loss, malabsorption, irritation and loss of normal bowel function.

DRUGS WITH SOCIAL USES

Few people other than pharmacologists consider alcohol, tobacco, tea, coffee or herbs to be drugs. However, they all contain pharmacologically active ingredients with known actions on the body. Alcohol, caffeine and nicotine have addictive properties as well as social effects on behaviour and personality. In moderation they may be beneficial but in excess they can cause physical damage. Alcohol, for instance, can be useful in the form of sherry as an appetite stimulant; whisky is a useful night sedative; and beer and stout provide useful energy and nutrients. However, excess use of alcohol may accompany loneliness or depression and can lead to liver or brain damage.

Alcohol has been consumed for thousands of years and early historical records refer to the beneficial effects of moderate consumption for medicinal purposes or 'to forget the sorrows of old age' (McKinn & Mishara 1987). Wine was recommended for health and vigour in old age and, as these authors note, the thirteenth-century inventor of brandy, Arnaud de Villeneuve, thought his discovery of 'aqua vitae' (the 'water of life') would increase longevity, maintain youth and relieve depression.

The beneficial effects of moderate alcohol consumption have been confirmed. Research studies have indicated that it is associated with reduced risk of heart disease compared with the risk for heavy drinkers and abstainers and has been found to promote well-being and to lift depression in older people (McKinn & Mishara 1987). These findings, recorded with older people in nursing homes, could have occurred either because of the beneficial effects of ethanol or because the residents responded to the psychosocial effects of drinking, especially being treated as individuals and allowed to mix in a social setting. The authors recommend the use of alcohol in a convivial environment rather than as medicine. Some people think that alcohol is a good sedative. In sufficient amounts, varying with the build, tolerance and other factors related to the make-up of the individual, it will certainly induce sleep, but this is not really a desirable use of alcoholic beverages. Alcohol depresses rapid eye movement sleep and many people wake up later in the night with rebound insomnia. The diuretic action of alcohol is also likely to disturb them. Many accidents among older people, especially frail people, are related to the use of alcohol or to sedatives, especially benzodiazepines, which should be prescribed with caution.

Herbalism has increased in popularity as an alternative to conventional medicine in recent years. For the most part it is considered safe but the tests used on these preparations and the arrangements for quality control are less stringent than for conventional drugs, although many contain pharmacologically active ingredients. Herbs reputed to act on the heart (adonis, false hellebore, yellow foxglove) all contain cardiac glycosides and will therefore potentiate the effect of prescribed drugs such as digoxin.

WHERE THE NURSE CAN HELP

Traditionally drugs have been prescribed by doctors, dispensed by pharmacists and administered by nurses, with the patient playing a passive role as the recipient. Today the boundaries of professional responsibility are becoming less distinct and increasingly it is recognized that patients themselves must be active partners in care, especially in the sphere of drug-taking, as the success or otherwise of medication will ultimately

rest on their intelligent participation. This chapter has drawn attention to the following important new trends:

- The role of the multidisciplinary team in the prescription, dispensing and administration of medication, with emphasis on the need for liaison between all members of that team. In future it is likely that the range and number of items in the nurses' formulary will be extended, so the nurse must have a sound knowledge of action and interaction and of side-effects
- The need to teach patients so that they are able to participate confidently in the self-administration of medication at home, so preserving independence for as long as possible
- The need in hospital to prepare patients to be responsible for all aspects of the management of their medication when they are discharged or, if this is not possible, to liaise with a member of the family or a friend who can share this responsibility. To this end many hospital units have introduced self-administration schemes with inpatients. These appear to be successful, although longer-term and more extensive evaluation would be helpful
- The need to remain abreast with innovations which encourage adherence to medication. These could include steps to simplify the drug regimen and the use of practical aids (special administration boxes, measures for dispensing liquid medication) which enable those with failing memory or physical disabilities to remain independent for as long as possible.

In the past patients of all ages received the bulk of their acute care in hospital. Many of the drugs which they received during this time had been discontinued by the time of discharge, hence there was no necessity for the patient or the nurse in the community to know about them. This is no longer the case. There is an increasing trend for patients to be managed in the community throughout the acute phases of ill health. The proportion of nurses employed in community settings compared with hospital is set to increase and they are required to monitor the effects of medication, assessing and reassessing the patient at regular intervals.

Nurse prescribing and the nurse formulary

Nurse prescribing in the UK has a long history. In 1986 the Cumberlege report proposed that community nurses should prescribe from a limited formulary of medicines, appliances and dressings. This report was followed by the Crown report in 1989 recommending that nurses with a district nursing or health-visiting qualification should be allowed to prescribe from a limited formulary. At the time most other specialist nurses were hospital-based and it was thought that they would not require prescribing powers because they would always be working with medical staff. As a result, the Medicinal Products: Prescription by Nurses Act, which passed through UK parliament as a private member's bill in 1992, was limited in scope. It enabled district nurses and health visitors to prescribe only from a very limited range of products, mainly OTC medicines, with just a few prescription-only items. These were listed in the *Nurses' Formulary*, which was appended to the *British National Formulary*. The Crown report also recommended collaboration between nurses and doctors preparing local protocols for drug administration. Qualified nurses were encouraged to administer and supply medicines under protocol. This is a general prescription that authorized the use of the drug in a community setting. This procedure became commonplace. For example, vaccines were often administered under protocol. However, issues arose relating to legality. The situation was again reviewed in 1992 and this resulted in the publication of two further reports. The Crown review in 1998 introduced the concept of patient-specific protocols. Group protocols were renamed 'patient group directives' and the legal position was clarified, although some problems remain, despite the use of guidelines to control prescription. The 1998 Crown review developed a more flexible approach to the powers of prescription. This was taken forward by the government in May 2001. It announced that nurse prescribers would be able to prescribe all the general sales list medicines and pharmacy medicines that general practitioners prescribe. They would also be able to prescribe from a list of prescription-only medicines to manage palliative care, minor injuries, minor ailments and health promotion. Patient safety is the key issue and the thrust of the reforms is to benefit patients by permitting more rapid access to medicines. The service is beneficial because professional time is freed for those with more complex needs. The extension of the nursing role which has resulted from nurse prescribing is in line with health care policy in the UK and extending professional roles. Nurse prescribing policy only applies to qualified nurses and midwives and they must first complete a training course with assessments.

Taking drug histories

The drug history should be completed with the patient, taking time to record and discuss all that is relevant and providing time for questions and explana-

tions. Checklists are often used to ensure that nothing is overlooked. However, a checklist is only of value if its role as an aide-mémoire is kept in mind; it will be of limited value if it is simply used to tick off items then discarded in an effort to complete the task mechanically. Frequently older people will tire or may need time to recall all relevant details so history-taking will require more than one session. It may be necessary to defer some aspects until a relative visits if they have been responsible for medication, or will need to be involved in future. Bearing these points in mind, the following checklists may be helpful for the nurse beginning to participate in patient assessment.

A checklist to record a drug history on admission to hospital

- *Information about prescribed drugs.* The medical staff will also obtain this information and record it in the medical case notes. When the nursing assessment is undertaken the information should be obtained directly from the patient or a relative and compared with the medical history. It should not be duplicated from one source to another because the purpose of the nursing history is to check and, when necessary, supplement information already given. Many patients are too ill when first admitted to tell the doctor everything, or they may feel overwhelmed
- *Information about the drug-taking routine.* This should include the times each drug is taken, the relationship between these times and other daily activities (e.g. sleep, meals). This may reveal unexpected problems which, with ingenuity, could be resolved. Thyroxine or diuretic drugs given too late in the day may lead to difficulty sleeping and a small alteration in routine may obviate the need for night sedation. A change in the routine of taking drugs either before or after meals may alter the pattern of absorption and response. Discussion of the routine will additionally give an indication of the degree of adherence and suggest problems which may arise after discharge
- *Information about OTC medication.* As pointed out earlier, mention of these drugs is frequently forgotten. Discussion should centre on medicines used routinely and occasionally and habits of use. This information may provide clues to symptoms such as diarrhoea when aperients are overused and may ensure that abnormal readings are not obtained in tests. Some surprising incidents have been recorded; for example, throat lozenges containing iodine

have made the thyroid test of a hypothyroid patient appear to fall within the normal range

- *The use of other substances.* This includes the use of alcohol, which may be valuable to some older people as an appetite stimulant, a use that may in many cases continue in hospital. The use of dietary supplements should not be overlooked. With the current trends in dietary fads, numerous misconceptions are possible; for instance, a patient may believe that the intake of supplementary vitamins is essential for health or think that the more 'slimmer's soups' they consume, the faster they will lose weight.

Monitoring medication-taking in hospital

Here the nurse is in an ideal position to monitor the patient's progress, to report response to treatment and to explain as many times as necessary how medication should be taken, answering questions as they arise. The patient can be observed for problems which may arise on discharge (e.g. poor vision, failing memory) and solutions can be sought and tested during hospital stay.

A checklist to record a drug history on discharge from hospital

Preparation for a smooth transition from hospital to home routine includes:

- Ensuring that patients (and relatives, if appropriate) have been given full verbal and written information about their medication
- Ensuring that the medication has been obtained from the pharmacy and given to the patient in good time before departure; hurriedly handing over a bag of medication as they are wheeled through the ward door is not reassuring
- Ensuring that the patient or relatives know where to obtain repeat prescriptions and the procedure that this will entail
- Liaison with health professionals in the community: the district nurse, general practitioner and pharmacist as necessary.

Monitoring medication-taking at home

Things are not so straightforward for the nurse in the community as in hospital. Visits may be intermittent and, even if they are made every day, it is unlikely that the administration of every dose of medication can be observed, even if the patient requires supervision. Liaison with other members of the multidisciplinary team remains of key importance, as discussed earlier.

However, the nurse is the health professional in closest and most constant contact with the patient and will probably be the person to notice a change or to be informed about any change by neighbours or relatives. There is a need for reassessment at regular intervals and this should form part of the patient's planned care. Clear documentation should be made of change in physical or cognitive function, of changes in response to medication and changes to the medication regimen. These may be discussed with the patient and family, promoting full participation in care.

Nurses are in an ideal position to take a major role in health education and in raising the awareness of older people and their families of the benefits and limitations of medication.

Value for money, medication and safety

Over the past 50 years the development of modern medication has made a major contribution to reducing the burden of ill health in the population, especially among older people, who take more drugs per head than younger people. This has had major implications for organizations providing health care, which have witnessed an enormous increase in the cost of medication. At the same time, patients' expectations have risen and the demand for new, effective medication is ever-increasing (National Audit Office 2001). As a result, the pharmaceutical industry is increasingly called to account for the costs of new drugs (Mason & Freemantle 1998). The National Institute for Clinical Excellence (NICE) stipulates criteria for establishing the value of new treatments and helping health service providers decide which products should be used routinely in clinical practice. As health care professionals, nurses should appreciate the role of organizations such as NICE. However, they should also recognize that expenditure on medicines is rising in response to the development of newer, more effective therapies and because more patients are receiving them (National Audit Office 2001). These pressures on costs need to be viewed as part of the overall package of patient care. It has been suggested, for example, that for some conditions expenditure ought to be increasing because such expenditure is a cost-effective and therefore desirable way of increasing health gain for the population. These effects should be viewed in a positive light. At the same time many products are routinely withdrawn from the market for safety reasons and the volume of medicines-related litigation continues to increase. Problems, when they occur, frequently attract wide publicity (Department of Health 2000). Nurses, as the health professionals in closest and most continuous contact with patients, can do much to allay anxieties by explaining the role of watchdog organizations in protecting patient safety, the pharmaceutical safeguards they take and the positive contribution that medication can have on health.

Recommended reading

Luker K, Austin L, Willock J, Ferguson B, Smith K 1997 Nurses' and GPs' views of the nurse prescribers' formulary. Nursing Standard 11: 33–38.
A useful research article which provides an account of nurse prescribing and the findings from an evaluation undertaken in eight demonstration sites. The authors examine nurses' prescribing patterns and the type of items which nurses and general practitioners would like to see added to the formulary.

Mannesse CK, Derx EH, Ridder M 1997 Adverse drug reactions in older patients as a contributing factor for hospital admissions. A cross-sectional study. British Medical Journal 315: 1057–1058.
A well-conducted research trial which clearly illustrates the problem of adverse drug reactions in the population of older people admitted to hospital.

National Audit Office 2001 A spoonful of sugar. Medicines management in hospitals. National Audit Office, London.
A valuable contribution to the literature which explains why the use of medicines in hospital should be optimized and the service pressures which can operate as significant barriers to service delivery.

Treloar A 2000 A pill in the sandwich: covert medication in food and drink. Journal of the Royal Society of Medicine 93: 406–411.
A thoughtful discussion concerning the troubled topic of covert medication. This article would be of interest to nurses both for their own information and to share with carers of older people.

Greenstein B, Gould DJ 2004 Trounce's clinical pharmacology for nurses, 17th edn. Churchill Livingstone, Edinburgh.
An introductory text on pharmacology and applied pharmacology suitable for nursing students which would also be a useful resource for qualified staff who are in need of updating. The book provides an up-to-date account of the action and use of drugs in the treatment of disease and explores the principles underlying medication. This edition contains an expanded section explaining in greater depth than formerly the regulation and control of drugs. In addition new sections deal with adverse drug reactions, the introduction of new drugs, clinical trials and the economic aspects of medicines.

References

Bird C, Hassall J 1993 Self-administration of drugs: a guide to implementation. Scutari Press, London

Britten N 2003 Does a prescribed treatment match a patient's priorities? British Medical Journal 327: 840

Britten N, Stevenson FA, Barry CA, Barber N, Bradley CP 2000 Misunderstandings in prescribing decisions in general practice: qualitative study. British Medical Journal 320: 484–488

Carey RL 1984 Compliance and related nursing actions. Nursing Forum 21: 157

Cargill JM 1992 Medication compliance in older people: influencing variables and interventions. Journal of Advanced Nursing 17: 422–426

Conn V 1991 Older adults: factors that predict the use of over the counter medication. Journal of Advanced Nursing 16: 1190–1196

Conn V 1992 Self-management of over-the-counter medications by older adults. Public Health Nursing 9: 29–36

Conn V 1995 Older adults and their caregivers: a transition to medication assistance. Journal of Gerontological Nursing 21: 33–38

Connolly MJ 1995 Inhaler technique of older patients: comparison of metered-dose inhalers and large volume spacer devices. Age and Ageing 24: 190–192

Coombes J, Horne R 1994 A checklist for medication discharge planning. Pharmaceutical Journal 253: 161–163

Crown J 1989 Review of prescribing and supply of medicines. Final report. Department of Health, London

Crown J 1998 Review of prescribing, supply and administration of medicines. A report on the supply and administration of medicines under group protocols. Department of Health, London

Cumberlege J 1986 Neighbourhood nursing. A focus for care. Report of the community nursing review. DHSS, London

Department of Health 2000 Pharmacy in the future. Implementing the NHS plan. Department of Health, London

Department of Health 2001 National service framework for older people. Department of Health, London

Department of Health 2002 National service framework for diabetes. Department of Health, London

Entwhistle B 1989 A problem of compliance. Nursing Standard 3: 32–34

Furlong S 1996 Do programmes of medicine self-administration enhance patient knowledge, compliance and satisfaction? Journal of Advanced Nursing 23: 1254–1262

Graveley EA, Oseasohn CS 1991 Multiple drug regimens: medication compliance among veterans 65 years and older. Research in Nursing and Health 14: 51–58

Griffiths H, Jordan S 2002 Corticosteroids: implications for nursing practice. Nursing Standard 17: 43–54

Haynes RB, Wang E, Da Mota Gomes M 1987 A critical review of interventions to improve compliance with prescribed medications. Patient Education and Counselling 10: 155–166

Haynes RB, McKibbon KA, Kanani R 1996 Systematic review of randomised trials of interventions to assist patients to follow prescriptions for medications. Lancet 348: 383–386

Kennedy S 1991 A safer alternative to drug dispensing. Nursing the Older 3: 30–31

Knapp P 2002 Can we help patients keep resolutions? Medicines Management 1: 9–11

Kolton KA, Piccolo P 1988 Patient compliance: a challenge in practice. Nurse Practitioner 12: 37–50

Lowe CJ, Raynor DK 2000 Intentional non-adherence in elderly patients: fact or fiction? Pharmaceutical Journal 265: R19

Mason J, Freemantle N 1998 The dilemma of new drugs – are costs rising faster than effectiveness? Pharmacoeconomics 13: 653–657

McGraw C, Drennan V 2000 District nurses and medication compliance devices. Pharmaceutical Journal 264: 368

McKinn WA, Mishara BL 1987 Drugs and ageing. Butterworth, Toronto

Montamat SC, Cusack BJ, Vestal RE 1989 Management of drug therapy in the older. New England Journal of Medicine 321: 303–309

Morrow D, Leirer V, Sheik J 1988 Adherence and medication instructions: review and recommendations. Journal of the American Geriatrics Society 36: 1147–1159

National Audit Office 2001 A spoonful of sugar. Medicines management in hospitals. National Audit Office, London

Oseasohn C, Graveley EA, Hudepohl NC 1989 Issues in medication compliance research. Canadian Journal of Nursing Research 21: 35–43

Otway C 2002 The development needs of nurse prescribers. Nursing Standard 16: 33–38

Parkin DM, Henney CR, Quirk J, Crooks SJ 1976 Deviation from prescribed treatment after discharge from hospital. British Medical Journal 200: 686–688

Pharmaceutical Journal 2002 Pharmacists take up offer of concordance project support. Pharmaceutical Journal 269: 598

Platzer H 1989 Post-operative confusion in the older. Nursing Times 85: 66–67

Pollock K, Blenkinsopp A, Grime J 2002 Concordance: a valuable contribution to make to debate. Pharmaceutical Journal 268: 837–838

Proos M, Reilly P, Eagan J et al. 1992 A study of the effects of self-medication on patients' knowledge and compliance with their medication regimen. Journal of Nursing Care Quality Special Report: 18–26

Ramsey R 1988 Adjusting drug dosages for critically ill older patients. Nursing 18: 47–49

Ramsey LE 1999 Guideline for the management of hypertension. Report of the third working party of the British Hypertension Society. Journal of Human Hypertension 13: 569–592

Ross FM 1991 Patient compliance: whose responsibility? Social Science and Medicine 32: 89–94

Townsend A, Hunt K, Wyke S 2003 Managing multiple morbidity in midlife: a qualitative study of attitudes to drug use. British Medical Journal 327: 837–840

Treloar A 2001 Concealing medication in patients' food. Viewpoint. Lancet 357: 62–64

United Kingdom Central Council for Nursing, Midwifery and Health Visiting 1992 Standards for the administration of medicines. UKCC, London

Wade B, Bowling A 1986 Appropriate use of drugs by older people. Journal of Advanced Nursing 11: 47–55

Watson V 1989 Drug compliance. Journal of District Nursing 7: 4–11

Westbury JL 2002 Concordance: forgotten or misunderstood? Pharmaceutical Journal 269: 358–361

SECTION 4

Current issues and reflections on caring for older people

Chapter 28

Assessment of older people

Fiona M. Ross and Claire O'Tuathail

INTRODUCTION

Assessment is the cornerstone of high-quality care upon which all subsequent interventions are based. The purpose and methods of assessment are as varied as the patients for whom it is intended. Older people do not form a homogeneous group and many are fit and healthy, therefore the purpose and methods of assessment must be flexible and sensitive. Assessment is a process whereby the actual and potential needs of individuals are identified and their impact on independent daily functioning and quality of life evaluated, within the context of their personal and social relationships, so that appropriate actions can be planned. Hughes (1995) highlights the complex nature of assessment in her definition, which emphasizes understanding the meaning and significance of problems for users in relation to prevailing knowledge, problem formulation, matching recommendations for action, identifying resources and specifying evaluation criteria. Assessment practice is then underpinned by a philosophy of health, a patient-centred or participative approach as well as knowledge of health and disease, assessment and decision-making skills.

Over the last 20 years governments have focused on challenging professionals from health and social care to improve assessment practice in order to tailor interventions and thus use resources more effectively. These political drivers are enshrined within the community care policies of the early 1990s (National Health Service (NHS) and Community Care Act 1990), the changes in the first general practitioner (GP) contract of 1990 (Department of Health 1989) and more recently in *The NHS Plan* (Department of Health 2000), the new targets established for general practice (Department of Health 2003) and importantly in the establishment of national standards for assessment outlined in the *National Service Framework for Older People* (NSFOP) (Department of Health 2001). The national standards for assessment laid down in the NSFOP require far-reaching systems change across institutional and community care that challenge organizational and professional cultures of practice, with important implications for nurses working in both institutional and community settings. This chapter discusses the scope of assessment, its role in different contexts of care and addresses questions that practitioners and nurses may ask: *Why* is an assessment needed? *Who* should be performing the assessment and *where*? *What*, if any, tools or frameworks should be used to carry out the assessment? *How* are the needs of patients formulated from assessment data? In answering these questions this chapter is presented in four parts. The first part begins by exploring a number of theoretical principles, which inform the process of assessment from which a conceptual framework is developed. This is then employed to examine the concept of need, multidisciplinary collaboration and self-assessment. The second part reviews current policy on assessment and its role in care management in social care, assessment of older people in primary care and recommendations for implementation of the single assessment process (SAP) recommended by *The NHS Plan* (Department of Health 2000). Selected assessment instruments are discussed in the third part of the chapter, in relation to their purpose, strengths and links with the conceptual framework. Finally we explore the connection between assessment data and planned interventions, with an emphasis on the collaborative interpersonal process between nurse and patient through which assessment data are interpreted and possible care options developed, drawing on case study material.

THE CONCEPTUAL BASIS OF ASSESSMENT

A primary function of assessment is the collection of data which describe an individual's attributes, behav-

iours and resources (Jarvis 1996). Secondary to this is an analysis of the data to form inferences and judgements concerning an individual's need for nursing and other health-related interventions (Savage 1991). There is however a lack of clarity in the literature concerning the means by which these functions are performed (Nolan & Caldock 1996). Models and frameworks are usually rooted in the professional identity of the assessor, resulting in self-limiting and often conflicting data (Vernon et al. 2000). It is necessary therefore to make explicit the assumptions which underpin any approach by examining the parameters and dimensions of the assessment process.

The scope of assessment

This section examines the health and illness dimensions as well as the interplay between objective and subjective perceptions of health and their relationship to, and influence on, assessment. The former contributes to understanding the focus of assessment and the latter to its process, which taken together provide a theoretical underpinning to defining the purposes and approaches to assessment of older people.

Health and illness

While it is commonplace to view health and illness as two ends of the same continuum, such a conceptualization suggests an oversimplification that belies the complex and multifaceted nature of health and illness. An alternative view is suggested by Downie et al. (1990), who describe the relationship between health and illness on two separate continua. One is a high-to-low well-being continuum and the other a high-to-low ill-health continuum. The relationship between the two is presented by crossing the two continua as axes (Fig. 28.1). Two important observations can be made about this relationship concerning the nature of an individual's health status. Firstly, it takes account of the context and is multidimensional. Secondly, if it is accepted that high well-being and low ill health reflect the positive poles of each continuum then they are negatively associated in the upper left and bottom right quadrants of Figure 28.1, while a more positive correlation exists between the two in the top right and bottom left quadrants. This reasserts the importance, both conceptually and in practice, of separating them, as the presence of health does not necessarily equate with the absence of illness. A fuller discussion of the multidimensional nature of health is given in Chapter 30.

Objectivity and subjectivity

The objective–subjective dimension to assessment rests on assumptions regarding our understanding about

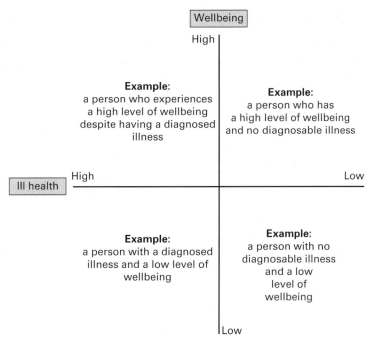

Fig. 28.1   The relationship between well-being and ill health. (Based on Downie et al. 1990.)

health and illness. In this respect it has implications for the method and process of assessment. Reed & Watson (1994) suggest that an objective or quantitative methodology dominates nursing practice and attribute this to the influence of the medical model. On this basis assessments are norm-referenced and identify need according to a set of predetermined attributes which must necessarily be attained to achieve self-sufficiency or to imply the absence of disease. The epitome of this approach is a mechanistic 'tick-box' type of assessment. Advantages of this method include the generation of data which may be used to compare patient profiles and aid communication between professionals who are familiar with the assessment tool. However overreliance on quantitative methods is likely to result in a limited understanding of an individual's health profile, because of a failure to take account of the person's wider context and relationships. A subjective or qualitative methodology can redress this balance through exploration and interpretation of the meaning of health and illness as experienced by the older person. Typically this approach will utilize less structured and more open-ended assessment schedules. At the very least it would advocate greater involvement and contribution to the assessment process by older people and their carers.

Throughout this chapter we return to consider the health–illness and objective–subjective dimensions in relation to principles of assessment of older people.

These provide a conceptual framework, which may be employed by nurses and other practitioners to guide their own assessments and facilitate understanding between and within professions regarding different assessment strategies. The intention is not to prescribe an approach that favours one element of each dimension over the other. Rather it is to offer some conceptual clarity regarding the nature, purpose and process of assessment.

The concept of need

The identification of need is one of the assumptions underlying assessment. As Christina Victor points out in Chapter 3, '*need* defines interventions/treatments or services from which people (either individuals or populations) would benefit'. However, the concept of need lacks clarity and is often utilized in an idiosyncratic way according to different professional groups. A number of useful typologies exist, however, by which the complexities of this concept can be better understood.

Bradshaw (1972) identifies four dimensions or types of need: (1) normative need, which is identified by the 'powers that be' who establish norms; (2) felt need, as stated by the individual; (3) expressed need, which may be inferred by observation, such as attendance rates at particular services; and (4) comparative need, which may be identified by examining different services or patient profiles (see Chapter 3 for more detail). It is useful to note that normative and comparative needs lie at the objective end of the objective–subjective continuum in so far as their identification is determined by assessing individuals in relation to other people. Conversely, felt and expressed needs are more subjective because their identification is determined by assessing people in relation to themselves.

Needs and risk assessment

The objective and subjective dimensions of need can be further illuminated by exploring problems in relation to needs and risk. Consider an older person living alone who has been assessed as needing institutional care because he or she is unable to get to the toilet unaided. Here the problem of incontinence has led to an identified need. However, from the patient's perspective the problem is not incontinence but rather a threat to independence. The continent but immobile older patient who chooses to wear a pad and use this as a receptacle in order to remain at home is not unfamiliar to district nurses. This emphasizes the interplay between health and social components of need and the extent to which the patient's perspective has to be considered in relation to, and balanced against, the objective, perhaps oversimplified assessment of health risk.

Pickin & St Leger (1993) highlight another feature of health and social need, arguing that assessment of need is a process of exploring the relationship between health problems and the resources available to meet those problems in order to achieve a desired outcome. Therefore, regardless of the problem, a need is only seen to exist so long as the necessary resource to meet that need, and thereby ameliorate the problem, is available. Needs are, of course, potentially limitless and there will inevitably be tensions between the problems experienced by individuals and the needs that the health and social care system is able to recognize and meet.

The concept of need also has implications for assessment of health as well as illness. The complexities of need together with the finite resources that have been discussed result in a tendency for nurses to focus primarily on deficits and illness. This is exacerbated by use of the term 'need', which places people in a dependent position, reinforcing the perception that they are problematic (Caldock 1994). While consideration of difficulties will remain central to definitions of need, a more holistic approach is warranted if assessments are to generate more than 'problem lists' and if solutions are to build upon an individual's strengths and coping strategies, rather than undermining them (Nolan & Caldock 1996). In practice this requires nursing assessments to describe skills, assets and other

positive features, as well as handicaps, disabilities and other dysfunctions (Fig. 28.2).

Carers' needs
The individual needs of older people are shaped to a large extent by their relationships with others and the potential for support. For example, two people with identical symptoms of Parkinson's disease may display different needs if one person lives alone and the other has a husband with time and energy to provide support. The Carers (Recognition and Services) Act 1995 makes provision for carers to have an independent assessment of their own needs. Regarding care of older people, the provisions of the Act cover those over 18 years of age who 'provide or intend to provide a substantial amount of care on a regular basis' (Department of Health 1996). Definitions of 'a substantial and regular amount of care' have been left to local authorities within the constraints of their available resources. Provision is therefore likely to be variable.

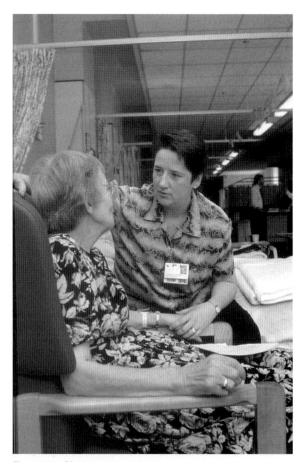

Fig. 28.2 Discharge assessment.

Despite introduction of this Act there remains a dearth of well-articulated methods to identify carers' needs, and the service options available to them are in a rudimentary state of development (Nolan & Caldock 1996). Furthermore, a predominant view persists in which carers are perceived by service providers as resources to be utilized. As a consequence their own needs have rarely been recognized (Twigg & Aitkin 1994). This is exacerbated by a requirement in the Act that an individual being cared for must agree to an assessment in order for the carer also to be assessed.

New approaches have emerged for assessing carers' needs, such as Nolan et al. (1994) framework which goes beyond the identification of practical difficulties to consider social and emotional needs, with particular emphasis placed upon the quality of the relationship between the carer and the cared-for. Further conceptual and empirical work is needed to develop reliable methods for assessing carer need, and increasingly social workers, care managers and others will be required to harness such developments to ensure carers receive the assessment of need which they deserve. Further information on carers is provided in Chapter 33.

Multidisciplinary assessment

If the concept of health is multidimensional then a prima facie case exists for multidisciplinary assessment. No one individual health or social care worker will possess the necessary repertoire of skills and knowledge to undertake such a task alone. A variety of assessment strategies reflecting different professional perspectives may be necessary to capture as comprehensive a picture as possible (Philp 1997). Multidisciplinary assessment can be understood as a combined approach to assessment, which involves specific diagnostic and assessment skills of various professionals involved in the care of a specific patient that contribute towards a holistic and collaborative care plan. It may be conducted in a variety of ways. Separate professional assessments may be integrated in a collaborative care plan as a result of a team meeting or case conference. Alternatively, and more rarely, a joint assessment may be made using a shared and even electronic record. Both the above approaches will require different professional disciplines to connect with each other in order to cultivate collaborative practice and improve health and social care outcomes. While variations in assessment between and within disciplines can be a source of conflict during the process, it can also strengthen the outcome by allowing for a broad and comprehensive account of an individual's condition to emerge that aims to encompass the following:

- identification of a broad range of health and social care needs and problems
- appropriate treatment, interventions and support
- multifaceted assessment of the potential for rehabilitation
- reducing dependency
- enhancing quality of life
- identifying services required by the client and his or her carer.

In practice, what does a multidisciplinary assessment mean? Throughout a period of contact with health and social services a number of assessments may be instigated for an individual. Hospital staff, for example, may identify the need for an occupational therapist to undertake assessment of an older person's functional abilities before discharge home is considered feasible. Similarly, once the patient has returned home, district nurses may be required to visit and monitor the patient's condition. From time to time the district nurse may need the skills of other professionals, such as the patient's GP or social worker, who will visit and perform assessments related to their own areas of care and expertise.

Although the principles of multidisciplinary assessment are accepted, there are often difficulties in the implementation. This is contested territory at a number of levels ranging from the frequently alluded- to lack of understanding of roles and responsibilities as well as the differences in organizational culture, professional ideology and training which influence the way in which individual professionals conceptualize health and illness and approach assessment (Pietroni 1992, Leathard 2003). There may be conflict regarding the conclusions drawn from a multidisciplinary assessment that flow from the different assumptions that underpin assessment approaches (Runciman 1989, Worth 2001). Ideally the team provides the forum for discussion and negotiation of an agreed plan. Studies that have compared social worker and district nurse assessment of older people have found that social workers are constrained by the system of fixed eligibility criteria in which they work, whereas district nurses have more flexibility, because health and nursing care is non-means-tested. Furthermore district nurses value their role in conducting holistic assessment, which is in contrast to the social worker's perspective on social and financial needs (Parry-Jones & Soulsby 2001, Worth 2001). Overcoming these tensions between professional approaches is a major challenge for the implementation of the SAP, which is discussed later in this chapter.

Self-assessment

Person-centred care is highlighted as a standard in the *NSFOP* (Department of Health 2001). Key themes of person-centred care are identified as proper assessment of potentially complex needs, integration of assessment, sharing of information between services and with clients and active involvement of older people in both health promotion and assessments. The SAP is one of the major innovations proposed to achieve these goals (Department of Health 2002a). User involvement and self-assessment are envisaged as forming an important aspect of this process.

Self-assessment refers to an assessment that is completed by the subject of the assessment without immediate professional involvement. This may range from structured questionnaires distributed by and returned to professionals for interpretation and further action where required, to systems that define need from the client's perspective and facilitate care-planning by clients themselves. Self-administered questionnaires have been used prospectively to identify risk across a number of domains, including functional decline (Balkrishnan & Anderson 2001, Hebert et al. 1996), to 'case-find' specific disorders such as Alzheimer's-type dementia (Ball et al. 2001) and to facilitate access to health services (Wasson et al. 1999). In the field of mental health some broader approaches to self-assessment have been developed in order to facilitate user identification of both need and services required to meet that need (Le Grand et al. 1996). In some cases self-assessment instruments may be construed as interventions in themselves, which identify specific actions to prevent or delay problems. An example of this is a home safety assessment that has been used extensively in the USA and includes environmental assessment for falls risk and other accidents in the home (Newton 1999).

Self-assessment in this context is an innovation that holds out considerable promise in terms of increased participation and ownership for potential service users. Potential benefits may be improved accuracy of assessment, proactive identification of unidentified need, and primary or secondary prevention of disorders and user enablement in relation to health and social care. However, whereas user involvement in professionally led assessment has been relatively well explored, self-assessment has not, particularly in the field of health care.

A multimethod systematic review of literature and practice of user-directed assessments to identify health and social care needs among older people is currently in progress. This review aims to address the following objectives.

- The scope of self-assessment – in what ways and for whom has it been used?
- The accuracy of self-assessment (where it is used in a screening or diagnostic manner)
- The effectiveness of self-assessment in terms of service and person-related outcomes including accessing services appropriate to need (including social support and medical treatments), uptake/engagement and satisfaction
- The acceptability of self-assessment from the perspective of both older people and professionals.

The review, funded by the NHS Service Delivery and Organization programme and led by Peter Griffiths at King's College London, is due for imminent report (www.sdo.lshtm.ac.uk/evaluatingmodels.htm#griffiths).

ASSESSMENT STRATEGIES

Care management

Assessment in care management is the process of the objective definition of needs by social services departments in the local authority, who are required to prioritize and target those in greatest need. Lewis et al. (1995) point out that this encapsulates the tension between identifying need and allowing choice on the one hand with rationing on the other. In other words, there are many potential conflicts arising from needs-led assessment within a resource-finite system that has to employ rationing. Therefore processes have been developed to determine eligibility for assistance against stated policy criteria.

Criteria of eligibility for social care assessment have been agreed by the local authority and health authority. This is to ensure that the assessment of need and the services that flow from it meet certain criteria. In some authorities these have been defined in terms of crisis management, such as avoiding imminent breakdown of care arrangements, risk of abuse or neglect, or the need for help and support with personal care. Other authorities have defined the eligibility criteria more broadly to encompass psychosocial needs, e.g. living alone, presence of serious physical or mental illness and disability or degree of stress unacceptable to person, carer or community.

Victor (1997) has carried out some secondary analysis of a survey of eligibility criteria undertaken by the Association of County Councils and Association of Metropolitan Authorities. Ten case studies based on real examples were used to ask a sample of 108 local authorities whether the individual would qualify for care and, if so, what type of care would be provided. Although there are difficulties in ensuring reliability of response from hypothetical vignettes used in a postal questionnaire, the study raises some interesting questions. Victor points out that the study revealed considerable agreement between the local authorities on eligibility, but that there was divergence on the amount of care that would be provided, which may reflect resource variation or different priorities for spending across different authorities. It is clear from this that assessment is part of the process of targeting need. Therefore, because of resource constraints, assessment cannot be value-free.

The extent to which assessment is used to ration and to limit services is a matter for difficult but important debate, and one that affects practitioners, managers and, inevitably, users of services (Parry-Jones & Soulsby 2001). For example, before October 2001, some people had to pay for their nursing care. Now everyone in need, regardless of setting and means, is eligible for NHS-paid care from a registered nurse. This gets rid of the anomaly of people having to pay for care in a nursing home that would be provided free in residential accommodation or at home. From February 2004 the payment was set at £40.00, £77.50, or £125.00 per week, according to nursing need assessed as low, medium or high respectively. Payments are made direct to the nursing home because the NHS cannot reimburse individuals directly; the NHS must pay nursing homes for care provided to patients. From April 2003, local authority-supported residents in nursing homes have also been receiving NHS-funded care, rather than from the local council.

In theory the aim of assessment in care management is that it should be a participative process involving the applicant, the carers and other relevant agencies. The policy defines need as the requirements of individuals to enable them to achieve, maintain or restore an acceptable level of social independence or quality of life, as defined by the particular agency or authority (Department of Health 1990). Thus 'need' is a personal and relative concept, which is to be defined and assessed at the local level. Local authorities have put in place systems to ensure that they can carry out a range of assessments, from simple to complex. Some assessments also require specialist skills, for example in mental health or learning disabilities. The way in which assessments should be defined and approached has been variously interpreted by different local authorities and is now being reviewed and modified to integrate with the developments around the SAP.

Care management practice flowing from the NHS and Community Care Act 1990 required staff to work collaboratively in the provision of care for older and disabled people; for example, nursing assessments formed part of the wider process of care management and were integral to an overall plan of care. Integrated, coordinated and collaborative working between agencies and professions was seen as a prerequisite to a well-functioning assessment system, although the extent to which this happened in practice was variable and often linked to pilot initiatives that were not sustained (Ross & Tissier 1997). Finding practical and comprehensive methods of assessment which avoid duplication but allow a holistic perspective to emerge has challenged those concerned with health and social care. The learning from the care management experience has contributed to the development of the SAP.

Integrated working

The term 'integration' commonly describes joined-up working between agencies, for example local authorities and health organizations, which aims to lead to the effective integration of services for the benefit of users and carers. This is also referred to as collaborative, partnership and joint working (see Chapters 6 and 7 for further discussion).

Older people want services to be flexible to their needs, coordinated and focused on helping them to remain in control and independent for as long as possible. But too often the response they receive is confused and disjointed. Working as a whole system in an integrated way requires that services are organized around the user (the term 'user' covers local-authority users, NHS patients and carers). In practice this should mean a reduction in the duplication of assessments, a coordinated approach to having an assessment done and the implementation of the action recommended.

Key principles of integrated working are that:

- All those involved recognize their interdependence
- Vision, action, resources and risks are shared
- Users experience services as seamless (Audit Commission 2002).

This approach is beneficial because crisis is avoided when individuals have their whole range of needs considered at one time. Partner agencies are able to focus on what they do best and have a better understanding of who else should be involved and as a result of this the whole system becomes more managed. By introducing new powers, the 1999 NHS Flexibilities Act removed legal and financial constraints that enabled the NHS and local authorities to provide and commission more integrated services. These included:

- Pooled budgets – packages of care tailored to individual needs supported by health and local authorities' pooled resources
- Lead commissioning – one authority takes the lead in commissioning a range of services for a particular group; this could be either health or local authority
- Integrated provision – health and social care services are provided by a single agency.

It is these far-reaching changes at a systems level that will in time lead to new thinking on service development, redesigned workforce roles and responsibilities as services are designed around need rather than historical practice.

The single assessment process

The NHS Plan (Department of Health 2000) set out a programme of investment and reform for a twenty-first-century health and welfare service. The underpinning principles of *The NHS Plan* are essential in ensuring that a modern care system for older people is provided (Box 28.1). *Modernising Social Services* (Department of Health 1998) set out the government's aim to ensure that social services promote people's independence, improve protection for vulnerable people and raise standards across the board. The *NSFOP* (Department of Health 2001) lies at the heart of this reform system. NSFs were established to improve services by setting national standards to improve quality and tackle variations in care. There are four themes and eight standards in the NSFOP (Box 28.2).

The aim of standard 2, person-centred care, is to:

ensure that older people are treated as individuals and they receive appropriate and timely packages of care which meet their needs as individuals,

---

Box 28.1   The NHS Plan *(Department of Health 2000)*

This reform programme will be taken forward through:
- Assuring standards of care
- Extending access to services
- Ensuring fairer funding
- Developing services that promote independence
- Helping older people to stay healthy
- Developing more effective links between health and social services and other services such as housing, and partners in the voluntary and private sectors

---

Box 28.2   National Service Framework for Older People *(Department of Health 2001)*

Respecting the individual
Standard 1: Rooting out age discrimination
Standard 2: Person-centred care

Intermediate care
Standard 3: Intermediate care

Providing evidence-based specialist care
Standard 4: General hospital care
Standard 5: Stroke
Standard 6: Falls
Standard 7: Mental health in older people

Promoting an active healthy life
Standard 8: The promotion of health and active life in older people

---

regardless of health and social services boundaries (Department of Health 2001: p. 23).

The standard states that:

NHS and social care services treat older people as individuals and enable them to make choices about their own care. This is achieved through the single assessment process, integrated commissioning arrangements and integrated provision of services, including community equipment and continence services (Department of Health 2001: p. 23).

The SAP was introduced as part of standard 2 of the NSFOP. The purpose of SAP is to ensure that older people receive appropriate, effective and timely responses to their health and social care needs, and that professional resources are used effectively. The drive to improve assessment was influenced by the experience of community care and care management policies, and from evidence that delays in hospital discharge can be attributed to lengthy and often duplicated assessment procedures (Victor et al. 2000), and on the other side of the coin of positive results from multicentre studies of comprehensive assessment processes, which have demonstrated reduced rates of decline in function, cognition and nutritional parameters, with improvements in mood, general well-being and health (Stuck et al. 1993). Economic appraisals have also suggested decreased direct costs of hospitalization and cost savings in a primary care setting (Philp et al. 2001). There is also some evidence that interdisciplinary comprehensive geriatric assessment has an impact on improving decision-making by professionals and the coordination of care (O'Tuathail et al. 2000). Building on this evidence and in relation to the aims of SAP it is important that:

- individuals are placed at the heart of assessment and care planning
- processes are timely and proportionate with need
- professionals are willing, able and confident to use their judgement
- care plans are routinely produced and users receive a copy
- professionals contribute to assessments in the most effective way
- information is collected, stored and shared as effectively as possible
- assessments are not duplicated by professionals and agencies.

The implementation of the SAP has been staged in recognition of its ambitious objectives, which require bringing together organizations with different values, cultures and professional disciplines that use different assessment frameworks and language. Superimposed on these constraints is the enormous challenge of moving paper-based records to electronic systems. By April 2005 local health and social care organizations should be ready to implement SAP fully, which, if the aspirations can be met, will lead to a huge transformation for older people – through multidisciplinary, interagency assessment of needs, interpreting information and ensuring that relevant services (support or treatment) is provided in an integrated way. We give some examples of progress with the development agenda later in this chapter.

The components of the single assessment process

The domains and subdomains of the SAP cover the user perspective, clinical history, health behaviour, personal care and physical well-being, the senses, mental health, relationships, safety and the environment (Box 28.3). According to policy recommendations, it should be conducted at four levels: (1) contact; (2) overview; (3) specialist; and (4) comprehensive assessment.

Contact assessment

This assessment refers to a contact between an older person and health and social services where significant needs are first described or suspected. It does not refer to each contact between, for example, a GP and an older person coming to the surgery. Basic personal information and the nature of the presenting need are identified and the potential presence of wider health and social care needs is explored.

The following seven key issues should be addressed in the contact assessment:

1. the nature of the presenting need
2. the significance of the need for the older person
3. the length of time the need has been experienced
4. potential solutions identified by the older person
5. other needs experienced by the older person
6. recent life events or changes relevant to the problem(s)
7. the perceptions of family members and carers.

Examples of contact assessment are given in Case study 28.1.

Overview assessment

An overview assessment is carried out when the individual's needs are such that a more detailed assessment is necessary. At overview assessment all or some of the domains of SAP, such as personal care and physical well-being, senses and mental health, are explored (Case study 28.2). The overview assessment is a holistic assessment, identifies needs from the older person's perspective, is undertaken using a standardized assessment instrument and may or may not lead to a more complex assessment. For many it will be the gateway to a more complex assessment and access to support to maintain independence. Implementation of the overview assessment system will prove to be a major organizational challenge. The Department of Health has established an accreditation process for off-the-shelf assessment tools that have been developed by independent researchers for national use. The accredited tools are as follows:

- EASYcare Version 2004 aims to provide a broad picture of physical, mental and social well-being from the perspective of the service user and includes contact and overview assessment (Philp et al. 2000). It has been translated into 15 languages and has accompanying manuals for assessors and training. The University of Sheffield has the copyright and further information can be obtained from J.Marriott@sheffield.ac.uk
- FACE for Older People V.3 stands for the Functional Assessment of the Care Environment for Older People. It has been developed by FACE Recording and Management Systems; it is not clear how far the tool has been tested for reliability and validity. The developers of FACE can be contacted at: Piclifford@aol.com
- MDS Home Care Version 2.3 is a standardized assessment system for assessing care needs. It collects the minimum amount of data necessary to be both comprehensive in its scope and reliable. The data are collected as part of the normal,

Box 28.3 The domains and subdomains of the single assessment process

Users' perspective
- Needs and issues in the users' own words
- Users' expectations, strengths, abilities and motivation

Clinical background
- History of medical conditions and diagnoses
- History of falls
- Medication use and ability to self-medicate

Disease prevention
- History of blood pressure monitoring
- Nutrition, diet and fluids
- Vaccination history
- Drinking and smoking history
- Exercise pattern
- History of cervical and breast screening

Personal care and physical well-being
- Personal hygiene, including washing, bathing, toileting and grooming
- Dressing
- Pain
- Oral health
- Foot care
- Tissue viability
- Mobility
- Continence and other aspects of elimination
- Sleeping patterns

Senses
- Sight
- Hearing
- Communication

Mental health
- Cognition and dementia, including orientation and memory
- Mental health, including depression, reactions to loss and emotional difficulties

Relationships
- Social contacts, relationships and involvement in leisure, hobbies, work and learning
- Carer support and strength of caring arrangements, including the carer's perspective

Safety
- Abuse and neglect
- Other aspects of personal safety
- Public safety

Immediate environment and resources
- Care of the home and managing daily tasks such as food preparation, cleaning and shopping
- Housing: location, access, amenities and heating
- Level and management of finances
- Access to local facilities and services
Reproduced from The domains of the single assessment process based on *Guidance on the Single Assessment Process*, Annex F: Department of Health 2002a.

www.opsi.gov.uk

Case study 28.1:   Contact assessment

Mr Smith visits his GP with a sore throat. There are no other health or social problems.

It is unnecessary for him to be entered into the single assessment process.

Mr Smith visits the GP. He is complaining of increasing difficulty getting up and down the stairs and has lost weight in the last 6 months.

A contact assessment is required by professionals who will explore health and social care problems where the presenting problems are not clear-cut and other potential problems will be identified.

Case study 28.2:   Overview assessment

Mr Smith lives alone since his wife died 4 years ago. He has been finding it increasingly difficult to manage his own personal care. He is complaining of tiredness and dizziness following any exertion. He says he feels quite miserable at times.

An overview assessment is required here where consideration is given to personal care, medical and mental health issues.

working routine. Software and training manuals are available. The developers of MDS Home Care can be contacted at: G.I.Carpenter@ukc.ac.uk

Specialist assessment

Specialist assessment provides a method of exploring specific needs and may be suggested following a contact or overview assessment. The specialist assessment enables the professional to identify the presence, extent, cause and likely development of a health condition or problem or social care need, and establish links with other conditions, problems and needs. Specialist assessments rely on the involvement and judgement of appropriately qualified and competent professionals, such as occupational therapists, physiotherapists, qualified social workers, registered nurses, geriatricians, old-age psychiatrists, other consultants working with older people, podiatrists, dieticians, dentists, housing and benefits professionals, and so on. Specialist assessments may rely on the use of assessment scales in support of professional judgement. Those carrying out specialist assessment may draw on information collected at contact or overview assessment, where these have been carried out.

Comprehensive assessment

A comprehensive assessment may arise in a number of ways. For example, it may be obvious to a doctor or other health professional that, based on his or her professional judgement, the needs and circumstances of an older person are such that a comprehensive assessment should be commenced. An overview assessment would be unnecessary in this situation and could delay the process of getting help to the older person.

On the other hand, at the initial contact assessment there could be uncertainty and an overview assessment may be carried out to investigate concern. When an overview assessment and specialist assessment are carried out the result is also a comprehensive assessment.

Comprehensive assessments are completed for people where the level of support and treatment is intensive or prolonged and includes permanent admission to a care home, intermediate care services or complex packages of care at home (Case study 28.3).

Comprehensive assessments will involve a range of different professionals or specialist teams, with relevant skills and knowledge. Geriatricians or old-age psychiatrists and their teams would play a key role in comprehensive assessment.

Tools for comprehensive assessment:

- Camberwell Assessment for the Needs of the Elderly (CANE)
- Functional Assessment of the Care Environment (FACE)

Case study 28.3: Comprehensive assessment

Mr Smith has had repeated admission to hospital following referral by his GP. He has many health problems contributing to his increasingly poor mobility. Social services provide a package of care with home care three times a day which includes personal care. He pays privately for someone to clean for him. During this admission Mr Smith says he cannot manage any more and wants to be looked after.

Mr Smith requires a comprehensive assessment including several specialist assessments.

- Minimum Data Set for Home Care (MDS Home Care)
- Sheffield 'Rainbow Assessment'
- Minimum Data Set – Resident Assessment Instrument
- The Royal College of Nursing (1997) *Assessment Tool for Nursing Older People* (Department of Health 2002b)

The single assessment summary

It is essential that local health and social services providers work towards an agreed single assessment summary for the collection of information on older people who are assessed, whether or not they go on to receive services. There are three components to the single assessment summary covering basic personal information, health needs and a summary of the care. This information should be stored in a systematic way and shared between agencies to avoid duplication.

Assessment scales

The Department of Health has provided a list of assessment scales that may be used to explore the domains and subdomains of the SAP (Box 28.4). The intention is to avoid being prescriptive: rather, to propose a menu of instruments from which health and social care organizations can select those most appropriate to the local context (Department of Health 2002b). However, anecdotal evidence suggests that organizations are struggling to discriminate between the strengths of relative instruments and a recent study of 26 local authorities in Warwickshire found that almost half had developed their own measures or significantly modified existing tools, thereby compromising reliability (Glasby 2004). The lack of clear central guidance and paucity of practical evidence-based information on accessible websites suggest that implementation may be uneven and problematic.

Box 28.4   Assessment scales of potential use for the single assessment process

Users' perspective of their needs and priorities
Life Satisfaction Index (Neugarten et al. 1961)
Schedule for the Evaluation of Individual Quality of Life
   (full or shortened form) (O'Boyle & McGee, 1992)
Sections on 'Personal fulfilment' and 'Spiritual
   fulfilment' from the Royal College of Nursing
   Assessment Tool for Nursing Older People (Royal
   College of Nursing 1997)
Mayers' Lifestyle Questionnaire (Mayers 1998)
Life Goals Questionnaire and Goal Planning Record
   (Wade 1999)
The Quality of Life in Later Life (QuiLL) Assessment
   (Evans et al.)

Nutrition
Subjective Global Assessment (Detsky et al. 1987)
Mini-nutritional assessment (Guigozy et al. 1997)
Screening tool for adults at risk of malnutrition
   (Malnutrition Advisory Group 2000)

Activities, and instrumental activities, of daily living
The Index of Activities of Daily Living (Katz et al. 1963)
Barthel Self-Care Index (Mahoney & Barthel 1965;
   see Shah et al. 1989 for a revised version) with the
   OARS Multidimensional Functional Assessment
   Questionnaire (Fillenbaum 1988)
Functional Independence Measure (Keith et al. 1987)
Community Dependency Index (Eakin & Baird 1993)
Canadian Occupational Performance Measure, 2nd
   edn (Law et al. 1994)

Pain
McGill Pain Questionnaire (Melzack 1975)
Oswestry Low Back Pain Disability Questionnaire
   (revised version) (Fairbank et al. 1980)
Brief Pain Inventory (BPI) (Cleeland 1994)
Palliative Outcome Scale (Hearn & Higginson 1999)

Tissue viability
Waterlow Pressure Sore Assessment (Waterlow 1996)

Mobility and balance
Performance Oriented Assessment of Mobility Prob-
   lems in Elderly Patients (POAM) (Tinetti 1986)
Balance Scale (Berg et al. 1992)

Falls
Falls Efficacy Scale (Tinnetti et al. 1990)
Falls Handicap Inventory (Rai et al. 1995)

Communication, visual and hearing disability
Four questions from the Lambeth Disability Screening
   Questionnaire (Peach et al. 1980):

1. Do you have difficulty seeing newsprint, even with
   glasses?
2. Do you have difficulty recognizing people across
   the road, even with glasses?
3. Do you have difficulty hearing a conversation,
   even with a hearing aid?
4. Do you have difficulty in speaking?

Frenchay Aphasia Screening Test (Enderby et al. 1987)
Assessment of Communication and Interaction Skills
   (ACIS) (Salamy et al. 1993)
Sheffield Screening Test for Acquired Language Disor-
   ders (Syder et al. 1993)

Cognitive impairment/memory
Mini-Mental State Examination (MMSE) (Folstein
   et al. 1975)
Short orientation–memory–concentration test of
   cognitive impairment (six items) (Katzman et al. 1983)
Gujarati version of the MMSE (Lindesay et al. 1997)

General mental health
General Health Questionnaire (12 or 28 items)
   (Goldberg 1978)

Depression/anxiety/mood
Philadelphia Geriatric Center Morale Scale (anglicized
   version, 17 items) (Challis and Davies 1986) (see
   Lawton 1975 for the original version)
Geriatric Depression Scale (15 items, or the four-item
   scale for overview assessment) (Yesavage et al.
   1983; Yesavage 1988)
Brief Assessment Schedule Depression Cards (BASDEC)
   (Adshead et al. 1992)
Hospital Anxiety Depression Scale (Zigmond & Snaith
   1994)

Relationships
Significant Others Scale (Power et al. 1988)
Practitioner Assessment of Neighbourhood Type
   (Wenger 1994)

Impact of caring on family carers
Cost of caring index (Kosberg & Crail 1986)
Relative stress scale (Zarit et al. 1998)
COPE Index (Nolan & Philp 1999)

Housing
Housing Options for Older People (HOOP) (Heywood
   et al. 1997)

Progress on the implementation of the single assessment process and some good practice examples

The policy timetable for the implementation of the SAP is short and progress towards achieving targets is patchy, with some recognition of the need for training and development (Department of Health 2004). However, the policy guidance seems to overlook the enormous change management agenda required to support grass-roots initiatives to enable one-stop shop, genuine user-focused assessment, within the context of agreed overarching strategic partnerships between health and local authorities. Inevitably, by the time this book is published, the sands will have shifted once again. Only time will tell how far the SAP meets the needs of older people, professionals and organizational effectiveness. The following two examples from London illustrate different methods of identifying older people who have fallen or are at risk of falling to prevent the associated functional decline that can often result.

The Wandsworth Project (the Battersea Model)

- Aimed to improve outcomes for older people who had fallen or were at risk of falling through timely intervention
- Focused on the relationships between practitioners to produce speedier and more appropriate outcomes
- Identified where services overlapped, were duplicated or were fragmented
- Used the validated Queen Mary's and Westfield screening tool
- Developed a comprehensive screening tool which doubled up as a resource for contact information
- Developed a multiagency falls care pathway that was capable of risk identification, screening, referral, treatment, rehabilitation and monitoring.

The Greenwich Project

A simple five-question screening tool was used to identify older people who fall, either face to face or over the phone, by the following:

- social services initial contact team
- district care managers
- in-house home care service
- community alarm service
- a multidisciplinary team in accident and emergency (A&E).

If users scored three or more on the screening tool they were referred to the newly formed community falls team (with user consent). The falls team carried out an overview assessment and referred on for specialist assessment where necessary within the team and to other services. User-held records meant that the information was available in the person's home.

This model works because:

- It identifies those at risk before they end up in A&E
- It finds 'cases' that may not have been referred to mainstream services
- It enables those in social services readily to access multidisciplinary service and advice
- It helps older people who otherwise may not be able to stay at home
- It demonstrates that some falls are preventable and not a natural consequence of ageing
- It raises the profile of falls and fracture prevention, leading to ongoing funding

Successes from both projects

- development of an integrated falls pathway
- falls assessment tool widely used
- encouraged whole system working and better communication – professionals were able to think outside their own boundaries
- implementation of the SAP
- developing forms of information about services and how to refer to them for users, carers and staff.

Assessment of older people in primary care

The expectations for assessment of older people in primary care are that it will provide a route to case-finding and access an assessment pathway. In the 1990s the health check for people over 75 years was introduced in primary care, which was designed to uncover unmet need. Under the terms of the 1990 GP contract (Department of Health 1989), those who are 75 and over were invited to participate in an annual consultation in order to assess whether medical services are required. Assessments focused on social needs, mobility, mental health, sensory needs, continence, physical functioning and medication. Community nursing staff, including practice nurses, health visitors and district nurses, carry out a large proportion of these health checks. Professionals undertaking the assessment need a thorough knowledge of:

- the generational characteristics and life experiences of older people
- the normal ageing process
- common pathologies in older age
- psychological adjustment to change in later life
- the purpose of the assessment
- the general practice
- services and resources available to older people.

Increasingly the literature confirms that concerns about an iceberg of unmet need among those not in receipt of health or social care are largely unwarranted (Jagger et al. 1996) and that many older people are a fit and low-risk group. Universal checks may not ultimately prove to be the most useful way of identifying those older people in greatest need of health and social support. Further, they employ a normative conceptualization of need in which aggregate data are used to establish norms. However, the data do have the potential to provide a picture of the health and social status of older people in the UK which could ultimately inform service provision and provide the opportunity for health promotion.

In the most recent GP contract (Department of Health 2003) chronic disease management targets are the main focus. Although the policy expectations around health assessments for older people remain rather unclear, the SAP is intended to link to primary care and to improve coordination of assessment practice. However, the challenges of making this happen while primary care is experiencing major change are huge (see Chapter 7 for a discussion of policy developments in primary care).

Health screening and case-finding

The term 'screening' is used in a variety of ways. It has been used interchangeably and somewhat misleadingly with the term 'assessment'. According to McKeown (1966), screening is the early identification of treatable disease. It may indeed form part of a health check or health assessment. Screening aims to identify those who have a particular problem or risk factor. General principles of screening are outlined in Box 28.5. It has also been argued that health promotion is effective into very old age, enabling an increased sense of well-being and delaying disability and premature death (Grimley Evans 1992), although ageist and untested assumptions about the physical and psychological costs and benefits of treatments have probably contributed to the exclusion of many old people from screening programmes (e.g. for breast and cervical cancer).

There are some recent examples of screening tools being incorporated in wider assessment systems such as the SAP. In this method validated tools are used to screen older people for risk. Risk is identified and the older person is then assessed using single assessment tools and referred on appropriately for early preventive health, social care, voluntary sector or other intervention to promote their independence and prevent deterioration. One of the difficulties with screening is the high numbers of people involved. Case-finding enables more detailed 'whole-person' single assessments to be offered to people who are most likely to be

---

Box 28.5 General principles of screening

- The condition screened for should pose an important health problem and the natural history of the condition should be well understood
- There should be a recognizable latent or early stage and the treatment of the disease at an early stage should be of more benefit than treatment started at a later stage
- There should be a suitable test or examination and the test or examination should be suitable to the population
- For diseases of insidious onset, screening should be repeated at intervals determined by the natural history of the disease and there should be adequate facilities available for the diagnosis and treatment of any abnormalities detected
- The chance of physical or psychological harm should be less than the chance of benefit and the cost of case-finding (including diagnosis and subsequent treatment) should be economically balanced against the benefit it provides

Source: Based on Austoker (1990).

---

at risk. This in turn reduces the number of people involved and enables more time to be spent with people who are most likely to need it. This method of targeting allows screening to be more manageable and cost-effective. Case-finding has been used, for example to target older people in areas of high deprivation, or for those not in contact with a GP in the previous 12

Case study 28.4: Case-finding from A&E attendance

An older lady was identified after she attended A&E following a fall. She says she feared she would have to go into nursing care. She was screened by a community liaison nurse and referred on to a 'virtual' community falls team and had multiple problems attended to. Temporary home care was put in place. After her problems were sorted out she was able to stay in her own home without any additional care input. Previously she had been looking at care homes as she felt that she would not be able to stay in her home any longer. She is currently managing to live independently in her own home.

months. Further examples are given in Case studies 28.4 and 28.5.

ASSESSMENT MEASURES

A confusing array of evidence-based assessment tools are available that are variable in quality and reliability. The research literature in this field can be seen to be complex and rather intimidating and not easy to apply to practice. The following section sets out some of the better known and established measures for assessing need: health and well-being, social support and relationships, physical and mental function. We discuss them in relation to their quality and person-centred nature.

Health and well-being

The World Health Organization (1946: p. 3) defines health as a 'state of complete physical, mental and social well-being and not merely the absence of disease or infirmity'. This definition incorporates both negative and positive conceptualizations of health and is both useful and potentially limiting. In the former it is the absence of something, i.e. disease or infirmity, while the latter is concerned with the presence of certain qualities, i.e. well-being, which supports our earlier discussion of the multidimensional nature of health and highlights the difficulties of measurement. In this respect quality of life is a key, but elusive and subjective concept in the assessment of individuals in health care, which is inherently difficult to measure (McKevitt et al. 2002). Bowling (2001a: p. 9) describes it as 'representing individual responses to the physical, mental and social effects of illness on daily living which influence the extent to which personal satisfaction with life circumstance can be achieved'. Specific instruments which measure quality of life include the Philadelphia Center Geriatric Morale

Scale (Lawton 1975) and the Life Satisfaction Indices A and B (Neugarten et al. 1961). The former has been developed specifically for older people and contains 17 items covering three main dimensions of agitation, attitudes towards own ageing and lonely dissatisfaction. The Royal College of Physicians and the British Geriatrics Society (1992) recommended this instrument as one of four standardized assessment measures in the care of older people. The Life Satisfaction Indices are concerned with capturing a respondent's feelings. Index A contains a series of 20 statements with which the respondent is asked to either agree or disagree; index B contains 17 open-ended questions to capture qualitative responses.

A number of instruments are also available which measure self-esteem, including the Self-Esteem Scale (Rosenberg 1965) and the Self-Esteem Inventory (Coopersmith 1967). Both these instruments interpret self-esteem in terms of self-acceptance or positive self-regard and require respondents to rate attitudinal statements. Rosenberg's is very quick to administer, containing only 10 items. These instruments are summarized in Table 28.1.

Social support and relationships

A further dimension of health is the extent to which individuals perceive their social environment to be supportive (Tudor 1996). The Perceived Social Support from Family and Friends instrument, developed by Procidano & Heller (1983), can be employed to capture this information and does so by asking the respondent to assess the functions of social networks.

Physical function

Assessment of illness amongst older people will be necessary during episodes of acute illness or when chronic illness becomes severe enough to affect an individual's capacity to care wholly for him- or herself. The level of individuals' ability to perform a variety of social roles free of physically or mentally related limitations is referred to as their functional status (Bowling 2001a). Assessment to establish functional status amongst older people has largely centred on their ability to perform the activities of daily living in three main areas:

1. social: activities outside the home
2. domestic: activities within the home
3. personal: self-care.

In turn these areas are influenced by mental, psychosocial and physical health functioning as well as

Table 28.1 Instruments for the assessment of health, well-being and quality of life

Instrument	Method of assessment	Key characteristics
Measures of well-being and quality of life		
Quality of Well-being Scale (Kaplan et al. 1976)	Self- or interviewer-administered	Requires respondents to rate their perceived ability to cope with symptoms and problems in the preceding 6 days
Philadelphia Center Geriatric Morale Scale* (Lawton 1975)	Self- or interviewer-administered	Assumes that well-being is multidimensional. Developed specifically for older people. Revised edition contains 17 items and covers three main dimensions: agitation, attitudes towards own ageing and lonely dissatisfaction. Popular scale amongst gerontologists internationally. Part of the battery of tests suggested by the Royal College of Physicians and the British Geriatrics Society
The Life Satisfaction Indices A and B* (Neugarten et al. 1961)	Self- or interviewer-administered	Developed to produce a short self-report measure of life satisfaction based on respondent's feelings. Life satisfaction scale A has a checklist of 20 items. The respondent either agrees or disagrees with the series of statements. Scale B contains 17 open-ended questions. May be used separately or together
Measures of self-concept and self-esteem		
Self-esteem scale (Rosenberg 1965)	Self- or interviewer-administered	A brief 10-item scale requiring the respondent to rate attitudinal statements
Self-esteem inventory (Coopersmith 1967)	Self- or interviewer-administered	Respondent rates attitudinal statements
Measures of social support		
Perceived social support from family and friends (Procidano & Heller 1983)	Interviewer-administered	Seeks the respondent's view on the extent to which needs for support, information and feedback are fulfilled by friends and family

Sources: Bowling (2001a, 2001b); Ross & Bower (1995); Tudor (1996).
*Instruments proposed by the Department of Health for consideration in the single assessment process (Department of Health 2002b).

the economic resources available (Krach et al. 1996). The interdependent nature of functional ability highlights a limitation of many of the instruments. Certain factors have to be considered when assessing older people, such as fluctuations in their energy levels, which occur through the day. Older people are also more likely to be taking medication. Some drugs can have transient effects on performance (e.g. diuretics, hypotensives and hypoglycaemics). The use of analgesia is also likely to make an important contribution to levels of performance.

Any number of contextual influences will need to be taken into account when selecting an instrument and interpreting its results. The following section reviews a range of common instruments that are commonly applied to assess physical and mental functioning in clinical practice and research. Their strengths and weaknesses are summarized, highlighting the relevance for nursing practice, in Table 28.2.

Physical function in older people has traditionally been assessed by measuring the person's ability to carry out personal self-care activities. The Barthel Activities

Table 28.2 Instruments for the assessment of physical function

Instrument	Method of assessment	Key characteristics
Measures of functional ability		
Index of Activities of Daily Living* (Katz et al. 1963)	Completion by observer (therapist or other)	One of the oldest of the disability scales. Assesses independence in four main areas: bathing, dressing, continence and feeding
Barthel Activities of Daily Living Index* (Mahoney & Barthel 1965)	Completion by observer (therapist or other)	Originally designed for use with long-term hospital patients with neuromuscular or musculoskeletal disorders. Covers nine dimensions of function. Does not cover activities of daily living such as cooking or shopping. Quick and easy to use, but based on performance rather than ability and less suited to community settings. Part of the battery of tests suggested by the Royal College of Physicians and the British Geriatrics Society
Townsend's Disability Scale (Sainsbury 1973)	Completion by interviewer or respondent	Frequently used in community surveys of older people. Covers a narrow range of self-care activities and has undergone numerous adaptations
Clifton Assessment Procedures for the Elderly (Pattie & Gilleard 1979)	Completed by a third party who knows the respondent well	Developed for use with older people in institutions. Consists of two schedules designed to measure behaviour and cognitive performance. The most extensively used measure of dependence in use in the UK. Despite widespread testing the evidence of reliability and validity is limited and has an institutional bias
Measures of psychological status and mood		
Abbreviated Mental Test (Hodkinson 1972)	Administered by an interviewer	Contains 10 items designed to assess orientation to time and place. Part of the battery of tests suggested by the Royal College of Physicians and the British Geriatrics Society
Mini-Mental State Examination* (Folstein et al. 1975)	Administered by an interviewer	A brief test of cognitive mental state. The scale has two parts, verbal and performance. The reading and writing involved might present difficulties for respondents with visual difficulties. Results can be influenced by respondent's level of education

Table 28.2 *Cont'd* Instruments for the assessment of physical function

Instrument	Method of assessment	Key characteristics
Geriatric Depression Scale* (Yesavage et al. 1983)	Administered by an interviewer	A 30-item scale designed to measure depression. Developed in order to overcome confounding effects of physical illness and presence of dementia. Part of the battery of tests suggested by the Royal College of Physicians and the British Geriatrics Society. Tested for reliability and validity, the Geriatric Depression Scale has been applied in a range of cultures
Measures of psychological status and social functioning		
Camberwell Assessment of Need* (Phelan et al. 1995)	Completed by therapist (or other) and respondent	Developed for use among individuals with severe mental illness. Measures level of need across 22 items related to physical, psychosocial, economic and mental functioning
Health of the Nation Outcome Scales (Wing et al. 1995)	Completed by third party who knows the respondent well	Measures an individual's health and social functioning across 12 areas related to mental illness. Intended for mandatory use across secondary and specialist psychiatric services from 1998

Sources: Bowling (1991, 1995); Ross & Bower (1995).
*Instruments proposed by the Department of Health for consideration in the single assessment process (Department of Health 2002b).

of Daily Living Index (Mahoney & Barthel 1965) covers the following dimensions: feeding, mobility from bed to chair, personal toilet (washing, etc.), getting on and off the toilet, bathing, walking on a level surface, going up and down stairs, dressing and incontinence. The instrument is completed by the nurse or therapist and was originally designed for use with long-term hospital patients. It therefore omits daily living tasks such as shopping and cooking and largely ignores the impact of the environment. In a feasibility study of its use in community settings, Ross & Bower (1995) found it required modification to take account of context and personal support.

One of the oldest and most popular indices of activities of daily living was developed by Katz et al. (1963). It was designed specifically for use with older patients and the authors claimed to have constructed a measure of fundamental biological functions. Using a rating form, patients are graded by the nurse or other therapist in relation to their ability in bathing, dressing, transferring (e.g. to chair), toileting, continence and feeding. Ratings are made on a three-point scale of independence for each operationalized activity. These scales are translated into a dependent–independent classification and the patient's overall performance is then summarized on an eight-point scale. Although a popular instrument, there is relatively little evidence for its reliability and validity (Bowling 2001a). The scale does not take into account adaptation to the context and relationships and therefore fails to capture the minor variations which can occur within categories in individual cases. This may be highly significant in terms of a person's ability to cope in a particular care setting.

Townsend's Disability Scale (Sainsbury 1973) is frequently used in community surveys of older people. It differs from the Activities of Daily Living Indices described above, as it relies upon self-reports which may be gathered by an interviewer or entered on the schedule by the respondent. It has undergone numerous adaptations but covers only a narrow range of self-care activities.

As well as those instruments that measure one dimension of functional status, a number attempt to cover several areas – for example, the Clifton Assessment Procedures for the Elderly (CAPE) (Pattie & Gilleard 1979). Designed specifically for use with older people, it consists of two schedules which measure behavioural and cognitive performance. It is completed by a third party who knows the respondent well.

Mental function

Assessment of mental functioning in older people often focuses upon their cognitive processes. A vast array of psychological tests is available to measure both global and specific elements of cognitive function. Many of these can only be administered either by qualified psychologists or under their supervision. This section will review a selected number of instruments available for use by nursing staff. Selected instruments are summarized in Table 28.2.

The Abbreviated Mental Test (AMT) (Hodkinson 1972) is a brief 10-item schedule of questions. It aims to assess orientation to time and place and offers a global measure of cognitive functioning. The Mini-Mental State Examination (MMSE) (Folstein et al. 1975) is also an instrument for measuring cognitive mental state. The interview schedule consists of two parts, one which requires patients to answer questions and the other requiring them to perform cognitive and behavioural tasks. A difficulty with the assessment of cognitive functioning is that, throughout the lifespan, it is influenced by both genetic factors and scholastic achievement (Plomin & Thompson 1993). Therefore, where the MMSE has been used to assess for evidence of dementia, false positives have occurred among patients with a history of high educational achievement and false negatives among those with a history of low educational achievement (Ritter & Watkins 1996).

Cognitive functioning in older people can also be affected by mood. The Geriatric Depression Scale (GDS) (Yesavage et al. 1983) is a useful instrument to assess mood and contains a 30-item scale. It was developed specifically to overcome confounding influences such as physical illness and dementia and is based on a person's self-reports. Depression is more often missed or misdiagnosed among older people. Particular experiences associated with old age, such as bereavement and the loss of social networks, can mask the symptoms. Depression can also be confused with early dementia, as older people often deny they are depressed and focus instead on their memory problems (Mottram et al. 1996). The identification of cognitive dysfunction among older people needs therefore to be interpreted with caution.

While there is a tendency in the literature to focus on mental health deficits in mood and cognition among older people, they are equally vulnerable to the consequences of other psychiatric disorders. The Camberwell Assessment of Need (CAN) (Phelan et al. 1995) has been designed to measure levels of need among individuals with a severe mental illness across 22 items related to physical, psychosocial, economic and mental functioning. Although not validated for use among an older population, it requires the patient and nurse each to rate the items. Data are also gathered on the perceived value of existing support, including established health care interventions, from which unmet needs are identified.

In a similar vein the Health of the Nation Outcome Scales (HoNOS) (Wing et al. 1995) rate an individual's health and social functioning across 12 areas related to mental illness. The scores are summed, giving an overall measure of present state. HoNOS is quick to use and is intended to be acceptable to any qualified mental health professional. However the ratings are scored solely by the professional. The HoNOS and CAN instruments incorporate items which consider an individual's level of risk both to themselves and to others.

Clearly there is a range of assessment instruments available for use with older people, although the use of different measures means that comparisons are often difficult to make, particularly when patients move between care settings (Ross & Bower 1995). It is for these reasons that the Department of Health is urging practitioners to use standardized assessment measures in SAP.

Once again, having reviewed these instruments, which are summarized in Table 28.2, the conceptual framework can be employed to appraise their suitability. Those instruments which measure physical aspects of illness, with the exception of the Townsend Disability Scale (Sainsbury 1973), are completed from observations made by someone other than the patient. Added to this, the observations are applied to specific operationalized scales which attempt to quantify functional deficits and overlook the patient experience. An overreliance on these instruments to plan care is therefore limited.

Those instruments which assess mental functioning rely predominantly upon self-reports, as the phenomenon of interest is not amenable to direct observation. However, they too are limited by the scope and precision of their content. There are exceptions, such as the

CAN (Phelan et al. 1995), which incorporates a more subjective methodology. In addition to including a respondent's rating the schedule invites the documentation of qualitative data concerning each item that is scored. This offers the potential for more sensitive interpretations to be formulated concerning the problems experienced by an individual.

In summary, when appraising those instruments that measure both health and illness, a common feature has been their tendency to rely on objective and reduced data to complete a checklist. This is of course an inevitable consequence of instrumentation and to some degree is desirable, as health and illness both have objective attributes, as reflected in the conceptual framework. However, as we have discussed earlier, there are other dimensions of health and illness, which are subjective in nature and which require sensitive discussion and exploration with the patient concerning the nature of the problem. This involves a broader analysis of the specific problem area. Its purposes include the formulation of need and the selection of possible interventions in collaboration with the patient. It therefore links assessment to the planning of care and will now be considered.

LINKING ASSESSMENT TO PLANNING CARE

As we have noted above, it is vital that assessments take into account the objective measures of health, but also focus on the quality, content or context of a person's health concerns and how these are related to other contributing factors. This means describing the patient's perspective and can only be done in collaboration with the patient through exploration and discussion.

The quality of the relationship between the professional and the patient will, in part, determine the validity of this process. A pragmatic approach to eliciting information is advised in which professionals demonstrate positive regard for the patient and do not attempt to interpret the information offered according to their own particular world view. The use of 'accurate empathy' is an important component, which underpins this interpersonal process (Rogers 1957). This should not be confused with the definition of empathy that implies identification with the patient or the sharing of similar experiences. Accurate empathy involves skilful reflective listening which seeks to clarify and amplify the patient's own perspective in terms of his or her experience and the meaning attributed to it. In this sense the process is concerned with eliciting felt and expressed need.

In this final part of the chapter two approaches to exploring the patients' perspective are explored. This is not to suggest that other methods do not exist or that they are any less effective. However the two approaches have been selected to reflect the dimensions of health within the conceptual framework. The first, a problem-centred approach, is concerned with deficits and dysfunctions and lends itself more readily to the assessment of illness. The second, a solution-focused approach, explores exceptions to deficits and dysfunctions and is therefore more closely aligned with health.

Problem–centred care planning

The first stage of care planning is to formulate specific problems. Predominantly open-ended questions will need to be employed to capture contextual data. Questions should facilitate a broad and meaningful exploration of the antecedents to the problem and its consequences. The interviewer will need to demonstrate flexibility as the problem may be perceived differently by the patient. Case study 28.6 illustrates some key issues. Mrs Brown's problem can be perceived at different levels. Medically it could be said that hypertension caused congestive heart failure and has subsequently contributed to oedema of the lower limbs with attendant ulceration. Normative or comparative needs might be identified, such as the prescribing of appropriate medications. The assessment using the Barthel index indicated that mobility problems have resulted in an inability to get in and out of bed, which exacerbates the oedema and ulceration, which suggests help from the 'putting to bed' service. Further exploration generates an alternative account of the problem from Mrs Brown's perspective. Attention is now focused on her desire not to be in bed, or more accurately, not to be in a position that restricts her mobility. To Mrs Brown this is the crux of the problem. Antecedents include heart disease and the resultant mobility problems but also her wish to preserve independence. The feared consequences of being in bed include a compromised ability to undertake self-care tasks and a reliance on others to restore her mobility. On this basis the nurse can now offer alternative interventions which take into account Mrs Brown's felt need. For example, the acquisition of a chair with a foot rest or spending short periods of time on her bed during the day when a nurse or home help will be available to assist her. The nurse might also offer to represent Mrs Brown's perspective in a referral to a social services care manager or a community occupational therapist to identify any additional resources that may be available to meet this problem. Whatever the outcome, this level of assessment allows a plan of care to be developed which is tailored to the individual needs of the patient.

Case study 28.6:   Problem-centred assessment

Mrs Brown is an 83-year-old widow who lives alone. She has experienced few health problems in her life, although over the course of the last 6 months, following several investigations and a brief stay in hospital, congestive heart failure has been diagnosed. More recently she has developed oedema in her lower limbs with superficial bilateral ulceration and has been referred to her local district nursing service for a home assessment.

The nurse undertakes an assessment using the Barthel index which highlights a mobility problem in transferring to and from bed. Alert to the possible connections between this deficit, oedema, ulceration and heart disease, the nurse shares her concerns with Mrs Brown and suggests they explore the problem in greater detail together. Mrs Brown feels there is little to discuss since her heart condition makes it very difficult to get in and out of bed. She gets breathless and her lounge chair is comfortable for sleeping in and sufficiently upright to allow her to sit and stand without too much strain.

The nurse agrees that Mrs Brown does appear to have found a solution but explains the consequences of remaining in an upright position both day and night and suggests she refers Mrs Brown to the 'putting to bed' service. This suggestion is met with clear disapproval. Puzzled by the degree of resistance, the nurse reflects this back to Mrs Brown in a neutral way and asks whether there are other concerns which might be important for her to know about if they are to find a better way of overcoming this difficulty.

Mrs Brown explains that since her husband died she has struggled to maintain her independence. Her daughter had thought a nursing home would be a sensible solution but this represents another loss to her: the loss of her home and the memories it holds for her of her late husband. The nurse reflects back the importance of independence to Mrs Brown and asks if she could say something more about how this might be affected by a 'putting to bed' service. Mrs Brown is fearful of being stranded in bed until someone comes to get her up. She doesn't sleep right through the night and often needs to use the toilet in the early hours of the morning. In short, being in bed is seen by her as an erosion of her independence.

Person-centred care

Person-centred care places the older person at the centre of the assessment and decision-making process. Person-centred care planning utilizes a patient's own aptitudes and strengths and is based on the premise that exceptions to problems can form the basis for solutions (George et al. 1990). Take, for example, an older man who complains of low mood and social isolation. A solution-focused approach would concentrate not on the problem but on those times or circumstances when low mood and social isolation were not so severe or were not present at all. These exceptions are then employed to construct solution interventions which, in their simplest form, may only require the patient to do more of what is already being done in order to solve the problem. Our older man may, for example, experience a greater sense of well-being when he undertakes activities or interests that he enjoys, such as reminiscing with others about his adventures in the war or visiting local beauty spots and spending time in the open air. The challenge for the professional is to identify, in collaboration with the patient, imaginative interventions which enable the promotion of these exceptions. In our example this might include negotiating attendance at a local old people's club or liaising with a charity for older people to see what organized events or trips they offer. Alternatively the man might accept assistance in writing to a war veterans'

association to put him in touch with like-minded people, or even placing an advertisement in his local paper or at the old people's club, inviting others with similar interests to contact him. He may also welcome the opportunity to visit historic sites or premises associated with the armed forces. If the professional carer who attends this man is unable to accompany him on such visits, he or she could network with his relatives or friends or even explore the possibility of students on placement undertaking the task as a health promotion exercise.

The process by which this type of care planning is undertaken will again involve predominantly qualitative enquiry. George et al. (1990) suggest two broad approaches which allow the identification of solution patterns. The first involves reflective questions which reflect a curiosity on the part of the professional to understand the times and context when the problem is not so severe. The second involves constructive questions which are employed to identify what the individual believes to be necessary for change to occur. For example: What will you need to improve your well-being? How will you know when things are better? What will be different when you no longer feel so low and socially isolated?

Constructive questions therefore begin to elicit the overall goal for a plan of care. The identification of objectives to attain this goal can be achieved by asking step-defining questions (George et al. 1990). For example: What will be the first sign that you are overcoming the problem? How will you know when it starts to happen? It is in relation to these step-defining questions that possible interventions can be identified and a meaningful plan of care developed which is tailored to an individual's felt need. Recently new approaches, such as the discovery interview (Wilcock et al. 2003), are being used to obtain the perspective of patients using narrative or stories to develop understanding grounded in experience. This is a powerful way of collecting views and for informing quality improvements.

SUMMARY

Assessment is a complex but central part of all care for older people, which in practice often falls short of the ideal. Although there will always be resource and organizational constraints, the aspirations to move towards more interprofessional approaches that take account of the experience and perspective of older people are goals worth pursuing.

Acknowledgements

We would like to thank the previous authors of this chapter in the third edition of *Nursing Older People*, Iain Ryrie and Margaret Edwards, as well as Ruth Harris for her ideas on self-assessment.

Recommended reading

Bowling A 2001a Measuring health: conceptual frameworks and the theory of measurement. Open University Press, Milton Keynes.
A comprehensive and updated review of quality-of-life measurement scales that have been selected for inclusion either because they have been well tested for reliability and validity or because considerable interest has been expressed in their content area. The author provides a useful discussion of the conceptualization of functioning, health and quality of life. Includes the measurement of functional ability, broad measures of health status, measures of psychological well-being, the measurement of social networks and social support and measures of life satisfaction and morale.
Bowling A 2001b Measuring disease. Open University Press, Buckingham.
This second edition complements Bowling's review of generic quality-of-life scales (see above). Most of the commonly used disease- and condition-specific measures of health-related quality of life are reviewed. The text attempts to present the strengths, weaknesses and coverage of each of the scales.
Bowling A 2002 Research methods in health: investigating health and health services. Open University Press, Buckingham.

There is a useful section in this book written by Ian Rees-Jones on health needs assessment, which articulates the important link with evaluation methods and health services research.
Grimley Evans J 1990 Quality of life assessments in older people. In: Hopkins A (ed) Measures of the quality of life and the use to which such measures may be put. Royal College of Physicians, London.
This chapter provides an interesting riposte to those who argue that the lives of younger people are of more value than those of older people. Grimley Evans argues for the principle that all life should be given equal weight. The chapter highlights the potential conflicts in the different measurements of quality of life, i.e. between subjective and objective assessments.
McDowell I, Newell C 1996 Measuring health: a guide to rating scales and questionnaire. Oxford University Press, Oxford.
This is the second edition of a reference book, which provides indepth reviews of the quality of leading health measurements. It provides a critical overview of the field, and each scale is discussed in terms of its purpose, conceptual basis, reliability and validity.

References

Adshead F, Day Cody D, Pitt B 1992 BASDEC: a novel screening instrument for depression in elderly medical inpatients. British Medical Journal 305: 397

Audit Commission 2002 Integrated services for older people. Audit Commission, London

Austoker J 1990 Breast cancer screening: a guide for primary health teams. National Health Service Screening Programme, Nottingham

Balkrishnan R, Anderson RT 2001 Predictive power of a risk-assessment questionnaire across different disease states: results in an elderly managed care enrolled population. American Journal of Managed Care 7:145–153

Ball LJ, Ogden A, Mandi D, Birge SJ 2001 The validation of a mailed health survey for screening of dementia of the Alzheimer's type. Journal of the American Geriatrics Society 49: 798–802

Berg K, Wood-Dauphinee S, Williams JI, Maki B 1992 Validation of an instrument. Canadian Journal of Public Health July/Aug (suppl. 2): 304–311

Bradshaw J 1972 The concept of social need. New Society 21: 640–643

Caldock K 1994 Policy and practice, fundamental contradictions in the conceptualization of community care for elderly people. Health and Social Care in the Community 2: 133–143

Carers (Recognition and Services) Act 1995 HMSO, London

Challis D, Davies B 1986 Matching resources to needs in community care. Ashgate, Aldershot

Cleeland CS, Ryan KM 1994 Pain assessment: global use of the Brief Pain Inventory. Annals of the Academy of Medicine, Singapore 23(2) 129–38

Coopersmith S 1967 The antecedents of self-esteem. WH Freeman, San Francisco

Department of Health 1989 The terms of service for doctors in general practice. HMSO, London

Department of Health 1990 The care programme approach. Circular: HC(90)23/LASSL(90)11. HMSO, London

Department of Health 1996 Carers (recognition and services) act 1995: policy guidance and practice guide. Department of Health, Wetherby

Department of Health 1998 Modernising social services. Stationery Office, London

Department of Health 2000 The NHS plan: a plan for investment. A plan for reform. Department of Health, London

Department of Health 2001 National service framework for older people. Department of Health, London

Department of Health 2002a Guidance on the single assessment process. Health services circular/local authority circular. Department of Health, London

Department of Health 2002b The single assessment process: tools and scales. Department of Health, London

Department of Health 2003 Delivering investment in general practice: implementing the new GMS contract. Department of Health, London

Department of Health 2004 Single assessment process for older people: dear colleagues letter 26/04/2004. Department of Health, London

Detsky AS, McLaughlin JR, Johnston N et al. 1987 What is subjective global assessment of nutritional status? Journal of Parenteral and Enteral Nutrition 11: 8–13

Downie RS, Fyfe C, Tannahill 1990 Health promotion models and values. Oxford University Press, Oxford

Eakin P, Baird H 1993 The community dependency index: a standardized assessment of need and measure of outcome for community occupational therapy. British Journal of Occupational Therapy 58: 1

Enderby P, Wood VA, Wade DT, Hewer RL 1987 The Frenchay aphasia screening test: a short, simple test for aphasia appropriate for non-specialists. International Rehabilitation Medicine 8: 166–170

Evans S, Hurley P, Gately C, Smith A, Banerjee A (in press) Assessment of Quality of Life in Later Life: Development and Validation of the QUILL. Quality of Life Research

Fairbank JCT, Couper J, Davies JB, O'Brien JP 1980 Oswestry: low back pain disability questionnaire. Physiotherapy 66: 271–273

Fillenbaum GG 1988 Multi-dimensional functional assessment of older adults: the Duke older Americans resources and services procedures. Lawrence Erlbaum Associates, New Jersey

Folstein MF, Folstein SE, McHugh PR 1975 'Mini-mental state': a practical method for grading the cognitive state of patients for the clinician. Journal of Psychiatric Research 12: 189–198

George E, Iveson C, Ratner H 1990 Problem to solution: brief therapy with individuals and families. BT Press, London

Glasby J 2004 Social services and the single assessment process: early warning signs? Journal of Interprofessional Care 18: 129–139

Goldberg D 1978 General health questionnaire. Nfer-Nelson, Windsor

Grimley Evans J 1992 Health and function in the third age. Nuffield Provincial Hospital Trust, London

Guigozy Y, Vellas B, Garry PJ 1997 Mini-nutritional assessment – evaluation of protein/energy malnutrition in the elderly. Facts and Research in Gerontology Newsletter (suppl. 2): 15–59

Hearn J, Higginson I 1999 Development and validation of a core outcome measure for palliative care. Quality and Health Care 8

Hebert R, Bravo G, Korner-Bitensky N, Voyer L 1996 Predictive validity of a postal questionnaire for screening community-dwelling elderly individuals at risk of functional decline. Age and Ageing 25: 159–167

Heywood F, Pate A, Means R, Galvin J 1997 Housing options for older people (HOOP), elderly accommodation counsel. The HOOP assessment tool may be downloaded, together with the report of its development, from http://www.housingcare.org/choice/decision/tools/hoop/hoop.asp

Hodkinson HM 1972 Evaluation of a mental test score for the assessment of mental impairment in the elderly. Age and Ageing 1: 233–238

Hughes B 1995 Older people and community care: critical theory and practice. Open University Press, Buckingham

Jagger C, Clarke M, O'Shea C, Gannon M 1996 Annual visits to patients over the age of 75 – who is missing? Family Practitioner 13: 22–27

Jarvis C 1996 Physical examination and health assessment. WB Saunders, Philadelphia

Kaplan R, Bush J, Berry J, Berry C 1976 Health status; types of validity and the index of well-being. Health Services Research 11: 478–507

Katz S, Ford A, Moskowitz R, Jackson B, Jaffe M 1963 Studies of illness in the aged. The index of ADL: a standardized measure of biological and psychosocial function. Journal of the American Medical Association 185: 914–919

Katzman R, Brown T, Fuld P et al. 1983 Validation of a short orientation-memory-concentration test of cognitive impairment. American Journal of Psychiatry 140: 6

Keith RA, Granger CV, Hamilton BB, Sherwin FS 1987 Functional independence measure: a new tool for rehabilitation. Advances in Clinical Rehabilitation 1, 6–18

Kosberg JI, Crail RE 1986 Cost of caring index. Gerontologist 26: 273–278

Krach P, De Vaney S, De Turk C, Zink MH 1996 Functional status of the oldest-old in a home setting. Journal of Advanced Nursing 24: 456–464

Law M, Baptiste S, Carswell A et al. 1994 Canadian Occupational Performance Measure, 2nd edn. Canadian Association of Occupational Therapists, Toronto

Lawton M 1975 The Philadelphia center geriatric morale scale: a revision. Journal of Gerontology 30: 85–89

Leathard A (ed) 2003 Interprofessional collaboration. Brunner Routledge, Hove

Le Grand D, Kessler E, Reeves B 1996 The Avon mental health measure. Mental Health Review 1: 31–32

Lewis J, Bernstock P, Bovell V 1995 The community care changes: unresolved tensions in policy and issues in implementation. Journal of Social Policy 24: 73–94

Lindesay J, Jagger C, Mlynik-Szmid A et al. 1997 The mini-mental state examination (MMS) in an elderly immigrant Gujarati population in the United Kingdom. International Journal of Geriatric Psychiatry 12: 1155–1167

Mahoney F, Barthel D 1965 Functional evaluation; the Barthel index. Maryland State Medical Journal 14: 61–65

Malnutrition Advisory Group 2000 Screening tool for adults at risk of malnutrition. British Association for Parenteral and Enteral Nutrition, Maidenhead

Mayers CA 1998 An evaluation of the use of Mayers' lifestyle questionnaire. British Journal of Occupational Therapy 61: 393–398

McKeown T 1966 An introduction to social medicine. Blackwell Science, Oxford

McKevitt C, Wolfe C, LaPlaca V 2002 Comparing professional and patient perspectives on quality of life. Research findings 2. Economic and Social Research Council, Slough

Melzack R 1975 The McGill pain questionnaire: major properties and scoring methods. Pain 1: 277–299

Mottram P, Hamer C, William J, Wilson K 1996 Sad screening. Nursing Times 92: 38–39

Neugarten B, Havighurst RJ, Tobin SS 1961 The measurement of life satisfaction. Journal of Gerontology 16: 134–143

Newton R 1999 Fall prevention project. Temple University. Philadelphia, Pennsylvania

NHS and community care act 1990. HMSO, London

NHS flexibilities act 1999 HMSO, London

Nolan M 1994 Geriatric nursing: an idea whose time has gone? A polemic. Journal of Advanced Nursing 20: 989–996

Nolan M, Caldock K 1996 Assessment: identifying the barriers to good practice. Health and Social Care in the Community 2: 77–85

Nolan M, Philp I 1999 COPE: towards a comprehensive assessment of caregiver need. British Journal of Nursing 8: 20

Nolan M, Grant G, Caldock K, Keady J 1994 A framework for assessing the needs of family carers: a multidisciplinary guide. BASE, Stoke-on-Trent

O'Boyle CA, McGee H 1992 The schedule for the evaluation of individual quality of life: administration manual. Department of Psychology, Royal College of Surgeons in Ireland Medical School, Dublin

O'Tuathail C, Ross F, Stubberfield D, Driscoll C 2000 Standardized multidisciplinary assessment of older people on discharge from hospital. South Thames evidence based practice. St George's Hospital Medical School, Kingston University, London

Parry-Jones B, Soulsby J 2001 Needs-led assessment: the challenges and the reality. Health and Social Care in the Community 9: 414–428

Pattie AH, Gilleard CJ 1979 Manual of the Clifton assessment procedures for the elderly. Hodder & Stoughton, Sevenoaks

Peach H, Green S, Locker D et al. 1980 Evaluation of a postal screening questionnaire to identify physical disability. International Rehabilitation Medicine 2: 189–193

Phelan M, Slade M, Thornicroft G et al. 1995 The Camberwell assessment of need: the validity and reliability of an instrument to assess the needs of people with severe mental illness. British Journal of Psychiatry 167: 589–595

Philp I 1997 Can a medical and social assessment be combined? Journal of the Royal Society of Medicine 32(Suppl): 11–13

Philp I 2000 EASY-Care: a systematic approach to the assessment of older people. Geriatric Medicine 30: 15–19

Philp I, Newton P, McKee K 2001 Geriatric assessment in primary care: formulating best practice. British Journal of Community Nursing 6: 290–295

Philp I, Lonles RV, Armstorong GK, Whitehead C 2002 Repeatability of standardized tests of functional impairment and well-being in older people in a rehabilitation setting. Disability and Rehabilitation 24: 243–249

Pickin C, St Leger S 1993 Assessing health need using the life cycle framework. Open University Press, Milton Keynes

Pietroni P 1992 Towards reflective practice: the languages of health and social care. Journal of Interprofessional Care 6: 7–16

Plomin R, Thompson L 1993 Genetics and high cognitive ability. Ciba Foundation Symposium 178: 67–84

Procidano M, Heller K 1983 Measures of perceived social support from family and friends: three validation studies. American Journal of Community Psychology 11: 1–24

Rai GS, Kinirons M, Wientjes H 1995 Falls handicap inventory: an instrument to measure associated with repeated falls. Journal of American Geriatrics Society 43: 723–724

Reed J, Watson D 1994 The impact of the medical model on nursing practice and assessment. International Journal of Nursing Studies 31: 57–66

Ritter S, Watkins M 1996 Assessment of older people. In: Norman I, Redfern S (eds) Mental health care for elderly people. Churchill Livingstone, Edinburgh, pp 99–130

Rogers C 1957 The necessary and sufficient conditions for therapeutic personality change. Journal of Consulting Psychology 21: 95–103

Rosenberg M 1965 Society and the adolescent self image. Princeton University Press, Princeton, NJ

Ross FM, Bower P 1995 Standardized assessment for elderly people (SAFE): feasibility study in district nursing. Journal of Clinical Nursing 4: 303–310

Ross F, Tissier J 1997 The care management interface with general practice: a case study. Journal of Health and Social Care 5: 153–161

Royal College of Nursing 1997 Assessment tool for nursing older people. Royal College of Nursing, London

Royal College of Physicians, British Geriatrics Society 1992 Standardized assessment scales for elderly people. A report of the joint workshops. Research Unit of RCP and BGS, London

Runciman P 1989 Health assessment of the elderly at home: the case for shared learning. Journal of Advanced Nursing 14: 111–119

Sainsbury S 1973 Measuring disability. Bell, London

Salamy M, Simons S, Keilhofner G 1993 Assessment of communication and interaction skills (ACIS) (the full assessment). Department of Occupational Therapy, University of Illinois, Chicago

Savage P 1991 Patient assessment in psychiatric nursing. Journal of Advanced Nursing 16: 311–316

Shah S, Cooper B, Maas F 1989 Improving the sensitivity of the Barthel index for stroke rehabilitation. Journal of Clinical Epidemiology 42: 703–709

Stuck AE, Siu AL, Wieland GD et al. 1993 Comprehensive geriatric assessment – a meta-analysis of controlled trials. Lancet 342: 1032–1036

Syder D, Body R, Parker M, Boddy M 1993 Sheffield screening test for acquired language disorders. Sheffield Health Authority, Nfer-Nelson, Sheffield

Tinetti ME 1986 Performance oriented assessment of mobility problems in elderly patients. Journal of American Geriatrics Society 34(2): 119–126

Tinnetti ME, Richman D, Powell L 1990 Falls efficacy as a measure of falling. Journal of Gerontology 45(6): 239–243

Tudor K 1996 Mental health promotion: paradigms and practice. Routledge, London

Twigg J, Aitkin K 1994 Carers perceived. Open Univerity Press, Milton Keynes

Vernon S, Ross F, Gould M 2000 Assessment for older people: politics and practice. Journal of Advanced Nursing 31: 282–287

Victor C 1997 Community care and older people. Thorne, Cheltenham

Victor C, Healy J, Thomas A, Seargeant J 2000 Older patients and delayed discharge from hospital. Health and Social Care in the Community. 8: 443–452

Wade DT 1999 Goal planning in stroke rehabilitation. Topics in Stroke Rehabilitation 6(2): 37–42

Wasson JH, Stukel TA, Weiss JE et al. 1999 A randomized trial of the use of patient self-assessment data to improve community practices. Effective Clinical Practice 2: 1–10

Waterlow J 1996 Pressure sore assessment. Nursing Times 92: 29

Wenger GC 1994 Support networks for older people: a guide for practitioners. Centre for Social Policy Research and Development, University of Wales, Bangor

Wilcock P, Stewart Brown GC, Bateson J, Carver J, Machin S 2003 Using patient stories to inspire quality improvement within NHS modernization collaborative programmes. Journal of Clinical Nursing 12: 422–430

Wing J, Curtis R, Beevor A 1995 HoNOS Health of the nation outcome scales: version 4. Royal College of Psychiatrists Research Unit, London

World Health Organization 1946 Constitution of the World Health Organization. WHO, New York

Worth A 2001 Assessment of the needs of older people by district nurses and social workers: a changing culture. Journal of Interprofessional Care 15: 257–266

Yesavage J 1988 Geriatric depression scale. Psychomopharmacological Bulletin 24: 709–711

Yesavage J, Brink T, Lum O et al. 1983 Development and validation of a geriatric depression scale: a preliminary report. Journal of Psychiatric Research 17: 37–49

Zarit SH, Stephens MA, Townsend A, Greene R 1998 Relative stress scale. Journal of Gerontology 53: 5

Zigmond AS, Snaith RP 1994 The hospital anxiety and depression scale. Nfer-Nelson, Windsor

Chapter **29**

Health care for older homeless people

Maureen Crane and Anthony M. Warnes

INTRODUCTION

A principal concern of public health analysts for several decades has been the persistence and growth of health inequalities. As early as 1842, Chadwick established a link between the appalling living conditions of the poor and their ill health (Wright 2002). Numerous studies and reports have since shown clear correlations between the standard of living, morbidity and life expectancy (British Medical Association 2003). Poor housing affects health, and people who are homeless are seriously affected. Homelessness causes health problems and aggravates existing conditions: 'risks to health are likely to increase the further a homeless person gets from being in adequate housing . . . infectious disease rises as soon as accommodation is cramped, overcrowded or insanitary, and the risks to physical health are likely to be at their most extreme when people are living on the streets' (Pleace & Quilgars 1996: p, 35).

Homelessness occurs among men and women of all ages, and both families and single people. In the UK, around 15–20% of single homeless people are in the older age groups (Warnes et al. 2003). Although the official retirement age recognizes 'older' as women aged 60 years and over and men when they reach the age of 65 years, it is widely agreed that the threshold of 'older' homelessness is 50 years of age. People of that age who have been homeless for many years tend to have physical health problems and disabilities that are comparable to non-homeless people who are 10–20 years older (Cohen & Sokolovsky 1989). Many British voluntary-sector organizations that work with homeless people and the UK Coalition on Older Homelessness accept this lower age limit. Many statutory service providers, however, still apply the official pensionable age (60 for women and 65 years for men) when assessing whether a homeless person is entitled to services.

This chapter describes the provision of health care for older homeless people in the UK. It has six main sections. The first describes the backgrounds of older homeless people, their numbers, reasons for homelessness and circumstances while homeless. The next two summarize their health problems and use of mainstream health care services. The third also discusses the problems associated with providing health care to the group. The fourth section describes the ways in which health care is being delivered to homeless people through specialist services, while the fifth concentrates on meeting the health care needs of older homeless people. This is followed by a discussion of the training needs of health staff working with homeless people, and the chapter concludes with a reflective commentary on health care arrangements for homeless people and the role of nurses in the delivery of services.

THE BACKGROUNDS OF OLDER HOMELESS PEOPLE

There are no reliable figures of the number of older homeless people in the UK at any given time, or about the number who become homeless and are rehoused over a period. According to official statistics, in 2002 almost 4500 households were accepted by local-authority housing departments in England as homeless and in priority need for rehousing because of old age (Office of the Deputy Prime Minister 2003). In addition, many older homeless people sleep on the streets, or stay in hostels and night-shelters. They have either not approached a local-authority housing department for help or have had their application rejected. They are generally known as 'non-statutory' or single homeless people. The number of older people in this group is unknown. In London, 700 people aged 50 years and over were in hostels on one night in 2000, while 569 people of a similar age slept rough in the city at some time between April 2001 and March 2002 (Crane & Warnes 2001a, Broadway 2002). An estimated 482 hostel residents in Scotland are aged 60 years and over, 13% of the total (Rosengard et al. 2001).

Reasons for becoming homeless

The backgrounds of older homeless people are diverse. Crane's (1999) study shows that some people became homeless in early adulthood. For them, homelessness was triggered variously by the break-up of childhood homes, marital breakdown or discharge from the army. A second group have been homeless since their 40s or early 50s. Some had always lived at home with their parents and when they died could not cope. Others had worked as merchant seamen or building labourers and for years had travelled around and stayed in missions, lodgings or work-camps. When they could no longer find work or ill health prevented them from working, they had no settled base. A third group became homeless for the first time in old age, having had stable accommodation, raised a family and worked until retirement. For many, homelessness was triggered by widowhood or the breakdown of a long-standing marriage or intimate relationship. For example, after becoming widowed, some older men gave up their accommodation and slept on the streets because they found it too painful and upsetting to remain in the home, while some became depressed, drank heavily, neglected themselves and their home, and were eventually evicted for rent arrears (Crane 1999).

Health problems, particularly the onset or increased severity of a mental illness, can also trigger homelessness among people who live alone. Dementia and paraphrenia (late-onset schizophrenia) are forms of mental illness that present in later life. Paraphrenia most often occurs in people who have lived alone for years and have few friends (Morley & Sellwood 1997). These illnesses affect a person's ability to cope at home and are sometimes undetected. This can lead to eviction because of squalid living conditions or a failure to renew housing-benefit claims and pay rent. A study in Dublin in the mid-1990s found that 163 people over the age of 65 years were living in filthy conditions. They were reported as reclusive, suspicious, verbally aggressive, hoarders and refusing help from services (Hurley et al. 2000). Some older people with a paranoid illness develop persecutory ideas about relatives or neighbours, and such ideas lead them to abandon their accommodation. Others who are confused or mentally disturbed drift into homelessness, because they wander away from their accommodation and stay on the streets.

The pathways leading to homelessness for older people are therefore complex. Although a single incident, such as widowhood, may be the direct trigger or proximate cause of a person being evicted or leaving home, other underlying factors are usually involved.

These include stresses and traumatic events, poor coping and social skills, a deficient support network and mental illness and alcohol problems. British and American studies have found that older men tend to have become homeless at all ages, whereas older women are more likely to have become homeless in old age (Crane & Warnes 2001b, Hecht & Coyle 2001).

Circumstances while homeless

Some older people are homeless for just a short while and receive help to find alternative housing, while others remain on the streets or in hostels for years. This is illustrated in Figure 29.1, which shows the duration of homelessness among 64 older homeless people in London, Sheffield and Leeds who were about to be rehoused (Crane & Warnes 2002a). Some older rough sleepers are reluctant to use services for homeless people because of their fear of intimidation from young homeless people. Many are estranged from their relatives and have no friends apart from their contacts with other homeless people. This is particularly true for those with long histories of homelessness. Some have had no family contact for more than 20 years and are unaware if their parents and siblings are still alive. Around one-tenth of older homeless men are extremely unsettled and frequently move from town to town. Some associate this behaviour with depression and an attempt to escape from painful memories.

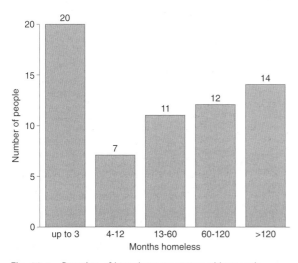

Fig. 29.1 Duration of homelessness among older people. Sample: 64 homeless people aged 50 years and over in London, Sheffield and Leeds. (Reproduced from Crane & Warnes (2002a) with permission.)

HEALTH PROBLEMS

Physical health problems

Physical health problems are common among older homeless people. In Glasgow, 65% of hostel residents aged 55 years and over had long-standing physical illnesses, while two studies of older hostel residents in London found that 47% and 55% had physical health problems (Crane & Warnes 2000, 2002b, Kershaw et al. 2000). The London figures are likely to underrepresent the prevalence of medical conditions, because some residents left the hostels before their problems could be assessed. In a study of 131 newly homeless older people in several English cities, 71% of the sample reported physical health problems (Crane et al. 2004).

Health problems are exacerbated by age, lack of treatment and lifestyle. Older people sleeping rough are exposed to dampness and the elements, and are at risk of exposure, hypothermia and frostbite. Some sleep on dirty streets or in filthy old buildings, and are susceptible to skin infestations, such as scabies and lice. Some use crowded and badly ventilated day centres, shelters and bed-and-breakfast hotels, where infection is rife. Many have foot problems such as blisters and corns caused by persistent walking and ill-fitting shoes, and musculoskeletal and circulatory problems such as arthritis, leg ulcers, oedema and cellulitis. Malnutrition is common (Wright 2002). Some older rough sleepers do not claim state benefits, have no income and eat discarded food from litter bins. Studies in London and in several American cities found that the food intake of most homeless people does not meet normal dietary requirements and is inadequate to maintain good health (Burt & Cohen 1989, Evans & Dowler 1999).

Chronic respiratory disorders and gastrointestinal problems are widespread. During the early 1990s, high rates of active tuberculosis were reported among homeless people in London, and the most vulnerable were middle-aged and older men who were heavy drinkers (Citron et al. 1995). Health problems are aggravated by heavy drinking (discussed later). Alcohol abuse leads to nutritional deficiencies, neurological disorders and seizures, peripheral vascular disease, cirrhosis of the liver, upper respiratory infections, gastrointestinal and pancreatic disorders, memory problems and brain damage (Wernicke–Korsakoff's syndrome). The latter is caused by a lack of thiamine (vitamin B_1), often through malnutrition and stomach or liver damage. It occurs in about 2% of the general population but 12.5% of those who are dependent drinkers (Alcohol Concern 2003).

Injuries from accidents and assaults are common. Rough sleepers are reported to be 50 times more likely than the general population to be fatally assaulted, and twice as likely to die accidentally (Grenier 1996). Those who are frail, have poor mobility, and whose senses are impaired by lack of sleep, heavy drinking or a mental illness are exceptionally vulnerable to violence and accidents. American studies have found that at least one-third of older homeless people are attacked and injured each year (Douglass et al. 1988, Cohen & Sokolovsky 1989).

Mortality rates

Mortality rates among homeless people are very high relative to those in the general population (Barrow et al. 1999, Nordentoft & Wandall-Holm 2003). British studies of the age of death in small samples of those recorded as homeless on coroners' reports have found average ages between 42 and 53 years, which compares with the late 70s for the general population (Keyes & Kennedy 1992, Grenier 1996). The figures have to be interpreted carefully, however, as a coroner's designation 'homeless' tends to be reserved for rough sleepers who cannot be linked to an address. Deaths to single homeless people who are residents of hostels and other temporary accommodation are generally ascribed to the address.

Mental health problems

Homelessness is associated with demoralization, depression, loss of self-esteem and feelings of hopelessness and despair (Belcher & Diblasio 1990, La Gory et al. 1990). Mental health problems ranging from depression to psychoses and dementia are common among older homeless people. Among 70 older hostel residents in London, three-fifths reported feeling depressed some or most of the time, and 27% perceived their future as hopeless and said that they expected to be dead within 6 months (Crane & Warnes 2000). Similarly, in New York city, two-fifths of older men on the streets were reported to be depressed and nearly one-third wished that they were dead (Cohen & Sokolovsky 1989: p. 166).

According to British and American studies, 40–68% of older homeless women and one-third of older homeless men have a psychotic illness or marked memory problems (Kutza 1987, Cohen et al. 1997). A study in London in 2000 found that three-quarters of homeless women aged 60 years and over in hostels and on the streets had mental health problems (Crane & Warnes 2001a). For some, a mental illness distorts reality and influences their capacity to seek and accept services. One man aged in his 60s slept rough in London for 7 years and refused to use hostels and day centres for homeless people. He believed that the staff

were terrorists and that they would cut off his arms and legs if he accessed the services (Crane 1999). A high proportion of older women who sleep rough are exceptionally disturbed and hostile.

Some older homeless people have severe memory problems which only become apparent when they leave the streets and move into hostels or are admitted into hospital. They require regular assistance or prompting with everyday tasks, such as personal hygiene, eating, budgeting and taking medication. Some are disoriented for place and time, and sometimes wander away from a hostel and get lost.

Alcohol problems

Only a small proportion (less than 5%) of older homeless people take illegal drugs, but around two-fifths of the men and 20% of the women have alcohol problems (Ladner 1992, Cohen et al. 1997, Hecht & Coyle 2001). For some, heavy drinking preceded homelessness and is associated with traumatic experiences, while others use alcohol as a means to cope with the physical conditions and stresses of being homeless. Some drink alcohol to keep warm, to help them sleep, or as a way of alleviating boredom and loneliness by socializing with other drinkers. Some have been drinking heavily for years and neglect their self-care, repeatedly fall, and are incontinent when drunk. They are more likely than non-drinkers to report depression, sleep disturbances, poor appetite and pessimism (Table 29.1).

Table 29.1 Self-reports of problems and aspirations among older hostel residents

Problems and aspirations	Alcohol consumption	
	Less than once a week (%)	Most days (%)
Depressed	44	72
Nightmares	10	50
Poor appetite	13	59
Pessimistic about the future	46	69
Hopes to be rehoused within 6 months	45	16
Expects to be dead within 6 months	3	41
Number of subjects	39	32

Reproduced with permission from Crane & Warnes (2000).
Sample: Older hostel residents at St Mungo's Lancefield Street Centre in London, 1997–1998.

Among 101 homeless and formerly homeless people of all ages at 'wet day centres' (where alcohol can be consumed on the premises) in four British cities in 2003, 84% reported being depressed and low in mood (Crane & Warnes 2003).

It is very difficult to break the cycle of heavy drinking, deteriorating health and low morale among older homeless people. Many have lost their family, home, job and friends, have serious physical health problems, and have little motivation to stop drinking. Moreover, giving up drinking means avoiding companions who are generally their only social contacts, and finding alternative ways to occupy their time. Some older heavy drinkers are admitted to detoxification units and undergo a withdrawal programme but subsequently resume drinking. Others find the prospect of abstaining too daunting. In a few towns and cities, there are specialist hostels and supported housing which help heavy drinkers but do not require them to abstain. They promote harm minimization and encourage heavy drinkers to reduce their alcohol intake, to change to less harmful substances (many consume strong beers), to eat nutritious food, and to address their health problems. These services are not however widespread.

Mental health and alcohol problems

A small proportion of older homeless people have both mental health and alcohol problems, commonly referred to as 'dual diagnosis' (Fig. 29.2). Among older rough sleepers, 18–25% of men and up to 9% of women are reported to have the dual problems (Crane & Warnes 2001a, 2002b). There is a complex relationship between the two problems. For some, heavy drinking induces psychotic thoughts and disturbed behaviour, while others drink heavily to mask the symptoms of a mental illness. Alcohol misuse may also worsen or alter the course of a psychiatric illness, while withdrawal may lead to psychiatric symptoms or illnesses (Department of Health 2002b). Older homeless people with combined problems are especially vulnerable and difficult to help, and many have been homeless for years. Some display disturbed or aggressive behaviour and are evicted from hostels for violence. They move from hostel to hostel, and end up sleeping rough because they are barred from all hostels in a town or city.

ACCESSING MAINSTREAM HEALTH CARE SERVICES

Although health problems are common among older homeless people, many are not registered with general

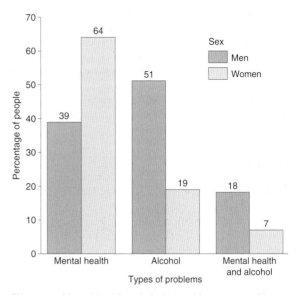

Fig. 29.2   Mental health and alcohol problems among older rough sleepers in London, 1999–2000. Sample: 834 people aged 50+ years. (Reproduced from Crane & Warnes (2001a) with permission.)

practitioners (GPs) and do not seek medical help when they are ill. Among 61 older rough sleepers admitted to a London hostel, several had serious health problems yet had not sought help. This included one man who had a carcinoma of the mouth, and another who had cataracts in both eyes and was nearly blind. There were also cases of untreated tuberculosis, jaundice and ascites from liver and renal failure, severe anaemia and fractured limbs. Some 41% were not registered with a GP and three-fifths had had no GP contact for more than 5 years, including some for over 20 years (Crane & Warnes 2000). In contrast, 97% of the UK general population is registered with a GP (Crisis 2002).

A minority of older homeless people use hospital accident and emergency (A&E) departments for medical care instead of a GP. A 1994 study of presentations to A&E at the Royal London Hospital found that 42 single homeless people had used the service at least four times during the previous 6 months (Hinton 1995). The frequent users tended to be men aged in their 50s with physical health and alcohol problems, and men and women aged in their 30s with mental health and alcohol problems. Using A&E is a costly way of obtaining health care. In 1999, an A&E visit cost an estimated £70 and a GP consultation just £18 (Finn et al. 2000). Some older homeless people use medical services dedicated to homeless people, which they find more accessible and the staff more sympathetic and understanding (described later).

Instead of receiving primary health care, some older homeless people end up being admitted to hospital during crises. They are more likely than the general population of a similar age to be admitted to hospital. A national survey in 2000 by the UK Department of Health found that 14% of the general population aged 65–79 years had been admitted to hospital during the previous year (Department of Health 2001a). In contrast, among 171 residents at a hostel in London for rough sleepers aged 50 years and over, 29% were admitted on 107 occasions over a 21-month period (Crane & Warnes 2001c). The principal reasons for admission were epileptic seizures, kidney and liver failure, ruptured oesophageal varices, pneumonia, tuberculosis, asthmatic attacks and injuries from falls. Likewise, 26% of 113 older homeless people who presented at a primary health care project in Manchester had had at least one admission to a general hospital during the previous 12 months (Blood 2003).

Problems in accessing and delivering health care

Some older homeless people do not seek medical help because they are poorly motivated and depressed. Several have mental health or literacy problems, poor social skills or chaotic lifestyles. They find it hard to cope with GP registration forms, appointment systems, busy waiting rooms and long waits. Others do not recognize the severity of their illness, or mistrust doctors. Some report being embarrassed about seeking help because they are dirty or unkempt, and fear being stigmatized by staff and other patients.

Some older homeless people refuse to comply with medical care. They decline to attend medical appointments or accept treatment, or discharge themselves from hospital before treatment is completed. Many live on the streets or in night shelters and bed-and-breakfast hotels where they receive minimal support and have to leave the premises during the day. There is nobody to ensure that they regularly take medication, attend doctors' appointments, and have dressings changed. In some hostels, the staff lack the skills or the time to ensure that the residents comply with medical treatments.

Many GPs are reluctant to register homeless people, particularly those sleeping rough, because they tend to have multiple health problems and some are disruptive or aggressive and upset other patients (Fisher & Collins 1993, Pleace et al. 2000). GPs are concerned about their ability to provide intensive health care to a high-needs and difficult-to-treat group alongside a 'normal' caseload. Some homeless people move around and do not stay in the area, and many do not cooperate with health promotion and screening targets. There is therefore a financial disincentive for GPs to offer permanent registration. Some GPs accept hostel residents as temporary patients, but this means that medical records are not transferred from the previous GP, making it hard to provide continuity of care. In Westminster in central London, the Health Support Team (a specialist homeless health care team) used 'client-held' records for homeless people, but found that they were not well maintained (Gorton 2003).

According to one London GP who provided medical care to older hostel residents, treating their illnesses was problematic because most were unable to provide a medical history and had little insight into their health problems. The GP was unaware of past illnesses, investigations and treatments. Many residents required extensive hospital investigations but some only stayed in the hostel for a short while. It was therefore difficult to arrange outpatient appointments and provide continuity of care, and to know if there were underlying and undetected problems. The work was more crisis management than the control of illnesses (Crane & Warnes 2001c).

Homeless people are sometimes discharged from hospital without due attention being given to their housing and social circumstances. This may result from: a lack of understanding by hospital staff about homelessness and insufficient information about a person's living conditions; pressure on hospital beds and staff; ineffective communication and coordination between health, housing and social services; a shortage of appropriate accommodation for homeless people with complex needs; and homeless people's own premature discharge.

There are also difficulties in obtaining mental health assessments for older homeless people and linking them to appropriate services. This is particularly true for those with dual mental health and alcohol problems, who commonly fall between the specialist services. Mental health teams will not work with clients who continue to drink alcohol, while alcohol services are reluctant to treat people who are poorly motivated to stop drinking or have disturbed behaviour (Warnes et al. 2003). A *Dual Diagnosis Good Practice Guide* describes the deficiency of current services for people with both severe mental health and substance misuse problems and concludes:

> Substance misuse is usual rather than exceptional amongst people with severe mental health problems and the relationship between the two is complex. Individuals with these dual problems deserve high quality, patient-focused and integrated care.

This should be delivered within *mental health services* . . . Patients should not be shunted between different sets of services or put at risk of dropping out of care completely (Department of Health 2002a: p. 4).

Case study examples

The complexities of providing health care to older homeless people therefore derive from both their personal characteristics and several shortcomings in the organization and delivery of services. With encouragement and support, however, many do accept health care and other services, and over time their circumstances improve. This is illustrated in the case study of Frank (Case study 29.1). He was sleeping rough, not in contact with services, and had serious health problems. When workers found him, however, he was persuaded to accept help, and his health and housing state improved. In contrast, the difficulties of helping some older homeless people is apparent from the case study of Harry (Case study 29.2). In his situation, the problems arose partly because of his chaotic behaviour and reluctance to accept support, and partly because appropriate services are unavailable to meet his high care needs. The next sections describe ways in which health care services are changing in response to the unmet needs of homeless people, and the services that are required to meet the particular needs of older homeless people.

SPECIALIST HEALTH CARE SERVICES FOR HOMELESS PEOPLE

The particular problems of delivering health care services to homeless people have been widely recognized over a long period. In 1981, the Acheson Report recommended additional funds to meet the health care needs of homeless people in inner London. In April 1998, the Department of Health introduced personal medical services (PMS) pilot schemes and local development schemes (LDS) with a view to the development of services for special-needs groups. Through flexible contractual arrangements, PMSs encourage health professionals to deliver accessible primary health care services to people in deprived communities, and to underserved and disadvantaged groups, including mentally ill and homeless people. By April 2002, there were 1750 PMS pilots (www.doh.gov.uk/pricare/pca.htm). Through LDSs, additional payments are available for GPs and members of the primary care team to provide services in deprived areas with high-morbidity populations and challenging practice workloads. The extra funding enables, for example, GPs to register homeless people in hostels and to provide comprehensive medical care supported by nursing interventions.

In 2002, the Department of Health published *Addressing Inequalities: Reaching the Hard-to-Reach Groups*, which noted that, 'improved access, improved

---

Case study 29.1

Frank became homeless for the first time at the age of 53 years. He had never married and had always lived with his parents in a council flat in south London. After they died, Frank found it difficult to manage at home and pay bills, and was evicted 2 years later for rent arrears. He had no siblings or close relatives, did not know what to do, and so slept on the streets. He stayed in a secluded place on the outskirts of the city for 5 years, during which time he had no contact with services. He did not claim social security benefits and survived by eating food from litter bins.

He was found by a street outreach team that had been newly formed by St Mungo's to seek out older rough sleepers in outer London. St Mungo's is a voluntary-sector organization that works with homeless people in London. Frank did not like sleeping rough, and was easily persuaded to move into a hostel. On admission, the hostel staff arranged for him to be seen by a local GP as he had a large sore on his lips. According to Frank, the sore had been there for some time. He was referred by the GP as an emergency to a hospital consultant, tests were carried out, and the diagnosis was a carcinoma of the mouth. Frank was given a course of radiotherapy at the hospital as an outpatient, and has since had hospital check-ups every few months.

The hostel staff helped him with a claim for social security benefits, and encouraged him to attend his medical appointments. At first Frank was wary of seeing a doctor and accepting treatment, partly through fear. The hostel workers initially accompanied him to the hospital, but after a few visits he attended alone. The staff liaised with the hospital workers to make sure that he kept his appointments and to get feedback on his progress. After Frank's treatment was completed, the hostel staff discussed with him his long-term housing options. He recognized that he would find it hard to live independently, and was therefore resettled in supported housing. At the time of writing, Frank has settled and has been in his accommodation for 3 years.

Case study 29.2

Harry was 64 years old and had been sleeping for 4 months in an old car in north London when he was found by a street outreach worker from St Mungo's. He had been evicted from his accommodation for rent arrears. He had been a heavy drinker for many years, had poor mobility, and suffered from severe back pains – he fell from a roof years ago. His hygiene and short-term memory were poor, and he had skin problems in his groins and strong body odour. Since sleeping rough, he had not claimed social security benefits, had no income and most of his clothes had been stolen.

The outreach worker arranged for Harry to be seen by a local GP and the local-authority social services' elderly team. The GP prescribed medication for his skin infection, and the duty social worker arranged an emergency admission to a registered care home. After a few weeks in the home, there was concern about Harry's behaviour. He was drinking heavily in the grounds and on the streets, and was threatening some of the vulnerable residents. The social worker transferred him to another registered care home, but Harry stayed only one night and then returned to the streets. He was then placed by the social worker in a bed-and-breakfast hotel.

At the time of writing, Harry has been in the bed-and-breakfast hotel for 3 months. His room is neglected and infested with flies, and he spends most days drinking with friends on the streets. He cannot cook and scavenges for food in litter bins. His legs are very swollen, but he refuses to visit his GP and therefore has no medication. His hygiene is extremely poor and he is incontinent of urine, which with the untreated skin infection causes a great deal of groin pain.

The local-authority social services team and the street outreach worker are trying to link him into appropriate care services. The bed-and-breakfast hotel where he currently lives is unsuitable as it does not provide meals or support. He requires a residential home which provides a high level of care and also has staff who are skilled to manage his difficult behaviour. Unfortunately, there is a severe shortage of such accommodation throughout the UK.

---

prevention and early intervention in primary care are central to reducing inequalities in health' (Department of Health 2002b: p. 1). It recommended that primary care trusts (PCTs) encourage the further development of PMS and LDS schemes. The Royal College of General Practitioners also produced in 2002 a revised statement on homelessness and primary care which has implications for the developing role of nurses in this area of work. Among its recommendations were that:

- Primary care practitioners should provide a welcoming and sensitive service to homeless people and enable them to access the full range of health and social services required to meet their needs
- Homeless people should be registered permanently (with the NHS and a specific practice) wherever possible and integrated into all health prevention and promotion activity in a practice
- PCTs should acquire a good understanding of the number of homeless people in their area and the problems they face, as well as the range of local agencies equipped to meet their needs
- PCTs should provide resources for ongoing and substantive [sic] support for homelessness services and develop diverse, well-resourced and locally appropriate services
- The new GP contract negotiations should address structural barriers that may affect the permanent registration of homeless people,

including the removal of perverse incentives such as deprivation and target payment anomalies (Royal College of General Practitioners 2002).

Primary care services under the new GP contract

After long negotiations, the new GP contract for general medical services was agreed in June 2003, and involves a major reorganization of general medical services. Primary health care will be divided into essential, additional and enhanced services, and the funding arrangements rationalized in this framework. Enhanced services are 'essential or additional services delivered to a higher standard, or extra, specialised services, such as drug and alcohol misuse clinics or minor injury services' (NHS Confederation 2003: p. 1). For further discussion of developments in primary care, see Chapter 7. National enhanced services are optional, but must be delivered according to national minimum standards. One such service is care of the homeless. A detailed specification of the requirements is available (see Box 29.1 for extract).

Primary health care services for homeless people

In many British towns and cities, dedicated health care services for homeless people have been developed which are flexible, easily accessible and popular.

Box 29.1   National Enhanced Service: Enhanced Care of the Homeless

The aims and service elements of Enhanced Care of the Homeless were published in July 2003 by the Department of Health (www.doh.gov.uk/gmscontract/supportingdocs.htm).

Aims

To ensure that:

- Homeless people have equal access to appropriate levels of service from practices designed to ensure that their health needs are effectively tackled
- GPs are provided with the knowledge, training and resources to enable them to deal effectively with homeless people's health needs
- GP services are empowered to tackle the health needs of homeless people holistically by working with relevant services (e.g. housing and social services) to integrate homeless people into local communities

Service outline

The National Enhanced Service identifies 15 service elements providing enhanced primary health care to homeless people. These include:

- The development of an up-to-date register of patients who are homeless and organizations to whom they provide services
- Liaison with local statutory services and homelessness agencies, and where appropriate the development of joint protocols, e.g. with the local homeless persons unit
- Flexible registration procedures, allowing for permanent registration to people who so wish
- Flexible appointment systems, including walk-in surgeries and longer appointments for people with multiple needs
- Provision for regular screening assessments based on research into the health needs and problems of homeless people
- Provision of outreach services
- Specialist assessment of the physical and mental health of homeless people when registering. Key elements should include a high index of suspicion for conditions of tuberculosis, hepatitis B and C and human immunodeficiency virus (HIV) and of substance abuse
- An annual review of the service

Among the PMS pilots developed after 1998, 25 have a special interest in primary care for homeless people (Wright 2002). The specialist health care services take various forms. A few 'walk-in' clinics have been established that provide medical, nursing and allied professional services, such as dentistry and chiropody (Table 29.2). Some are also multiagency centres or 'one-stop shops' with housing, social security benefits and social services advisers.

Some GP practices are funded to work with homeless people. Established in 1998, the Edith Cavell Practice in south London serves refugees, homeless people and substance misusers. Another, the Morley Street Surgery in Brighton and Hove, provides health care to homeless and insecurely housed people (Warnes et al. 2003). Other examples include the Hanover Medical Centre in central Sheffield which has provided treatment and support to homeless people and families as well as general patients for many years, and the

Homeless Advocacy Project in Manchester, which was established in 1997 at a GP surgery. The Homeless Advocacy Project became a PMS pilot site in April 2000, and anecdotal evidence claims that there has since been a marked reduction in presentations by homeless people at the local A&E department (Allen 2000).

Several towns and cities in the UK, including Birmingham, Blackpool, London and Southampton, now have peripatetic teams of nurses, health visitors, doctors and allied workers who provide health care to homeless people on the streets and at hostels, shelters, bed-and-breakfast hotels, and drop-in and day centres. In Glasgow, for example, a physical health team was established in 2001 to provide health screening, chronic disease management and support to homeless people in hostels and at day centres, and to help them register or re-establish contact with a GP. The team is led by a nurse practitioner and has nurses with district

Table 29.2 Examples of specialist medical clinics for homeless people

Clinic	Services provided at the clinic	Services provided outside the clinic
Great Chapel Street Medical Centre, central London	Medical and nursing; mental health; substance misuse; dentistry; chiropody; benefits advice; social work	Outreach service on the streets and at day centres. Residential care-home sick bay (Wytham Hall)
Luther Street Medical Centre, Oxford	Medical and nursing; mental health; substance misuse; needle exchange; drug and alcohol detoxification (with other projects); dentistry; chiropody; acupuncture	Outreach service on the streets, in hostels, day centres, and at night-shelter. Nursing support to detoxification unit
Joseph Cowen Healthcare Centre, Newcastle-upon-Tyne	Medical and nursing; mental health; sexual health promotion; needle exchange; bathing and deinfestation services; clothes' store; social services	Outreach service on the streets and at drop-in centres. Includes information on injection-based injuries and pregnancy advice and support
Primary Care Centre for Homeless People, Leeds	Medical and nursing; mental health; substance misuse; dentistry; chiropody; condom distribution; volunteer befriending scheme; hepatitis B immunization	Outreach service on the streets, in hostels, at day centres. Volunteers escort people to court

or practice-nurse qualifications and five nursing assistants. Box 29.2 describes the operation of the Leicester Homeless Primary Health Care Service.

A few teams have link workers and hospital discharge coordinators. The link workers visit projects used by homeless people, help clients register with GPs and provide advice about accessing other health services, such as dentists, counselling, and mental health and substance misuse services. They also advocate with housing, health and benefit agencies on behalf of clients, and accompany them to appointments. There are link workers attached to the Homeless Advocacy Project in Manchester, and the Primary Care for Homeless People scheme in north London. The latter team also has two hospital discharge coordinators who cover four hospitals. Their role is to assess the needs of homeless people in hospital, and assist them with accessing housing, substance misuse and social security benefits. They also liaise with the local homeless person's unit about pending discharges

---

Box 29.2   The Leicester Homeless Primary Health Care Service

Dedicated primary health care for homeless people in Leicester dates back to 1990, when two clinics a week were arranged by a GP. In 1998, an assessment of the needs of homeless people confirmed considerable unmet health needs. In response to these findings, a personal medical services (PMS) pilot was set up in March 2000 for 3 years, after which it continued with PMS status. It now has $1^1/_2$ full-time GPs, a full-time specialist nurse practitioner, a practice nurse for 25 h a week, an administrator and a receptionist. The full-time GP and the specialist nurse practitioner are clinical management partners.

The team has an administrative base, where clients' notes are kept and telephone queries answered, and a clinical base at a day centre. It also operates an outreach service, and provides open-access sessions five days a week at each of the two local day centres for homeless people, and medical cover at six hostels and at the city's night-shelter. Computerized information about the clients is recorded, and can be accessed at any time. Twenty-four-hour medical care is provided. The project staff provide cover Monday to Friday from 8 a.m. to 6.30 p.m., and subscribe to the local out-of-hours service which can contact them at any time if difficulties arise.

The service has worked with around 5000 clients, and has an active list of 1000 patients at any given time. A full range of primary care services is provided, including vaccinations, minor surgery, health promotion, maternity and contraceptive services, treatment for drug misuse, community alcohol detoxification and a chronic disease management programme for asthma, diabetes and hypertension. The GPs have completed the Royal College of General Practitioners Certificate in the Management of Drug Misuse, and one has attended acupuncture training, while the full-time nurse is trained in extended nurse prescribing (Leicester Homeless Primary Health Care Service 2002).

of homeless people, and undertake homelessness assessments in hospital on behalf of the unit. Occasionally they receive referrals from A&E staff of older people who have arrived in the department but are confused and unable to confirm whether they are homeless or the address of their accommodation. The workers try to link them back into hostels or existing tenancies (Blood 2003).

Medical respite care services

There are very few medical facilities for homeless people on the streets or in night-shelters who are ill or recovering from an injury but do not require hospital admission. A medical respite care service, the only one known in the UK, was established in 1984 at Wytham Hall in north-west London. It is a 'sick-bay' for homeless people who are ill and is staffed by doctors and care workers, many of whom live on site. It provides temporary accommodation, health care treatment, convalescent care and eventual rehousing (www.wythamhall.co.uk).

Similar medical respite care has been provided in Boston, Massachusetts, USA since 1985 by Boston Health Care for the Homeless. Two projects, Barbara McInnis House (72 beds for men and women) and Betty Snead House (18 beds for women), provide temporary accommodation for homeless people who are too ill to manage on the streets or in shelters. Twenty-four-hour nursing staff are available and there is daily input from physicians and nurse practitioners. The services provided include: recuperative care for people recovering from surgery or fractures or other trauma; nursing care for people with illnesses, such as cancer or heart disease, or infections such as pneumonia; and end-of-life care for terminally ill people who have no family (www.bhchp.org).

Mental health services for homeless people

Mental health services for homeless people have developed rapidly since 1990 when the Mental Health Foundation and the Department of Health launched the Homeless Mentally Ill Initiative to fund services in London. From 1996 the scheme was extended to other cities and towns. Local-authority social services departments receive funding for support services for the mentally ill from the Department of Health through the Mental Health Grant. Since 2000, the Department of Health has required local authorities with a rough-sleeping problem to target funds on specialist services for rough sleepers (Department of the Environment, Transport and the Regions 1999).

Hostels and supported housing have been developed exclusively for mentally ill homeless people, and in Birmingham, Brighton, Glasgow, London, Manchester, Nottingham and Oxford, community mental health teams now provide services to homeless people on the streets, at day centres and in hostels and bed-and-breakfast hotels. The teams comprise community psychiatric nurses, psychiatrists and drug and alcohol workers, while some have social workers and allied staff (Warnes et al. 2003). In London, qualified social workers from Westminster City's Social Services Department undertake intensive street work with the mental health team to arrange mental health assessments for isolated and chronic rough sleepers who resist help. Several, whom it had previously been impossible to engage, have been admitted to hospital under the Mental Health Act (Randall & Brown 2002). Similar teams operate in Madrid, Spain, and several US cities (Maldonado & Romano 1997, Vázquez et al. 1999).

MEETING THE HEALTH CARE NEEDS OF OLDER HOMELESS PEOPLE

This section describes ways of meeting the health care needs of older homeless people, paying particular attention to the role of nurses. Little has previously been written about delivering health care to this client group. The *National Service Framework for Older People* does not specifically refer to older homeless people, although it does acknowledge the importance of the early identification of health problems, and a holistic and multidisciplinary approach to assessing needs (Department of Health 2001b).

Engaging with older homeless people

Many older homeless people neglect their general health and do not seek treatment when they are ill. Nurses and other health care staff therefore need to work proactively with them, find out about their circumstances, and persuade them to have a health check-up and accept necessary treatment. Some nurses will first come into contact with older homeless people because they are admitted into an A&E department or a ward. It is important that they engage with this client group and gain their trust. Many are fearful of doctors and nurses, and worried about what will happen to them. Some will have had little or no contact with health professionals or other formal services for a long time. Reassurance and encouragement to accept help are crucial if the health needs of this group are to be addressed.

Nurses working in specialist health care projects for homeless people should take the opportunity to meet older clients when they conduct surgeries in hostels and day centres. It should not be assumed that the older clients will ask for medical care. It may take several weeks of repeated contact before some are willing to accept help. A few homeless health teams have link workers (described earlier), who can play a crucial role in engaging with isolated older homeless people in temporary accommodation or at day centres.

Assessing needs

Comprehensive assessments are required of older homeless people's health and social needs. Besides a medical history and thorough screening for physical health problems and injuries, information is needed about: their mental health and cognitive states; current housing situation; daily living and personal care skills; contact with relatives and with support services; whether in receipt of social security benefits; and use of alcohol and illegal drugs. Further discussion of the single assessment process can be found in Chapter 28. Consideration should be given to the risks posed by self-neglect, poor physical health, mobility problems, mental health problems, confusion, heavy drinking, poor daily living skills, unsuitable accommodation and insufficient support (Warnes & Crane 2000).

Nurses and medical staff should undertake the health elements of the assessment, and refer to a mental health team if depression, cognitive impairment or other mental health problems are suspected. Some clients may be depressed, never having come to terms with the losses or traumas that caused them to become homeless. Appraisal of functional capabilities, and of housing and social support needs, requires the skills of occupational therapists and social workers. Hospital-based and community nurses need to be aware of other agencies working with vulnerable people and what they offer, and of their referral procedures.

Hospital admissions are a unique opportunity to assess the medical, mental and social care needs of older homeless people who otherwise rarely use services. The initial assessments carried out by nurses therefore need to be thorough, so that older patients who are homeless can be quickly identified and promptly referred to hospital social workers and other services. The Department of Health has recommended that all acute hospitals should have formal admission policies which can easily detect whether a person is homeless (Department of Health 2003).

Assessing the needs of older homeless people is not easy. Some will have mental health problems or cognitive deficits and be unable to give accurate details about physical illnesses and treatment, and their housing circumstances. Some may be reluctant to provide information or deliberately mislead. They may be too embarrassed to admit that they are having difficulty with self-care tasks, or that they are forgetful or have an alcohol problem. As trust is built over time, more truthful information may be ascertained. Wherever possible, and with the person's consent, details should also be obtained from other agencies who have had contact with the individual.

Providing health and personal care

Because of severe physical, mental health or alcohol problems, many older homeless people have high care needs. They require assistance with personal hygiene and bathing, and prompting to eat. Some are confused or poorly motivated and need supervision to take medication, and encouragement to attend appointments and comply with medical treatments. Some need to be escorted to appointments as they are distrustful of service providers, and may not comprehend information that is given to them. It is important that care is delivered flexibly, as some may refuse treatment one day but can later be persuaded to accept it. Although this may be frustrating in a busy ward or clinic, persistence has nevertheless proved effective for many who initially have been reluctant to accept help.

Hospital discharges

Much attention has recently been focused on hospital discharges. An inspection of discharge arrangements for older people in eight local authorities was conducted in 1997 (Horne 1998). In 2003 the Department of Health published a report, *Discharge From Hospital: Pathway, Process and Practice*, and one appendix concentrates on the discharge of homeless people. It stresses the importance of an agreement between the local homeless person's unit, the acute hospital and the PCT to ensure appropriate accommodation and continuity of care for homeless people on discharge. A 2003 report by Help the Aged focused on older homeless people's discharge from hospital (Blood 2003).

For many older homeless people, a stay in hospital is an opportunity to improve their housing situation and ensure that they have accommodation on discharge. Many are unable to live independently and require supported housing or a registered care-home. This takes time to arrange and it is therefore essential that they are referred to hospital social workers as early as possible after admission. Some will have been staying in hostels, and one option is for them to return to the hostel to await more permanent housing. This will however depend on the capacity of the hostel to meet the health and support needs of the individual. Close liaison with the hostel manager about the person's needs and treatment plan is therefore necessary.

No older homeless person should be discharged from hospital back to the streets. It is also unacceptable only to provide individuals with a list of hostels or bed-and-breakfast hotels and expect them to make their own arrangements. While there is pressure to free hospital beds and to discharge patients as soon as possible, this should not apply to older homeless people, one of the highest risk groups in society.

Health promotion

Little health promotion work is undertaken with homeless people, even though many have poor diets, misuse substances, and neglect their general and dental health. In 1996, the Health Education Authority proposed that flexible health promotion programmes should fill this gap and be delivered by mainstream health service workers because many homelessness agencies lack the required time, resources and skills (Power et al. 1999). A 2001 study of over 70 residential projects for single homeless people in London found that most admitted that their health promotion activity was 'marginal', ad hoc and a function of staff interests (Hinton et al. 2001).

Older homeless people require encouragement to access dentists, chiropodists and opticians. Many will not have had an eye test for some time. Compared to their housed contemporaries, older homeless people have poor dental health and are unlikely to be registered with a dentist (Khan 2000). Some hostels and day centres for homeless people arrange for chiropodists and opticians to visit at regular intervals. In some areas, community or personal dental services have been established to provide dental treatment to homeless people and other groups who would not otherwise access dental services. Further discussion of health promotion issues and older people is given in Chapter 30.

THE TRAINING NEEDS OF HEALTH STAFF WORKING WITH HOMELESS PEOPLE

There is a lack of understanding among many health care workers about homelessness and the complex problems of homeless people, and the need for staff training in the field is increasingly acknowledged. In a revised statement on homelessness and primary care, the Royal College of General Practitioners noted: 'the extent and pervasive nature of negative stereotyping is recognized as an important barrier to good quality primary care ... all front-line staff in general practice –

and particularly receptionists–must be trained in non-discriminatory practice with regards to homeless people' (Royal College of General Practitioners 2002: pp. 7, 11). The Royal College of General Practitioners recommends that education around homelessness issues should be multidisciplinary and include methods of risk assessment and dealing with complex needs, such as alcohol and drug misuse and mental illness.

Several training initiatives have been developed. A homelessness training unit, managed by the South Thames Assessment, Resource and Training Team (START) at the South London and Maudsley NHS Trust, delivers a training programme to front-line staff working with homeless people. It is funded by the Homelessness Directorate and offers various courses, including: understanding and working with personality disorder; dealing with bereavement and death while working with homeless people; and reminiscence work. The Croydon Homeless Health Team provides training for practice managers and receptionists in general practice on registering homeless people and their vulnerabilities, and Primary Care for Homeless People in north London offers training to hospital staff on the needs of homeless people and available services (Blood 2003, Gorton 2003).

Training for nurses

Nurses play a key role in delivering health care services to homeless people. In 2000, the London Standing Conference for Nurses, Midwives and Health Visitors was established to give nurses a voice in decision-making on professional and health care issues (details at www.london.nhs.uk). Fourteen work themes were identified, one of which was nursing and homelessness. A homeless working group was established in March 2000 of representatives from health care services and the voluntary sector, to examine health care provision for homeless people in London. Among its findings were that most nurses who work with homeless people have previously worked in community settings but that there is no formal mechanism for them to develop appropriate skills and knowledge. Most learn through experience and peer support. In addition, there are few career progression opportunities (London Standing Conference for Nurses, Midwives and Health Visitors 2001).

The Homeless Working Group recommended that a modular diploma or degree in social exclusion nursing be developed, with opportunities for nurses with community experience to progress to rotational posts in various homeless settings, then to nurse practitioner or clinical nurse specialist, and finally to expert practitioner or consultant nurse. The latter would work across health and social services. The Royal College of General Practitioners also recommended that itself and the Royal College of Nursing should 'collaborate to acknowledge that the aspiration of nurses in the field of homelessness should be recognized as a specialism with a core curriculum, training opportunities and qualification' (Royal College of General Practitioners 2002: p. 6).

Started in 2003, Middlesex University runs a part-time Masters Degree, an Advanced Diploma and a Postgraduate Certificate in Social Inclusion, which is designed for nurses and other health and social care professionals who work with socially excluded people. The topics include: concepts and current issues in social inclusion; current social policy initiatives; health needs assessment of socially excluded groups; meeting health needs; and research methods in health care services.

CONCLUSIONS

Since the late 1990s, British health care services have undergone rapid reorganization, reform and expansion. Service and practice innovations have been introduced to reach out to marginal groups, including homeless people, who previously had been inadequately helped. As part of these reforms, nurses have undertaken significant and often lead roles in developing services for 'special-needs' and 'hard-to-reach' groups, and several PMSs are nurse-led. Multidisciplinarity and proactive case work distinguish the new approach. Close working relationships are developed with social workers, housing providers, specialist substance abuse services and community mental health teams. The external links are the first step towards a proactive approach to helping people with serious untreated health problems, but there is more work to do.

Although there have been few recent substantial studies of homeless people's utilization of health care services (not even hospital A&E), early reports from individual specialist projects suggest that a large number of homeless people have benefited from the new reforms. Specialist and dedicated health services reduce the prevalence of untreated health problems among older homeless people, and sympathetic and tenacious responses help some older people regain a sense of being valued and of self-worth. Specialist primary care staff often work with a client in close cooperation with housing, social service and benefits agencies, and in this way play a valuable role in both the reduction of homelessness and the prevention of returns to homelessness. While to date the dedicated services remain an unusual rather than a normal feature of a city's primary and community health care services, they are spreading and the scope for further development and improvements in effectiveness and coordination is large.

Acknowledgements

We thank the older homeless people and the staff and managers of organizations that have participated in our research over the years. Particular thanks are sent to the outreach workers from St Mungo's who provided information for the case studies. We are also grateful to the Henry Smith's Charity, the Sir Halley Stewart Trust, and the Leverhulme Trust for their support of our research programme on homelessness.

Recommended reading

Cohen C, Sokolovsky J 1989 Old men of the Bowery: strategies for survival among the homeless. Guilford Press, New York.
A detailed account of older homeless men on the Bowery in New York City, describing their backgrounds, health problems, social networks and strategies for survival.
Crane M 1999 Understanding older homeless people: their circumstances, problems and needs. Open University Press, Buckingham.
This book traces in detail the histories and pathways into homelessness of older people, and the problems and needs among those who are homeless.
Gorton S 2003 Guide to models of delivering health services to homeless people. Crisis, London.
Using examples in London, this guide describes models of health care services for homeless people by mainstream and specialist providers.
Warnes AM, Crane M 2000 Meeting homeless people's needs: service development and practice for the older excluded. King's Fund, London.
This book describes effective ways of helping older homeless people, and has first-hand accounts of services in the UK, USA and Australia.
Warnes AM, Crane M, Whitehead N, Fu R 2003 Homelessness factfile. Crisis, London.
This factfile provides comprehensive information about homeless people in the UK, and policy and service responses to homelessness and its prevention.
Wright N 2002 Homelessness: a primary care response. Royal College of General Practitioners, London.
This book presents an overview of the health problems of homeless people, and is written as a practical manual to help professionals deliver high-quality primary care to this population.

Useful websites

www.bhchp.org
Boston Health Care for the Homeless

www.nhchc.org
National Health Care for the Homeless Council
www.olderhomelessness.co.uk
UK Coalition on Older Homelessness
www.sheffield.ac.uk/sisa/Research_Field_5.shtml
Sheffield Institute for Studies on Ageing, University of Sheffield

References

Acheson D 1981 Primary healthcare in inner London: report of a study group commissioned by the London Planning Consortium. Department of Health and Social Security, London

Alcohol Concern 2003 Factsheet 6: Wernicke-Korsakoff syndrome. Alcohol Concern, London

Allen M 2000 Homelessness and health in Manchester: health needs assessment. Part one. Homeless Advocacy Project, Manchester

Barrow S, Herman D, Cordova P, Struening E 1999 Mortality among homeless shelter residents in New York City. American Journal of Public Health 89: 529–534

Belcher J, DiBlasio F 1990 The needs of depressed homeless persons: designing appropriate services. Community Mental Health Journal 26: 255–266.

Blood I 2003 The discharge of older homeless people from hospital. Help the Aged, London

British Medical Association 2003 Housing and health: building for the future. British Medical Association, London

Broadway 2002 CHAIN activity report: April 2001–March 2002. Broadway, London

Burt M, Cohen B 1989 Differences among homeless single women, women with children, and single men. Social Problems 36: 508–524

Citron K, Southern A, Dixon M 1995 Out of the shadow: detecting and treating tuberculosis amongst single homeless people. Crisis, London

Cohen C, Sokolovsky J 1989 Old men of the Bowery: strategies for survival among the homeless. Guilford Press, New York

Cohen C, Ramirez M, Teresi J, Gallagher M, Sokolovsky J 1997 Predictors of becoming redomiciled among older homeless women. Gerontologist 37: 67–74

Crane M 1999 Understanding older homeless people: their circumstances, problems and needs. Open University Press, Buckingham

Crane M, Warnes AM 2000 Lessons from Lancefield Street: tackling the needs of older homeless people. National Homeless Alliance, London

Crane M, Warnes AM 2001a Single homeless people in London: profiles of service users and perceptions of needs. Report for Bondway, St Mungo's and Thames Reach. Sheffield Institute for Studies on Ageing, Sheffield

Crane M, Warnes AM 2001b Older people and homelessness: prevalence and causes. Topics in Geriatric Rehabilitation 16: 1–14

Crane M, Warnes AM 2001c Primary health care services for single homeless people: defects and opportunities. Family Practice 18: 272–276

Crane M, Warnes AM 2002a Resettling older homeless people: a longitudinal study of outcomes. Sheffield Institute for Studies on Ageing, University of Sheffield, Sheffield

Crane M, Warnes AM 2002b Harrow Road Hostel: a review of the first twelve months. St Mungo's, London

Crane M, Warnes AM 2003 Wet day centres in the United Kingdom. A research report and manual. Sheffield Institute for Studies on Ageing. University of Sheffield, Sheffield

Crane M, Warnes AM, Fu R 2004 Building homelessness prevention practice: combining research evidence and professional knowledge. Sheffield Institute for Studies on Ageing. University of Sheffield, Sheffield

Crisis 2002 Critical condition: vulnerable single homeless people and access to GPs. Policy brief. Crisis, London

Department of the Environment, Transport and the Regions 1999 Annual report on rough sleeping. Department of the Environment, Transport and the Regions, London

Department of Health 2001a 2000 Health survey for England: the health of older people (aged 65+). Department of Health, London

Department of Health 2001b The national service framework for older people. Department of Health, London

Department of Health 2002a Mental health policy implementation guide: dual diagnosis good practice guide. Department of Health, London

Department of Health 2002b Addressing inequalities: reaching the hard-to-reach groups. Department of Health, London

Department of Health 2003 Discharge from hospital: pathway, process and practice. Department of Health, London

Douglass R, Atchison B, Lofton W et al. 1988 Aged, adrift and alone: Detroit's elderly homeless. Final report to the Detroit Area Agency on Aging. Department of Associated Health Professions, Eastern Michigan University, Ypsilanti, Michigan

Evans N, Dowler E 1999 Food, health and eating among single homeless and marginalized people in London. Journal of Human Nutrition and Dietetics 12: 179–199

Finn W, Hyslop J, Truman C 2000 Mental health, multiple needs and the police: findings from the Revolving Doors Agency link worker scheme. Revolving Doors Agency, London

Fisher K, Collins J 1993 Access to health care. In: Fisher K, Collins J (eds) Homelessness, health care and welfare provision. Routledge, London, pp. 32–50

Gorton S 2003 Guide to models of delivering health services to homeless people. Crisis, London

Grenier P 1996 Still dying for a home. Crisis, London

Hecht L, Coyle B 2001 Elderly homeless: a comparison of older and younger adult emergency shelter seekers in Bakersfield, California. American Behavioral Scientist 45: 66–79

Hinton T 1995 Measuring Up? A study of how A&E services respond to single homeless people. Health Action for Homeless People and Crisis, London

Hinton T, Evans N, Jacobs K 2001 Healthy hostels: a guide to promoting health and well-being among homeless people. Crisis, London

Horne D 1998 Getting better? Inspection of hospital discharge care management arrangements for older people. Department of Health, London

Hurley M, Scallan E, Johnson H, De La Harpe D 2000 Adult service refusers in the Greater Dublin area. Irish Medical Journal 93: 207–211

Kershaw A, Singleton N, Meltzer H 2000 Survey of the health and well-being of homeless people in Glasgow. Office for National Statistics, London

Keyes S, Kennedy M 1992 Sick to death of homelessness. An investigation into the links between homelessness, health and mortality. Crisis, London

Khan A 2000 Dental health, attitudes and behaviour: a comparison between elderly homeless people and non-homeless people. Annual report 1999–2000. Great Chapel Street Medical Centre, London

Kutza E 1987 A study of undomiciled elderly persons in Chicago: a final report. Retirement Research Foundation, Chicago

Ladner S 1992 The elderly homeless. In: Robertson M, Greenblatt M (eds), Homelessness: a national perspective. Plenum Press, New York, pp 221–226

La Gory M, Ferris R, Mullis J 1990 Depression among the homeless. Journal of Health and Social Behaviour 31: 87–101

Leicester Homeless Primary Health Care Service 2002 Annual report: April 2001–March 2002. Leicester Homeless Primary Health Care Service, Leicester

London Standing Conference for Nurses, Midwives and Health Visitors 2001 Nursing and homelessness: a review of nursing and the provision of health care services for homeless people within the London region. London Standing Conference for Nurses, Midwives and Health Visitors, London

Maldonado JL, Romano MTL 1997 European observatory on homelessness: annual report on homelessness in Spain 1977. European Federation of National Organizations Working With the Homeless (FEANTSA), Brussels

Morley M, Sellwood W 1997 Schizophrenia in later life. In: Norman I, Redfern S (eds) Mental health care for elderly people. Churchill Livingstone, New York, pp 223–245

NHS Confederation 2003 Managing workload. GMS contract negotiation factsheet 3. NHS Confederation, London

Nordentoft M, Wandall-Holm N 2003 10 year follow up study of mortality among users of hostels for homeless people in Copenhagen. British Medical Journal 327: 81

Office of the Deputy Prime Minister 2003 Statutory homelessness: England fourth quarter 2002. News release 2003/0037. Office of the Deputy Prime Minister, London

Pleace N, Quilgars D 1996 Health and homelessness in London: a review. King's Fund, London

Pleace N, Jones A, England J 2000 Access to general practice for people sleeping rough. Centre for Housing Policy, University of York, York

Power R, French R, Connelly J et al. 1999 Promoting the health of homeless people: setting a research agenda. Health Education Authority, London

Randall G, Brown S 2002 Helping rough sleepers off the streets. A report to the Homelessness Directorate. Office of the Deputy Prime Minister, London

Rosengard A and associates with Scottish Health Feedback 2001 The future of hostels for homeless people. Scottish Executive Central Research Unit, Edinburgh

Royal College of General Practitioners 2002 Statement on homelessness and primary care. Royal College of General Practitioners, London

Vázquez C, Muñoz M, Rodriguez-Gonzales A 1999 Spain. In: Helvie C, Kunstmann W (eds) Homelessness in the United States, Europe and Russia. Bergin and Garvey, Westport, CT, pp 169–205

Warnes AM, Crane M 2000 Meeting homeless people's needs: service development and practice for the older excluded. King's Fund, London

Warnes AM, Crane M, Whitehead N, Fu R 2003 Homelessness factfile. Crisis, London

Wright N 2002 Homelessness: a primary care response. Royal College of General Practitioners, London

Chapter 30

Health promotion for older people

Sarah Cowley

INTRODUCTION

The nursing role with older people who are ill or dependent is widely accepted, but for nurses and health visitors to engage in health promotion work with this age group has been regarded as a 'challenge' (McClymont et al. 1991). It is, however, a key standard within the *National Service Framework (NSF) for Older People* (Department of Health 2001) which aims to extend the healthy life expectancy for older people. Key standard 8 requires that: 'The health and well-being of older people is promoted through a coordinated programme of action led by the NHS and supported by local councils' (Department of Health 2001: p. 107). Health inequalities are a particular concern, being associated with socioeconomic status and the amount of social support available (Grundy & Sloggett 2003). More recently, attention has been drawn to the wide disparities in the health experiences of older people internationally (World Health Organization 2003), and the need for governments to ensure they take account of a growing proportion of older people when planning health care.

Around one in five of the UK population is over 60 years old, a ratio that has remained fairly steady since 1971 (Grundy 1996). Even so, at the 2001 census the significant milestone was passed in which, for the first time, people aged 60 years and over (approaching 21%) formed a larger part of the population than children under 16 (20%) (National Statistics Online 2004a). Also, the total number of older people has grown in keeping with an expanding population, and the numbers of very elderly (over 85 years) has doubled from 0.9% of the population in 1971 to 1.9% of the population in 2001 (National Statistics Online 2004b). Table 30.1 summarizes figures from these different sources. In some parts of the country, this rate may be even

Table 30.1 Population aged 60 and over as a percentage of total UK population by age

Age group	1971	1981	1991	2001
60–64	5.8	5.2	5.0	4.9
65–69	4.9	5.0	4.8	4.4
70–74	3.6	4.2	3.9	4.0
75–79	2.4	3.0	3.2	3.3
80–84	1.4	1.7	2.2	2.2
85–89	0.6	0.8	1.1	1.3
90+	0.2	0.3	0.4	0.6
60+	19.0	20.2	20.7	20.7
65+	13.3	15.0	15.7	15.8
75+	4.7	5.8	7.0	7.4
85+	0.9	1.1	1.6	1.9

higher; Worthing was identified as the local authority with the highest percentage (4.6%) of residents over 85 years in 2001. For further detailed discussion of epidemiological trends, see Chapter 3.

In 2001, there were about 336 000 people aged 90 and over, but the census identified nearly 4000 of these as providing 50 h or more of unpaid care per week to another family member or friend. Although only 26% of people aged 90 and over living in households are men, they make up just over half of the carers in this age bracket (National Statistics Online 2004a). This information is a useful counterpoint to concerns about the cost of caring for an increasing number of older people, when there is a shrinking population of working age. Awareness of these continuing contributions from older people to the community in which they live accounts for the celebratory approach encouraged by the World Health Organization, who comment that:

> Population ageing is one of humanity's greatest triumphs. It is also one of our greatest challenges. As we enter the 21st century, global ageing will put increased economic and social demands on all countries. At the same time, older people are a precious, often ignored resource that makes an important contribution to the fabric of our societies. The World Health Organization argues that countries can afford to get old if governments, international organizations and civil society enact 'active ageing' policies and programmes that enhance the health, participation and security of older citizens. The time to plan and to act is now (World Health Organization 2002a: p. 6).

The idea of an active, positive approach to ageing (Figs 30.1 and 30.2) will underpin much of this chap-

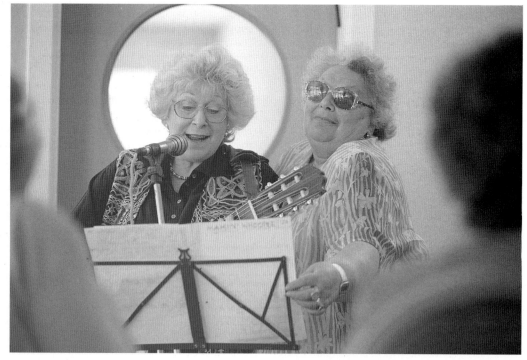

Fig. 30.1 Singing. (Photograph by Jon-Paul Davis, courtesy of Age Concern Scotland.)

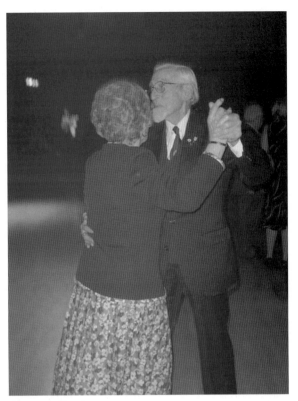

Fig. 30.2   Dancing.

ter, which will be presented in two main parts. First, it will examine the different ideas about how health might be viewed and will critically consider the suitability of these alternative formulations for older people. Great significance is attached to personal health beliefs, so much of this section will concentrate on lay explanations of health and illness as a contrast to the more traditional medical focus on concepts of disease. Table 30.1 draws attention to the diversity of perceptions to be expected; the 'population over 60 years old' encompasses an age range of some 40 years. Few 20-year-olds would appreciate being expected to think about their health in the same way as someone approaching retirement, and it would make little sense. Similarly, the difference in experiences and personal histories between a generation born early in the twentieth century and those who were small children during the Second World War is likely to be quite great; there is no reason to believe their expectations and perceptions of health will all be the same.

Different approaches to promoting health will be explained in the second section. An important theme running through the chapter is the importance of enabling people in later life to retain autonomy and dignity; approaches to health promotion will be con-

sidered with this in mind. The use of the term 'older people' is intended to focus on this human face of a wide and diverse population; as individuals they might take on the role of client, patient, consumer, customer or service user for a temporary period, but their permanent status is that of a 'person'. This section incorporates some practical examples of ways for nurses to carry out health-promoting work with older people.

The chapter aims to persuade any doubters that health is a resource that remains relevant from the beginning of life to its end. Despite the undoubted difficulties faced by older people, the extent of severe disability in old age appears to be reducing. In 1991, 80% of men and 79% of women aged over 85 years and living in private households were able to bathe themselves, feed themselves, get in and out of bed and get to the toilet without help from another person (Grundy 1996). Furthermore, nurses have many of the key skills required for health promotion and many opportunities to engage in preventive care. There is good reason to be optimistic that nurses will continue to develop new and interesting ways to promote the health of older people.

HEALTH

At a surface level, everyone understands and uses the word 'health' quite readily without causing confusion or needing recourse to a dictionary. On closer inspection, though, it becomes apparent that 'health' is a word that rarely stands alone. It is much easier to explain what is meant by 'health care' or a 'health club', or to use the adjective to describe things such as a 'healthy diet' or 'healthy living' than it is to consider what is meant by 'health' in an abstract sense. Even attaching descriptors, as in phrases like 'good health' or 'poor health', seems to make the term easier to grasp. However, each addition alters the meaning of the word 'health', and demonstrates the huge diversity of understanding and the multitude of very different connotations and underlying assumptions associated with the term. These meanings change over time as well; some definitions are included in Box 30.1.

In part, the shift in thinking from when the World Health Organization was first constituted in 1946 to when it drew up the Ottawa Charter for Health Promotion in 1986 illustrates a greater sophistication of understanding. These varied definitions also show that there are different ways of conceptualizing health and of considering what kind of entity it is. An international review of health promotion practices and concepts identified the various ways that health may be viewed (Anderson 1984); these are summarized in

---

Box 30.1   Defining health

'health is a state of complete physical, mental and social well-being and not merely the absence of disease or infirmity' (World Health Organization 1946)

'health is created and lived by people within the settings of their everyday life; where they learn, work, play and love. Health is created by caring for oneself and others, by being able to take decisions and control over one's life circumstances, and by ensuring that the society one lives in creates conditions that allow the attainment of health by all its members' (World Health Organization 1986)

'a person's health is equivalent to the state of the set of conditions which fulfill or enable a person to fulfil his or her realistic and chosen biological potentials' (Seedhouse 1986: p. 72)

'by health, I mean the power to live a full adult, living, breathing life in close contact with what I love – the earth and the wonders thereof – the sea – the sun, all that we mean when we speak of the external world. I want to enter into it, to be part of it, to live in it, to learn from it, to lose all that is superficial and acquired in me and to become a conscious, direct human being. I want, by understanding myself, to understand others. I want to be all that I am capable of becoming so that I may be ... a child of the sun ... but warm, eager, living life – to be rooted in life – to learn, to desire, to feel, to think, to act. That is what I want. And nothing less. That is what I must try for' (Mansfield 1977: pp, 278–279)

Box 30.2   Concepts of health

Health can be considered:
- as an outcome or product
- as a potential or capacity
- as a process

Health may be:
- something experienced by individuals
- identified by outside observers, particularly clinicians

Health may be:
- a fixed state
- a dynamic relationship
- an attribute of one element of the individual, such as physical fitness
- a characteristic of the whole person representing social, spiritual, emotional and physical aspects

---

Box 30.2. Since that review was completed, the spiritual dimension of health has been widely recognized (World Health Organization 1998). None of the different ways of considering the concept of health are entirely satisfactory if used alone, although some are given greater credence in our society and within the National Health Service (NHS) than others. Evaluating the different viewpoints with an eye to the health of older people is a good way of examining how useful they might be as a basis for practice.

Health as a product

In the traditional medical formulation, health is viewed as a 'product', bound up with notions of disease and measurable deviations from a biological norm. Such biomedical measurements give rise to the widely accepted idea of health as a 'state', as suggested in the World Health Organization (1946) definition in Box 30.1. That definition has been thoroughly

criticized for seeming static and fixed, as well as far too idealistic and unattainable for most people (Anderson 1984, Seedhouse 1986, Aggleton 1990). Even so, it remains useful in drawing attention to the fact that health is not the same as an 'absence of disease', an idea that still has wide currency. Often, this is presented by describing a continuum, with absolute health placed at the positive end and total disease, or even death, at the other negative extreme. It is easy to see how readily such a linear view could portray health as associated with youth and fitness, with any deterioration towards the 'disease' end of the continuum being almost inevitably linked in people's minds with ageing and a pessimistic outlook.

Such an 'all-or-nothing' view of health would be quite detrimental to older people who may be healthy in some respects but not others. People living at home with a well-managed long-term condition like diabetes or arthritis, for example, may not wish to characterize themselves as 'ill'. It is entirely possible for a person of any age to be healthy in one aspect of their lives and unhealthy in another. This suggestion implies that health is a characteristic of the whole person, which may be affected in part without being radically changed by a single unhealthy element.

A large, nationwide Health and Lifestyle survey demonstrated wide agreement with the idea that health could be identified as the absence of disease, but for most people it was more than that (Blaxter 1990). Most people considered health to be a relative state that differed throughout the life course. The researchers interviewed over 9000 people, and discovered clear differences between the perceptions of health held by women and men, according to the age of the respondents and to their social class. Beliefs about the causes of health and illness will be considered again, as they need taking into account when planning health promotion activities. The survey showed that health was viewed as a multifaceted concept, as Blaxter explains:

> The negative definition of health as 'not ill, no disease' has within itself at least two dimensions: the absence of symptoms, or feeling ill, and 'wholeness' or absence of diagnosed pathology. Sometimes these are clearly separate, as when a respondent defined health as being without aches and pains even though chronic disease was present (Blaxter 1990: p. 31).

This explanation draws attention to the idea of 'diagnosed pathology'. In turn, this emphasizes the difference between health as a personal experience and as something that can be identified by an outside observer, like a nurse or doctor. The older World Health Organization definition (World Health Organization 1946) supports the idea that 'disease' and 'infirmity' are clearly demonstrated by recourse to a medical diagnosis, while its more recent formulation (World Health Organization 1986) stresses the importance of personal control and decision-making as essential components of health.

Certainly, however it is recognized, an absence of disease seems considerably more attainable than the somewhat utopian ideal presented by the World Health Organization (1946) definition. It may also be easier to envisage, although negative health states encompass far more than disease alone; illness, disability, injury, deformity and disorder are all variations on the theme of negative health states (Downie et al. 1990). Not all are amenable to medical treatment, but an awareness of them may be useful for purposes of planning health services, since it may be possible to effect and measure a change for the better.

This way of looking at health, again, concentrates on the end-state or 'product' and is closely aligned to the emphasis on 'outcomes' stressed in much health policy. It has also become closely associated with the recent idea that health can be viewed as a 'commodity' to be supplied (Seedhouse 1986). However, equating health with a series of clearly definable and measurable qualities (even if they are health measures, like blood pressure or cholesterol levels) tends to imply that they can be obtained from others, by being bought, sold or somehow acquired. There is a danger that restoring health is viewed as little more than a technical matter, and control for it is likely to be removed from the person (Aggleton 1990).

The way in which health is viewed remains a very personal matter. Perhaps the most negative aspect of the view of health as a product is its association with the idea that health is best 'owned' and controlled by health care professionals rather than the people whose health is under discussion. This is a particular problem for older people, whose views may be disregarded in favour of those expressed by doctors, nurses or social workers. In turn, this is linked with a tendency to underplay the importance of the practical, social and cultural context for health.

However, the view of health as a state underpins most of the surveys that illustrate the extent of ability and disability within the older age group; these continue to provide very helpful information to discredit stereotyping perceptions of older people. Moreover, the traditional view of health that underpins the biomedical approach remains significantly useful when illness occurs. The clarity that can be lent to a confusing or frightening situation by identifying a specific diagnosis or measurable basis for reassurance should not be underestimated. The extent to which health promotion practice can capitalize on these positive aspects without undermining the self-determination of older people will be considered further, once the formulations of health as a 'potential' or as a 'process' have been explained.

Health as potential

The idea of health as a 'potential' is proposed by Anderson (1984), who links it with an ability to cope with, or adapt to, environmental challenges as well as an ability to realize personal goals and aspirations. Seedhouse (1986) is perhaps the writer most recently associated with promoting this view; he has described health as the 'foundation for achievement' (Box 30.3). He suggests that regarding health as a potential can integrate a number of different ways of looking at health, including the ideas described above that it can be regarded as an 'ideal state' or as a 'commodity' that can be bought or given. He also incorporates two other ideas that will be considered further; these are the group of theories that hold that health is a personal strength or ability, whether physical, metaphysical or intellectual, and the theory that health is the physical and mental fitness to do socialized daily tasks.

The idea that health consists of the physical and mental fitness to do socialized daily tasks is usually ascribed to the sociologist Talcott Parsons, who defines health as the: 'optimum capacity of an individual for the effective role and tasks for which he has been socialised' (Parsons 1981: p. 69).

Box 30.3   Health as potential

The idea of health as the 'foundation for achievement' incorporates theories that health is:

- an ideal state
- the physical and mental fitness to do socialized daily tasks
- a commodity that can be bought or given
- a personal strength or ability: physical, meta-physical or intellectual

Approaches designed to increase health:

- sociological approach
- medical science
- humanist approach

This forms part of a wider theory of how society functions, and is intended to show how health and illness are relevant to this. As part of the theory, it is supposed that people whom society recognizes as 'sick' (usually by formal medical diagnosis, although self-diagnosis and family recognition may be sufficient) are afforded relief from their daily duties and responsibilities – the functions they are generally expected to contribute to their own social world. In return, they are expected to take on a 'sick role' which holds certain alternative responsibilities, such as making clear attempts to recover, and obeying approved advice like 'medical orders' or prescribed routines.

Although that was not its intention, it is easy enough to see how this theory can suggest that people exist only for the purpose of serving society – and that once they are too old or infirm to carry out their 'socialized roles' they have no further 'function'. Furthermore, the theory offers no help in explaining those aspects of negative health that are long-standing, like disability, long-term conditions or the kind of non-specific frailty that often accompanies great age. As with the utopian ideal of a state of complete well-being, this theory brooks no variations on the theme of health as 'optimum capacity' and appears to offer no individual choice or autonomy.

Even so, as with most of these different ways of considering health, it is possible to recognize elements of this theory in the lay descriptions offered to researchers. Williams (1983) spoke to 70 older people in Aberdeen about how they perceived their health. When he analysed the interviews, he found that most uses of the word 'fit' were synonymous with 'healthy' or 'strong', but a clear link with the idea of what a person might be considered fit *for* was implicit in much of the dialogue. The idea of sickness as being unfit for

normal duties or unable to care for oneself was readily recognized; however the existence of weakness in their constitutions did not imply being unfit for normal duties, for example:

> where a constitutional weakness existed unaccompanied by current disabling disease. In such cases, the sufferer might indeed feel vulnerable; but vulnerability on its own, unaccompanied by a recognised disease, was felt as inadequate grounds for excusing oneself from normal obligations (Williams 1983: p. 193).

This view was held so strongly that many of Williams' informants reversed the association, implying that being accepted as unfit to carry out 'normal obligations' (which included social activities as well as employment or work-related activities like shopping and cooking) indicated the presence of an illness or disabling disease. In the nationwide Health and Lifestyle survey, women were more likely than men to associate health with the ability to carry out daily activities; this included descriptions of older people who were considered healthy because they were able to carry out everyday tasks such as housework (Blaxter 1990).

In similar vein, Cribb & Dines (1993) broaden the concept to 'functioning within normal limits', an approach that explicitly includes the diversity of expectation at different ages – although it begs the value-laden questions of what constitutes 'normal', and who should decide. Further, Cribb & Dines (1993) suggest that fitness may be an implicit part of the concept of functional ability. This illustrates something of the complex, overlapping and confusing nature of health. It is possible to identify separate aspects and concepts embedded in the idea of health, but such components are not truly separable, and various commentators may categorize them differently.

Seedhouse (1986), for example, places notions of fitness under the group of theories that describe health as a personal strength or ability; he lists physical, metaphysical and intellectual abilities. The idea of strength, as opposed to weakness, featured strongly in the ideas of what constituted health in the eyes of the older Aberdonians interviewed by Williams (1983). Physical fitness, vitality and energy were considered important. Weaknesses were often anatomically located, perhaps by referring to painful joints or weakened organs, although medical attention was not necessarily required for these problems. This was a category of disorder echoed in a study of health perceptions held by women in East London (Cornwell 1984). 'Health problems that are not illness' included ageing, reproduction and problems that were not considered amenable to medical intervention. This category included a long list of health problems that are regarded as a normal part of growing old, such as rheumatism, arthritis, digestive disorders, varicose veins, palpitations and feeling the cold, as well as loss of hearing and vision. The informants clearly distinguished 'health problems that are not illness' from the notion of 'real illness' that required medical intervention, and 'normal illness', which covered self-limiting conditions, childhood ailments and everyday infections such as fevers and flu.

These coping abilities and the capacity to care for oneself or distinguish when to call in expert help may be considered as intellectual or metaphysical strengths, although they were not identified as such by the lay informants in these studies. Seedhouse (1986) associates the group of theories that consider health in terms of strengths or abilities with humanism. The emphasis they place on individual responses clearly supposes that everyone will have a unique and personal reaction to any given situation. In this formulation, health is described as a way of responding appropriately – as a means to an end, which is how Seedhouse justifies incorporating this viewpoint into his idea that health is a potential. He argues that 'potential' is the common factor that links the various ideas about health and approaches to increase it (listed in Box 30.2) and goes on to emphasize both choice and being realistic:

> A person's health is equivalent to the state of the set of conditions which fulfil or enable a person to work to fulfil his or her realistic chosen and biological potentials. Some of these conditions are of the highest importance for all people. Others are variable dependent upon individual abilities and circumstances (Seedhouse 1986: p. 76).

With its emphasis on potential, this theory is very 'future-oriented'. This may be a disadvantage for some older people, especially those who prefer to focus on their past with fondness and pride more than on a future that could seem comparatively limited. Alternatively, they may feel that striving for further achievement when they are coping with increasing disability or disease is too heavy a responsibility. However, Seedhouse suggests that people may continue to develop new potentials throughout life and in the face of quite serious disabilities or illnesses. He explains this in terms of maintaining a positive balance between 'liabilities' and 'obstacles' that threaten health (particularly adverse living conditions and diseases) and central conditions for maintaining health; his examples particularly emphasize personal control, understanding and autonomy in present situations.

This 'situational' emphasis is even more central in the third view of health to be considered – that of health as a process.

Health as process

The third way of looking at health emphasizes health as an ever-changing, dynamic phenomenon or process which:

> may relate to optimum physical growth and body development. The health process may be cumulative in relation, for example, to learning and development or cyclical in phases of creation and destruction. The point appears to be that health is a continuing pattern of change occurring over the lifetime in all dimensions of the individual (Anderson 1984: p. 61).

This viewpoint emphasizes that choices are greatly influenced by self-concept, environment and culture; likewise the ability (or not) to cope with stress or flow with experience. Regarding health as a process emphasizes seeing it as a means rather than an end in itself. Although this is similar in many respects to the idea of health as 'potential', a key difference lies in the fact that 'processes' require context and meaning to make sense of them – so linkages, patterns, interconnections and actions are emphasized more than separate factors or events. If health is viewed as a process, it is not possible to conceive any aspect of it that can stand alone, or be under the control of anyone other than the people whose health is under discussion; the whole sociocultural context is important (Cowley 1995).

This integration is central to autonomy and self-care; people act in certain ways because of the meanings they attach to those actions, according to what they regard as 'normal' and to the power they have to make choices (Kickbusch 1989). These three points are drawn from the seminal work of Giddens (1976); ascribed meanings, norms and power relate to the particular context of a person's life and the experiences he or she has had in the past and expects to have in future. Health is not often the central reason for deciding on a particular course of action. Indeed, Kickbusch (1989) suggests that increasing control over one's life is more important than considering health as an outcome and end in itself. However, everyday choices (such as what to eat for lunch or where to live) may be forced on older people in the name of health, particularly when they are in a 'crisis' situation following an acute illness, sudden hospitalization, increased disability or the dependency that often accompanies advanced years.

There is a view enshrined in medical science that all diseases and disorders have a single or specific cause; much medical research is directed at determining which factor causes a particular disease (Neihoff & Schneider 1993). Taken to its extreme, this view can be used to suppose that health is best promoted by focusing on identifying and preventing these determinants of disease, rather than taking into account individual healing processes. One of the most significant 'process' theories opposes this view, stressing the importance of starting from a consideration of how health is created and maintained, rather than focusing on the negative aspects of illness and disorder (Antonovsky 1987).

This health-creating, 'salutogenic' theory (which is the opposite of 'pathogenic' theories that focus on causes of disease) has been singled out as particularly useful for promoting older people's health (Sidell 1997) since it challenges the notion that older people are somehow a 'high-risk' group. Health-visiting practice is based in a philosophy of salutogenesis, so Rogers (2003) argues that there is a need for more health visitors to work with older people, but that workforce is gradually getting smaller. All human beings face pathogenic challenges and risks from disease but, by virtue of having survived the challenges for a greater number of years than their young relatives, older people have demonstrated their salutogenic ability. Instead of asking what stops them from being sick, Sidell (1997) suggests we should be asking how they remain healthy. There were 8560 people over the age of 100 years in England and Wales in 2001 (National Statistics online 2004c), compared to only 300 in 1951 (Population Statistics, OPCS & Government Actuary's Department 1994). Fewer than half of these centenarians (47%) live in communal establishments, with the rest remaining in ordinary households. Presumably they have learned something about maintaining their health during the course of their long lives!

Antonovsky's (1987) idea is that life experiences produce 'generalised resistance resources', which are positive methods of responding and adapting to situations. These resistance resources promote the development and maintenance of a strong 'sense of coherence', which is described as the extent to which one has a pervasive, enduring and dynamic feeling of confidence that things will work out as well as can reasonably be expected. This explanation locates the theory very closely in the person's own context, expectations and culture, but it incorporates practical and physiological aspects as well. These are explained in the three central components of a sense of coherence, which are manageability, meaningfulness and com-

prehensibility, and are explored below. Table 30.2 summarizes the fundamental differences between salutogenesis and preventive approaches drawn from the more usual pathogenic paradigm (after Cowley & Billings 1997).

The idea of *manageability* refers to the extent to which people feel they have the resources to meet demands that arise in their daily lives. This includes resources that are under direct individual control or those accessible from family, friends or the community. For older people, this may involve having the confidence that they can obtain suitable treatment or learn coping strategies for dealing with a long-term sickness or distressing symptoms, for example. Health care professionals may serve as 'resources' if they are able to help in practical ways or teach ways of coping. The idea depends quite closely on people experiencing a practical and physical sense of self-empowerment in coping with their own biology and threats to health.

Comprehensibility refers to the extent to which sense and order can be drawn from the situation, and the world seems understandable, ordered, consistent and

Table 30.2 Alternative perspectives on health

Pathogenesis	Salutogenesis
Main focus: disorder, i.e. treatment of disease, problems, difficulties, dysfunction	Main focus: order, i.e. sense of coherence, of well-being and personal experience
Concerned with: professional knowledge; medical science and objective understanding: empirical measurements	Concerned with: lay knowledge; personal experience and subjective understanding: human values
Prevention involves identifying risk factors, e.g. of disease, disability, delayed development; identifying and removing barriers to health	Prevention involves creating resources for health, e.g. caring, trust, autonomy, growth, development; promoting healthy activities, e.g. participation, involvement
Essentially reactive: only looks to the future if it can be scientifically predicted	Essentially proactive: looks at the potential for improving the future
Individual emphasis: separateness and single focus (e.g. germ theory of disease, medical prescription, single patient)	Social focus: sociocultural context and integration – meaningfulness, comprehensibility and manageability

clear. In translating an exceptional experience such as illness, disability or unpleasant symptoms into the 'normal' context of their everyday lives, people make sense of what is happening to them and can gain strength to deal with the situation. Williams & Popay (1994) explain that personal knowledge borne of what they term the 'privilege of experience' may differ from the scientific knowledge held by health care professionals. Nevertheless, they stress that lay knowledge is generally internally consistent, logical and rational. This is especially important for older people, whose wealth of personal experience may be a source of individual strength to cope with health problems in a way that is unique and meaningful to them.

The sense of *meaningfulness* individuals can gain from a situation refers to their ability to participate fully in the processes shaping their future. This participation is central to the definition of health outlined in the Ottawa Charter (World Health Organization 1986) which links health to an ability to take decisions and control over one's life; as such, health cannot be separated from the psychosocial context in which the person lives. To be fully engaged in the health-creating processes of their own lives, people need to 'make sense' of events in an emotional as well as a cognitive sense. This means setting symptoms, experiences, treatments and coping mechanisms in the context of their own family, friends, personal contacts and reasons for living. Social relationships are significantly implicated in enhancing health (House et al. 1988). They may be linked to the extent to which life continues to hold a positive meaning for older people and are a useful marker for health inequalities, in that those with fewer sources of such support have poorer health (Grundy & Sloggett 2003).

'Health as process' theories favour concentrating on salutogenic approaches that create or enable health to develop, which may avoid some of the negative stereotyping that automatically assumes that older people have poor health. Alternatively, this viewpoint may be criticized on the grounds that it is unrealistic only to think about the positive aspects of health, given the patterns of morbidity and raised incidence of both acute and long-term sickness among older people. Even so, there is much to be said for assuming that people accumulate certain personal strengths and wisdom in the course and process of their everyday lives that can serve as resources to enable them to cope with health problems that may arise in old age.

Summary: the concept of health

This section has reviewed three different ways of looking at health: as a product, as potential and as a process. There are some aspects in common between each view and they are better regarded as complementary rather than as competing. Health is not the opposite of disease, but sickness does occur and has a significant impact on health; this is never more important than in the later years, when disabling symptoms, diagnosed illnesses and long-standing disabilities occur with increased frequency (Tinker 1997). Illnesses and disabilities may be best acknowledged through the notion of health as a state, or product.

However, only looking at illness and disability patterns across a group of people can undermine individual aspirations and perceptions. In a study of over-90-year-olds, for example, only 8% rated themselves as either unfit or very unfit, despite the fact that some 93% of them had a chronic disorder or health problem (Bury & Holme 1991). Personal perceptions may be better acknowledged in the concept of health as individual potential. Also, there is a paradox, 'that health is a goal that is desired universally, but which does not have a universally shared meaning, and so cannot be desired universally' (Seedhouse 1986: p. 10).

It is important to acknowledge that health is a social rather than a medical concept. This is particularly strongly acknowledged in the view of health as a process, since it emphasizes the inseparability of health from the context in which it occurs. This is significant for older people, whose health is demonstrably affected by their psychosocial context, including the amount of autonomy and social support they have (Rowe & Kahn 1987). Reviewing a wide range of research about health, Rijke (1993) has identified several characteristics of health that help to integrate the different aspects of the overall concept; they are summarized in Box 30.4.

Health is regarded by the World Health Organization as a fundamental human right, which suggests that all people should have access to the basic resources for health (World Health Organization 1998). The challenge for nurses is to decide how to

---

Box 30.4   Characteristics of health

- Autonomy
- Will to live
- Experience of meaning and purpose in life
- Creative expression of meaning
- Body awareness
- Consciousness of inner development
- Individuality: the experience of being part of a greater whole
- Vitality, energy

promote health for older people. Theories of health promotion explain the different approaches and give some guidance in selecting suitable frameworks for practice. These are considered next.

HEALTH PROMOTION

The definition of health promotion offered by the Ottawa Charter on Health Promotion (World Health Organization 1986) has been criticized at least as vigorously as the World Health Organization's initial definition of health (discussed earlier). However, it offers a useful starting point for discussion by stating that:

> Health promotion is the process of enabling people to increase control over, and to improve, their health. To reach a state of complete physical, mental and social well-being, an individual or group must be able to identify and to realize aspirations, to satisfy needs and to change or cope with the environment. Health is, therefore, seen as a resource for everyday life, not the objective of living. Health is a positive concept, encompassing social and personal resources as well as physical capacities. Therefore, health promotion is not just the responsibility of the health sector, but goes beyond healthy life-styles to well-being (World Health Organization 1986 reproduced in Cribb & Dines 1993: p. 206).

The main criticisms centre on the fact that the definition is so broad that it can incorporate almost any activities and lead to so many interpretations that the idea of 'health promotion' could become almost meaningless (Tannahill 1985). Indeed, health promotion is probably far too complex and dynamic to be viewed as a single concept or be encompassed within a single definition, despite valiant attempts to clarify its meaning (Maben & Macleod Clark 1995).

Health promotion is an essentially contested term, with the concepts of 'health' and 'promotion' both being open to fierce debate and controversy (Dines & Cribb 1993). A selection of the different, sometimes conflicting and convoluted views of health has already been examined above. While they offer some clues about different approaches to enhancing health, there is no straightforward pathway from the various concepts of health to action in health promotion. Furthermore, new approaches, strategies and models are being developed all the time, in line with new ideas, innovations and changing government policies.

Health promotion has become a significant discipline, having developed initially from the public health movements of the nineteenth and twentieth centuries (Bunton & Macdonald 1992). Understanding is made more difficult by the fact that health promotion shares many of its roots, aims, beliefs and principles with a number of kindred disciplines such as public health, primary health care, community development and environmental health. Furthermore, it encompasses both a guiding philosophy and a set of activities that are undertaken across agencies and by many professionals, who may each interpret the term differently and feel varying degrees of ownership of the concept of health promotion.

This part of the chapter will unravel some of these complexities and explore the potential for health-promoting approaches when nursing older people in a variety of different situations. First, some of the background will be given about how old-fashioned approaches to health education fell into disrepute, leading to a modernizing of the concept as one vital part of health promotion. This discussion will lead on to a consideration of health protection, which is closely associated with public health work and is another of the concepts incorporated under the umbrella term of health promotion. Prevention is the third key aspect of health promotion, and the terminology and approaches used in that sphere will be explained.

There have been many debates and controversies about what counts as health promotion, so this part of the chapter will conclude by detailing the important principles that need to underpin all the work. It will explain that recognizing and evaluating health promotion requires a consideration of both the activities of health promotion and the principles that informed their planning and implementation.

Health education

The new ideals embedded in the term 'health promotion' were developed, in part, to challenge the supremacy of the rather didactic approach to health education that was prevalent before the 1970s. Health education had developed before and after the Second World War; during this period people were expected to respect authority and obey orders without question. It was a great age of discovery as countless new so-called 'wonder drugs' such as antibiotics, steroids and effective immunizations were developed; this led to a growing belief in the almost magical power of medicine to prevent, treat and cure an ever-increasing range of illnesses. In keeping with this period of history, the 'traditional approach' to health education assumed that people should obey doctors' orders in order to become healthy. A further assumption of this approach was that people had only to be given information about what they needed to do to persuade them to change their behaviour.

Inevitably, this 'health persuasion' approach failed, as shown by a huge mass of research (Beattie 1991). Because it was so professionally led, people were often unable to follow the instructions given to them. People with inadequate incomes were unable to eat the special diets they were advised to, for example, or to heat damp homes to prevent hypothermia. Written instructions, in the ubiquitous and still popular 'health education leaflet', assume that people are able to see and to read the sometimes complex language used. Leaflets are often available in only one language (English) and assume cultural homogeneity among the people reading them. If that was ever true of UK society, it is certainly no longer the case. In 2001, just 91.7% of pensioners in England and Wales were born in the UK (National Statistics online 2004c), and both the percentage and absolute numbers of people from minority ethnic groups are expected to rise noticeably over the coming decades (Tinker 1997). The old-fashioned approach to health education fell into disrepute partly because it was shown to be ineffective and insensitive but also because it supports professional knowledge and discredits people's own personal beliefs and experience (Beattie 1991). A more serious charge than ineffectiveness concerns the claim that it actually does harm by disempowering people (Illich 1976) and by holding them responsible for things that they are unable to change; this has been termed 'victim-blaming' (Crawford 1977). Unfortunately, health persuasion and giving firm advice remain remarkably prevalent and popular amongst some professionals (including nurses, who often believe they 'know better' than their patients) and politicians. The former policy of the *Health of the Nation* (Department of Health 1992) had stressed lifestyles and advising individuals about how they should behave, in order to be healthy. There has been some change, in that the more recent public health policy, *Choosing Health: Making Healthy Choices Easier* (Department of Health 2004) stressed the importance of partnership-working and taking account of the experience of people whose health is to be promoted. A major criticism of this, and of much recent government policy, is the lack of attention paid to the older population, only partly mitigated by the production of the *NSF for Older People* (Department of Health 2001). There is still a tendency, too, for information about health to be given in a way that implies firm direction.

In the context of this chapter, it is worth bearing in mind that the older population of today grew up in the time when this kind of directive approach was expected. That is not to say either that they approved of it or that they felt it to be a benefit, although some might have done. However, they may not voice objections to being 'told what to do' by professionals as much as younger people who have grown up in a consumerist society, expecting to be consulted and have their views taken into account. Illich (1976) led the attack on what he called 'the expropriation of health' by the medical profession. He suggested that placing doctors in charge of decisions about all important aspects of social life (for example, deciding who should be classified as 'disabled' and therefore entitled to welfare benefits) is essentially harmful because it destroys the potential of people to recognize their own needs (like deciding for themselves if they are disabled or not) and to deal with their own vulnerability and human weaknesses in a unique and personal way.

Modern approaches to health education, developed in response to these criticisms, take into account the physical, practical, social and psychological context of people's lives, and aim to enable them to develop this autonomy (Weare 1992). Health education is now defined as comprising 'consciously constructed opportunities for learning, involving some form of communication designed to improve health literacy, including improving knowledge, and developing life skills which are conducive to individual and community health' (World Health Organization 1998: p. 14). Approaches may aim to help people individually by enabling them to develop the skills they need, or they may focus on whole groups and communities with a view to changing cultural expectations where these serve as a constraint (Tones 1993). To make autonomous and empowered choices, individuals need social, psychomotor and self-regulatory skills and other competencies; they also need to live in a supportive and healthy society that provides the practical, psychosocial and cultural environment that is needed for them to exercise such choices (Tones 1997). The key differences between traditional and modern approaches to health education are summarized in Table 30.3.

In health promotion circles, the traditional approach to health education is often disparagingly called an 'individualistic approach', which may seem confusing to nurses who generally strongly approve of strategies that either allow or insist on 'individualized care' (Gallagher & Burden 1993, Pursey & Luker 1995). However, a failure to recognize that very few individuals are in a position to exercise a completely free choice in the way they behave is the major problem. It is partly to overcome such constraints that the older people's NSF suggests that the NHS and councils should work to develop 'healthy communities which support older people to live lives which are as fulfilling as possible. This will include working with

Table 30.3 Health education

Traditional approach	Modern approach
• Assumes that health educators are the experts, and they know which relevant and appropriate information to pass on	• Respects and values the beliefs, culture and knowledge of the recipient of health education as well as the educator
• Concentrates on health educators giving information to passive recipients	• Assumes education is participatory and communication is two-way
• Information may be transmitted by verbal instruction or written leaflets	• Concentrates on developing life skills, self-esteem and autonomy
• Concentrates on prevention of disease and negative health	• Explicitly aimed at both positive health and prevention of negative aspects
• Emphasizes physical disease and medical risk factors	• Physical, social and mental aspects are all considered equally important
• Assumes people are free to choose their behaviour	• Recognizes sociopolitical context and major constraints to health-related behaviour
• Efforts are targeted at individuals	• Efforts may be targeted at individuals, groups and/or communities
• The collective and social context of health is not addressed	• Addresses both the individual and collective (social) context of health

council services such as leisure and lifelong learning' (Department of Health 2001: p. 107).

Some observers might argue that emphasizing the importance of rational choices, defined as such because they meet the views and requirements of professional experts, could relegate anyone who is unable or unwilling to behave in an approved manner to the stigma of being considered irrational, ignorant or non-compliant (Case study 30.1). However, most people have a store of personal wisdom and health beliefs upon which to draw; the role of the health educator is to enable the development of life skills and self-esteem, in order to promote autonomy and self-empowerment. While this may be achieved by one-to-one education, it often involves working with wider groups who support and learn from each other, or to help change culturally entrenched patterns of behaviour and health belief. These may be linked with formal religious or ethnic groupings, but more often simply relate to personal experience and the habits of a lifetime.

Tinker (1997) reviews a number of surveys about the eating patterns of the older population, for example. These show that most older people eat a similar diet to the rest of the population, but generally consume smaller quantities. Malnutrition is an occasional problem, but obesity and overweight are prevalent. Older people are more likely to eat fresh vegetables, salad and fruit than those between the ages of 16 and 44 years old, but are also more likely to use solid fat,

drink whole milk and add salt when cooking. Home refrigeration was not widely available when the current retired population were youngsters developing their eating habits, so salted food was a more significant part of a normal diet. Likewise, frozen vegetables, skimmed-milk products and vegetable oils have only become usual during the last 30 years or so – long after most 70–90-year-olds formed their cooking and eating preferences.

While health education can target a wide audience (for example, by campaigns in the mass media) to create changes in culture, expectations and health beliefs, this does nothing to remove many of the structural barriers to change or causes of ill health. In addition to creating a more modern approach to health education, it was necessary for health promoters to find new ways of removing some of these barriers. The sphere of 'health protection' is considered next.

Health protection

The nineteenth century was a period of huge public health reform; slums were cleared and replaced with safe housing, sewage systems installed in the large cities to ensure a clean water supply and regulations enacted about the slaughter of animals to secure a safe supply of food. Once these major reforms had been achieved, there was a tendency for the public at large and the medical profession as a whole to believe that there were no other really important barriers to public

Case study 30.1   Different styles of health education in practice

When the district nurse visited 82-year-old Mrs Mary Davies to follow up her visit to the accident and emergency department, she found her upset, miserable and in pain. She had been walking back home from the paper shop, when her bad knee gave way. She fell and could not get up; someone had called an ambulance. First Mrs Davies felt silly, then relieved, because they were kind and checked her over, which made her feel safe. But then that nurse had told her she was far too heavy and she must lose weight or she might not be so lucky next time; she should do more exercise, the nurse said. She didn't know how she was supposed to exercise when she could hardly move – her bad knee was swollen and bruised and the bandages they had put on felt too tight.

At times like this she missed her first husband, who had always been very practical and would have known what to do. Not that he liked skinny women, mind you – he used to say he liked a bit of meat to get hold of! Bert, her second husband, was kind in his way, as well, and had made some sausages and bacon for her dinner before he went out. Fried food had always given her indigestion, but she had always done all the cooking so he didn't know how to make stews and pies like she did. She had always been on the large side, and had never had time for exercise, what with having to walk all the way to shops and carry the things back two or three times a week. It used to be better when there was a greengrocers at the end of the road. You couldn't get fresh vegetables now like you used to, and she missed having a natter to her neighbours while she waited to be served. Mind you, her old friends had nearly all moved away or had to go into homes now – she didn't like to think about when that would happen to her. The paper shop sold most of what you needed and the milkman delivered some tinned food, but it was too far to walk to the shops at the other end of the estate, and they cost a fortune too.

Mary felt much better by the time this nurse had left and Bert had come home. She couldn't really recall that the nurse had said much, but she had stayed some time and put the bandage on her leg right, which eased the pain. Mary wasn't sure why she had told the nurse so much about herself – just nattering, she supposed. She had never thought of walking to the shops as 'exercise' before – it was just what you had to do. Of course, she had always known about good home cooking, and she was sure she could find some recipes that used less fat – like in the war, when you couldn't get it anyway. She said she would look some of them out for the nurse, who was too young to remember rationing but was interested in it. Mind you, it would be good to be able to get some fresh vegetables again. She hadn't heard about that 'dial and ride' to the shops idea. The nurse said it was like a minibus that came right to your door and took you to the shops, but you had to share it with other people going in the same direction and sometimes it meant waiting for a while for everyone to get together. That would be like the old days, talking to friends while you waited, and you could get a whole batch of vegetables in one go, so you would save money there. It did make sense too, to think that her bad knee might not hurt so much if she was less heavy – and she won't mind talking to that nurse about her weight when she comes again.

As she left the house, the district nurse recalled the number of meetings she had attended with voluntary organizations and the local council to get the 'dial and ride' scheme off the ground. Her manager had sometimes been a bit peeved about her involvement, because he did not see what it had to do with nursing. But she had been able to explain the importance of choice and mobility in health terms, which had helped convince the councillors that their investment in the scheme was worthwhile – and it was certainly proving to be a really useful community resource for so many proud and independent older people on her caseload, like Mrs Davies.

---

health, and the whole movement shifted its attention to developing personal preventive measures and therapeutic treatments for illness (Ashton & Seymour 1988). However, just as the limitations of the traditional approach to health education became apparent, it soon became obvious that there was a continuing need to ensure that society as a whole provided the kind of environment that made healthy choices not just possible, but easier and preferable to the alternatives.

Health protection can, therefore, be seen as the descendant of the old, regulatory approach to public health, although it too has been infused with a modernizing vigour. Public health is considered further below, but health protection is its political wing, and still an essential part of health promotion. It has been defined as follows:

> Health protection comprises legal and fiscal controls, other regulations and policies and voluntary codes of practice aimed at the enhancement of positive health and the prevention of ill-health (Downie et al. 1990: p. 51).

Fiscal policies that influence the wealth, employment situation and availability of housing and welfare benefits for the whole population clearly have an impact on health, since poverty and inequalities are closely implicated as causes of ill health (Townsend et al. 1988, Blackburn 1991, Benzeval et al. 1995). Lifelong limitations on health choices have an accumulative and adverse impact in old age, to the extent that Rowe & Kahn (1987) have suggested that the usual picture gives a distorted image of how successful ageing might be. The impact of living in an unequal society is believed to have an adverse effect in itself, as there are measurable increases in crime and a lack of social cohesion in countries that experience the greatest inequalities in health (Wilkinson 1996). This, too, is significant for many older people living in a society in which they no longer feel safe and health inequalities are discernible at all ages (Grundy & Sloggett 2003).

It is not only the economic situation that is important; general legislation is significant in the sphere of health protection. Personal choice may be sacrificed for the benefit of the health of the public in general. In some cases, this is to protect vulnerable people from exploitation, as in laws that control the sale and use of dangerous drugs, setting age limits for the sale of alcohol and tobacco or providing protection to children from abuse at the hands of their parents and adult caretakers. There is no legislative equivalent to protect older people from family violence, although dependency may render them as vulnerable as small children (Biggs & Phillipson 1992).

Indeed, there is increasing concern about abuse within residential care settings and nursing homes too (UKCC 1997) and regulation in this sphere may be seen as one form of 'health protection'. In a move designed to provoke policy developments, the World Health Organization supported the Toronto Declaration on Elder Abuse in 2002. This declaration defines elder abuse as 'a single or repeated act, or lack of appropriate action, occurring within any relationship where there is an expectation of trust, which causes harm or distress to an older person. It can be of various forms: physical, psychological/emotional, sexual, financial or simply reflect intentional or unintentional neglect' (World Health Organization 2002b: p. 3). Chapter 32 provides a wide discussion of abuse of older people. Placing the issue of elder abuse within a framework of universal human rights, the Toronto Declaration stresses that preventing elder abuse in an ageing world is everybody's business. This is intended to encourage all governments to develop systems to deal with this major problem. Key requirements of an effective preventive system, agreed in Toronto, are reproduced in Box 30.5.

Box 30.5 Toronto declaration on elder abuse (www.who.int/hpr/ageing)

- A cultural perspective is mandatory in order to understand fully the phenomenon of elder abuse, i.e. the cultural context of any particular community in which it occurs
- Equally important is to consider a gender perspective, as the complex social constructs related to it help to identify the form of abuse inflicted by whom
- In any society some population subgroups are particularly vulnerable to elder abuse, such as the very old, those with limited functional capacity, women and the poor
- Ultimately elder abuse will only be successfully prevented if a culture that nurtures intergenerational solidarity and rejects violence is developed
- It is not enough to identify cases of elder abuse. All countries should develop the structures that will allow the provision of services (health, social, legal protection, police referral) to respond appropriately and eventually prevent the problem

---

Sometimes regulation is used effectively to 'protect people from themselves'. Examples of such laws include the compulsory use of seat belts in cars and crash helmets by motor cyclists, the banning of smoking on the London Underground system, numerous health and safety regulations in the workplace, laws concerning the control of communicable diseases and the mental health provisions that allow care to be imposed on people who are legally deemed unable to maintain their own safety.

Some health protective regulations are intended to 'facilitate' rather than compel. Improving uptake of influenza vaccine was one of the key targets to come from the *NSF for Older People* (Department of Health 2001). This is not a compulsory requirement but, by making the vaccination available free to all over the age of 65 years, it is hoped that the annual morbidity and mortality from this disease will be reduced. By 2003, the number of over-65s taking up this health protective measure had risen to 68% (Department of Health 2003).

Even though, in the developed world, the major causes of death in the older population are from noncommunicable diseases, older people can still be particularly vulnerable to the impact of infectious disease. A warning to the world to avoid complacency about communicable diseases came in 2003, when sudden acute respiratory syndrome (SARS) made international headlines. SARS was a newly identified human infection caused by a coronavirus and transmitted during face-to-face exposure to infected droplets expelled during coughing or sneezing (World Health Organization 2003). The disease spread rapidly, with the international outbreak eventually causing more than 8000 cases and 900 deaths in 30 countries. Overall, around 11% of those infected died, but this ratio was much higher in the older population (World Health Organization 2003).

Concentrating on the national and legislative aspects of this sphere of health promotion activity tends to distract from its importance for nurses, who may feel that, since they are not in a position to enact laws, it holds no relevance for them. However, gathering evidence that helps to make a case for legislation is part of health protection. Nurses may usefully provide health-related information for policy reviews and serve as a resource to campaigning groups or voluntary organizations concerned with the welfare of older people. Professional nursing associations are a useful forum for debate, and they are generally involved in contributing to the formulation of policy, particularly in relation to health service provision.

Local policies can enable or inhibit healthy choices too, and there is a clear role for nurses in contributing to these plans (Case study 30.2). Health visitors adopted the idea of 'the influence on policies affecting health' as one of their key principles during the 1970s (Council for the Education and Training of Health Visitors (CETHV) 1977), and drew attention to the significance of strategies and plans that operate at a more local level (Twinn & Cowley 1992). Furthermore, the principles that are intended to apply to developing policies at a broader level are generally just as applicable to a strategy planned at the level of a hospital ward, local clinic or general practice. These were initially set out by the World Health Organization when they developed a strategy to establish Health for All by the Year 2000 in 1977 (Kickbusch 1987), then clarified and developed through later discussions and

---

Case study 30.2   A health-promoting strategy

Janis Jones is the senior nurse and manager on a busy medical ward. She had become really frustrated with trying to cope with new contract requirements, constantly raising expectations and the ever-faster speed of throughput. Actually, when she reflected on why she felt so irritated by it all, she realized that was part of the problem. Not only was the ward constantly busy all the time, but she hated the depersonalizing language, the need to move people on as if they were bits of baggage and the constant pressure to clear beds. It worked all right, of course; they worked with the liaison nurses and followed the hospital discharge policy, so they got people out as quickly as they could, but she had a constant, nagging feeling that it could be better.

As she reflected on this state of affairs, Janis realized that even though she could not control all the pressures and outside influences, she could develop a way of coping with them in her ward. She decided to consult the nurses on her staff about discharge planning for older people in the ward, because they were often the most vulnerable or in need of special help when they returned home. After some discussion, the nurses decided to review the procedure for everyone, because it would be fairer and easier to implement across the board; in any case most of their patients were in the older age range. Janis arranged for the community nurse liaison, occupational therapist, ward social worker and medical consultant to come to the

next meeting. She was quite anxious about that because there had been some angry phone calls in the past, when she had had to send someone home rather quickly to clear a bed or if communications had gone astray for some reason. But when the meeting happened they were all very supportive and interested in developing ways of making the process smoother and agreed to help her and the ward nurses to work on the new discharge planning system.

It took a lot longer than she had thought it would to develop a really effective and workable system. However, once they had begun to involve the other professionals, some patients and their families (Janis felt a bit embarrassed at not thinking of them first) it gradually started to fall into place. They had to get used to working with so many people beyond the ward staff, but it seemed natural now; as did talking with patients about discharge as soon as they arrived. After all, they knew they would not be staying in that ward permanently, and mostly they were very pleased to be discussing going home. They were not so happy if it was likely that they would need transferring to a care home, but at least their relatives and social workers got involved sooner, and could support the patients when they needed it. The whole ward team felt quite proud of their system once they had started to use it, and it was much easier to liaise with the community staff and social worker now they knew them better.

Continued

Case study 30.2   A health-promoting strategy (*Continued*)

Perhaps it was just coincidence that the patients seemed more relaxed, but Janis was sure she was getting fewer anxious telephone calls from relatives. The new system seemed far more satisfying for the nurses, because they started considering discharge earlier, documented what they had asked and who they had spoken to on the care plan and discussed with the patients whenever they could. They felt confident that their care was taking individual circumstances and personal preferences into account as far as possible, even though emergency pressure still arose. Now, when

there were sudden demands for a bed to be cleared, the nurses felt much better able to decide, in conjunction with the patient, whether an earlier discharge was feasible or not.

Janis was keen to see if it was really making the kind of difference she thought it was. She decided her next move was to arrange to have the system audited properly, and to see if the approach could be fully incorporated into the hospital policy instead of just being an 'optional extra' on her ward.

---

conferences about the importance of primary health care at Alma-Ata (World Health Organization 1978) and health promotion in Ottawa (World Health Organization 1986). The principles are summarized in Box 30.6.

Prevention

The widespread criticisms that have been made about problems arising from a concentration *only* on medically dominant approaches to health promotion should not distract from the significant contribution that medicine makes to the prevention of disease. The key issue is that health promotion should be wider

than disease prevention alone; indeed, prevention is not only concerned with illness. Nevertheless, a number of the most clearly measurable benefits to health have come from advances in this sphere and nurses have a major role in contributing to the prevention of disorders, dependency and other unwanted states in older people. In each of the NSFs, prevention is highlighted as a priority, not only in terms of preventing the problem from arising in the first place, but also to minimize the effects of the disease once it has occurred. Preventive work is often described using a typology drawn from work on preventive psychiatry (Caplan 1969), which classifies prevention according to which stage of disease development is targeted (Box 30.7).

Primary prevention aims to avoid the onset of a disorder in the first place, as in the *NSF for Coronary Heart Disease* (Department of Health 2000a). Standards 1 and 2 are concerned with reducing heart disease in the population, indicating that the NHS and partner agencies should, first, develop, implement and monitor policies that reduce the prevalence of coronary risk factors in the population, and reduce inequalities in risks of developing heart disease and, second, contribute to a reduction in the prevalence of smoking in the local population. Secondary prevention aims to minimize harm by early identification and treatment, as in the extension of screening for breast and cervical cancer notified in *The NHS Cancer Plan* (Department of Health 2000b), which was the first NSF to be published. Sadly, the NSFs do not, in the main, focus on primary or secondary prevention in the older population, despite the potential for huge improvements in the health of this age group. The key target for reducing deaths from coronary heart disease focuses on those under the age of 70 years, as does routine cancer screening, although it is available on request for older people. However, there is a strong focus on tertiary

---

Box 30.6   Guiding principles for health strategies

Five principles are critical in developing health promotion policy:

1. Equity, particularly equity of access to the prerequisites for health, but also in accessing health care provision and services
2. Participation to affirm the right of people to define health in their own terms and build on individual, social and cultural diversity
3. Collective responsibility, accepting that health is primarily a social enterprise. Development at grassroots level is as significant as central policy; emphasizes multidisciplinary, collaborative actions and healthy alliances
4. 'Ecological vision' means taking full account of the impact of physical and social environments on people's health
5. Increasing options through policies, so that healthy choices are easier than unhealthy ones

> **Box 30.7   Prevention**
>
> **Primary prevention**
> - Prevention of the first onset or first manifestation of a disease process, or some other first occurrence. May involve reduction of risk factors or strengthening of personal resources for health
>
> **Secondary prevention**
> - Prevention of the progression of a disease process or other unwanted state, through early detection when this affects outcome favourably. Screening and ready access to health care are both important
>
> **Tertiary prevention**
> - Prevention of avoidable complications of an irreversible, manifest disease or some other unwanted state. Includes rehabilitative aspects of care and management of incurable or chronic disorders and of disabilities
>
> **Also consider:**
> - Prevention of the recurrence of an illness or other unwanted phenomenon

prevention, which is concerned with rehabilitation and avoidance of complications of disease, in all of the NSFs. The target for people with diabetes to be offered screening for the early detection (and treatment if needed) of diabetic retinopathy (Department of Health 2004), a key cause of blindness in older people, was carried forward as a major priority for all primary care trusts (Department of Health 2002).

Some commentators, such as Downie et al. (1990), extend prevention to incorporate unwanted states other than diseases. In practice, it is extremely difficult to separate activities as precisely as the typology in Box 30.7 suggests, particularly once the idea is extended beyond disease to include unwanted states. The prevalence of obesity among older people has been noted, for example; this is not only an unwanted state in itself, but it may be relevant to the onset of heart disease, worsening of mobility and joint problems and various other disorders. Should a weight reduction programme, therefore be classified as 'primary prevention' of a heart disease that is not yet manifest? Or would it be better to regard obesity as a 'disease' in itself, being treated to avoid the unwanted further complications that may arise if it is left unchecked by this 'tertiary prevention'? The actual designation does not really seem to matter too much;

what is important is for people to achieve the end result of preventing avoidable disorders.

The idea of 'risk factors' that contribute to diseases or problems is important in primary prevention. However, identifying the patterns of risk factors is not the same as knowing the causes of disease. Indeed, Rijke (1993) claims that much of the research into risk factors is seriously flawed, because so many of the samples are drawn from treatment centres and clinics that are not representative of the healthy population as a whole. Many of the studies are retrospective, which is to say that they note factors held in common by people who have already developed the disease. These are not predictive in the sense of being able to tell who among the people that have those factors will identify the disorder; they generally disregard the protective factors and salutogenic influences that may serve as powerful resources for health.

Indeed, Skrabenek (1992) goes so far as to suggest that risk-factor epidemiology should be viewed as a non-science. From a list of 246 different factors implicated as risks for coronary heart disease by 1981, Skrabenek selected 46 to compare to a list of risk factors for scurvy, compiled before the lack of vitamin C was known to be the cause. Risk factors nominated (but not proven) as significant for heart disease included widowhood, illegitimate birth, no church attendance, alcoholism and slow beard growth; for scurvy, factors implicated included bad butter, debauchery, dampness, distilled spirits and gluttony. While Skrabanek's scepticism should be recognized as quite extreme, it does help to point out how often risk factors are targeted on grounds of 'moral approval' rather than necessarily because they offer a clear direction for preventive action.

However, some studies offer clear and helpful directions about which factors could be most usefully focused for change. From a prospective study, for example, Luukinen et al. (1996), identified being female, urinary urgency, a poor pulse rise after standing up, frequent fear of falling and one or more falls in the previous year as risk factors for falls among people over 70 years old and living at home in Finland. It would be possible to arrange for someone with urinary urgency to be investigated and possibly treated (see Chapter 17 on eliminating). Otherwise, provision of a home commode or advice about timing trips to the toilet may be sufficient to avoid falls caused by hurrying. Older people who fear falling may restrict their activities, thus reducing their functional ability and exposing themselves to even greater risk when they do move. Arranging a protected programme of activity to ensure the person retains, and possibly improves, mobility would be a useful preventive response.

There is a division between the medically oriented strategies for prevention and the more recent salutogenic approaches that mirror the traditional and modern approaches in health education. In contrast to the 'risk-factor approach' that emphasizes removing the threat of disease, for example, Rowe & Kahn (1987) review a wide range of research into ageing to reveal a more positive, health-oriented approach that would emphasize developing strengths and health potential. They question the view that impaired carbohydrate metabolism and osteoporosis are natural consequences of ageing, and suggest that exercise has the potential to improve the glucose intolerance, insulin resistance and bone loss often seen in this age group. In addition to these benefits, Dawe & Moore-Orr (1995) showed that mild exercise programmes improved memory, independence and mental health; the programmes were run by nurses for institutionalized patients aged 70 years and over, and consisted of 15 min stretching, flexing and walking. Regular, moderate activity has been shown to reduce the risk of cardiac death by 20–25% among people with established heart disease (Merz & Forrester 1997) so it is worth starting to exercise even after a medical problem has been diagnosed.

Rowe & Kahn (1987) also emphasize psychosocial factors in health and disease among older people. They suggest that providing help, care and material assistance to older people may be directly protective because of the physiological effects of social support and care. Like Rowe & Kahn (1987), Rijke (1993) emphasizes the importance of autonomy and choice in preventing health problems from developing in the first place. Psychosocial resources may also enable people to get better and earlier medical care, which is significant in relation to secondary prevention.

The sphere of tertiary prevention seems a natural extension of the nursing role, and many clinical nurse specialists (Wilson-Barnett & Beech 1994, Forbes et al. 2003) and practice nurses (Stilwell 1995, Smail 1996) have achieved high levels of expertise in enabling people to live fulfilled and active lives despite quite impaired functional ability or significant chronic illness (Case study 30.3).

On the whole nurses probably spend more time directing their health-promoting practice at individuals who already have established health problems, particularly when they come into contact with older people. This is hardly surprising given the nature of their role; it draws attention to the extensive opportunities that nurses have to undertake preventive work using the good assessment and communication skills which should now form part of their basic education and training (Macleod Clark et al. 1997).

However, there is a need for them to exercise their nursing skills in a health-promoting way. Some nurses appear inclined to communicate in ways that justifiably invoke all the criticisms directed at the traditional approaches to health education and prevention, while others appear able to implement what Macleod Clark (1993) terms 'health nursing'. This involves allowing people the opportunity to contribute and participate in decisions about their own health and preventive care; it draws attention to the principles that underpin and define health promotion work. These are considered next.

Case study 30.3 Tertiary prevention

Mr Brown had been attending outpatients on and off for more than 20 years, so he had seen some changes, especially when his old specialist left and the new one came. His rheumatism had started before he retired, but now it was getting more and more of a problem; he supposed it was what you had to expect when you were nearly 80.

It was different at the hospital now, though; instead of always seeing the doctor, he sometimes saw a nurse specialist. He was a bit uncertain about that at first, but now he had got to know her he was very happy about it – she really seemed to understand what he needed. She always put him through his paces, checking his tablets and how well he could walk, and got him moving joints that he didn't know moved any more! It wasn't just that,

though; he could talk to her. He didn't know how she knew which questions to ask, but she did – like this morning. He wasn't going to mention getting to the toilet – it was too embarrassing, like a child always with a dribble on his trousers. Perhaps that was why she asked him about how he was managing – but in such a matter-of-fact way that it just seemed natural to answer and not difficult at all. It might be easier to use a urinal, as she said; at least then he wouldn't be worn out with pain by the time he got to the toilet. He could give it a try, as she had arranged for him to borrow one from the hospital store. He wasn't too sure about having a home assessment though; he would think about it and let her know next time, like she suggested. Perhaps it would be a good idea but he would take his time to decide.

Principles of health promotion

Health promotion is continually developing and expanding. An updated definition explains that:

> Health promotion represents a comprehensive social and political process. It not only embraces actions directed at strengthening the skills and capabilities of individuals, but also action directed towards changing social, environmental and economic conditions so as to alleviate their impact on public and individual health. Health promotion is the process of enabling people to increase control over the determinants of health and thereby improve their health. Participation is essential to sustain health promotion action (World Health Organization 1998: p. 11).

This definition implies that almost all activities that are intended to improve health could conceivably be regarded as health promotion. However, as the above discussion has hinted, even some activities that are designated as such actually seem more likely to cause harm. Trying to classify different health promotion activities under particular headings seems doomed to failure, since so many facets of the work are interlinked and dependent on each other. This classification practice seemed important when proponents of health promotion were trying to emphasize its distinctive features in relation to the strategies that were prevalent until the early 1980s. Much energy was devoted to trying to decide whether a particular action was actually 'health promotion', or if it was 'only health education', or 'only disease prevention'.

Eventually it became clear that the tasks were less important than the intentions that informed their planning and the manner in which they were carried out. Some of the more harmful attitudes still prevail in nursing as elsewhere, so it may be important to ask of our practice, as Dines & Cribb (1993) suggest, 'is this being done in a health promoting way?' To answer that question it is necessary to apply the principles that inform health promotion; these have been advanced and developed since the World Health Organization established its health-for-all policy (World Health Organization 1986, Labonte 1997). The principles are summarized in Box 30.8.

These principles are not supposed to restrict, but the point is to ensure that health-promoting activities do not contravene them. In nursing, it may be that there still exists a directive, controlling and medicalized approach to 'traditional nursing'. This would clearly contravene the health-promoting principles and undermine the intent to promote health whatever nursing activities are involved. Alternatively, a more

---

Box 30.8   Principles of health promotion

Health promotion action means:

- building healthy policy
- creating supportive environments
- strengthening community action
- developing personal skills
- reorienting health services to primary care

Health promotion practice involves:

- enabling
- mediating
- advocacy

Health promotion:

- places a high value on citizen participation and collectivism
- questions the dominance of economic rationalism in public policy
- rejects professional dominance in favour of common understanding between lay and professional spheres of knowledge

---

participative, enabling and holistic 'modern' approach to nursing appears to be developing. This would be consistent with the principles of health promotion, and activities undertaken in this manner would promote health even if that was not their stated intention.

Public health

Health promotion sits within a wider framework of public health, which has been defined as the 'science and art of promoting health, preventing disease, and prolonging life through the organized efforts of society' (Acheson 1998). Public health is a social and political concept aimed at improving health, prolonging life and improving the quality of life among whole populations through health promotion, disease prevention and other forms of health intervention. In its glossary of terms, the World Health Organization (1998) points to the distinction that has been made in the health promotion literature between public health and a new public health, to emphasize significantly different approaches to the description and analysis of the determinants of health, and the methods of solving public health problems. As with the 'old and new' divisions in all other aspects described in this chapter, there is an expanded understanding in the more modern approach.

The new public health seeks a comprehensive understanding of the ways in which lifestyles and living conditions determine health status. It recognizes the need to mobilize resources and make sound investments in policies, programmes and services that create, maintain and protect health by supporting healthy lifestyles and creating supportive environments for health. Taking a new public health approach, the World Health Organization policy framework (World Health Organization 2002a) identifies the positive determinants of active ageing. These apply at all ages and interact to such an extent that it is rarely possible to identify a single factor that will predict how well an individual or population will age. Box 30.9 summarizes the determinants and key statements about them. Increasingly, health promoters are concerned with trying to influence health determinants, rather than concentrating on the individuals alone. Nurses need to be aware that these wider factors may be very influential in the health of older people in the long term, so they can take them into account and possibly influence them, should the occasion arise. Some nurses choose to work in public health departments, where there is likely to be a greater opportunity to work in partnership between the NHS and other agencies, developing projects and programmes directed at the determinants of health for a wider population, not just individuals.

CONCLUSION

This chapter has reviewed a selection of different ways of looking at the much-contested concept of 'health' and has considered different approaches to promoting health, with the older population in mind. Throughout, particular emphasis has been placed on the importance of autonomy, choice and enabling people to create health on their own terms. This is not only important as a philosophical basis for health promotion and for nursing; it is a necessary way of working if health promotion is to be successful and active ageing of older people is to become the norm. Taking a wide social and political approach to health promotion will lead nurses into the field of public health, with its emphasis on improving the health of the whole population.

Box 30.9   Determinants of active ageing

Cross-cutting determinants: culture and gender
- Culture, which surrounds all individuals and populations, shapes the way in which we age because it influences all of the other determinants of active ageing
- Gender is a 'lens' through which to consider the appropriateness of various policy options and how they will affect the well-being of both men and women

Determinants related to health and social service systems
- To promote active ageing, health systems need to take a lifecourse perspective that focuses on health promotion, disease prevention and equitable access to quality primary health care and long-term care
- Health promotion, disease prevention, curative services, long-term care and mental health services all need considering

Behavioural determinants
- The adoption of healthy lifestyles and actively participating in one's own care are important at all stages of the lifecourse. One of the myths of ageing is that it is too late to adopt such lifestyles in the later years

- Tobacco use, physical activity, healthy eating, oral health, alcohol, medications, iatrogenesis and adherence all need considering

Determinants related to personal factors
- While genes may be involved in the causation of disease, for many diseases the cause is environmental and external to a greater degree than it is genetic and internal
- Biology and genetics and psychological factors need considering

Determinants related to the physical environment
- Physical environments, safe housing, avoiding falls, clean water, clean air and safe foods all need considering
- The great majority of injuries are preventable; however, the traditional view of injuries as 'accidents' has resulted in historical neglect of this area of public health

Determinants related to the social and economic environment
- Social support, violence and abuse, education and literacy are all relevant
- Income and social protection are significant economic determinants of active ageing

Recommended reading

Kendall S (ed) (1999) Health and empowerment: research and practice. Arnold, London.
A collection of research about empowerment through different approaches to health promotion, including a chapter by Andrée le May (see Chapter 10 of this volume) about empowering older people through communication.

Raeburn J, Rootman I (1998) People-centred health promotion. Wiley, Chichester.
Clear, practice-focused text about health promotion, explaining the particular philosophy highlighted in the title.

Tones K, Green J (2004) Health promotion: planning and strategies. Sage, London.
Comprehensive text with lots of clear examples, explanations and research to illustrate the points made.

World Health Organization (2002) Active ageing: a policy framework. WHO, Geneva.
Can be downloaded from the World Health Organization website, at http://www.who.int/hpr/ageing, which also has a wealth of other papers and information about healthy ageing.

References

Acheson D 1998 Public health in England. HMSO, London

Aggleton P 1990 Health. Routledge, London

Anderson R 1984 Health promotion: an overview. European Monographs in Health Education Research 6: 4–119

Antonovsky A 1987 Unraveling the mystery of health: how people manage stress and stay well. Jossey Bass, San Francisco

Ashton J, Seymour H 1988 The new public health. Open University Press, Milton Keynes

Beattie A 1991 Knowledge and control in health promotion: a test case for social policy and social theory. In: Gabe J, Calnan M, Bury M (eds) Sociology of the health service. Routledge, London, pp 162–202

Biggs S, Phillipson C 1992 Understanding elder abuse: a training manual for helping professionals. Longman, Harlow

Blackburn C 1991 Poverty and health. Open University Press, Buckingham

Blaxter M 1990 Health and lifestyles. Tavistock/Routledge, London

Benzeval M, Judge K, Whitehead M (eds) 1995 Tackling inequalities in health: an agenda for action. King's Fund, London

Bunton R, Macdonald G 1992 Health promotion: disciplines and diversity. Routledge, London

Bury M, Holme A 1991 Life after ninety. Routledge, London

Caplan C 1969 An approach to community mental health. Tavistock Publications, London

Cornwell J 1984 Hard earned lives: accounts of health and illness from East London. Tavistock Publications, London

Council for the Education and Training of Health Visitors (CETHV) 1977 An investigation into the principles and practice of health visiting. CETHV, London

Cowley S 1995 Health-as-process: a health visiting perspective. Journal of Advanced Nursing 22: 433–441

Cowley S, Billings J 1997 Family health needs project research report. Department of Nursing Studies, King's College, London

Crawford R 1977 You are dangerous to your health: the ideology and politics of victim-blaming. International Journal of Health Services 7: 633–680

Cribb A, Dines A 1993 Health promotion: concepts. In: Dines A, Cribb A (eds) Health promotion: concepts and practice. Blackwell Scientific Publications, Oxford, pp 3–63

Dawe D, Moore-Orr R 1995 Low-intensity, range-of-motion exercise: invaluable nursing care for elderly patients. Journal of Advanced Nursing 21: 675–681

Department of Health 1992 Health of the nation: a strategy for health in England. HMSO, London

Department of Health 2004 Choosing health: making healthy choices easier. HMSO, London

Department of Health 2000a National service framework for coronary heart disease. Department of Health, London

Department of Health 2000b The NHS cancer plan: a plan for investment, a plan for reform. Department of Health, London

Department of Health 2001 National service framework (NSF) for older people. Department of Health, London

Department of Health 2002 Improvement, expansion and reform: the next 3 years. Priorities and planning framework 2003–2006. Department of Health, London

Department of Health 2003 National service framework (NSF) for older people: a report of progress and future challenges. Department of Health, London

Department of Health 2004 National service framework for diabetes – one year on. Department of Health, London

Dines A, Cribb A 1993 Health promotion: concepts and practice. Blackwell Scientific Publications, Oxford

Downie R, Fyfe C, Tannahill A 1990 Health promotion: models and values. Oxford Medical Publications, Oxford

Forbes A, While A, Dyson L, Grocott T, Griffiths P 2003 Impact of clinical nurse specialists in multiple sclerosis – synthesis of the evidence. Journal of Advanced Nursing 42: 442–462

Gallagher U, Burden J 1993 Nursing as health promotion – a myth accepted? In: Wilson-Barnett J, Macleod Clark J (eds) Research in health promotion and nursing. Macmillan Press, Basingstoke, pp 51–60

Giddens A 1976 New rules of sociological method. Hutchinson, London

Grundy E 1996 Population review: (5) The population aged 60 and over. Population Trends 84: 14–20

Grundy E, Sloggett A 2003 Health inequalities in the older population: the role of personal capital, social resources and socio-economic circumstances. Social Science and Medicine 56: 935–947

House J, Landis K, Umberson D 1988 Social relationships and health. Science 241: 540–545

Illich I 1976 The epidemics of modern medicine. Excerpts reproduced in: Davey B, Gray A, Seale C (eds) Health and disease: a reader, 2nd edn. Open University Press, Buckingham, pp 237–242

Kickbusch I 1987 Issues in health promotion: Dr Ilona Kickbusch. Health Promotion International 1: 437–442

Kickbusch I 1989 Self-care in health promotion. Social Science and Medicine 29: 125–130

Labonte R 1997 The population health/health promotion debate in Canada: the politics of explanation, economics and action. Critical Public Health 7: 7–27

Luukinen H, Koski K, Kivela S-L, Laippala P 1996 Social status, life changes, housing conditions, health, functional abilities and lifestyle as risk factors for recurrent falls among the home-dwelling elderly. Public Health 110: 115–118

Maben J, Macleod Clark J 1995 Health promotion: a concept analysis. Journal of Advanced Nursing 22: 1158–1165

Macleod Clark J 1993 From sick nursing to health nursing: evolution or revolution? In: Wilson-Barnett J, Macleod Clark J (eds) Research in health promotion and nursing, Macmillan Press, Basingstoke, pp 256–270

Macleod Clark J, Maben J, Jones K 1997 Project 2000: perceptions of the philosophy and practice of nursing: shifting perceptions – a new practitioner? Journal of Advanced Nursing 26: 161–168

Mansfield K 1977 Letters and journals. Pelican Books, London

McClymont M, Thomas S, Denham M 1991 Health visiting and elderly people: a health promotion challenge, 2nd edn. Churchill Livingstone, Edinburgh

Merz C, Forrester J 1997 The secondary prevention of coronary heart disease. American Journal of Medicine 102: 573–580

National Statistics Online 2004a http://www.statistics.gov.uk/census2001/press_release_uk.asp (accessed 5 January 2004)

National Statistics Online 2004b http://www.statistics.gov.uk/census2001/pop2001/united_kingdom.asp (accessed 5 January 2004)

National Statistics Online 2004c http://www.statistics.gov.uk/census2001/pop2001/england_wales.asp (accessed 5 January 2004)

Neihoff J-U, Schneider F 1993 Epidemiology and the criticism of the risk factor approach. In: Lafaille R, Fulder S (eds) Towards a new science of health. Routledge, London, pp 118–128

Parsons T 1981 Definitions of health and illness in the light of American values and social structure. In: Caplan AL, Engelhardt HT, McCartney JJ (eds) Concepts of health and disease: interdisciplinary perspectives. Addison-Wesley, Reading, MA

Population Statistics, OPCS and Government Actuary's Department 1994 Centenarians: 1991 estimates. Population Trends 75: 30–32

Pursey A, Luker K 1995 Attitudes and stereotypes: nurses work with older people. Journal of Advanced Nursing 22: 547–555

Rijke R 1993 Health in medical science; from determinism towards autonomy. In: Lafaille R, Fulder S (eds) Towards a new science of health. Routledge, London, pp 74–83

Rogers E 2003 Health visitors and older people: thinking out of the box. Community Practitioner 76: 381–385

Rowe J, Kahn R 1987 Human ageing: usual and successful. Science 237: 143–149

Seedhouse D 1986 Health: the foundations for achievement. John Wiley, Chichester

Sidell M 1997 Older people's health: applying Antonovsky's salutogenic paradigm. In: Sidell M, Jones L, Katz J, Peberdy A (eds) Debates and dilemmas in promoting health: a reader. Macmillan Press, Basingstoke, pp 9–15

Skrabenek P 1992 Risk-factor epidemiology: science or non-science? Health, lifestyle and environment: countering the panic. Social Affairs Unit, London

Smail J 1996 Shifting the boundaries in practice nursing. In: Gastrell P, Edwards J (eds) Community health nursing: frameworks for practice. Baillière Tindall, London, pp 259–271

Stilwell B 1995 Developing experts: the nurse in general practice. In: Littlewood J (ed) Current issues in community nursing. Churchill Livingstone, Edinburgh, pp 127–146

Tannahill A 1985 What is health promotion? Health Education Journal 44: 167–168

Tinker A 1997 Older people in modern society, 4th edn. Longman, London

Tones K 1993 Changing theory and practice: trends in methods, strategies and settings in health education. Health Education Journal 52/53: 126–139

Tones K 1997 Health education as empowerment. In: Sidell M, Jones L, Katz J, Peberdy A (eds) Debates and dilemmas in promoting health: a reader. Macmillan Press, Basingstoke, pp 33–42

Townsend P, Davidson N, Whitehead M 1988 Inequalities in health: the Black report/the health divide. Penguin Books, Harmondsworth

Twinn S, Cowley S 1992 The principles of health visiting: a re-examination. Health Visitors' Association and UK Standing Conference on Health Visiting Education, London

UKCC 1997 The continuing care of older people: the nursing, community nursing and health visiting contribution in hospital/residential/domiciliary settings. UKCC, London

Weare K 1992 The contribution of health education to health promotion. In: Bunton R, Macdonald G (eds) Health promotion: disciplines and diversity. Routledge, London, pp 66–85

Wilkinson R 1996 Unhealthy societies: the afflictions of inequality. Routledge, London

Williams R 1983 Concepts of health: an analysis of lay logic. Sociology 17: 185–205

Williams G, Popay J 1994 Lay knowledge and the privilege of experience. In: Gabe J, Kelleher D, Williams G (eds) Challenging medicine. Routledge, London, pp 118–139

Wilson-Barnett J, Beech S 1994 Evaluating the clinical nurse specialist: a review. International Journal of Nursing Studies 31: 561–571

World Health Organization 1946 Constitution. WHO, Geneva

World Health Organization 1978 Alma-Ata 1978: primary health care. WHO, Geneva

World Health Organization 1986 Ottawa charter for health promotion. WHO, Ontario, Canada. (Reproduced as an appendix in Dines A, Cribb A (1993) Health promotion: concepts and principles. Blackwell Scientific Publications, Oxford)

World Health Organization 1998 Health promotion glossary. WHO, Geneva

World Health Organization 2002a Active ageing: a policy framework. WHO, Geneva

World Health Organization 2002b The Toronto declaration on the global prevention of elder abuse. WHO, Geneva

World Health Organization 2003 World health report. WHO, Geneva

Chapter 31

Complementary therapies

Helen Brett

INTRODUCTION

There appear to be potential benefits in the use of complementary therapies with older people and this chapter will set out to explore some of the opportunities available to them. The aim of this chapter is to add to the professional debate around the integration of complementary therapies into nursing practice concerned with care of older people. The chapter begins with a discussion on the role of the nurse in the safe use of complementary therapies as well as some evaluation of its evidence base. It will not attempt to be comprehensive, but instead will introduce those therapies most frequently used by nurses and discuss how they may be safely applied. Debate inevitably rages around whether or not there is a need for such therapies and even whether nurses should provide them alongside orthodox care. Whilst guidance and 'expert' opinion from bodies such as the Nursing and Midwifery Council (NMC), the Royal College of Nursing (RCN) and the House of Commons Select Committee and other authors will be discussed, inevitably more questions may be raised than are answered.

Holism will be explored in relation to nursing and complementary therapies. The literature will be explored to identify conceptual links that might validate the use of complementary therapies within nursing practice. It is important to explore claims that such use is evidence of expanded nursing practice that develops existing skills and knowledge, or whether they are new nursing activities for which specialist training and supervision are needed. These are key issues and will inform the approach taken when seeking to integrate therapies into practice.

Complementary therapies in general will be set in context by briefly reviewing methods of classification. This process will help to clarify the focus of intent when using a therapy as a nursing activity, which is embedded in the context of a developing nursing rationale. There will be a brief discussion of the literature to determine if the increased interest of nurses in using complementary therapies is mirrored by a corresponding interest by patients/clients – the consumers.

Four complementary therapies – massage, aromatherapy, Bach flower remedies and t'ai chi – have been chosen for discussion, because each raises different issues in terms of its applicability and appropriateness for integration into the nursing care of the older person. They are also different in terms of the level and complexity of training required and its relation to current nurse education.

Massage is an example of a complementary therapy that is used in practice, including nursing care of older people (Rankin-Box 2001). Massage will be discussed in some depth, including its history and links with contemporary nursing practice. The use of massage in current nursing practice will be explored using the relevant literature.

Aromatherapy often incorporates massage but the addition of the use of pharmacologically active essential oils makes its use more problematic, particularly in the level of competence required in prescription of oils. Bach flower remedies are introduced as an oral remedy that may also be used in conjunction with massage and aromatherapy, but also, like t'ai chi, may encourage patients to take back the locus of control for their own recovery. T'ai chi is a therapy that has its origins in a different paradigm and its use in care is usually offered by an external practitioner or a nonnursing member of the care team, such as a physiotherapist.

Before such notions can be addressed it is essential to identify what the generic term 'complementary therapies' may mean.

WHAT ARE COMPLEMENTARY THERAPIES?

There appear to be over 300 different techniques and therapies available from which to choose and because of this several authors have sought to categorize them. But to do so meaningfully is very difficult, especially as so many of the therapies are based on unfamiliar cultural and belief systems, many of which emanate from eastern as opposed to western medical practices (Brett 2002). Pietroni (1992) has grouped them according to how they may be used:

1. Complete systems of healing, which include osteopathy and acupuncture, traditional Chinese medicine, herbal medicine, osteopathy, chiropractic, homeopathy, naturopathy and ayurvedic medicine. These systems of healing describe therapies that have a diagnostic, investigative and therapeutic understanding of the process of disease. These are therapies that all have an application in the care of the older person but are unlikely to be delivered by nurses, as they require considerable training. In the case of therapies such as osteopathy and acupuncture, training lasts 3–4 years. The therapies are also less amenable to integration into clinical nursing practice and are mostly offered as a supplementary service

2. Diagnostic practices that use methods not usually linked to orthodox medicine, for example, kinesiology, iridology, hair analysis, aura diagnosis and crystals. The problem with these therapies is that they are not supported by research and are regarded as verging on 'quackery'

3. Therapeutic modalities such as massage, aromatherapy, reflexology, therapeutic touch and shiatsu. These therapies are primarily used in nursing to address problems such as pain and stress. They also have the potential to enhance communication because of the amount of focused time usually involved in the therapy

4. Self-help measures such as relaxation and yoga, breathing and relaxation techniques, meditation, visualization, nutrition and t'ai chi. The self-help measures that are included in this group are skills that patients/clients are encouraged to undertake to diminish their symptoms, improve their health or maintain their well-being. Here the nurse acts as an educator or facilitator and the therapies listed could all play a part in caring for the older person. Yoga and t'ai chi in particular are useful for improving flexibility and mobility. Breathing and relaxation techniques, meditation and visualization all have the potential to enhance quality of life and empower older people to take control of their health and well-being.

An alternative classification has been provided by Bell & Sikora (1996), who divided complementary therapy into only three categories

1. psychological: including counselling, healing, radionics and rebirthing
2. physical : including massage, aromatherapy and chiropractic
3. pharmacological: including dietary interventions, homeopathy and the use of shark's cartilage.

As can be seen, within the above categories there is a tremendous diversity of therapies listed and many of them are little-known. So, rather than just look at systems, however varied, Vickers (1993) thought it best to categorize them into headings that broadly indicate their mode of delivery:

- touch therapies
- structural therapies
- functional therapies
- oriental therapies
- therapies that involve movement and stillness.

The benefit of such categories is that, like Pietroni's (1992) classification, they offer a framework with which to make sense of the claims made for each therapy and to try and distinguish the theoretical basis for these claims. This process also helps to identify and clarify the characteristics of the relationship between the practitioner and the patient/client. The examples in the various groups are not exhaustive as nurses have used other therapies such as humour, music, art therapy and reflexology (Wells & Tschudin 1994, Rankin-Box 2001). The effectiveness of any complementary therapy as a nursing intervention seems to depend as much on the attitudes and values that the practitioner holds about the chosen therapy as on the therapeutic skills he or she performs. In Pietroni's scheme, groups 3 and 4 are the therapies that are seen as complementing or supplementing orthodox care and are the therapies that nurses are using in their practice, whereas the other two groups are seen as having the potential to be 'alternative' to orthodox treatments (Gates 1995).

The distinction is important, particularly in terms of the use of 'complementary' therapies within nursing practice, because it is their use as a 'supplement' to orthodox care that is both their strength and weakness. The therapies most commonly used, such as massage and aromatherapy, offer the reflective practitioner the opportunity to explore the nursing needs of their patients/clients, to push at the boundaries of care and to find innovative and complementary ways of addressing long-standing problems (Dossey et al. 1995, Rankin-Box 2001).

But the definition of 'supplement' in the *Oxford Paperback Dictionary* (1988) is of 'a thing added as an extra' and it is this aspect that is usually relevant to the management of nursing resources and provides one of the major stumbling blocks to the widespread integration of complementary therapies into nursing. There is a tendency to equate the use of complementary therapies within nursing with giving more time to individual patients/clients. So, for example, giving a back massage for relaxation may take 30 min. But time is a finite resource and if the nurse is giving a back massage to one patient then in all probability there are some other 'nursing' tasks that are not being done and other patients not being cared for. There is a need to prioritize the use of a range of care skills and, because massage is often time-consuming and seen as an extra, it can be difficult to justify its use as a nursing activity.

Inevitably, in any classification there will be some overlap of treatment type and therapy and the expression 'complementary therapy' can only serve as an umbrella term to introduce a huge variety of differing techniques. The term 'complementary', as opposed to alternative therapy, does appear to be the most acceptable one to use because of how the words are perceived by others. Alternative suggests that a therapy will be used instead of, whilst complementary suggests that it will be used as an adjunct to, conventional treatment (Norton 1995). Therefore, for the purpose of this chapter a complementary therapy is one that is used for its potential to complement and enhance current nursing practice (Rankin-Box 2001). Whilst the term 'alternative' once dominated the literature, Kendrick (1999) and Wright (1995) both feel that 'complementary' has overtaken it and suggest that this makes such procedures less confrontational to other health care professionals (Brett 2002). In reality the two terms are often used interchangeably and the combined term 'complementary and alternative medicine' (CAM) now seems to be most often adopted within the literature. This has been defined as:

> diagnosis, treatment and/or prevention which complements mainstream medicine by contributing to a common whole, by satisfying a demand not met by orthodoxy or by the conceptual frameworks of medicine (Ernst & Cassileth 1998).

As well as the different usage of the above terminology, in any discussion involving such therapies the concept of holism may well be included, especially when seeking a justification for their promotion. Because of the immense debate within the literature as to whether or not complementary therapies are any more holistic than orthodox care (Brett 2002), it is necessary to consider holism now.

HOLISM

McMahon (1991) suggests that for some nurses 'holistic nursing care' is synonymous with complementary therapy and, whilst Long et al. (2000) note that the concept of holism is extremely difficult to measure, Owen & Holmes (1993) describe it as a 'turbid, amorphic term', the meaning of which alters according to the context in which it is used. They maintain that nurses have failed to recognize the complexity of the concept, failed to distinguish its different meanings, overlooked their implications and ignored their philosophical susceptibilities. Cribb et al. (1994) identify how aspiring to give holistic care opens up philosophical and practical problems. As this debate continues it may be useful to consider Griffin's (1993) preconditions for holistic care:

- respect for persons
- openness and receptivity
- reflection
- seeing comprehensively.

Buckle (1993) therefore insists that complementary therapies may only encompass holistic ideologies if the patients' whole needs and such aspects of care, as listed above, are fully addressed. Without doing this, she asserts that we are just performing other tasks.

Whether or not complementary therapies are holistic, or people really appreciate their underlying philosophies, it does appear that more and more people are demanding to use them (Ernst & White 2000, Thomas et al. 2001). For example, it has been estimated that approximately one-quarter of the British population have accessed some type of CAM and, of those, 80% are pleased with them (Furnham 2000). Approximately 90% of these consultations are funded by the public themselves (Fox 2001) and furthermore, recently, almost 67 % of local health authorities have been purchasing at least one form of CAM for their patients (White & Ernst 2000). Sharma (1992) suggests that consumers of the health service are taking a more critical attitude to orthodox medicine. They are searching more actively for relevant information and there is evidence of increased confidence in the ability to make effective choices for their own health care (Pietroni 1996). Although consumers are becoming more disillusioned with orthodox medicine and want access to complementary therapies, they also want reassurance that these therapies are safe (Dickinson 1996). Interestingly, consumers seem more confident of a successful outcome in relation to complementary medicine than the evidence supports (Dickinson 1996, Vickers 1996). Whether this is the same for older people is unclear, although Sidell (1995) felt there is potential in offering such therapies to older people, especially when they are seeking care rather than cure and symptomatic relief from emotional and physical pain.

Some of this is reflected in Furnham's (2002) work. After reviewing several studies, he concluded that the key factors, listed below, influenced the reasons people chose to try complementary therapies:

- They were not 'brand-loyal' to one type of care and wanted to be able to choose from a variety of therapists
- Orthodox care did not provide enough time and advice to meet their needs
- They were searching for a cure that was painfree and without side-effects
- Some therapies were accessed as a 'last-hope' attempt to help chronic, palliative and terminal conditions
- They believed that such therapies offered 'holistic' care and also that they emphasized 'wellness', not illness.

Furnham (2002) noted that, whilst such users often have different values and beliefs to non-users and that some of their desires may not be realistic, there is a need to challenge the widely held myth that, because they choose such treatments, they are:

> especially gullible or naïve, or have unusual (neurotic) personalities or bizarre values or belief systems (p. 230).

Evidence also suggests that nurses are as keen to use complementary therapies, both within and outside their conventional practice, as patients are to access them. Kendrick (1999) asserted that whilst over the last 20 years complementary therapies have re-emerged as an obvious adjunct to allopathic medicine, nurses have been impeded in practising them, as to do so has been made so politically sensitive. Although he admits that there are challenges ahead, he feels that health care could be enriched by their usage, as patients would have more choice in the type of treatment they receive.

Yet there is disagreement as to whether nurses should, or even want to (Hoban 2003), integrate complementary therapies within their current practice as concerns have been raised that many nurses are not adequately trained and thus just 'dabble' (Hoban 2003, Stevenson 1995). Wright (1995) has suggested that creating levels of competence to practise may just be supporting old reductionist perspectives when part of the rationale for complementary therapies is the holistic approach they offer. This is too simplistic an approach; it assumes universality of application when the provision of any complementary therapy is as complex as the application of orthodox nursing care. Previous discussion in this chapter has also cautioned against supposing that offering complementary therapies means that care is 'holistic'. If complementary therapies are a legitimate part of nursing work then nurses wishing to use them in their practice to benefit patients have a corresponding professional responsibility to gain appropriate knowledge that is based on appropriate and rigorous evidence.

Whilst Wright (1989) feels that, as carers, nurses possess the skills to enable them to take on these extra roles, Johnson's (2000) literature review suggests that, where complementary practitioners were more skilled than the nursing staff, it would be preferable for them to perform the treatments. She holds a strong view about this as her work also identified that nurses tended to qualify in and practise the therapies according to their own wishes and not in accordance with the needs of their individual patients. This is supported by Chadwick (1999), who surveyed a small sample of nurses to establish why they wished to integrate complementary therapies into practice and found that most respondents had been more interested in expanding their own clinical roles as opposed to enhancing patients' care.

Major concerns about integrating complementary therapies into nursing practice centre on the correct use of appropriate therapies and the training and regulation of those delivering them. Avis notes in her forward to the RCN's (2003) guidance on integrating complementary therapies into clinical care that because the regulation of so many individual therapies is so unclear, both the NMC and the RCN cannot give definitive advice for those seeking to practise such therapies.

It therefore befalls us all to abide by the Code of Professional Conduct (NMC 2002a), which briefly states:

> You must ensure that the use of complementary or alternative therapies is safe and in the interests of patients and clients. This must be discussed with the team as part of the therapeutic process and the patients or clients must consent to their use (clause 3.11; p. 6.).

Within the *Guidelines for the Administration of Medicines* (NMC 2002b) there is a further brief paragraph, which notes:

> Complementary and alternative therapies are increasingly used in the treatment of patients. Registered nurses, midwives and health visitors who practise the use of such therapies must have successfully undertaken training and be competent in this area (please refer to the scope of professional practice). You must have considered the appropriateness of the therapy to both the condition of the patient and any co-existing treatments. It is essential that the patient is aware of the therapy and gives informed consent (p. 9).

Nurses are encouraged to enhance their roles, but only if the guidance within *The Scope of Professional Practice* (NMC 2002c) is adhered to. It clearly states that each registered nurse, midwife or health visitor:

must ensure that any enlargement or adjustment of the scope of personal professional practice must be achieved without compromising or fragmenting existing aspects of professional practice and care and that the requirements of the Council's Code of Professional Conduct [2002a] are satisfied throughout the whole area of practice (p. 6).

But, whilst some nurses welcome the opportunity to embrace more flexible working practices, others may feel it is too risky to take on complementary practices as the guidance given is not specific enough to afford them sufficient protection. In an endeavour to help nurses practise such therapies safely, the RCN (2003) has devised a framework for guidance. These guidelines are set out very clearly and advise you to consider the following before attempting to integrate any CAM initiative within an orthodox clinical setting:

- the therapy must be appropriate, relevant and meet the needs of and 'be in the best interests and safety of patients/clients'
- informed consent is obtained, as patients/clients must fully understand what is to be done and also be aware that they may withdraw from this treatment at any time
- there must be collaboration with all professionals involved in the care
- a policy within your employing authority needs to be in place before any intervention is initiated. This may mean that you will have to develop one
- there must be clarity over how those who wish to deliver the therapies will be resourced, trained and appropriately supervised
- it reminds nurses practising such therapies that they remain personally and professionally accountable for their actions
- the effectiveness of all interventions needs to be evaluated (Ersser 1995).

Undoubtedly, as complementary therapies become more popular amongst both nurses and patients/clients, there is:

> a growing need to develop a rigorous systematic and sustained evidence base (Brett 2002 p. 239).

and whilst it is not within the remit of this chapter to debate such issues, Ernst & Fialka (1994) state that patients have a right to choose from adequate options, therefore health care professionals have the duty to determine what is safe and effective. In principle it means that nursing interventions should be based on facts rather than personal opinion. There is good reason for subjecting them to the same critical scrutiny applied in other areas of nursing as evidence-based practice does not necessarily curtail freedom of choice but allows freedom to select from appropriate, safe and effective options (Ernst & Fialka 1994).

In addition to the guidance given by the NMC and RCN, the sixth report from the House of Lords Select Committee on Science and Technology on CAM (2000), endorsed by the Department of Health in 2001, will influence the way in which many therapies continue to be practised. The 15-month inquiry noted that, as the use of CAM was now both widespread and increasing, issues relating to its evidence base, regulation of therapies and the status of those who provide them needed to be addressed urgently. This report classified the therapies under the three main groups:

1. Group 1 comprises professionally organized, discrete alternative systems of assessment and treatment, which include 'the big five' therapies of chiropractic, homeopathy, osteopathy, acupuncture and herbal medicine. These were deemed to have already developed a substantial evidence base, are effective, well-regulated, have a proper educational footing and are sought after by the general public
2. Group 2 contains those therapies that are deemed to be developing a reasonable body of knowledge, are addressing training issues and are the ones most often used to complement orthodox practice as they appear to aid comfort and support readily. They include aromatherapy, massage, shiatsu, Bach flower remedies and reflexology, which are the therapies also favoured by most nurses, especially when treating older people and those requiring chronic, terminal and palliative care
3. Group 3 is deemed to have no established evidence base yet and includes therapies such as ayurvedic medicine, Chinese herbal medicine and traditional Chinese medicine, which have been used for centuries by other cultures. There has been some unrest within the 'professions' over this, as the possibility for attracting research funding or being able to access them through the National Health Service is now questionable.

So that the public could both benefit from some of the above therapies and be protected from the potential risks of poor practice, the report strongly urged that there should be more integration and open-mindedness between CAM and orthodox practitioners. Attention particularly focused on the fact that those practising complementary therapies should recognize when they needed to refer their patient to another health care professional (Rankin-Box 2002). It also recommended that the NMC and RCN should provide more guidance about differing therapies and ensure that nursing recruits have a basic level of knowledge. It will be interesting to watch how all of this unfolds, and whilst this crucial debate continues, there are many instances of – often lone – nurses who have successfully helped others to use such therapies in their everyday practice (Brett 1999, Hoban 2003, RCN 2003).

THE TACTILE THERAPIES

Before introducing tactile therapies it is necessary to consider the role of touch.

Touch

Although the use of touch is an inherent component of the provision of nursing care (Lawler 1991, Estabrooks & Morse 1992, McCann & McKenna 1993) and its potential benefits are widely documented, some patients can initially find the tactile therapies alarming (Vortherms 1991). A number of studies have explored touch within nursing practice and have emphasized its complexity as a powerful and essential means of communication (Weiss 1979, Sims 1988, Bottorff 1993), which may or may not involve acts of great significance. Touch has been identified as the earliest sense to develop in humans, providing a fundamental means of interacting with the environment and others (Montague 1986). Tactile stimulation is deemed necessary for physical survival and has biological significance in nurturing and the healthy, behavioural development of any individual (Bowlby 1984). It has the potential both to enhance verbal communications and to facilitate social interaction, including information-giving and the expression of feelings (Savage 1995). Unlike verbal communication, the message conveyed through touch cannot be easily changed or corrected (Argyle 1975) so there is potential for misinterpretation. Pratt & Mason (1981) suggest that touch is used by the majority of people in a ritual form to indicate a relationship existing between one person and another and requires some kind of contract between the people concerned.

Seemingly nurses have the permission of society to violate norms, as touching is regarded as part of the day-to-day relationship between any patient and nurse (Estabrooks & Morse 1992). 'Nursing touch' is categorized variously by different authors. For example, Routasalo (1996) describes two different types of touching: necessary and non-necessary. Taken at face value this is a simplistic classification but pragmatically it is convenient and is the most common framework found in nursing theory. The categories can be further subdivided to uncover the complexities of a key nursing skill. 'Necessary touch' can encompass procedural (Barnett 1972), instrumental (Watson 1975, Sims 1986) and task-related touch (Estabrooks & Morse 1992), or functional touch (Vickers 1996). 'Non-necessary touch' is defined as 'spontaneous physical contact between nurse and patient' (Routasalo 1996) and can include expressive (Watson 1975), comforting (Morse et al. 1994), reassuring (Teasdale 1995), caring touch (Seaman 1982) or affective touch (Vickers 1996).

Traditionally, nursing has tended to focus on 'instrumental' acts of touching (Sims 1986), such as helping a patient to eat, dress or take medication. Such practices are easily observed and measured but this approach appears to suggest that nurses only help people by caring for them and doing manual techniques, associated with specific diagnoses (Wright 1995). There is currently a move away from this view and a swing towards a softer, yet more difficult to define, expressive type of nursing practice.

As the amount of physical contact exercised in a society is governed by sets of fairly well-defined behavioural norms which determine the individual's role and the situation in which he or she is (Pratt & Mason 1981), it has been observed that touching within western society declines after childhood (Jourard 1966). Montague (1986) found that, whilst the need for touch does not necessarily diminish with age, older patients may think that touch should only be used for the 'proper' treatment of specific conditions. Barnett (1972) suggested that this heightened need for touch in childhood may return during sickness and perhaps outweigh these notions of 'proper' behaviour. Yet Hollinger (1980) stresses that to generalize that all older people have an increased need for touch during illness is foolish as their perception of touch is influenced by prior experience and 'touch socialization'. Any older person may therefore like or dislike such touch.

In a small study by McCann & McKenna (1993), patients' perceptions of comfort and being touched by nurses appear to be linked to the part of the body touched and the gender of the nurse initiating that touch. Day (1973) also noted that patients needed to know 'their' nurse before they felt supported and comforted by touch. Touch and lack of touch are intriguing and complex entities because the meaning of touch varies from one person to another and from one situation to another. Various studies have looked at the significance of age, sex, culture and social class of patients in relation to touch but it is the overriding principle of individualized, patient-centred care that, combined with theoretical insights, will ensure that the care given is appropriate.

Massage

Massage has been described as an extension of purposeful touch, which may enable nurses to use touch to its full potential (Tutton 1991) and is generally defined as a systematic form of touch which:

> involves the manipulation of soft tissue for therapeutic purposes and may be performed on most parts of the body utilizing a variety of techniques, all involving different degrees of pressure (Brett 2002).

As a generic term, massage covers a range of actions that include body rubbing. The word 'massage' is thought to mean 'press softly' in Arabic or 'knead' in Greek but also has derivations from Hindi and French (Hildebrand 1994, Horrigan 1995). In the west, the first written records of massage are found in Greece. Hippocrates wrote about its value in, among other things, improving muscle tone and relieving muscular tension and thought that the 'physician must be experienced in many things, but assuredly also in rubbing' (Vickers 1996). Evidence suggests that massage was used in China around 3000 BC (Trevelyan & Booth 1994) and in India around 1800 BC. Early Japanese, Persian, Egyptian, Roman and Greek texts offer further evidence that massage was valuable in the cure and relief of many conditions (Hildebrand 1994). One of the most famous people to benefit from a daily massage for his asthma was said to be Julius Caesar.

There was some decline in the use of massage after the Middle Ages as it was seen to be sinful but, with a resurgence of interest in all things bodily, during the Renaissance, massage became popular once again. Mercurialis (1530–1606 AD), the attending physician to Mary Queen of Scots, encouraged this as he had started to use massage alongside his orthodox practice. By the early nineteenth century, John Grosvenor trained 'rubber nurses' at the Radcliffe Hospital, Oxford, to massage stiff joints and fractured limbs and, whilst it was normally only available to the wealthy, the Radcliffe allowed poor patients to benefit from this 'friction' (massage). By 1894, some nurses who had received massage training, with which they could endorse their nursing certificates, formed the Society of Trained Masseurs, which eventually became the Chartered Society of Physiotherapy, with registration in 1964.

Whilst many attribute the development of modern-day massage to Per Henrik Ling (1776–1839), Goldstone (2000) disputes this as he felt that there were many other physicians before and after Ling who contributed to the wealth of information now available on massage. He felt that it was really Mezgar, the Dutch physician, rather than Per Ling, the movement therapist, who should be credited with the introduction of modern massage. Even so, Per Ling has been very influential in encouraging massage and is credited with the modern-day term 'Swedish massage'. Goldstone (2000) asserted that, whilst massage was once the province of the medically trained, it is now mainly carried out by lay personnel as an alternative procedure.

Technique

Massage is deemed to be effective in alleviating painful and chronic conditions, such as arthritis, stroke and multiple sclerosis. One has only to witness how someone in pain will, almost without thinking, stroke or rub the affected part of the body in order to ease and aid healing (Brett 2002). Massage involves using touch with patients in, perhaps, a very different way than they may have experienced before and the media's promotion of it as a sexual rather than a therapeutic procedure may create unnecessary alarm amongst patients. In this sense massage is seen as comprising, amongst others, the following specific strokes or techniques.

- Effleurage, which is a longitudinal stroke, where the hands are placed flat on the area to be massaged, usually the back, and moved slowly in a gliding motion with light to moderate pressure
- Pétrissage, which involves deeper pressure applied by the fingers and thumb, often in a circular movement. I would suggest that these strokes or techniques are part of the conventional understanding of what 'massage' might mean in the context of nursing care.

The therapeutic intervention used in the methodology of the studies by Sims (1986), Fraser & Ross Kerr (1993) and Tutton (1987) was a back massage that included the strokes described above. The therapeutic benefits identified were the relief of anxiety and tension, promotion of relaxation, improved communication with patients and their increased well-being. Yet the integration of massage into clinical nursing practice may be troublesome because there is a variety of techniques that might constitute the term 'massage' (Vickers 1996). 'Massage' is often used in the literature in such a loose way as to suggest that there is a single, standardized technique that would form the therapeutic intervention and the literature does not go into great detail as to what techniques were used (Farrow 1990).

Even though studies have tried to identify how massage works, it is still unclear, and the way it is practised and the length of time taken are often described very differently. For example, some of the literature selected for this chapter, while specifying the part of the body massaged and giving an indication of the duration of the massage, does not give enough detail on the techniques used (Farrow 1990). Fraser & Ross Kerr (1993: p. 241) describe the intervention as being:

> back massage consisting of 5 minutes of slow, rhythmic massage, using a combination of light to moderate pressure from the crown of the head to the sacral area in a circular motion with no crossing over of hands and continuous contact.

In contrast, Ferrell-Torry & Glick (1993: pp. 96–97) describe:

> the massage as consisting of 30 minutes of effleurage and pétrissage to the feet, back, neck and shoulders using warmed cocoa butter lotion as a skin lubricant. In conjunction with this, myofascial trigger-point therapy was utilised ... once the TPs were located slow, milking strokes of increasing pressure were utilised along the length of the affected muscle.

It is apparent from these descriptions that if nurses were to try and replicate these interventions for the legitimate nursing goals of promoting relaxation and improving communication with patients in the first example, and modifying anxiety and the perception of pain in the other, they would need differing levels of skill and knowledge in massage practice. Further studies in general do not explore in depth the nature of the relationship between the nurse and the patient although, in some cases, this was part of the rationale for using massage. More work needs to be done to establish whether the length of time the massage takes is related to the level of knowledge and skills required and the outcomes.

Why use massage in nursing?

Anecdotally it would seem that massage has the potential to benefit most, if not all, of the systems of the body and, whilst Vickers (1996) asserts that there is still a paucity of rigorous research studies to support this view, others would argue that there is now a growing body of evidence to support its use.

In the previous edition of this book Angela Avis (1999) discussed a study that she had undertaken, which had set out to encourage the development of safe and efficacious use of essential oils and massage by nurses in one health authority. The remit involved critical scrutiny and monitoring of practice and the communication of relevant information to nurses working within the health authority. As part of this process a survey was conducted to ascertain the extent to which essential oils and massage were being used in terms of geographical spread and clinical integration. The reasons given for using massage include: as an aid to sleep, to help relaxation, to promote comfort, to improve movement in the care of patients with osteoarthritis, and to enhance communication between nurse and patient. Four broad categories were identified in relation to the:

1. therapeutic potential of massage in promoting relaxation
2. therapeutic potential of massage for a specific nursing problem
3. therapeutic potential of massage for a group of patients/clients
4. enhancement of nursing care by using massage.

A high proportion of the nurses in the survey were quite specific about the use of massage in their clinical practice. Specific nursing problems, together with the promotion of relaxation, were the main reasons put forward. Promoting relaxation, taken in a general sense, was the main motivation for nurses using massage. Relaxation is also one of the most widely discussed benefits of massage in the general literature (Vickers 1996). The respondents identified quite specific nursing problems for which massage had therapeutic potential. Only a small proportion of the respondents articulated the general concept of enhancing patient care. The analysis showed that when nurses were using massage in their clinical practice it was for a wide spectrum of nursing problems and in a broad range of specialized clinical areas. The analysis highlighted some reasons why massage might be used as a therapeutic intervention but it did not indicate exactly what the 'massage' being used entailed in terms of its physical technique or the complexity of the context of care. Nevertheless the results of the survey do give an indication of the reasons for using massage as a nursing intervention and are relevant to the care of older people.

An analysis of the literature revealed 17 sources that identified the potential for the use of massage within clinical practice. There was considerable agreement between the responses from the survey and the references in the literature. The rationale for using massage within three categories is shown in Table 31.1. Analysis of the survey and literature indicates that there are some patient-centred concerns and problems within nursing practice, such as reducing anxiety and stress and the relief of pain, which might legitimately be addressed by using massage as a therapeutic intervention. Promoting relaxation was the single most common justification for using massage in both the survey and the literature.

In two other studies by Tutton (1987) and Fraser & Ross Kerr (1993), it was demonstrated that back massage could be an effective, non-invasive technique to incorporate into the care of the older person for promoting relaxation and improving communication. In particular, Fraser & Ross Kerr highlight the dehumanizing effects of a health care system where technological advance and cure dominate, that has serious and profound implications for the older person who is chronically ill, and that the effects of human touch and interaction are important factors in caring for older people. Fraser & Ross Kerr saw massage as a valuable nursing technique.

Other studies have also identified that soothing massage may aid relaxation and reduce tension (Kaada & Torsteinbo 1989); abdominal massage

Table 31.1 Rationale for using massage within three categories

Survey	Literature
Therapeutic potential in promoting relaxation	
Promotes relaxation	Relaxation (Farrow 1990, Fraser & Ross Kerr 1993, Foster 1994, Stevenson 1994, Corner et al. 1995, Davies & Riches 1995)
Reduces stress	Stress (Farrow 1990, Dunn et al. 1995)
Alleviates anxiety	Anxiety (Farrow 1990, Ferrell-Torry & Glick 1993, McNamara 1994, Malkin 1994, Corner et al. 1995, Dunn et al. 1995, Wilkinson 1995)
Therapeutic potential for a specific nursing problem	
Aids to sleep	Insomnia (Farrow 1990)
Relieves pain	Pain (Farrow 1990, Ferrell-Torry & Glick 1993, Fordham & Dunn 1994, McNamara 1994, Malkin 1994, Wilkinson 1995)
Enhancing nursing practice	
Promotes holistic nursing	Holistic approach (Foster 1994; Malkin 1994)
Enhances basic care	Enhance nursing practice (Tutton 1991)
Enhances communication between nurse and patient	Improve communication with patients (Fraser & Ross Kerr 1993)

increases peristaltic action (Beard & Wood 1994); and, as long ago as 1945, Scull noted that, after neck massage, patients experienced a reduction in both muscle tension and spasm.

Many have advocated that only a total body massage will effect relief but, in current busy practice settings, because of reasons already stated earlier in the chapter, this may be impracticable. Because of this I sought to help nurses in two continuing care wards to integrate hand massage into their everyday practice (Brett 1999). At that time, there were only two small-scale studies (Snyder et al. 1995a, 1995b) to inform the work, but they did suggest that it could help bring some relaxation to those exhibiting agitated behaviour. The initial evaluation revealed that both patients and clients gained pleasure from this small procedure. Cox & Hayes (2000) sought ways in which they could massage critically ill patients and they found that a 5-min foot massage induced relaxation and reduced their patients' stress. They also noted how pleasurable it was for patients, as opposed to some of the other treatments they had to endure. It may be that we need to consider some of these smaller-scale interventions.

As the current older generation have, on the whole, been bought up to be very private, they may initially shun such procedures. Yet it is apparent that such activities and skills relating to touch and massage may be eminently suitable to develop in the care for older people. Yet it is essential that they are clearly defined so that they can be supported by appropriate education and training. But if massage is introduced appropriately and respectfully into the care of older people they may both enjoy and benefit from these techniques.

Aromatherapy

The ancient Greek, Roman, Indian, Chinese, Egyptian, Australian aboriginal and Persian civilizations were using plant extracts for healing centuries ago. Records dating back to 4500 BC show how such plants were used in the preparation of perfumes, cosmetics, medicine and embalming the dead (Hopkins 1995). The early Egyptian hieroglyphics also show their use and oils such as cinnamon, frankincense and myrrh are referred to in the Bible. The term 'aromatherapy' (aromatherapie) was first coined by Gattefosse in 1928 whilst working in the cosmetics industry, but it was Marguerite Maury who most famously blended essential oils so that they could be used therapeutically. Aromatherapy was hardly used in the UK until the 1960s and in health care probably much later (Case study 31.1).

A simple definition of aromatherapy is that it is a treatment using aromatic substances or essential oils

for therapeutic effect. A definition of the therapy becomes more complex when the mode of delivery is explored. The main focus of the therapy is the inhalation of the oils but the mode of administration of these oils is varied and also includes absorption via the skin and internal dosage. Currently the aromatherapy organizations do not allow non-medically trained therapists to administer essential oils internally because of fears over their potential toxicity (Brett 2002). It is thought that chemical properties of the essential oils, when absorbed by the body, by any route, have certain therapeutic benefits (Stevenson 1995). In the UK the main form of administration is via massage, although many individuals may also scent their baths or rooms with the oils, while in France they are prescribed orally by trained doctors.

Vickers (1996) has highlighted several inconsistencies in the aromatherapy literature. A wide range of different properties have been ascribed to each essential oil, a plethora of conditions are thought to be amenable to each therapy and there is a general lack of consistency between the sources. These issues are important when nurses consider using aromatherapy within their clinical practice. Is the intended therapeutic effect physical or psychological? Where is the evidence that the use of a particular oil will produce a specific effect? What is the role of massage as a form of administration? In the previous section the power of touch and massage was discussed, so in an aromatherapy massage, how can the nurse know if it is the use of the essential oil that is significantly therapeutic or does it simply add a pleasing aroma to a massage session? A study by Dunn et al. (1995), which evaluated the use of aromatherapy, massage and periods of rest in an intensive care unit, showed that the patients who received aromatherapy reported significantly greater improvement in their mood and perceived levels of anxiety. The study showed that massage could offer a useful therapy for nurses to consider when planning psychological care of patients in this particular setting and that the addition of 1% essential oil of lavender appeared to enhance the effects of the massage and might have contributed to the patients' well-being.

The results of this study cannot be generalized to other settings but there are two other studies that were undertaken with cohorts of older people and these suggest that lavender essential oil may have a part to play in promoting relaxation, particularly with regard to sleep disturbance. Hudson (1996) emphasized that inadequate sleep in older people can produce symptoms of tiredness, lack of muscle coordination, dysarthria and difficulty in maintaining attention, and that these symptoms may be

Case study 31.1   Aromatherapy

David, aged 89, fell last year and fractured his pubic rami. After a painful week he was admitted to hospital where he suffered a series of strokes. Whilst he had no visible paralysis, the strokes left him with limited speech and comprehension and also very restricted mobility. After a 6-month stay in hospital, he returned home to the care of his wife and has been home for just over 8 months. Because he is only bed- or chair-bound he finds his body aches all of the time and, whilst co-dydramol does give him some relief, he is reluctant to take it as it makes him so very constipated.

Three months ago, once his condition had stabilized, I was asked to treat him with aromatherapy massage to help ease both his stiffness and aching joints. Upon examination he was deemed to be too frail to be able to tolerate a full body massage. His skin was also very friable as he had received topical steroid treatment for long-standing eczema. Instead I chose to treat him with very gentle massage to his arms and legs, paying extra attention to his hands and feet, using the essential oils lavender (*Lavandula angustifolia*) and Roman chamomile (*Anthemis nobilis*).

The essential oils were chosen because of their analgesic and sedating properties and they are also safe and soothing in chronic skin conditions. All topical applications are administered in a carrier oil and I chose to use the non-nut-based grapeseed oil to minimize the possibility of further allergic skin reactions. Because of his age and frailty I used a very low concentration mix and added only two drops of each essential oil to 15 ml of the grapeseed oil (more information about dosage may be found in Brett 2002).

David was positioned comfortably (in bed) and each arm and leg was massaged in turn, taking extra care around the joints as 'where there is reduced tone in their stabilizing muscles [if massaged] too vigorously subluxation of the joint could occur' (Brett 2002: p. 181). I therefore used gentle and upward effleurage strokes and applied pétrissage and stretching exercises to his hands and feet. Whilst initially he was only able to tolerate a few strokes on each limb he immediately benefited from the stretching movements.

These procedures were taught to his wife and she continues to perform them on a twice-weekly basis. Although his mobility is hardly improved, he does seem to be able to hold his cup and spoon more easily and is also able to propel himself for short bursts in his wheelchair. The biggest benefit he notes is that as his arms ache less he no longer takes his co-dydramol and is therefore less constipated. He rates this as the biggest success. I continue to make up and supply the oils and advise where necessary.

It will be useful to see, longer term, whether his wife will also receive some benefit from performing such activities, as there is some evidence that suggests that the carer as well as the patient may benefit because of the symbiotic relationship built up during this time (Brett 2002).

---

wrongly labelled as part of the ageing process and ignored. A small study was undertaken by Hudson (1996) that compared one group of patients where a drop of lavender oil was applied to their pillow and a control group who continued with their normal calming preparations. A record was kept which categorized sleep, dozing, wakefulness and alertness according to nursing observation over a 2-week period and this indicated that there was consistent improvement in both the quality of sleep and day-time activity in the group that received the lavender oil. There seemed to be considerable methodological problems with this study and the author acknowledged the number of variables that might dilute the findings, but it was an effort at systematic introduction of a complementary therapy that incorporated evaluation, indicating that lavender oil might play a part in promoting sleep.

The second study, by Cannard (1996), addressed the problem of sleep disturbance in the older patient in a nursing development unit. The study recorded the sleep patterns of the patients before the use of aromatherapy and after its introduction. Instead of a single oil this study used a blend of basil, juniper, lavender and sweet marjoram oils. Another difference from the previous study was that, if the inhalation of oils was not effective in inducing sleep, then a 5-min hand massage was given, using the blend of oils in a sweet almond carrier oil. The study showed that the particular blend of oils used appeared to be effective in improving the sleep patterns of the patients. But there were limitations to the study: when hand massage was used, no evaluation of the effect of hand massage with no aromatherapy was undertaken. This raises the point made earlier as to whether it was the massage itself rather than the oils used during the massage that was effective. Both studies had a small sample size and relied on self-report data, from either the nurse or patient. In addition there was a wide range of variables that may have influenced the intervention. Therefore the finding that essential oils play a part in caring for older patients with sleep disturbance must be accepted cautiously.

Van Toller (1996) has demonstrated that the part of the brain associated with olfaction is intimately connected with the limbic system, which is associated with motivation, emotion and non-verbal thought. It is reasonable to think that nurses can manipulate these basic physiological functions by using the sense of smell for therapeutic benefit.

Although Mantle (1997) and Vickers (1996) stress there is some confusion within the literature as to the therapeutic worth or toxicity of essential oils and therefore a need for caution, the use of aromatherapy in the care of the older person has great potential. But good practice requires sound knowledge of the chemical properties of the essential oils and their therapeutic indications and contraindications (Stevenson 1995). Patients or clients of whatever age are not a homogeneous group and any therapeutic intervention must be planned and delivered in a way that takes into account individual difference, i.e. the importance of respect. Further nursing research on aromatherapy in the care of the older person will improve understanding and guide patient-centred approaches.

FLOWER REMEDIES

Flower remedies are an oral therapy, which is useful to consider as it so readily combines with massage, aromatherapy and reflexology. Flower remedies are becoming increasingly popular and appear to have a place in the emotional care of older patients. Whilst I have not seen these widely practised in conventional settings, I feel they could be a valuable adjunct to the use of other therapies with either older people themselves and/or their carers. But flower remedies are not to be regarded as a magic potion that will cure all ills, although they may act as a catalyst in the healing process.

Using flowers for emotional healing began centuries ago by the ancient Egyptians and Australian aboriginal people (Hakanson 1998), but it was the work in the 1930s by Edward Bach (pronounced Batch) that brought such treatments into everyday use. Because of their success, Bach gave up his medical practice in 1930 to concentrate on further developing remedies to combat negative emotions, as he was sure such emotions badly affected the healing process. By 1936 he had identified all 38 remedies and the composite Rescue Remedy (Howard 1990). Rescue Remedy is possibly the most widely known of his remedies and has probably been used by many of us in 'emergency situations'.

Whilst the underlying principle behind their action is unknown it is promulgated that the remedies work by entering:

> into direct contact with the Higher Self of Man ... and act as divine energy impulses, across all energy levels (Scheffer 1990: p. 24).

As they appear to have no side-effects they may be taken internally even by the very old and, if used with caution, are safe. It is essential, prior to use, to assess not only patients' symptoms, but also their entire lifestyle, in order that the appropriate remedy may be selected. It is usual to use a combination of two or three remedies, taken up to four times a day, singly, dropped straight into the mouth, or mixed in a glass of water A combination of drops may be added to the bathwater, a massage oil blend and even when performing reflexology. This is an effective, easily used therapy that encourages patients to take back some responsibility for their own healing (Mantle 1997).

The few examples given below are remedies that are particularly helpful for older people (more can be read about other remedies in Howard 1990, Scheffer 1990, Brett 2002). *Aspen* helps those who are fearful for no apparent reason, as it helps them cope, and put their fears into perspective (Scheffer 1990). It seems particularly useful in older people who may be afraid of death and dying.

Gorse is particularly helpful for despairing, distrustful and despondent people searching for hope. These traits are particularly noted for those suffering from chronic and terminal disease, especially when their conventional treatments appear ineffective or disagreeable. Whilst not offering false hope, some reasonable hope may help lift their spirits and help them cope with any palliative care or even be able to refuse care in their terminal stages more readily.

Honeysuckle is considered good for those who live in the past in order to avoid reality, perhaps when they are newly bereaved or when they have to leave their home to enter an institution. Honeysuckle can help them to 'move on' from the past, into their changing life, and make their memories less painful (Scheffer 1990). It combines well with walnut or star of Bethlehem, especially when there is unresolved grief and shock.

Olive is valuable because it has such calming properties and is said to relate to 'the principle of regeneration, peace and restored balance' (Scheffer 1990). It is especially useful for people who are worn out and lacking in energy because it has the potential to replenish these depleted stocks, encourage individuals to listen to their own needs, and then regulate their actions accordingly. Such mental or physical exhaustion may be experienced not only by those enduring lengthy illness or treatments, but also by those who are caring for such people. Once a greater peace of mind is established it may be easier for them to cope with what lies ahead.

Whilst the Bach flower remedies remain the best-known essences, there are many others, from around the world, including the Australian bush and flower remedies and the Californian poppy essences, most of which are now readily available in the UK.

T'AI CHI

T'ai chi is a complementary therapy that has its roots in eastern traditions and has particular relevance for the health of the older person. As movement is an integral part of life, we take it for granted, but loss of mobility is a common problem for older people (Abrams 1978). As physical exercise is positively associated with an active, healthy lifestyle (Haskett 1984), increased habitual activity or exercise patterns are likely to improve functional ability, lifestyle and independence (Adams & de Vries 1973). However, Blair & Garcia (1996) highlight the link between levels of physical inactivity and low physical fitness with morbidity and mortality levels in industrialized countries. The risk of death associated with functional limitation is high in older adult populations. There are at least three separate components of physical fitness that appear to be important for the preservation of function: (1) muscular strength; (2) aerobic power; and (3) balance (Blair & Garcia 1996), but Wolf et al. (1996) describe how many group activities undertaken for the total physiological benefit of older people fail to stress balance control mechanisms.

T'ai chi can be described as a moving meditation, comprising a slow sequence of meditative exercises which emphasize gentle rotation and stretching of the spine. The arm movements are slow, circular, continuous, smooth and controlled and weight is shifted regularly from one foot to the other (Dennis 1996, Fugh-Berman 1996). T'ai chi is based on the Taoist philosophy that teaches that the world is a manifestation of the interplay of two forces, yin and yang. The movements in t'ai chi reflect this belief as each move is seen to be created naturally by its predecessor so that no effort is required to enact the complete form (Vickers 1993).

There are various studies indicating that t'ai chi can improve balance in older people. Tse & Bailey (1992) found that well older people who practised t'ai chi had significantly better postural control compared to an equivalent sedentary group, but the study was not controlled for other types of exercise so the results may simply show the difference between out-of-shape people and relatively fit people. Judge et al. (1993) included t'ai chi in a programme of lower-extremity strengthening, walking and postural control exercises designed to improve the balance of healthy older people and reduce the risk of falls and fall-associated injuries. The study sample was small but the results suggest that there were improvements in balance. Wolf et al. (1996) conducted a study that evaluated the effects of two exercise approaches, t'ai chi and computerized balance training, on specified primary outcomes that included functional indicators of frailty, and secondary outcomes which included the occurrence of falls. The participants were 200 persons aged 70 and older living in the community. The interventions were conducted over 15 weeks and the study found that the t'ai chi intervention significantly reduced the risk of multiple falls. The studies described above have been conducted using 'healthy, able-bodied' older people but Vickers (1993) and Dennis (1996) describe situations where t'ai chi has been used in the sitting position using the bottom as the point for centring the distribution of weight and energy. Kirsteins et al. (1991) evaluated the safety and potential use of t'ai chi as a weight-bearing exercise for older people with rheumatoid arthritis. They found that there was no significant exacerbation of joint symptoms and, because t'ai chi is a weight-bearing exercise, there were the advantages of strengthening the connective tissue surrounding the joint and the stimulation of bone formation.

When thinking about the practicalities of introducing any form of exercise within National Health Service or community health care schemes, the need for expensive and technically sophisticated equipment requiring the supervision of a high proportion of qualified staff is a substantial deterrent. An advantage of t'ai chi exercise is that it is a low-technology approach to exercise that is performed in groups, making it cost-effective in terms of resources. Another benefit is that the exercises allow people to become more aware of their bodies and how they move. Thus mobility is improved not only by greater strength and suppleness but by greater efficiency and awareness. T'ai chi develops ease and grace in movement and promotes a sense of well-being (Vickers 1993, Dennis 1996).

The possible use of t'ai chi in the care of older people highlights interprofessional issues in the use of complementary therapies. Although this book is aimed at nurses, they do not have a monopoly on the use of complementary therapies within clinical practice, and physiotherapists are often taking the initiative with t'ai chi. A fundamental requirement of an activity or intervention that is claimed to be therapeutic for the patient is that the patient's needs inform the rationale for its use.

CONCLUSION

There are many areas that need to be addressed in relation to the safe and systematic integration of complementary therapy into practice that it has not been possible to cover in detail. This chapter has provided some insight into safe approaches to integrating therapies into practice, but also the pitfalls along the way. These are obviously just the first steps toward integration but they give an indication of the seriousness of the undertaking and the depth of commitment needed.

Bay (1995) cautions that complementary therapies are not for everyone. Informed consent is about people being able to make choices about the use of complementary therapies, based upon their own individual values, without undue interference. This provides a challenge for nurses caring for older people who may be suffering from confusion or dementia. Norman (1999) points out that these patients are often unable to express their wishes and inflexible care routines may fail to respond to their individual needs and preferences.

It would seem that the integration of complementary therapies into nursing practice can be challenging and its success seems to be reliant upon the support of the multidisciplinary team. It is important therefore to work collaboratively with others and institute meticulous protocols and procedures, which will support the change process.

This chapter ends with the story of Procrustes, a highwayman from Greek mythology who invited travellers to spend the night before resuming their journey. The unfortunate traveller was tied to a bed and, if too tall, limbs were chopped off and, if too short, they were stretched to fit (Marks-Maran 1995). Paradoxically, such inflexibility can also arise from nurses with well-meant intentions who are determined to use complementary therapies such as holistic care. Their zeal can override their ability to be receptive to their patients' wishes and sensibilities. But:

there is – [also] – a danger that the phenomenon may, like the butterfly that is pinned down for closer inspection, be destroyed in the attempts to understand it (Janet Quinn 1995, cited in Brett 2002).

Recommended reading

Brett H 2002 Complementary therapies in the care of older people. Whurr, London.
This book gives an insight into using complementary therapies safely with older people. It also uses several case studies and has an extensive glossary, which includes information on essential oils, flower remedies and complementary therapy terminology

Dossey B, Keegan L, Guzzetta C, Kolkmeir L 1995 Holistic nursing: a handbook for practice, 2nd edn. Aspen, Maryland.
A comprehensive book that includes theoretical and practical aspects of holistic nursing

Ingham E (1991) The original works of Eunice D. Ingham. Stories the feet can tell thru reflexology – stories the feet have told thru reflexology (with revisions by Dwight C. Byers). Ingham Publishing, St Petersburg, USA.
Whilst not written in an academic style it is deemed to be one of the 'classical' reflexology texts.

Rankin-Box D (ed) 2001 The nurses' handbook of complementary therapies. Baillière Tindall, London.
A book which is designed to answer queries about some of the complementary therapies and also gives some advice about competent practice.

Royal College of Nursing 2003 Complementary therapies in nursing, midwifery and health visiting practice. Royal College of Nursing, London.
Royal College of Nursing guidance on integrating complementary therapies into clinical care.

Sayre-Adams J, Wright S 1995 The theory and practice of therapeutic touch. Churchill Livingstone, Edinburgh.
This book explores the history and conceptual basis of therapeutic touch (TT) and introduces a critical appraisal of the associated literature and practice research.

Stone J, Mathews J 1996 Complementary therapies and the law. Oxford University Press, Oxford.
The authors discuss legal issues that concern therapists.

Vickers A 1996 Massage and aromatherapy: a guide for health professionals. Chapman & Hall, London.
Whilst rather an old text now, it documents the problems in establishing a research base in complementary therapies.

Willison K, Andrews G 2004 Complementary medicine and older people: past research and future directions. Complementary Therapies in Nursing and Midwifery 10: 80–91.
Very useful review of CAM and older people.

Zollman C, Vickers A 2001 ABC of complementary medicine. London, BMJ Books.
Useful introductory guide to CAM.

Useful websites

www.elsevier.com
Complementary Therapies in Nursing and Midwifery Journal and International Journal of Aromatherapy.
www.fimed.org
Prince of Wales's Foundation for Integrated Health.
www.icmedicine.co.uk
Institute for Complementary Medicine.
www.ifparoma.org
International Federation of Professional Aromatherapists (IFPA).
www.nccam.nih.gov
National Centre for Complementary and Alternative Medicine.

www.nccan.nih.gov
Complementary and alternative medicine on PUBMed.
www.nmc-uk.org
Nursing and Midwifery Council.
www.parliament.the-stationary-
office.co.uk/pa/id/idsctech/htm
*Sixth report from the House of Lords Select Committee on science
and technology (HL paper 123).*
www.rccm.org
Research Council for Complementary Medicine.
www.rcn.org.uk
*Royal College of Nursing online (Complementary Therapies in
Nursing Forum).*
www.the-cma.org.uk
Complementary Medical Association.

References

Abrams M 1978 Beyond three score years and ten. Age
Concern, London

Adams GM, de Vries HA 1973 Physiological effects of an
exercise programme upon women aged 52–79. Journal of
Gerontology 28: 50–55

Argyle M 1975 Bodily communication. Methuen, London

Avis A 1999 Complementary therapies. In: Redfern SJ, Ross
FM (eds) Nursing older people, 3rd edn. Churchill
Livingstone, Edinburgh, pp 215–232

Barnett J 1972 A survey of the current utilisation of touch by
health team personnel with hospitalised patients.
International Journal of Nursing Studies 9: 195–209

Bay F 1995 Complementary therapies – just another task?
Complementary Therapies in Nursing and Midwifery 1:
34–36

Beard G, Wood G 1994 Massage principles and techniques.
WB Saunders, Philadelphia, PA

Bell L, Sikora K 1996 Guest editorial. Complementary
therapies and cancer care. Complementary Therapies in
Nursing and Midwifery 2: 57–58

Blair S, Garcia M 1996 Get up and move: a call to action for
older men and women. Journal of the American
Geriatrics Society 44: 599–600

Bottorff J 1993 The use and meaning of touch in caring for
patients with cancer. Oncology Nurse Forum 20: 1531–1538

Bowlby J 1984 Attachment and loss, vol. 1: Attachment, 2nd
edn. Penguin, London

Brett H 1999 Aromatherapy in the care of older people.
Nursing Times 95: 33, 56–57

Brett H 2002 Complementary therapies in the care of older
people. Whurr Publishers, London

Buckle J 1993 When is holism not complementary? British
Journal of Nursing 2: 744–745

Cannard G 1996 The effect of aromatherapy in promoting
relaxation and stress reduction in a general hospital.
Complementary Therapies in Nursing and Midwifery 2:
38–40

Chadwick L 1999 What are the reasons for nurses using
complementary therapy in practice. Complementary
Therapies in Nursing and Midwifery 5: 144–148

Corner J, Cawley N, Hildebrand S 1995 An evaluation of the
use of massage and essential oils on the wellbeing of
cancer patients. International Journal of Palliative
Nursing 1: 67–73

Cox C, Hayes J 2000 Immediate effects of a five minute foot
massage on patients in critical care. Complementary
Therapies in Nursing and Midwifery 6: 9–13

Cribb A, Bignold S, Ball S 1994 Linking the parts: an
exemplar of philosophical and practical issues in holistic
nursing. Journal of Advanced Nursing 20: 233–238

Davies S, Riches L 1995 Healing touch. Nursing Times 91:
42–43

Day F 1973 The patient's perception of touch. In: Anderson
E et al. (eds) Current concepts in clinical nursing. Mosby,
St Louis

Dennis M 1996 Gently does it. Therapy Weekly April 18: 7

Dickinson DPS 1996 The growth of complementary therapy:
a consumer-led boom. In: Ernst E (ed) Complementary
medicine: an objective appraisal. Butterworth
Heinemann, London, pp 150–161

Dossey B, Keegan L, Guzzetta C, Kolkmeier L 1995 Holistic
nursing, 2nd edn. Aspen, Maryland

Dunn C, Sleep J, Collett D 1995 Sensing an improvement: an
experimental study to evaluate the use of aromatherapy,
massage and periods of rest in an intensive care unit.
Journal of Advanced Nursing 21: 43–50

Ernst E, Cassileth B 1998 The prevalence of complementary/
alternative medicine in cancer – a systematic review.
Cancer 83: 777–782

Ernst E, Fialka V 1994 Evidence-based complementary
medicine. Complementary Therapies in Nursing and
Midwifery 3: 42–45

Ernst E, White A 2000 The BBC survey of complementary
medicine use in the UK. Complementary Therapies in
Medicine 8: 32–36

Ersser S 1995 Complementary therapies and nursing
research: issues and practicalities. Complementary
Therapies in Nursing and Midwifery 1: 44–45

Estabrooks C, Morse J 1992 Toward a theory of touch: the
touching process and acquiring a touching style. Journal
of Advanced Nursing 17: 448–456

Farrow J 1990 Massage therapy and nursing care. Nursing
Standard 4: 26–28

Ferrell-Torry A, Glick O 1993 The use of therapeutic
massage as a nursing intervention to modify anxiety
and the perception of cancer pain. Cancer Nursing 16:
93–101

Fordham M, Dunn V 1994 Alongside the person in pain.
Baillière Tindall, London

Foster H 1994 Supportive therapies: a reflection on practice.
Journal of Clinical Nursing 3: 4–5

Fox M 2001 Access to complementary health care: why the
NHS is the key. Complementary Therapies in Nursing
and Midwifery 7: 123–125

Fraser J, Ross Kerr J 1993 Psychological effects of back
massage on elderly institutionalised patients. Journal of
Advanced Nursing 18: 238–245

Fugh-Berman A 1996 Alternative medicine: what works?
Odonian Press, Tuscon, AZ

Furnham A 2000 How the public classify complementary medicine: a factor analytic study. Complementary Therapies in Medicine 8: 111–118

Furnham A 2002 Complementary and alternative medicine. Psychologist 15: 228–231

Gates B 1995 The use of complementary and alternative therapies in health care: a selective review of the literature and discussion of the implications for nurse practitioners and health-care managers. Journal of Clinical Nursing 3: 43–47

Goldstone L 2000 Massage as an orthodox medical treatment past and future. Complementary Therapies in Nursing and Midwifery 6: 169–175

Griffin A 1993 Holism in nursing: its meaning and value. British Journal of Nursing 2: 310–312

Hakanson D 1998 Oracle of the dreamtime. Aboriginal dreamings offer guidance for today. Connections Book Publishing, London

Haskett W 1984 Overview: health benefits of exercise. In: Matarazzo J (ed) Behavioural health: a hand-book of health enhancement and disease prevention. Wiley, New York

Hildebrand S 1994 Therapeutic massage. In: Wells R, Tschudin V (eds) Well's supportive therapies in health care. Baillière Tindall, London, pp 103–128

Hoban V 2003 Integrating complementary therapies. Nursing Times 99: 20–23

Hollinger L 1980 Perception of touch in the elderly. Journal of Gerontological Nursing 6: 741–746

Hopkins C 1995 Aromatherapy: remedies for everyday ailments. Parallel Books. Bristol

Horrigan C 1995 Massage. In: Rankin-Box D (ed) The nurses' handbook of complementary therapies. Churchill Livingstone, Edinburgh

House of Lords Select Committee on Science and Technology 2000 The 6th report on complementary and alternative medicine (HL paper 123). Stationery Office. London

Howard J 1990 The Bach flower remedies step by step. Saffron Walden, CW Daniel

Hudson R 1996 The value of lavender for rest and activity in the elderly patient. Complementary Therapies in Medicine 4: 52–57

Johnson G 2000 Should nurses practise complementary therapies? Complementary Therapies in Nursing and Midwifery 6: 120–123

Jourard SM 1966 An exploratory study of body accessibility. British Journal of Social and Clinical Psychology 5: 221–231

Judge J, Lindsey C, Underwood M, Winsemius D 1993 Balance improvements in older women: effects of exercise training. Physical Therapy 73: 254–265

Kaada B, Torsteinbo O 1989 Increase of plasma beta endorphin levels in connective tissue massage. General Pharmacology 20. 487–489

Kendrick K 1999 Challenging power, autonomy and politics in complementary therapies: a contentious view. Complementary Therapies in Nursing and Midwifery 5: 77–81

Kirsteins A, Dietz F, Hwang S 1991 Evaluating the safety and potential use of a weight-bearing exercise, tai chi chuan, for rheumatoid arthritis patients. American Journal of Physical Medicine and Rehabilitation 70: 136–141

Lawler 1991 The body in nursing. Churchill Livingstone, Melbourne

Long A, Mercer G, Hughes K 2000 Developing a tool to measure holistic practice: a missing dimension in outcome measurement with complementary therapies. Complementary Therapies in Medicine 8: 26–31

Malkin K 1994 Use of massage in clinical practice. British Journal of Nursing 3: 292–294

Mantle F 1997 Bach flower remedies. Complementary Therapies in Nursing and Midwifery 3: 142–144

Marks-Maran D 1995 Procrustes in the ward: fitting people into models. In: Jolley M, Brykczynska G (eds) Nursing: beyond tradition and conflict. Mosby, London, pp 55–70

McCann K, McKenna H 1993 An examination of touch between nurses and elderly patients in a continuing care setting in Northern Ireland. Journal of Advanced Nursing 18: 836–846

McMahon R 1991 Therapeutic nursing: theory issues and practice. In: McMahon R, Pearson A (eds) Nursing as therapy. Chapman & Hall, London, pp 1–25

McNamara P 1994 Massage for people with cancer. Wandsworth Cancer Support Centre, London

Montague A 1986 Touching: the human significance of the skin, 3rd edn. Perennial Library, New York

Morse JM, Bottorff J, Hutchinson S 1994 The phenomenology of comfort. Journal of Advanced Nursing 20: 189–195

Norman I 1999 Person centred dementia care. In: Redfern S, Ross F (eds) Nursing elderly people. Churchill Livingstone, Edinburgh, pp 525–564

Norton L 1995 Complementary therapies in practice: the ethical issues. Journal of Clinical Nursing 4: 343–348

NMC 2002a Code of professional conduct. Nursing and Midwifery Council, London

NMC 2002b Guidelines for the administration of medicines. Nursing and Midwifery Council, London

NMC 2002c The scope of professional practice. Nursing and Midwifery Council, London

Owen M, Holmes C 1993 'Holism' in the discourse of nursing. Journal of Advanced Nursing 18: 1688–1695

Pietroni P 1992 Beyond the boundaries: relationship between general practice and complementary medicine. British Medical Journal 305: 564–566

Pietroni P 1996 The greening of medicine. In: Innovations in community care and primary health. Churchill Livingstone, Edinburgh, pp 15–18

Pratt J, Mason A 1981 The caring touch. Heyden, London

Rankin-Box D (ed) 2001 The nurses' handbook of complementary therapies. Baillière Tindall, London

Rankin-Box D 2002 Ethics and quality in complementary therapy education. Nursing Times 98: 40–42

RCN 2003 Complementary therapies in nursing, midwifery and health visiting practice. Royal College of Nursing, London

Routasalo P 1996 Non-necessary touch in the nursing care of elderly people. Journal of Advanced Nursing 23: 904–911

Savage J 1995 Nursing intimacy. Scutari Press, London

Scheffer M 1990 Bach flower therapy. Theory and practice. Thorsons, London

Scull C 1945 Massage – physiologic basis. Archives of Physical Medicine 26: 159–167

Seaman L 1982 Affective nursing touch. Geriatric Nursing 3: 162–164

Sharma V 1992 Complementary medicine today. Routledge, London

Sidell M 1995 Rethinking ageing: health in old age, myth, mystery and management. Open University Press, Buckingham

Sims S 1986 Slow stroke back massage for cancer patients. Nursing Times 82: 47–50

Sims S 1988 The significance of touch in palliative care. Palliative Medicine 2: 58–61

Snyder M, Egan E, Bums K 1995a Efficacy of hand massage in decreasing agitation behaviors associated with rare activities in people with dementia. Geriatric Nursing March/April: 60–63

Snyder M, Egan E, Bums K 1995b Interventions for decreasing agitation behaviors in persons with dementia. Journal of Gerontological Nursing July: 35–40

Stevenson C 1994 The psychological effects of aromatherapy following cardiac surgery. Complementary Therapies in Medicine 2: 27–35

Stevenson C 1995 Aromatherapy. In: Rankin-Box D (ed) The nurse's handbook of complementary therapies. Churchill Livingstone, Edinburgh, pp 51–58

Teasdale K 1995 Theoretical and practical considerations on the use of reassurance in the nursing management of anxious patients. Journal of Advanced Nursing 22: 79–86

Thomas K, Nicholl J, Coleman P 2001 Use and expenditure on complementary medicine in England: a population based survey. Complementary Therapies in Medicine 9: 2–11

Trevelyan J, Booth B 1994 Complementary medicine for nurses, midwives and health visitors. Macmillan, Basingstoke

Tse S, Bailey DM 1992 Tai chi and postural control in the well elderly. American Journal of Occupational Therapy 46: 295–300

Tutton E 1987 The effect of slow-stroke back massage on the perceived well-being of elderly female patients in a nursing unit. MSc thesis. University of London, London

Tutton E 1991 An exploration of touch and its use in nursing. In: McMahon R, Pearson A (eds) Nursing as therapy. Chapman & Hall, London, pp 142–169

Van Toller S 1996 Introduction to the sense of smell. In: Vickers A (ed) Massage and aromatherapy. Chapman & Hall, London, p 35

Vickers A 1993 Complementary medicine and disability. Chapman & Hall, London

Vickers A 1996 Massage and aromatherapy: a guide for health professionals. Chapman & Hall, London

Vortherms R 1991 Clinically improving communication through touch. Journal of Gerontological Nursing 17: 5

Watson W 1975 The meanings of touch: geriatric nursing. Journal of Communication 25: 104–112

Weiss S 1979 The language of touch. Nursing Research 28: 76–80

Wells R, Tschudin V 1994 Supportive therapies in health care. Baillière Tindall, London

White A, Ernst E 2000 Economic analysis of complementary medicine. Complementary Therapies in Medicine 8: 111–118

Wilkinson S 1995 Aromatherapy and massage in palliative care – does it improve patients' quality of life? International Journal of Palliative Nursing 1: 15–20

Wolf SI, Barnhart HX, Kutner NG et al. 1996 Reducing frailty and falls in older persons: an investigation of t'ai chi and computerised balance training. Journal of the American Geriatrics Society 44: 489–497

Wright S 1989 Changing nursing practice. Edward Arnold, London

Wright S 1995 The competence to touch: helping and healing in nursing practice. Complementary Therapies in Medicine 3: 49–52

Chapter 32

Abuse of older people

Claudine McCreadie and Bridget Penhale

INTRODUCTION

In November 1965 the following letter, written by three members of the House of Lords and a number of other concerned people, appeared in the correspondence columns of *The Times*:

> Sir, We, the undersigned, have been shocked by the treatment of geriatric patients in certain mental hospitals, one of the evils being the practice of stripping them of their personal possessions. We have now sufficient evidence to suggest that this is widespread.
>
> The attitude of the Ministry of Health to complaints has merely reinforced our anxieties. In consequence, we have decided to collect evidence of ill-treatment of geriatric patients throughout the country, to demonstrate the need for a national investigation. We hope this will lead to the securing of effective and humane control over these hospitals by the Ministry which seems at present to be lacking.
>
> We shall be grateful if those who have encountered malpractices in this sphere will supply us with detailed information which would of course be treated as confidential (Martin 1984).

The Nursing and Midwifery Council professional code of conduct provides nurses with unambiguous guidance about professional standards. It states that:

> As a registered nurse, midwife or specialist community public health nurse, you must:
>
> - Protect and support the health of individual patients and clients
> - Protect and support the health of the wider community
> - Act in such a way that justifies the trust and confidence the public have in you
> - Uphold and enhance the good reputation of the professions.
>
> You are personally accountable for your practice. This means that you are answerable for your actions and omissions, regardless of advice or directions from another professional.
>
> You have a duty of care to your patients and clients, who are entitled to receive safe and competent care.
>
> You must adhere to the laws of the country in which you are practising (Nursing and Midwifery Council, 2004).

This sets the framework for the profession's response to abuse, as it does to any other condition that they face in the course of work. Any abuse of an older person contradicts those standards. A document from the UKCC (forerunner of the Nursing and Midwifery Council) concerning practitioner–client relationships is absolute in its assertion:

> 'Zero tolerance of abuse is the only philosophy consistent with protecting the public' (UKCC 1999, p. 4). This document covers the practitioner's responsibilities in terms of relationships with clients and is essential reading for students and practitioners alike.

Apart from routine care on the wards, the hospital setting provides highly significant opportunities for the identification and prevention of abuse. Nurses working in accident and emergency departments may be among the first to encounter severe cases of physical abuse and neglect and to identify the non-accidental from the accidental injury (Kingston & Penhale 1995, Vernon 1995). Nurses contributing to decisions about the discharge of patients may understand, and are certainly in a position to explore, the nature of the home circumstances to which an older person is returning – circumstances which may be critical in relation to possible abuse.

In the community, nurses are also in the front line as far as possible abuse goes (Harrison 1994, Kingston & Phillipson 1994, Richardson 1998, Kitchen et al. 2002; Fig. 32.1). It is important, therefore, that in whatever position they hold, nurses are aware of the existence of abuse (it can and does occur) and of the possible effects of abuse. Community nurses visit older peoples' homes regularly. Their knowledge of the older person, his or her social network, the relationships in the family, the way people come and go, the older person's state of mind, something probably of his or her history, make them amongst the foremost experts on people's family circumstances. As a regular visitor, the observant and listening nurse may come to know things that other professionals, involved on a less regular basis, never get to know (Phair & Goodman 2003). Nurses are frequently managers or owners of residential or nursing homes, as well as members of staff. Community nurses also visit residential and nursing homes. So here also nurses may be expert on the communal household. They may know where the quality of care is doubtful, know their staff's difficulties and stresses, know the personalities and disabilities of residents and the demands that can be made, and the way that staff respond to these demands. In the context of communal settings, nurses can be instrumental in promoting good practice and high standards of care. Finally, nurses are active in the registration and inspection of communal settings, are involved in the training and supervision of students and junior nurses and undertake key management tasks such as appointments and the letting of contracts for nursing-home placements. In all these contexts knowledge and awareness of abuse issues are important.

This chapter begins by examining definitions of abuse and then looks at prevalence and research in both community and communal settings. Wherever possible, research specifically involving nurses is

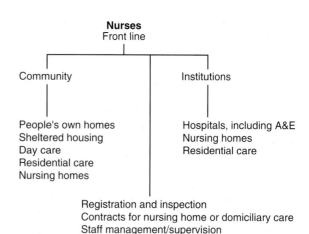

Fig. 32.1 Nurses are in the front line. A&E, Accident and Emergency.

drawn on. Issues around intervention are discussed very largely in the context of the community, reflecting the lack of research into abuse in communal settings. However, for nurses working in acute wards the reality is that their patients are discharged to community settings and they can play a potentially crucial role in being alert to the safety of those settings. Intervention is discussed, with particular reference to assessment of older people, legal and professional issues and multi-disciplinary working. Attention is given to financial abuse, confidentiality and education and training. The issues arising in communal settings are considered in the sections voicing concerns about abuse and the regulation of nursing homes. The chapter concludes with a brief consideration of policy development and a note on the organization Action on Elder Abuse. Although writing from the perspective of developments in the UK, these developments have been substantially influenced by research from abroad, and particularly the USA. There is now an interesting literature available from Canada and Australia as well as continental Europe and much that can be learnt, along with proper recognition of differences in service provision, culture and legal systems between the countries.

Although there have been a number of overview articles about elder abuse in the nursing literature (Mowbray 1989, Fagg 1994, Harrison 1994, Kingston & Penhale 1994, Kingston & Phillipson 1994, Penhale & Kingston 1995, Pritchard 1996), little research specifically with nurses has been undertaken. However, there have been several small studies (Lowe 1993, Clarke & Ogg 1994a, 1994b, Kitchen et al. 2002) and helpful research has been done in Sweden, which is reported in some detail in this chapter. This research examined how district nurses defined abuse (Saveman et al. 1993a, 1995), the nature of the cases they encountered (Saveman et al. 1993b, 1996) and the problems they faced in addressing abusive situations (Saveman et al. 1992).

DEFINITIONS

The word 'abuse' has no legal meaning, nor is it clear that older people would naturally use this word. Some kinds of behaviour that are defined as abuse are criminal acts, such as assault and theft; others, such as verbal abuse, or the restraint of someone who is aggressive, may seem much more contingent upon particular circumstances. Gilleard (1994) points out that in communal settings a conflict may often exist between the need to get a care task done, for example, bathing a patient, and respect for the autonomy of the patient, who may not wish to have a bath. What is abuse in these circumstances? At what point does it

differ from poor-quality care? Hughes & Wilkin (1987) found that toileting routines in a home where over 50% of patients were incontinent were:

> regimented, dehumanising and completely without privacy, although this is not to say that staff were brusque, cold or uncaring. The characteristics of the toileting process have to be seen as a consequence of the need to toilet large numbers of disabled people in a very short space of time (Hughes & Wilkin 1987: p. 414).

Studies of individual nursing homes have found that psychological abuse, in the form of infantilization, demeaning and humiliating attitudes and ignoring of patients, is common (Hockey 1990, Foner 1994, Lee-Treweek 1994). But how far is this, as one of them comments: 'a reflection of the complex tangle of attachments, obligations, and antagonisms involved in nursing home care'? (Foner 1994: p. 250). Further, when is restraint abuse, given that the patient may be violent, that either the patient or somebody else may need protection, and that the reality of care in communal settings may be a shortage of staff? If someone is over-sedated or given inappropriate medication, is this abuse? Dr Baker, in his original article, clearly thought so in the example given in Case study 32.1. Further attention has been paid to this area in recent years (Chambers 1999) and the issue was raised as

Case study 32.1

An elderly widow lived alone and was regularly visited by her children ... she complained of tightness in the chest. The GP was asked to visit, found some evidence of early heart failure and [prescribed] digitalis and a diuretic. Relatives visiting a few months later thought her condition had deteriorated and the GP was asked to visit again. She was somewhat tremulous and he prescribed medication for early parkinsonism. Soon after this the old lady became rather more agitated and was put on a day-time tranquillizer. [The relatives were still concerned and took her to stay with relatives. The move unsettled her and she became depressed.] The local GP was asked to call and he prescribed antidepressants [as well as her other medication] and when she did not improve the dose was increased. She then developed some nocturnal restlessness, so she was given sedatives at night. The dose of these was also increased. A domiciliary visit revealed a very confused old lady, drowsy by day, restless by night, incontinent and having occasional falls. Source: Baker (1975: p. 21).

part of a wider enquiry into elder abuse by the House of Commons Health Committee in 2004 (House of Commons Health Committee, 2004).

Under the general umbrella of elder abuse, therefore, a great many different situations may be subsumed. There is also room for considerable debate about where to draw the line in distinguishing abuse from poor-quality care, or unkindness, or mistaken strategies for coping, or poor relationships, or even slipping the change from the shopping into your pocket.

Despite the lack of standard definitions, it is easier to be clear about the meaning of abuse if the different types of abuse are spelt out. There is now widespread agreement about five types of abuse:

1. physical violence
2. psychological abuse
3. financial abuse
4. sexual abuse
5. neglect.

Sometimes sexual abuse is subsumed under physical abuse, although it has been increasingly recognized as a form of abuse in its own right.

Abuse involves both behaviour by someone, and the effect that this has on the other person. That is, it occurs in the context of a relationship. Self-neglect is generally regarded as a distinct phenomenon in the UK, although in the USA it is often included (McCreadie 1996). The following definitions, taken from McCreadie (1996: p. 11) and UKCC (1999: p. 6) incorporate both behaviour and effect.

Physical abuse

'The non-accidental infliction of physical force that results in bodily injury, pain or impairment' (Stein 1991: p. 97). This type of abuse may also cause psychological harm to the individual.

Examples of behaviour
These include hitting, slapping, pushing, burning, 'poor application of manual handling techniques or unreasonable physical restraint' (UKCC 1999, p. 6).

Examples of effects
Such effects include bruises, fractures, burns, broken teeth, sprains, cuts, hair loss, bleeding, fear, anxiety and depression.

Psychological abuse

'Any verbal or non-verbal behaviour which demonstrates disrespect for the client and could be emotionally or psychologically damaging' (UKCC 1999, p. 6).

Psychological abuse includes the use of threats, humiliation, bullying, swearing and other verbal conduct, and any other form of mental cruelty, that results in mental or physical distress.

Examples of behaviour
Such behaviour includes treating an elderly person as a child, blaming, swearing, intimidating, mocking, name-calling, threatening violence or physical harm, coercing, isolating the elder and denying privacy.

Examples of effects
Effects include fear, depression, confusion, loss of sleep and loss of appetite.

Financial abuse

'The unauthorised and improper use of funds, property or any resources of an older person' (Stein 1991: p. 97). This includes not only illegal acts such as theft, but the inappropriate use of funds, property or resources.

Examples of behaviour
Examples include misappropriating money, valuables or property, forcing changes to will, denying the elder the right to access personal funds and inappropriate withholding or handling of a client's money or possessions.

Examples of effects
Such effects include loss of money, inability to pay bills, deterioration in health or standard of living, lack of amenities, unusual activity in bank accounts, signatures on documents uncertain, lack of solid arrangements for financial management, eviction or house sale notices.

Sexual abuse

'Forcing, inducing or attempting to induce the client to engage in any form of sexual activity' (UKCC 1999). Direct or indirect involvement in sexual activity without consent is a key element here.

Examples of behaviour
Non-contact sexual abuse includes looking, photography, indecent exposure, harassment, serious teasing or innuendo, pornography. Contact sexual abuse includes touch (e.g. of breasts, genitals, anus, mouth), masturbation of either or both persons, penetration or attempted penetration of vagina, anus or mouth, with the penis, fingers or other objects (Brown & Turk 1992: p. 47).

Examples of effects

Such effects include difficulty in walking or sitting, bruises, bleeding, venereal disease and psychological trauma.

Neglect

'The repeated deprivation of some assistance that the older person needs for important activities of daily living' (Clarke & Ogg 1994b: p. 4). It is considered to be the failure or refusal by the caregiver (formal or informal) to meet the essential needs of the individual older person.

Examples of behaviour

Neglect includes failure to provide food, fluids, personal hygiene, shelter, clothing, medical care (aids, assistance or equipment), hygiene and personal care, as well as the inappropriate use of medication (under- or overmedication).

Examples of effects

Effects include malnutrition, pressure sores, oversedation, untreated medical problems, depression and confusion.

It is helpful to consider some dimensions of abuse, particularly the severity of effect upon individuals and the extent of their distress. However, it may also be useful to consider how frequently abuse is occurring and how long it has been going on (McCreadie 1996). Some of the answers to these questions may provide clues to the nature of the abusing situation and to the appropriateness of intervention. Having noted all this, for the practitioner, the definitions provided for the purposes of academic research can have limited value. Real life is far more complicated and the practitioner faces complex situations when suspecting abuse. As seen elsewhere, the search for standard definitions, applicable to all settings and situations, is unlikely to be easily achieved. It is probably better to recognize that a number of different definitions exist and to acknowledge the differences that exist between them in an open manner that means that appropriate actions can then be taken (Penhale 1993). It is also important to note the following explicit statements by the UKCC:

> Registered nurses, midwives and health visitors have a responsibility to protect clients from all forms of abuse (UKCC 1999: p. 7)

and:

> If in the course of their professional practice, registered nurses, midwives and health visitors suspect or believe that a client is or has been abused, they must report this as soon as practical to a person of appropriate authority (UKCC 1999: p. 7).

What this means in practice is that practitioners must know about their local practice guidelines relating to abuse and to whom and at what point they should report concerns or suspicions.

NURSES' EXPERIENCES OF WORKING WITH ABUSE

It has been stated that abuse is one of the most difficult problems encountered by nurses (Phillips 1988). A small survey of 24 district nurses and two community psychiatric nurses working with older people in Tower Hamlets, London, found that 'several . . . had misgivings or reservations over the "labelling" of the interaction, communication and behaviours in relationships as being "abusive". The community psychiatric nurses in particular were apprehensive of reducing the complexities of family relations and the care of a disabled elderly person to morally laden terms such as 'abuser', 'victim' or 'perpetrator', resulting in connotations of blame and judgement' (Clarke & Ogg 1994b: p. 6). When the researchers talked to four of the respondents in greater detail, they found that the nurses invariably saw the carer as the vulnerable party in the relationship. They also thought that, within a particular household, behaviour might not be perceived as abusive. Intervention by a third party might only make matters worse. They also associated the term 'elder abuse' with physical abuse, whereas in practice they encountered many types of behaviour which had a harmful impact on the older person.

In the Swedish research, 21 district nurses, all with experience of a case of abuse, were asked in tape-recorded interviews to describe a case from their own personal experience and then they were asked about how they defined abuse and how they recognized it when it was occurring (Saveman et al. 1993a). The authors suggest that for these district nurses four salient factors in defining abuse were:

1. the actual act of abuse (i.e. the behaviour)
2. the relationship between the two parties
3. the impact of the abuse on the abused person
4. the intention of the abuser.

Acts of abuse appeared to be ranged on a continuum, as shown in these examples:

> If you beat somebody, for instance to get money or something like that (Saveman et al. 1993a).

> You ignore what the sick person wants (Saveman et al. 1993a: p. 1395).

As has been widely reported in other research, abusers were not just carers, but could be relatives living together without family responsibilities, professional caregivers, or the abuse could result from the way services were run. This is an important point, as it is a commonplace in the literature to see the word 'carer' used, as though only carers can be abusers. The nurses tried to think themselves into the situation of the abused person:

> Having to give your keys to the home help service and having just anyone coming and going in your home, looking for things in your drawer and entering your bedroom. I think many regard this as abuse (Saveman et al. 1993a: p. 1395).

> And then there's also the kind of psychological abuse you know, where you make them understand how stupid they are (Saveman et al. 1993a: p. 1395).

Finally, the nurses referred to the intentions of the abuser. This was sometimes seen as a deliberate act to inflict harm, sometimes actions which the abuser knew harmed the older person but did not want to believe that this was the case. Although intention is clearly relevant to an understanding of the abusive situation, and to the nature of any intervention, many commentators consider that it should not be part of a definition of abuse, as essentially it is the effect on the person who is abused that is important (McCreadie 1991).

The authors of the Swedish report note that 'the district nurses had no distinct, easily formulated definition of abuse ... instead they reasoned around it using intuition, concrete descriptions, sometimes with examples and abstract terms to explain the abuse' (Saveman et al. 1993a: p. 1397):

> Taking their identity away from them somehow. They can't even decide about their own lives, possessions or existence (Saveman et al. 1993a: p. 1396).

> Everything is a question of losing one's respect for the person you beat or the person you rob or terrorize psychologically (Saveman et al. 1993a).

Thus the replies of these nurses, like those of their counterparts in London (Clarke & Ogg 1994a, 1994b), reflect the rather blurred nature of the boundaries of abuse. The Swedish authors suggest, however, that the common theme running through all the examples the nurses cited was that of 'overriding the boundaries of a person's integrity/autonomy' (Saveman et al. 1993a: p. 1397).

PREVALENCE

Table 32.1 gives details of the four major studies on the prevalence of abuse that have taken place in the last 10 years. The Boston study (Pillemer & Finkelhor 1988) was a stratified random sample survey of people over the age of 65 living in the community. Respondents were asked either in a telephone interview, or in person, about their experience of physical violence, verbal aggression and neglect. These categories of abuse were defined as follows:

- Physical: at least one act of physical violence against the respondent since he or she was 65
- Psychological: chronic verbal aggression – being insulted, sworn at or threatened at least 10 times or more in the preceding year
- Neglect: deprivation of some assistance important to daily life 10 times or more during the preceding year.

Table 32.1   Prevalence of elder abuse in Boston USA, 1986; Canada, 1990; UK, 1992; and Amsterdam, the Netherlands, 1994

Type of abuse	Boston, USA, 1986 (%)	Canada, 1990 (%)	UK, 1992 (%)	Amsterdam, the Netherlands 1994 (%) (Comijs 1999)
Physical	2	0.5	1.5	1.2
Psychological*	1.1	1.1	5.4	3.2
Financial	Not in study	2.5	1.5	1.4
Neglect	0.4	0.4	Not in study	0.2
Multiple	Not in study	0.8	Not in study	Not in study
Base	2020	2008	593	1797

*Persistent verbal abuse.
Source: McCreadie & Tinker 2003, and drawn from Comijs 1999.

In order to include older people who were too physically or mentally impaired to be interviewed, an interview was conducted with a proxy respondent, who was the primary carer of the designated respondent. Interestingly, the rates of reported maltreatment were higher in the proxy interviews than in those with the 'independent' older people. Overall, a 72% response rate was achieved. As can be seen from Table 32.1, the most frequent type of abuse reported was physical violence, reported by 2% of respondents, followed by chronic verbal aggression, reported by 1% of respondents, and neglect, by less than 0.5% of respondents.

The Canadian survey, funded as part of a federal government initiative against family violence, was a national sample survey of people over the age of 65 living in the community. The sample size, 2008, was large enough to generalize the findings to the older Canadian population. The survey, by telephone only, used the same definitions as the Boston one, but also included financial abuse. This was defined by asking respondents whether anyone they knew had tried to: persuade them to give them money; cheat or trick them into giving money; persuade them to relinquish control over their finances; influence them to change their will; make them give up something of value; or persuade them to sign over their house to them.

As can be seen from Table 32.1, financial abuse turned out to account for more than one-half of the cases, while verbal abuse accounted for another third. The significantly lower rates of physical violence, compared with the Boston study, are attributed by the authors to the generally lower rate of violence in Canadian society. However, the authors stress that the estimates of prevalence should be regarded as the minimum, for three main reasons:

1. The criteria for what constituted abuse were relatively strict
2. Not all forms of abuse would necessarily be included in these definitions. The authors quote their own finding that 4% of older Canadians with grandchildren had been denied access to them at least once since they were 65 and question whether this is another form of abuse or could be seen as psychological abuse. They make the point that there are forms of maltreatment other than the four strictly defined categories of this study (Podnieks 1990)
3. The findings report what victims themselves admitted to the interviewer, and the authors suggest that there may well have been some underreporting.

The only survey in the UK (Ogg & Bennett 1992) made use of a government national sample survey: the Office of National Statistics omnibus survey. This covered 2130 people of all ages, of whom 593 were over the age of 60 (women) or 65 (men). Individuals were asked questions as part of the wider Omnibus survey. To do this, older people were given cards with the following definitions of abuse:

- Physical abuse: whether a close family member or relative had pushed, slapped, shoved or been physically rough with them in any other way
- Verbal abuse: whether a close family member or relative had recently frightened them by shouting, insulting or speaking roughly to them
- Financial abuse: whether a close family member or relative had taken money or property from them without their consent.

The different levels of abuse reported, compared with the North American studies, are more likely to reflect these definitions than the actual levels of abuse in the community. Ogg & Bennett also asked younger adults if they had abused older people. This produced higher rates of verbal, but not of physical, abuse.

One particular difficulty for prevalence studies using the general population is that people who are highly dependent on another person, and particularly people who have significant mental impairment, are unable to participate, except by proxy. The Boston study addressed this (Pillemer & Finkelhor 1988) but neither the Canadian nor the British study did. Yet it is precisely these people whom practitioners would identify as most at risk (Decalmer & Glendenning 1993). The large-scale study conducted in Amsterdam, the Netherlands, found that psychological abuse was more than twice as common as any other form of abuse, but there was not much difference between financial abuse and physical abuse. As seen in Table 32.1, reports of neglect appeared to be relatively uncommon. However, in this study, non-response appeared to be quite high for older women as well as for those with mental and physical incapacity. In Australia, the medical records of all patients over the age of 65 referred to an area-based geriatric and rehabilitation service were examined retrospectively over a 1-year period using very similar definitions to the two North American studies (Kurrle et al. 1992). The results of this study were similar to those from other countries. There have also been a number of studies in countries such as Finland (Kivela et al. 1993), which have established comparable overall rates of abuse (in the region of 5%). In addition, countries such as Spain, Israel and Japan are currently undertaking national studies.

In 1996 in the USA, the US National Elder Abuse Incidence Study (NEAIS) was designed to try and discover national estimates of reported and unreported cases of elder abuse and neglect (Tatara & Thomas 1998, Thomas 2000). The definitions used in this study included abandonment, and psychological abuse was defined in terms of emotional upset rather than behaviour, as found within the prevalence studies, for example, persistent verbal abuse. The study findings estimated that 450 000 older people in domestic settings were abused or neglected by other people in the USA in 1996. This amounts to 1.01% of people over the age of 60 years. Physical abuse appeared to relate to only a small proportion of the total. The principal forms of abuse by others were neglect and psychological abuse. In comparison with the prevalence studies, the overall rate was low and the incidence of neglect (after self-neglect was excluded) was high. These differences probably partly reflect differences between random community sampling in the prevalence research and reports by agencies and 'sentinels' (these were agency staff who did not officially report cases) within the incidence study.

There have also been studies of prevalence in specific populations, notably by questioning the carers of patients with dementia and those who were receiving respite care. These have been based on asking questions of carers and show substantially higher reported rates of three types of abuse. The researchers have in general expressed surprise at the willingness of carers to admit to abuse. Table 32.2 shows the results of three UK studies. These studies all employed the same definitions, which were the same as those used by Pillemer & Finkelhor in the Boston community prevalence study. Not only is more abuse reported, but verbal abuse in particular is much higher.

There has been very little research on prevalence in institutions and none on abuse in hospital settings.

Research in 57 residential and nursing homes in the USA found that 10% of staff (i.e. nursing assistants, not professionally trained nurses) admitted to at least *one* act of physical abuse in the preceding year; excessive restraint was the most frequently recorded form of abuse. Just over a third (36%) of respondents had observed at least one act of physical abuse by others in the preceding year; restraint accounted for around two-thirds of all reports. Respondents reported a very much higher rate of verbal than of physical abuse (Pillemer & Moore 1989).

Understanding abuse in the community

The Boston prevalence study (Pillemer & Finkelhor 1988) produced a number of interesting findings. Abuse was not related to age, or to ethnic, religious, educational or economic background. Table 32.3 shows the rates of abuse per 1000 older people as they related to gender, co-residence and health for the three different kinds of abuse. The first fact to notice is that the risk of physical and verbal abuse is higher for co-resident older people – an obvious but important point when it comes to the awareness of risk of abuse by others. As can be seen, perhaps surprisingly, the rate of physical and verbal abuse towards men is higher than towards women. This partly reflects the fact that there are fewer older men overall: in absolute terms the numbers abused were very similar – 52% men to 48% women. However, the difference in relative risk appears to result from the fact that older men are more likely to be living with someone else than older women – in this study 83% compared with 58%. It is also qualified by a further finding, from follow-up data, that women appeared to be more seriously abused. Another striking finding is the one relating to

Table 32.2 Prevalence of abuse in specific populations

Type of abuse	Percentage of carers admitting abuse		
Physical	14	12	10.5
Verbal	41	52	34
Neglect	12	12	–
All	45	55	37
Base	51 carers of respite patients, London 1989	67 carers of dementia patients, London 1992	38 carers of dementia patients, Northern Ireland 1992–1994
Method	Interviews	Postal survey: 33.5% response	Interviews
Authors	Homer & Gilleard (1990)	Cooney & Mortimer (1995)	Compton et al. (1997)

Table 32.3   Rates per 1000 of elder abuse by characteristics of victim: Boston survey of prevalence

Factors	Rates per 1000 by victim characteristics		
	Physical	Verbal	Neglect
Gender			
Male	37*	21	1
Female	13*	9	5
Living arrangements			
Lives alone	7*	6	5
Lives with spouse	33*	19	2
Lives with child only	25*	18	4
Lives with spouse and child	42*	23	11
Other	16*	–	–
Overall health			
Excellent	12	5	–
Good	24	13	–
Fair	18	12	8**
Poor	47	30	22**

*P = 0.01, **P = 0.0001.

Source: Pillemer & Finkelhor (1988).

the stereotype of elder abuse which prevailed during the 1980s – of abuse as behaviour perpetrated by an adult child who was the main carer of the older person – this research shows the higher prevalence of marital abuse in old age, thereby reflecting the fact that older people, if they are living with anyone, are more likely to be living with their spouse.

Some results from the Canadian national survey (Podnieks 1990) are shown in Table 32.4. Here the proportions of victims of different types of abuse are shown in relation to non-victims, thus highlighting some of the differences between them. As can be seen, the abuse is gendered, but again in an unexpected way. Recently we have begun to see much-needed attention given to the needs of older men who experience abuse (Mouton et al. 2001, Pritchard 2001). In the Podnieks study, more men were found to be victims of physical violence, although not of the other forms of abuse, while substantially more women were victims of neglect. Considerable differences occurred between the different types of abuse; the risk of financial abuse increased markedly for those living on their own, just as the risk of physical and verbal abuse declined. In terms of health, it is notable that the health of non-victims was in general better than that of victims but, as in the Boston study, there were differences between the types of abuse. More than half of victims of verbal aggression, and just under half of those who reported physical violence, reported that their health was good to excellent. In contrast to non-victims, victims also reported

health. There are no statistically significant associations between health status and physical and verbal abuse, although highly significant ones (P = 0.0001) for neglect. Clearly this is just as likely to be an effect of the neglect as it is to be its cause. Finally, contrary to

Table 32.4   Characteristics of victims of different types of elder abuse compared with non-victims

Factors	% of victims and non-victims				
	Physical	Verbal	Neglect	Financial	All non-victims
Gender					
Male	64	39	13	38	39
Female	36	61	87	62	67
Living arrangements					
Lives alone	–	8	38	58	39
Lives with spouse	73	69	12	31	45
Lives with child only	–4	13	8	7	
Lives with spouse and child	18	11	25	–	5
Other	9	8	12	4	4
Overall health					
Excellent	9	15	–	6	18
Good	36	39	25	31	45
Fair	36	31	25	47	29
Poor	18	15	50	16	8

Source: Podnieks (1990).

greater unhappiness and a greater sense of hopeless-ness, and nearly a third of victims of all types of abuse had wished that their life might end (Podnieks 1990). The picture therefore is one of considerable suffering, but also marked by a degree of coping and resilience – overall only 1 in 10 victims had felt hopeless about the future very often during the past week – a finding that Podnieks followed up in some further research, which is reported in the next section (Podnieks 1992).

However, these large prevalence studies mainly tell us about one side in the abusive relationship – the victim – and it is necessary to turn to the smaller and more intensive pieces of research to learn more about the wider household and the factors which seem to discriminate abusive from non-abusive situations. These display considerable consistency in relation to physical and verbal abuse, which are the types of abuse that have been the subject of most research (McCreadie 1996). Apart from the importance of co-residence, abusive situations appear, on current knowledge, to be discriminated from non-abusive situations by, first, the characteristics of the abuser and most notably any problems they may have in their own right, and, second, the quality of the long-term relationship between the two parties. Abuse is therefore not a product of the illnesses and disabili-ties of old age so much as a manifestation of longer-term problems in personalities and relationships, which may be exacerbated by behaviour arising from illness or disability. The picture which prevailed for some time of the implicitly well-meaning and younger carer, who is stressed by the demands of car-ing, and hits out at the dependent and implicitly demanding older person, is a drastically simplified and to a large extent inaccurate picture of the com-plexities of abusive situations.

The study by Homer & Gilleard (1990) illustrates this, as does the Swedish research (Saveman et al. 1996). Homer & Gilleard examined the factors that dis-tinguished those carers who admitted abuse (physical or verbal abuse or neglect) from those who did not. They found that all carers who admitted abuse were co-resident with their relative.

The factors most significantly associated with abuse were alcohol consumption by the carer and abuse by the patient. The circumstances triggering physical violence in the seven carers who admitted to it were physical abuse or threats of violence by the patient in four cases, incontinence in one, and both in one, and one carer 'could not identify the trigger' (Homer & Gilleard 1990: p. 1361).

Surprisingly, there was no association between abuse and the volume of services received by the household. Also, significantly, Homer & Gilleard (1990), using the Clifton Assessment Procedures for the Elderly, found no difference in the level of physical dependency between abused and non-abused patients, and no association between abuse and the diagnosis of dementia or degree of mental impairment in the patient. They comment: 'The presence or absence of disruptive behaviour may be more impor-tant than cognitive impairment' (Homer & Gilleard 1990: p. 1361).

There have been a number of studies specifically on the relationship between dementia and abuse (McCreadie 1996, Penhale & Kingston 1997). What emerges most strongly from this research is that the carer, who may also be older and in poor health, may in some circumstances, be most at risk. In the study by Compton and his fellow psychiatrists in Northern Ire-land (Compton et al. 1997), 38 carers were asked about abuse toward the patient with dementia. A third admitted to verbal abuse and 10% to physical abuse. The significant factors predicting the abuse were co-residence, poor health in the carer, poor pre-morbid relations, abuse or problem behaviour by the patient, and carer dissatisfaction with the help received. In contrast to many studies (McCreadie 1996), there was no association between alcohol consumption and abuse; the authors ascribe this to the probable rate of abstinence in Northern Ireland.

In the Swedish research, the 21 district nurses par-ticipated in detailed interviews in which they described at least two cases of abuse known to them (Saveman et al. 1995, 1996). The 44 cases were then subjected to very detailed analysis by the researchers, who distinguished four different scenarios in which the abuse was occurring. These were:

1. There are demands from one party, which the other is unwilling or unable to meet. These led to abuse of either one person, or the other, or both. There were 14 cases of this kind; and the following example taken from the original report (Saveman 1994: 119) illustrates the com-plexity of this kind of situation:

   It is just that the mentally retarded son, who is living at home, thinks that it is very difficult with his mother being in bed all the time . . . She had been in bed the whole of the previous week and she had not eaten or anything. He had taken her food. He was so tired because of this and did not know where to turn. Clearly, there we are again – her just lying and lying there, and of course, it's that he has been going around the house getting worked up about it. He has to do everything for her.

2. The demands implicit in a caring situation led to abuse of the patient, or the carer, or both. There were 12 cases of this kind:

> Sometimes she does not recognize her husband and sends him out ... he described how ashamed he was of her, had been for a long time, for the way she behaved and for her illness, and how he lost his patience and got very nasty with her ... How hard he finds it to suddenly have a wife that he does not know any more. He is old and does not understand what it is all about and he has landed in something the very existence of which is quite alien to him (Saveman et al. 1996: p. 220).

3. The perpetrator exercised power over the older person and abused him or her. There were 13 such cases:

> His wife had forbidden him to contact any of his relatives at all ... If he, as it were, disobeyed, say he spoke to his brothers and his relations, then she beat him up, she really hit him hard. He was never allowed to be home by himself so that he could get to a telephone. She held him in an iron grip. 'I have been beaten, I get beaten every day', he said, when he suddenly met his brother. He never dared to show anyone. Yes, they [his relatives] also think that she is strange in some way. I think he was beaten to death, I really do (Saveman et al. 1996: p. 227).

4. There has been a history of violence in the relationship. There were five such cases, which were graphically described by Homer & Gilleard (1990) as the 'elderly graduates of domestic violence':

> The wife has always been violent towards him. Today they are both handicapped and he cares for her, but he also gets help from their daughter. In spite of her handicap, she is still able to be aggressive and mentally abusive.

The cases described by these nurses were therefore complex and mostly defied any simple construct of perpetrator and victim:

> In the narrated cases, the relationships were characterized by a dependency that may have created negative feelings of being isolated, trapped and unable to manage efficiently by oneself:

> in some there seemed to have been a long-lasting dependency that had now become full of conflict ... the long-lasting conflicts concerning dependency seemed to be related to two phenomena. Firstly, the parties appeared to see each other primarily as a means to fulfilling the other's purposes, not as an end in her/himself. When one party could no longer fulfill his or her role, it threatened the other. Secondly, this apparently sometimes made the perpetrators try very hard to exercise their power over the failing party. This implied abuse, an important part of which was the fact that the parties strove to isolate each other (Saveman et al. 1996: p. 229).

Further, the authors mention the financial dependency of many carers and therefore the need to stay in the relationship. Benefits augment household income and, where incomes are very low, can create such financial dependency (Glendinning 1989). Moreover, the costs of long-term residential care, now more fully subject to means-testing, and the impact on inheritance, can also create powerful incentives for those who are better off to carry on caring at home.

UNDERSTANDING ABUSE IN COMMUNAL SETTINGS

Communal settings comprise residential homes, nursing homes, hospital and day care. In these settings, there is an organizational context to the delivery of care, so that something more may often be at issue than the behaviour of a particular individual towards a resident or patient. As the numerous inquiries into grave deficiencies in institutional care have shown, abuse may flourish within a culture which allows it to be acceptable (Martin 1984, Secretary of State for Health 1992, Clough 1999, Stanley et al. 1999).

These interwoven aspects of abuse and standards of care are illustrated in the following examples of abuse in the UKCC's report into professional misconduct cases (UKCC 1994): a report which, it has been said, should be 'mandatory reading for all nurses' (Nolan 1994). Between 1990–1991 and 1993–1994 the number of allegations involving older people rose, both absolutely and as a proportion of all cases. The UKCC draws particular attention in the report to the rise in the number of misconduct cases in nursing homes which, by 1994, constituted the highest single group of cases:

> Whilst the complaints reveal serious professional misconduct such as physical and verbal abuse, they also identify wholly inadequate systems of drug administration, ineffective management systems, lack of systematic care-planning or effective record-keeping and almost non-existent induction or in-service training ... Financial controls and audit procedures designed to safeguard residents' finances appear to be woefully inadequate (UKCC 1994: p. 7).

Table 32.5 indicates how these factors affected older people in different communal settings. However, this is indicative of a problem and not a measure of the extent of abuse or the reasons for it. There is 'extremely limited empirical evidence' (Gilleard 1994: p. 195), particularly about nurses, as what research there is has concentrated on nursing-home assistants, rather than professionally qualified staff.

The best-known research is a survey by telephone undertaken in the USA in 1987 of 577 nursing assistants in 57 residential and nursing homes (Pillemer & Moore 1989, 1990, Pillemer & Bachman-Prehn 1991). Respondents were asked to report both their own actions and observations of other people involving physical abuse of patients in the past year. Physical abuse covered excessive use of restraints, pushing, grabbing, shoving or pinching, slapping or hitting, throwing something at a resident and hitting or trying to hit a resident with an object. Only a very small number of staff (1%) admitted to using physical force more than 10 times, always in the context of excessive restraint, although 6% had observed others doing so. When the reasons for physical abuse were examined, the significant factors were staff burnout, patient aggression and conflict between staff and patients (Pillemer & Bachman-Prehn 1991). Gilleard (1994) questions the value of always defining restraint or forced feeding as abusive, because invariably they may be the outcome of 'conflicting principles' (e.g. the view that a terminally ill patient needs to be fed or that patients need restraining in the interests of other patients or of themselves). He suggests that there needs to be 'much more thought put into determining the context in which such potentially harmful procedures are undertaken' (Gilleard 1994: p. 99).

From their research, Pillemer & Moore (1990) found that psychological abuse by the nursing-home assistants was much more frequently reported and observed than physical abuse. This was defined to include:

- yelling at the patient in anger
- insulting or swearing at the patient
- isolating the patient inappropriately
- threatening to hit or throw something at the patient
- denying the patient food or privileges.

Eighteen per cent of their 577 respondents admitted to yelling at the patient in anger between two and 10 times in the previous year, although only 1% admitted to yelling more than 10 times. Five per cent had insulted the patient. However, 44% had observed others yelling at a patient in anger between two and 10 times, 30% had observed patients being insulted or sworn at and 8% had seen the patient denied food, or isolated, or threatened. Five per cent had seen others yelling at the patient in anger and 11% had seen patients insulted or sworn at more than 10 times. The factors which most accurately predicted psychological abuse, like physical abuse, were staff burnout and patient aggression. As patient aggression increased, the probability of the nursing-home assistant psychologically abusing patients increased. Patient aggression appeared to be more important than staff burnout (Pillemer & Bachman-Prehn 1991).

Pillemer & Moore (1989) expressed themselves 'surprised' by the generally high levels of staff–patient conflict over patients' unwillingness to eat, personal hygiene, unwillingness to dress and toileting. Coupled with these high rates of conflict was patient aggression towards staff.

Table 32.5 Cases investigated by UK Professional Conduct Committee, 1991–1994

Sphere of practice	Numbers of cases, and as % of total number of cases investigated			
	1990–1991	1991–1992	1992–1993	1993–1994 (provisional)
Elderly care	16 (8)	22 (4)	12 (9)	2 (2)
Elderly mentally ill	(included under elderly care and mental illness)	11 (9)	18 (14)	
Nursing home	15 (8)	28 (15)	27 (21)	35 (26)
Total elderly	40 (16)	50 (27)	46 (36)	60 (45)
All cases	195 (100)	183 (100)	127 (100)	133 (100)

Values in parentheses are percentages of total number of cases investigated.
Source: UKCC (1994: p. 5)

Eastley and colleagues (1993) investigated staff experience of aggression from older residents in different care settings. This included 36 staff in psychogeriatric hospital wards and 72 staff in homes for elderly mentally infirm people. In total, 204 care staff in four units in each setting completed a questionnaire, a response rate of 72%. From the results, it appeared that patients had assaulted 81% of staff in the hospital wards in the week prior to the survey, Almost two-thirds (65%) of staff in the homes for elderly mentally ill people also reported assaults. Sixty-one per cent of the staff in the hospital wards had formal qualifications, but only 39% had any training in managing aggression. Interestingly, the comparable figures in the homes for the elderly mentally ill were 28% formal qualifications and 28% training in managing aggression.

In a study of violent behaviour among patients on an acute psychogeriatric admission ward, Shah (1992) emphasized the importance of trained staff. In this study, the incidence of violent behaviour by patients was very much lower. Shah concluded that 'such patients could be maintained in the community, e.g. social service institutions, provided there is adequate provision of well-trained staff' (Shah 1992: p. 43). However, this study was based on recorded violence, and such incidents tend to be significantly under-reported (Department of Health and Social Security 1988, Freyne & Wrigley 1996, Goodridge et al. 1996). In an Irish study, a special reporting system was set up in a long-stay ward for patients with dementia (Freyne & Wrigley 1996). During a 3-month period, 47 incidents were reported, although one patient accounted for nearly half of these reports. Three-quarters of these episodes occurred when staff members were assisting patients with activities of daily living. Eight patients accounted for the remaining 24 incidents, 80% of which were rated by the nursing staff as not so serious, although in half of these cases the staff sustained minor injuries, such as bruises, abrasions or scratch marks. Respondents stated the frequency of aggressive incidents as 'numerous' and all, not surprisingly, found aggressive behaviour difficult to deal with. However, there was no statistically significant difference between those with and without training in managing aggression. The issue, of course, in relation to the abuse of the patient is whether, in some circumstances, aggressive behaviour by the patient leads to aggressive responses.

Additional factors to be taken into account are whether those individual staff members who responded aggressively are trained in managing aggression and what the management response is towards incidents, individual staff members, the staff

group as a whole and also towards those patients/residents who act aggressively. The issues raised concerning violence towards care staff has received some attention (McCreadie 2000); staff from both health and social care may be affected and need to be aware that abuse can occur as a result of provocation by residents/patients. Practitioners also need to know how to deal with such situations and be mindful of the existence of zero-tolerance policies towards abuse (UKCC 1999).

Intervention in the community

Elder abuse undoubtedly presents nurses with some of their most difficult professional dilemmas. Yet, as has been suggested earlier, due to their position in the community and their role within it, community nurses are in an ideal position to detect abuse. Nurses are generally very well placed to observe and be aware of the potential for abuse to occur in the community setting. As there has been major growth in independently supplied home care over the last decade, until recently an area where regulation and inspection of standards have been lacking, nurses may well be visiting older people in situations where there is no involvement from other statutory agencies. Thus they may be in an ideal position to monitor situations carefully and to report abusive situations to social services as the lead agency in co-ordinating local responses to abuse (see Department of Health 2000 for further discussion of this).

One of the few pieces of research in the UK which has specifically involved community nurses was undertaken for West Lambeth Community Care National Health Service Trust, London (Lowe 1993). Fifty-four community nurses were asked about their experience of elder abuse over a year. Table 32.6 shows a breakdown by eight different categories of abuse. The nurses suspected nearly twice as many cases as they actually knew of. Overall, emotional and financial abuse and categories of neglect accounted for over half of the actual cases and more than three-quarters of the suspected cases. There were considerable differences in recall between nurses working in different neighbourhoods, which the researcher ascribed to differences in awareness and interpretation of abuse. Interestingly, the neighbourhood with the highest incidence of recorded abuse also recorded a considerably higher number of contacts with clients in the same period. The nurses lacked confidence and were unsure about the skills they possessed or needed to develop to deal with cases of abuse. As we have seen, this finding is similar to views expressed by nurses (Trevitt & Gallagher 1996) and other professionals, such as social

Table 32.6 Actual and suspected cases of abuse recorded by 54 community nurses, West Lambeth, London, 1992–1993

Type of abuse	Actual	Suspected
Emotional	6	7
Deprivation of nutrition	3	6
Inadequate care	3	4
Inappropriate drugs	2	1
Financial	2	8
Assault	1	1
Involuntary isolation	1	5
Sexual	0	1
Total	18	33

Source: Lowe (1993).

workers (Pritchard 1995). Most significantly, only three out of all these cases of abuse were discussed with a manager by the nurses. The reasons given for this were:

- The patient did not want action taken
- The patient requested confidentiality
- There was insufficient evidence
- Resolution occurred without intervention
- The nurse did not know how to tackle the difficult issues involved.

Similar reasons were given by members of a community psychiatric team in a study of 74 assessments in Cambridge. Only one abuse case was documented, although on further investigation six other cases (all serious) were identified as 'at risk' (Kerr et al. 1994). However, setting may be important. In a study of 26 nurses in an accident and emergency department, 96% indicated that they would consult with a senior colleague if they suspected abuse and 94% with a doctor (Vernon & Bennett 1996).

Lowe (1993) found that community nurses were reluctant to follow the local procedure for elder abuse, which, as a first step, required them to ask the relative/carer for an explanation of the injury or situation. As in the Swedish research quoted above, the reality of most of the situations was not as straightforward as this suggests and their desire to act was based on growing concern over a period of time. 'Rushing in' did not appear appropriate. Lowe suggested a close link between this and the care assessment procedures of the local authority, with risk assessment also built into these procedures (Lowe 1993). The single assessment process introduced under the *National Service Framework for Older People* also contains such guidance

and emphasizes that assessment concerning abuse needs to take place, particularly within complex assessments (Department of Health 2001a, 2001b). Further information on the single assessment can be found in Chapter 28.

The over-75 health assessment offers an important opportunity to members of the primary care team to assess possible risks of abuse to the older person (Amiel & Heath 2003, Phair & Goodman 2003). In the USA, Shugarman and colleagues (2003) have evaluated the incorporation of routine screening for potential abuse within more standardized health assessment of older people and found this to be successful. A helpful and practical guide to the UK health assessment process recognizes that the assessment is more than a health check and should also be used to prevent difficulties and to examine carer needs (Heath 1995). Heath suggests that there are three levels of assessment. There is the initial check, which can 'alert the practitioner to problems which require further assessment' (Heath 1995: p. 30); secondly, there is a more detailed assessment; and finally, for a small minority of patients there may be a full interdisciplinary assessment. This is indicated 'when the identified problems are complex, when health or social breakdown is imminent, when high-dependency patients are discharged from hospital, and when an older person is being considered for transfer to long-term care' (Heath 1995: p. 31). Under social functioning, most of the concerns are raised which should elicit, at the very least, some warning signals for the nurse who is aware that abuse is a possibility:

It is helpful to ask who the older person sees in the course of a week. Can the person do what he or she wishes socially and recreationally? If not, what are the difficulties? Is the person able to handle his or her own affairs at home, such as paying bills? Family relationships are a central aspect of social functioning, and it is important to be sensitive to varying family structures and the roles assumed within these. The needs of carers may be different from those of the older person. Carers should ideally be seen alone so that they can raise any problematic issues. It is also important to recognize family dysfunction, which may precede inadequate care or abuse (Heath 1995: p. 33).

Under the terms of the Carers (Recognition and Services) Act, 1995, if an individual is in receipt of community care services or is having either an assessment or reassessment of need then the carer is eligible in his or her own right to an assessment of any needs for assistance. In relation to caring, it is worth noting that during the 1990s more men than women took on the role of spouse carer; currently there are equal numbers of male and female spouse carers, both generally and, more importantly, those providing 20 h or more care a week for a person (Hirst 2001). This trend is expected to continue for the foreseeable future. Further details on carers are discussed in Chapter 33.

It should also be added here that, as part of good practice, it is important to see the older person alone. And in any situation that may involve abuse, separate interviews for the elder and others involved in the situation are not just good practice, but are likely to be essential. If there is any reluctance on the part of carers for this to happen, this should obviously be noted and, if possible, further explored. Bennett (2000) maintained that if this situation arose in practice it was always likely to provide useful clues about the situation for the assessment.

PROFESSIONAL AND LEGAL ISSUES

A difficult issue for nurses and other health professionals is the professional and legal framework that exists to protect individuals who have experienced abuse. In the majority of cases narrated by the district nurses in Sweden, the abused party did not want to change the situation. This could be attributed to a variety of reasons, including the powerful one of protection for the perpetrator. There are a number of reasons why an older person might not wish to report or acknowledge an abusive situation (see Penhale 1993 for further discussion of this). It has been said that when it concerns an adult child, elder abuse is the most complex of all forms of domestic violence and that the attachment of parent to child is a critical factor in an older person's desire to remain in a given situation (Lambert 1992).

One of the most obvious and important factors about abuse of an older person is that it occurs in the context of a person's history: 'How any particular instance of mistreatment fits into that life story is critical' (Holstein 1995: p. 181). One interesting piece of research, a follow-up study of victims of different types of abuse in Canada, showed how older people coped with their situation, and that their whole life experience was relevant to that ability to cope (Podnieks 1992).

The legal issues around abuse are very considerable. Although there is no specific law which relates to abuse and protection of older people or vulnerable adults, sections from a large number of laws in different fields, including domestic violence, community care and mental health legislation, might apply. There are a number of specialized books, which offer guidance concerning this aspect. Readers who wish to pursue this will find a detailed list of references in McCreadie (1996). There has been a major overview of the law in relation to people who are not competent to take their own decisions, including financial decisions, and in relation to adults who are at risk of abuse and neglect (Law Commission 1995), although specific legislation relating to incapacity is still awaited in England and Wales. However, following government statements (Lord Chancellor's Department 1999), it is anticipated that such legislation, when implemented, will not explicitly cover issues of abuse and protection. In Scotland, the Adults with Incapacity Act was passed in 2000 and this contains helpful material relating to older people as well as clear guidance to be followed concerning incapacity.

In practice, nurses should always consult with their manager about the best course of action to take in a situation. They will also need to consider what the local procedures and guidance for their agency require them to do. It is likely that social services who are mandated locally to be the lead agency for coordinating responses to abuse (Department of Health 2000), will need to be involved. There may also need to be involvement with the police and other agencies such as housing or the registration and inspection units of the Commission for Social Care Inspection if the situation concerns a residential or nursing home. Therefore, nurses should be aware of and prepared for the possibility of involvement and liaison with different organizations when dealing with abusive situations.

Importantly, the conclusions drawn from the Swedish research (Saveman et al. 1996) are that district nurses need support in dealing with situations where they think or know abuse is happening. In general, the respondents were prone to side with the weaker party in the relationship, rather than being able to assess with some objectivity the moral and ethical issues that they needed to address. The consequence of this was that their intervention risked making the situation worse. Saveman et al. (1996) argue that it is a strength to view the abusive family system from a wider perspective, to analyse the situation in order to understand its complexity and find suitable interventions. To do this, nurses must be able to step outside the system and reflect on it as a whole in order to find solutions.

The conflict between respecting the expressed wishes of patients and protecting them from harm is one of the most difficult of the issues encountered. Kingston & Phillipson (1994: p. 1189) comment:

> It is important to remember that elderly people have the right to reject offers of assistance: they can, and do, say no to interventions. This right may only be ignored in certain circumstances, for example, if the elderly person is mentally incapable of making a decision as assessed by colleagues from psychiatric or psychological disciplines.

We must acknowledge, however, that at times an older person may be intimidated into a position of rejecting help. Although it can be very difficult to assess this type of situation, the involvement of other professionals within the assessment can be helpful in confirming or refuting this. And even within such situations it is not likely that the individual can be forced to accept help, but it may be that a system of ongoing monitoring can be established for the person.

It has been suggested, in the context of nurses' help to younger abused women, that their contribution lies both in the ability to provide 'holistic, wellness-focused care' (Henderson & Eriksen 1994: p. 12) and in their role as an advocate (Kingston & Phillipson 1994, Evans 1996). Henderson & Eriksen (1994) point out that, in relation to younger women, where there is no issue over mental capacity, it can be comforting for nurses to recognize that they are not responsible for making changes happen in the abused woman's life. Nurses can be helped to understand that the abused woman is the expert and the only one qualified to decide what is right for her. The individual nurse's responsibility is to ensure that there is a supportive environment in which the woman is empowered to explore her options and to take control of her life.

This is equally true for older people (Wetle & Fulmer 1995). Even in the most intractable circumstances, when the parties do not want help, 'every effort should be made to "keep the door open", to continue to communicate and to offer options' (Wetle & Fulmer 1995: p. 42). It is important also to remember that situations can and do change over time. A person who is reluctant to accept help at one point in time may accept it at a later date. Older people therefore need to know that it is possible to change their mind and that if they initially refuse offers made, the possibility of help will remain open to them should they need it. In order to do this, they will need to have information about how to access help in future and whom to contact. And of course, this information should be provided in a sensitive way: a leaflet announcing services for abused people may not be appropriate for a vulnerable person in a difficult and unsafe situation.

Inter-professional and inter-agency approaches to managing abuse

No one professional is likely to have a comprehensive picture of the household in which an older person is living. Moreover, there is a wide range of resources and expertise available and services for helping will be found in a variety of agencies. The number and type of agencies and services will vary from area to area. For these reasons it is widely agreed that nurses need to work closely with colleagues in other services in both the statutory and the voluntary sectors (Kingston & Penhale 1994, Kingston & Phillipson 1994). The discharge of older people from hospital offers a clear, if demanding, opportunity to develop communication with other professionals. The appropriateness of providing any particular service will depend on the type of abuse, the reasons for the abuse and the views and decision-making capacity of the parties involved. There is a danger that victims of abuse may just be provided with the same services as other frail older people, without proper regard for the wider household perspective which the research suggests is so important. In many cases it may be necessary to think in terms of services to both abuser and abused.

Attention has been drawn in the research literature to the success of victim support groups and advocacy programmes (Wolf & Pillemer 1994), to mediation (Craig 1994) and to volunteer support, either face-to-face or on the telephone (Podnieks 1992, Filinson 1993, Gillen 1995). Where physical or psychological abuse is occurring in a relationship involving the care of a dependent person, education or anger management may be an appropriate form of intervention (Garcia & Kosberg 1992, Reay & Browne 2002). Research has also indicated that psychological stress in carers of people with dementia can be reduced by an intensive training programme (Brodaty & Gresham 1989). The Mental Health Foundation (1995) has funded research which has applied this approach specifically to the management of difficult or irritating behaviour in dementia patients with considerable success, although it has involved substantial professional input (Hinchliffe et al. 1992). It is often thought that respite care is the most valuable service in the prevention of abuse but, while there is evidence of the considerable benefits of respite care to carers (Levin et al. 1994), its impact on physical and psychological abuse is questionable (Homer & Gilleard 1994).

In order for nurses to respond appropriately to abuse, they need three kinds of support: support from education and training, from the setting in which they work and from their professional body: 'It is only when nurses have this firm base of support that they will be at ease with their role [of helping] and feel able to intervene consistently and effectively' (Henderson & Eriksen 1994: p. 15).

FINANCIAL ABUSE

Dimond gives a useful account of the nurse's responsibility in handling patients' money and the legislation by which other people can take responsibility for older people's finances if they are unable to do so for themselves (Dimond 1995: Chapter 25). An example illustrates the dilemmas that can arise for nurses (Case study 32.2). In this instance, apart from letting the relative know that the nurse is concerned there is little that can be done.

The UKCC (1994) observed the weakness of controls over residents' finances in some misconduct cases. Beaulieu (1992), in Canada, received 'many accounts' from the 30 residents she interviewed about the loss of money, pension cheques and belongings. Research which bears on financial abuse in residential care has raised a whole important range of issues around the handling of older people's finances, particularly those suffering from dementia, and has raised questions about how useful it is to discuss such a wide range of issues under a heading of financial abuse (Langan & Means 1996). In respect of residential as opposed to nursing-home settings, the researchers drew on data from both statutory (two specialist homes) and voluntary and private homes (23, response rate 33%) in a local authority in the north of England. Two particular issues relevant to financial abuse arose. One was the extent to which the proprietors of homes had legal responsibility for the older person's financial affairs, thereby opening up opportunities for abuse. The second related to financial abuse of some older people by their relatives. Three homes in the private and voluntary sectors and both the specialist statutory homes expressed concern about this.

The Social Services Inspectorate (1993: p. 16) stresses that 'particular thought must be given to the most appropriate service provision in cases of financial abuse'. As a result of their work, Langan & Means (1996) recommend an improved advocacy and advice strategy, with a view to ensuring that older people have financial arrangements that are legal and appropriate.

CONFIDENTIALITY

A major issue that has to be thought through and addressed in any guidance for nurses is confidentiality. It is a basic precept of the professional Code of Conduct for nurses that they respect any information that is given to them in confidence by a patient. Dimond (1995) lists the exceptions to the code as: consent of the patient, interests of the patient, court orders, statutory duty to disclose, the public interest and where the police can require information. If the patient is not willing for information to be disclosed to another professional, the patient's interests must be the paramount consideration. Abuse by family members presents the nurse and other professionals with difficult issues of confidentiality. Since it is invariably bound up with relationships and dispositions within a whole household, it is often the case that vital information may be held by another professional, or the nurse may hold a piece of this essential information that is lacking elsewhere, the possession of which would make it easier to assess the best course of action in the interests of the patient and the wider household. The disasters which can ensue from withholding information in the supposed interests of the patient were graphically illustrated in the report on Christopher Clunis, which should be mandatory reading for anyone working in the health and social care services (North East Thames Regional Health Authority 1994).

Another aspect of confidentiality relates to information about the working of health services. Some of this may be legitimately confidential, for example certain kinds of financial and personnel information. However, information about standards of care, and how these are affected by resources, is not confidential in any real sense of the word as understood by professionals (Hunt 1995). The issues arising when a nurse is concerned about possible abuse of a patient, particularly by a colleague, are discussed below.

Education and training

It is now being recognized that it is essential for nurses, whether working in communal or community settings, to have some training around the issues of elder abuse. In 1994 around 81% of nursing colleges responding to a survey (representing 48 nursing colleges) provided some teaching on elder abuse (Kingston et al. 1995). The amount of time given to this varied from 1 h to 1 day (median 3.5 h). The authors

---

Case study 32.2

Mary B was visited regularly by her daughter Jean and each week the ward sister noticed that Jean brought the pension book in for her mother to sign. However, it was noticeable that Mary never seemed to have any money for purchases from the ward trolley, and if the ward had not supplied her with the fruit squash, tissues and soaps, she would not have had any of those items. Janice, the ward sister, mentioned it to Jean who flushed a little and said that she did not have anything to do with her mother's money and by the time she had personally paid for the bus fare to the hospital she did not have any funds for such purchases and anyway the hospital provided that, did they not? Source: Dimond (1995: p. 355).

suggested that there should be a systematic component in all nursing curricula addressing issues of family violence throughout the life-course. In particular, basic awareness training concerning the different forms of abuse and neglect is fundamental for all health and social care practitioners, together with more advanced courses provided for those who are specializing in work with vulnerable older people. An introductory level of knowledge and awareness for all practitioners would increase the likelihood that abuse, when and wherever it occurs, will be detected and reported, within local guidelines and procedures, so that appropriate action can then be taken. Nurses are central within this and are a key professional group to include within such training. Educational curricula at pre- and post-registration levels also need to include relevant modules concerning abuse and neglect.

However, it is also thought important that nurses should join other professionals in training initiatives as part of a holistic inter-professional approach for health and social care provision (Bennett & Kingston 1993). In addition, the Department of Health has consistently advocated for education and training about abuse to be provided on a multi-agency, multi-disciplinary basis (Department of Health 1993, 2000). A number of commentators have also suggested that abuse should be seen as a wider issue in the care of older people and that the nursing 'profession needs to address the lack of education and skills in dealing with older people's needs' (Castledine 1994: p. 676). Recent research on the effect of education on knowledge and management of elder abuse suggests that, whilst educational courses for professionals assist in improving the identification and reporting of abusive situations, courses need to be specifically planned and targeted in order to take into account the baseline knowledge about abuse, as this appears to affect receptiveness to training courses and the amount of learning that takes place (Richardson et al. 2002).

VOICING CONCERNS ABOUT ABUSE

Placing concern about the well-being of patients first can be extremely difficult for nurses, as for other staff. Action on Elder Abuse and Counsel and Care are voluntary-sector organizations that have issued advice to people who are concerned about the possible abuse of an older person and feel they should do something about it (Action on Elder Abuse 1994, Counsel and Care 1994, Mullan 1995). These people may be a member of the public, or a professional in contact with older people in their own homes, or a member of staff in a hospital, or nursing home, or other communal setting who may be concerned about a fellow member of staff's, or about a relative's, behaviour towards the patient. Additionally, contact can be made with the organization Public Concern at Work, a legal charity that provides assistance to those individuals who wish to raise concerns but do not know how best to do this and who may require some support in order to do so. More recently, introduction of legislation in the form of the Public Interest Disclosure Act 1998 has provided some protection for individuals who whistle-blow. Information about this Act and of other forms of assistance is available on Public Concern at Work's website (for details, see useful addresses listed at the end of this chapter).

The report of the inquiry into abuse at Ashworth Special Hospital, which in many ways parallels earlier reports of ill treatment, cited four reasons why nurses 'do not ordinarily report untoward events involving professional malpractices' (Secretary of State for Health 1992). These are: (1) peer-group loyalty; (2) fear of not being believed; (3) a conviction that it is futile to complain; and (4) fear of intimidation and reprisals. Martin (1984), in his review of abuse in long-term care in the 1960s and 1970s, identifies some of the 'key questions' raised by Pilgrim (1995) when he writes:

> It is almost impossible to exaggerate the power of the working group – usually for our purposes the staff of a ward, or sometimes even the members of a shift. The confined circumstances in which they work, their common problems, their interdependence in work, the isolation from staff on other wards and sometimes their feelings of being forgotten or neglected all foster a strong sense of group identity. Awareness of the group, and loyalty to it, rapidly gain strength until its cohesion becomes a pervasive influence on individual behaviour (Martin 1984: pp. 242–243).

Although these words were written in the context of the long-term large institutions which have been closing down as part of public policy, they are relevant to the care of older people, as of other dependent groups, in smaller homes where isolation, shift work, conflict with residents, the demanding nature of the daily care routines and so on, all promote the need for moral support from colleagues. Support involves loyalty to the group:

> Loyalty offers many reasons for people to do nothing, say nothing and put up with situations of which they may not approve ... but hidden behind that comprehensible face of inaction is the more pervasive feeling of fear ... it may be fear of being forced out of the job by colleagues and losing that

all important income to the family's stretched finances. It may be fear that the owner, in hearing what has been said, will make the decision, not liking the message, to shoot the messenger, or fear that one will not be believed and therefore be regarded as at best unreliable or incapable of making sound judgements. It may be fear that in saying and doing nothing, one is contaminated and thus just as much a part of the problem as anybody else. To protest is to become a troublemaker; at least that is one way in which organizations respond to the difficult issues raised by outspoken or unorthodox individuals (Counsel and Care 1995: p. 9).

REGULATION

However, the wider context in which care is provided is also of crucial importance in relation to the prevention of abuse. In so far as nursing homes are concerned, those authorities involved in registration and inspection are in the forefront of this wider context. It is their responsibility to make sure that homes reach certain standards before they are opened, and that these are maintained once they are. This includes checks to establish that owners and managers of homes are 'fit' to run care establishments. Some nurses work for the Commission for Social Care Inspection (formerly the National Commission for Care Standards or NCSC), which is the organization concerned with this area of work. The role of nurses as registration and inspection officers therefore provides them with the opportunity to 'ensure that homes are the safest possible environment for vulnerable older people' (Counsel and Care 1995: p. 23). Counsel and Care (1995) suggests that all care homes should devise and adopt policies outlining how to identify and act upon suspicions of abuse.

Regulation of standards is now recognized as central to good-quality services in health and social care. However, a topical report on the regulation and inspection of social services concluded:

> The relationship of regulation to the quality of care is unclear. At the least it establishes a minimum standard – a safety net below which care standards should not be able to fall ... but in the end some of the most important factors are outside the direct scope of regulation – the motivation of providers, the attitudes of care staff, the supportive involvement of friends and relatives. Regulation can never substitute for these but at its best it can serve to encourage and reinforce them (Burgner 1996: p. 117).

A Royal College of Nursing (1992) survey of nurses working with older people in residential and nursing homes covered 134 nurses in communal settings, 68 in community nursing, 15 inspectors and 16 'others'. It was widely thought that registration and inspection requirements were not being met or enforced. The report recommended that the workload of inspectors should be such that they are able to maintain close contact with each home and that they should have powers to enforce the standards required by the health authority. A further survey (Royal College of Nursing 1994) of inspectors in 70 health authorities reaffirmed wide variations between areas in both the quantity and quality of inspections. While all respondents met the statutory requirement of two visits a year, those with fewest resources did not undertake unannounced visits. The resources allocated to registration and inspection apparently bore no relationship to the provision of nursing-home beds in an area (Royal College of Nursing 1994).

Following these reports and other concerns, the government decided that the registration and inspection functions of local authorities and health authorities (for residential and nursing-home provision, respectively) should be altered. Accordingly these functions were removed from local authorities and formed part of the National Care Standards Commission, which was established following implementation of the Care Standards Act 2000. This was then amalgamated with the social care inspection function of the Social Services Inspectorate (part of the Department of Health) to form the Commission for Social Care Inspection, operational from 2004. This also covers the regulation and inspection of nursing homes and those units that provide joint provision (i.e. residential and nursing-home care on the same site). Many of the former inspectors who had worked within the various authorities transferred to work within the Commission, whose brief was extended to include the regulation of domiciliary as well as residential provision.

Legislation, in the form of the Registered Homes Act 1984 and the Care Standards Act, stipulates the grounds on which homes may be de-registered. This includes provision for emergency action to be taken, if necessary, in order to provide protective measures for residents. Clearly abusive situations are likely to be covered by such provision. Generally, however, actions such as home closures are not undertaken lightly. This is in part, perhaps, due to the distress that this will almost inevitably cause for those residents who are already frail and vulnerable. Bennett et al. (1997) suggested an alternative model, whereby instead of instigating closure in the case of investigations, management of a home could be transferred, at least on a temporary basis, to the relevant local authority. Within this situation, an existing, experienced manager could be introduced to manage the home for an interim period, if not on an ongoing basis.

In the absence of such a model being implemented, however, it is likely that careful and sensitive planning and coordination between a number of different agencies are necessary to try and ensure that, if residents have to be moved, the transition period runs as smoothly as possible and any traumatic effects are minimized. An example of this was evident in the actions taken by the regional office of the NCSC in conjunction with the police and local social services department on closing a residential home in East Anglia and transferring the residents. This followed investigations over several months concerning abuse of a number of residents (physical, financial and psychological). Whilst the investigations were ongoing, thorough contingency planning between the regional office of the NCSC and local health and social care agencies had to take place, so that when the police were ready to act, closure of the home and transfer of residents could take place at the same time (Bines 2003). Such collaboration, although difficult to attain, is clearly essential within such situations if good practice is to be achieved.

POLICY DEVELOPMENT

The development of appropriate policies relating to abuse and protection is a difficult and problematic area. Certainly, since 1990, there has been a considerable development, particularly by social services departments, and to a lesser extent by health purchasers and providers of policies to address the abuse of older people. These have increasingly been framed in terms of adult protection, most recently, by the publication of the government guidance document, *No Secrets* (Department of Health 2000). This clearly stated that abuse in communal settings was to be included and addressed within local policies relating to abuse and protection. Within the community, a policy which is framed only in terms of protection may not recognize adequately that older people may be at risk of harm, although not necessarily frail and vulnerable, and that they may very well need the help of services because the person with whom they are living has the capacity to inflict harm upon them. This needs to be clearly reflected within policies at the local level.

In 1991, the Royal College of Nursing issued guidelines for nurses (Royal College of Nursing 1991) and these were updated in 1996 (Royal College of Nursing 1996). A number of valuable points are made, including the suggestions for nurses to keep accurate written records and to record telephone conversations with other professionals (Royal College of Nursing 1996). The Royal College of Nursing also contributed to new guidelines on the abuse of older people in the community, along with a number of other concerned organizations, including Action on Elder Abuse, Age Concern England, the British Geriatrics Society, the Carers National Association and the Royal College of General Practitioners. These give guidance on what to do if concerned about a possible case of abuse (Action on Elder Abuse 1996).

It is essential that nurses working with older people, from the range of possible settings, are aware of and familiar with the national framework provided within *No Secrets* and more crucially, perhaps, with the local policies and procedures in their localities. Familiarity means not just awareness of, but also knowledge and understanding of the guidance and relevant roles and responsibilities within the processes that are established at local level to deal with abuse and neglect.

NATIONAL AND INTERNATIONAL DEVELOPMENTS

Action on Elder Abuse is a national charity which was launched in 1992 with the aims of preventing elder abuse by raising awareness, education, promoting research and the collection and dissemination of information (Mullan 1995, Penhale & Kingston 1995). Membership is open, on payment of an annual subscription, to anyone sympathetic to these aims and many members are nurses. An information bulletin is issued six times a year to members and an annual conference is held. The charity runs an information and enquiry service, including information provided for students. Information leaflets and training material, including videos, have been produced. In the late 1990s, the charity was involved in the piloting of a telephone helpline in four areas of England. Following evaluation of the pilot, this helpline was subsequently established on a national basis in 1998 and is staffed by trained volunteers. The helpline is open to anyone who is concerned about elder abuse and offers advice, information and guidance in relation to situations of elder abuse and/or neglect. Calls from professionals, including nurses, who are concerned about actual or potential situations of abuse are regularly taken. The helpline does not offer a referral or counselling service, however. The charity has been supported financially by Age Concern England, as well as by the Department of Health and other charitable sources. It is the only UK-based charity to focus entirely on elder abuse, although, as seen earlier in this chapter, there are other voluntary organizations involved in aspects of the problem.

The International Network for the Prevention of Elder Abuse was established in 1997 as a global initiative to combat, alleviate and prevent elder abuse. There are six regional sectors (Europe, North America, Latin America, Asia, Africa and Oceania). Interested individuals and groups can join or affiliate to the network, which provides regular information about global responses to abuse. Further details can be obtained through the website for the network (see useful addresses, below).

CONCLUSION

> The challenge is to make sure that efforts on behalf of mistreated older persons do more good than harm and do not lead to the neglect of other societal needs (Wolf 1992: p. 429).

Rosalie Wolf was a leading campaigner against elder abuse in the USA throughout the 1980s and 1990s. Her words here are profoundly important. The unease of many nurses – and other professionals – in intervening in abusive situations is connected to the fear of making things worse. It is probably the first rule of practice that older people must be listened to, whether they are carer or cared-for, abuser or abused, whether they are in hospital or in community settings. Second, awareness that abuse can and does exist is essential to dealing with it, although it is always important to discuss concerns with managers and not to 'rush in' without a careful plan of action. Finally, the current legitimate and necessary interest in the ill treatment of older people should have the effect of making us all think about the general way that we as a society treat our elders and the ways in which discrimination against older people might exacerbate situations of abuse and neglect. Prevention of abuse should be our main priority. Abuse, whether by paid staff or by family members, is the extreme end of a continuum covering the care of older people. It is most likely to be prevented by the strengthening of a whole range of other services which bear on household and family relationships and the provision of communal health and social care.

Recommended reading

Amiel S, Heath I 2003 Family violence in primary care. Oxford University Press, Oxford.
A general text on family violence, including five chapters relating specifically to older people. Although written specifically for general practitioners, nurses would find it useful.

Bennett G, Kingston P, Penhale B 1997 The dimensions of elder abuse: perspectives for practitioners. Macmillan, Basingstoke.
This is a helpful background text written from an integrated health and social care perspective for a multidisciplinary audience of practitioners. The book includes chapters on the law, on key healthcare issues, on different aspects of interventions and on abuse in care settings as well as international perspectives.

Clarke M, Ogg J 1994 Identifying the elderly at risk. Journal of Community Nursing 8: 4–9.

Clarke M, Ogg J 1994 Recognition and prevention of elder abuse. Journal of Community Nursing 8: 4–6.
These two articles are based on research with a small group of district nurses in Tower Hamlets, London, and provide valuable data about the nurses' knowledge and experience of elder abuse.

McCreadie C 1996 Elder abuse: an update on research. Age Concern Institute of Gerontology, King's College, London. Although out of print it is available on www.kcl.ac.uk/kis/schools/life_sciences/health/gerontology
The aim of this update is to provide an easily accessible source of research on elder abuse for practitioners, students and teachers. Although written primarily with a social services audience in mind, it provides a useful source of data for a wide range of readers. After an introduction, the chapters cover definitions, current research findings, both in the UK and abroad, abuse in communal settings, issues of financial abuse and interventions. Each chapter is divided into specific sections, which have their own list of references. There are also a number of tables, providing summaries of research findings by topic.

Pritchard J 1996 Working with elder abuse. Kingsley, London.
This is a practical training manual which has been written for home care, residential and day care staff, but which nurses would find very useful in thinking about elder abuse. It has a range of exercises and photocopiable work sheets, and is valuable both for those in training positions as well as nursing students and front-line practitioners.

Royal College of Nursing 1996 Combating abuse and neglect of elderly people: guidelines for nursing. Royal College of Nursing, London.
The Royal College of Nursing first published guidelines in 1990, but in recognition of the changing knowledge of the field, these have been substantially revised and updated.

Saveman B-I, Norberg A, Hallberg IR 1992 The problems of dealing with abuse and neglect of the elderly: interviews with district nurses. Qualitative Health Research 2: 302–317.

Saveman B-I, Hallberg IR, Norberg A 1993 Identifying and defining abuse of elderly people, as seen by witnesses. Journal of Advanced Nursing 18: 1393–1400.

Saveman B-I, Hallberg IR, Norberg A, Eriksson S 1993 Patterns of abuse of the elderly in their own homes as reported by district nurses. Scandinavian Journal of Primary Health Care 11: 111–116.

Saveman B-I, Hallberg IR, Norberg A 1996 Narratives by district nurses about elder abuse within families. Clinical Nursing Research 5: 220–236.

These four articles all report on a detailed research project with district nurses in Sweden. They throw light not only on how the nurses think about abuse, but also on the nature of the cases they have encountered and the professional issues they face in dealing with them. They are particularly valuable in enabling the nurses' experience to be understood and in the way they illustrate the complexity and diversity of elder abuse.

Stanley N, Manthorpe J, Penhale B (eds) 1999 Institutional abuse: perspectives across the lifecourse. Routledge, London.

A useful volume concerning institutional abuse. Contains three chapters relating to elder abuse as well as other chapters about vulnerable adults. Useful material concerned with user perspectives.

United Kingdom Central Council for Nursing, Midwifery and Health Visiting 1994 Professional conduct – occasional report on standards in nursing homes. UKCC, London.

This report gives a graphic indication of some of the ill-treatment that has occurred in nursing homes. It is a valuable document about abuse and some of the steps necessary to prevent abuse.

United Kingdom Central Council for Nursing, Midwifery and Health Visiting 1999 Practitioner–client relationships and the prevention of abuse. UKCC, London.

This is an important and constructive document which not only highlights the responsibilities of nurses in relationships with clients, but also emphasizes some of the key issues relating to abuse and its prevention.

Useful addresses

Action on Elder Abuse Astral House 1268 London Road London SW16 4ER; www.elderabuse.org.uk

Counsel and Care Twyman House 16 Bonny Street London NW1 9PG; www.counselandcare.org.uk

International Network for the Prevention of Elder Abuse (INPEA): www.inpea.net

Public Concern at Work UK office: Suite 306, 16 Baldwins Gardens, London EC1N 7RJ; www.pcaw.co.uk

References

Action on Elder Abuse 1994 Elder abuse in care homes: who to contact and what to do. Action on Elder Abuse, London

Action on Elder Abuse 1996 The abuse of older people at home: information for workers. Action on Elder Abuse, London

Amiel S, Heath I 2003 Family violence in primary care. Oxford University Press, Oxford

Askham J, Bary C, Grundy E, Hancock R, Tinker A 1992 Life after 60. A report from the gerontology data service. Age Concern Institute of Gerontology, King's College, London

Baker AA 1975 Granny-battering. Modern Geriatrics 5: 20–24

Beaulieu M 1992 Elder abuse: levels of scientific knowledge. Journal of Elder Abuse and Neglect 4: 135–149

Bennett G 2000 Personal communication to B. Penhale

Bennett G, Kingston P 1993 Elder abuse: concepts, theories and interventions. Chapman & Hall, London

Bennett G, Kingston P, Penhale B 1997 The dimensions of elder abuse: perspectives for practitioners. Macmillan, Basingstoke

Bines J 2003 Personal communication to B. Penhale

Brodaty H, Gresham M 1989 Effect of a training programme to reduce stress in patients with dementia. British Medical Journal 299: 1375–1379

Brown H, Turk V 1992 Defining sexual abuse as it affects adults with learning disabilities. Mental Handicap 20: 44–55

Burgner T 1996 The regulation and inspection of social services. Department of Health/Welsh Office, London

Burston GW 1975 Granny battering. British Medical Journal 3: 592

Castledine G 1994 Elder abuse by nurses is on the increase. British Journal of Nursing 3: 675–676

Chambers R 1999 Potential for abuse of medication for the elderly in residential and nursing homes in the UK. Journal of Elder Abuse and Neglect 10: 79–90

Clarke M, Ogg J 1994a Identifying the elderly at risk. Journal of Community Nursing 8: 4–9

Clarke M, Ogg J 1994b Recognition and prevention of elder abuse. Journal of Community Nursing 8: 4–6

Clough R 1999 Scandalous care: interpreting public enquiry reports of scandals in residential care. Journal of Elder Abuse and Neglect 10: 13–28

Comijs H 1999 Elder Mistreatment: prevalence, risk indicators and consequences. Vrije Universiteit, Amsterdam

Compton SA, Flanagan P, Gregg W 1997 Elder abuse in people with dementia in Northern Ireland: prevalence and predictors in cases referred to a psychiatry of old age service. International Journal of Psychiatry 12: 632–635

Cooney C, Mortimer A 1995 Elder abuse and dementia: a pilot study. International Journal of Social Psychiatry 41: 276–283

Counsel and Care 1994 Older people at risk of abuse in a residential setting. Fact sheet 2. Counsel and Care, London

Counsel and Care 1995 Care betrayed. Counsel and Care, London

Craig Y 1994 Elder mediation: can it contribute to the prevention of elder abuse and the protection of the rights of elders and their carers? Journal of Elder Abuse and Neglect 6: 83–96

Decalmer P, Glendenning F 1993 The mistreatment of older people. Sage, London

Department of Health and Social Security 1988 Violence to staff. Report of the DHSS advisory committee on violence to staff. HMSO, London

Department of Health 1993 No longer afraid: the safeguard of older people in domestic settings. Department of Health, London

Department of Health 2000 No secrets: the protection of vulnerable adults – guidance on the development and implementation of multi-agency policies and procedures. Department of Health, London

Department of Health 2001a National service framework for older people. Department of Health, London

Department of Health 2001b National service framework for older people: single assessment process. Department of Health, London

Dimond B 1995 Legal aspects of nursing, 2nd edn. Prentice-Hall, Englewood Cliffs, NJ

Eastley R, Macpherson R, Richards H, Mian I 1993 Assaults on professional carers of elderly people. British Medical Journal 307: 845

Evans G 1996 Age-old concerns. Nursing Times 92: 58

Fagg J 1994 Detection of abuse. Nursing Times 90: 67–68

Filinson R 1993 An evaluation of a program of volunteer advocates for elder abuse victims. Journal of Elder Abuse and Neglect 5: 77–93

Foner N 1994 Nursing home aides: saints or monsters? Gerontologist 34: 245–250

Freyne A, Wrigley M 1996 Aggressive incidents towards staff by elderly patients with dementia in a long-stay ward. International Journal of Geriatric Psychiatry 11: 57–63

Garcia JL, Kosberg JI 1992 Understanding anger: implications for formal and informal caregivers. Journal of Elder Abuse and Neglect 4: 87–99

Gilleard C 1994 Physical abuse in homes and hospitals. In: Eastman M (ed) Old age abuse, 2nd edn. Age Concern England/Chapman & Hall, London, pp 93–110

Gillen L 1995 Elder abuse peer support partners: a family violence prevention strategy utilizing volunteers. Journal of Volunteer Administration Winter 27: 26–29

Glendinning C 1989 The financial circumstances of informal carers. Final report, DHSS 529. Social Policy Research Unit, University of York, York

Goodridge DM, Johnston P, Thomson M 1996 Conflict and aggression as stressors in the work environment of nursing assistants: implications for institutional elder abuse. Journal of Elder Abuse and Neglect 8: 49–58

Harrison S 1994 The need to be aware. Journal of Community Nursing 8: 22–23

Heath H 1995 Health assessment of people over 75. Nursing Standard 9: 30–37

Henderson AD, Eriksen JR 1994 Enhancing nurses' effectiveness with abused women. Journal of Psychosocial Nursing 32: 11–15

Hinchliffe AC, Hyman I, Blizard B, Livingston G 1992 The impact on carers of behavioural difficulties in dementia: a pilot study on management. International Journal of Geriatric Psychiatry 7: 579–583

Hirst M 2001 Trends in informal care in Great Britain during the 1990s. Health and Social Care in the Community 9: 348–357

Hockey JL 1990 Experiences of death: an anthropological account. Edinburgh University Press, Edinburgh

Holstein M 1995 Elder mistreatment: ethical issues, dilemmas and decisions. Multidisciplinary ethical decision-making: uniting differing professional perspectives. Journal of Elder Abuse and Neglect 7: 169–182

Homer A, Gilleard CJ 1990 Abuse of elderly people by their carers. British Medical Journal 301: 1359–1362

Homer A, Gilleard CJ 1994 The effect of inpatient respite care on elderly patients and their carers. Age and Ageing 23: 274–276

House of Commons Health Committee 2004 Elder Abuse. Second report of session 2003–04. The Stationery Office, London

Hughes B, Wilkin D 1987 Physical care and quality of life in residential homes. Ageing and Society 7: 399–426

Hunt G 1995 Whistleblowing in the health service. Edward Arnold, London

Kerr J, Dening T, Lawton C 1994 Elder abuse and the community psychiatric team. Psychiatric Bulletin 18: 730–732

Kingston P, Penhale B 1994 A major problem needing recognition: assessment and management of elder abuse and neglect. Professional Nurse February: 9: 343–347

Kingston P, Penhale B 1995 Elder abuse and neglect: issues in the accident and emergency department. Accident and Emergency Nursing 3: 122–128

Kingston P, Phillipson C 1994 Elder abuse and neglect. British Journal of Nursing 3: 1171–1172, 1189–1190

Kingston P, Penhale B, Bennett G 1995 Is elder abuse on the curriculum? The relative contribution of child abuse, domestic violence and elder abuse in social work, nursing and medicine qualifying curricula. Health and Social Care in the Community 3: 353–362

Kivela S-L, Köngäs-Saviaro P, Kesti E, Pahkala K, Ijäs M-L 1993 Abuse in old age – epidemiological data from Finland. Journal of Elder Abuse and Neglect 4: 1–18

Kitchen G, Richardson B, Livingston G 2002 Are nurses equipped to manage actual or suspected elder abuse? Professional Nurse 17: 647–650

Kurrle SE, Sadler PM, Cameron ID 1992 Patterns of elder abuse. Medical Journal of Australia 157: 673–676

Laing W, Buisson E 1995 Care of elderly people – market survey 1995. Laing & Buisson, London

Lambert C 1992 The dysfunctional family and elder abuse. Violence Update, 2: 6–8

Langan J, Means R 1996 Financial management and elderly people with dementia in the UK: as much a question of confusion as abuse? Ageing and Society 16: 287–314

Law Commission 1995 Mental incapacity. Law Com. Report no. 231. HMSO, London

Lee-Treweek G 1994 Bedroom abuse: the hidden work in a nursing home. Generations Review 4: 2–4

Levin E, Moriarty J, Gorbach P 1994 Better for the break. HMSO, London

Lord Chancellor's Department 1999 Making decisions: helping people who have difficulty making decisions for themselves. HMSO, London

Lowe C 1993 Elder abuse. West Lambeth Community Care (NHS) Trust, London

Martin JP 1984 Hospitals in trouble. Blackwell, Oxford

Martin J, Meltzer H, Elliot D 1988 The prevalence of disability among adults. OPCS survey of disability in Great Britain, report 1. HMSO, London

McCreadie C 1991 Elder abuse: an exploratory study. Age Concern Institute of Gerontology, King's College, London

McCreadie C 1996 Elder abuse: an update on research. Age Concern Institute of Gerontology, King's College, London

McCreadie C 2000 Violence towards social care staff. Report to DOH task force. Available online at: www.doh.gov.uk/violencetaskforce/knowledge.htm

McCreadie C, Tinker A 2003 Elder abuse. In: Tallis R, Fillit H (eds) Brocklehurst's Textbook of geriatric medicine and gerontology, 6th edn. Churchill Livingstone, Edinburgh, pp 1399–1406

McCreadie C, Bennett G, Gilthorpe MS, Houghton G, Tinker A 2000 Elder abuse: do GPs know or care? Journal of the Royal Society of Medicine 93: 67–72

Mental Health Foundation 1995 Making life better: mental health for older people. Mental Health Foundation, London

Mouton C, Talamantes M, Parker R, Espino D, Miles T 2001 Abuse and neglect in older men. Clinical Gerontologist 24: 15–26

Mowbray CA 1989 Shedding light on elder abuse. Journal of Gerontological Nursing 15: 20–24

Mullan C 1995 'It doesn't happen here . . .' Elderly Care 7: 36

Nolan M 1994 Deregulation of nursing homes: a disaster waiting to happen? British Journal of Nursing 3: 595

North East Thames Regional Health Authority 1994 The report of the inquiry into the care and treatment of Christopher Clunis. HMSO, London

Nursing and Midwifery Council 2004 The NMC code of professional conduct: standards for conduct, performance and ethics. Nursing and Midwifery Council, London

Ogg J, Bennett G 1992 Elder abuse in Britain. British Medical Journal 305: 998–999

Penhale B 1993 Abuse of elderly people: considerations for practice. British Journal of Social Work 23: 95–112

Penhale B, Kingston P 1995 Recognising and dealing with the abuse of older people. Nursing Times 91: 27–28

Penhale B, Kingston P 1997 Elder abuse, mental health and later life: steps towards an understanding. Ageing and Mental Health 1: 296–304

Phair L, Goodman W 2003 The role of the community nurse. In: Amiel S, Heath I (eds) Family violence in primary care. Oxford University Press, Oxford, pp 391–395

Phillips LR 1988 The fit of elder abuse with the family violence paradigm and the implications of a paradigm shift for clinical practice. Public Health Nursing 5: 222–229

Pilgrim D 1995 Explaining abuse and inadequate care. In: Hunt G (ed) Whistleblowing in the health service. Edward Arnold, London, pp 77–85

Pillemer KA, Bachman-Prehn R 1991 Helping and hurting: predictors of maltreatment of patients in nursing homes. Research on Aging 13: 74–95

Pillemer KA, Finkelhor D 1988 The prevalence of elder abuse: a random sample survey. Gerontologist 28: 51–57

Pillemer KA, Moore D 1989 Abuse of patients in nursing homes: findings from a survey of staff. Gerontologist 29: 314–320

Pillemer KA, Moore D 1990 Highlights from a study of abuse of patients in nursing homes. Journal of Elder Abuse and Neglect 2: 5–29

Podnieks E 1990 National survey on abuse of the elderly in Canada. The Ryerson study. Ryerson Polytechnical Institute, Toronto

Podnieks E 1992 Emerging themes from a follow-up study of Canadian victims of elder abuse. Journal of Elder Abuse and Neglect 4: 59–111

Pritchard J 1995 The abuse of older people, 2nd edn. Jessica Kingsley, London

Pritchard J 1996 Darkness visible. Nursing Times 92: 26–31

Pritchard J 2001 Abuse of older men. Jessica Kingsley, London

Reay A, Browne K 2002 The effectiveness of psychological interventions with individuals who physically abuse or neglect their elderly dependents. Journal of Interpersonal Violence 17: 416–431

Richardson J 1998 Detection of elder abuse. Journal of Community Nursing 12: 8

Richardson B, Kitchen G, Livingston G 2002 The effect of education on knowledge and management of elder abuse: a randomized controlled trial. Age and Ageing 31: 335–341

Royal College of Nursing 1991 Guidelines for nurses. Abuse and older people. Royal College of Nursing, London

Royal College of Nursing 1992 A scandal waiting to happen? Royal College of Nursing, London

Royal College of Nursing 1994 An inspector calls? Royal College of Nursing, London

Royal College of Nursing 1996 Combating abuse and neglect of older people. RCN guidelines for nurses. Royal College of Nursing, London

Saveman B-I 1994 Formal carers in health care and the social services witnessing abuse of the elderly in their homes. Medical dissertations, New series no. 403. Umea University, Umea, Sweden

Saveman B-I, Norberg A, Hallberg IR 1992 The problems of dealing with abuse and neglect of the elderly: interviews with district nurses. Qualitative Health Research 2: 302–317

Saveman B-I, Hallberg IR, Norberg A 1993a Identifying and defining abuse of elderly people, as seen by witnesses. Journal of Advanced Nursing 18: 1393–1400

Saveman B-I, Hallberg IR, Norberg A 1993b Patterns of abuse of the elderly in their own homes as reported by district nurses. Scandinavian Journal of Primary Health Care 11: 111–116

Saveman B-I, Norberg A, Anders G, Oden B 1995 The trustworthiness of the stories of elder abuse narrated by district nurses. Scandinavian Journal of Caring Sciences 9: 29–34

Saveman B-I, Hallberg IR, Norberg A 1996 Narratives by district nurses about elder abuse within families. Clinical Nursing Research 5: 220–236

Secretary of State for Health 1992 Report of the committee of enquiry into complaints about Ashworth hospital. CM 2028-1. HMSO, London

Shah AK 1992 Violence and psychogeriatric inpatients. International Journal of Geriatric Psychiatry 7: 39–44

Shugarman LR, Fries BE, Wolf RS, Morris JN 2003 Identifying older people at risk of abuse during routine screening practices. Journal of the American Geriatrics Society 51: 24–31

Social Services Inspectorate 1993 No longer afraid: the safeguard of older people in domestic settings. Department of Health, London

Stanley N, Manthorpe J, Penhale B 1999 (eds) Institutional abuse: perspectives across the lifecourse. Routledge, London

Stein KF 1991 A national agenda for elder abuse and neglect research: issues and recommendations. Journal of Elder Abuse and Neglect 3: 91–108

Tatara T, Thomas C 1998 National elder abuse incidence study. Available online at: http://www.aoa.dhhs.gov/abuse/report/default.htm

Thomas C 2000 The first national study of elder abuse and neglect: contrast with results from other studies. Journal of Elder Abuse and Neglect 12: 1–14

Trevitt C, Gallagher E 1996 Elder abuse in Canada and Australia: implications for nurses. International Journal of Nursing Studies 33: 651–659

United Kingdom Central Council for Nursing, Midwifery and Health Visiting 1994 Professional conduct – occasional report on standards of nursing in nursing homes. UKCC, London

United Kingdom Central Council for Nursing, Midwifery and Health Visiting 1999 Practitioner–client relationships and the prevention of abuse. UKCC, London

Vernon M 1995 A & E – why so complacent? Nursing Times 91: 28–30

Vernon MJ, Bennett GCJ 1996 Elder abuse: nursing awareness, attitudes and professional experience in accident and emergency departments. Age and Ageing 25 (suppl. 1): 138

Wetle TT, Fulmer TT 1995 Elder mistreatment: ethical issues, dilemmas and decisions. A medical perspective. Journal of Elder Abuse and Neglect 7: 31–48

Wolf RS 1992 Making an issue of elder abuse. Gerontologist 32: 427–429

Wolf RS, Pillemer K 1994 What's new in elder abuse programming? Four bright ideas. Gerontologist 34: 126–129

Chapter 33

Carers and lay caring

Ann Mackenzie and Diana T. F. Lee

Lay caring has become an issue in the provision of health care as a result of longevity, the health and social care reforms that emphasize care by the community and changes in family composition. This chapter addresses some of the major aspects of lay caring, drawing on research and examples from clinical practice. Lay caring is interpreted as informal or unpaid care by family, friends and neighbours, as distinct from the care offered by statutory services, professionals or organized volunteers. Other terminology, such as informal carers, is used synonymously in specific references to policy and research.

BACKGROUND TO LAY CARING

The ageing population has posed many new challenges for societies throughout the world. Longevity does not necessarily mean extra years of active and healthy life. Longer life associated with chronic ill health often brings additional years of high morbidity, senescence and dependency. The 2001 General Household Survey (Office for National Statistics 2002a) found that 64% of older respondents over 75 years old reported a longstanding illness, disability or infirmity, with 47% indicating that such a condition limited their activities. It also pointed out that the proportion of respondents reporting health problems increased steadily with age. Indeed, the care and support of older people have attracted much research and policy attention worldwide over the past 20–30 years. In the UK, where community care reforms have emphasized that 'the great bulk of care is provided by friends, family and neighbours' (Department of Health 1989: para 1.9), these lay carers have become central to policy development, and there has been a recognition of the contributions that carers make to the support of older dependent people who live outside institutions. The National Strategy for Carers acknowledges that 'Carers play a vital role – looking after those who are sick, disabled, vulnerable or frail' (Department of Health 1999: 11). It notes three key approaches to supporting people who choose to be carers: (1) giving information on the means to provide care and about available help and services; (2) support from communities in planning and provision of services; and (3) care that promotes choice, maintains health and recognizes the carer's role.

In most countries, meeting the care needs of older people is a shared responsibility involving both formal and informal or lay caring support systems. Formal care generally means institutional care provided by statutory or voluntary organizations to meet specific needs, while informal care refers to home-based, non-professional informal care provided by family, friends and neighbours (Lea 1994). This distinction between formal and informal care has become blurred, with overlapping responsibilities resulting from the development of home help and community nursing and the consequent introduction of formal support systems into the traditional domain of the informal sector (Lingsom 1993). While meeting the care needs of older people is seen as a balance of responsibility between informal and formal care, there has been a tremendous growth in informal care over the past decades for various economic and social reasons. Informal care has been considered to be more economic, with savings to the public funds. The value of unpaid care in monetary terms has been estimated by the Institute of Actuaries as £33.9 billion per annum (British Medical Association 1995) which, despite being a rough calculation, indicates a high economic saving to the state. Informal care is also considered to be socially desirable because it accords with the wish of older people for closeness with family and friends, while at the same time maintaining autonomy and independence in the community. Informal care is at different stages of debate in different countries, owing to differences in family structures and traditions of welfare provision, such as availability of institutional care and adequate pension provision (Twigg 1993). In the USA the majority of disabled people use informal care but not all informal caregivers receive formal support in the same measure and the role of carers is unclear in relation to that of professionals and formal government services (Lyons & Zarit 1999). In the UK, explicit policy of care by the community, noted in the community care reforms (Department of Health 1989), has encouraged a diversity of care available, including statutory, independent and voluntary, with specific attention being paid to the issue of informal or lay caring (Department of Health 1999). More recent policy initiatives call for greater patient

and public involvement and demonstrate government commitment to patient-centred care. The Commission for Patient and Public Involvement in Health (CPPIH) will oversee the new system for patient and public involvement at both macro and micro level. The promise by the government of greater involvement will enable patients and other users to put forward their views and gain information about services. The functions of the patient advice and liaison services (PALS), set up in some trusts, will be incorporated into the new system of patient and public involvement and the monitoring functions of community health councils (CHCs), which will be abolished, will be taken over by the CPPIH. At community level patient and public involvement fora (PPIFs) will be set up in every National Health Service and primary care trust. It is at this level that informal carers are most likely to get involved. This initiative is welcome but it is a complex and rather cumbersome system and will need increased resources and a change in attitude of staff as well as policy to make it work (Gillespie et al. 2002).

TYPES AND PREVALENCE OF LAY CARERS

The General Household Survey of 2000 (Office for National Statistics 2002a) reports that there has been little change in the prevalence of adults caring in the past decade, estimating that there are 6.8 million adults caring for a sick, disabled or older person living in the UK. While women are most likely to provide care in the age group 45–64 (27% of women compared to 19% of men), men are more likely to be caring for someone aged over 65 (18% compared with 15%). One reason is that there are more likely to be a high proportion of women in the very old group and they are more likely to be disabled. Additional information on carers is available from the 2001 census (Office for National Statistics 2002b) which has, for the first time, included a question about people providing unpaid care and the number of hours spent caring. The census reports that there are 5.2 million informal carers in England and Wales and that the majority of these look after someone who is over pensionable age. Over a million provide care for more than 50 hours a week. In the USA it is also estimated that about 80% of health care for older people is being provided by family members (Whitlach & Noelker 1996). In addition, over half of all care provided is given by other older persons. Several reasons are suggested why older persons are serving as caregivers to other older adults. While life expectancy is increasing and the size of the older population is escalating, societal changes, caused by factors such as women returning to work, a lower birth rate and migration of family members away from their older relatives have resulted in fewer adult children being available for caregiving to parents. Therefore, care provided to an older dependant has to be given by another older person, who is usually the spouse of the dependent person. Also, the non-availability of a continuum of health care services has further limited the personnel and agency support available to the older dependants. As a consequence, caring responsibilities are left to older family members.

A survey undertaken in Derbyshire (Mudge 1995) has found that 37% of carers were in the age range 60–74 years. These older carers may be ill and disabled themselves and therefore providing care to another older person may be overwhelming. Older caregivers may thus be called the 'hidden patients' (Hills 1998). Older carers were more likely to be providing domestic and practical assistance rather than personal and physical care and the person being cared for was likely to be receiving visits from health and social services personnel (Parker 1993).

The informal care sphere designates a wide spectrum of unpaid forms of support and interaction, from voluntary, to self-help, to neighbour, to familial and personal friendship systems. A detailed analysis of the carers of older people in the UK (Parker 1993) shows a variety of caring situations. People caring for their parents or parents-in-law are unlikely to be doing so in the same household, and those caring for older family members, friends and neighbours are even less likely to be caring in the same household. They are also likely to be carrying out less personal and/or physical care than those involved in the care of their relatives. In comparison, in-household care is associated with a degree of mental impairment, with or without physical disability, in the dependent person. Those dedicated to in-household care tend to be more heavily involved with significantly longer hours of care.

Spouses are most likely to be in-household carers, are older than other groups of carers, are likely to be carrying sole responsibility in the provision of care and are much more likely to be involved in providing personal or physical care, or both. Given that in the 2000 General Household Survey (Office for National Statistics 2002a) 50% of older people lived just with their spouse, this group of carers is bound to be substantial. A similar pattern is seen in other European countries and, in some instances, caring may be devolved to nieces and nephews, when there is an extended family with no immediate, first-degree relative (Mestheneos & Triantafillou 1993).

This overall picture of different people being involved in the informal care of older persons has highlighted the danger of seeing carers as a homogeneous group and not acknowledging that there are important differences within this group. The difficulties encountered in taking up the caring role and the needs of these carers are certainly different. Gender, age, marital and economic status and regional variations all have an influence on the prevalence of caring and implications for government policies. Previously emphasizing gender as the only explanatory variable in understanding informal care has been found to be problematic in the UK (Ross & Mackenzie 1996) and the USA (Kane et al. 1999) and one is likely to lose sight of other important factors that mediate the experience of caring. Graham (1991), for example, has strongly argued for the need to recognize factors such as race and culture, which may affect the different ways in which carers respond to the experience of caring, yet little is known about the caring patterns of minority ethnic groups in the UK.

Needs of ethnic and minority groups

Often the needs of black and ethnic-minority groups are overlooked, or the assumption is made that they have strong kinship networks and do not need the help of other services (Gunaratnum 1993). The increasing emphasis on informal care and large-scale provision may mean that small group needs are not visible (Gunaratnum 1993). This is particularly true for Chinese populations, who make up the third largest ethnic community in the UK (Fig. 33.1). Although they have traditionally strong family and filial obligations, they are likely to suffer just the same difficulties as other populations in looking after older relatives (Mackenzie & Holroyd 1996). Research on a sample of Chinese elders in Liverpool suggested that older carers are isolated and hesitant to express their caring

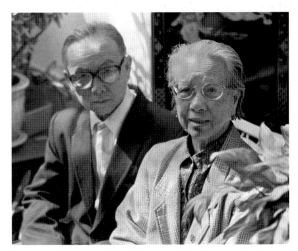

Fig. 33.1 Chinese elders. (Photograph by Jon-Paul Davis, courtesy of Age Concern Scotland.)

needs about caring responsibilities even within their own Chinese community (Au & Au 1994). A national survey on the health and lifestyles of Chinese people living in England found that, in comparison with the general population, they had comparatively poor social support networks (Sprotson et al. 1999). With a large increase of people aged over 60 years in the general population (Office for National Statistics 2002b), this lack of social support networks is likely to affect older Chinese caregivers. Despite government attention to carers, there is still a need for better information to be given to black and ethnic-minority communities (Banks 1999), who frequently do not have knowledge of National Health Service and local-authority services or are unable to access them due to cultural and linguistic factors. To overcome some of these problems, Tameside employed bilingual workers to identify carers and invite them to meetings to find out their information and other needs. Bilingual contact points were also offered on an ongoing basis (Banks & Cheeseman 1999).

NATURE OF LAY CARING

Formal and informal care differs as regards the motivation of the caregivers. The desire to do good, which embodies the moral dimension of caring, motivates and sustains lay carers, who interrupt their personal lives to tolerate possibly difficult circumstances arising from the lay caring relationship (Lea 1994). This commitment, an important factor that determines the development, maintenance and success of the lay caring relationship, defines to a large extent the behaviour and attitudes of both the carers and the recipients (Kitson 1987). While formal carers are paid for their services, informal caregivers are assumed to be motivated by altruism or moral obligations to the care recipient. As the carers are usually family members of the recipient, the lay caring relationship is therefore further defined by the familiarity and intimacy of the relationship between these participants. Such relationships, however, may paradoxically create problems.

While it cannot be assumed that caring by family members is always problematic, stressful or burdensome, a great deal of literature has identified the difficulties and personal costs of caring by lay carers, whether they be family, neighbours or friends.

BURDENS AND COSTS OF CARING

Caring has been described as a duty without a break which requires the use of appropriate knowledge and skills to help in the performance of caring activities that are directed to meet the physical, mental and emotional needs of the recipient (Kitson 1987). In a review of the literature on the outcome of lay caring, Browning & Schwirian (1994: p. 17) found that 'aversive impact on physical and mental health, psychological disorders and emotional distress, feelings of burden, personal strain and social isolation' were associated with home caregiving. Various studies (Dewey et al. 2002, Pickard & Glendinning 2002) have indicated how this involvement restricts the personal freedom and the quantity and quality of social contacts of the carer. Obviously, there are 'costs' to carers in the maintenance of their caring role. Caregiver costs are defined as potential or actual negative changes in the caregiver's life or feelings (Picot 1995). They include both the caregiver's subjective perception of the care recipient's impairments and the objective impact of the caregiving situation. In a study across four geographical areas of England, costs of informal care for older people who are mentally and physically frail are described in areas of financial, time and social (Resource Implications Study of Medical Research Council Cognitive Function and Ageing 1998). Costs in all areas were reported, with the highest percentage of subjects reporting at least one social cost. Four main costs of caring are widely discussed in the literature on informal caring: (1) emotional and psychological; (2) physical; (3) social; and (4) financial.

Emotional and psychological costs

Although commitment is an important basis for the development and maintenance of informal care, this can have the consequence that people underestimate and may deny the emotional burdens of caregiving and try to deny such burdens. Using a grounded theory approach to gain a better understanding of the caregiving experience from the perspective of the caregivers, Boland & Sims (1996) concluded that the central idea emerging from the data was caregiving as a solitary journey, with burden, responsibility and commitment shaping the context of this journey. Also of importance is that commitment to care appeared to moderate descriptions of burden and responsibility in this journey.

The passive dependent position of the dependant has also helped to induce emotional stress in the carer, as the carer has to protect the dependant's self-esteem and make decisions on the dependant's behalf. Emotional distress may be further exacerbated by the fact that both carers and dependants are also forced into unfamiliar roles or role reversal and that, very often, carers are required to provide intimate care. This can produce complex and conflicting feelings of frustration, embarrassment, guilt, anger, fear, love and hate, in both the carers and the dependants (Sharp 1992). For instance, guilt may be experienced from wishing the loved one dead, which may eventually lead to emotional exhaustion (Lea 1994). Furthermore, dependants can be manipulative and occasionally aggressive but are very adept at giving an entirely different picture to outsiders (Nolan & Grant 1989). In these circumstances, there may be no satisfaction in the caring role. When the carer cannot obtain satisfaction, because the carer–dependant relationship is one that is too demanding, with difficult or upsetting dependant behaviour, carer burden is further pronounced. Helplessness and depression may develop if all these feelings are not being resolved.

In a review of the caregiving literature, Schultz et al. (1990) report that carers experience a higher incidence of psychiatric conditions and that depression in older carers is not uncommon. Clipp (1991) also found that carers of persons with Alzheimer's disease took more psychotropic drugs than other older adult community-dwellers and as much as those who were in institutions. In fact, cognitive impairment in the care recipient has been found to cause increased stress in the carer because the cognitively impaired older persons are suffering from both loss of self-care ability and progressive loss of memory. The carers not only have to assume the care responsibility, but also experience the 'loss' of a spouse or friend.

Indeed, caring consists of two interdependent, complementary dimensions of love and labour (Graham 1983). Love is concerned with affective aspects of caring, while labour is the task or activity involved in the caring role. It has been demonstrated that the objective circumstances of the caring task contribute only a small part to carer stress and that emotional elements are more significant (Nolan & Grant 1989). Feelings of love and affection for the recipient may make it easier for the carer to provide care, and yet these same feelings may paradoxically prevent people from caring (Lea 1994). Carers suffer the pain too when they witness the growing debilitation and increasing handicap in their beloved dependent relatives or friends. The emotional stress of carers may also be linked to the uncertainty of caregiving outcomes and the frustration of being unable to visualize any sort of future, as one carer expressed (Nolan & Grant 1989: p. 956):

> Each year it gets a little bit harder, a little bit
>   worse, a lot more soul destroying.
> When will it end? How will it end?
> What traumas lie ahead before it ends?
> HOW WILL IT END??? [original emphasis]

It has been found that the life-cycle state at which caregiving occurs may be an important factor in understanding carers' stress. Younger carers are found to have significantly higher stress because they are still involved in working outside the home and child-rearing duties (Schwarz & Roberts 2000).

Physical costs

Caregiving activities also take a toll on carers' physical well-being. The degree of physical help required from the carers is variable, depending on the unique problems of the dependants. In examining carer burden, Nolan et al. (1990) found that such physical help may include assisting the dependants with dressing, washing, toileting, mobilizing, bathing, feeding and other personal care. Carers undoubtedly experience a high level of physical exertion in their daily lives and it is natural that they feel physically tired and exhausted. Moreover, informal care of older people is often provided by spouses and children who are often themselves older (Sharp 1992). With increasing age there is greater potential for physical challenge. These older carers have immense difficulty in performing caring activities such as lifting, bathing and dressing. Their physical well-being is certainly affected.

Various studies have looked into the physical health of carers. Caregivers, who had an average age of 60 years, looking after a family member who had suffered a stroke, had relatively poor health compared to the general population (Bugge et al. 1999). Nolan et al. (1990) also reported that carers in their study found that caring threatens physical health and they felt physically tired. In their review of the caring literature, Schultz et al. (1990) conclude that, in most studies, carers reported an increased vulnerability to physical illness. In a more recent study, Picot (1995) has identified that the most frequently perceived cost of caring among 83 caregivers is physical fatigue. Out of 650 carers with an average age of 63 who were looking after frail older people, one-third felt that their general health had been affected. Daughters were more likely to report ill health than other female carers (Resource Implications Study of Medical Research Council Cognitive Function and Ageing 1998). However, Pollock (1994) argues that ill health in most carers cannot be directly attributed to their caring duties because the average age of most of the carers was 61, and two-thirds of all people over 45 years of age already have chronic health problems. Studies may also define general health as including both mental and physical aspects of health. Hence, while it is widely acknowledged that carers experience a level of physical exertion in their daily living far above that experienced by other people, it is debatable whether or not the relationship between caring and ill health is a causal one.

Social costs

Caregiving activity is also to some degree routinized and carers often have to be close to the recipient of care for many hours a day because of the unpredictability of the needs of the frail older person and because they are afraid of leaving their dependants alone safely at home. Friends and social opportunities, previously obtained from employment and leisure activities, may thus gradually disappear (Sharp 1992). Carers may become restricted in their personal freedom and in the amount and quality of their social contacts. Shrinking of their social circle, with reduced contact with friends and entertainment, may contribute to an increasing sense of isolation. Through interviews with 17 families providing lay care to a dependant at home, Boland & Sims (1996) found that feelings of isolation or aloneness were evident in the majority of caregivers, described as 'in a small little world – isolated' (Boland & Sims 1996: p. 57). It was found that these feelings of isolation also included neglecting one's personal needs, being unable to have or maintain an outside job, and decreasing family or social contacts. Carers in Nolan et al.'s (1990) study also reported having no time for friends, social life and holidays and no private time. This decrease of social contact outside the home is further pronounced when there is a lack of family support or when little help can be offered by other family members and relatives (Lewis & Meredith 1988). Restrictions on social life may threaten carers' emotional health, and the lack of freedom may lead carers to feel that they are trapped and that life opportunities have been lost. Of the five main needs for carers of older people in Ireland, companionship, someone to talk to when family support is lacking, was the most prevalent (Clifford 1990). The impact of caregiving on unwaged time was reported by around one-third of supporters of frail older people as restricting social activities and reducing time for holidays (Resource Implications Study of Medical Research Council Cognitive Function and Ageing 1998).

Financial costs

In caring for a dependant at home, extra expenditure may be required to cover heating, laundry, special diet and transportation, in addition to the 'normal' medical treatment fee and the cost of aids. These financial constraints are all the more onerous for people who may have been forced to give up paid work altogether or to take on part-time work in order to become full-time carers (Sharp 1992). Picot (1995) found that the financial cost was the second most frequently perceived cost of caring described by the 83 family carers in her study. Financial costs are especially relevant in the older carers' group, because many older adults live on a fixed pension and are often unable to obtain paid employment. The recent trend of older people who are past retirement age continuing to work part-time will be curtailed if they are caregivers and have little opportunity for extra money to supplement pensions. Lack of finances is also reported as contributing to the stress and burden of caring. The British Medical Association (1995) recommends improved financial support in the form of a carers' allowance to replace earnings and compensate for time spent caring, guaranteed respite care for 2 weeks a year and regular time out.

Costs to the family

To the above costs might be added 'costs to the family'. While most research has focused on the individual who is providing care, one should not lose sight of the important fact that the stresses and strains associated with caregiving will affect the family as a unit. Although one individual in the family generally takes the role of primary caregiver, changes in that person's role and the consequences of the burden or strains of caregiving can affect the family unit. The extent to which providing care to an older dependant creates strains in the family unit is influenced by the family's overall demands, as well as by the resources available to the family. Fink (1995) found that it is the process by which care is provided, rather than the amount of care, that influences family strains. For example, lack of privacy and increased tension among family members may be intensified if the dependent person lives with the family. However, while families experience difficulties when a member is physically or emotionally challenged, most families do not abandon the person. The stresses of caring do not stop even if the older person has to be admitted to institutional care. Families continue to visit and show concern about the welfare of their relatives. Interestingly, in a study about Chinese elders who were living in institutions it was found that the dependent elders were themselves supporting the families by protecting them and not burdening them with difficulties that elders themselves experienced in the residential care home (Lee et al. 2002).

In summary, each of these 'costs' can act as a cause of stress and burnout in lay caring. If they are not being attended to, they may gradually erode the caring relationship, resulting in anxiety and depression in both the carers and the dependants.

SATISFACTION AND REWARDS OF CARING

The emphasis on the burden and costs of caring has frequently overshadowed the satisfaction and benefits that carers gain from caring. A number of research studies in different cultures identify the satisfaction as well as the burden of caring, even though the caring situation continues to be stressful (Motenko 1989, Clifford 1990, Grant & Nolan 1993, Mackenzie & Holroyd 1996).

Grant & Nolan (1993) examined the sources of rewards and satisfaction by analysing qualitative data from a questionnaire sent to carers. Three main dimensions of the sources of satisfaction were identified. First, satisfaction is derived from the interpersonal dynamics, which include the act of giving and seeing the dependant's appreciative response. This reciprocity of mutual giving and receiving is described in terms of seeing the dependent person smile, say thank you and touching each other, all regarded as small but appreciative responses. Reciprocity was also perceived by way of repayment for past services. Second, satisfaction is derived from intrapersonal or intrapsychic orientation, described in terms of the caring act improving the quality of life and heightening awareness of what the carer could achieve and, in addition, seeing caring as a worthwhile challenge. The third source of satisfaction is protecting the dependent person from institutional care, much of which is not regarded as a good alternative to care at home.

These sources of satisfaction were also noted in a study carried out in Chinese populations, where duty and obligation are not seen as negative but as repayment for services or support provided in the past. Small reciprocal acts, such as good humour, thanks and physical improvements, made the act of caring worthwhile. In addition, repayment for past kindness and providing an alternative to institutional care sustained the carer through the burden and stress of caring (Mackenzie & Holroyd 1996).

A study in Ireland (Clifford 1990) explored the rewards of caring by interviews with carers of frail older people. Family obligation and a sense of duty seen as a normal part of family life, expressions of love, religious conviction and altruism were all reasons given for caring, each being perceived as a positive reason. Expressions of affection and appreciation were seen as motivating factors that gave satisfaction and sustained the caring relationship. A sense of achievement at having kept the relative at home and a feeling of personal fulfilment are also benefits. Achievement was also frequently reported by caregivers in a study in the USA (Kane et al. 1999), together with a sense of affection and seeing the older person's health improve or remain stable.

Enduring relationships that are meaningful and that continue to offer companionship and affection, even if the spouse is suffering from dementia (Motenko 1989), provide a form of social support for the caregiver and offer gratification as well as frustration.

The few studies that have identified satisfaction as a part of caring raise awareness about the similarities of carers' experiences as well as the differences. The differences may be more to do with an emphasis on what is important and may be related to the different lifestyles that people are used to. Given that older people find it difficult to change their habits, traditional practices may affect the priority of need. Clifford (1990) compares studies on loneliness and notes that in Ireland people rely on the extended family and close-knit community support, whereas in Denmark, where people value privacy and are used to being alone, they are less lonely and more independent than in the USA or UK. For the older Chinese population living in Hong Kong, the change in family composition has been rapid over the past 10 years. Previously the extended family provided support and help with decision-making, but now the kinship networks are reduced, leading to isolation and loneliness for old people. Community care programmes that are intended to support family carers will need to be sensitive to the cultural characteristics of older Chinese carers in order that benefits of caregiving and valued traditions of the Chinese family are sustained (Lui et al. 2000). Apart from giving financial help, increasing the benefits of caregiving are concerned with enhancing caregivers' sense of achievement (Resource Implications Study of Medical Research Council Cognitive Function and Ageing 1998) and providing greater recognition of caregivers' roles by government, society, professionals and the community (British Medical Association 1995).

For lay carers the caring situation has been found to be both burdensome and rewarding. From a selected review of the literature some conclusions can be drawn about the characteristics of lay carers of older dependants and of their situation.

CHARACTERISTICS OF LAY CARERS

- Carers are not a homogeneous group. Kinship ties and ethnic background are two differentiating elements (Atkin 1992)
- The main lay carer of older people in married couples is most often the spouse, who is also older, and frequently female (Parker 1992)
- Once responsibility for the caring role has been accepted, little further help is offered by family or outside services (Twigg 1992, Mackenzie & Holroyd 1996)
- High involvement in personal tasks and other caring responsibilities is experienced by those who care for dependants in the same household and by spouses
- Caring for older dependants is burdensome and demands emotional, psychological, physical, social and financial costs from the carer that

result in isolation, reduced social networks and physical and mental ill health (Lewis & Meredith 1988, Nolan & Grant 1989, Clifford 1990)

- Caring offers satisfaction and rewards that lead to a sense of achievement and fulfilment, while at the same time the act of caring is burdensome and frustrating (Clifford 1990, Grant & Nolan 1993)
- Carers have a number of common needs but there are also differences that reflect individual lifestyles and family practices that shape priorities.

As a result of our knowledge from the extensive literature on carers, identifying carers' needs is the first step in planning interventions and offering services.

SUPPORT FOR CARERS

The burdens of informal caring, which involve feelings of loss, grief, depression, physical and emotional exhaustion, having very little time for oneself, worrying about financial aspects and obtaining needed services, have been discussed. While critics have said that the negative aspects of caring have been overemphasized in the literature, it cannot be denied that the knowledge thus obtained is of great value in identifying the specific and particular needs of carers, especially the large number of older adults who are caring for their older dependants.

While it is recognized that the carer–recipient interaction is multidimensional and requires many disciplines to be involved in providing appropriate services and support, nursing is the most highly utilized service and nurses are able to serve in a variety of roles (Baines & Oglesby 1992). The support of informal carers must therefore be seen as a legitimate and important focus for nursing intervention. In fact, there is evidence to suggest that there is a significant relationship between carers' distress levels and the subsequent long-term institutionalization of their older dependants (Gilleard 1987). Without appropriate support carers may find the burden of caring too difficult. Therefore, it is reasonable that informal carers should demand that the limits to their responsibilities are acknowledged and addressed.

Because of the heterogeneity of informal carers, it is important to realize that the needs of different informal carers are not the same. Older carers, for example, may encounter more difficulty in providing physical care than those who are younger. Consideration of such differences will enable nurses to provide support that is sensitive to individual needs. Nurses should also be aware that different types of support may be needed at different stages of the caring process. It has

been demonstrated that the very early period of caring can be very stressful (Clarke & Watson 1991).

Awareness of the needs of informal carers in the very early stages of caring is therefore important. In the USA a longitudinal study of 307 caregivers revealed that professionals involved in hospital discharge may underestimate the amount of post acute-care tasks carried out by families and called for more careful assessment of the capacities and abilities of families to cope at an early stage (Kane et al. 1999). The importance of assessing the needs of potential caregivers or, indeed, whether or not the caregiver is suitable to take on the role of caring at all, is part of discharge planning from hospital and an important task for nurses in acute-care settings (Nolan & Grant 1992). Factors such as the physical tasks of lifting, which may be impossible for older carers to carry out, may lead to frustration, elder abuse or breakdown of caregivers' health and consequently to unplanned readmission.

Different needs of carers

Carers' needs change as the rehabilitation of the cared for person progresses (Kelson et al. 1999). Many carers' needs are unmet even though the services are available (Anderson et al. 1995). In reviewing the literature on what carers would like to receive from professional service providers, Nolan & Grant (1989) found that there is a remarkable consensus with regard to what services are important but currently not provided by health professionals. These are discussed in terms of four areas of deficiency – the lack of: (1) information; (2) skills training; (3) emotional support; and (4) sufficient, regular, respite services.

Information needs

Carers want accurate, appropriately timed and accessible information and are often overwhelmed and swamped by all the information they are given (Banks & Cheeseman 1999).

Many carers need information on a variety of areas, such as the condition of the dependant's health and the treatment regimen, advice about the physical as well as the psychosocial aspects of caring and about sources of financial or legal aid, availability of community services, healthy coping and adjustment strategies. With relevant information, carers are offered a degree of informed choice and this might increase their sense of control over the caring situation. Information is needed both before and after discharge (Wolfe et al. 1996). However information is not always appropriate or given at the right time or in the right form. For instance, stroke survivors and their carers have identified gaps in knowledge and information about their treatment and stroke condition (Wellwood et al. 1994) and services (Pound et.al. 1994). The Carers' National Association (1996) surveyed carers' experiences of the National Health Service and found that only 11% reported they had been given any information that would enable them to care more safely. Also carers from black and minority ethnic communities identified difficulties in finding out about services and support (Katbamna et al. 1998). Evidence from a systematic review indicates that structured individual information-giving may help stroke patients and their family carers cope with stroke (Forester et al. 2002). Nurses are the main providers of information (Nolan & Grant 1989, Richardson et al. 1989, Gunaratnum 1993, Yee 1995), and are key to meeting this need, particularly for older people and those from black and ethnic-minority backgrounds.

Skills training

As informal carers are not professional health care providers, they are untrained to handle the different tasks of caring, such as dealing with incontinence or lifting. They would certainly benefit from training and education with regard to different caring skills, such as lifting and moving techniques, use of disability aids, observing for side-effects of medications and care of the incontinent dependant. Older men who are carers may have different skills requirements to women, and the relationship between the carer and the dependant may also influence the activities that carers perform such as bathing, toileting and other intimate hygiene activities. Yet, focusing only on the physical aspects of caring is not enough. As discussed earlier, it is dealing with the emotional aspects of caring that has created the stress and turmoil for informal carers.

Emotional support

There is abundant evidence in the literature (Nolan & Grant 1989, Sharp 1992, Pollock 1994) to show that emotional support is perceived by carers as being most important. Carers must be listened to. Very often lending a sympathetic ear can be helpful because carers usually lack a confidant to share their emotions. Being recognized and valued for their work is the fundamental platform for support and it has been found that the absence of such perceptions adds to the stresses of caring (Nolan & Grant 1989). Nurses need to appreciate the work of the carers by giving more explicit recognition to them. Carers should be acknowledged and valued through both explicit and implicit channels. They should be praised for their efforts, and both they and the care recipients, as well

as other significant persons in the caregiving situation, should be included in the development and implementation of the plan for nursing care. It is also important that carers' needs are attended to as much as those of the dependants. Carers have to be helped to recognize and deal with a number of emotions arising from the caring experience and to find meaning in their situation. Therapeutic use of communication and interpersonal skills is important here. Some nursing strategies that may benefit elder caregivers and their care recipients in dealing with their emotions include life review, pet therapy, group interactions, hobbies and music therapy (Baines & Oglesby 1992). At times when the emotional distress is not easy to cope with, referral to more intensive counselling, such as bereavement counselling, may be needed. If necessary, referral to formal services such as mental health sources may assist the older caregiver to cope with the responsibilities of caregiving.

Respite services

Carers also need to address their own needs. Some form of regular respite from the role as a carer, by short stays in hospital or nursing home for the dependant, should be made available to relieve carers from the day-to-day demanding caring responsibilities. Offering chances for carers to attain 'normality' for themselves has been shown to reduce their negative perceptions and hostile feelings towards the dependant (Clarke & Watson 1991) and to maintain and promote the caring relationship. In studying their experiences of informal caring in late life, older carers supported the idea of a home-based respite care because they see this alternative as less distressing and disruptive to the care recipient (McGarry & Arthur 2001).

Social support

Provision of social support for the carers is also important. The desire for a support group has also been expressed by the carers themselves (Mudge 1995). Social support can buffer or cushion the stressful and negative effects of caregiving by conveying to the carers that they are esteemed, valued and cared for in a mutually obliging communication network. This can be made up of informal or formal sources. Informal sources of support include relatives, friends and neighbours and the relationship between the carer and the dependant, while formal sources of support include professional helpers, such as nurses and counsellors. Social support can also be given by carers' self-help groups. Being supported and valued was one of the positive aspects that came from a small study carried out in one of the inner London boroughs (Morton & Mackenzie 1994). This sort of response highlights the fact that caring is a tiring and isolating activity, leaving little energy for other things. These carers appreciated having someone else to organize activities for them and saw the group as a recognition of the contribution they were making to health care. Another interesting finding of this research was the fact that the group's needs changed over time. When first established, the group's needs concentrated on information, friendship and social contact. The members said it provided 'structure to the week' and 'something to look forward to'. For a longer-established group, with an average membership of 2 years, members were concerned with lobbying for change and trying to raise awareness about the problems of carers (Morton & Mackenzie 1994). Involving carers in a self-help programme early on helps to reduce the crisis of subsequent emotional burnout. Nurses are appropriate facilitators for the development and subsequent maintenance of self-help groups. Chapman (1995) describes the setting-up of a carers' support group by district nurses as a result of asking carers what they needed. The objectives of the group included enabling carers to share information, to provide a forum for meeting other carers in an informal atmosphere and to provide information about voluntary and statutory services. Other topics for discussion in the group were gardening, bird-watching and cooking. In this situation the professionals acted as a resource and facilitator to the group and arranged sitters for the dependent person. Social support is especially important to older carers because they may not have adequate transport, and many are not able to leave the dependant for whom they have been caring for an extended period (Baines & Oglesby 1992). They may need help with transport and respite services before they are able to socialize.

ASSESSMENT AND INVOLVEMENT OF CARERS

Involvement of carers in assessing their needs can be carried out at different levels: at the local-authority or health-authority level, at a local community level, for instance based on general practice populations, and at an individual level. Probably all are needed, and most certainly there needs to be sharing of the information in order to achieve a coordinated service. Evaluation of new projects is crucial if such initiatives are to be of any value (Powell & Kocher 1996). The consumer focus of the community care reforms in the UK assumes that users, both carers and clients, will have a choice and be active participants in their care. The vulnerable, such as disabled and frail older people, may have very little

choice. For example, they may not be able to choose private-sector services because of financial cost or they may not have enough information about what is on offer. Explicit strategies will need to be developed if social service departments are to involve service users, including carers (Social Services Inspectorate 1995). The articulate, mobile and informed may represent the majority and those who are busy, isolated and devoid of energy after the demands of caring will not get involved. Getting users involved in assessment and planning is an expensive business if little more than a cursory questionnaire is to be distributed. An effective assessment will mean collecting information from carer groups and professionals. The Carers' National Association are advocates and can be used as advisers at national and local level (Carers' National Association 1996).

Wistow & Barnes (1993) reported on a project that involved carers in a formal consultation with the local authority that was carried out in Birmingham – the Community Care Special Action Project (CCSAP). As part of this project providers of services sought to consult carers, identified as the users of the service, about the carers' experiences of the service and to elicit suggestions for improvement. This project included older people and was intended to make the services more sensitive and to inject consultation into the organization. As a result of this consultation there have been improvements to existing services, such as improved transport to day centres and the setting-up of a taskforce to look at improved access to public buildings, transport and in the home (Wistow & Barnes 1993). This level of consultation requires large-scale organization and intersectoral working. Similarly, the new system of involving patients and the public will require intersectoral working and organizational change (Gillespie et al. 2002). It will require incorporating the values of partnership into a system driven by policy outcomes and will not be an easy process. The meaning of public involvement is likely to be different depending on which perspective is taken into account. Organizational outcomes and patient outcomes are not easy to combine. Agendas of patients and their families are different to those of organizations. Carers may be identified as users or providers of the service, with differing priorities depending on how the group is defined. Their views will be important whether they are identified as users or as providers. However, individual carers do not always have the time or the energy to contribute to local voluntary groups and will be reliant on professionals to put forward their views. Comprehensive assessment and the careful gathering of information will be crucial to the success of public involvement.

The White Paper on community care, *Caring for People,* emphasizes that people should be assisted to live independently in their own homes (Department of Health 1989) and that the family may choose to look after their relatives at home. On the one hand it appears that carers have a choice whether or not to care at home but, on the other hand, the policy for social and health care agencies is to support people in their own homes and avoid institutionalization. Therefore carers will be expected to look after relatives at home irrespective of their choice. A report from the King's Fund (Robinson & Batstone 1996) emphasizes the importance of a focus on individual need for older people and their carers in terms of rehabilitation, rather than wholesale provision based on facilities or disease categories. Empowering carers to take part in decision-making is an approach that professionals and policy-makers should be embracing (Askham 1997). The Carers (Recognition and Services) Act entitles carers to an assessment of their needs by local authorities (Department of Health 1995). However this is still not routine social service practice and carers are not clear about their entitlement (Department of Health 1998, Banks & Cheeseman 1999). The needs of those who are caring for someone with dementia are inadequately understood due to deficient assessment (Ferguson & Keady 2002). Also, urgent attention is needed for assessment of carers of older people with mental health problems, particularly in black and ethnic-minority communities (Audit Commission 2000). The practice of carrying out assessments by telephone is not appropriate for many older caregivers who need time to consider their needs and feel bombarded by questions.

Given that carers are not a homogeneous group and have different needs, this notion of individual assessment applies to carers as well as dependants and should be part of the normal work of community nurses.

One form of assessment is to ask carers themselves what they need, so acknowledging that they are experts and should participate in decision-making. This may not be easy to do while the carer is at home and nurses may offer to meet outside the home to talk about personal needs separate from relatives' needs. However, assessments of older caregivers must take into account gender and culture and the nature of the health problem of the dependant. For example, professionals carrying out assessment of caregivers who are looking after someone with a mental health problem are urged to visit the home (Audit Commission 2000). Taking account of the needs of both carers and users is important as there are likely to be needs in common (Banks 1999).

A further difficulty is encountered by the demand for evidence-based commissioning, where effectiveness and efficiency are sought in return for services. Measurable outcomes in practice and research that demonstrate improvement are difficult to find and make it all the more important to evaluate new projects and to disseminate the findings. A guide to help local support services check and improve quality of services for carers will be useful to check the quality standards set out by the government (Blunden 2002). Research outcomes for carers are frequently measured in terms of burden and stress. However, while objective measures are important, the perspectives of the individuals involved are even more important. Older caregivers interpret the outcomes of care and service provision in terms of their personal and social context and their outcomes are inextricably linked with that of the person they care for (Banks & Cheeseman 1999). The satisfactions and benefits of caregiving are subjective and tied up with the feeling of doing something worthwhile and meaningful. Nurses and other professionals will need to identify and use measures for outcomes determined by the caregiver as well as the more traditional measures decided by professionals (Askham 1997).

TARGETING SERVICES FOR CARERS

Services are offered in the context of the reforms in *The NHS Plan* (Department of Health 2000) to support carers and their families in the community. The difficulty may be that carers are often seen as part of the service and not as clients. Community nurses remain the main direct providers of care with access to families and are therefore in a position to carry out assessments and to act as advocates on behalf of carers. Twigg (1989) raises questions about the responsibilities that social and health agencies have towards carers, depending on whether they are clients themselves with their own needs or whether they are expected to be a resource for professionals to use. She states that agencies can perceive carers in terms of resources, co-workers and co-clients (Twigg & Atkin 1994). The community nurse may regard the carer as a resource, helping with the tasks of caring when the nurse is not able to provide full nursing care. Hearn (1993), in a small study of the family, regarded carers more as co-workers who understood community nurses' inability to control the referral of resources from other agencies, or even their own visiting times. The carers recognized the limitations that the district nursing service put on nurses who had insufficient time to do the job and so they joined the nurses to help out with the work. The difficulty that this kind of commitment poses for carers is that they may not be seen as having health care needs of their own; instead they are regarded as part of service provision. Clearly, identifying their needs separately from those of the dependants would have advantages (Ross & Mackenzie 1996).

How professionals perceive the carers' position in terms of their contribution to the care of the dependent person will determine to some extent the ways in which carers' needs are identified and met. District nurses seem to see carers as a resource and to feel that carers need to be supported in order that they can look after the patient. Twigg & Atkin (1994: p. 75) quote a manager as saying: 'without carers we couldn't run the community nursing service . . . so we've got a vested interest, if you like, to keep the carer as well as possible'.

Assessing how much help carers get, and which carers get help, is another factor. Nurses, for instance, seem to offer support to carers not so much on the basis of the relationship between carer and dependant but on the household in which they live. If there is a married daughter to help with the care then district nurses are less likely to offer care (Arber & Gilbert 1993). Community nurses have to make adjustments to their caseloads, differentiating those who need more care from others and not keeping people on the caseload unnecessarily (Badger et al. 1989).

A major contribution to the targeting of resources can be made by community nurses completing a community profile. Many carers will only be known through the nurses' contacts with patients who, in many cases, are referred to nurses by the general practitioner. Identifying those carers who do not receive services for their relatives in the local population is a first step. Otherwise, many carers in the local community will be missed. Mawby (1993) described an initiative by district nurses to find carers based on the general practice population. Having identified carers by using the general practice age–sex register, 50 were interviewed. The result was a support group set up for carers who were hitherto unknown to the district nurse. There is a comprehensive literature that highlights carers and their needs (Richardson et al. 1989, Banks & Cheeseman 1999: p. 1). Carers want a good quality of life for the person they care for and some control over their lives. They want:

- to be fully informed
- to be recognized and have their own health and well-being taken into account
- to use high-quality services, both for the person cared for and for themselves, which they can depend upon
- to have some time off and a break from caring
- emotional support and relief from their isolation
- training, advice and support to care
- financial security
- their voice to be heard, both in their individual situations and in the development of local services.

CONCLUSION

Since the 1980s, lay caring and carers have occupied an increasingly high profile in the UK, due mainly to a policy agenda that has emphasized caring in the community, and also to the feminist movement and related research about women carers, and strong lobbying from articulate and politically aware interest groups. A large volume of literature has drawn attention to carers' needs as a group and as individuals. More knowledge is needed about how these needs can be met effectively and any new initiatives should be properly evaluated to this end. Nurses who work in the community, particularly, have the privilege of entry to private lives and can see at first hand the difficulties for carers. This knowledge, together with their access to a wide range of resources, enables nurses to make a major contribution, along with other providers, to assessing, planning and providing care. Such a key position means they are able to identify need for commissioners and purchasers of services.

Recommended reading

Gallagher SK 1994 Older people giving care: helping family and community. Auvurn House, London.
This book, based on a research study, explores ways in which age, gender and marriage affect the amount, range and types of informal care given by older people. It also provides succinct discussion of the implications of these caring patterns for theories of ageing, gender and marriage as well as public policy, emphasizing the role of older people in providing unpaid care to kith and kin. There are useful summaries and discussions at the end of each chapter.

Powell M, Kocher P 1996 Strategies for change: a Carers Impact resource book. King's Fund Publishing, London.
Based on the findings of the Carers Impact project's development work with social services and health agencies, this book gives practical advice on how agencies can work together to provide a high-quality service for carers, drawing on examples of practice from case studies across England. A useful bibliography is included.

Twigg J 1992 (ed) Carers research and practice. HMSO, London.
This book summarizes research in readable form from an extensive literature on lay carers and draws conclusions for practice. The contributors are well known to research in the field of caring. There are useful summaries at the end of each chapter.

Yee L 1995 Improving support for black carers: a sourcebook of information, ideas and service initiatives. King's Fund, London.
The difficulties for black carers in accessing services are discussed in this short and readable paperback. There is background to some of the problems of access and why they have arisen, dispelling some of the myths about carers in black populations. Chinese carers are also mentioned. There is much in this book

that nurses need to be aware of in their work with black populations and other ethnic groups.

References

Anderson CS, Linto J, Stewart-Wynne EG 1995 A population-based assessment of the impact and burden of caregiving for long-term stroke survivors. Stroke 16: 843–849

Arber S, Gilbert N 1993 Men: the forgotten carers. In: Bornat J, Pereira C, Pilgrim D, Williams F (eds) Community care: a reader. Macmillan, Basingstoke, pp 134–142

Askham J 1997 Supporting caregivers of older people: an overview of problems and priorities. Australian Journal on Ageing 17: 5–7

Atkin K 1992 Similarities and differences between informal carers. In: Twigg J (ed) Carers: research and practice. HMSO, London, pp 59–94

Audit Commission 2000 Forget me not: Mental health services for older people. Audit Commission, London

Au WKL, Au KPK 1994 Care in the Chinese community: the way ahead. Merseyside Chinese Community Development Association, Liverpool

Badger F, Cameron E, Evers H 1989 District nurses' patients: issues of caseload management. Journal of Advanced Nursing 14: 518–527

Baines EM, Oglesby FM 1992 The older as caregivers of the older. Holistic Nurse Practitioner 7: 61–69

Banks P 1999 Carer support: time for a change of direction? A policy discussion paper. King's Fund, London

Banks P, Cheeseman C 1999 Taking action to support carers. A Carers Impact guide for commissioners and managers. Kings Fund, London

Blunden R 2002 How good is your service to carers? A guide to checking quality standards for local carer support services. King's Fund, London

Boland DL, Sims SL 1996 Family caregiving at home as a solitary journey. Image: Journal of Nursing Scholarship 28: 55–58

British Medical Association 1995 Taking care of the carers. BMA, London

Browning JF, Schwirian PM 1994 Impact of care recipient health problems and mental status. Journal of Gerontological Nursing 20: 17–21

Bugge C, Alexander H, Hagen S 1999 Stroke patients' informal caregivers: patient, caregiver, and service factors that affect caregiver strain. Stroke 30:1517–1523

Carers' National Association 1996 New rights for carers: how to get my carer's assessment – a carer's guide. Carers' National Association, Edinburgh

Chapman H 1995 Carers group. In: Ross F, Elliott M (eds) Innovations in community nursing. Community and District Nursing Association, Edinburgh

Clarke C, Watson D 1991 Informal carers of the dementing older: a study of relationships. Nursing Practice 4: 17–21

Clifford D 1990 The social costs and rewards of caring. Avebury, Aldershot

Clipp E 1991 Social problems in aging. In: Baines E (ed) Perspectives on gerontological nursing. Sage, Newbury Park, pp 198–214

Department of Health 1989 Caring for people: community care in the next decade and beyond. Cmd 849. HMSO, London

Department of Health 1995 Carers' Recognition and Services Act: policy and practice guidance. Department of Health, London

Department of Health 1998 A matter of change for carers? Inspection of local authority support for carers. Department of Health, London

Department of Health 1999 Caring about carers: a national strategy for carers. Stationery Office, London

Department of Health 2000 The NHS plan: a plan for investment, a plan for reform. Cm 4818-1. Stationery Office, London

Dewey HM, Thrift AG, Mihalopoulos C et al. 2002 Informal care for stroke survivors: results from the North East Melbourne Stroke Incidence Study (NEMESIS). Stroke 33: 1028–1033

Ferguson C, Keady J 2002 The mental health needs of older people and their carers. In: Nolan M, Davies S, Gordon G (eds) Working with older people and their families: key issues in policy and practice. Open University Press, Buckingham, pp 120–138.

Fink SV 1995 The influence of family resources and family demands on the strains and well-being of caregiving families. Nursing Research 44: 139–146

Forester A, Smith J, Young J et al. 2002 Information provision for stroke patients and their caregivers (Cochrane review) In: The Cochrane Library, issue 4. Update Software, Oxford

Gilleard CJ 1987 Influence of emotional distress among supporters on the outcome of psychogeriatric day care. British Journal of Psychiatry 150: 219–233

Gillespie R, Florin D, Gillam S 2002 Changing relationships findings from the patient involvement project. King's Fund, London

Graham H 1983 Caring: a labour of love. In: Finch J, Groves D (eds) A labour of love: women, work and caring. Routledge, London

Graham H 1991 The concept of caring in feminist research: the care of domestic service. Sociology 25: 61–78

Grant G, Nolan M 1993 Informal carers: sources and concomitants of satisfaction. Health and Social Care 1: 147–159

Gunaratnum Y 1993 Breaking the silence: Asian carers in Britain. In: Bornat J, Pereira C, Pilgrim D, Williams F (eds) Community care: a reader. Macmillan, Basingstoke, pp 114–123

Hearn J 1993 An exploration of carers' perceptions of their participation in care of their relatives in the community and the district nurses' role in this participation. Unpublished dissertation, Department of Nursing Studies, King's College, London

Hills GA 1998 Caregivers of the older: hidden patients and health team members. Topics in Geriatric Rehabilitation 14: 1–11

Kane RA, Reinardy J, Penrod JD, Huck S 1999 After hospitalisation is over: a different perspective on family care of older people. Journal of Gerontological Social Work 31: 119–141

Katbamna S, Baker R, Parker G 1998 Guidelines of primary health care teams. South Asian Carers Project. University of Leicester Nuffield Community Care Studies Unit, Leicester

Kelson M, Ford C, Rigge M 1999 Stroke rehabilitation. Patient and carer views. Royal College of Physicians, London

Kitson AL 1987 A comparative analysis of lay-caring and professional (nursing) caring relationships. International Journal of Nursing Studies 24: 155–165

Lea A 1994 Defining the roles of lay and nurse caring. Nursing Standard 9: 32–35

Lee TFD, Woo J, Mackenzie A 2002 The cultural context of adjusting to nursing home life: Chinese elders' perspectives. Gerontologist 42: 667–675

Lewis J, Meredith B 1988 Daughters who care: daughters caring for mothers at home. Routledge, London

Lingsom S 1993 Paying informal carers. In: Twigg J (ed) Informal care in Europe. Social Policy Research Unit, University of York, pp 171–190

Lui HL, Lee TFD, Mackenzie AE 2000 Community care of older Chinese People in Hong Kong: a selective review. Australasian Journal on Ageing 19: 180–184

Lyons KS, Zarit SH 1999 Formal and informal support: the great divide. International Journal of Geriatric Psychiatry 14: 183–196

Mackenzie A, Holroyd E 1996 An exploration of the carers' perceptions of caregiving and caring responsibilities in Chinese families. International Journal of Nursing Studies 33: 1–12

Mawby D 1993 Support for carers. Nursing Times 89: 67–68

McGarry J, Arthur A 2001 Informal caring in the late life: a qualitative study of the experiences of older carers. Journal of Advanced Nursing 33: 182–189

Mestheneos E, Triantafillou J 1993 Dependent older people in Greece and their family carers. In: Twigg J (ed) Informal care in Europe. Social Policy Research Unit, University of York, ch 9

Morton AJ, Mackenzie AE 1994 An exploratory study of the consumer's views of carer support groups. Journal of Clinical Nursing 1: 63–64

Motenko AK 1989 The frustrations, gratifications, and well-being of dementia caregivers. Gerontologist 29: 166–172

Mudge K 1995 Considering the needs of carers: a survey of their views on services. Nursing Standard 9: 29–31

Nolan MR, Grant G 1989 Addressing the needs of informal carers: a neglected area of nursing practice. Journal of Advanced Nursing 14: 950–961

Nolan MR, Grant G 1992 Mid-range theory building and the nursing theory–practice gap: a respite care case study. Journal of Advanced Nursing 17: 217–223

Nolan MR, Grant G, Ellis NC 1990 Stress is in the eye of the beholder: reconceptualizing the measurement of carer burden. Journal of Advanced Nursing 15: 544–555

Office for National Statistics 2002a Living in Britain: results from the 2001 general household survey. Stationery Office, London

Office for National Statistics 2002b. Census 2001: national report for England and Wales. Stationery Office, London

Parker G 1992 Counting care: numbers and types of informal carers. In: Twigg J (ed) Carers: research and practice. HMSO, London, pp 6–29

Parker G 1993 Informal care of older people in Great Britain: the 1985 general household survey. In: Twigg J (ed) Informal care in Europe. Social Policy Research Unit, University of York, ch 10

Pickard S, Glendinning C 2002 Comparing and contrasting the role of family carers and nurses in the domestic health care of frail older people. Health and Social Care in the Community 10: 144–150

Picot SJ 1995 Rewards, costs and coping of African American caregivers. Nursing Research 44: 147–152

Pollock A 1994 Carers' literature review. Nursing Times 90: 31–33

Pound P, Gompertz P, Ebrahim S 1994 Patients' satisfaction with stroke services. Clinical Rehabilitation 8: 7–17

Powell M, Kocher P 1996 Strategies for change: a Carer's Impact resource book. King's Fund, London

Resource Implications Study of Medical Research Council Cognitive Function and Ageing 1998 Mental and physical frailty in older people: the costs and benefits of informal care. Ageing and Society 18: 317–354

Richardson A, Unel J, Aston B 1989 A new deal for carers. King's Fund, London

Robinson J, Batstone G 1996 Rehabilitation. A development strategy. A King's Fund working paper. King's Fund, London

Ross F, Mackenzie A 1996 Nursing in primary health care. Routledge, London

Schultz R, Visintainer P, Williamson G 1990 Psychiatric and physical mobility effects of caregiving. Journal of Gerontology 45: 181–191

Schwarz KA, Roberts BL 2000 Social support of strain of family caregivers of older adults. Holistic Nursing Practice 14: 77–90

Sharp T 1992 Listening to carers. Nursing Times 88: 29–30

Social Services Inspectorate 1995 A way ahead for carers. Department of Health, London

Sprotson K, Pitson L, Whitefield G, Walker E 1999 Health and lifestyles of the Chinese population in England. Health Education Authority, London

Twigg J 1989 Models of carers: how do social care agencies conceptualise their relationship with informal carers? Journal of Social Policy 18: 53–66

Twigg J (ed) 1992 Carers: research and practice. HMSO, London

Twigg J 1993 Introduction. In: Twigg J (ed) Informal care in Europe. Social Policy Research Unit, University of York, York, p 1

Twigg J, Atkin K 1994 Carers perceived: policy and practice in informal care. Open University Press, Buckingham

Wellwood I, Dennis MS, Warlow CP. 1994 Perceptions and knowledge of stroke among surviving patients with stroke and their carers. Age and Ageing 23: 293–298

Whitlach CJ, Noelker LS 1996 Caregiving and caring. Encyclopedia of Gerontology 1: 253–268

Wistow G, Barnes M 1993 User involvement in community care: origins, purposes and applications. Public Administration 71: 279–299

Wolfe C, Rudd T, Beech R (eds) 1996 Stroke services and research. Stroke Association, London

Yee L 1995 Improving support for black carers: a sourcebook of information, ideas and service initiatives. King's Fund, London

Chapter 34

Reflections

Fiona M. Ross and Sally J. Redfern

INTRODUCTION

In this chapter we return to and reflect on themes running through the book, which are not the subject of separate chapters because of their relevance to many. We draw on material from our contributors and listen to 'voices' of older people raised in earlier chapters and from literature in an attempt, where possible, to integrate these with the themes. Themes that we highlight are concerned with images of ageing, valuing personal care and relationships, balancing rights and risks, rehabilitation and empowerment of older people, critical care, inter-professional issues and developing roles in nursing, and questions about raising the quality of practice and education.

IMAGES OF AGEING

In this book we have sought to convey a positive image of ageing (Figs 34.1–34.3) by emphasizing individual activity and social engagement as well as the nurse's role in contributing to maximizing the potential for improvement and maintenance of function for people challenged by chronic disease. This emphasis runs counter to that of institutionalized ageism, common in so many western societies. The old person with failing faculties and diminished control of physical function so often continues to be the butt of ridicule in the media, in cartoons and literature:

> An ageing man is but a paltry thing,
> A tattered coat upon a stick (Yeats 1928).

And in self deprecation:

> You know you're getting old when you stoop to tie
> your shoes and wonder what else you can do while

you're down there (George Burns, cited in Katz 1988: 14).

Factors contributing to ageism are complex and have been alluded to in a variety of contexts in this book. Christina Victor, in Chapter 2, discusses the various theoretical and empirical positions that influence our thinking, the questions we ask and the responses we make to older members of our own families and to

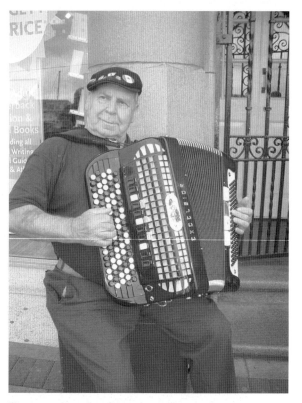

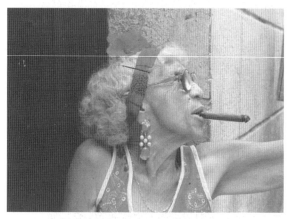

Fig. 34.1   Smoking in Havana.

Fig. 34.2   Accordion player.

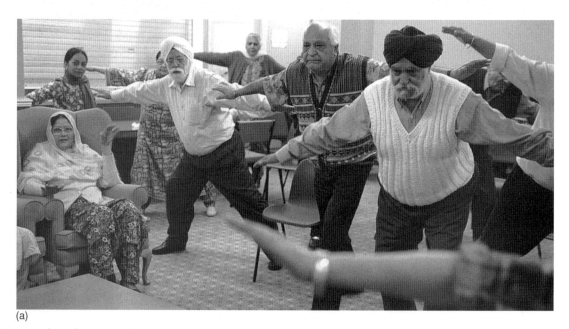

(a)

Fig. 34.3   (a, b, c) Keeping fit. (Photographs a and b by Jon-Paul Davis, courtesy of Age Concern Scotland.)

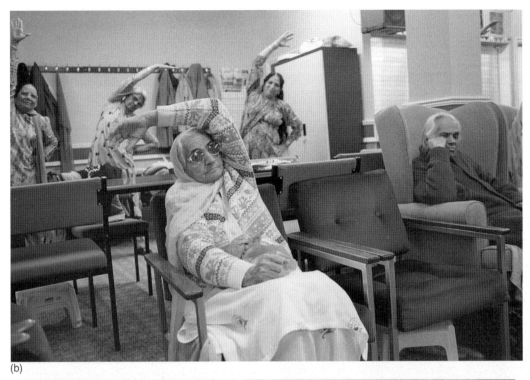

(b)

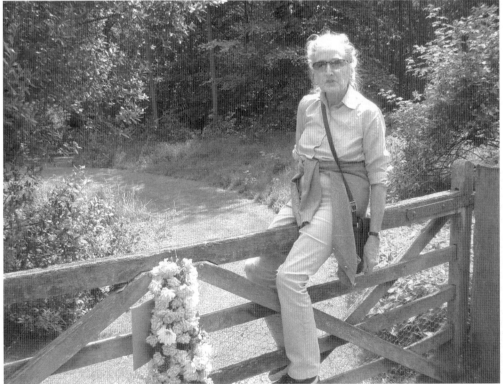

(c)

Fig. 34.3 *(Continued)*

people in our care. The biological model of ageing has been and continues to be pervasive and influential in policy and practice. It depicts ageing as a process of continual and inexorable decline with the onset of pathological changes in physical health. Deterioration of mental health is seen to be part of the same process, making important links with loss of role and status. Figure 34.4 challenges stereotypes of old age through images developed to counter ageism by the London Standing Conference of Nurses, Health Visitors and Midwives. Ageing in these terms is often viewed as physical and mental degeneration, with increasing incidence of illness and dependency. Thus old people, whose ages span 40 years from 60 to 100 years old and more, are stereotyped as a homogeneous group with problems. These ideas have often been the underpinning for ageism, labelling, institutionalization and an absence of innovation in care.

I'm an old woman now
And nature is cruel,

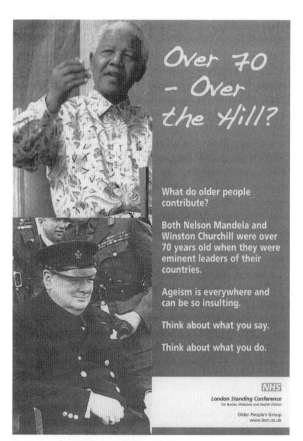

Fig. 34.4 Over 70 – over the hill? (Reproduced with permission: London Standing Conferences supports origins and roles of practitioner initiatives.)

Tis her jest to make
Old age look like a fool.
The body it crumbles
Grace and vigour depart (Elder 1977: 8).

The concern of much sociological theoretical development and research has been the social context of old people's lives, in particular housing, health, poverty and isolation. The social construction of old age is discussed in Chapter 2 and developed by Christina Victor through analysis of empirical findings from demographic and epidemiological studies in Chapter 3. The notion that old age and dependence are social constructions and that society reinforces class, gender and income differentials in old age is an important theme that is picked up by Sue Davies and her colleagues in the discussion of dementia in old age (Chapter 24) and by Debbie Tolson and Iain Swan in Chapter 11 with reference to the services provided for people with hearing difficulties. Maria Ponto in Chapter 4 discusses the work on disengagement from the perspective of psychology and some of its unfortunate consequences for policy and practice that have reinforced the biological model of ageing. The biological model justifies a laissez-faire and passive response from practitioners and condones the warehousing and institutionalizing of older people, so denying individuality and discouraging professional initiative. Countering ageism at system, professional and individual levels is being addressed through the *National Service Framework for Older People* (Department of Health 2001) standard 1. This standard aims to tackle concerns relating to reports of 'poor, unresponsive, insensitive and discriminatory' services by driving up standards and reducing regional variations in the provision of health and social services. The *National Service Framework* raises many challenges for the National Health Service and for nursing in the way in which resources are allocated to services for older people, recruitment and retention of staff into the speciality, the extent to which the age of service user influences clinical decision-making and attitudes and behaviours expressed towards older people, which can be demeaning or, at the very least, thoughtless.

The life history and biographical approach to ageing is introduced in Chapter 2. This has its origins in both psychology and sociology. It takes account of how people see and value their own lives and the meaning of social events, thereby promoting self-esteem:

I'll tell you who I am . . .
I'm a small child of ten,
with a father and mother

brothers and sisters who
love one another (Elder 1977: 7).

We hope that what is coming through the pages of this book, articulated by the different subject specialists, is the view that assumptions should not be made about old people as a homogeneous group with needs easily categorized into problems. We have tried to avoid age- and gender-biased language. We want to convey our views that older people have their own memories, experiences and outlook on the future. People now in their 80s and 90s have lived through immense social change, two world wars and massive technological innovation. They have reared children without the crutch of the welfare state. For many they are characterized by a stoicism, pride and forbearance that needs no condescending professional attitude. As Doris Lessing puts it:

> They have already been felled several times, and picked themselves up, put themselves back together, each time with more and more difficulty, and their being on the pavement with their hands full of handbag, carrier bag, and walking stick is a miracle (Lessing 1983: 174).

No strangers to hard work, some old people have memories of leaving school on their 14th birthday to start work:

> In the cardboard factory, it was very tiring, standing all day from half past seven to six o'clock . . . I swore I would never let my children do the same

and memories of the war:

> when I had my son I went into the Nelson Hospital and that was tough when the bombing and doodle bugs started . . . one morning when I thought I've had enough of this, the sirens went and the nurse ran away. I'm in the ward with about 20 babies and I thought, well I can only save one and that is mine. I lay over the top of his cradle and held the other baby the nurse had left. When the bomb came down, there was flying glass, all in my hair, but at least we were safe.

It is not just the indigenous population of white elders who have seen and endured tough times over the decades since World War I. The groups of older people from ethnic minorities are also diverse in terms of their reasons for settling in this country, class, religion, culture as well as ethnicity. Chronological age itself is determined by cultural systems and, in some communities, people are regarded as 'elders' from their mid-50s, which has implications for how those individuals who were part of the inward migration to the UK in the 1950s are treated. The experience of ageing in black and ethnic minorities is context-specific with collective opportunities for enjoyment and prayer, but may also feature loneliness, as illustrated by the following interview extract with a Hindu woman in her 80s:

> *Mrs A was brought up in a high-caste family in India and was active in the independence movement. She came to London in the swinging 60s and worked in a middle-ranking post in the civil service:*

> The men I realized do not want a woman as their equal . . . I became an alcoholic, because of the extreme loneliness of London, whereas in Delhi I was somebody, I had a group of friends and my own family, with a purpose in life . . . even though I got the job in the civil service, it meant nothing, because there was nobody to talk to, nobody to bother, suddenly this complete anonymity.

Ageism is not just expressed in social and professional attitudes, but is often unfortunately an entrenched part of institutional policies and practice. The organization of health services for older people and its development as a medical specialty have been less well recognized and resourced than, for example, paediatric care. It was only in the 1950s that Marjorie Warren pioneered the work that made geriatrics a respectable specialty in medicine. Even so, in many medical schools, departments of ageing are small and often peripheral to the mainstream specialties. A career in the medicine of old age for a young graduate is still perceived as a worthy but low-status choice. To some extent these attitudes have also prevailed in nursing care of older people, in that there are often difficulties in recruiting staff to work in care settings for older people and the demand for post-registration training in gerontological nursing is always lower than for popular areas such as critical care. There are signs that this is changing, but perhaps too slowly, as a result of the work of Alan Pearson at Burford, who pioneered models of primary nursing and 'nursing beds', which influenced the growth of nursing development units and nurse-led units in the care of older people. Andrei Dunn discusses primary nursing in Chapter 8 in the context of hospital care, and Claire Goodman and Sally Redfern trace the history of nursing development units and nurse-led units in Chapter 9.

Accessibility of services for old people is another example of the institutionalization of ageism. Issues such as rationing, use of services and uptake are vital considerations in present policy for old people. The ageing population, with its increasing need for care, combined with reductions in length of stay in hospital and often inadequate community care provision available on discharge, has resulted in the pejorative but common term of 'bed-blocker'. This term implies that it is the individual who is responsible for being an obstacle and preventing others from receiving necessary care, rather than the system being faulty. Christina Victor discusses in Chapter 3, and later with Fiona Ross in Chapter 7, the issues of accessibility and utilization of services. The increasing shift towards a mixed economy of care and the escalating costs of long-term care have serious implications for the choices and care alternatives available for individuals.

INDIVIDUAL CARE AND THE PATIENT EXPERIENCE

We hope that the book has conveyed our own beliefs about the importance of valuing individuals, their history, their concerns and needs within the caring relationship. Good communication is central to this, as Andrée Le May describes in Chapter 10. Perhaps what is often overlooked is the emotional and challenging nature of the work for nurses, who need to be supported by a cohesive team and positive organizational culture. There is increasing evidence from patients' surveys of perceived shortcomings in the delivery of 'essential nursing care', including nutritional support and basic personal care, such as help with toileting (Ross et al. 2004). Case study 34.1 is based on a true story that illustrates a failure in communication. Names have been changed to protect confidentiality.

What is striking about Janet's story is the apparent lack of attempts to involve the patient on setting nursing care goals. Again, the tendency for society and professionals to display an alarming arrogance in asserting that they know what is best for older people is illustrated, this time from literature:

> Our campaign for Annie is everything that is humane and intelligent. There she is, a derelict old woman, without friends, some family somewhere but they find her condition a burden and a scandal and won't answer her pleas; her memory going, though not for the distant past, only for what she said five minutes ago; all the habits and supports of a lifetime fraying away around her, shifting as she sets a foot down where she expected firm ground to be . . . and she sitting in her chair suddenly surrounded by well wishing faces who know exactly how to put the world to rights (Lessing 1983: 162).

Patronizing attitudes conveyed by knowing how 'to put the world to rights' are one thing, but even those professionals who are trying their best to offer appropriate services and to communicate sensitively in a 'humane and intelligent' way may still miss the mark. It is frequently the case that 'off-the-shelf' services are not acceptable to the old person. When this happens it is important that other solutions are explored using approaches to assessment and care planning discussed in Chapter 28. Situations where the balance between rights and risks are at their starkest are in the care of people with dementia. Attempts to keep people living

---

Case study 34.1 A failure in communication

Janet is 75 years old and married to a retired general practitioner. She has ovarian carcinoma, for which she has had intensive treatment. Over a period of time she experienced increasingly frequent episodes of intermittent bowel obstruction which, exacerbated by a fever and cellulitis, precipitated her admission to a local acute hospital unit. Her medical management was faultless but the nursing care was seen to have serious shortcomings, some of which are summarized below:

- Although on admission a nutritional assessment was completed by the dietician, the recommendations were not implemented by the catering staff – time went by before anyone did anything about it
- The intravenous infusion was frequently interrupted, requiring recannulation, which on one

occasion was delayed for 7 h – a message was given, but not followed up
- Constant disruption of her sleep due to late administration of intravenous medications – task-centred drug rounds meant that individual needs for sleep were overlooked
- An attempt to take a blood sugar from Janet was stopped as she had the foresight to ask the right question and establish that they had the wrong patient – this error was averted by her alertness, but what else might have happened?

Janet's husband did not wish to complain formally, preferring to make a 'series of observations and concerns which are more difficult and painful to ignore than to articulate'. His view was that 'failure of communication was probably the root of all the problems, compounded by pressure of work and understaffing'.

in the community for as long as possible mean that many old people are deteriorating within their own homes. However, it is the family and neighbours who are faced with an old lady going out in a nightgown to look for her dead daughter, forgetting to lock up, losing keys, forgetting to eat or leaving the gas on. Introducing paid carers to support people with dementia in their homes is not always the easy solution, because strangers (and a series of different faces) may further confuse or be the subject of suspicion. Innovative approaches to dementia care, discussed in Chapter 24, must be disseminated widely to lay as well as professional audiences. Frequently it is the community, neighbours, shopkeepers as well as families who remonstrate for admission to care, because they can no longer cope with the anxiety and feeling of responsibility if something were to go wrong. On the other hand, for those who are looked after successfully, it is the community network and families who have made it work.

Old people themselves are the best judge of their capabilities and limits. Why should it be any different than for the rest of us? There are plenty of examples of elder statesmen and figures from the world of literature and the arts, both women and men, who in their 80s continue in public life with vigour and vision. We would not assume to give 'we-know-best' advice to Archbishop Tutu or Nelson Mandela, who both continue to provide inspirational leadership around the globe (Fig. 34.5). For the most part people know when and how to develop personal strategies to minimize risk and maintain as far as possible their normal activities. A 78-year-old woman, for example, who was travelling to Norfolk weekly to care for her dying brother told us: 'there will be nobody to look after me.

This doesn't worry me very much, because I want to look after myself, but I think that there is an insidious carefulness that has crept into my activities'. This woman was deciding to take fewer personal risks because of her knowledge of potential consequences.

REHABILITATION AND EMPOWERMENT OF OLDER PEOPLE

The concept of rehabilitation is a complex, but continuous thread running through this book. We take it to mean 'the whole process of enabling and facilitating the restoration of a disabled person to regain optimal functioning (physically, socially and psychologically) to the level they are able or motivated to achieve' (Waters 1996: 242). Some chapters are more explicit in their attention to rehabilitation than others – the chapters on mobility, care of the foot, sight, hearing, nutrition, elimination, maintaining healthy skin, coping with pain, depression and confusion, for example. In this section we bring together features of rehabilitation raised in earlier chapters, so demonstrating its importance throughout the book. We identify aspects to which nurses could usefully give more attention, with the aim of enhancing feelings of empowerment and maximizing people's independence.

Autonomy, choice and enabling people to create health on their own terms are important features of health promotion and are emphasized by Sarah Cowley in Chapter 30. The principles of health promotion she outlines – enabling, mediating, advocacy, creating supportive environments, developing personal skills, valuing citizen participation – are fundamental to provision of autonomy, choice and empowerment of older

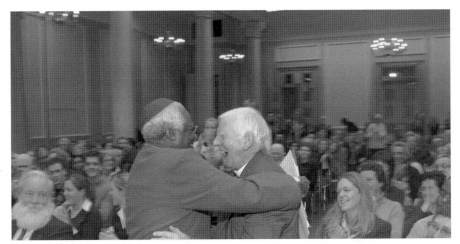

Fig. 34.5 Meeting of old friends – Archbishop Desmond Tutu and Reverend Professor Christopher Evans.

people and to their potential for rehabilitation. This means allowing people to make their own informed decisions.

Maximizing people's well-being and rehabilitation potential requires skilled therapeutic intervention by nurses to overcome the many challenges to communication that occur for older people, particularly people with visual impairment, hearing loss, speech impairment, cognitive impairment and social isolation. Andrée le May, in Chapter 10, looks at these challenges and the process of therapeutic care that skilled nurses provide. The aim of therapeutic nursing care is to define every person's potential for rehabilitation, so maximizing his or her independence. This applies to all potential and actual health deficits covered in this volume and their consequences, be they pain, depression, immobility, breathing difficulties, malnutrition or incontinence. Separate chapters cover each of these conditions. Promoting rehabilitation and self-determination and maximizing independence are fundamental to nursing, whatever the focus. These principles apply equally to promotion and maintenance of health, care of people who are ill or disabled, and care of people who are dying.

Empowerment is a concept that we believe is important in every care setting for older people. Although this book does not deal specifically with critical care nursing, it is our view that the principles of holistic nursing care apply equally to the seriously ill person. The challenges in critical care are different, the pace of decision-making is rapid, the emotions and anxiety of families and carers are raw and exposed and the medical and nursing needs of older people complex. Nurses working in critical care need knowledge of the management of acutely ill people as well as an understanding of the different needs of the older person.

There is evidence to show the benefits of therapeutic, rehabilitative nursing care. For example, time spent by nurses in promoting continence is inversely related to the prevalence of incontinence (see Chapter 17 by Christine Norton). Nurses who concentrate on prevention increase patients' independence and reduce the misery of what many regard as a degrading and stigmatizing condition. The outcome is better for nurses and care workers too. No longer do they see the job principally in terms of cleaning up after incontinence has occurred.

Another example is the potential nurses have in detecting, remedying and preventing depression in older people – a problem that is easily missed and often goes unreported, as discussed by Colin Hughes in Chapter 25. Nurses see older people in a variety of settings and are in a unique position to improve the quality of life of people with depression. Adequate assessment which takes a comprehensive, inter-professional approach and involves the patient and family will detect problems that are so often missed and will maximize the potential for rehabilitation and well-being (see Chapter 28).

Deafness, which is often linked to depression, causes feelings of powerlessness and rejection. Hearing loss is an invisible handicap so different to the handicap of blindness. The stigma is therefore far greater, especially when linked, as it so often is erroneously, to the notion of 'senility' and mental decay. Deaf people can be helped through rehabilitation but they refrain from seeking help because they fear being stigmatized or they take the ageist view that to be deaf is part of being old and nothing can be done about it. As we learn from Debbie Tolson and Iain Swan in Chapter 11, there are many environmental hearing aids on the market now, such as alarm light systems and telephone, television and radio attachments that do not disturb other people. Also, public recreational halls are now often wired with the loop system for the benefit of people with hearing loss. Extending this requirement to locations frequented by older people, like hospital wards and nursing and residential homes, would benefit many more people.

There is no doubt that giving patients information about their treatments and medication increases the likelihood of adherence to the prescription even when faced with unpleasant side-effects. People cope with side-effects if they know what these are and can balance them against the benefits of the treatment (see Chapter 27 by Dinah Gould). Encouraging self-medication for people who want to and can manage their own regimens reduces errors and increases concordance and the patient's sense of control over the recovery process. Nurses have a major role in promoting rehabilitation in this way.

Intermediate care schemes provide individual packages of care for people wanting to stay at home even when their need for nursing care is substantial. If more schemes were available, so that people could be offered a real choice, this would increase the potential for maintaining independence. On the other hand, some older people prefer to live in a residential home or a nursing home, rather than struggling to cope with activities of daily living at home. We know of a woman in her 90s who was impatient to move from her bungalow into a care home, but she had to wait 5 years before a bed became available.

Residents deteriorate and rehabilitation is impossible if they lose a sense of personal autonomy and control over their daily lives and are denied opportunities for self-help. Oversupportive environments in care homes exert too few demands on an old person and encourage apathy, boredom and submissiveness. Care homes that offer residents genuine choice, freedom and privacy, and have the minimum of rules and regulations, are often rich in facilities and resources and have open access to the outside world. These environments promote rehabilitation, empower residents to take initiatives themselves and maximize their independence. Care home managers who recognize the need for continuing education and training for their staff, and invest in training, provide a residential environment that optimizes the balance between ensuring security and safety for residents and encouraging them to make choices, take control and be independent. As discussed in Chapter 9, the same applies to sheltered-housing schemes when wardens are over-controlling.

Nursing homes are not, traditionally, seen as centres of rehabilitation for their permanent residents but they could be developed in this way. The outcomes would be better resident and staff morale, reduced morbidity of residents, the possibility of enabling some people to be discharged home and enhanced quality of life of those remaining (Nazarko 1997). It is disturbing to learn that some care staff in long-stay settings prefer to look after submissive, dependent old people because they are easier to 'manage' than more independent residents who make their wishes known. When applied to people with dementia, as discussed in Chapter 24, any potential for rehabilitation and choice is lost from the start, well before total dependence need occur.

The story in Case study 34.2 is intended to illustrate the support, advocacy and care that can be found in nursing-home settings, despite the fact that increasing dependency unwittingly occurred.

Far-sighted health care professionals, who know their clients and their life histories well, encourage family carers, as well as people they care for, to demand the kind of support they need – for information, for training in skills and tasks, for emotional support, for social support, for respite services and for culturally sensitive services, for example (see Chapter 33 by Ann Mackenzie and Diana Lee). If carers' demands for support are met, they are likely to want to continue caring and the rewards of caring will increase. Raising the level of the service user's voice will maximize the rehabilitation potential of cared-for people and will increase the range of choices open to carers. However, family carers can be forgiven if they feel they have little choice. Current policies on community care promote the notion that it is better for social and health care agencies to support people in their own homes, so avoiding the negative effects of institutionalization. This can mean, for carers, very little choice in fact. They are expected to look after relatives at home whatever their preference. It also suggests that care at home is never 'institutional'. Yet the worst features of institutionalization – unwanted routines, rules and regulations, depersonalization, emotional distance from carers, segregation from the outside world and so on – can be just as much a feature of care at home.

Case study 34.2   A positive experience

Peggy was admitted to a private nursing home about 15 miles from the small seaside village she had lived in for the last 30 years of her life. In her early 80s and without any close relatives, she had worked indefatigably as a volunteer for meals on wheels, nursed her mother and husband (both in their 90s) through their terminal illnesses and cared in numerous ways for friends and neighbours. She began to have difficulty living alone because of a rapidly failing memory. When admitted to a private nursing home she deteriorated, yet recognized friends with a sparkle in her eyes, but without apparently making connections that they could understand. All her life she had given tremendous warmth to all around her and it was remarkable to see her do this in an unfamiliar place when living at close quarters with strangers. The care staff did more than they should have for her, feeding

and helping her to the toilet when, given time and encouragement, she could do these things for herself. Essentially a gregarious person, she responded with smiles and giggles to the staff and they loved her.

Over the last few months of her life she became increasingly frail and dependent. Although the general practitioner recommended admission to hospital, the matron of the home insisted that she could be cared for in the home. The nursing care was excellent with attention to detail and there was someone with her when she died peacefully. For those looking on, the decision to admit her to a home seemed a compromise. However, the warmth and companionship she found, despite her mental confusion during her final frail months, was perhaps just what she needed and allowed her to continue to give in the only way she could, with her smiles, right to the end.

INTERPROFESSIONAL WORKING

Care of older people frequently requires a collaborative approach between different professionals. This should be at both interagency and interprofessional levels. There is a growing literature on the problems that exist with converting the policy rhetoric, that interprofessional work is a good thing, into reality. In the care of older people there are some good models of multiprofessional care-planning and discharge arrangements, but often these break down in practice when the system is under pressure. The reasons are to do with speed of patient turnover, lack of organizational and professional commitment, inadequate resourcing or communication failure. In Chapter 8 Andrei Dunn emphasizes the importance of multi-professional discharge planning for older people and, in Chapter 28, models of multiprofessional assessment between health and social care are reviewed. A question that continues to arise from this debate is how far the patient or carer is involved in the decision-making with the professional team. A pervading theme in this book is that, despite the professional rhetoric about empowerment and involving the patient and carer in the process of care, too often in reality this falls short. The way in which services are professionally defined is addressed in Chapter 33 on carers and lay caring. Too often personal sacrifice is the outcome, as described by this woman in her late 70s a year after her husband died:

> I don't say this in any way with regrets, you get an inner strength, you just do go on. I look back now and think how on earth did I . . . and you do reach the end of your tether . . . I shouted you know . . . I'm not a shouting person, we never quarreled and yet it got to a pitch and then I would shout. There was one occasion and I shouted I don't want to be doing this, and that still keeps coming back to me and makes me feel terrible and I can never undo it, because it's done. But I was so tired and I couldn't get down on the floor any more to mop up the mess.

As well as trying to ensure that the clients' and carers' needs are centre stage, we need to carry out research to investigate what methods of inter-professional team-working make a difference to the outcomes of care for older people and their families. There is some work from the USA that supports the effectiveness of inter-professional teams working in care of older people in relation to functional outcomes and reduced levels of care (Page et al. 2003). In this book various chapters cover interprofessional work for older people, for example, nurses and physiotherapists collaborating on a rehabilitation programme, referred to by Janet Simpson and Elaine New in Chapter 13, and nurses and social workers working together to develop strategies to identify early signs of abuse, discussed by Bridget Penhale and Claudine McCreadie in Chapter 32.

EMERGING ROLES FOR NURSES WORKING WITH OLDER PEOPLE

There is much debate in the professional literature about developing specialist practice and nurse practitioner roles. There are a number of factors that contribute to this debate, such as the changing boundaries between medicine and nursing resulting from the reduction in working hours for junior doctors, the shift of services from acute to primary care, and professional aspirations. There has always been a central role for nursing and nurses in the care of older people. For reasons referred to earlier on the low status ascribed to the medical specialty of geriatrics, nursing has tended to play a reactive provider role rather than leading and innovating from the front. There is tremendous scope both in institutional and community settings for nurses to lead the way in giving patient- and family-centred care that does not lose sight of the people, their memories and the significance of these to their lives.

Examples of innovative roles developed over recent years in the UK are the consultant nurse and modern matron that have been added to clinical nurse specialist and nurse practitioner roles, as discussed in Chapters 8 and 9. A recent research study on the consultant nurse role has demonstrated the impact consultant nurses have in making care more user-focused, developing new nurse-led services and improving current practice by developing procedures, processes and protocols in health care (Guest et al. 2004). The findings showed that the consultant nurses demonstrated their impact, in what was only their first 2–3 years in the job, more in terms of improving the processes of care than in showing a clearly defined impact on health outcomes for patients and clients. More research is needed to investigate their impact on health outcomes of older people when consultants have been in the job for a few more years. Demonstrating the impact of a new role is not easy when consultant nurses work, by definition, as leaders and influential members of an interprofessional team. One of the consultant nurse respondents in the study summed up the difficulties of impact measurement:

> I'm [keen to have an impact on] outcomes for people. The only thing is . . . but I suppose that is going to be an aim of the job . . . is to prove that it's myself that has that outcome, you know. I mean I have to ask myself 'what would happen if I wasn't here?' And I don't think those things would've happened. But the outcome's going to be shared, very much,

with direct clinicians. So it's . . . I can't do anything without other people working with me can I?

Demonstrating an impact is possible, however, as the extract in Case study 34.3 shows. This extract has been drawn from a series of interviews conducted over time with a consultant nurse in care of older people (Guest et al. 2004). It conveys the job as demanding but exciting and extremely satisfying in the success with which the consultant was able to make a major impact on the quality of care. We have traced her progress on

---

Case study 34.3   Making an impact as a consultant nurse

Service development
On her first anniversary in the role, at the second interview, the consultant described herself as feeling good with respect to the service development activities that she had initiated:

> It's starting to crystallize now, for me. Ummm. It still feels very positive . . . I really just hope that . . . you know it's one of these roles that gets the opportunity to grow and to blossom, and that people recognize that that does take time . . . it's not one of those things that people look at in 3 years and say, 'Oh well, consultant nurses haven't been able to do anything, let's just forget all about them,' you know. This is 3 years out of 50 or 60 years of the NHS, so you have to put things into some kind of perspective.

At the third interview, she mentioned four service development projects she was working on. The first was an education project on incontinence of patients which was led by a community colleague and involved all medical staff (house officers, registrars and consultants) as well as herself and all nurses, with the result, she said, that 'we're getting consistent education right the way through, which is great'. She had been given responsibility for leading this project in the directorate together with the medical consultant. The project was designed initially to involve audit and education of all new medical staff although she was keen for other professionals to share the learning opportunity too, so as to promote multidisciplinary learning.

The second project was a re-evaluation of a nurse-led transient ischaemic attack (TIA) service for which funds had been acquired from the trust. By the fourth interview, the consultant said that the project had been set up and was progressing well. They had integrated medical and nursing documentation and sent out publicity material to the primary care trust and general

practitioners with a view to starting data collection the following month.

The third project was a service development designed to ensure rapid access to health services for potential stroke patients. This will, the consultant told us, enable nursing practice to be more holistic, interdisciplinary and preventive. The trust had accepted the business plan and agreed to fund a 6-month pilot evaluation and audit facilitator. At the same time, the research group was bidding for a research grant to take the evaluation further jointly with medical and university colleagues; their bid had got through the first round. If successful, the university would provide research support in the trust and nurses would be seconded to be involved in the research as data collectors.

The fourth project was a multidisciplinary outreach team project due to start soon. The consultant, who was co-leader of the project with the consultant geriatrician and was coordinating it jointly with the superintendent physiotherapist, described the huge amount of work required to get the multidisciplinary team going. Following a successful bid for funds to the Modernization Agency, they had to work very hard to set up the team of nurses, physiotherapists, geriatrician and primary care colleagues to meet the deadline for 'going live' in a couple of weeks. Funds would cover appointment of an audit administrator to evaluate the outreach work using preset performance indicators. The consultant was looking forward to getting started:

> I think we've got a very forward-thinking team, they don't have a lot of problems with boundaries, they don't get very territorial.

At the fourth interview, the consultant described herself as having to troubleshoot in the outreach project, with a particular emphasis on advising how best multidisciplinary teams can learn to handle defensive staff in improving standards of care. Her approach was to

Continued

Case study 34.3   Making an impact as a consultant nurse (*Continued*)

encourage discussion of the difficulties amongst all staff, support the staff, engage in teamwork, act as a role model in providing good care and learn from each other. She was able to report a number of achievements: the clinical inter-professional pairs of staff were working well (nurses were paired for outreach work with physiotherapists, occupational therapists, speech and language therapists and social workers), they were well received and accepted by clients; they were overcoming challenges without difficulty; and improvement in patient care in the wards and in discharge arrangements was already apparent. The evaluation was continuing through audit and the consultant's doctorate work, both of which she said were going well. She hoped to demonstrate effectiveness of the project and get more funds from the trust for a further year.

By the fifth interview, the new outreach team had been set up but the consultant was facing the problem of being unable to get adequate staffing cover:

> I think I told you – on the basis of ummm the senior nurses around the unit would be seconded on to the team, so of course that means that they still have their ward commitments as well..And it's very, very difficult to get replacements for them when they're not able to do outreach work...It needs to be somebody with expertise. So it's something we've struggled with a little bit over the last month...we've been a bit of a victim of our own success, because it's been going very well...Which is great, it's very positive...At the same time it's quite frustrating because it's not about...it's not about money. It's actually about people with the right skills, the right expertise, and the authority to make decisions.

The problem was quickly resolved, however, when two part-time workers were employed to do outreach work. As mentioned earlier, the consultant hoped to capitalize on the success of winning funds from the Modernization Agency by persuading the trust to continue the funding for a second year:

> We've got funding from the Modernization Agency for a year...The plan is at the end of the...well in September to start writing, you know to write a business plan to put to the trust to see whether or not they will continue funding.

Impact and effectiveness
By the second interview, the project on implementing the multidisciplinary outreach team for older people was

moving forward following the successful bid for funds from the Modernization Agency. By the fifth interview, baseline data collection had been completed and the consultant was pleased with progress:

> I've done all the baseline audits against [established performance indicator] standards, so in 3 months' time we'll be looking to see where we've been, who we've visited, what input we've been able to do. And I've been collecting sort of vignettes from each team, for sort of a newsletter to go out next week – we do a 3-monthly newsletter...And to make people sort of aware that this is where we can help, this is the sort of thing that we've been able to do...So that's been quite good.

Later on the consultant reported success in acquiring funding from the trust to enable consolidation of the outreach work and to expand its influence:

> We were successful in bidding for another 2 years' funding for the outreach team [this came from the Department of Health *National Service Framework* standard 4 implementation fund] – the team will now be full-time and focus on practice development as well as supporting inpatient management.

At the third interview, the consultant mentioned the progress achieved on a project evaluating nurse-led beds. The evaluation report had been particularly well received by the trust, which is to continue funding the project for another year. A positive outcome from the study was identified as a saving of some £134 000 by 24% of patients being discharged home rather than to a care home, as had been expected at the start. Also, the quality of care was better than before, she told us, with some patients destined for continuing care gaining sufficient improvement in their level of independence that an alternative discharge destination became a possibility:

> So we're all feeling sort of quite, you know that all of the work that we've been trying to do and push forward, is starting to come together now, with some support as well. So I think that's quite positive for people.

At the fifth interview, the consultant was jubilant about the progress made in developing the new TIA service. The stroke unit had been trying for 4 years to get this new service going and only now, since she had been in post, was it moving ahead:

> Fantastic! Up and running. Started on the 2nd of June. Ummm. Got patients coming through. Every-

Continued

Case study 34.3   Making an impact as a consultant nurse (*Continued*)

body seems to be happy with that. We've had one or two minor glitches with radiography, trying to sort of book our CT scan sessions and things like that. So I've sort of again you know been wheeled in to try to iron those out, and am negotiating furiously. But things seem to be going all right at the moment. But the great thing is that the stroke unit actually feels as though it's achieving something that it's been trying to do for the last 4 years, and get this TIA service off the ground... they're getting the patients in through the doors and they're doing what they wanted to do – which is give people an easy-access, one-stop service.

After the final interview, she was delighted to be able to report continued good news: 'the TIA service is going really well – and the trust may well extend this next year'. It became clear that the consultant's work was being recognized as an important innovation by the trust when she was asked to advise on setting up more consultant posts in care of older people. She identified the need for two more – one in stroke care and the other in implementing the Department of Health's policy drive to improve standards of basic care, which is so often left to junior nurses and health care assistants:

I've been talking to one of our associate directors of nursing about developing consultant nurses' roles for Essence of Care [Department of Health policy initiative], which I think would just give that a kind of – I don't know – the kind of kudos that it really needs. Because so much of the sort of fundamentals of care is always devolved down to the most junior

member of staff, and yet it's one of the most important things that we need to be doing...And she's very keen and [wants me to get on and develop] a business plan for that, and a sort of role description.

Conclusion

This consultant's profile marks her out as an achiever who thrives on challenge and has the skills to overcome problems, as occurred in turning a resistant ward sister into an enthusiastic and cooperative colleague. There are many more examples of achievements than problems in her story and she was blessed with strong managerial and medical support. She seems to have developed a good balance between the different components of the job, including research and evaluation which she integrated into service development initiatives and her professional doctorate. She seems to thrive on the continued opportunities for expanding the role rather than seeing them as an added burden to an already overstretched workload. Although she was active in clinical practice, this profile of the role suggests more of a 'designer-developer' than a 'superspecialist'. That is to say, rather than focusing the nurse consultant role on expert clinical practice working directly with patients, this consultant is more likely to act as a troubleshooter when complex clinical problems arise and leave the day-to-day clinical work in the hands of her nursing colleagues. Instead, her approach takes a broader, organization-wide, more strategic focus which is facilitative and supervisory in working towards her main goal of developing and improving practice

her considerable achievements over time and we conclude by classifying her as occupying a certain type of consultant role, that of designer-developer for services for older people.

RAISING QUALITY OF CARE

Maintaining high quality of care occurs as an underlying thread throughout the book. Assessment is the cornerstone of high-quality care and leads to successful care planning when all professionals – medical, nursing, therapy and social care practitioners working collaboratively – are involved in the assessment, planning and purchasing of care. This is embodied in the single multiprofessional assessment approach discussed in Chapter 28. The outcome of interprofessional collabo-

rative working is that duplication of effort is avoided and patients benefit.

Assessment of carers' needs is as important as that of patients' needs. Where services are good, carers are asked during the assessment process about their own needs, as discussed in Chapter 33. Attention to the needs of ethnic-minority groups and others with specialist or out-of-the-ordinary needs is often overlooked. Ensuring individual attention of this kind, though, can be difficult to achieve in today's climate of evidence-based commissioning when purchasers demand efficiency and cost-effectiveness from service providers.

There is a need for development work with staff, and also residents, of care homes to help them examine what they do and how their approach to care affects residents and direct care staff. This kind of scrutiny is important at all levels, from top management to direct care staff, and including residents. As discussed in Chapter 9, action research can ensure that staff are involved in identifying their training and development needs and in taking decisions about making improvements. When direct care workers are given recognition and are respected for the job they do, as occurred in domus units for older mentally frail residents (Lindesay et al. 1991), their self-esteem will rise, they will value themselves as having status in health care work and the quality of care to residents will improve. It will not if direct care workers are deprived of the recognition they deserve.

Research that links quality of care to outcomes in terms of health and well-being of care home residents and service users generally is thin on the ground. Standardized questionnaire surveys are not very effective at discovering older people's true feelings about their living accommodation, their care and their quality of life. Depth studies using conversational interviews are more revealing and older people do say what they really feel if asked in the right way. Use of the critical incident technique helps older people to reveal their true feelings about the quality of their care (Norman et al. 1992, Ford et al. 1997, Redfern & Norman 1999).

Nurses are having, more than ever before, to demonstrate their worth and this is a particular challenge for nurses working in low-tech care of older people, a field that many policy-makers and management consultants believe can be left to unqualified or minimally qualified health care workers. There is no doubt that health care assistants are indispensable in the care of older people but the benefits of a high ratio of nurses to health care workers are well-established (Audit Commission 1991, Buchan & Ball 1991, Bagust 1992, Carr-Hill et al. 1992, Harrington 2001). Expert nursing is as important in the care of older people as it is for any age group and for any condition. The definition of an expert nurse described by Benner et al (1996: 145) still holds true as someone who has '(1) clinical grasp and response-based practice; (2) embodied know-how; (3) [sees] the big picture; and (4) [sees] the unexpected'. The expert nurse intuitively understands a situation and its solution without having to rely on rules or guidelines and so goes straight to the heart of the problem, uncluttered by having to consider other fruitless possibilities, as Kennedy (2002, 2004) describes in district nursing. Nurses with this level of expertise exist and work with older people and their families. They are specialists in their field. More research is needed, not so much on whether nurses make a difference – it is known that they do – but on what it is that is different and how this is achieved. The knowledge gained and lessons learned would then be available for nurses and their colleagues to make improvements in areas of their practice they know to be weak.

Examples of bad practice do exist but the media do not help with their sensationalist style of reporting cases of abuse. Examples of good practice do not often get publicized. Nurses could do more to publicize good care, using evidence, not just in the nursing press but also in national and local newspapers, in women's and men's magazines, and on local radio and television. Codes of practice and regular auditing of hospitals and care homes are important too and are practised and welcomed by good centres. Research is needed to identify the predictors of high quality and to use these as levers to promote good practice in all settings. Much better to discover the correlates of high quality and apply them widely than to concentrate on rooting out the bad apples and going through the lengthy and often unsuccessful process of hospital closure, deregistering care homes and sacking staff.

Rotating students through long-stay settings can help to raise standards of practice and is happening regularly. All settings need a budget for continuing education and training for staff and this is particularly important for staff of nursing homes and care homes, given the increasing frailty and nursing needs of their residents.

A person who complains of a health problem is likely to be correct in identifying that something is wrong. The complainant should always be listened to. There will always be something wrong, even if it turns out to be different to what was first thought or that fears are unfounded. We are told that the user's voice is being heard increasingly in this consumer age, but how much are individual needs really being met, given the relentless drive for efficiency and cost-effectiveness? The unglamorous areas of care are ones in which nurses can do much to improve practice – in hearing loss, vision, foot disorders, tissue viability, dentition, nutrition, elimination, confusion, depression, for example. More research is needed into effectiveness of care of older people in these areas. Nurses can do much to improve care by evaluating the effectiveness of different therapies, thereby enhancing patients' independence, comfort, dignity and well-being through rehabilitation and therapeutic programmes.

The importance of informed, evidence-based and skilled care has been emphasized throughout this book. For example, Susan McLaren in Chapter 16 describes the importance of using research findings to shape nutritional assessments. The increasing problem of malnutrition in some hospitals is evidence of the poor practice in this area. Education at pre- and post-registration levels is a key to good practice. Continuing education is crucial to ensuring the workforce maintains current and relevant knowledge and skills. The commissioning relationship between National Health Service trusts and education providers may mean that priorities for purchasing education sideline courses on care of older people. Staff find it increasingly difficult to take time off when clinical areas are hard-pressed and understaffed. Recent initiatives in education are, however, taking account of the multi-professional care team and are offering inter-professional training. There are increasing opportunities for students from different health professions to engage in joint clinical problem-solving and decision-making and together find solutions in the care of older people.

FUTURES

What then should be the proper focus of the nurse's care? We need to improve communication and information-giving and we need above all to be supported to respect, understand and address the needs of old people as diverse and individual. This is easier said than done, particularly in hard-pressed organizations facing continuous demands to implement fast-moving policy and meet new service targets. Nurses need support and space to express their own feelings, in order, as Margaret Johnson states in the conclusion to Chapter 26, just to be there with someone's distress and pain. We hope that this book will help nurses work with others to gather and integrate the knowledge necessary to give sensitive and appropriate care to all older people in every setting:

> Do not go gentle into that good night,
> Old age should burn and rave at close of day;
> Rage, rage against the dying of the light (Thomas 1952).

References

Audit Commission 1991 The virtue of patients: making the best use of ward nursing resources. HMSO, London

Bagust A 1992 Ward nursing quality and grade mix. Health Economics Consortium, University of York, York

Benner P, Tanner CA, Chesla CA 1996 Expertise in nursing practice: caring, clinical judgment and ethics. Springer, New York

Buchan J, Ball J 1991 Caring costs: nursing costs and benefits. Institute of Manpower Studies, Brighton

Carr-Hill R, Dixon P, Gibbs I et al. 1992 Skill mix and the effectiveness of nursing care. Centre for Health Economics, University of York, York

Department of Health 2001 National service framework for older people. Department of Health, London

Elder G 1977 The alienated: growing old today. Writers' and Readers' Publishing Co-operative, London

Ford P, Health H, McCormack B, Phair L 1997 What a difference a nurse makes: an RCN report on the benefits of expert nursing to the clinical outcomes in the continuing care of older people. Royal College of Nursing, London

Guest D, Peccei R, Rosenthal P et al. 2004 An evaluation of the impact of nurse, midwife and health visitor consultants. King's College London. Available online at www.kcl.ac.uk/nursing/nru/nru.html

Harrington C 2001 Strengthening the care giving workforce: improving the quality of long term care. American Journal of Nursing 101: 55–56

Katz E 1988 Old age comes at a bad time: wit and wisdom for the young at heart. Special edition for Past Times, Robson Books, London

Kennedy C 2002 The work of district nurses: first assessment visits. Journal of Advanced Nursing 40: 710–720

Kennedy C 2004 A typology of knowledge for district nurse assessment practice. Journal of Advanced Nursing 45: 401–409

Lessing D 1983 The diaries of Jane Somers. Penguin, London

Lindesay J, Briggs K, Lawes M, Macdonald A, Herzberg J 1991 The domus philosophy: a comparative evaluation of a new approach to residential care for the demented elderly. International Journal of Geriatric Psychiatry 6: 727–736

Nazarko L 1997 Restoring independence. Nursing Management 4: 21–23

Norman IJ, Redfern SJ, Tomalin DA, Oliver S 1992 Developing Flanagan's critical incident technique to elicit indications of high and low quality nursing care from patients and their nurses. Journal of Advanced Nursing 17: 590–600

Page A et al. 2003 Keeping patients safe: transforming the work environment of nursing. National Readiness Press, Washington, DC

Redfern S, Norman I 1999 Quality of nursing care perceived by patients and their nurses: an application of the critical incident technique. Parts 1 and 2. Journal of Clinical Nursing 8: 407–421

Ross F, Smith E, Mackenzie A, Masterson A 2004 Identifying research priorities in nursing and midwifery service delivery and organization: a scoping study. International Journal of Nursing Studies 41: 547–538

Thomas D 1996 Do not go gentle into that good night. In: The nation's favourite poems. BBC Books, London, p 63

Waters K 1996 Rehabilitation. In: Wade L, Waters K (eds) A textbook of gerontological nursing: perspectives on practice. Baillière Tindall, London, pp 238–257

Yeats WB 1973 Sailing to Byzantium. In: Oxford book of twentieth century verse (compiled by Larkin P). Oxford University Press, London, pp 82–83

Index

Page numbers in italics refer to figures and boxes.

M

O